Clinical Medicine

Clinical Medicine

A textbook for medical students and doctors

Edited by

Parveen J Kumar

Senior Lecturer
St Bartholomew's Hospital Medical College, London

and

Michael L Clark

Consultant Physician
St Bartholomew's Hospital, London

with the assistance of

William F Jackson

Honorary Consultant Physician
Guy's Hospital, London

Baillière Tindall
London Philadelphia Toronto
Sydney Tokyo

Bailliére Tindall
WB Saunders
24-28 Oval Road,
London NW1 7DX.

The Curtis Centre
Independence Square West,
Philadelphia, P.A. 19106–3399, USA.

1 Goldthorne Avenue
Toronto, Ontario M8Z 5T9, Canada

Harcourt Brace Jovanovich Group (Australia) PTy Ltd.,
32–52 Smidmore Street, Marrickville, NSW 2204, Australia

Harcourt Brace Jovanovich (Japan) Inc
Ichibancho Central Building, 22–1 Ichibancho
Chiyoda-ku, Tokyo 102, Japan

First published 1987

Reprinted 1988 and 1989

DISCARDED

Printed in Great Britain by
Mackays of Chatham PLC, Letchworth.

British Library Cataloguing in Publication Data

Clinical medicine
    1. Pathology   2. Medicine
    I. Kumar, PJ   II. Clark, ML
    616   RB111

ISBN 0–7020–1137–1

Contents

LRI Baker MA, MD, FRCP,
Consultant Physician,
Department of Nephrology,
St Bartholomew's Hospital,
London
Renal disease

A John Camm BSc, MD, FRCP, FACC,
Professor of Clinical Cardiology,
St George's Hospital Medical School,
London
Cardiovascular disease

WR Cattell MD, FRCP, FRCP(E),
Physician and Senior Consultant Nephrologist,
St Bartholomew's Hospital,
London
Renal disease; Water, electrolyte and acid–base homeostasis

AW Clare MD, FRCPsych, FRCPI,
Professor of Psychological Medicine,
Medical College of St Bartholomew's Hospital,
London
Psychological medicine

ML Clark MD, FRCP,
Senior Lecturer and Consultant Physician,
Department of Gastroenterology,
St Bartholomew's Hospital,
London
Nutrition; Gastroenterology; Liver, biliary tract and pancreatic diseases; Environmental disorders

Charles RA Clarke MB, BChir, FRCP,
Consultant Neurologist,
St Bartholomew's Hospital,
London
Environmental disorders; Neurology and muscle disease

Robert J Davies MA, MD, FRCP,
Reader in Respiratory Medicine,
Academic Department of Respiratory Medicine,
Medical College of St Bartholomew's Hospital,
London
Immunology; Respiratory disease

PL Drury MA, MRCP,
Consultant Physician,
Diabetic Unit,
King's College Hospital and Greenwich District Hospital,
London
Endocrinology

List of Contributors

MJG Farthing MD, MRCP,
Wellcome Senior Lecturer and Honorary Consultant Physician,
Department of Gastroenterology,
Medical College of St Bartholomew's Hospital,
London
Infectious diseases and tropical medicine

EAM Gale MA, MB, MRCP,
Senior Lecturer and Consultant Physician,
Director, Department of Diabetes and Immunogenetics,
St Bartholomew's Hospital Medical College,
London
Diabetes and other disorders of metabolism

RN Greenwood BSc(Eng), ACGI, MSc, MBChB, MRCP,
Senior Registrar,
Department of Nephrology,
St Bartholomew's Hospital,
London
Renal disease

CJ Hinds MRCP, FFARCS,
Consultant and Senior Lecturer,
Department of Anaesthesia and Intensive Care,
St Bartholomew's Hospital,
London
Intensive care

EC Huskisson MD, FRCP,
Senior Lecturer and Consultant Physician,
Department of Rheumatology,
St Bartholomew's Hospital,
London
Rheumatology and bone disease

JDT Kirby FRCP,
Consultant Physician,
Department of Dermatology,
St Bartholomew's Hospital,
London
Dermatology

Parveen J Kumar BSc, MD, MRCP,
Senior Lecturer and Honorary Consultant
Physician,
Department of Gastroenterology,
Medical College of St Bartholomew's Hospital,
London
*Genetics and molecular biology; Gastroenterology;
Liver, biliary tract and pancreatic diseases*

JS Malpas DPhil, FRCP, FRCR,
Professor of Medical Oncology and
Director, Imperial Cancer Research Fund
Department of Medical Oncology,
Medical College of St Bartholomew's Hospital,
London
Diseases of the blood; Medical oncology

RM Pearson MA, MB, MRCP,
Consultant Physician (Clinical Pharmacology),
Harold Wood Hospital;
Senior Lecturer,
Department of Clinical Pharmacology,
Medical College of St Bartholomew's Hospital,
London
Poisoning

WF Jackson MA, BChir, MRCP,
Honorary Consultant Physician,
Guy's Hospital, London;
Medical Producer, British Medical Television;
formerly Editorial Director,
Medicine International, Oxford
Editorial consultant

Marie Carling BM
Baillière Tindall
33 The Avenue
Eastbourne

Developmental editor

Jan Ross MSc
38 Marlow Bottom Road
Marlow
Bucks

Indexer

DDK Rolston MD, MNAMS, DM,
Associate Professor of Gastroenterology,
Department of Gastroenterology and Wellcome
Research Unit,
Christian Medical College Hospital,
Vellore, India
Infectious diseases and tropical medicine

Peter Story MD, FRCPath,
Consultant Haematologist,
Institute of Orthopaedics,
Royal National Orthopaedic Hospital,
London
Bleeding disorders

P Turner MD, FRCP,
Professor of Clinical Pharmacology,
Medical College of St Bartholomew's Hospital,
London
Adverse drug reactions

Preface

There must be a good reason to write a new textbook of medicine when there are already a number on the market. It seemed to us that none of those currently available adequately conveyed the detail and background needed for medical practice in the late 1980s and 1990s. We have tried to strike a balance between exciting new developments in medical research and the vast quantity of established fact that needs to be absorbed by today's student. For this reason each chapter attempts to link scientific advances with clinical practice so that the management of disease can be based on sound physiological concepts.

This book is designed for both medical students and practising doctors and we have tried to produce a detailed but comprehensible text that bridges the gap between the purely introductory and the larger reference works. Tropical diseases have been included, and because the book will have a worldwide distribution we have discussed the presentation of disease as seen in developing countries. Disorders seen only in childhood have been excluded as these are well covered in other texts and would make this book too large. However, there are chapters on intensive care, nutrition, adverse drug reactions, poisoning and environmental medicine, which are often neglected yet play an important role in modern medical practice. There is inevitably an enormous chapter on infectious diseases but we felt that a description of all infectious agents should be included for quick reference; this chapter also contains basic information on antibiotic chemotherapy and a section on epidemiology and host resistance. A short chapter on genetics, molecular biology and immunology provides the basic principles of these subjects. Today's clinical students will have covered much of this in their preclinical course, but we hope that established practitioners will find it a useful introduction. Specific genetic and immunological disorders are covered in appropriate chapters.

We have concentrated on the management of disease but, within the text, have highlighted details of practical procedures and emergency therapy so that this book will be an invaluable companion in clinical practice. The practising clinician can use the book for reference or as a quick and easy guide to the management of an individual patient. Each chapter contains many tables and figures as an aid to learning. There are many cross-references, so that it is easy to move through different parts of the book to pursue different aspects of a particular topic and repetition has been minimized.

The contributors are all actively engaged in both clinical and research work, so the text has been written by clinicians who are not only in the forefront of medical advance but who also do ward rounds and outpatient clinics. At the time of writing all the contributors were working at St Bartholomew's Hospital, London, and thus combine a unified teaching approach with high academic standards.

We would like to thank all our colleagues for their hard work and cooperation and also our families and the many friends who have supported us during the preparation of this book.

Parveen Kumar
Michael Clark

Acknowledgements

We would like to thank all our colleagues and medical students who have helped in the writing of this book. As well as the anonymous reviewers arranged by the publishers we would like to thank in particular Dr Clive Bartram, Miss Diana Cundell, Dr Anthony Dawson, Dr David Galton, Dr Joe Hall, Dr Craig Halliday, Dr David Leaver, Dr Anthony Mann, Dr Richard Meyrick-Thomas, Dr Mike Murphy, Professor Lesley Rees, Dr Rodney Reznik, Dr John Sachs, Dr David Scott, Dr Judith Webb, Dr David Westaby and Dr David White who have either read sections or generously provided material. Dr David Levison kindly reviewed the pathology in some of the chapters. We are also grateful to the medical illustration department of St Bartholomew's Hospital who have drawn the illustrations and given helpful and patient advice, in particular Mrs Theresa Lanigan, Wendy Proctor and Mark de Pienne who have done the artwork and Mrs Kathy Clench who has coordinated it.

We must also thank Ms Nikki Thomas, the gastroenterology department secretary, for considerable help in the preparation of the typescript. Marie Carling and Nicholas Dunton from Baillière Tindall have also given considerable, practical help and guidance and without their invaluable help this book would not have been completed.

Every effort has been made to check the drug dosages given in this book. However, as it is possible that some errors have been missed or that dosage schedules have been revised the reader is strongly urged to consult the drug companies' literature before administering any of the drugs listed.

1

Infectious Diseases and Tropical Medicine

has occurred since then has been largely due to improvements in:
- Sanitation, housing and water supply
- Nutrition

Nevertheless, the increase in world travel in the past 30–40 years has brought Westerners into contact with a number of diseases unusual in the West, such as malaria and schistosomiasis. The number of notifications of malaria in the UK has markedly increased during the past decade and tuberculosis is a common problem amongst immigrants.

Advances in modern technology have enabled a number of new infective agents to be identified and their role in disease to be studied. Important new enteric infections are those due to rotaviruses, *Campylobacter*, *Cryptosporidium* and *Clostridium difficile*. The new hepatitis viruses, non-A non-B and delta viruses, are as yet incompletely characterized, but will certainly become increasingly recognized in the future. Legionnaires' disease, Lyme disease, toxic shock syndrome and the acquired immunodeficiency syndrome (AIDS) have all presented recently as major clinical problems with a substantial mortality, the causative agent of each being identified within a few years of recognition of the disease.

The control of infectious diseases world-wide has been vastly improved by the use of effective vaccines

Introduction

Global impact

Infectious diseases are the commonest afflictions of mankind and are a major source of morbidity and mortality in both developed and developing countries. Table 1.1 shows estimated morbidity and mortality figures for the common infectious diseases.

The infant mortality due to diarrhoeal disease in the Western World at the beginning of the twentieth century was similar to that in many parts of the Third World today. The reduction in mortality rate which

Table 1.1 League table of infectious diseases world-wide.

Disease	Estimated morbidity (No. of cases in thousands per year)	Estimated mortality (No. of deaths in thousands per year)
Diarrhoeal disease	3 000 000 – 5 000 000	10 000
Respiratory infection	?	5 000
Malaria	150 000	1 500
Measles	80 000	1 000
Schistosomiasis	20 000	1 000
Whooping cough	20 000	400
Neonatal tetanus	?	150

and antimicrobial agents. Technological advances in molecular biology have also improved the diagnosis, treatment and control of infectious diseases. For example, monoclonal antibodies can now be used for immunodiagnosis and the genetic manipulation of virulent bacterial strains has allowed the development of effective, safe vaccine strains (e.g. Texas Star-SR vibrio for cholera).

Epidemiology

The prevalence of infectious diseases varies markedly throughout the world and depends on climatic conditions, sanitation, the quality of the water supply, and to some extent the specific disease resistance of the indigenous population at risk. The continuance of infectious diseases in a human population requires:
- Reservoirs of infection
- Effective modes of transmission

Reservoirs
Human reservoirs are necessary for the agents of those diseases which (under natural conditions) exclusively afflict humans. Specific examples of such diseases are hepatitis A and B, cholera, shigellosis and smallpox, the last of which has now been eliminated following aggressive vaccination programmes.

Many sites in the body are used by microorganisms to gain a permanent hold on the host. The skin and nasopharynx are populated by a wide variety of non-pathogenic and sometimes pathogenic microorganisms; for example, meningococci and corynebacteria may be found in the nasopharynx.

The intestinal tract serves as an important reservoir for enteropathogens such as *Giardia*, *Entamoeba histolytica* and *Salmonella*, all of which may continue to be excreted in the stool despite clinical recovery from an acute infection.

Viruses may remain in the body for many months or years, notable examples being hepatitis B virus and the neurotropic herpesviruses.

Helminths may remain in the circulation (e.g. schistosomes in the portal vein) or lymphatic system (e.g. filarial worms) for many years, the former constantly producing millions of ova, a high proportion of which are deposited back into the environment.

Animal reservoirs of human disease are also important both in the Western and Third Worlds. The following are common examples of zoonoses (infections which can be transmitted from animals, except arthropods, to man):
- From battery-farmed chickens—*Salmonella* or *Campylobacter* infection

- From domestic cats—*Toxoplasma gondii* infection
- From domestic and wild animals—*Giardia* infection
- From cattle—*Cryptosporidium* infection

Diseases which rely on arthropods for their transmission include malaria, yellow fever, Dengue fever and rickettsial infections.

Environment reservoirs may also act as a temporary lodging place for some bacteria, viruses and parasites.

Water contaminated with enteropathogens is a constant cause of concern in the tropics; water may also be a reservoir of hepatitis A virus. Cysts of some protozoa, notably *Giardia*, may remain viable despite apparently effective water purification procedures.

Soil is also a source of the agents of human disease, particularly spore-forming bacteria such as *Clostridium* and *Bacillus anthracis*, whose spores can remain viable under suitable climatic conditions for many months.

Transmission
Airborne spread. Some viruses, bacteria and bacterial spores can be carried directly by the wind. Some are generally spread by droplets in the air, e.g. influenza viruses, and other microorganisms such as *Legionella* are spread by aerosol, characteristically from air-conditioning units.

Spread by direct contact. This includes:
- Person-to-person spread, e.g. skin infections (impetigo, ringworm and scabies) and sexually transmitted diseases
- Faecal–oral spread, particularly amongst children in residential institutions, e.g. shigellosis, giardiasis and hepatitis A
- Inoculation of infection, e.g. transfusion of blood or blood products containing hepatitis B, non-A non-B or AIDS viruses or by contaminated needles (drug abusers, medical and paramedical personnel)
- Insect bites, e.g. mosquitoes (malaria), sand fly (leishmaniasis), ticks (babesiosis) and bugs (Chagas' disease)
- Entry through the skin, which occurs with the larval forms of some helminths which can survive in soil or water, e.g. *Schistosoma*, *Strongyloides* and hookworm

Spread by food and water. Contaminated food and water is the usual mode of transmission of enteropathogens. Some bacteria, such as *Shigella*, require as few as 10 organisms to initiate infection, whereas others like *Vibrio cholerae* require approximately 10^8 organisms. Cysts of parasites such as *Giardia* and *Entamoeba histolytica* can survive in water for many months and are relatively resistant to water treatment procedures.

Spread by fomites. Transmission of infection can occur between persons via an inanimate object, e.g. bed linen, books.

Principles and basic mechanisms

Fig. 1.1 summarizes the important steps which occur during the pathogenesis of infection.

Specificity
Microorganisms are generally highly specific with respect to the organ or tissue that they infect. This predilection for specific sites in the body relates partly to the *milieu extérieur*, i.e. the immediate environment in which the organism finds itself; for example, anaerobic organisms colonize the highly anaerobic colon, whereas aerobic organisms are generally found in the mouth, pharynx and proximal intestinal tract. Other organisms which clearly show selectivity are:

- *Streptococcus pneumoniae* (respiratory tract)
- *Escherichia coli* (urinary tract)
- *Chlamydia trachomatis* (genital tract)

Even within a species of bacterium such as *Escherichia coli*, different strains will show selectivity towards a particular organ, e.g. the enterotoxigenic *E. coli* causes acute diarrhoeal disease, whereas the uropathogenic *E. coli* is responsible for urinary tract infection.

Even within an organ a pathogen may show selectivity for a particular cell type. In the intestine, for example, rotavirus predominantly invades and destroys intestinal epithelial cells on the upper portion of the villus, whereas reovirus selectively enters the body through the specialized epithelial cells, known as M cells, which cover the Peyer's patches.

Epithelial attachment
Many bacteria attach to the epithelial substratum by specific organelles called pili (or fimbriae) which contain a surface lectin(s), a protein or glycoprotein that recognizes specific sugar residues on the host cell. Such is the specificity of this attachment mechanism that it limits enterotoxigenic *Escherichia coli* infection, for example, to certain species. Some viruses and protozoa (*Plasmodium*, *Entamoeba histolytica*) also interact with their target cell surface membrane by a similar mechanism. Other parasites such as hookworm have specific attachment organelles (buccal plates) which firmly grip the intestinal epithelium.

Multiplication and colonization
These follow epithelial attachment. Pathogens may

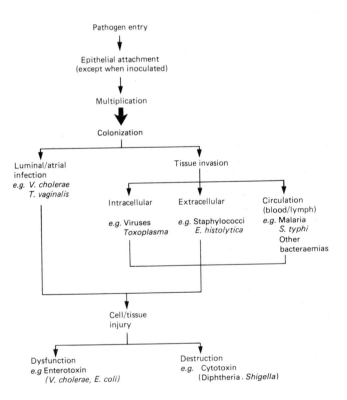

Fig. 1.1 The pathogenesis of infection.

then either remain within the lumen of the organ that they have colonized or may invade the tissues.

Invasion

Invasion may result in:
- An intracellular location for the pathogen (e.g. viruses, *Toxoplasma*, *Leishmania*, *Plasmodium*)
- An extracellular location for the pathogen (e.g. mycobacteria, staphylococci and *E. histolytica*)
- Invasion directly into the blood or lymph circulation (e.g. schistosome larvae, trypanosomes, *Leishmania* and *Plasmodium*)

Once the pathogen is firmly established in its target tissue, a series of events follow which usually culminate in damage to the host.

Tissue dysfunction or damage

The mechanism by which microorganisms produce disease has been the subject of intensive investigation and a number of well-defined mechanisms have now been described.

Exo- and endotoxins. Microorganisms may secrete exotoxins. These have many diverse activities, including inhibition of protein synthesis (diphtheria toxin), neurotoxicity (*Clostridium perfringens*, *C. tetani* and *C. botulinum*) and enterotoxicity, which results in intestinal secretion of water and electrolytes (*Escherichia coli*, *Vibrio cholerae*).

Endotoxins are lipopolysaccharides in the cell wall of gram-negative bacteria. They are responsible for many of the features of gram-negative shock, namely hypotension, fever, intravascular coagulation and, at high doses, death.

Tissue invasion. *Staphylococcus aureus* has both tissue invasive qualities, e.g. abscess formation and bacteraemia, as well as producing toxins causing diarrhoea and a toxin responsible for a widespread erythema (staphylococcal scalded skin syndrome). Similarly, some pathogenic *Escherichia coli* can produce tissue invasion without production of a specific toxin.

Secondary immunological phenomena. Enveloped viruses such as herpesviruses and poxviruses can induce antibody-mediated cytolysis of the host cell by depositing viral antigen on the cell surface, which is then recognized by host immunoglobulins (IgG or IgM) with subsequent activation of the classical complement pathway.

Microbial activation of the classical or alternative complement pathway yields the chemotactic factors C3a and C3,C5a, both of which attract inflammatory cells which then not only attack infected cells but also injure surrounding tissue.

Other immune phenomena which may occur include immune complex vasculitis (in viral hepatitis, malaria or leprosy), anaphylaxis (in aspergillosis or helminth infection), and delayed hypersensitivity (in tuberculosis or histoplasmosis).

Many infections are self-limiting, and immune and non-immune host defence mechanisms will eventually clear the pathogens. This is generally followed by tissue repair, which may result in complete resolution or leave residual damage.

Metabolic consequences

Infection not only causes local damage but also has important generalized effects.

Fever

Body temperature is controlled by the thermoregulatory centre in the anterior hypothalamus in the floor of the third ventricle. This centre is sensitive to endogenous pyrogen (now known to be interleukin I), which is released from a variety of cells involved in host defence, primarily blood monocytes and phagocytes, under the influence of microbial exogenous pyrogens. Interleukin I is thought to act on the thermoregulatory centre by increasing prostaglandin synthesis. The antipyretic effect of salicylates is brought about, at least in part, through its inhibitory effects on prostaglandin synthetase.

Fever production is thought to have a positive effect on the course of infection. However, for every 1°C rise in temperature, there is a 13% increase in basal metabolic rate and oxygen consumption. Fever therefore leads to increased energy requirements at a time when anorexia leads to decreased food intake. The normal compensatory mechanisms in starvation, e.g. mobilization of fat stores, are inhibited in acute infections. This leads to an increase in skeletal muscle breakdown, releasing amino acids which, via gluconeogenesis, are used as energy.

In chronic infection there is time for adaptation and the body is able to utilize fat stores more effectively and thus weight loss is much slower.

Protein metabolism

During acute infection major changes occur in protein metabolism:
- There is a diversion of synthesis away from somatic and circulating proteins such as albumin towards acute phase proteins such as C-reactive protein, haptoglobin, alpha-1-antitrypsin, caeruloplasmin and fibrinogen
- Protein synthesis is also directed towards immunoglobulin production and there is production of lymphocytes, neutrophils and other phagocytic cells
- There is a marked increase in nitrogen losses, which may reach 10–15 g per day

It is often impossible to meet these nutritional needs other than by intensive nutritional support.

Mineral metabolism and acid–base balance

Mineral metabolism and acid–base balance are disturbed during acute infection. In general, sodium and water are retained, principally due to the effects of increased levels of aldosterone and inappropriate secretion of antidiuretic hormone. During the convalescent period after acute infection, a diuresis may occur. Acid–base balance disturbance is common, and includes respiratory alkalosis following tachypnoea related to fever, respiratory acidosis and hypoxaemia associated with pneumonia, and metabolic acidosis associated with septicaemia.

In acute infection these changes are mild and resolve promptly without specific intervention. However, in situations where infections are prolonged and resolution is slow, supportive care may be necessary, particularly with respect to managing nutritional deficits and electrolyte and acid–base disturbances.

Host defence (see also Chapter 2)

The human body has natural resistance to infection as well as the ability to develop acquired resistance to specific pathogens when necessary.

Natural resistance

Body surface

The epithelial barriers of skin and mucous membranes are the primary lines of defence. In the bronchial tree, retrograde beating of cilia and intermittent coughing and expectoration provide a simple mechanism for keeping the upper airways free of invading pathogens. In the intestine, villus movement and peristalsis are usually antigrade, and tend to expel pathogens through the anus.

Chemical factors such as gastric acid are particularly active against certain enteropathogens, namely *Salmonella*, *Shigella* and *Vibrio cholerae*, while the low pH of the urine inhibits the growth of many urinary pathogens.

The gel-forming properties of mucus forms a sticky trap both for normal flora and for pathogens, and constant secretion of mucus results in a continuous shedding of organisms from a variety of body sites.

The normal microbial flora play a vital role in impeding the growth of certain pathogens; for example, certain non-pathogenic *E. coli* produce colicins which are lethal to *Salmonella* and *Shigella*.

Surface immunoglobulins are found on all mucous membranes and are active during the early phase of colonization. Secretory IgA is particularly important since it is resistant to the action of proteolytic enzymes. However, gonococci, meningococci and some streptococci produce IgA proteases able to cleave secretory IgA$_1$ (which accounts for approximately 40% of the IgA secreted).

Extracellular fluids

Natural antibodies are present in these fluids, some of which neutralize toxins, others act as opsonins and promote phagocytosis, while others activate complement, resulting in bacteriolysis. Beta lysin is released from platelets in inflammatory exudates and has the ability to kill gram-positive bacteria. C-reactive protein is also involved in complement activation. In the presence of viruses, some cells produce substances called interferons. These have broad-spectrum antiviral activity which is not limited to the invading virus.

Phagocytic cells

Organisms may be carried by lymphatics and trapped in lymph nodes where they become a target for phagocytosis by macrophages. Failing this they will ultimately enter the circulation and be ingested by circulating neutrophils or by phagocytic cells in the liver (Kupffer's cells), spleen, bone marrow, pituitary or adrenal gland.

Acquired resistance

Antibodies

The presence of foreign antigens leads to the transformation of B lymphocytes into plasma cells which produce immunoglobulin (Ig). The primary response is the production of IgM. IgM is an active cell agglutinin and also activates complement via the classical pathway. It is, however, a large molecule and does not cross the placenta. Within 10–14 days the IgG response begins, and IgG becomes the predominant antibody in the circulation. IgG antibodies can act:

- As opsonins by forming a bridge between the pathogen (Fab fragment) and the phagocytic neutrophil (Fc fragment)
- As antitoxins
- As complement activators
- By taking part in antibody-dependent cell-mediated cytotoxicity
- By blocking attachment of microbial pathogens to the substratum or preventing entry into the cell (e.g. blocking entry of the malarial parasite into the red cell)

Secretory immunity to specific organisms occurs in many luminal and atrial (e.g. vaginal) infections, which often involves blocking of the attachment of microorganisms (e.g. *Vibrio cholerae*, influenza virus —see p. 59) to the epithelium. Not all antibody production during infection is useful, as many antibodies have no protective function whatsoever, although they may be useful for serodiagnosis.

Cell-mediated immunity

T lymphocytes are particularly important in those diseases in which immunity is not acquired by circulating antibodies. Cell-mediated immunity is important in fungal and viral infections, in some bacterial infections (leprosy, brucellosis, tuberculosis and syphilis) and in some parasitic infections (leishmaniasis and schistosomiasis). Some T lymphocytes are cytotoxic, recognizing and destroying cells which bear a foreign antigen (virus-infected cells). In addition, sensitized T lymphocytes produce lymphokines which activate and attract macrophages to the site of infection.

T lymphocytes survive for long periods and therefore provide lasting protection against infection.

The immunological response to infection generally involves both humoral and cellular mechanisms; for example, specific antibodies may limit the spread of a virus, but sensitized T lymphocytes are required for its elimination.

Host susceptibility

Many factors are known to influence an individual's susceptibility to infection. Individuals at the extremes of life are more susceptible to infection. The infant has a relatively immature immune system and in the early neonatal period relies heavily on transplacental passage of immunoglobin (IgG) from its mother and of secretory immunoglobulin (sIgA) in colostrum and breast milk. Immune function in the elderly is less effective than in the younger adult and may be further modified by impaired nutrition. There are also some genetic determinants of susceptibility to infection, a good example being the relative resistance of individuals carrying the HbS gene (sickle-cell trait) to malaria.

Table 1.2 Opportunistic infections.

Predisposing factors	Infecting organisms (with special associations)
Primary immunodeficiency Antibody defects (hypo- or agammaglobinaemia, selective IgA deficiency)	Bacteria (respiratory, intestinal and urinary)
Cell-mediated defects (Swiss, Wiskott–Aldrich or DiGeorge's syndrome) Combined defects (severe combined immunodeficiency)	Viruses, bacteria and fungi (e.g. *Candida*)
Malignant disorders, e.g. leukaemia, lymphoma Diminished cell-mediated immunity, neutropenia	Viruses (CMV, VZV, HSV), gram-negative organisms (causing bacteraemia), fungi
Infection with HIV Diminished cell-mediated immunity	Viruses, *Pneumocystis*, *Cryptosporidium*
Allograft recipients (renal, bone marrow, heart) Diminished cell-mediated immunity	Enterobacteriaceae, *Pseudomonas* or gram-negative bacteria (all causing bacteraemia), herpesvirus, fungi
Bone marrow failure Neutropenia	Enterobacteriaceae, *Pseudomonas*, *Candida*, etc. (causing bacteraemia or disseminated infection), herpesvirus
Defective clearance of pathogens Splenectomy Fibrocystic disease	Pneumococcal and other bacterial pathogens
Gut motility disorders Endotracheal tube Liver disease	Gut aerobes and anaerobes, *Pseudomonas*, *Klebsiella*, Enterobacteriaceae
Tissue, vessel and organ implants Prosthetic heart valve CSF shunt Peritoneal dialysis catheter Central venous catheter	Bacteria and *Candida*. Often organisms of low pathogenic potential, e.g. *Staphylococcus epidermidis*

Diabetics have increased numbers of infections, particularly pyogenic infections, as do patients with both primary and secondary immunodeficiency.

Opportunistic infection
Opportunistic infection occurs in individuals with compromised host defence mechanisms. Sometimes the infecting agent is not a normal pathogen. The clinical presentation is often atypical, leading to diagnostic difficulty. The failure of local defence mechanisms leads to an absence of signs of infection, such as fever and pus.

Opportunistic infections are noted for their chronicity and for their resistance to conventional antimicrobial chemotherapy. Table 1.2 summarizes the important situations where opportunistic infection may arise and the infectious agents commonly associated with these diseases.

Interaction between nutrition and infection

Undernutrition impairs host defence (Fig. 1.2). Natural resistance to infection is lowered by alterations in the integrity of body surfaces, the reduced ability to repair epithelia, and the reduction in gastric acid production. In addition, immunological abnormalities are found:
- Tissue and circulating macrophage function is impaired
- T lymphocyte function is depressed
- The total lymphocyte count is below 1×10^9 cells per litre, which is indicative of a relatively immunocompromised host
- Cell-mediated immunity is in a state of anergy,

i.e. the body fails to respond to a recall antigen such as the Mantoux test
- Antibody production is less sensitive to undernutrition, but in severe malnutrition depression in both circulating and secretory immunity are detectable. This is of importance clinically in that vaccination (e.g. against polio) may have to be more aggressive in malnutrition before protective immunity is achieved
- Complement levels fall rapidly in severe acute malnutrition and remain low during long periods of established suboptimal nutritional status. Complement levels have been used as a biochemical marker of nutritional status

Diagnosis (Fig. 1.3)

HISTORY
Particular attention should be paid to the following:
- Foreign travel—remembering that certain diseases can exist both in the tropics and Europe, e.g. leishmaniasis, giardiasis
- Immigrants—country of origin
- Food and water—food poisoning is extremely common
- Occupation, e.g.
  sheep farmers—hydatid disease
  sewer workers—leptospirosis
  leather workers—anthrax
- Domestic pets, e.g.
  budgerigars—psittacosis
  cats—toxoplasmosis
  dogs—*Toxocara canis* infection, rabies
- Sexual activity—hepatitis B, non-A non-B hepatitis, mixed enteric infections and AIDS

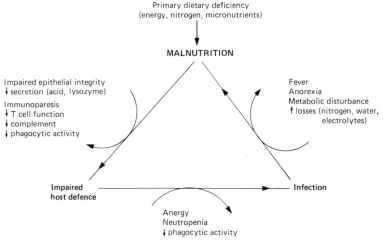

Fig. 1.2 Nutrition–infection–host defence: a complex interaction.

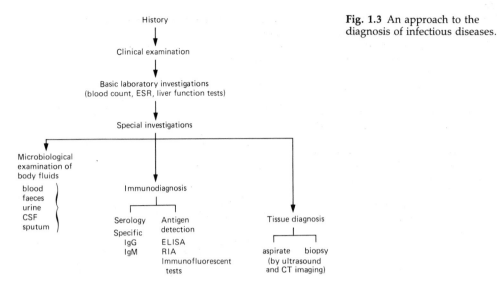

Fig. 1.3 An approach to the diagnosis of infectious diseases.

should be particularly considered in male homosexuals
● Drug addiction—consider hepatitis B and pyogenic infections, e.g. staphylococcal
● Tattooing—consider hepatitis B
● Injections and transfusions—may act as a route of transmission for infections

CLINICAL EXAMINATION

A general examination should be performed with particular attention to skin rashes, lymphadenopathy and hepatosplenomegaly. In cases of sexually transmitted diseases the perineum, rectum and vagina should be inspected. The presence of a fever is helpful, but less emphasis is now placed on fever patterns because of improved laboratory diagnosis. High swinging fevers are characteristically seen with localized pus.

INVESTIGATION

Tests should be performed as appropriate. If the diagnosis is obvious, e.g. a measles rash is present, no tests are necessary. The list below gives examples of situations where tests may be useful.

● *Full blood count and film* are usually performed and often give a guide to the type of infection, although the changes are not invariable:
   (a) Polymorphonuclear leucocytosis–bacterial infections
   (b) Neutropenia—viral infections, brucellosis, typhoid, overwhelming septicaemia
   (c) Lymphocytosis—viral infections, whooping cough
   (d) Atypical monocytes—infectious mononucleosis

   (e) Eosinophilia—parasitic infections, helminths
The ESR is usually raised.
● *Liver function tests* are slightly raised in infections but this is a non-specific sign. They will also be raised in hepatitis and other liver infections.
● *Urine analysis*   } These should also be performed, even in the absence of symptoms and signs.
● *Chest x-ray*

Further investigations are often required to make the specific diagnosis:
● Blood culture
● Microscopic examination and culture of appropriate body fluids, e.g. urine, faeces, CSF, sputum
● Viruses can be identified in the above body fluids by:
   (a) Electron microscopy
   (b) Tissue culture (cytomegalovirus)
   (c) Immunological antigen capture techniques (rotavirus)
● Immunodiagnosis—immunological techniques are now available for the identification of:
   (a) *Pathogen-specific antigens* using polyvalent antisera or monoclonal antibodies
   (b) *Specific serological responses* to infection using immunodiffusion, complement fixation, indirect haemagglutination, indirect immunofluorescence or enzyme-linked immunosorbent assay (ELISA)
A high titre of IgM specific to a pathogen (e.g. hepatitis A or B virus, cytomegalovirus) is diagnostic of a recent infection. In infection a single raised IgG is unhelpful as this only indicates a previous rather than a current infection. However, a rising titre can confirm the diagnosis (e.g. in brucellosis or mycoplasma infection).

These immunological techniques are particularly useful in the identification of pathogens that are difficult to culture by standard microbiological techniques or intracellular pathogens that require tissue culture

- Tissue diagnosis—biopsy/aspiration with isolation of pathogen:
  (a) Bone marrow/liver biopsy for generalized infections such as tuberculosis, leishmaniasis
  (b) Rarely, if the above technique is negative, splenic aspiration for leishmaniasis
  (c) Lung biopsy for *Pneumocystis carinii* infection
- Imaging procedures—ultrasound and CT scan (with needle aspiration) for abscesses in liver, lung, brain or abdomen

Pyrexia of unknown origin (PUO)

A major diagnostic problem is the patient who has a pyrexia, either intermittent or continuous, which lasts for three weeks or more and in whom routine investigations have failed to reveal a cause. PUO may merely be an unusual presentation of a common disease. Table 1.3 shows some of the common causes of PUO.

Infection is particularly likely in individuals who do not normally live in the UK and in travellers who have recently returned from tropical or subtropical regions. Tuberculosis, leishmaniasis, malaria and amoebic liver abscess are common findings in such individuals.

Age is another important pointer, since cancer and the connective tissue diseases are more common in the elderly.

Immunocompromised individuals are at particular risk of infectious disease and often present with a particularly unusual spectrum of infections (see p. 6).

An aggressive approach to the diagnosis of PUO is justified since there is a good chance that determination of a specific diagnosis will influence management and result in curative treatment. It is always worth repeating the history and examination since new signs may have evolved since the patient's initial admission to hospital. All drug therapy should be reassessed and, if possible, stopped.

INVESTIGATION

First-line investigations such as a full blood count, blood culture, urinalysis, routine blood chemistry and chest x-ray should be repeated.

Other investigations
- CT and ultrasound scanning are particularly valuable in revealing primary and secondary neoplastic diseases and also for showing occult abscesses.

Table 1.3 Common causes of pyrexia of unknown origin (PUO).

Infection (40%)
Pyogenic abscess
Tuberculosis
Urinary infection
Biliary infection
Subacute bacterial endocarditis
EBV infection
CMV infection
Q fever
Toxoplasmosis
Brucellosis

Cancer (30%)
Lymphomas
Leukaemia
Solid tumours, e.g.
  hypernephroma
  hepatoma
  pancreatic carcinoma

Immunogenic (20%)
Drugs
Connective tissue and autoimmune diseases, e.g.
  rheumatoid disease
  systemic lupus erythematosus
  polyarteritis nodosa
  polymyalgia/cranial arteritis
Sarcoidosis

Factitious (1–5%)
Switching thermometers
Injection of pyrogenic material

Remain unknown (5–9%)

- Aspiration or needle biopsy under imaging control provides a histological diagnosis.
- Laparoscopy may be required to confirm a gynaecological cause, e.g. pelvic inflammatory disease, multiple peritoneal metastases or tuberculous peritonitis.
- Needle biopsy of the liver may be required to confirm granulomatous hepatitis, tuberculosis or metastatic cancer.
- Scanning with gallium-59, which is taken up by polymorphs, can localize an abscess.

Laparotomy is rarely performed since the advent of more sophisticated imaging and guided-biopsy techniques.

Septicaemia

The term *bacteraemia* refers to the transient presence of organisms in the blood (generally without causing symptoms) as a result of local infection or penetrating injury.

The term *septicaemia*, on the other hand, is usually reserved for when bacteria or fungi are actually multiplying in the blood, usually with the production of severe systemic symptoms such as fever and hypotension.

Pyaemia describes the serious situation when, in a septicaemia, organisms and neutrophil polymorphs embolize to many sites in the body causing abscesses, notably in the lungs, liver and brain.

Septicaemia has an extremely high mortality and demands immediate attention.

CAUSES

The term *primary septicaemia* is used to describe the situation when the focus of infection is not apparent. Such patients are generally elderly, undernourished or suffering from chronic disease, particularly alcoholic cirrhosis and diabetes.

The common sites of infection and infective agents responsible for *secondary septicaemia* are shown in Tables 1.4 and 1.5. Pneumococcus and *Haemophilus influenzae* are common causes of septicaemia in children, whereas in neonates gram-negative rods and group B streptococci are the most likely aetiological agents. *Neisseria gonorrhoeae* is a common cause of septicaemia in young adults, but it is usually mild without serious effects. Intravenous drug abusers frequently suffer bacteraemia and septicaemia, often caused by *Staphylococcus aureus*, *Pseudomonas* and *Serratia*.

CLINICAL FEATURES

Fever, rigors and hypotension are the cardinal features of severe septicaemia. However, the illness may be preceded by less specific symptoms such as headache, lethargy, apprehension and subtle changes in conscious level. Other clinical features and their pathogenesis are shown in Table 1.6.

INVESTIGATION

Septicaemia is almost always treated initially on the basis of a clinical diagnosis after appropriate specimens have been sent to the laboratory. Probable origins of infection and likely pathogens must be sought on the basis of a careful history and examination. The type of infection will clearly differ in hospitalized and otherwise previously healthy adults (see Tables 1.4 and 1.5). Body fluids or other specimens (blood, urine, CSF, tissue or abscess aspirates) should be submitted to full microbiological examination. Imaging investigations such as ultrasonography and CT scan may be required.

Catheters or cannulae, which might be sources of infection, should be removed and sent for culture.

TREATMENT

Antibiotic therapy should be commenced immediately. If the organism and its antibiotic sensitivities

Table 1.4 Septicaemia in a previously healthy adult.

Site of origin	Usual pathogen(s)
Skin	*Staphylococcus aureus* and other gram-positive cocci
Urinary tract	*Escherichia coli* and other aerobic gram-negative rods
Respiratory tract	*Streptococcus pneumoniae*
Gallbladder or bowel	*Streptococcus faecalis*, *E. coli* and other gram-negative rods *Bacteroides fragilis*
Pelvic organs	*Neisseria gonorrhoeae*, anaerobes

Table 1.5 Septicaemia in hospitalized patients.

Clinical problem	Usual pathogen(s)
Urinary catheter	*Escherichia coli*, *Klebsiella*, *Proteus*, *Serratia*, *Pseudomonas*
Intravenous catheter	*Staphylococcus aureus* and *S. epidermidis*, *Klebsiella*, *Pseudomonas*, *Candida albicans*
Post-surgery:	
Wound infection	*Staphylococcus aureus*, *Escherichia coli*, anaerobes (depending on site)
Deep infection	Depends on anatomical location
Burns	Gram-positive cocci, *Pseudomonas*, *Candida albicans*
Immunocompromised patients	Any of the above

Table 1.6 Special clinical features of septicaemia.

Clinical feature	Cause
Hypotension ('endo-toxic shock')	Liberation of bacterial endo-toxin (cell-wall lipopolysaccharide) which reduces vascular tone and increases permeability
Pulmonary oedema and adult respiratory distress syndrome (ARDS)	Increased permeability of the alveolar capillary endothelium, impaired gas exchange and hypoxia
Disseminated intravascular coagulation (DIC)	Activation of blood coagulation by endothelial damage, endo-toxins and immune complexes

are unknown, a combination of drugs should be chosen to cover the likely pathogens. If there is an obvious site of skin sepsis, drugs such as flucloxacillin (1 g 6-hourly i.v.) and an aminoglycoside to cover *Staphylococcus aureus* should be used. If bowel sepsis is suspected then a broader-spectrum drug of the cephalosporin group (e.g. cefoxitin 1–2 g every 6–8 h i.m. or i.v.) would be advisable. In the absence of any helpful clinical guidelines a combination of a penicillin drug which is active against *Pseudomonas* (carbenicillin 5 g every 4–6 h by slow i.v. injection or ticarcillin 15–20 g in divided doses) with an aminoglycoside such as tobramycin (3–5 mg·kg^{-1} daily in divided doses every 8 h) should be given. Metronidazole (1 g every 8 h by rectum) is often added to provide additional cover against anaerobic organisms.

Shock should be treated (see p. 635).

Antimicrobial chemotherapy

Widespread and often inappropriate use of antibiotics has led to increasing numbers of organisms with multiple drug resistance. Antibiotics are not required for all infections, particularly minor skin infections or intestinal bacterial infections, the majority of which are self-limiting conditions. Nevertheless, in many countries of the world antibiotics are readily available 'over the counter', and are often used in inadequate amounts and for the wrong diseases.

Although the majority of antibiotics are relatively safe drugs, important toxic effects do occur when used in the incorrect dosage and in the presence of other disease states, notably renal disease. In addition, antibacterial therapy may result in secondary yeast or fungal infection or may facilitate the growth of a second bacterial pathogen, such as *Clostridium difficile*, an important cause of antibiotic-associated colitis.

Thus it is essential that a number of factors should be taken into account before commencing, and during, antimicrobial chemotherapy.

Choice of drug
Blind therapy. In the majority of clinical situations antimicrobial therapy is begun before the organism is identified and its antibiotic sensitivities known. The choice of drug(s) is therefore dependent on a clinical diagnosis and a knowledge of the organisms likely to be involved in a given situation. Before beginning 'blind' therapy it is essential to obtain appropriate body fluids or other specimens for microbiological examination. Adjustments to the antibiotic regimen can then be made, if necessary, when antibiotic sensitivities are available.

Spectrum of activity. The spectrum of antibacterial activity of the drug chosen should ideally be as narrow as possible, as it will then have fewer detrimental effects on the normal bacterial flora of the host. 'Blind' therapy, however, by necessity generally covers a broader spectrum than required.

Bactericidal vs. bacteriostatic. In the majority of infections there is no firm evidence that bactericidal drugs (penicillins, cephalosporins, aminoglycosides) are more effective than bacteriostatic drugs, but it is generally considered important to use the former in the treatment of bacterial endocarditis and in patients in whom host defence mechanisms are compromised.

Patient factors. In addition to age and pregnancy, the following factors should be considered:
- *The site of infection.* The chosen drug must be able to gain access to the part of the body involved. The brain, eye, biliary tract, prostate and loculated abscesses are inaccessible to many drugs.
- *Renal and hepatic function.* Impaired renal or hepatic function necessitates a major modification of the dose regimen or even complete avoidance of certain drugs. Care should be taken when using aminoglycosides, carbenicillin, ticarcillin, flucytosine and some antituberculous agents in patients with renal impairment. Other drugs, such as nalidixic acid, tetracycline and vancomycin, should be avoided altogether.

Dose
The dose of drug used is influenced by the type of infection to be treated and the age of the patient. Bacterial endocarditis and deep-seated abscesses (e.g. in brain or lung) generally require high-dose therapy for several weeks, generally beginning with intravenous administration of drugs. Dosages of individual drugs are given under the description of each disease.

Route of administration
Some drugs (e.g. some of the cephalosporins) are only available as intravenous preparations, but many antibiotics are well-absorbed by the oral route and generally there is no advantage to the patient for therapy to be administered by the more expensive parenteral route. Patient compliance must, however, be taken into account.

Duration of therapy
For some infections the arbitrary 7–10 days' treatment has now been dramatically reduced, as there is now good evidence that a 3-day course of antibiotics is quite sufficient to treat many lower urinary tract infections.

Monitoring

In serious infections (e.g. subacute bacterial endocarditis), monitoring of circulating drug concentrations is important for assessing efficacy of treatment. Drug concentrations can be measured directly in serum, but the efficacy of therapy is best determined by serum bactericidal assay just before and at a standard time after administration of antibiotics. The highest dilution of serum that completely kills the causative organism can then be determined.

Monitoring for toxicity is particularly important with the aminoglycoside antibiotics. Concentrations are determined immediately before ('trough' levels) and usually 15–30 minutes after intravenous administration of the drug. High 'trough' levels of $>2\ \mu g \cdot ml^{-1}$ are considered to be the most important factor in causing the oto- and nephrotoxicity commonly seen with these agents.

Combination antibiotic therapy

Combinations of antibiotics are commonly used in the empirical treatment of many serious infections such as septicaemia, meningitis, tuberculosis and endocarditis, but some care must be taken in the choice of drugs within such combinations. There is still some concern that a combination of a bactericidal and a bacteriostatic antibiotic may impair their therapeutic efficacy. However, this concept is by no

Table 1.7 Antibiotic chemoprophylaxis.

Clinical problem	Aim	Drug regimen
Rheumatic fever	To prevent recurrence and further cardiac damage	Phenoxymethylpenicillin 250 mg twice daily or benzathine penicillin 916 mg monthly
Infective endocarditis	To prevent infection on abnormal, prosthetic or homograft heart valves following potentially bacteriaemic procedures	*Dental/oropharyngeal procedures* Oral amoxycillin 3 g 1 h before (erythromycin for penicillin-sensitive individuals—1.5 g 1 h before and 500 mg 6 h after). Parenteral penicillin is used for procedures under general anaesthesia or for 'high-risk' patients with prosthetic valves *Genitourinary/gastrointestinal procedures* Ampicillin 1 g plus gentamicin 80 mg i.v. before and 8 and 16 h after procedure
Meningitis:		
Due to meningococci	To prevent infection in *close* contacts	Rifampicin 600 mg twice daily for 2 days or sulphadimidine 2 g daily for 5 days
Due to *Haemophilus influenzae*	To reduce nasopharyngeal carriage	Rifampicin 10–20 $mg \cdot kg^{-1}$ daily for 4 days
Tuberculosis	To prevent infection in exposed (close contacts) tuberculin-negative individuals, infants of infected mothers and immunosuppressed patients	Oral isoniazid 5 $mg \cdot kg^{-1}$ daily for 6–12 months
Malaria	To prevent infection	Oral chloroquine 400–500 mg as a single dose each week, 2 weeks before and for 6 weeks after leaving endemic area Where chloroquine resistance occurs (get advice): chloroquine 400–500 mg plus oral sulfadoxine/pyrimethamine (Fansidar) 1 tablet (500 mg and 25 mg respectively) each week, beginning 2–3 days before and continuing for 6 weeks after leaving endemic area, or oral dapsone/pyrimethamine (Maloprim) 1 tablet (100 mg and 12.5 mg respectively) each week as above
Recurrent urinary tract infection	To reduce morbidity	Oral co-trimoxazole, long-term low dose

means universally applicable since the bacteriostatic drug tetracycline and the bactericidal drug rifampicin are thought to be synergistic. Generally, combinations of bactericidal drugs are at least additive and in some situations are synergistic, whereas combinations of bacteriostatic drugs are generally only additive.

Antibiotic chemoprophylaxis
This is required in certain disease states (see Table 1.7).

Mechanisms of resistance to antimicrobial agents

The development or acquisition of resistance to an antibiotic by bacteria invariably involves a mutation at a single point in a gene or transfer of genetic material from another organism (see Fig. 1.4). Single-point mutations occur in *Escherichia coli*, for example, at the rate of approximately 1 per 10^5–10^7 cell divisions. A mutation resulting in antibiotic resistance by this mechanism would involve alteration of a single nucleotide base.

Larger fragments of DNA may be introduced into a bacterium either by transfer of 'naked' DNA or via a bacteriophage (a virus) DNA vector. Both the former (transformation) and the latter (transduction) are dependent on integration of this new DNA into the recipient chromosomal DNA. This requires a high degree of homology between the donor and recipient chromosomal DNA.

Finally, antibiotic resistance can be transferred from one bacterium to another by conjugation, when extra chromosomal DNA (a plasmid) containing the resistance factor (R factor) is passed from one cell into another during direct contact. Transfer of such R factor plasmids can occur between unrelated bacterial strains and involve large amounts of DNA.

Transformation is probably the least clinically important mechanism, whereas transduction and R factor transfer are probably the most important for the sudden emergence of multiple antibiotic resistance in a single bacterium.

ANTIBACTERIAL DRUGS

Naturally occurring compounds

Penicillins
Structure. Penicillins, like cephalosporins, have a beta-lactam ring associated with a peptide or peptide-like structure (see Fig. 1.5).

Relatively minor changes to the side-chain of benzyl penicillin render the phenoxymethyl derivative acid resistant and allow it to be absorbed well when given orally. The presence of an amino group in the phenyl radical of benzyl penicillin increases the antimicrobial spectrum of the native penicillin and makes it active against both gram-negative and gram-positive organisms. More extensive modification of the side-chain (e.g. as in cloxacillin) renders the drug insensitive to bacterial penicillinase, a major advance in treating infections caused by penicillinase (beta-lactamase)-producing staphylococci.

Mechanism of action. Penicillins block the terminal cross-linking reaction (between alanine and glycine) of bacterial cell wall mucopeptide formation.

Indications for use. Benzyl penicillin can only be given parenterally and is the drug of choice for serious infections, notably infective endocarditis, pneumococcal, meningococcal, streptococcal and gonococcal infections, clostridial infections (tetanus, gas gangrene), actinomycosis, anthrax, and spirochaetal infections (syphilis, yaws).

Procaine penicillin and benzathine penicillin are

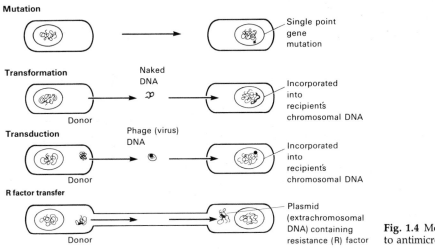

Fig. 1.4 Mechanisms of resistance to antimicrobial drugs.

Fig. 1.5 The structure of penicillins.

long-acting drugs whose effects last for 24 h and 3–4 weeks, respectively, after a single intramuscular injection. Procaine penicillin is used in the treatment of gonorrhoea and syphilis, and benzathine penicillin is used for rheumatic fever prophylaxis when regular administration of oral penicillin proves unreliable.

Phenoxymethylpenicillin (penicillin V) is an oral preparation which is chiefly used as maintenance therapy for rheumatic fever prophylaxis.

Flucloxacillin is used in infections caused by penicillinase-producing staphylococci. Methicillin is also effective but must be given by injection.

Ampicillin is susceptible to penicillinase, but its antimicrobial activity includes gram-negative organisms such as *Salmonella*, *Shigella*, *Escherichia coli*, *Haemophilus influenzae* and *Proteus*. It is useful in the treatment of urinary tract and upper respiratory tract infections. Amoxycillin has a similar sphere of activity to ampicillin, but is better absorbed when given by mouth.

Clavulanic aid is a powerful inhibitor of many bacterial beta-lactamases and when given in combination with an otherwise susceptible agent such as amoxycillin can broaden the spectrum of activity of the drug.

Carbenicillin and ticarcillin are active against *Pseudomonas* infection and the acylureido-penicillin derivatives (azlocillin, mezlocillin, piperacillin) have increased activity against gram-negative organisms, including *Pseudomonas*, compared with other penicillins.

Resistance. Bacteria producing penicillinase are resistant to some penicillins.

Interactions. Penicillins inactivate aminoglycosides when mixed in the same solution.

Toxicity. Hypersensitivity (skin rash, urticaria, anaphylaxis), encephalopathy and interstitial nephritis can occur. Ampicillin also produces a hypersensitivity rash in approximately 90% of patients with infectious mononucleosis who receive this drug. Generally, the penicillins are very safe.

Cephalosporins
The cephalosporins have major advantages over the penicillins in that they are innately resistant to staphylococcal penicillinases and have a broader range of activity which includes both gram-negative and gram-positive organisms. Like the penicillins they have a beta-lactam ring, but this is associated with a dihydrothiazine ring in place of the thiazolidine ring found in penicillins (see Fig.1.6). Side-chain modifications increase their potency and range of activity. Structural modifications have produced orally active drugs such as cephalexin and cephradine and a variety of highly potent parenteral preparations such as cefuroxime, cephamandole and cefoxitin.

Mechanism of action. Like penicillins, cephalosporins inhibit bacterial cell wall synthesis.

Indications for use. These potent broad-spectrum antibiotics are useful for the treatment of serious systemic infections, particularly when the precise nature of the infection is unknown. They are commonly used for serious postoperative sepsis and in immunocompromised patients, particularly during treatment of leukaemia and other malignancies.

Fig. 1.6 The structure of a cephalosporin.

Resistance. Cephalosporins generally resist the action of beta-lactamase-producing bacteria.

Interactions. Increased nephrotoxicity is seen when cephalosporins are used in conjunction with other nephrotoxic antibiotics such as aminoglycosides and some diuretics.

Toxicity. This is as for penicillin; some patients are allergic to both groups of drugs. The early cephalosporins caused proximal tubule damage, although the newer derivatives have less nephrotoxic effects.

Aminoglycosides
Structure. These antibiotics are derived from *Streptomyces* species and are polycationic compounds of amino sugars (see Fig. 1.7).

Mechanisms of action. Aminoglycosides interrupt bacterial protein synthesis by inhibiting ribosomal function (messenger and transfer RNA).

Indications for use. Streptomycin is bactericidal for susceptible organisms. In the past it was widely used for the treatment of tuberculosis, but its use has now been largely superseded by newer agents because it had to be given parenterally and had a high toxicity. Neomycin is also highly toxic when given systemically and therefore it is only used for the topical treatment of eye and skin infections and orally for preoperative 'bowel sterilization' and in the management of portosystemic encephalopathy. Even though it is poorly absorbed, prolonged oral administration can produce toxic effects such as ototoxicity.

Gentamicin and tobramycin are given parenterally. They are highly effective against many gram-negative organisms including *Pseudomonas*. They are active against *Streptococcus faecalis* and also the beta-lactamase-producing staphylococci. The newer aminoglycosides, netilmicin and amikacin, have a similar spectrum of antibacterial activity and are generally resistant to the aminoglycoside-inactivating enzymes produced by some bacteria. Their use should be restricted to gentamicin-resistant organisms.

Resistance. Some bacteria produce phosphorylating, adenylating or acetylating enzymes which inactivate

aminoglycoside antibiotics. These enzymes are coded for and transferred by R factors (extra-chromosomal DNA).

Interactions. Enhanced nephrotoxicity occurs with other nephrotoxic drugs, ototoxicity with some diuretics, and neuromuscular blockade with curariform drugs.

Toxicity. Aminoglycosides are nephrotoxic and ototoxic (vestibular and auditory), particularly in the elderly. Blood levels must be checked (p. 12).

Tetracyclines
Structure. These are bacteriostatic drugs possessing a four-ring hydronaphthacene nucleus (see Fig. 1.8). Variation of the native compound is obtained by different substitutions to give, for example oxy- and chlortetracycline, or doxycycline.

Mechanism of action. Tetracyclines inhibit bacterial protein synthesis by interrupting ribosomal function (transfer RNA).

Indications for use. Tetracyclines are active against gram-positive and gram-negative bacteria. They are particularly useful for the treatment of respiratory infections, notably acute and acute-on-chronic bronchitis, and of intestinal bacterial overgrowth, and as prophylaxis for traveller's diarrhoea (doxycycline). Doxycycline is also used for the treatment of acne and rosacea. Tetracyclines are also active against *Vibrio cholerae*, *Rickettsia*, *Mycoplasma*, *Coxiella burnetii*, *Chlamydia* and *Brucella*.

Resistance. Some bacteria possess reduced bacterial cell permeability to tetracycline, which is coded for by an R factor. Resistance is particularly important in infections with pneumococci and *Haemophilus influenzae*.

Interactions. The efficacy of tetracyclines is reduced by antacids, barbiturates and oral iron replacement therapy.

Toxicity. Tetracyclines are generally safe drugs, but they may enhance established or incipient renal failure, although doxycycline is safer than others in

Fig. 1.7 The structure of an aminoglycoside.

Fig. 1.8 The structure of tetracycline. Substitution of CH_3, OH or H at positions A to D produces variants of tetracycline.

this group. Brown discoloration of growing teeth (and thus these drugs are not given to children or pregnant women) and photosensitivity can occur.

Erythromycin
Structure. Erythromycin consists of a lactone ring with unusual sugar side-chains.

Mechanism of action. Erythromycin inhibits protein synthesis by interrupting ribosomal function.

Indications for use. Erythromycin has a similar antibacterial spectrum to penicillin and is useful in individuals with penicillin sensitivity. It can be given orally or parenterally. Recently it has been more widely used and is included in the treatment regimen of all pneumonias as many are due to *Mycoplasma*. It is effective in the treatment of infections due to *Bordetella pertussis* (whooping cough), *Legionella*, *Campylobacter*, *Chlamydia*, *Coxiella* and *Listeria*.

Toxicity. Erythromycin estolate may produce cholestatic jaundice after prolonged treatment.

Chloramphenicol
Structure. Chloramphenicol is the only naturally occurring antibiotic containing nitrobenzene (see Fig. 1.9). This structure is probably important for its toxicity in humans and for its activity against bacteria.

Mechanism of action. Chloramphenicol is structurally similar to uridine-5-phosphate and competes with messenger RNA for ribosomal binding. It also inhibits peptidyl transferase.

Indications for use. Despite its toxicity, chloramphenicol is indicated for the treatment of severe infection due to *Salmonella typhi* and *paratyphi* (enteric fevers) and infection due to *Haemophilus influenzae* (meningitis and acute epiglottitis). It is also active against *Yersinia pestis* (plague) and is used topically for purulent conjunctivitis.

Resistance. Bacterial R factors code for acetylating enzymes which can inactivate chloramphenicol and also reduce bacterial cell permeability to this agent.

Interactions. Chloramphenicol enhances the activity of anticoagulants, phenytoin and oral hypoglycaemic agents.

Toxicity. Severe irreversible bone marrow suppression is rare but nevertheless restricts the usage of this drug to the indications above and for ill patients. Chloramphenicol should not be given to premature infants or neonates because of their inability to conjugate and excrete this drug; high blood levels lead to circulatory collapse and the often fatal 'grey baby syndrome'.

Fusidic acid
Structure. Fusidic acid has a structure resembling that of bile salts.

Mechanism of action. It is a potent inhibitor of bacterial protein synthesis. Its entry into cells is facilitated by the detergent properties inherent in its structure.

Indications for use. Fusidic acid is mainly used for penicillinase-producing *Staphylococcus aureus* infections such as osteomyelitis or endocarditis, and for other staphylococcal infections associated with bacteraemia or septicaemia. The drug is well absorbed orally but is relatively expensive. It is well concentrated in bone.

Resistance. This may occur rapidly and is the reason why fusidic acid is given in combination with another antibiotic.

Toxicity. Fusidic acid is a safe drug and if necessary can be given during pregnancy.

Synthetic compounds

Sulphonamides
Structure. The sulphonamides were the first synthetic, systemically active agents. They are all derivatives of the prototype sulphanilamide. Variations in biological activity are obtained by different substitutions on the side-chain (see Fig.1.10).

Mechanism of action. Sulphonamides block thymidine and purine synthesis by inhibiting microbial folic acid synthesis.

Indications for use. Sulphamethoxazole is mainly used in combination with trimethoprim as co-trimoxazole for urinary tract infections and acute-on-chronic bronchitis. Sulphapyridine in combination with 5-

Nitrobenzene

Fig. 1.9 The structure of chloramphenicol.

Fig. 1.10 The structure of a sulphonamide.

aminosalicylic acid (i.e. sulphasalazine) is used in inflammatory bowel disease

Resistance. Bacteria may become resistant to sulphonamides by production of sulphonamide-resistant dihydropteroate synthetase and by altering bacterial cell permeability to these agents.

Interactions. Sulphonamides potentiate oral anticoagulants and hypoglycaemic agents.

Toxicity. Sulphonamides cause thrombocytopenia, folate deficiency and megaloblastic anaemia and haemolysis in individuals with glucose-6-phosphate dehydrogenase deficiency, and therefore should not be used in such people. Co-trimoxazole should be avoided in the elderly if possible, as deaths have been recorded, probably due to the sulphonamide component.

Nitroimidazoles
Structure. These agents are active against anaerobic organisms, notably anaerobic bacteria and some pathogenic protozoa. The most widely used drug is metronidazole (Fig. 1.11). Minor modifications in the structure of nitroimidazole have produced other related compounds such as tinidazole and nimorazole.

Mechanism of action. After reduction of their nitro group to a nitrosohydroxyl amino group by microbial enzymes, nitroimidazoles cause strand breaks in microbial DNA.

Indications for use. Metronidazole is of major importance in the treatment of anaerobic bacterial infection, particularly that due to *Bacteroides*. It is also used prophylactically in colonic surgery. It may be given orally, by suppository (entirely satisfactory blood levels can be obtained by this route) or intravenously (very expensive). It is also the treatment of choice for amoebiasis, giardiasis and infection with *Trichomonas vaginalis*.

Interactions. Nitroimidazoles can produce a disulphuram-like reaction with ethanol.

Toxicity. Nitroimidazoles are tumorigenic in animals and mutagenic for bacteria, although carcinogenicity has not been described in humans. They cause a metallic taste, and peripheral neuropathy with prolonged use. They should be avoided in pregnancy.

Vancomycin
Vancomycin is produced by *Streptomyces orientalis*.

Structure. Vancomycin is a complex and unusual glycopeptide primarily active against gram-positive bacteria.

Mechanism of action. Vancomycin inhibits cell wall synthesis and is bactericidal.

Indications for use. Vancomycin is given orally in pseudomembranous enterocolitis and intravenously in methicillin-resistant *Staphylococcus aureus* (MRSA) infections. It is expensive and its use should be restricted to these two conditions.

Toxicity. Vancomycin can cause oto- and nephrotoxicity. Care must be taken to avoid extravasation at the injection site as this causes necrosis and thrombophlebitis.

ANTIFUNGAL DRUGS

Naturally occurring compounds

Polyenes
The most potent of these is amphotericin B, which is used intravenously in severe systemic fungal infections. Nephrotoxicity is a major problem and dosage levels must take into account background renal function. Nystatin is not absorbed through mucous membranes and is therefore useful for the treatment of oral and enteric candidiasis and for vaginal infection. It can only be given orally or as pessaries. Polyenes react with the sterols in fungal membranes, increasing permeability and thus damaging the organism.

Griseofulvin
This naturally occurring antifungal is concentrated in keratin and is therefore useful for chronic fungal infection of nails, although treatment may be required for many months. It is also widely used for the treatment of ringworm.

Synthetic drugs

Imidazoles such as miconazole (Fig. 1.12), keto-

Fig. 1.11 The structure of metronidazole, a nitroimidazole.

Fig. 1.12 The structure of miconazole, an imidazole.

conazole and clotrimazole are all active against strictly aerobic organisms:

- Clotrimazole is used topically for the treatment of ringworm.
- Miconazole is a potent systemic antifungal which may be used with amphotericin B in severe systemic fungal infection and is active both orally and parenterally.
- Ketoconazole is the most recently introduced imidazole antifungal and is active orally. It can produce liver damage.

The fluorinated pyridine derivative, flucytosine is usually used in combination with amphotericin B for systemic fungal infection. Side-effects are uncommon, although it may cause bone marrow suppression. It is active when given both orally and parenterally.

ANTIVIRAL DRUGS

Idoxuridine
As a 5% solution with dimethyl sulphoxide (DMSO) this agent is active against herpes simplex virus (HSV), but to be effective it must be applied to the skin before the appearance of vesicles. It is also effective as a 0.1% solution when instilled into the eye for HSV keratitis. Similar topical use in herpes zoster probably alters the clinical course of the illness if given early.

Vidarabine (adenine arabinoside)
This agent may be given intravenously and is active against HSV and varicella zoster virus (VZV). It is also used in severe varicella infection (chickenpox). Its major toxic effects include bone marrow suppression and renal impairment.

Acyclovir
This agent is relatively free from side-effects and is effective against many herpes virus infections. Oral and topical preparations are available for the treatment of HSV infections. An intravenous preparation can be used for the treatment of systemic virus infection in the immunocompromised host, particularly VZV infections, and also for primary HSV infection.

Interferon
This is a naturally occurring substance produced by T lymphocytes during virus infection. Interferon production occurs in response to many different viruses and production stimulated by one virus may confer protection against a second viral invader. Recombinant DNA technology has enabled this substance to be produced commercially and it is currently being evaluated as a treatment for acute and chronic hepatitis, herpes virus infections and otherwise untreatable conditions such as Lassa fever.

Prevention

Although effective antimicrobial chemotherapy is available for many diseases, the ultimate aim of any infectious disease control programme is to prevent infection occurring. This may be achieved either by:

- Eliminating the source or mode of transmission of an infection
- Reducing host susceptibility to environmental pathogens

Control of sources and transmission

Water and food supplies constitute a major reservoir of infection by which a pathogen can reach large numbers of individuals very rapidly. Surveillance of water quality in the Industrialized World has led to the control of many acute diarrhoeal diseases such as cholera and enterotoxigenic *Escherichia coli* infection, although such diseases continue to be a major problem in the developing world. Surveillance of milk herds for tuberculosis and brucellosis has had a major impact on those parts of the world where such controls have been possible. Factory chickens, however, inevitably carry *Campylobacter*, which may have contributed in part to the increased reports of this infection in the West. Food handlers constitute an important potential source of enteric infection; therefore, epidemics of *Salmonella*, for example, should be fully investigated so that carriers can be identified.

Screening of blood donors has proved essential to control the spread of hepatitis viruses and will constitute an important control measure in limiting the spread of acquired immunodeficiency syndrome. Definition of high-risk carrier populations, such as male homosexuals and immigrants from endemic areas of infectious disease, may also be important.

Reduction of host susceptibility

Immunization has changed the course and natural history of many infectious diseases. Passive immunization by administering pre-formed antibody, either in the form of immune serum or purified gamma globulin, provides short-term immunity, and has been effective in both the prevention and treatment of a number of bacterial and viral diseases (Table 1.8). Long-lasting immunity is, however, only achieved by active immunization with a live attenuated organism, a dead organism or an antigen preparation of part of an organism. Active immunization may also be performed with microbial toxin (either native or modified), in which case the immunogen is called a toxoid. Important preparations available for active immunization are shown in Table 1.9. The active immunization schedule currently recommended in the UK is summarized in Table 1.10.

Table 1.8 Examples of passive immunization available.

Infection	Antibody	Indication	Efficacy
Bacterial			
Pertussis	Human pertussis immune globulin	Treatment	±
Tetanus	Human tetanus immune globulin	Prevention and treatment	+
Diphtheria	Horse serum	Prevention and treatment	±
Botulism	Horse serum	Treatment	±
Viral			
Hepatitis A			
Measles	Human normal immune globulin	Prevention	+
Rubella			
Hepatitis B	Human hepatitis B immune globulin	Prevention	+
Varicella zoster	Human varicella zoster immune globulin	Prevention	+
Rabies	Human rabies immune globulin	Prevention	+

Table 1.9 Preparations available for active immunization.

Live vaccines
Oral polio (Sabin)
Measles
Mumps
Rubella
Yellow fever
BCG

Dead organisms, crude or purified extracts
HBV
Pertussis
Typhoid
Polio (Salk)
Cholera
Meningococci (group A and C)
Rabies

Toxoids
Diphtheria
Tetanus

Table 1.10 Immunization schedule recommended in the UK.

Year of life	Vaccines	Dose schedule
1	DTP plus OPV *or* DT (if P contra-indicated)	At 3, 5 and 9–12 months
2	Measles	Single dose
School entry	Booster DT plus OPV	Single dose
10–14 (females)	Rubella	Single dose
11–13	BCG (tuberculin-negative individuals) (under reconsideration in UK)	Single dose
School leavers	T plus OPV	Single dose

DTP = diphtheria (D)/tetanus (T)/pertussis (P) (triple vaccine); OPV = oral polio vaccine; BCG = bacille Calmette-Guérin.

Bacterial infections

Gram-positive cocci

STAPHYLOCOCCAL INFECTIONS

Staphylococci are aerobic, facultatively anaerobic, gram-positive cocci. They contain a number of cellular antigens and produce enzymes such as coagulase as well as toxins such as enterotoxin. Their pathogenicity correlates most closely with the production of the coagulase enzymes. Coagulase-positive strains are referred to as *Staphylococcus aureus* and coagulase-negative strains as *Staphylococcus epidermidis*. While both strains are pathogenic to humans, infection is usually due to *S. aureus*. Staphylococci are part of the normal microflora of the human skin, the upper respiratory tract, especially the nasopharynx, and the intestinal tract. Twenty-five per cent of the population are permanent carriers of *S. aureus*.

Approximately 20% of all human staphylococcal

infections are autogenous. Transmission is most frequently by direct contact with an infected individual, but may be airborne or via fomites. Several predisposing host factors have been identified (Table 1.11).

The organism can cause a wide clinical spectrum of diseases. These are usually localized, but infection may spread, resulting in bacteraemia or metastatic infection. Table 1.12 shows a list of conditions due to *S. aureus*; a few of these will be considered below.

Skin infections
These are discussed on p. 921.

Osteomyelitis
Acute osteomyelitis is almost always due to staphylococcal infection. It occurs predominantly in males between the ages of 3 and 12 years, usually affecting the lower limbs. A history of trauma is often present. The diaphysis is initially involved, with subsequent spread of the infection to the periosteum and the subcutaneous tissues. Signs of inflammation are present. The child is usually irritable and febrile. There is leucocytosis and blood cultures are positive in about 75% of patients.

Table 1.11 Host factors which increase susceptibility to staphylococcal infections (predominantly *Staphylococcus aureus*).

Injury to skin or mucous membranes, e.g.
  abrasions
  trauma (accidental or surgical)
  burns
  insect bites

Metabolic abnormalities, e.g.
  diabetes mellitus
  uraemia

Foreign bodies*, e.g.
  intravenous and other indwelling catheters
  cardiac and orthopaedic prostheses
  tracheostomies

Abnormal leucocyte function, e.g.
  Job's syndrome
  Chédiak–Higashi syndrome
  steroid therapy
  drug-induced leucopenia

Post-viral infections, e.g.
  influenza

Miscellaneous conditions, e.g.
  excess alcohol consumption
  malnutrition
  malignancies
  old age

*Often *Staphylococcus epidermidis*.

Table 1.12 Clinical conditions produced by *Staphylococcus aureus*.

Due to invasion

Skin:
  Furuncles
  Cellulitis
  Impetigo
  Carbuncles

Lungs:
  Pneumonia
  Lung abscesses

Heart:
  Endocarditis
  Pericarditis

Central nervous system:
  Meningitis
  Brain abscesses

Bones and joints:
  Osteomyelitis

Miscellaneous:
  Parotitis
  Pyomyositis
  Septicaemia
  Enterocolitis

Due to toxin

Staphylococcal food poisoning

Scalded-skin syndrome:
  Generalized erythema
  Bullous impetigo
  Staphylococcal scarlet fever

Toxic shock syndrome

Osteomyelitis involving the vertebrae occurs in adults over 50 years of age. The onset is insidious, with pain; often there are no other features of infection.

Radiographs are usually normal in the first week after onset in both varieties of osteomyelitis.

Food poisoning (see Table 1.19, p. 33)
This results from ingestion of food contaminated with pre-formed heat-stable enterotoxin. *S. aureus* accounts for approximately 5% of all food poisoning in the UK. Contamination is usually from an infected individual.

Foods such as canned foods, processed meats, milk and cheese favour the growth of *S. aureus*. The illness is manifest within 6 h of ingestion of contaminated foods and affects close to 100% of individuals who have eaten such foods. In contrast to food poisoning due to other organisms, staphylococcal food poisoning is characterized by the presence of persistent vomiting. Fever, when present, is usually below 38°C. Abdominal discomfort, diarrhoea or dysentery may be present. Treatment is not necessary as the illness is short-lived (12–24 h). Antibiotics are of no value since the disease is due to toxin and not bacteria.

Toxic shock syndrome (TSS)

Staphylococci which produce the pyrogenic exotoxin C and enterotoxin F are believed to be responsible for this syndrome. TSS is seen most frequently in menstruating women below the age of 30 years who use tampons. However, it can occur in other situations and men and children are not exempt. It is characterized by the abrupt onset of fever, a diffuse macular erythema, vomiting, diarrhoea, severe myalgia and shock. Treatment is supportive. Antibiotics are usually given, although the syndrome is produced by the exotoxin.

Scalded skin syndrome (SSS)

Scalded skin syndrome is caused by staphylococci which elaborate the toxin exfoliatin. It is seen in children under 5 years of age and is characterized by a painful macular skin rash followed by bullae and generalized shedding of the epidermis.

TREATMENT

Any local lesion, e.g. an abscess, should be drained. Systemic infection is treated with antibiotics. Hospital-acquired infections are usually penicillin-resistant and therefore treatment is with flucloxacillin, methicillin or nafcillin, usually together with fusidic acid. Seventy per cent of infections acquired outside the hospital are penicillin sensitive and penicillin is the drug of choice. Increasing antibiotic resistance is still a problem and most hospitals have restrictions on the use of single antibiotics. The control of staphylococcal cross-infection is important.

Recently epidemic methicillin-resistant *S. aureus* (EMRSA) has accounted for 20–40% of all clinical isolates of *S. aureus* in some hospitals. EMRSA is resistant to most antibiotics, except vancomycin, and the treatment of serious infections is difficult. Isolation of patients and high standards of hygiene are required to control hospital epidemics.

STREPTOCOCCAL INFECTIONS

Streptococci are round or ovoid gram-positive, facultatively anaerobic, catalase-negative bacteria. Virulence is attributed to the cell wall M protein and the production by some streptococci of hyaluronidase, DNAses or streptokinase. The spread of streptococci is mediated by direct contact, fomites or airborne droplet infection. Group A beta-haemolytic streptococci (*Streptococcus pyogenes*) are responsible for the majority of human infections (Table 1.13). Group B streptococci frequently produce neonatal sepsis and meningitis, and Group C and G organisms occasionally cause pharyngitis and

Table 1.13 Diseases caused by streptococci.

Suppurative
Skin:
Impetigo
Pyoderma
Erysipelas
Cellulitis
Pharyngeal:
Pharyngitis
Tonsillitis
Peritonsillar abscess
Infections confined to women:
Puerperal sepsis
Endometritis
Pulmonary:
Pneumonia
Empyema
Others:
Osteomyelitis
Infective endocarditis
Meningitis
Peritonitis
Lymphangitis
Bacteraemia
Non-suppurative
Rheumatic fever
Glomerulonephritis
Scarlet fever

endocarditis. Alpha-haemolytic streptococci (known collectively as *S. viridans*) found commonly in the mouth, e.g. *S. sanguis* and *S. mitis*, as well as *S. mutans*, a non-haemolytic streptococcus, cause three-quarters of all streptococcal endocarditis.

S. pneumoniae is the commonest cause of pneumonia (see p. 594).

Scarlet fever

Scarlet fever occurs when the infectious organism (usually a group A streptococcus) produces erythrogenic toxin in an individual who does not possess neutralizing antitoxin antibodies. The disease is notifiable.

CLINICAL FEATURES

The incubation period of this relatively mild disease of childhood is 2–4 days following a streptococcal infection. The initial infection may be anywhere, but is usually in the pharynx. Regional lymphadenopathy, fever, rigors, headache and vomiting are present. The rash, which usually appears on the second day of illness, initially occurs on the neck but rapidly becomes punctate, erythematous and generalized. It is typically absent from the face, palms and soles, and is prominent in the flexures.

The rash usually lasts about 5 days and is followed by extensive desquamation of the skin. The face is flushed with characteristic circumoral pallor. Early in the disease the tongue has a white coating through which prominent bright red papillae can be seen ('strawberry tongue'). Later the white coating disappears, leaving a raw-looking, bright red colour ('raspberry tongue').

Scarlet fever may be complicated by the development of peritonsillar or retropharyngeal abscesses and otitis media.

DIAGNOSIS

The diagnosis is established by the typical clinical features and culture of throat swabs, where the organisms are usually found in abundance. Elevated anti-streptolysin O and anti-DNAse B levels in the serum are indicative of streptococcal infection.

TREATMENT

Treatment is directed at preventing the non-suppurative complications of streptococcal infections (see Table 1.13).

Penicillin is the drug of choice and may be given orally as phenoxymethylpenicillin 125 mg four times daily for 10 days or as a single intramuscular injection of benzathine penicillin 916 mg in adults. Individuals allergic to penicillin can be treated effectively with erythromycin 250 mg four times daily for 10 days.

The role of tonsillectomy in preventing further attacks of pharyngitis remains controversial.

PREVENTION

Chemoprophylaxis with penicillin or erythromycin should be given in epidemics.

Erysipelas

Erysipelas is an acute, rapidly progressive infection of the skin which is almost always due to group A streptococci. It usually occurs in the very young or the elderly. The onset is abrupt; fever, headache and vomiting are common. The erythematous skin lesion, which is usually on the face, enlarges rapidly and has a sharply demarcated raised edge. Vesicles and bullae appear within this lesion which then rupture, leaving crusts on the surface. Regional lymphadenopathy is common. Bacteraemia, when present, is associated with a high mortality rate. Treatment with penicillin is rapidly effective.

Rheumatic fever

This is discussed on p. 511.

Acute glomerulonephritis

This is discussed on p. 380.

Gram-negative cocci

NEISSERIAL INFECTIONS

Neisseria are gram-negative, non-motile, non-spore-forming, aerobic, round or oval diplococci. *N. meningitidis* and *N. gonorrhoeae* are the only two bacteria in this group which are commonly pathogenic to humans.

Meningococcal infection

Meningococci (*N. meningitidis*) are ubiquitous. However, group A is commonly found in Africa and group B on the European and American continents. The incidence of group C and Y infections appears to be steadily rising world-wide. Group A is responsible for epidemics of meningitis and group B and C for sporadic infections. Its virulence is attributed to the polysaccharide capsule (which resists phagocytosis) and the lipopolysaccharide–endotoxin complex (which is responsible for its clinical toxicity). Transmission is by droplet infection or direct contact. Humans are the only known reservoirs. Following transmission, *N. meningitides* colonize the nasopharynx preferentially because of the humidity, increased carbon dioxide tension and specific receptor substances synthesized by the nasopharynx to which they adhere. Invasiveness of the organism appears to be almost solely dependent on the amount of specific anti-meningococcal bactericidal antibodies in the host. A history of a recent viral respiratory infection is common.

CLINICAL FEATURES

Four major clinical syndromes due to meningococci are recognized:
- *Meningococcaemia* may occur alone or in association with meningitis. It is characterized by the presence of headache, fever, malaise and myalgia. The patient looks toxic, and has tachycardia and tachypnoea. Skin manifestations occur early and consist of a purpuric rash and/or petechiae which also affect the conjunctivae.
- *Fulminant meningococcaemia* (Waterhouse–Friderichsen syndrome) occurs in about 10% of patients. It is characterized by an extremely rapid downhill clinical course, with extensive haemorrhage into the skin, hypotension, shock, confusion, coma and death within a few hours of the onset of symptoms. Disseminated intravascular

coagulation, due to activation of the complement system, may further complicate the clinical picture. Haemorrhage into the adrenal glands may or may not be present. Without treatment, the mortality rate approaches 100%.

- *Meningococcal meningitis* presents with fever, nausea, vomiting, headache, photophobia, altered consciousness and neck rigidity. The clinical presentation is indistinguishable from other acute bacterial meningitides (see p. 835).
- *Chronic meningococcaemia* is rare. It is characterized by intermittent fever, a maculopapular rash, arthralgia and splenomegaly. Blood cultures are positive during bacteraemic episodes.

N. meningitidis may also rarely result in polyarthritis, pericarditis and nephritis.

DIAGNOSIS

This is established by demonstrating meningococci in body fluids such as blood, CSF, petechial or joint aspirates. The CSF is turbid with an increase in neutrophils and protein. Counterimmunoelectrophoresis to group A and C has recently been found useful.

TREATMENT

Benzylpenicillin is the treatment of choice, the dose being 1.2–2.4 g i.v. 4-hourly for adults. Ampicillin is equally effective. Chloramphenicol ($75–100\,mg\cdot kg^{-1}$) is the drug of choice in individuals allergic to penicillin. Treatment for shock (p. 635) and disseminated intravascular coagulation (p. 301) should be instituted.

PREVENTION AND CONTROL

Penicillin does not affect the carrier state. Family contacts of patients are protected effectively by rifampicin 600 mg two times daily for 2 days. Immunoprophylaxis with vaccines against group A and C organisms is effective and available.

Gonorrhoea

Gonorrhoea is caused by *N. gonorrhoeae*. It is discussed further on p. 44.

Gram-positive bacilli

CORYNEBACTERIA INFECTION

Corynebacterium diphtheriae is a gram-positive, pleomorphic, non-sporulating, aerobic, club-shaped bacillus. Three morphological varieties are recognized—*mitis*, *intermedius* and *gravis*. Of these, *mitis* is generally associated with mild infections. Only corynebacteria exposed to the bacteriophage beta which carries the *tox*$^+$ gene are capable of toxin production. The toxin has two subunits, A and B. Subunit A is responsible for clinical toxicity. Subunit B serves only to transport the toxin component to specific receptors, present chiefly on the myocardium and in the peripheral nervous system. Humans are the only natural hosts.

Diphtheria

Diphtheria caused by *C. diphtheriae* occurs worldwide. Its incidence in the West has fallen dramatically following widespread active immunization. Transmission is mainly through airborne droplet infection and rarely through fomites.

CLINICAL FEATURES

The incubation period varies from 2 to 7 days. Diphtheria is essentially a disease of childhood. The manifestations may be regarded as local (due to the membrane) or systemic (due to exotoxin). The presence of a membrane, however, is not essential to the diagnosis. The illness is insidious in onset, and is associated with tachycardia and low-grade fever. If complicated by infection with other bacteria such as *Streptococcus pyogenes*, fever is high and spiking.

Nasal diphtheria is characterized by the presence of a unilateral, serosanguinous nasal discharge which crusts around the external nares.

Pharyngeal diphtheria is associated with the greatest toxicity and is characterized by marked tonsillar and pharyngeal inflammation and the presence of a membrane. This tough greyish-white membrane is formed by fibrin, bacteria, epithelial cells, mononuclear cells and polymorphs, and is firmly adherent to the underlying tissue. Regional lymphadenopathy is prominent and produces the so-called 'bull-neck'.

Laryngeal diphtheria is usually a result of extension of the membrane from the pharynx. A husky voice, a brassy cough, and later dyspnoea and cyanosis due to respiratory obstruction are common features.

Clinically evident myocarditis occurs, often weeks later, in patients with pharyngeal or laryngeal diphtheria. Acute circulatory failure due to myocarditis may occur in convalescent individuals around the 10th day of illness and is usually fatal. Neurological manifestations may occur either early in the disease (palatal and pharyngeal wall paralysis) or several weeks after its onset (cranial nerve palsies, paraesthesias, peripheral neuropathy or, rarely, encephalitis).

Cutaneous diphtheria is being increasingly seen in association with burns and in individuals with poor personal hygiene. Typically the ulcer is punched-out with undermined edges and is covered with a greyish-white to brownish adherent membrane. Constitutional symptoms are uncommon.

DIAGNOSIS

This must be made on clinical grounds since therapy is usually urgent and bacteriological results of culture studies and toxin production cannot be awaited.

TREATMENT

The patient should be isolated and bed rest advised. Antitoxin therapy is the only specific treatment. It must be instituted rapidly to prevent further fixation of toxin to tissue receptors, since fixed toxin is not neutralized by antitoxin. Depending on the severity, 20 000 to 120 000 units of horse-serum antitoxin should be administered intravenously after an initial test dose to exclude any allergic reaction. There is a risk of anaphylaxis immediately after antitoxin administration and of serum sickness 2–3 weeks later. Antibiotics should be administered concurrently to eliminate the organisms and thereby remove the source of toxin production. Procaine penicillin, 1.2 g i.m., once daily for 7 days is usually effective.

The cardiac and neurological complications need intensive therapy, as described on p. 624.

PREVENTION

Diphtheria can be effectively prevented by active immunization in childhood (see p. 19).

All contacts of the patient should have throat swabs sent for culture; those with a positive result should be treated with penicillin or erythromycin and active immunization or a booster dose of toxoid given.

LISTERIAL INFECTION

Listeria monocytogenes is found world-wide. Listeriosis predominantly occurs perinatally, but may occasionally occur in immunocompromised adults. It causes abortions, septicaemia and meningitis. The mortality rate is high.

The diagnosis is established by culturing this gram-positive bacillus from blood, infected tissues or secretions. Treatment is with penicillin and tobramycin.

CLOSTRIDIAL INFECTIONS

Clostridium is a gram-positive, spore-forming, obligatory anaerobic bacillus. Some species, such as *C.*

botulinum and *C. tetani*, produce potent neurotoxins, whereas *C. perfringens* produces numerous enzymes and only occasionally an enterotoxin (see Table 1.19). All clostridia which are pathogenic to humans produce exotoxins and require a low redox potential for growth. They are normal commensals of human and animal gastrointestinal tracts, and are widely distributed in soil where, as spores, they may survive for many years in adverse conditions.

Tetanus

Tetanus occurs when a wound is contaminated by *C. tetani* in unimmunized individuals. The wound may be trivial and disregarded by the patient. The clinical manifestations of the disease are due to the potent neurotoxin, tetanospasmin. Tetanospasmin acts on both the alpha and gamma motor systems at synapses, resulting in disinhibition. It also produces neuromuscular blockade and skeletal muscle spasm, and acts on the sympathetic nervous system. The end result is marked flexor muscle spasm and autonomic dysfunction. The organism is not invasive.

CLINICAL FEATURES

The incubation period varies from a few days to several weeks. Four clinical varieties are recognized.

Generalized tetanus. This is the commonest form. Initially the patient complains of feeling unwell. This is followed by trismus (lock-jaw) due to masseter muscle spasm. Spasm of the facial muscles produces the characteristic grinning expression known as risus sardonicus. If the disease is severe, painful reflex spasms develop, usually within 24–72 h of the initial symptoms. The interval between the first symptom and the first spasm is referred to as the 'onset time'. The spasms may occur spontaneously, but are easily precipitated by noise, handling of the patient or by light. The frequency of spasms usually increases and respiration becomes impaired due to laryngeal spasm. Oesophageal and urethral spasm lead to dysphagia and urinary retention, respectively. Arching of the neck and back muscles occurs (opisthotonus). Autonomic dysfunction is evidenced by tachycardia, a labile blood pressure, sweating and cardiac arrhythmias. Patients with tetanus are mentally alert.

Death results from aspiration, hypoxia, respiratory failure, cardiac arrest or exhaustion. Mild cases with rigidity usually recover. Poor prognostic indicators are:
- Short incubation period
- Short onset time
- Cephalic tetanus
- Extremes of age
- 'Skin poppers' (narcotic addicts who inject drugs subcutaneously)

Localized tetanus. Pain and stiffness is confined to the site of the wound. The tone of the surrounding muscles is increased.

Cephalic tetanus. This is an uncommon form and usually occurs when the portal of entry of *C. tetani* is the middle ear. Cranial nerve abnormalities, particularly of the seventh nerve, are usual. Generalized tetanus may or may not develop.

Tetanus neonatorum. This occurs in neonates due to infection of the umbilical stump. Failure to thrive, poor sucking, grimacing and irritability are followed by rapid development of intense rigidity and spasms. Mortality approaches 100%.

DIAGNOSIS

Few diseases resemble tetanus in its fully developed form. The diagnosis is therefore a clinical one. Rarely *C. tetani* may be isolated from wounds.

Phenothiazine overdosage can mimic tetanus, but shows a dramatic response to benztropine 2 mg i.v.

TREATMENT

Nursing care. Improvement in nursing care techniques has contributed more than any other single measure to the decrease in the mortality rate from 60% to nearer 20%. Patients are nursed in a quiet, isolated, well-ventilated, darkened room. Intragastric feeds may be necessary; bladder and bowel care are also important.

Wound debridement. This should be carried out where indicated.

Antibiotics and antitoxin. Both antibiotics and antitoxin should be administered, even in the absence of an obvious wound. Intravenous penicillin is the drug of choice. Human antitetanus immunoglobulin 2000–3000 units should be given to neutralize any circulating toxin; it has no effect on fixed toxin. If human antitetanus immunoglobulin is not available, immune equine tetanus immunoglobulin 10 000–20 000 units i.v. should be given, after excluding allergy to this product.

Antitoxin administrations

Most antitoxins are heterologous and therefore dangerous hypersensitivity reactions are common.

Prior to treatment:
- Question patient about:
  (a) Allergic conditions, e.g. asthma, hayfever
  (b) Previous antitoxin administration
- Read instructions on antitoxin package carefully.
- Always give a subcutaneous test dose.

Control of spasms. Diazepam is the drug of choice. Up to 120 mg per 24 h may be required to control spasm and rigidity in adults.

The role of corticosteroids is controversial. Curarization and artificial respiratory support is best left to specialist units. The judicious use of a tracheostomy may be helpful in averting death.

Active immunization. Once recovery has occurred, active immunization should be instituted as immunity following tetanus is incomplete.

PREVENTION

Tetanus is an eminently preventable disease and all persons should be immunized regardless of age. Those who work in a contaminated environment, such as farmers, are particularly at risk. Active immunization with either plain toxoid or the alumadsorbed toxoid can be given. Of these, the latter is superior. Initially two doses of 0.5 ml of the toxoid are given intramuscularly at 8-week intervals. The third dose is given 6–12 months later as a booster. Subsequently boosters are required at 5-year intervals. Infant immunization schedules in the UK include tetanus (see p. 19).

Protection by passive immunization with either the equine or human antitetanus toxin is short-lived, lasting only about 2 weeks.

Botulism

Botulism is caused by *C. botulinum*. This organism is found in the soil and food is easily contaminated with the spores, which can survive heating to 100°C. The organisms proliferate in preserved canned foods and produce toxins. Only three types of neurotoxin—A, B and E—have consistently been shown to produce disease in humans. The toxins, which are the most potent known to man, result in marked neuromuscular blockade. They are heat-labile and are inactivated by heating at 80°C for 30 minutes or at 100°C for 10 minutes.

Rarely botulism can occur from wound infection. It is also seen in infants under 6 months and occasionally in adults following ingestion of the spores, the toxin being produced in vivo.

CLINICAL FEATURES

Nausea, vomiting and diarrhoea are early symptoms. Neurological symptoms dominate the clinical picture and include blurred vision, diplopia, laryngeal and pharyngeal paralysis, and later generalized paralysis; consciousness is not altered. Respiratory insufficiency may occur. The marked cholinergic blockade results in urinary retention and constipation. Fever is unusual.

DIAGNOSIS

The presence of toxin in faeces, serum or suspected food items is demonstrated by injecting the material into mice. The differential diagnosis includes the Guillain–Barré syndrome.

TREATMENT

Treatment is supportive and should be directed at maintaining adequate respiration, with assisted ventilation if necessary. Intravenous administration of 20 ml of antitoxin is followed by 10 ml 2–4 h later and then every 12–24 h as necessary. The role of antibiotics has not been adequately evaluated. Guanidine hydrochloride in doses of 15–40 $mg \cdot kg^{-1}$ improves botulism-induced paralysis by reversing the intramuscular blockage.

PROGNOSIS

The overall mortality rate for botulism is high (50–70%), but patients who survive the acute paralysis can recover completely.

Gas gangrene

Gas gangrene (clostridial myonecrosis) is commonly caused by *C. perfringens*. *C. novyi* and *C. septicum* are less frequently implicated. Gas gangrene occurs in lacerated wounds associated with fractures or retained foreign bodies. It is characterized by the onset of inordinately severe pain, with thickened induration and oedema at the injury site. When gas gangrene occurs in a limb, the part distal to the injury becomes cold and pulseless. Blebs appear and discharge a watery fluid, which later becomes haemorrhagic. The involved muscles at first appear pale and oedematous, but later they become beefy-red in colour and then brownish-black and frankly gangrenous. The characteristic crepitus of gas gangrene is a late feature. Systemic signs of toxicity are prominent. The patient is febrile, tachypnoeic and has a marked tachycardia. Hypotension and renal and hepatic failure develop as terminal events. Consciousness remains unaltered.

TREATMENT

Treatment consists of adequate surgical debridement, with parenteral penicillin combined with another antibiotic to cover aerobic and anaerobic organisms which are frequent wound contaminants. The role of anti-gas gangrene toxin and hyperbaric oxygen is controversial.

Pseudomembranous colitis

Pseudomembranous colitis is caused by *C. difficile*. It usually occurs a few days after institution of antibiotic therapy, although it has been known to occur even a month after discontinuing antibiotics. Clindamycin has been most frequently implicated, but ampicillin, tetracycline, lincomycin and the cephalosporins have also been causally related to some cases. Fever, diarrhoea (rarely with blood) and abdominal cramps are usual. Sigmoidoscopic examination reveals a markedly erythematous, ulcerated mucosa covered by a membrane-like material. The presence of this membrane is not essential to the diagnosis.

DIAGNOSIS

Identification of the toxin (by observing its cytopathic effect on cells in tissue culture) in stool specimens is diagnostic. Culture of the organism alone is insufficient.

TREATMENT

All suspected antibiotics should be discontinued. Vancomycin 125 mg orally, four times daily, for 10 days, has until recently been the drug of choice. Metronidazole is also effective and considerably less expensive.

BACILLUS INFECTIONS

Anthrax

Anthrax, a zoonosis, is caused by *Bacillus anthracis*, a slow-growing, gram-positive, non-motile, facultatively anaerobic, capsulated spore-forming bacillus. The spores are extremely hardy and withstand extremes of temperature and humidity. The organism is capable of toxin production and this property correlates most closely with its virulence. The disease occurs world-wide. Epidemics have been reported in the Gambia, in both North and South America and in southern Europe. Transmission is through direct contact with an infected animal and is seen in farmers, butchers and dealers in wool and animal hides. Spores can also be ingested or inhaled.

CLINICAL FEATURES

The incubation period varies from 1 to 5 days.

The cutaneous form is the commonest mode of presentation and is seen most frequently in the tropics. It is self-limiting in the majority of patients. Typically, a small erythematous, maculopapular lesion is present which subsequently vesiculates and undergoes ulceration, with formation of a central black eschar. Occasionally the perivesicular oedema is marked and toxaemia may be present.

Respiratory involvement (woolsorter's disease) due to inhalation of spores results in a non-productive cough, fever and retrosternal discomfort. Pleural effusions are common. In some patients there is apparent clinical improvement followed by the abrupt onset of dyspnoea, marked cyanosis and death.

DIAGNOSIS

Diagnosis is established by demonstrating the organism in smears or by culture. Detection of a four-fold increase in antibodies measured by indirect microhaemagglutination in paired sera (i.e. acute and convalescent samples) is diagnostic.

TREATMENT

Penicillin is the drug of choice. In mild cutaneous infections, phenoxymethylpenicillin 500 mg four times daily for 2 weeks is adequate. In more severe infections, e.g. when septicaemia is present, up to 24 g of intravenous crystalline penicillin is required daily. Sulphonamides, chloramphenicol and tetracycline have also been used successfully. The role of steroids in fulminant anthrax infections is questionable.

Any infected animal that dies should be burnt and the area in which it was housed disinfected. Where animal husbandry is poor, mass vaccination of animals may prevent widespread contamination.

Vaccination of exposed workers is effective.

Bacillus cereus infection

This gram-positive, aerobic, spore-forming bacillus can cause food poisoning and wound sepsis.

Gram-negative bacilli

BRUCELLOSIS (MALTA FEVER, UNDULANT FEVER)

Brucella is an intracellular, non-spore-forming, non-capsulated, gram-negative coccobacillus. Three species are recognized—*abortus*, *melitensis* and *suis*. Brucellosis is a zoonosis and has a world-wide distribution (Table 1.14), although it has been virtually eliminated from cattle in the UK. The organism does not withstand pasteurization. The brucella endotoxin (a cell wall lipopolysaccharide) is responsible for systemic symptoms and host hypersensitivity accounts for formation of granulomas. The organisms usually gain entry into the human body via the mouth, though less frequently they may enter via the respiratory tract, genital tract or abraded skin. The bacilli travel in the lymphatics and infect lymph nodes. This is followed by haematogenous spread with ultimate localization of the bacilli in the reticuloendothelial system. Spread is by the ingestion of raw milk from infected cattle. The disease often occurs in workers in close contact with animals or carcasses.

Table 1.14 Main geographical distribution and natural hosts of the *Brucella* species.

Organism	Geographical distribution	Natural host
B. abortus	World-wide, except northern Europe, Japan, Yugoslavia	Cattle
B. melitensis	Mediterranean region (especially Malta), Middle East	Goats and sheep
B. suis	Far East, USA	Pigs
*B. canis**		Beagles

*Rarely causes disease in humans.

CLINICAL FEATURES

The incubation period varies from 1 to 3 weeks. The onset of *acute brucellosis* is insidious, with malaise, headache, weakness, generalized myalgia and night sweats. The fever pattern is classically undulant, although continuous and intermittent patterns are frequent. Lymphadenopathy, hepatomegaly and spinal tenderness may also be present. The presence of splenomegaly is indicative of severe infection. Arthritis, spondylitis, bursitis, osteomyelitis, orchitis, epididymitis, meningoencephalitis and endocarditis have all been described, especially in infections with *B. melitensis* or *B. suis*.

Chronic brucellosis is characterized by easy fatiguability, myalgia, occasional bouts of fever and depression, which may persist for several months. Splenomegaly is present. It needs to be distinguished from other causes of prolonged fever (p. 9).

DIAGNOSIS

Blood cultures are positive during the acute phase of illness in 50% of patients. Serological tests are of greater value. The *Brucella* agglutination test which demonstrates a four-fold or greater rise in titre over a 4-week period is highly suggestive of brucellosis. A single titre greater than 1 in 60 is also suggestive of brucellosis in the appropriate clinical setting. An elevated serum IgG level detected by extraction with 2-mercaptoethanol (2-ME) is evidence of current or recent infection. A negative 2-ME test excludes chronic brucellosis. Specific *Brucella* immunoglobulins can be detected by the ELISA technique.

TREATMENT

Tetracycline 500 mg orally four times daily is given, but relapses occur. Co-trimoxazole 960 mg two times daily is also effective.

PREVENTION AND CONTROL

Prevention and control involves careful attention to hygiene when handling infected animals, eradication of infection in infected animals, and pasteurization of milk. No vaccine is available for use in humans.

BORDETELLA INFECTIONS

Bordetella is a non-motile, non-spore-forming, gram-negative coccobacillus. *B. pertussis* causes pertussis (whooping cough). *B. parapertussis* and *B. bronchiseptica* produce milder infections.

Pertussis

Pertussis occurs world-wide. Humans are both the natural hosts and reservoirs of infection. Pertussis is highly contagious and is spread by droplet infection. In its early stages it is indistinguishable from other types of upper respiratory tract infection and hence spread occurs easily. Epidemics are common and have increased in the UK since the safety of the whooping cough vaccine was questioned.

CLINICAL FEATURES

The incubation period varies from 7 to 14 days. It is a disease of childhood, with 90% of cases occurring below 5 years of age. However, no age is exempt. During the *catarrhal stage* the patient is highly infectious, and cultures from respiratory secretions are positive in over 90% of patients. Malaise, anorexia, mucoid rhinorrhoea and conjunctivitis are present. The *paroxysmal stage*, so called because of the characteristic paroxysms of coughing, begins about a week later. Paroxysms with the classic inspiratory whoop are seen only in younger individuals in whom the lumen of the respiratory tract is compromised by mucus secretion and mucosal oedema. The whoop results from air being forcefully drawn through the narrowed tract. These paroxysms usually terminate in vomiting. Conjunctival suffusion and petechiae and ulceration of the frenulum of the tongue are usual. Lymphocytosis due to the elaboration of lymphocyte promoting factor by *B. pertussis* is characteristic; lymphocytes may account for over 90% of the total white blood cell count. This stage lasts approximately 2 weeks and may be associated with several complications, including bronchitis, lobar pneumonia, atelectasis, rectal prolapse and inguinal hernia. Cerebral anoxia may occur, especially in younger children, resulting in convulsions. Bronchiectasis is a late sequel.

DIAGNOSIS

The diagnosis is suggested clinically by the characteristic whoop and a history of contact with an infected individual. It is confirmed by growing the organism in culture. Cultures of swabs of nasopharyngeal secretions result in a higher positive yield than cultures of 'cough plates'.

TREATMENT

If the disease is recognized in the catarrhal stage, erythromycin will abort or decrease the severity of the infection. In the paroxysmal stage antibiotics have little role to play in altering the course of the illness.

PREVENTION AND CONTROL

Affected individuals should be isolated to prevent contact with others. This is particularly important in hostels and boarding schools. Pertussis is an easily preventable disease and effective active immunization is available (p. 19).

HAEMOPHILUS INFECTIONS

Haemophilus is a gram-negative pleomorphic, facultatively anaerobic coccobacillus. Those pathogenic to humans include *H. influenzae*, *H. ducreyi* and *H. parainfluenzae*. In general, non-encapsulated forms produce luminal infections, e.g. bronchitis, and encapsulated organisms produce invasive disease, e.g. meningitis. *Haemophilus* is a normal commensal of the upper respiratory tract and is found in about 80% of healthy individuals.

Of the six antigenic types of *H. influenzae* identified, type B is the most important in humans and demonstrates the greatest pathogenicity, especially in children below 5 years of age. It can produce disease in several human organs (Table 1.15). Infec-

Table 1.15 Major clinical syndromes associated with *Haemophilus influenzae*.

Respiratory system Sinusitis Bronchitis Pneumonia
Central nervous system Meningitis Brain abscess
Cardiac system Endocarditis Pericarditis
Miscellaneous Septic arthritis Cellulitis Epiglottitis Otitis media

tion is generally autogenous and hence sporadic cases are common.

There is evidence of increasing immunity to *Haemophilus* with age. This is related to the presence of anticapsular and specific bactericidal antibodies. Cross-reacting antibodies to other gram-negative bacteria can also contribute to immunity. Adults with impaired host defence mechanisms, e.g. alcoholics, appear to have an increased risk of infection. A history suggestive of an antecedent viral fever is usual.

Infections with *Haemophilus influenzae*

H. influenzae infections have a world-wide distribution.

Meningitis
H. influenzae is the commonest cause of meningitis in the second year of life. The clinical features are described on p. 836.

Generally the response to treatment is slow. About 25% of children have permanent residual neurological deficits such as deafness.

Epiglottitis
This is characterized by a dramatically rapid course and fatal outcome in children if appropriate treatment is not instituted. The onset is acute with high fever, pooling of oropharyngeal secretions, dysphagia and marked respiratory distress. Examination reveals a markedly swollen and inflamed epiglottis.

Pneumonia
H. influenzae type B accounts for about 30% of all childhood bacterial pneumonias and 3–6% of pneumonias in adults.

DIAGNOSIS

This is made by isolation and culture of the organism.

TREATMENT

This is urgent as delay may result in a high mortality, especially in patients with meningitis and epiglottitis. In these conditions the drug of choice is chloramphenicol 50–100 mg·kg^{-1} per day i.v. for children and 4 g per day i.v. for 7–10 days for adults. Ampicillin can be used for less severe cases, but resistance to this drug is increasing.

PREVENTION

Children in close contact with an infected individual are at an increased risk of developing the disease. Unfortunately chemoprophylaxis is not helpful. Recently, a purified capsular antigen vaccine has been tried.

CHOLERA

Cholera is caused by the curved, actively motile, flagellated gram-negative bacillus, *Vibrio cholerae*. The organism is killed by temperatures of 100°C in a few seconds, but can survive in ice for up to 6 weeks. The El Tor biotype has replaced the classical biotype as the major cause of cholera. This is because the El Tor *V. cholerae* is a hardier organism. Infection with the El Tor biotype is frequently unrecognized as it produces milder clinical symptoms; a chronic gall-bladder carrier state can result in about 3% of all infected adults. All three strains (Inaba, Ogawa and Hikojima) are pathogenic. The fertile, humid Gangetic plains of West Bengal have traditionally been regarded as 'the home of cholera'. However, the seventh and most recent pandemic of cholera, which was caused by the El Tor biotype, affected large areas of Asia, North Africa and Southern Europe. Humans are the only known natural hosts. Transmission is by the faecal–oral route. Contaminated water plays a major role in the dissemination of cholera, although contaminated foods and contact carriers may be instrumental in the spread during epidemics.

Achlorhydria or hypochlorhydria facilitates passage of the cholera bacilli into the small intestine where they proliferate and elaborate an exotoxin with A and B subunits. The B subunit binds to specific GM1 ganglioside receptors and the A subunit activates the intracellular enzyme adenylate cyclase. This produces elevation of 3'5'-cyclic AMP, which in turn produces massive secretion of isotonic fluid into the intestinal lumen (see p. 196). The toxin is bound irreversibly to the receptor site where it exerts its effect for 24–48 h. The clinical effects are produced by the toxin and the organism is not invasive.

CLINICAL FEATURES

The incubation period varies from a few hours to 6 days. The majority of patients with cholera have a mild illness which cannot clinically be distinguished from diarrhoea due to other infective causes. Classically, however, three phases are recognized in the untreated disease. The *evacuation phase* is characterized by the abrupt onset of painless, profuse, watery diarrhoea, associated with vomiting in the severe forms. 'Rice water' stools, so called because of mucus flecks floating in the watery stools, are characteristic of this stage. If appropriate supportive treatment is not given, the patient passes on to the *collapse phase*. This is characterized by features of circulatory shock (cold clammy skin, tachycardia, hypotension and peripheral cyanosis) and dehydration (sunken eyes, hollow cheeks and a diminished urine output). The patient, though apathetic, is usually lucid. Muscle cramps may be severe. Children may, in addition, present with convulsions due to hypoglycaemia. At this stage renal failure and aspiration of vomitus present major problems. Should the patient survive this stage, he then enters into the *recovery phase*, with a gradual return to normal of clinical and biochemical parameters in 1–3 days.

Cholera sicca is an uncommon but severe form of cholera. It presents with massive outpouring of fluid and electrolytes into dilated intestinal loops. Diarrhoea and vomiting do not occur and hence the disease is frequently not recognized. The mortality rate is high.

DIAGNOSIS

Diagnosis is largely clinical. Examination of freshly passed stools may demonstrate rapidly motile organisms. This is not diagnostic as *Campylobacter* may also give a similar appearance. However, demonstration of the rapidly motile vibrios by dark-field illumination and subsequent inhibition of their movement with type-specific antisera is diagnostic.

Stool and rectal swabs should be taken for culture.

TREATMENT

With appropriate and effective rehydration therapy, mortality has decreased to less than 1%. Rehydration may be given orally or intravenously. Intravenous rehydration is required only for severely dehydrated individuals with features of collapse. Intravenous solutions recommended by the World Health Organization (WHO) include Ringer's lactate solution and the 'Diarrhoea Treatment Solution' (sodium chloride 4.0 g, sodium acetate 6.5 g, potassium chloride 1.0 g and glucose 9.0 g per litre). Several litres of intravenous fluid are usually required to overcome the features of shock. Maintenance of hydration is effectively carried out by oral rehydration solutions (ORS).

Oral rehydration, for maintenance therapy or for correction of mild to moderate dehydration, is best carried out by giving a glucose–electrolyte solution. WHO ORS and numerous commercial preparations of varying composition are available (Table 1.16). Mildly dehydrated individuals should be given ORS 50 ml·kg^{-1} in the first 4 h followed by a maintenance of a 100 ml·kg^{-1} daily until the diarrhoea stops. For moderate dehydration ORS 100 ml·kg^{-1} is given within the first 4 h followed by 10–15 ml·kg^{-1} per hour. Antibiotics such as tetracycline 250 mg four times daily for 3 days or doxycycline help eradicate the infection, decrease stool output and shorten the duration of the illness dramatically.

PREVENTION AND CONTROL

Immunization with currently available vaccines results in poor immunity and is no longer recommended. Attenuated live cholera vaccines are under intensive evaluation. Chemoprophylaxis with tetracycline 500 mg two times daily for 3 days for adults and 125 mg daily for children is effective. The most effective preventive measures, however, are good hygiene and sanitary living conditions.

Table 1.17 compares the pattern of infection caused by *Vibrio cholerae* with the patterns of infection caused by other gut organisms.

ENTEROBACTERIACEAE INFECTIONS

The Enterobacteriaceae is a diverse group of aerobic and facultatively anaerobic gram-negative organisms. Included in this category are *Escherichia coli*, *Salmonella* and *Shigella*.

Escherichia coli infection

E. coli is commonly responsible for urinary tract infections, pneumonia, bacteraemia, neonatal meningitis, and peritoneal and biliary infections. Such infections are indistinguishable from similar clinical conditions caused by other bacteria.

Table 1.16 Oral rehydration solutions available in the UK.

	Sodium (mmol·l^{-1})	Potassium (mmol·l^{-1})	Chloride (mmol·l^{-1})	Bicarbonate (mmol·l^{-1})	Glucose (mmol·l^{-1})	Sucrose (mmol·l^{-1})
WHO/UNICEF	90	20	80	30	111	—
Sodium chloride and oral glucose powder compound	35	20	37	18	200	—
Dioralyte	35	20	37	18	200	—
Rehidrat*	50	20	50	20	91	94
Dextrolyte†	35	13.4	30.5	—	200	—

*Plus fructose 2 mmol·l^{-1} and citric acid 9 mmol·l^{-1}.
†Plus lactate 7.7 mmol·l^{-1}.

Table 1.17 Patterns of gut infection.

	Non-inflammatory	Inflammatory	Penetrating
Major location:	Jejunum	Colon	Ileum
Clinical presentation:	Watery diarrhoea	Dysentery	Enteric fever
Common pathogens:	*Vibrio cholerae* Enterotoxigenic *Escherichia coli*	*Shigella* Enteroinvasive *Escherichia coli* *Salmonella* *Clostridium difficile* *Campylobacter* *Entamoeba histolytica* (see p. 79)	*Salmonella typhi* *Yersinia enterocolitica*
Pathogenetic mechanisms:	Enterotoxin (CT, LT, ST) production causing intestinal secretion of water and electrolytes	Invasion of gut epithelium ± cytotoxin release	Invasion and bacteraemia

CT = cholera toxin; LT and ST = *E. coli* heat-labile and heat-stable toxins.

E. coli responsible for enteric disease have different serotype characteristics from those which cause disease elsewhere in the body. Three main categories of *E. coli* capable of producing human diarrhoeal disease are recognized.

Enterotoxigenic E. coli (ETEC) produces a diarrhoeal illness which is mediated through a heat-labile toxin (LT) and/or a heat-stable toxin (ST). Toxin production is genetically encoded by transferable DNA plasmids. LT resembles cholera toxin in its mode of action since it also acts via cyclic AMP and is associated with massive secretion of water and electrolytes into the intestinal lumen. ST activates guanylate cyclase with elevation of cyclic GMP levels and subsequent secretion of water and electrolytes (see Fig. 4.24a, p. 196). Clinically ETEC produces three syndromes:
- An illness indistinguishable from severe cholera
- 'Traveller's diarrhoea', a milder disease (other causes are shown in Table 1.18)

Table 1.18 Causes of traveller's diarrhoea.

Pathogen	Proportion of cases (%)
Enterotoxigenic *Escherichia coli*	40–75
Shigella	0–15
Salmonella	0–10
Rotavirus	0–10
Giardia lamblia, Entamoeba histolytica	0–3
Unknown	22–25

- Diarrhoea of varying severity in children, especially in the Third World

Enteroinvasive E. coli (EIEC) produces an illness similar to that produced by *Shigella* (see below).

Enteropathogenic E. coli (EPEC) attaches to and damages intestinal epithelium, producing diarrhoea, primarily in children below 2 years of age. Toxins are thought to be involved in the production of diarrhoea. Epidemics are common especially in nurseries.

TREATMENT

Many *E. coli* gut infections are self-limiting and require no specific antimicrobial therapy. For severe infection, particularly with colitis and a systemic illness, ampicillin 2 g daily or co-trimoxazole 960 mg twice daily can be given. Gentamicin 2–5 mg·kg^{-1} daily or tobramycin 3–5 mg·kg^{-1} daily in divided 8-hourly doses are effective alternatives in severe illness with septicaemia.

Co-trimoxazole 480 mg twice daily is effective prophylaxis against traveller's diarrhoea due to ETEC, and early treatment with the standard therapeutic dose of 960 mg two times daily will shorten the duration of the illness.

Salmonellosis

Salmonella is a gram-negative, flagellated, non-capsulated and generally motile bacillus. Biochemically three species are recognized—*S. typhi* and *S. paratyphi, S. choleraesuis* and *S. enteritidis*. Their thermal death point is 60°C but they can withstand freezing and dry conditions for prolonged periods of time. Although salmonellae have a world-wide distribution, they usually result in disease only where there is poor hygiene and overcrowding. Transmission occurs by ingestion of contaminated foods (particularly eggs and poultry products) or water. In the UK, spread is often by carriers, usually food handlers, who contaminate the food. Following ingestion, the salmonellae colonize the small intestine and proliferate in Peyer's patches. They are then carried through the lymphatics, enter the bloodstream, and are thereby transported to the reticuloendothelial system.

A spectrum of clinical syndromes due to *Salmonella* is recognized:
- Enteric fever (typhoid or paratyphoid fever)
- Enterocolitis
- Extra-intestinal focal infections, e.g. osteomyelitis
- Food poisoning
- Carriers

Typhoid fever

This is caused by *S. typhi*. Humans are the only known reservoirs. The incubation period is usually 10–14 days. The onset is insidious, with headache being a prominent symptom. The fever is remittent and gradually increases in severity in a step-ladder fashion over 3–4 days. Cough, sore throat and altered behaviour may also be present. Constipation is usually present initially and diarrhoea occurs only late in the disease. Physical examination during the first week reveals a toxic individual with a relative bradycardia. During the second week several physical signs can be elicited. An erythematous maculopapular rash which blanches on pressure and is referred to as 'rose spots' appears, chiefly on the upper abdomen and thorax, and lasts for only 2–3 days. These spots are not easily visible on dark-skinned patients. A soft splenomegaly occurs in about 75% of patients. Cervical lymphadenopathy, hepatomegaly (present in about 30% of patients) and right iliac fossa tenderness are other physical signs which may be present. The third week of illness, aptly referred to as 'the week of complications', is the time when the majority of complications occur. These include lobar pneumonia, haemolytic anaemia, meningitis, peripheral neuropathy, acute cholecystitis, urinary tract infection and osteomyelitis. Intestinal perforation occurs in 2–3% and intestinal haemorrhage in 2–8%. The fourth week of illness ('the week of convalescence') is characterized by a gradual return to health.

Diagnosis. Leucopenia is present. Blood cultures are positive in about 80% during the first week and 30% in the third week. Urine cultures are helpful during the second week and stool cultures during the second to fourth week. Marrow cultures are occasionally helpful. Of the serological tests the Widal test, which measures serum agglutinins against the O and H antigens, is most helpful, a fourfold increase in titre in sequential blood samples being suggestive of *Salmonella* infection.

Carriers. Carriers can be divided into chronic carriers, defined as individuals who excrete *Salmonella* for at least 1 year, and convalescent carriers. The presence of Vi agglutinin in the serum in a dilution greater than 1:10 is suggestive of a carrier state. Since the gallbladder is frequently the focus of infection, duodenal aspirates for culture of the bile-containing duodenal juice may yield useful information.

Treatment. Chloramphenicol (75 mg·kg^{-1} daily in four divided doses) remains the drug of choice. It is 4–6 days before the temperature shows signs of diminishing, although subjective improvement is noted earlier. Treatment should be continued for 2 weeks. Co-trimoxazole 960 mg daily is also effective; again therapy should be continued for 2 weeks. Ampicillin 6 g daily is a useful alternative. Complications such as intestinal perforation or haemorrhage may occur despite adequate treatment and require surgical intervention.

Eradication of a carrier state can be difficult, but ampicillin 4–6 g daily with probenicid 2 g daily for 6 weeks may be effective. If chemotherapy does not effect a cure, cholecystectomy remains the only mode of treatment.

Prevention and control. This includes provision of safe drinking water, sanitary disposal of excreta and proper attention to hygiene by those who handle food. Monovalent typhoid vaccine is used as it is less likely to produce local and systemic reactions. No vaccine has so far given complete protection.

Paratyphoid fever

Paratyphoid fever is due to *S. paratyphi* A, B or C. They result in an illness clinically indistinguishable from typhoid fever. However, paratyphoid fever is a milder illness. Treatment is with co-trimoxazole two tablets daily.

Enterocolitis

This is an acute, short-lived infection, and is usually due to *S. enteritidis* serotype *typhimurium*. It is generally mild, lasting 2–3 days, and presents with fever, malaise, cramping abdominal pain, bloody diarrhoea and vomiting. Occasionally a cholera-like picture may be present. Treatment is symptomatic. This *Salmonella* is an important cause of food poisoning; other organisms responsible are shown in Table 1.19.

As with typhoid fever, a chronic carrier state may develop. Treatment is as described for *S. typhi* carriers.

Shigellosis (bacillary dysentery)

Shigellosis is an acute self-limiting intestinal infection caused by one of four species of gram-negative,

Table 1.19 Bacterial causes of food poisoning.

Organism	Source	Incubation period	Symptoms	Diagnosis	Recovery
Staphylococcus aureus	Contaminated food, usually by humans	2–6 h	Diarrhoea, vomiting and dehydration	Culture organism in vomitus or remaining food	Rapid (few hours)
Bacillus cereus	Spores in food survive boiling	1–6 h	Diarrhoea, vomiting and dehydration	Culture organism in faeces and food	Rapid
Clostridium perfringens	Spores in food survive boiling	8–22 h	Watery diarrhoea and cramping pain	Culture organism in faeces and food	2–3 days
Clostridium botulinum	Spores survive cooking but only germinate in anaerobic conditions, e.g. canned or bottled foods	18–36 h	Brief diarrhoea and paralysis due to neuromuscular blockade	Demonstrate toxin in food or faeces	10–14 days
*Salmonella enteritidis**	Bowels of animals, especially fowl	12–24 h	Abrupt diarrhoea, fever and vomiting	Culture organism in stool	Usually 2–5 days, but may be up to 2 weeks
Campylobacter	Bowels of animals, especially fowl; also in milk	48–96 h	Diarrhoea ± blood, fever, malaise and abdominal pain	Culture organism in stool	3–5 days

*Many strains, including *S. typhimurium*.

Non-microbial toxins such as dinoflagellate plankton toxin in shellfish ('red tide'), scrombotoxin from some varieties of spoiled fish (see p. 671) and red kidney bean toxin (haemagglutinin) from partially cooked beans also cause acute diarrhoea.

non-spore-forming bacilli. These include *Shigella dysenteriae*, *S. flexneri*, *S. boydii* and *S. sonnei*. While all of them are enteroinvasive, *S. dysenteriae* type I and some strains of *S. flexneri* and *S. sonnei* have been demonstrated to elaborate a toxin which is enterotoxic, neurotoxic and cytotoxic. Like salmonellosis, shigellosis is found world-wide and is more prevalent in areas with poor hygiene and overcrowding. Transmission is by the faecal–oral route.

CLINICAL FEATURES

The incubation period is short, usually being 2 days. The onset is acute, with fever, malaise, abdominal pain and diarrhoea. As the disease increases in intensity, bloody diarrhoea with mucus, tenesmus, faecal urgency and severe cramping abdominal pain becomes prominent. Nausea, vomiting, headache and convulsions (in children) may occur and have been attributed to the neurotoxin. When the disease is due to *S. dysenteriae*, which is responsible for the more fulminant forms of shigellosis, a cholera-like picture is occasionally seen. Sigmoidoscopy shows the presence of a markedly hyperaemic and inflamed mucosa, with transversely distributed ulcers with rugged undermined edges. The appearances are often indistinguishable from other dysenteric infections and from non-specific inflammatory bowel disease. Complications such as colonic perforation,

septicaemia and the haemolytic uraemic syndrome may occur.

DIAGNOSIS

The diagnosis is made on the basis of a stool culture.

TREATMENT

Treatment is symptomatic. In severe illness, ampicillin 50–100 mg·kg^{-1} daily in children and 2 g daily in adults may decrease the severity of illness.

Public health measures, particularly the disposal of excreta and the provision of clean water, prevent infection. Outbreaks in schools can only be controlled by good hygiene.

CAMPYLOBACTER INFECTIONS

Campylobacter is a gram-negative, motile, curved spiral rod which is microaerophilic and thus fails to multiply under aerobic or strict anaerobic conditions. *Campylobacter* causes acute diarrhoea, sometimes with blood, and is now one of the most common causes of acute gastroenteritis in the UK. *Campylobacter pyloridis* has recently been implicated in the causation of non-specific antral gastritis and possibly peptic ulceration.

CLINICAL FEATURES

Symptoms begin 2–5 days after eating infected material (usually chicken or milk), the commonest being fever, headache and malaise. These are followed rapidly by diarrhoea, often with blood and quite severe cramping abdominal pain. The patient generally appears unwell. Sigmoidoscopy can show the changes of acute colitis, which may be indistinguishable from those of ulcerative colitis.

DIAGNOSIS

Direct phase microscopy of a wet mount of stool may reveal the motile curved rods resembling 'flying birds'. The organism may be cultured on special media within 48 h. In severe infections the organism may be cultured from the blood.

TREATMENT

In the majority of cases, *Campylobacter* enteritis is a self-limiting illness, resolving in 5–7 days. Although the organism is sensitive to erythromycin, there is no evidence that treatment with this antibiotic alters the natural history of the infection. However, if systemic symptoms continue in association with persistent bacteraemia, antibiotics are usually administered.

YERSINIA INFECTIONS

The only two major human pathogens are *Yersinia pestis*, which causes plague, and *Y. enterocolitica*, which causes mesenteric lymphadenitis and enterocolitis.

Y. enterocolitica infection

Y. enterocolitica results in a number of clinical syndromes depending on the host's age and immune status. Patients may present with enterocolitis, acute mesenteric lymphadenitis or terminal ileitis. Enterocolitis is characterized by the presence of fever, diarrhoea and severe abdominal pain, which may lead to a mistaken diagnosis of appendicitis. Arthritis (sometimes with Reiter's syndrome—see p. 350) and erythema nodosum are seen and are immunologically mediated.

This is usually a self-limiting disease and no treatment is required. In very severe cases tetracycline 1 g daily may be given.

Plague

Plague is caused by *Y. pestis*, a gram-negative, non-motile, non-spore-forming, pleomorphic bacterium. Nowadays it is mainly limited to animals, but sporadic cases of plague, as well as occasional epidemics, occur world-wide in humans. The major

reservoirs are woodland rodents which transmit infection to domestic rats (*Rattus rattus*). The vector is the rat flea, *Xenopsylla cheopis*. These fleas bite humans when there is a sudden decline in the rat population. Occasionally, spread of the organisms may be through infected faeces being rubbed into skin wounds or through inhalation of droplets.

Virulence is attributed to the presence of the endotoxin, exotoxin and fraction I (a soluble protein which prevents phagocytosis of the organism). Clinical manifestations are attributed to the lipopolysaccharide endotoxin.

CLINICAL FEATURES

Three clinical forms are recognized—Bubonic, pneumonic, and septicaemic plague.

Bubonic plague is the commonest form and occurs in about 90% of infected individuals. The incubation period is about a week. The onset of illness is acute, with high fever, chills, headache, myalgia, nausea, vomiting and, when severe, prostration. This is rapidly followed by the development of lymphadenopathy, most commonly involving the inguinal lymph nodes (buboes). Characteristically these are matted and tender, and suppurate in 1–2 weeks. Petechiae, ecchymoses and bleeding from the gastrointestinal tract, the respiratory tract and the genitourinary tract may occur. Mental confusion follows the development of toxaemia.

Pneumonic plague is characterized by the abrupt onset of features of a fulminant pneumonia with bloody sputum, marked respiratory distress, cyanosis and death in almost all affected patients.

Septicaemic plague presents as an acute fulminant infection with evidence of shock and disseminated intravascular coagulation. If left untreated, death usually occurs in 2–5 days. Lymphadenopathy is unusual.

DIAGNOSIS

The diagnosis is easily established by demonstrating the organism in lymph node aspirates, in blood cultures or on sputum examination.

TREATMENT

Treatment is urgent and should be instituted before the results of culture studies are available. Several antimicrobial drugs are effective, including streptomycin 0.5 g i.m. every 4 h for 48 h followed by 0.5 g every 6 h for 5 days, or tetracycline 2–3 g daily for 14 days.

PREVENTION AND CONTROL

Prevention of plague is largely dependent on the control of the flea population and the use of potent antiflea agents such as 2% aldrin. Outhouses, huts, etc. should be sprayed with insecticides effective against the local flea. Rodents should not be killed until the fleas are under control as the fleas will leave dead rodents to bite humans. Tetracycline 500 mg four times daily or sulphonamides 2–4 g daily for 7 days are effective chemoprophylactic agents. Patients themselves can be infective when the buboes break down; patients with pneumonic plague can spread the organism by droplet spread. A partially effective formalin-killed vaccine is available for use by travellers to plague-endemic areas.

TULARAEMIA

Tularaemia is due to infection by *Francisella tularensis*, a gram-negative organism. It is primarily a zoonosis, affecting mainly rodents, including rabbits and squirrels. Vectors are ticks, flies and mosquitoes. Humans are infected by handling infected animals or from vector bites. The microorganisms enter through the skin or through minor abrasions in the mouth or conjunctivae. Occasionally infection occurs from contaminated water or from eating uncooked meat. The disease occurs world-wide and is frequently seen in the USA, particularly in hunters and butchers.

CLINICAL FEATURES

The incubation period of 2–7 days is followed by a generalized illness. A number of clinical syndromes can be seen:
- The ulceroglandular form is the commonest. A papule occurs at the site of inoculation. This ulcerates and is followed by tender, suppurative lymphadenopathy. Infected material entering the eye is followed by a purulent conjunctivitis with periauricular lymphadenopathy.
- Pneumonic forms present with cough, chest pain and eventually a pneumonia, sometimes accompanied by a pericarditis.
- The septicaemic form presents with the sudden onset of a fever, myalgia, headache and shock.

DIAGNOSIS

Diagnosis is by culture of the organism or by a rising titre seen on a bacterial agglutination test.

TREATMENT

Treatment is with streptomycin or more usually gentamicin. The patient should be isolated.

PREVENTION

In endemic areas all wild animals should be handled using gloves. Infected meat and water should be adequately cooked. A vaccine is available for laboratory staff handling possibly infected animals.

GLANDERS

Glanders is caused by a gram-negative bacillus, *Pseudomonas mallei*. It affects mainly horses but can be transmitted to man, mainly horse handlers. The disease is acquired by inhalation or inoculation of infected material. In the acute state, the patient is toxic with a high fever and delirium. There is an ulceration of the upper respiratory tract with eventual pneumonia, empyema and lung abscess. Septicaemia develops, which was fatal prior to antibiotics becoming available. Treatment is with sulphonamides.

MELIOIDOSIS

Melioidosis is due to the gram-negative bacillus, *Pseudomonas pseudomallei*, which is a soil saprophyte. It infects humans (particularly diabetics or traumatized patients) by penetrating through skin abrasions, occasionally by inhalation, or via ingestion of contaminated water. It is found world-wide, but occurs mainly in South-East Asia.

Septicaemia with abscesses in the lung, kidney, liver and spleen may occur. The central nervous system may be involved. The prognosis is poor. A chronic form, usually presenting with an unresolved pneumonia, also occurs.

Diagnosis is by culture of the organism. An indirect haemagglutination test is positive after 1 week.

TREATMENT

The patient should be barrier-nursed and treated with chloramphenicol and tetracycline.

PASTEURELLOSIS

Pasteurelloses are infections primarily of animals. Three species are known to infect man, the commonest being *Pasteurella multocida*, which is also the most virulent. All these organisms are commensal in the nasopharynx and gastrointestinal tract of a number of domestic and wild mammals. Transmission to humans may occur through a bite or scratch.

CLINICAL FEATURES

Focal soft tissue infection with marked erythema, severe tenderness and regional lymphadenopathy may be present. These organisms are also responsible for chronic respiratory infections, bacteraemia, and brain and renal abscesses.

TREATMENT

Penicillin is the drug of choice and should be given parenterally as benzylpenicillin 1–2 g every 4 h.

LEGIONNAIRES' DISEASE

This is caused by the fastidious *Legionella pneumophila*, a weakly gram-negative, catalase-positive bacillus. It is described on p. 596.

BACTEROIDES INFECTION

Bacteroides is an obligatory anaerobic, non-spore-forming, gram-negative bacillus. *B. fragilis* is the most important anaerobic human pathogen and is a normal commensal in the human large gut. It does not produce an endotoxin and because of its polysaccharide capsule it resists phagocytosis. *B. fragilis* also produces heparinase, which may be involved in the development of thrombophlebitis, and beta-lactamases, which inhibit the action of penicillin. It is not a highly invasive organism and grows best in necrotic tissues.

CLINICAL FEATURES

Seventy-five per cent of all intra-abdominal infections, particularly postoperative infections, are caused by anaerobes. *Bacteroides* is a frequent cause of hepatic, subhepatic, pelvic and splenic abscesses. The pus has a characteristic putrid smell. *Bacteroides* also causes pelvic infections and may result in endometritis, Bartholin's abscess and pelvic peritonitis. Bacteraemia and Fournier's gangrene are also caused by *B. fragilis*.

DIAGNOSIS

This depends on strict anaerobic culture with special media. Recently gas–liquid chromatography has been used to detect the volatile fatty acids produced by anaerobic bacteria.

TREATMENT

Surgery is usually required as well as chemotherapy. Metronidazole (1–2 g daily by mouth or 1 g 8-hourly by rectum) is the drug of choice; it is also used prophylactically in colorectal surgery, with a dramatic reduction in postoperative infections.

Actinomycetes

Actinomycetes are gram-positive, branching higher bacteria (not fungi) and include *Actinomyces israelii*, *Nocardia asteroides* and *N. brasiliensis*.

Actinomyces is a normal mouth and intestine commensal, but *Nocardia* is a soil saprophyte. *Actinomyces* produces an illness characterized by chronicity and poor infectivity. It has a world-wide distribution. Disease due to *N. asteroides* is frequently seen in the USA and Europe, whereas *N. brasiliensis* gives rise to disease more commonly in southern Asia.

Actinomycosis

In actinomycosis, characteristic clusters of organisms referred to as 'sulphur granules' are formed. *Actinomyces* is a rare cause of disease in the Western World. Three clinical forms of disease are recognized:
- The *cervicofacial variety* usually occurs following dental extraction. It is often indolent and slowly progressive, associated with little pain, and results in induration and localized swelling of the lower part of the mandible ('lumpy jaw'). Lymphadenopathy is uncommon. Occasionally acute inflammation occurs.
- The *thoracic variety* follows inhalation of these organisms into a previously damaged lung. The clinical picture is not distinctive and is often mistaken for malignancy or tuberculosis. Symptoms such as fever, malaise, chest pain and haemoptysis are present. Empyema occurs in 25% of patients and local extension produces chest wall sinuses with discharge of sulphur granules.
- *Abdominal actinomycosis* most frequently affects the caecum. Characteristically, a hard indurated mass is felt in the right iliac fossa. Later, sinuses develop. The differential diagnosis includes malignancy, tuberculosis, Crohn's disease and amoeboma. Pelvic actinomycosis appears to be increasing with wider use of intrauterine contraceptive devices.

TREATMENT

Treatment involves surgery, and penicillin is the drug of choice. High-dose i.v. penicillin is given for 4–6 weeks followed by oral penicillin for some weeks after clinical resolution. Tetracyclines are also effective.

Nocardiosis

CLINICAL FEATURES

Nocardia gives rise to two distinct clinical entities:
- *Pulmonary disease* presents with cough, fever, and haemoptysis. Pleural involvement and empyema may occur.
- *Mycetoma* is the result of local invasion by *Nocardia* and presents as a painless swelling, usually on the sole of the foot (Madura foot). The swelling of the affected part of the body continues inexorably. Nodules gradually appear from which purulent fluid containing characteristic 'grains' of the organisms are discharged. Systemic

symptoms and regional lymphadenopathy are distinctly uncommon. Sinuses may occur several years after the onset of the first symptom.

Mycetoma may also be produced by several other members of actinomycetes, including *Actinomadura* and *Streptomyces*. It is then referred to as an actinomycetoma. When caused by true fungi belonging to Eumycetes, e.g. *Madurella mycetomi* or *Petriellidium boydii*, it is referred to as eumycetoma. The clinical presentation, with the exception of different coloured 'grains', is similar to that of mycetoma.

DIAGNOSIS

This is often difficult to establish as *Nocardia* is not easily detected in sputum cultures or on histological section.

TREATMENT

Treatment consists of adequate surgical drainage of the pus combined with prolonged chemotherapy. The drug of choice is sulphadiazine in doses of up to 9 g daily. Co-trimoxazole may also be used.

Mycobacteria

Mycobacteria are acid-fast, aerobic bacilli which grow extremely slowly. The cell wall contains complex lipids and glycolipids, one of which—the cord factor—is responsible for producing granulomas. No extracellular enzyme or toxins have been identified. The capacity of mycobacteria to produce disease is therefore attributed to their ability to multiply within phagocytic cells and to withstand intracellular enzymatic digestion.

A clinical classification of mycobacteria is shown in Table 1.20.

Tuberculosis

Tuberculosis is largely due to *Mycobacterium tuberculosis*.

EPIDEMIOLOGY

Tuberculosis is present world-wide, with an extremely high prevalence in Asian countries, where 60–80% of children below the age of 14 years are infected. Tuberculosis is spread predominantly by droplet infection.

The prevalence of tuberculosis increases with poor social conditions, inadequate nutrition and overcrowding.

Table 1.20 Classification of *Mycobacterium* species based on their capacity to produce disease.

Species	Disease produced
Obligate intracellular bacteria:	
M. leprae	Leprosy
Facultative intracellular bacteria:	
M. tuberculosis	Most cases of human tuberculosis
M. bovis	Cattle and rarely human tuberculosis
Rare forms:	
M. avium–intracellulare	Fowl and human tuberculosis
M. scrofulaceum	Lymph node infection
M. kansasii	Human tuberculosis

PATHOLOGY

The characteristic lesion is a granuloma with central caseation and Langhans' giant cells.

The primary infection usually involves the lungs, but can involve other areas such as the ileocaecal region of the gastrointestinal tract. It is almost always accompanied by lymph node involvement.

In most people the primary infection heals leaving some surviving tubercule bacilli. With a lowering of host resistance, these are reactivated, producing local spread as well as haematogenous spread to all organs of the body, including the lungs, bones and kidneys. This particularly occurs in the elderly, in alcoholics, in patients with diabetes mellitus, lung disease, or after gastrectomy, as well as in patients who are on corticosteroids or immunosuppressed.

Occasionally the primary infection progresses locally to a more widespread lesion; haematogenous spread can also occur.

Tuberculosis in the adult is therefore usually the result of reactivation of old disease, occasionally a primary infection, or, more rarely, re-infection.

CLINICAL FEATURES

Pulmonary tuberculosis is the commonest form; this is described on p. 599, along with the chemotherapeutic regimens.

Tuberculosis also affects other organs, including:
- The gastrointestinal tract—mainly the ileocaecal area, but occasionally the tongue is affected and also the peritoneum, producing ascites (see p. 202)
- The genitourinary system—the kidney is mainly involved, but tuberculosis is also the cause of

painless, craggy swellings in the epididymis, and salpingitis, tubal abscesses and infertility in females
- The central nervous system—tuberculous meningitis and local tuberculomas within the brain itself can occur
- The skeletal system—arthritis and osteomyelitis with cold abscess formation can occur
- The skin—inducing lupus vulgaris
- The eye—producing choroiditis, iridocyclitis or phlyctenular keratoconjunctivitis
- The pericardium—producing constrictive pericarditis
- The adrenal glands—causing destruction and producing Addison's disease
- The lymph nodes—this is a common mode of presentation, especially in young adults and children. Any group of lymph nodes may be involved, but hilar and paratracheal lymph nodes are the commonest. Initially the nodes are firm and discrete, but later they become matted and can suppurate and form sinuses.

Scrofula is the term used to describe massive cervical lymph node enlargement. It is most often due to *M. tuberculosis*, and rarely due to *M. scrofulaceum* or *M. kansasii*. Signs of acute inflammation are absent.

Leprosy (Hansen's disease)

The causative organism is the acid-fast bacillus *M. leprae*. Unlike other mycobacteria, it does not grow in artificial media or even in tissue culture. While inability to culture the organism obtained from lesions and secretions is suggestive of *M. leprae*, it is not diagnostic. The following additional properties have recently been found to be useful in its identification:
- Loss of acid fastness following pyridine extraction
- The ability of the organism to grow slowly in the foot-pad of mice. Other mycobacteria also grow in the foot-pad of mice, but these produce distinct histological changes
- The ability of *M. leprae* to oxidize 3,4-dihydroxy-phenylalanine to pigmented products
- The ability of this organism to invade peripheral nerves, a property not demonstrated by other mycobacteria

Leprosy is found primarily in Asia and Africa (Fig. 1.13). Endemic foci are still present in the USSR and parts of the USA. Of the 15 million people with leprosy world-wide, about two-thirds are in Asia. The precise mode of transmission is unknown; it is likely that nasal secretions play an important role.

Once an individual has been infected, subsequent progression to clinical disease appears to be dependent on several factors:
- Sex—males appear to be more susceptible than females. In India, the ratio of affected males to females is 2:1.
- Genetic susceptibility—studies in twins have shown a concordance in identical but not in non-identical twins.
- The immunological response of the individual to the bacillus

CLASSIFICATION

Two polar types of leprosy are recognized:
- *Tuberculoid leprosy*—a localized disease which

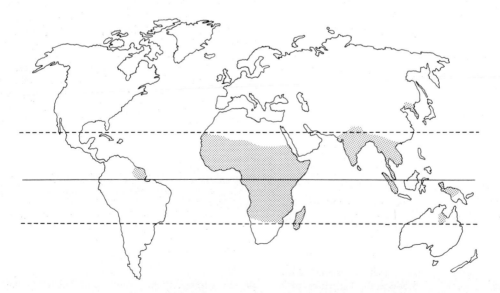

Fig. 1.13 The geographical distribution of leprosy, showing areas where the prevalence is 5 in 1000 or greater.

occurs in individuals who exhibit a marked immunological resistance to the organism
- *Lepromatous leprosy*—a generalized disease which occurs in individuals with impaired cell-mediated immunity

The following types are also recognized:
- *Borderline leprosy* has features of both the polar varieties.
- *Indeterminate leprosy* is characterized by one or more hypopigmented, sometimes erythematous, ill-defined macules of variable size. Sensation, sweating and hair growth over the macules are usually normal.
- *Neuritic leprosy* is not associated with skin lesions. The affected nerve is enlarged and firm and sensory loss in the area of the nerve's distribution is present.

Two subdivisions of lepromatous leprosy have recently been included in the classification. The patient is said to have the 'subpolar' lepromatous (LL_s) form when he has passed through a borderline phase before becoming lepromatous, and the polar lepromatous (LL_p) form where the patient is lepromatous throughout. Borderline disease has also been further classified as borderline tuberculoid (BT) and borderline lepromatous (BL), depending on which features of the polar forms predominate.

Two indices are currently in use to evaluate the response to treatment of patients in whom the skin-smear test for acid-fast bacilli is positive:
- *Bacteriological index (BI)*. This index is an objective way of evaluating the response to treatment. The skin-smear is graded from 1+ to 6+ depending upon the number of bacilli present per high power field. The BI is calculated by taking the mean result of four slide examinations. For example, a decrease in BI from 6 to 3.5 on therapy indicates a good response to treatment.
- *Morphological index (MI)*. This is the percentage of solid staining acid-fast bacilli on smears (solid bacilli represent viable bacteria). A patient with an MI of 0% is not infectious.

CLINICAL FEATURES

The incubation period varies from 2 to 6 years, although it may be as short as a few months or as long as 20 years. Leprosy should be considered in any individual who presents with hypopigmented skin patches associated with loss of sensation, especially to touch or temperature, and evidence of nerve involvement (thickening or tenderness), in whom non-cultivable acid-fast bacilli have been identified in skin smears.

The onset of leprosy is generally insidious. However, acute onset is known to occur and patients may present with a transient rash, with features of an acute febrile illness, with evidence of nerve involvement, or any combination of these.

Tuberculoid leprosy (TL)
In tuberculoid leprosy the infection is localized because the patient has unimpaired cell-mediated immunity. The characteristic skin lesion is a hypopigmented, anaesthetic patch with thickened, clearly demarcated edges, central healing and atrophy. The face, gluteal region and extremities are most commonly affected. Frequently the nerve leading to this hypopigmented patch and the regional nerve trunk are thickened and tender. Unlike other parts of the body, a tuberculoid patch on the face is not anaesthetic. Nerve involvement leads to marked muscle atrophy. Tuberculoid lesions are known to heal spontaneously.

Lepromatous leprosy (LL)
Although practically every organ can be involved, the changes in the skin are the most obvious manifestation. Peripheral oedema and rhinitis are the earliest symptoms. The skin lesions predominantly occur on the face, the gluteal region and the upper and lower limbs. They may be macules, papules, nodules or plaques. Of these, the macule is the earliest lesion. Infiltration is most noticeable in the ear lobes. Thinning of the lateral margins of the eyebrows is characteristic. The mucous membranes are frequently involved, resulting in nasal stuffiness, laryngitis and hoarseness of the voice. Nasal septal perforation with collapse of the nasal cartilages produces a saddle-nose deformity. With progression of the disease, the typical leonine facies due to infiltration of the skin becomes apparent. Glove and stocking anaesthesia, gynaecomastia, testicular atrophy, ichthyosis and nerve palsies (facial, ulnar, median and radial) develop late in the disease. Neurotrophic atrophy affecting the phalanges leads to the gradual disappearance of fingers. Nerve involvement is less pronounced than in tuberculoid leprosy.

Lucio's phenomenon is seen only in Mexico and Central America, where lepromatous leprosy is associated with an endarteritis which results in skin ulceration. The ulcers are large, with undermined edges and markedly necrotic bases. Smears from the base generally reveal numerous acid-fast bacilli. Healing is by scar formation. Treatment is wide surgical excision with skin grafts. Chemotherapy alone is ineffective in healing ulcers.

Borderline leprosy
Borderline (dimorphous) leprosy is most frequently encountered in clinical practice. The lesion is neither as localized as in tuberculoid leprosy nor as widespread as in lepromatous leprosy. The skin lesions may be macules, plaques, annular or punched out. Patients may remain borderline or may develop the lepromatous form.

The lepromin test
This is a measure of host resistance to leprosy and not a test for detecting leprosy. 0.1 ml of a suspen-

sion of dead bacilli (either Mitsuda lepromin or the Dharmendra lepromin) is injected intradermally. Two reactions are observed:

- The early Fernandez reaction becomes positive in 48 h and reflects the *sensitivity* of the tissue to the leprosy bacilli protein.
- The late (Mitsuda) reaction develops in 4–5 weeks and reflects the resistance of the host to the bacteria. This reaction is strongly positive in tuberculoid leprosy and is negative in lepromatous leprosy.

Lepra reactions

Lepra reactions are immunologically mediated acute reactions which occur in patients with the borderline or lepromatous spectrum of disease. Two forms are recognized.

Erythema nodosum leprosum (ENL; type II lepra reaction), is a humoral antibody response to an antigen–antibody complex (i.e. a type III hypersensitivity reaction). It is seen in 50% of patients with treated LL. It is characterized by fever, arthralgia and crops of painful, subcutaneous erythematous nodules. It may last from a few days to several weeks.

The *borderline reaction* (type I lepra reaction) is seen in patients with borderline disease; it is a type IV delayed hypersensitivity reaction. Both upgrading or reversal reactions (i.e. a clinical change towards a more tuberculoid form) and downgrading reactions (i.e. a change towards the lepromatous form) can occur. The borderline reaction is characterized by acute inflammation of pre-existing borderline lesions. Neurological deficits such as an ulnar nerve palsy may occur abruptly.

DIAGNOSIS

The diagnosis of leprosy is essentially clinical. Patients should be examined in adequate natural light. The demonstration of acid-fast bacilli in smears from the skin or nasal mucosa is highly suggestive. Occasionally nerve biopsies are helpful. The definitive diagnosis is established by cultivating the organisms in the foot-pad of mice.

TREATMENT

Leprosy should be treated in specialist centres with adequate physiotherapy and occupational therapy support. Multi-drug therapy is now essential because of developing drug resistance (up to 20% of cases are resistant to dapsone).

Dapsone (DDS), a folate synthetase inhibitor, is bacteriostatic. It has the advantage of being cheap and well tolerated. Side-effects are few and include haemolytic anaemia and sulphaemoglobinaemia. In 1982 the World Health Organization recommended that it should be taken on a daily basis (100 mg) along with rifampicin 600 mg once monthly and clo-

fazimine 100 mg daily with an extra dose of 300 mg monthly. The monthly doses are given under supervision. This triple therapy should be given for a minimum of 2 years or continued until a patient's skin smears become negative for acid-fast bacilli. However, in TL or BT, 6 months' therapy is acceptable.

The major disadvantage with clofazimine is that it is a dye and causes a generalized reddish-brown pigmentation in light-skinned individuals and a slaty grey pigmentation in dark-skinned individuals. Ethionamide is a suitable alternative. More recently acedapsone (DADDS), a depot sulphone, has been used with some success.

Surgery and physiotherapy play an important role in the management of trophic ulcers and deformities of the hands, feet and face.

Treatment of lepra reactions

Treatment of lepra reactions is urgent, as irreversible eye and nerve damage can occur with amazing rapidity. Anti-leprosy therapy must be continued. Type II lepra reactions (ENL) are effectively treated with analgesics, chloroquine, clofazimine and antipyretics. Thalidomide, a drug known for its potent teratogenic effects, is by far the most effective in the ENL reaction, but must be used with caution. Prednisolone 30–40 mg daily for a few weeks is effective in type I reactions.

PREVENTION AND CONTROL

This depends on rapid treatment of infected patients, particularly those with LL and BL, to decrease the bacterial reservoir. It is spread by close contact, but only a small proportion of contacts—approximately 1%—develop the disease. Anti-leprosy vaccines are under clinical trial; the efficacy of the BCG vaccine against leprosy is debatable. Mass chemoprophylaxis is impractical and its efficacy in household contacts has not been established.

Mycobacterial ulcer

Also known as Buruli ulcer, after the Buruli region in Uganda, this condition occurs in tropical, rural areas near rivers, e.g. in Zaire, Nigeria and Malaysia. It is caused by *M. ulcerans*. The disease is contracted by swimming in infected water. Initially a small subcutaneous nodule develops. This undergoes ulceration which involves the subcutaneous tissue, muscle and fascial planes. The ulcers are usually large, with undermined edges and markedly necrotic bases. Smears taken from necrotic tissue generally reveal numerous acid-fast bacilli. Treatment is wide surgical excision with skin grafts. Antituberculous therapy is ineffective.

Mycoplasma

Mycoplasma is a small free-living, motile bacterium which lacks a cell wall. *Mycoplasma pneumoniae* is found world-wide and may cause up to 20% of pneumonias. Infection is endemic but epidemics also occur, the infection being spread by airborne droplets between close contacts. *M. pneumoniae* infection is found most commonly in childhood, adolescence and early adulthood.

The oropharynx, trachea and bronchi are commonly involved, but there is frequently infiltration into the lung, causing pneumonia.

The clinical features and treatment are described on p. 594.

Sexually transmitted diseases (STDs)

The incidence of many sexually transmitted diseases has increased substantially during the last 30 years. Even syphilis, which had shown a gradual decline in the first half of this century, is increasing again, largely in the male homosexual population. The rising rates of gonorrhoea, non-specific urethritis and herpes simplex virus 2 (HSV-2) infection are largely due to the increased numbers of sexual contacts (homosexual and heterosexual) that many individuals make during adolescence and early adulthood. Other factors which contribute to increased transmission rates relate to the fact that women and homosexual men may carry STD without symptoms, and that venerophobia is less pronounced since the advent of effective treatment for many sexually transmitted diseases. The most widely used contraceptives (intrauterine devices and oral contraceptives) do not limit the spread of infectious disease, unlike the sheath and to some extent the diaphragm.

The organisms responsible for specific STDs are summarized in Table 1.21. Full clinical features of the illnesses they cause are given elsewhere.

HISTORY

In addition to the general medical history it is important to take a detailed history of sexual contacts (heterosexual and homosexual), with particular emphasis on whether these were regular or casual and the specific nature of the sexual activity, namely, genital, orogenital, oroanal or anogenital. It is also important to know whether there is a past history of STD and whether any specific antimicrobial therapy has been received recently.

Table 1.21 Sexually transmitted diseases and their causative organisms.

Sexually transmitted disease	Causative organism
Syphilis (see p. 42)	*Treponema pallidum*
Gonorrhoea (see p. 44)	*Neisseria gonorrhoeae*
AIDS (see p. 62)	Human immuno-deficiency virus

Non-specific genital infection:
 Men
   Non-specific urethritis (NSU) and non-specific proctitis
   Reiter's disease (NSU, conjunctivitis and seronegative arthritis) (see p. 350)
 Women
   Cervicitis
   Pelvic inflammatory disease
	Chlamydia trachomatis, Ureaplasma urealyticum and others

Trichomoniasis (see p. 81)	*Trichomonas vaginalis*
Candidiasis (see p. 67)	*Candida albicans*
Genital herpes (see p. 52)	Herpes simplex virus
Genital warts (see p. 926)	Papovavirus
Granuloma inguinale (see p. 45)	*Calymmatobacterium granulomatis*
Lymphogranuloma venereum (see p. 44)	*Chlamydia trachomatis* (LGV strain)
Chancroid (see p. 45)	*Haemophilus ducreyi*

EXAMINATION

General examination should include a search for neurological or cardiovascular evidence of advanced syphilis, and for lymphadenopathy, Kaposi's sarcoma and opportunistic infection in patients suspected of acquired immunodeficiency syndrome (AIDS) or the AIDS-related complex. In men with urethral discharge, a gram-stain for leucocytes and organisms should be made and a wet preparation should be examined for *Trichomonas vaginalis*. Material should also be dried on a slide for examination by an immunofluorescent technique for *Chlamydia*. Microbiological culture for gonococci and, if possible, *Ureaplasma* should be performed. Smears from the urethral meatus of women should also be examined by gram-stain and cultured for gonococci. Smears should also be taken from the lateral wall and posterior fornix of the vagina and from the cervical os for examination by gram-stain and culture.

In men with balanitis and balanoposthitis (inflammation of the glans penis and prepuce), smears should be taken for gram-staining and for microbiological culture of *Candidu* and aerobic and anaerobic bacteria, including *Haemophilus ducreyi*.

Careful examination should be made for the vesicles of HSV; if in doubt, material should be sent in transport medium for virus culture.

When anorectal infection is suspected, proctoscopy should be performed and rectal smears examined by gram-stain and cultured, particularly for gonococci. Similarly throat swabs should be performed when there has been orogenital contact. Blood should be taken for syphilis serology (VDRL test and TPHA), for hepatitis B surface markers, particularly in high-risk individuals (male homosexuals, bisexuals, intravenous drug abusers), and also for antibody to HIV in individuals suspected of AIDS or the AIDS-related complex.

TREATMENT, PREVENTION AND CONTROL

Treatments for individual sexually transmitted diseases are given elsewhere.

Prevention of STD must be tackled on many fronts, including health education at school and through the media, the use of protective measures, particularly the sheath, avoidance of sexual contact with individuals known to have STD or in high-risk groups, and ultimately by vaccine development, which will probably be particularly important for the control of AIDS.

Historically, contact tracing has been an important community-based approach to the control of STD, but the rising incidence rates would suggest that this method is failing, largely because of the increased numbers of casual sexual contacts that now commonly occur. Many individuals, particularly male homosexuals, regularly present themselves to STD clinics for regular check-ups, since it is now widely known that asymptomatic carriage of infection, particularly in the rectum, is common.

Many diseases not classically regarded as STDs are transmitted by sexual contact in male homosexuals (Table 1.22). These should be searched for in patients presenting at an STD clinic, particularly individuals with diarrhoea or other bowel symptoms, and those with weight loss, intermittent fever and malaise.

'Gay bowel disease' is the term used to describe diarrhoea occurring in homosexuals. Diarrhoea may be related to a variety of infecting organisms, which are often multiple. Protozoa as well as bacteria can be found. *Giardia* and *Cryptosporidium* can involve both the small and large bowel.

Syphilis

Treponema pallidum is a motile spirochaete which is generally acquired by close sexual contact, the organism entering the new host through breaches in squamous or mucous epithelium. Primary infection of non-genital sites may occasionally occur in medical personnel. A fetus can acquire the infection by transplacental passage of the organism from an

Table 1.22 Additional organisms which are sexually transmitted in male homosexuals.

Viruses:
  Human immunodeficiency virus (HIV)
  Hepatitis B virus and delta virus
  Hepatitis A virus
  Non-A non-B hepatitis virus(es)
  Cytomegalovirus

Bacteria:
  Salmonella
  Shigella
  Campylobacter

Protozoa:
  Giardia lamblia
  Entamoeba histolytica
  Cryptosporidium

Helminths:
  Strongyloides stercoralis
  Trichuris trichiura
  Enterobius vermicularis

infected mother during the later stages of pregnancy, giving rise to congenital syphilis.

Both congenital and acquired syphilis have early and late stages, each of which has classical clinical features (Table 1.23).

Primary
Two to four weeks after exposure to the pathogen a papule develops, usually on a genital site (penis, labia or cervix), which soon ulcerates to become the painless, hard chancre. This is associated with painless, regional lymphadenopathy. One of the commonest sites to see a chancre nowadays is in the anus of homosexual men. The primary chancre heals, usually within a few weeks.

Secondary
Two or three months after the chancre has healed, variable combinations of fever, sore throat, malaise and arthralgia occur. Signs include:
- Generalized lymphadenopathy
- Generalized skin rashes involving the whole body with the exception of the face, but including the palms and soles of the feet—common
- Condylomata lata—warty, plaque-like lesions found in the perianal area and other moist body sites
- Superficial confluent ulcers—found in the mouth and on the external genitalia

After a few months the features of secondary syphilis abate, but in up to 20% of individuals may recur during a period known as early latency. After 1 year the period of late latency is entered; this may continue for many years before the late stages of syphilis become apparent.

Table 1.23 Classification and clinical features of syphilis.

	Clinical features
ACQUIRED	
Early stages	
Primary	Hard chancre
	Painless, regional lymphadeno-pathy
Secondary	*General:* Fever, malaise, arthralgia, sore throat and generalized lymphadenopathy
	Skin: Red/brown maculopapular, non-itchy, sometimes scaly rash; condylomata lata
	Mucous membrane: Mucous patches, 'snail-track' ulcers in oropharynx and on genitalia
Late stages	
Tertiary	*Late benign:* Gummas (bone and viscera)
	Cardiovascular: Aortitis and aortic regurgitation
	Neurosyphilis: Meningovascular involvement, general paralysis of the insane (GPI) and tabes dorsalis
CONGENITAL	
Early stages	Stillbirth or failure to thrive
	'Snuffles' (nasal infection with discharge)
	Skin and mucous membrane lesions as in secondary syphilis
Late stages	*'Stigmata':* Hutchinson's teeth, 'sabre' tibia and abnormalities of long bones
	Keratitis, uveitis, facial gummas and CNS disease

Tertiary
Late benign syphilis generally involves the skin and the bones. Gummas (granulomatous, sometimes ulcerating lesions) can occur anywhere in the skin, frequently at sites of traumas. They are commonly found in the skull, tibia, fibula and clavicle, although any bone may be involved. Visceral gummas occur mainly in the liver (hepar lobatum) and the testes. Cardiovascular and neurosyphilis are discussed in detail elsewhere (see p. 548 and p. 838).

Congenital syphilis
Congenital syphilis usually becomes apparent between the second and sixth week after birth, early signs being nasal discharge, skin and mucous membrane lesions, and failure to thrive. Signs of late syphilis generally do not appear until after 2 years of

age and take the form of 'stigmata' relating to early damage to developing structures particularly teeth and long bones. Other late manifestations parallel those of adult tertiary syphilis (see Table 1.23).

DIAGNOSIS

Treponemas may be identified by dark ground illumination and are present in chancres and in the mucosal patches of secondary infection. Individuals with either primary or secondary disease are highly infectious.

Serological tests are helpful in the diagnosis of syphilis. The Wassermann reaction (WR) has now been superseded. The VDRL (Venereal Disease Research Laboratory) test is a useful screening test and is positive within 3–4 weeks after the primary infection. It generally becomes negative by 6 months after treatment. However, this test also becomes negative in untreated patients (50% of patients with late stage syphilis).

False-positive results may occur in other infectious diseases, particularly:
- Infectious mononucleosis
- Hepatitis
- Mycoplasma infections
- Some protozoal infections

They may also occur in some patients with:
- Cirrhosis
- Malignancy
- Autoimmune disease

The *T. pallidum* immobilization (TPI) test is the most specific test. It remains positive for years after successful treatment. However, it is an expensive test and is now becoming replaced by the *T. pallidum* haemagglutination assay (TPHA) and fluorescent treponema antibodies absorbed (FTA-ABS) test, both of which are highly specific. The FTA-ABS test is positive in more than 90% of patients with primary infection and in all patients with latent and late syphilis. It remains positive for life, even after treatment. Activity on the VDRL test correlates most closely with active infection.

Examination of the CSF for evidence of neurosyphilis (p. 838) and a chest x-ray to determine the extent of cardiovascular disease (p. 463) should also be performed.

TREATMENT

Early syphilis (primary or secondary) should be treated with long-acting procaine penicillin 1.2 g daily by intramuscular injection for 10 days. When compliance is in doubt, a single injection of benzathine penicillin 2.4 g will maintain adequate levels of drug for approximately 2 weeks. For late stage syphilis, particularly when there is cardiovascular or neurological involvement, the treatment course should be extended to between 2 and 3 weeks. For patients sensitive to penicillin, tetracycline or erythromycin, 500 mg four times daily for 2 weeks, is effective.

The Jarisch–Herxheimer reaction is due to release of endotoxin when large numbers of organisms are killed by antibiotics, and is seen in 50% of patients with primary syphilis. It occurs about 8 h after the first injection and usually consists of mild fever, malaise and headache lasting a few hours. In secondary syphilis, 90% of patients are affected. In tertiary syphilis a severe reaction, although rare, can occur so that prednisolone is often given 24 h before the antibiotic treatment. Penicillin should not be withheld because of the Jarisch–Herxheimer reaction; since it is not a dose-related phenomenon, there is no value in giving a smaller dose.

Gonorrhoea

Gonorrhoea, which is caused by *Neisseria gonorrhoeae*, occurs world-wide but has reached epidemic proportions in the USA. Transmission is commonly through sexual contact, although non-sexual transmission is possible; for example an infected mother may pass on the infection to a newborn child, usually resulting in gonococcal conjunctivitis.

CLINICAL FEATURES

A small percentage of males and 30–40% of females with gonorrhoea are asymptomatic. Symptomatic males usually present within 3–5 days with urethritis characterized by a purulent urethral discharge, meatal oedema, dysuria and frequency of micturition. Local complications are rare, but periurethral abscesses and epididymitis can occur. In symptomatic females, gonorrhoea results in a purulent vaginal discharge, frequency of micturition and anorectal discomfort; bartholinitis may occur. Male homosexuals are often asymptomatic, but anal and pharyngeal involvement is not uncommon. Disseminated gonococcal infection produces fever, malaise, myalgia and a diffuse pustular and erythematous rash. Joint involvement with an asymmetrical tenosynovitis and arthritis, meningitis and perihepatitis have also been reported.

Pelvic inflammatory disease is the commonest complication of gonorrhoea in women. There is ascending infection leading to endometritis and salpingitis. This presents acutely with lower abdominal pain, tenderness and fever. Treatment should be started quickly to avoid the late complication of infertility.

DIAGNOSIS

Though the clinical presentation is suggestive, definitive diagnosis can only be made by identifying the organisms in smears or by culturing them in special media (Thayer–Martin or New York City medium). No serological tests have been found useful. Other sexually transmitted diseases such as syphilis should be looked for and treated appropriately (see p. 43).

TREATMENT

Procaine penicillin (2.4 g in men, 4.8 g in women i.m.) with 1 g of probenicid orally as a single dose, ampicillin 2 g as a single oral dose with 1 g probenicid orally (repeated for women), or tetracycline 0.5 g by mouth four times daily for 7 days is usually effective. The procaine penicillin/probenicid regimen has the advantage of being effective against syphilis, but has no effect on *Chlamydia trachomatis* infections. Tetracycline, however, effectively eradicates *Chlamydia trachomatis* infection but not syphilis. Anorectal gonorrhoea should be treated only with a procaine penicillin/probenicid combination. Spectinomycin (2 g in men, 4 g in women, as a single intramuscular dose) and cefotaxime are useful for treating penicillinase-producing *N. gonorrhoea* and in patients who are allergic to penicillin.

Post-gonococcal urethritis should be treated with tetracycline. Contacts should be traced and treated appropriately.

Lymphogranuloma venereum (LGV)

Chlamydia trachomatis (p. 51) is responsible for this sexually transmitted infection. It is endemic in the tropics, with the highest incidences in Africa, India and South-East Asia.

CLINICAL FEATURES

The primary lesion is a painless ulcerating papule on the genitalia and only occurs in one-quarter of the patients. A few days after this heals, regional lymphadenopathy develops. The lymph nodes are painful and fixed and the overlying skin develops a dusky erythematous appearance. Finally, nodes may become fluctuant (buboes) and may rupture. Acute LGV may present as proctitis with perirectal abscesses, the appearances sometimes resembling anorectal Crohn's disease.

DIAGNOSIS

The diagnosis is made on the basis of:
- The characteristic clinical picture
- Isolation of an LGV strain of *C. trachomatis* (only possible in specialized laboratories)
- Immunofluorescence using specific monoclonal antibodies for identifying organisms in pus from a bubo
- A rising titre in a complement fixation test

The intradermal Frei test is non-specific and unreliable. Great care must be taken to exclude syphilis and genital herpes.

TREATMENT

Early treatment with oxytetracycline 500 mg four times daily for at least 2 weeks is generally necessary. Chronic infection may result in extensive scarring, abscess and sinus formation and surgical drainage may be required. Sexual partners should also be treated.

Urethritis and cervicitis

Chlamydia trachomatis is an important cause of urethritis (non-gonococcal or non-specific urethritis, NSU). Symptoms of burning pain on micturition and urethral discharge begin a variable time after exposure. Chronic infection can lead to urethral stricture. The same organism may also infect the uterine cervix, but in many cases cause no symptoms. It is also a cause of proctitis in homosexuals.

Treatment with oxytetracycline 250 mg four times daily for 2–3 weeks is best given to both partners, followed by a 2-week course of erythromycin if symptoms recur.

Chancroid

Chancroid (soft chancre) is an acute sexually transmitted disease caused by *Haemophilus ducreyi*. It occurs chiefly in tropical countries, with occasional outbreaks in the USA and Europe.

CLINICAL FEATURES

The incubation period is 2–7 days. Initially a papule forms, which then ulcerates and in about 3 days results in an irregular, variably sized, tender ulcer with undermined edges and a necrotic base. It is not unusual for multiple ulcers to coalesce to form a giant ulcer. Lesions are generally on the penis in men and on any part of the perineum in women. Regional lymphadenopathy is usual and may, if left untreated, result in abscess formation and suppuration. A feeling of being unwell and mild fever are common.

DIAGNOSIS

Clinical differentiation of chancroid from other sexually transmitted diseases such as syphilis, herpes simplex and lymphogranuloma venereum is difficult. The diagnosis is confirmed only when the organism is isolated in culture from the ulcer or from enlarged lymph nodes, but not all clinical cases are culture-positive.

TREATMENT

H. ducreyi is sensitive to tetracycline (500 mg four times daily for 1–3 weeks) and sulphonamides.

Other useful drugs include co-trimoxazole, erythromycin, streptomycin and kanamycin.

Granuloma inguinale

Granuloma inguinale is the least common of all sexually transmitted diseases in North America and Europe, but is endemic in the tropics and subtropics, particularly the Caribbean, South-East Asia and South India. Infection is caused by *Calymmatobacterium granulomatis*, a short, encapsulated gram-negative bacillus. The infection was also known as Donovanosis, the organism originally being known as Donovan's body. Although sexual contact appears to be the most important mode of transmission, the infection rates are low, even between sexual partners of many years' standing.

CLINICAL FEATURES

In the vast majority of patients, the characteristic, heaped-up ulcerating lesion with prolific red granulation tissue appears on the external genitalia, perianal skin or the inguinal region within 1–4 weeks of exposure. However, almost any cutaneous or mucous membrane sites can be involved, including the mouth and anorectal regions. Extension of the primary infection from the external genitalia to the inguinal regions produces the characteristic lesion, the 'pseudo-bubo'.

DIAGNOSIS

The clinical appearance usually strongly suggests the diagnosis, but *C. granulomatis* (Donovan bodies) may be identified intracellularly in scrapings or biopsies of an ulcer. Culture or serological methods of diagnosis are not available.

TREATMENT

Antibiotic treatment should be given for at least 10–14 days. Tetracycline 500 mg four times daily, streptomycin 1 g twice daily i.m., or ampicillin 500 mg four times daily are the three most commonly used drugs. Alternatives include erythromycin and chloramphenicol.

Spirochaetes

Important spirochaetal infections include those due to *Treponema* (syphilis, bejel, yaws and pinta) and *Borrelia* (the relapsing fevers, tropical ulcer and cancrum oris) (Table 1.24).

Table 1.24 Spirochaetal infections.

Disease	Organism
Syphilis	*Treponema pallidum*
Bejel (endemic non-venereal syphilis)	*Treponema pallidum* variant
Yaws	*Treponema pertenue*
Pinta	*Treponema carateum*
Leptospirosis (Weil's disease)	*Leptospira icterohaemorrhagiae*
Canicola fever	*Leptospira canicola*
Louse-borne relapsing fever	*Borrelia recurrentis*
Tick-borne relapsing fever	*Borrelia duttonii*
Cancrum oris	*Borrelia vincentii*
Lyme disease	*Borrelia burgdorferi*
Rat-bite fever	*Spirillum minus*
	Streptobacillus moniliformis

Syphilis

This is described on p. 42.

Bejel (endemic non-venereal syphilis), yaws and pinta

These diseases are endemic throughout the tropical and subtropical regions of the world (see Fig. 1.14).

Bejel
A variant strain of *Treponema pallidum*, sometimes referred to as *T. pallidum endemicum*, is responsible for this infection and is spread by non-venereal routes in situations where hygiene is poor. The organism enters through abrasions in the skin. The disease is found in children and differs from venereal syphilis in that a primary lesion is not commonly seen, although the late stages are indistinguishable from syphilis. Specific treponemal serology tests cannot differentiate these conditions and treatment is the same as for syphilis.

Yaws
Apart from syphilis, yaws is the most widespread of the treponemal diseases. It is spread by direct contact, usually in children, the organism again entering through damaged skin. After an incubation period of weeks or months, a primary inflammatory reaction occurs at the inoculation site, from which organisms can be isolated. Dissemination of the organism leads to multiple papular lesions containing treponemas; these skin lesions usually involve the palms and soles. There may also be bone involvement, particularly the long bones and those of the hand.

In late yaws bony lesions may progress to cause gross destruction and disfigurement, particularly of the skull and facial bones, the interphalangeal joints and the long bones. Plantar hyperkeratosis is characteristic. Like syphilis, there may be a latent period between the early and late phases of the disease, but visceral, neurological and cardiovascular problems do not occur. Serological tests for syphilis are positive. Treatment is with long-acting penicillin which, together with improved hygiene, has substantially reduced the prevalence of this disease.

Pinta
Pinta is restricted mainly to Central and South America but otherwise closely resembles endemic

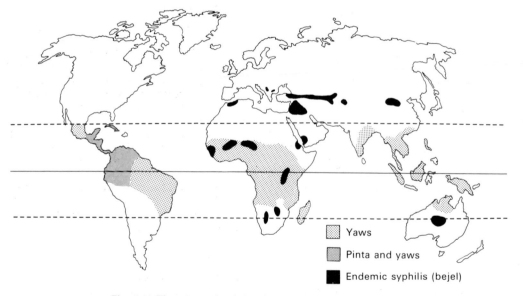

Fig. 1.14 The geographical distribution of bejel, yaws and pinta.

syphilis. The primary lesion is a pruritic red papule, usually on the hand or foot. It may become scaly but never ulcerates and is generally associated with regional lymphadenopathy. In the later stages similar lesions can continue to crop for up to 1 year associated with generalized lymphadenopathy. Eventually the lesions heal, leaving hyperpigmented or depigmented patches. Syphilis serology is positive and treatment is as for other treponemal infections by long-acting penicillin.

Leptospirosis

This zoonosis is most commonly caused by *Leptospira icterohaemorrhagiae* (from rodents), when infection is known as Weil's disease, or *L. canicola* (from dogs and pigs). Leptospires are excreted in the animal urine to which humans may then be exposed. Certain occupational groups are particularly at risk, namely veterinarians, those involved in animal husbandry, abattoir workers and, in the past, miners and sewer workers. Pet owners and those who swim in rural waters may also be exposed to the infection. Weil described a disease which consisted of jaundice, haemorrhage and renal impairment due to *L. icterohaemorrhagiae* but, fortunately, only 10–15% of patients suffer such a severe illness, the majority escaping with a benign self-limiting illness without jaundice.

CLINICAL FEATURES

The incubation period is usually 10 days (range 2–26 days). Leptospirosis has two phases: a leptospiraemic phase lasting up to a week, followed by an immune phase, which is generally separated from the former phase by an asymptomatic period of 1–3 days.

The leptospiraemic phase is similar to many acute systemic infections, and is characterized by severe headache, fever, malaise, anorexia and myalgia. The majority of patients have suffusion of the conjunctivae. Infrequently there is hepatosplenomegaly, lymphadenopathy and various skin rashes.

During the immune phase of the illness 50% of patients have meningism, about one-third of whom have CSF lymphocytosis and a modest elevation of CSF protein concentration. The majority recover uneventfully at this stage. However, a small proportion go on to develop tender hepatomegaly, jaundice, haemolytic anaemia, oliguric renal failure with microscopic haematuria, and occasionally cardiac involvement characterized by atrial and ventricular dysrhythmias and congestive cardiac failure. The mortality of Weil's disease is still unacceptably high at between 5–20%.

DIAGNOSIS

- Leptospires can be cultured from blood or CSF

during the first week of the illness. A minority of patients excrete the organism in the urine during the second week of the illness and may continue to do so for a further 2–4 weeks.
- Specific IgM leptospiral antibodies appear by the end of the first week and are useful diagnostically.
- Blood tests show a polymorpholeucocytosis and a raised ESR.
- Other laboratory investigations may be abnormal depending on the organs involved.

TREATMENT

Leptospires are sensitive to penicillins, erythromycin, tetracycline and chloramphenicol. Penicillin is most commonly used (2.4 g daily for 1 week), although the course of the illness is unlikely to be altered if treatment is begun after the fifth day of the illness. Complications, e.g. renal or liver failure, are treated appropriately.

The relapsing fevers

These conditions are so named because after apparent recovery from the initial infection, one or more recurrences may occur after a week or more without fever. The disease is caused by members of the genus *Borrelia*. *B. recurrentis* is spread by body lice and *B. duttonii* by soft ticks. The disease is found in Africa, India, the Middle East, Mediterranean Europe and South America. The louse-borne variety occurs in epidemics when humans live in close contact in impoverished conditions and the tick-borne disease is found in areas where traditional mud huts are the form of shelter for both humans and the tick.

CLINICAL FEATURES

Symptoms begin 7–10 days after infection and consist of a high fever of abrupt onset with rigors, generalized myalgia and headache. A petechial or ecchymotic rash may be seen. The general condition then deteriorates, with delirium, hepatosplenomegaly, jaundice, haemorrhagic problems and circulatory collapse. Although complete recovery may occur at this time, the majority experience one or more relapses of diminishing severity approximately 1 week after the initial illness. Without specific treatment, approximately one-third of patients will die.

Louse- and tick-borne relapsing fevers are clinically similar, although louse-borne fever tends to have a shorter initial illness with more frequent relapses.

DIAGNOSIS

Spirochaetes can be demonstrated microscopically in the blood during febrile episodes.

TREATMENT

Penicillin or tetracycline can be used, although both give rise to a severe Jarisch–Herxheimer reaction (see p. 44). Some strains of *Borrelia duttoni* are resistant to penicillin, so it is advisable to use tetracycline for this type of infection in the first instance.

PREVENTION

Ticks live for years and remain infected, passing the infection to their progeny. These reservoirs of infection should be controlled by spraying houses with insecticides such as 2% benzene hexachloride and by reducing the number of rodents. In contrast, patients infested with lice should be deloused by washing with 1% Lysol or dusting with 10% dicophane (DDT).

Cancrum oris

Cancrum oris is caused by *Borrelia vincentii* in association with anaerobic bacteria, commonly a member of the fusobacteria. The disease occurs in deprived and undernourished individuals with poor hygiene.

Cancrum oris usually occurs in children who are recovering from a debilitating illness, commonly measles. Rapidly progressive gangrenous destruction of the inner aspect of the mouth and cheek occurs, which may continue to progress even after treatment with penicillin. The mortality is high, probably reflecting the underlying poor physical state of the patient.

Lyme disease

This disease was first recognized in 1975 and the causative agent, *Borrelia burgdorferi*, was finally identified in 1983. The disease is transmitted by *Ixodes dammini* or related ixodid ticks. It was originally described in Lyme, Connecticut, but is now known to occur in many parts of the USA, in Europe and in Australia.

CLINICAL FEATURES

The first stage of the illness consists of the unique and characteristic skin lesion—erythema chronicum migrans, often accompanied by headache, fever, malaise, myalgia, arthralgia and lymphadenopathy. The second stage follows weeks or months later, when some patients develop neurological (meningoencephalitis, cranial or peripheral neuropathies) or cardiac (myocarditis) problems. Finally, the third stage of the disease consists of arthritis, which recurs in attacks for several years, often with associated erosion of cartilage and bone. Arthritis has not been seen in patients in the UK.

DIAGNOSIS

The clinical features and epidemiological considerations are usually strongly suggestive of infection with this spirochaete, but the diagnosis can be confirmed by isolation of the organisms from blood, skin lesions or CSF. The yield is low by this technique; however, serological testing, particularly for specific IgM antibodies, is highly effective.

TREATMENT

Penicillin or tetracycline given early in the course of the disease shortens the duration of the illness in approximately 50% of patients. High-dose parenteral penicillin (benzathine penicillin, 2.4 g weekly for 3 weeks) or intravenous benzylpenicillin (2 g daily for 10 days) should be given.

Rat bite fevers

Two spirochaetes, *Spirillum minus* and *Streptobacillus moniliformis*, produce similar febrile illnesses following rat bites. Although the wound initially heals, 1–3 weeks later a local inflammatory response occurs which may be associated with swelling and ulceration. Systemic sequelae of generalized infection are then evident and periodic fevers may continue for several weeks. *Spirillum minus* causes a milder illness with a shorter incubation period and less prolonged sequelae.

DIAGNOSIS

Spirochaetes can be identified in aspirates from the inflammatory site, from a regional lymph node (*Spirillum minus*), or from the blood (*Streptobacillus moniliformis*). Serological tests are available and may be helpful in diagnosis.

TREATMENT

Both organisms are sensitive to penicillin and tetracycline.

Rickettsiae and similar organisms

Rickettsiae are small bacteria which are spread to humans by arthropod vectors, namely, human body lice, fleas, ticks and larval mites. Rickettsiae inhabit the alimentary tract of these arthropods and the disease is spread to the human host by inoculation of their faeces through human skin, generally by irritation and scratching. Rickettsiae multiply intracellularly and can enter most mammalian cells, although the main lesion produced is a vasculitis due to invasion of endothelial cells of small blood vessels. Thus multi-system involvement is usual. The causative organisms and arthropod vectors for rickettsial infections are shown in Table 1.25.

CLINICAL FEATURES

Epidemic typhus

This is the most important rickettsial infection. Major outbreaks of typhus fever have occurred, mainly during famines and wars. It is found in Africa, Mexico, South America and Asia.

The incubation period is 1–3 weeks followed by an abrupt febrile illness associated with profound malaise and generalized myalgia. After 2 or 3 days the fever remains constant at around 40°C. Headache is severe and there may be conjunctivitis with orbital pain. A measles-like eruption appears around the fifth day, the macules increasing in size and eventually becoming purpuric in character. At the end of the first week, signs of meningoencephalitis are evident and CNS involvement may progress to stupor or coma, sometimes with extrapyramidal involvement. At the height of the illness, splenomegaly, pneumonia, myocarditis and gangrene at the peripheries may be evident. Oliguric renal failure occurs in fulminating disease, which is usually fatal. Recovery begins in the third week but is generally slow.

The disease may recur many years after the initial attack due to rickettsiae that lie dormant in lymph nodes. The recrudescence is known as Brill–Zinsser disease. The factors which precipitate recurrence are not clearly defined, although other infections may be important.

Endemic (murine) typhus

This is a rat infection which is inadvertently spread to man by a rickettsiae-carrying rat flea. The disease closely resembles epidemic typhus but is much milder and rarely fatal.

Rocky Mountain spotted fever.

Infected hard ticks transmit this infection to humans,

the same arthropod vector being responsible for other tick-borne typhus fevers in Africa, India and the Mediterranean (*Rickettsia conorii*), in Central Asia and the Far East (*Rickettsia siberica*), and in Australia (*Rickettsia australis*).

Rocky Mountain spotted fever is limited to North and South America. As in other tick-borne typhus fevers, many patients will be able to give an account of tick bites or exposure to ticks. Clinical features closely resemble those of epidemic typhus, although the incubation period may be shorter and an eschar (crusted necrotic papule) may develop at the site of the bite in association with regional lymphadenopathy. The typical, generalized maculopapular rash occurs, which includes the palms and soles of the feet. The rash eventually becomes petechial. Neurological, haematological and cardiovascular complications occur as in epidemic typhus.

Scrub typhus

Found throughout Asia and the Western Pacific, this disease is spread by larval trombiculid mites (chiggers). Like tick-borne typhus, an eschar can often be found. Again the clinical illness resembles that of epidemic typhus, with an abrupt onset febrile illness, rash and severe toxaemia. Bronchitis and interstitial pneumonia occur commonly, but physical findings in the chest are minimal. The infection may recur despite treatment with antibiotics.

Rickettsial pox and trench fever

Rickettsial pox is an urban disease described initially in New York City in 1946. A rodent mite was responsible for the spread of the infection to humans, the epidemic being related to massive expansion of the mouse community in large apartment buildings. The disease is mild, but similar in character to other rickettsial infections. *Trench fever* is also a relatively mild illness, but multiple relapses are common. Although the causative agent of both these diseases, *Rochalimaea quintana*, was originally classified with the rickettsiae, it is now known that the organism does not demand an intracellular existence and may

Table 1.25 Rickettsial infections.

Disease	Organism	Vector
Typhus fevers:		
Epidemic typhus	*Rickettsia prowazekii*	Human lice
Endemic (murine) typhus	*Rickettsia typhi* (*R. mooseri*)	Rat flea
Rocky Mountain spotted fever	*Rickettsia rickettsii*	Tick
Scrub typhus	*Rickettsia tsutsugamushi*	Larval mite
Rickettsial pox	*Rickettsia akari*	Mite
Trench fever	*Rochalimaea quintana*	Human lice
Q fever	*Coxiella burnetii*	None

be cultured on bacteriological media. Both of these diseases are now rare and rickettsial pox may have disappeared completely.

DIAGNOSIS

The diagnosis is generally made on the basis of the history and clinical course of the illness. Although the causative organisms can be isolated by inoculation of infected blood into laboratory animals, this is laborious and may take several weeks.

Serodiagnosis using the Weil–Felix *Proteus* agglutination test, which relies on the fact that *Rickettsia* and *Proteus OX* strains have common antigens, has been used for more than 50 years. Typical results of this test in different rickettsial infections are shown in the Table 1.26.

TREATMENT

Chloramphenicol 50 mg·kg^{-1} is given as an initial dose, followed by the same total dose given daily in three or four divided doses. Improvement generally occurs in 48 h; treatment should continue for at least 24 h after the fever has abated. Alternatively, tetracycline 2 g daily may be given. Corticosteroids are also used in severely ill patients.

CONTROL

This is achieved by control of vectors, namely lice, fleas, mites and ticks. Lice and fleas can be eradicated from clothing, etc. by insecticides (0.5% malathion or dicophane [DDT]). Chemical repellants are also useful. Control of rodents is vital.

Bites from ticks and mites should be avoided by wearing protective clothing on exposed areas of the body, especially in high-risk regions. Mites can also be destroyed by chemical spraying from the air.

Table 1.26 Weil–Felix reaction* in rickettsial infections.

Rickettsial infection	*Proteus* strain	
	OX19	OXK
Typhus fevers:		
Epidemic typhus	+	−
Endemic typhus	+	−
Rocky Mountain spotted fever	+	−
Scrub typhus	−	+
Rickettsial pox	−	−
Trench fever	−	−
Q fever	−	−

*Agglutination of *Proteus* strains by patients' serum.
+ = positive result (i.e. agglutination occurs);
− = negative result.

Q fever

Q fever is a zoonosis due to the rickettsia-like organism *Coxiella burnetii*. This organism is smaller than true rickettsiae, more resistant to physical and chemical injury and has a negative Weil–Felix reaction since it does not share common antigens with *Proteus*. Clinically, Q fever differs from rickettsial illnesses as the rash is not a major feature and transmission of the disease to humans is independent of an arthropod vector. Important modes of spread to man are thought to be dust, aerosols and milk from infected cows. *Coxiella burnetii* is widespread in domestic and farm animals. It is spread between them by ticks, which constitute an important arthropod reservoir of the disease.

CLINICAL FEATURES

Fever begins insidiously, together with other symptoms of an influenza-like illness, 1–2 weeks after exposure. The acute illness may resolve spontaneously without treatment, but with persisting infection, symptoms and signs of an atypical pneumonia may develop, followed by endocarditis. A petechial rash may be apparent at this stage. Occasionally epididymo-orchitis, uveitis and osteomyelitis may be present. Untreated chronic infection is usually fatal.

DIAGNOSIS

Serodiagnosis by complement fixation tests is important since *C. burnetii* is an obligate intracellular organism and does not grow on standard microbiological culture media. The organism possesses two classes of antigens, phase I and phase II. Antibodies to the phase I antigens appear later in the illness than antibodies to the phase II antigens; high titres are diagnostic in endocarditis. Persistently high titres of both antibodies confirm chronic infection.

TREATMENT

Tetracycline is the treatment of choice for acute infection. For endocarditis a prolonged course of treatment is required, clindamycin often being given in association with tetracycline. Co-trimoxazole and rifampicin may also be useful.

Chlamydiae

Although chlamydiae were once thought to be large viruses, it is now clear that they are true intracellular bacteria with a cell wall and both DNA and RNA, and are susceptible to a range of antibiotics. They are

Table 1.27 *Chlamydia* infections.

Disease	Organism
Trachoma	*C. trachomatis*
Lymphogranuloma venereum	*C. trachomatis* (LGV strain)
Urethritis, cervicitis, proctitis	*C. trachomatis* (non-LGV strain)
Psittacosis	*C. psittaci*

ubiquitous and found in almost every avian and mammalian species and it has been estimated that up to 20% of the human population is infected with this organism. They are highly infectious, but rarely kill their host. There are two species—*Chlamydia trachomatis* and *C. psittaci*; Table 1.27 shows the diseases produced.

Trachoma

This is the commonest cause of blindness in the world and is found in the tropics and the Middle East. It is entirely preventable. It commonly occurs in children and is probably spread by direct transmission or possibly by flies.

Infection is bilateral and begins in the conjunctiva, with marked inflammation and scarring. Scarring of the upper eyelid causes entropion, leaving the cornea exposed to further damage. The corneal scarring that eventually occurs leads to blindness. The changes in the eye are sometimes accompanied by an upper respiratory tract infection.

Trachoma may also occur as an acute ophthalmic infection in the neonate.

DIAGNOSIS

The diagnosis is generally established by:
● The typical clinical picture
● The presence of intracytoplasmic inclusion bodies in conjunctival cells

TREATMENT

Tetracycline ointment applied locally each day for 2–3 months is effective, as is systemic therapy with oral tetracycline or sulphonamide. Once infection has been controlled, surgery may be required for eyelid reconstruction and for treatment of corneal opacities. Community health education with respect to hygiene and earlier case reporting could make a substantial impact on disease prevalence.

Genital infections

Lymphogranuloma venereum (LGV) is caused by a different strain of *C. trachomatis* and is described on p. 44.

Other genital infections are caused by non-LGV-producing strains (see p. 45).

Psittacosis (ornithosis)

Although originally thought to be limited to the psittacine birds (parrots, parakeets and macaws), it is now known that the disease is widely spread amongst many species of birds, including pigeons, turkeys, ducks and chickens, hence the broader term 'ornithosis'. Human infection is related to exposure to infected birds and is therefore a true zoonosis. The causative organism, *C. psittaci*, is excreted in avian secretions; it can be isolated for prolonged periods from birds who have apparently recovered from infection. The organism gains entry to the human host by inhalation.

CLINICAL FEATURES AND TREATMENT

These are discussed on p. 595.

Viral infections

Viruses are much smaller than other microorganisms and contain either DNA or RNA. Since they are metabolically inert they must live intracellularly, using the host cell for synthesis of viral proteins and nucleic acid. Viruses have a central nucleic acid core surrounded by a protein coat which is antigenically unique for a particular virus. The protein coat (capsid) imparts a helical or icosahedral structure to the virus. Some viruses also possess an envelope consisting of lipid and protein (Fig. 1.15).

Hepatitis viruses are discussed on p. 224.

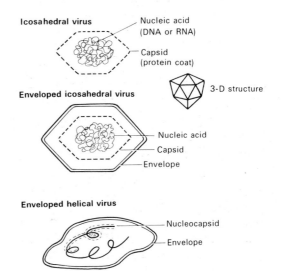

Fig. 1.15 The basic structure of viruses.

DNA viruses

Details of the structure, size and classification of DNA viruses are shown in Table 1.28.

ADENOVIRUSES

Adenovirus infection commonly presents as an acute pharyngitis. By school age the majority of children show serological evidence of previous infection. Certain subtypes produce an acute conjunctivitis associated with pharyngitis. In adults, adenovirus causes acute follicular conjunctivitis and rarely pneumonia which is clinically similar to that produced by *Mycoplasma* (see p. 594). Adenovirus has also been implicated as a cause of gastroenteritis (p. 196) without respiratory disease and may be responsible for acute mesenteric lymphadenitis in children and young adults.

Herpesviruses

Herpes simplex virus (HSV) infection

Two types of HSV have been identified: HSV-1 is the major cause of herpetic stomatitis, herpes labialis ('cold sore'), keratoconjunctivitis and encephalitis, whereas HSV-2 causes genital herpes and may also be responsible for systemic infection in the immuno-compromised host. These divisions, however, are not rigid, for HSV-1 can give rise to genital herpes.

Primary inoculation of the infection is via skin or mucous membrane. The initial infection may go unnoticed or may produce a severe inflammatory reaction. The virus then remains latent, most commonly in the trigeminal nerve, but may be reactivated by trauma, febrile illnesses and ultraviolet radiation, producing the recurrent form of the disease known as herpes labialis ('cold sore'). Recurrent infections occur in one-third of patients.

In genital herpes the primary infection is usually more severe and recurrences are inevitable. The virus remains latent in the sacral ganglia and during recurrence can produce a radiculomyelopathy, with pain in the groin, buttocks and upper thighs. Primary anorectal herpes infection is now common in male homosexuals.

Immunocompromised patients such as those receiving intensive cancer chemotherapy or those with the acquired immunodeficiency syndrome (AIDS) may develop disseminated HSV infection involving many of the viscera. In severe cases death may result from severe hepatitis and encephalitis.

Neonates may develop primary HSV infection following vaginal delivery in the presence of active genital HSV infection in the mother. Caesarean section should therefore be performed in the presence of active genital HSV infection.

Humoral antibody levels increase following primary infection, but mononuclear cell responses are probably more important in preventing dissemination of disease.

The clinical picture, diagnosis and treatment are described on p. 924.

Varicella zoster virus (VZV) infection

VZV produces two distinct diseases—varicella (chickenpox) and herpes zoster (shingles). The primary infection is chickenpox. It usually occurs in childhood, the virus entering through the mucosa of the upper respiratory tract. The primary infection almost never occurs twice in the same individual. The virus then remains latent in sensory and motor nerve cells for many years. It may recur as localized disease limited to a dermatome innervated by a single spinal or cranial sensory ganglion (shingles)

Table 1.28 Human DNA viruses.

| Structure | | Approximate size | Group | Viruses |
Symmetry	Envelope			
Icosahedral	–	80 nm	Adenovirus	Adenoviruses
Icosahedral	+	100 nm	Herpesvirus	Herpes simplex virus types 1 and 2 Varicella zoster virus Cytomegalovirus Epstein–Barr virus
Icosahedral	–	50 nm	Papovavirus	Human papillomavirus Polyomavirus
Complex	+	300 nm	Poxvirus	Variola virus Vaccinia virus

and/or may affect a motor nerve such as the facial nerve, causing facial palsy. Shingles is never the result of a primary infection. Patients with chickenpox or shingles are infective, the virus being spread from fresh skin lesions by direct contact or airborne transmission.

CLINICAL FEATURES

Fourteen to twenty-one days after exposure to VZV, a brief prodromal illness of fever, headache and malaise heralds the eruption of chickenpox, characterized by the rapid progression of macules to papules to vesicles to pustules in a matter of hours. In young children the prodromal illness may be very mild or absent. The illness tends to be more severe in older children and can be debilitating in adults. The lesions occur on the face, scalp and trunk, and to a much lesser extent on the extremities. It is characteristic to see skin lesions at all stages of development on the same area of skin. Fever subsides as soon as new lesions cease to appear. Eventually the pustules crust and heal without scarring.

Important complications of chickenpox include pneumonia, which generally begins 1–6 days after the skin eruption. Pulmonary symptoms are usually more striking than the physical findings, although a chest radiograph usually shows diffuse changes throughout both lung fields. Central nervous system involvement occurs in about 1 per 1000 and most commonly presents as an acute truncal cerebellar ataxia. The immunocompromised are susceptible to disseminated infection with multi-organ involvement.

Shingles (p. 925) occurs in adults, particularly the elderly, producing an identical skin lesion to chickenpox, although restricted to a sensory nerve distribution.

TREATMENT

Chickenpox requires no treatment in healthy children and infection results in life-long immunity. However, the disease may be fatal in the immunodeficient or the immunosuppressed, when it is reasonable to use passive immunization with varicella zoster immunoglobulin (VZIg).

Cytomegalovirus (CMV) infection

Infection with CMV is found world-wide and has its most profound effects as an opportunistic infection in the immunocompromised. A large proportion of the adult population has serological evidence of previous exposure to the virus, although infection is generally symptomless.

CLINICAL FEATURES

In healthy adults CMV causes an illness similar to infectious mononucleosis, with fever, lymphocytosis with atypical lymphocytes, and hepatitis. Infection may be spread by blood transfusion. Disseminated fatal infection with widespread visceral involvement occurs in the immunocompromised.

Intrauterine infection may have serious consequences on the fetus; there is generally CNS involvement causing microcephaly and motor disorders, often associated with jaundice, hepatosplenomegaly, thrombocytopenia and haemolytic anaemia. In older children CMV infection presents as hepatitis with or without jaundice.

DIAGNOSIS

Serological tests can identify past (IgG) or current (IgM) infection. The virus can also be identified in tissue culture by the presence of characteristic intranuclear 'owl's eye' inclusions.

Epstein–Barr virus (EBV) infection

This virus causes an acute febrile illness known as infectious mononucleosis (glandular fever), which occurs world-wide in adolescents and young adults. EBV is probably transmitted in saliva.

CLINICAL FEATURES

The predominant symptoms are fever, headache, malaise and sore throat. Palatal petechiae and a transient macular rash are common, the latter occurring in 90% of patients who have received ampicillin for the sore throat. Cervical lymphadenopathy, particularly of the posterior cervical nodes, and splenomegaly are characteristic. Mild hepatitis is common, but other complications such as myocarditis, meningitis, mesenteric adenitis and splenic rupture are rare. Although some young adults remain debilitated and depressed for some months after infection, the evidence for the occurrence of latency and reactivation of the virus in healthy individuals is controversial, although these are thought to occur in immunocompromised patients.

DIAGNOSIS

EBV infection should be strongly suspected if atypical mononuclear cells (glandular fever cells) are found in the peripheral blood. It can be confirmed during the second week of infection by a positive Paul–Bunnell reaction. Specific EBV IgM antibodies indicate recent infection by the virus. The Monospot test is a sensitive and easily performed screening test. Clinically similar illnesses are produced by CMV and toxoplasmosis but these can be distinguished serologically.

TREATMENT

The majority of cases require no specific treatment and recovery is rapid. Corticosteroid therapy is advised when there is neurological involvement, e.g. encephalitis, meningitis or the Guillain–Barré syndrome, or when there is marked thrombocytopenia or haemolysis. Corticosteroid therapy has also been used with good effect when malaise and intermittent fever are prolonged.

EBV is also considered to be the aetiological agent responsible for Burkitt's lymphoma and nasopharyngeal carcinoma.

PAPOVAVIRUSES

These small viruses tend to produce chronic infections, often with evidence of latency. They are capable of inducing neoplasia in some animal species and were among the first viruses to be implicated in tumourigenesis. Human papillomavirus is responsible for the common wart. The human BK virus, polyomavirus, is the only other human virus of importance in this group. It is generally found in immunosuppressed individuals and may be detected in the urine of between 15 and 40% of renal transplant patients, in patients receiving cytotoxic chemotherapy and in those with immunodeficiency states, notably the Wiskott–Aldrich syndrome.

POXVIRUSES

Smallpox (variola)

This disease has now been eradicated following an aggressive vaccination policy and careful detection of new cases.

CLINICAL FEATURES

Variola major has a 12-day incubation period in the majority of patients, followed by a prodromal febrile illness. Early lesions appear in the oropharynx, then on the skin, where the classic evolution of macule to papule to vesicle and finally to pustule occurs. Unlike chickenpox, when the lesions appear in crops, smallpox lesions are all at the same stage at any moment in time. In addition, smallpox lesions tend to predominate in the periphery, whereas in chickenpox they occur mainly on the trunk. Smallpox lesions heal with scars.

An uncommon but usually fatal type of smallpox is the haemorrhagic variety, in which coagulopathy leads to haemorrhage into mucous membranes and the viscera.

Variola minor (alastrim) was a mild form of smallpox confined to Africa and South America which had a very low mortality.

Vaccinia virus

This is a laboratory virus and does not occur in nature in either man or animals. Its origins are uncertain but it is thought to be a derivative of the variola or cowpox virus used by Jenner for vaccination against smallpox. Vaccination is now not recommended, except for laboratory personnel handling the virus for experimental purposes. Should the disease reappear, herd immunity would be very low and widespread dissemination of the disease might result.

RNA viruses (Table 1.29)

PICORNAVIRUSES

Poliovirus infection (poliomyelitis)

Poliomyelitis occurs when a susceptible individual is infected with poliovirus type I, II or III. These viruses have a marked propensity for the nervous system, especially the anterior horn cells of the spinal cord and cranial nerve motor nuclei. Poliomyelitis is found world-wide but its incidence has decreased dramatically following improvements in sanitation, hygiene and the widespread use of polio vaccines. Spread is usually via the faecal–oral route, as the virus is excreted in the faeces.

CLINICAL FEATURES

The incubation period varies from 10 to 14 days. Although polio is essentially a disease of childhood, no age is exempt. The clinical manifestations vary considerably:
- *Inapparent infection* is common and occurs in 95% of infected individuals.
- *Abortive poliomyelitis* occurs in approximately 4–5% and is characterized by the presence of fever, sore throat and myalgia. The illness is self-limiting and of short duration.
- *Non-paralytic poliomyelitis* has features of abortive poliomyelitis as well as signs of meningeal irritation, but recovery is complete.
- *Paralytic poliomyelitis* occurs in approximately 0.1% of all infected individuals. This form of the disease is characterized initially by features simulating abortive poliomyelitis. Symptoms subside for 4–5 days, only to recur in greater severity with signs of meningeal irritation and muscle pain, which is most prominent in the neck and lumbar region. These symptoms persist for a few days and are followed by the onset of asymmetric paralysis without sensory involvement. The paralysis is usually confined to the lower limbs in children under 5 years of age and the upper limbs in older children, whereas in adults it manifests as paraplegia or quadriplegia.
- *Bulbar poliomyelitis* is characterized by the

Table 1.29 Human RNA viruses.

Structure		Approximate size	Group	Viruses
Symmetry	Envelope			
Icosahedral	−	30 nm	Picornavirus	Poliovirus ⎱ Coxsackievirus ⎬ Enterovirus Echovirus ⎰ Enterovirus Rhinovirus
Icosahedral	−	80 nm	Reovirus	Reovirus Rotavirus
Icosahedral	+	50–80 nm	Togavirus	Rubella virus Alphaviruses ⎱ Arbovirus Flaviviruses ⎰
Helical	+	80–120 nm	Orthomyxovirus	Influenza viruses A, B and C
Helical	+	100–300 nm	Paramyxovirus	Measles virus Mumps virus Respiratory syncytial virus
Helical	+	60–175 nm	Rhabdovirus	Rabies virus Vesicular stomatitis virus
Helical	+	100 nm	Retrovirus	Human immunodeficiency virus (HIV)
Helical	+	100–300 nm	Arenavirus	Lassa virus Lymphocytic chorio- meningitis virus
Pleomorphic	+	Filaments or circular forms; 100 × 130–2600 nm	—	Marburg virus Ebola virus

presence of cranial nerve involvement. Soft palate, pharyngeal and laryngeal muscle palsies are common.

Aspiration pneumonia, myocarditis, paralytic ileus and urinary calculi are late complications of all types of poliomyelitis.

DIAGNOSIS

The diagnosis is a clinical one. Distinction from the Guillian–Barré syndrome is easily made by the absence of sensory involvement and the asymmetrical nature of the paralysis in poliomyelitis.

TREATMENT

Treatment is symptomatic. Bedrest is essential during the early course of the illness. Respiratory support with intermittent positive pressure respiration is required if the muscles of respiration are involved. Once the acute phase of the illness has subsided, occupational therapy, physiotherapy and occasionally surgery play an important role in patient rehabilitation.

PREVENTION AND CONTROL

Immunization has dramatically decreased the prevalence of this disease world-wide. Trivalent oral poliovaccine (TOPV) (active virus) is used (see Table 1.10); occasionally inactivated poliovirus vaccine is used intramuscularly.

Coxsackie-, echo- and enterovirus infection

These viruses are spread by the faecal–oral route. They each have a number of different types and are responsible for a broad spectrum of disease involving the skin and mucous membranes, muscle, nerves, the heart (see Table 1.30), and rarely other organs, such as the liver and pancreas.

Skin and oropharyngeal disease
There is a vesicular eruption on the fauces, palate and uvula (herpangina). The lesions eventually evolve into aphthous ulcers. The illness is usually associated with fever and headache, but is short-lived, recovery occurring within a few days.

Table 1.30 Picornavirus infections (excluding poliovirus and rhinovirus).

Disease	Coxsackievirus A (types A_1–A_{22}, A_{24})	Coxsackievirus B (types B_1–B_6)	Echovirus (types 1–9, 11–27, 29–33)	Enterovirus (types 68–71)
Cutaneous and oropharyngeal				
Herpangina	+++	+	+	
Hand, foot and mouth	+++	+		+
Erythematous rashes	+	+	+++	
Neurological				
Paralytic	+		±	+
Meningitis	++	++	+++	+
Encephalitis	++	++	±	+
Cardiac				
Myo- and pericarditis	+	+++	+	
Muscle				
Myositis (Bornholm disease)	+	+++	+	

Hand, foot and mouth disease

Oral lesions are similar to those seen in herpangina but may be more extensive in the oropharynx. However, vesicles and a maculopapular eruption also appear on the palms of the hands and the soles of the feet. This infection commonly affects children; recovery occurs within a week.

Neurological disease

Other enteroviruses in addition to poliovirus can cause a broad range of neurological disease, including meningitis, encephalitis, and a paralytic disease characteristic of poliomyelitis.

Heart and muscle disease

Viruses are an important cause of acute myocarditis and pericarditis, from which, in general, there is complete recovery. However, these viruses can also cause chronic congestive cardiomyopathy and rarely constrictive pericarditis.

Skeletal muscle involvement, particularly of the intercostal muscles, is an important feature of Bornholm disease, a febrile illness usually due to coxsackievirus B. The infection affects both children and adults and may be complicated by meningitis or cardiac involvement.

Rhinovirus infection

Rhinovirus is responsible for the common cold (p. 572); peak incidence rates occur in the colder months, especially spring and autumn. There are multiple rhinovirus immunotypes, which makes vaccine control impractical.

REOVIRUS

Reovirus infection

Reovirus infection occurs mainly in children, causing mild respiratory symptoms and diarrhoea. A few deaths have been reported following disseminated infection of brain, liver, heart and lungs.

Rotavirus infection

Rotavirus (Latin *rota* = wheel) is so named because of its characteristic circular outline with radiating spokes. It is responsible world-wide for both sporadic cases and epidemics of diarrhoea, and is presently one of the most important causes of childhood diarrhoea. The prevalence is higher during the winter months.

Clinically the illness is characterized by vomiting, fever, diarrhoea, and the metabolic consequences of water and electrolyte loss. Histology of the jejunal mucosa in children shows shortening of the villi, with crypt hyperplasia and mononuclear cell infiltration of the lamina propria.

Treatment is directed at overcoming the effects of water and electrolyte imbalance with adequate oral rehydration therapy and, when indicated, intravenous fluids. Antibiotics should not be prescribed.

Adults may become infected with rotavirus but symptoms are mild or absent.

TOGAVIRUSES

These can be divided into the rubella virus and the arboviruses.

Rubella

Rubella ('German measles') is caused by a spherical, enveloped fragile RNA virus which is easily killed by heat and ultraviolet light. While the disease can occur sporadically, epidemics are not uncommon. It has a world-wide distribution. Spread of the virus is via droplets; maximum infectivity occurs during the time the rash is present.

CLINICAL FEATURES

The incubation period varies from 14 to 21 days, averaging 18 days. The clinical features are largely age-determined, with symptoms being mild or even absent in children under 5 years of age. The peak incidence of the disease is at 15 years.

During the prodrome the patient complains of malaise and fever. Mild conjunctivitis and lymphadenopathy may be present. The distribution of the lymphadenopathy is characteristic and involves the suboccipital, postauricular and posterior cervical groups of lymph nodes. Small petechial lesions on the soft palate (Forchheimer spots) are suggestive but not diagnostic. Splenomegaly may be present.

The eruptive or exanthematous phase usually occurs within the first 7 days of the initial symptoms. The rash first appears on the forehead and then spreads to involve the trunk and the limbs. It is pinkish-red, macular and discrete, although some of these lesions may coalesce. It usually fades by the second day and rarely persists beyond the third day after its appearance.

COMPLICATIONS

Complications are rare; they include superadded pulmonary bacterial infection, arthralgia, haemorrhagic manifestations due to thrombocytopenia, encephalitis and the *congenital rubella syndrome*. Rubella affects the fetuses of 50–70% of all women who contract the infection during the first trimester of pregnancy. The incidence of congenital abnormalities diminishes in the second and third trimesters. Congenital rubella syndrome is characterized by the presence of fetal cardiac malformations, especially patent ductus arteriosus and ventricular septal defect, eye lesions, especially cataracts, microcephaly, mental retardation and deafness. The *expanded rubella syndrome* consists of the manifestations of the congenital rubella syndrome plus hepatosplenomegaly, myocarditis, interstitial pneumonia and metaphyseal bone lesions.

DIAGNOSIS

This is usually clinical. It can be confirmed by culturing the virus from throat swabs or urine or by demonstrating an increased antibody titre (measured using the sensitive haemagglutination inhibition test) in the second of two successive blood samples taken 14 days apart.

TREATMENT

Treatment is symptomatic.

PREVENTION

Prevention of rubella is important. Human immunoglobulin can decrease the symptoms of this already mild illness, but does not prevent the teratogenic effects. Several live attenuated rubella vaccines have been used with great success in preventing this illness and these have been successfully combined with the measles and mumps vaccine. The side-effects of vaccination have been dramatically decreased by using vaccines prepared in human embryonic fibroblast cultures (RA 27/3 vaccine). Use of the vaccine is contraindicated during pregnancy or if there is a likelihood of pregnancy within three months of immunization.

Arbovirus (arthropod-borne) infection

Arboviruses are zoonotic viruses, with the possible exception of the O'nyong-nyong fever virus of which humans are the only known vertebrate hosts. They are transmitted through the bites of insects, especially mosquitoes and ticks, although infection can result from the ingestion of contaminated foods or inhalation of these organisms. Over 385 viruses are classified as arboviruses. *Culex*, *Aedes* and *Anopheles* mosquitoes account for the transmission of the majority of these.

Although the majority of arbovirus diseases are generally mild, epidemics are frequent and when these occur the mortality is high. In general, the incubation period is less than 10 days. The illness tends to be biphasic and, as in other viral fevers, pyrexia, conjunctival suffusion, a rash, retro-orbital pain, myalgia and arthralgia are common. Lymphadenopathy is seen in dengue. Life-long immunity after an infection is usual. In some of these viral fevers, haemorrhage is a feature (Table 1.31), although its pathogenesis is speculative. Increased vascular permeability, capillary fragility and disseminated intravascular coagulation have been implicated. Encephalitis may be prominent in some fevers.

Alphaviruses

The 24 viruses of this group are all transmitted by mosquitoes; eight result in human disease. These viruses are globally distributed and tend to acquire their names from the location where first isolated (such as Ross River, Eastern Venezuelan, and Western encephalitis viruses) or by the local expression for a major symptom caused by the virus (such as chikungunya meaning 'chronic bleeding'). Infec-

Table 1.31 Viral infections associated with haemorrhagic manifestations.

Arbovirus
Mosquito-borne:
    Yellow fever (urban and sylvan)
    Dengue haemorrhagic fever
    Chikungunya
    Rift Valley fever
Tick-borne:
    Congo and Crimean haemorrhagic fevers
    Kyasanur Forest disease
    Omsk haemorrhagic fever

Arenavirus
Argentinian haemorrhagic fever
Bolivian haemorrhagic fever
Lassa fever
Epidemic haemorrhagic fever

Picornavirus
Acute haemorrhagic conjunctivitis

Paramyxovirus
Atypical measles

tion is characterized by fever, skin rash, arthralgia, myalgia and sometimes encephalitis.

Flaviviruses
There are 60 viruses in this group, some of which are transmitted by ticks and others by mosquitoes.

Yellow fever

Yellow fever, caused by a flavivirus, results in an illness of widely varying severity. It is a disease confined to Africa and South America between latitudes 15° north and 15° south of the equator. For poorly understood reasons, yellow fever has not been reported from Asia, despite the fact that climatic conditions are suitable and the vector, *Aedes aegypti*, is common. The infection is transmitted in the wild by *A. africanus* in Africa and the *Haemagogus* species in South and Central America. These mosquitoes are responsible for maintaining infection in monkeys, which form the sylvan reservoir. *A. aegypti* and the *Haemagogus* species are responsible for transmission of this disease from monkeys to humans in Africa and South and Central America, respectively. Once infected a mosquito remains so for its whole life.

CLINICAL FEATURES

The incubation period varies from 3 to 6 days. When the infection is mild, the disease is indistinguishable from other viral fevers such as influenza or dengue. Classically, however, jaundice, proteinuria and haemorrhage occur.

Three phases in the illness are recognized. Initially the patient presents with a high fever of acute onset, usually 39–40°C, which then returns to normal in 4–5 days. During this time headache is prominent. Retrobulbar pain, myalgia, arthralgia, a flushed face and suffused conjunctivae are common. Epigastric discomfort and vomiting are present when the illness is severe. Relative bradycardia (Faget's sign) is present from the second day of illness. The patient then makes an apparent recovery and feels well for several days. Following this 'phase of calm' the patient again develops increasing fever, deepening jaundice and hepatomegaly. Ecchymosis, bleeding from the gums, haematemesis and melaena may occur. Coma, which is usually a result of uraemia or haemorrhagic shock, occurs for a few hours preceding death. The mortality rate is up to 40% in severe cases.

DIAGNOSIS

The diagnosis is established by isolating the virus (when possible) from blood during the first 3 days of illness, by demonstrating increasing neutralizing antibody titres, or by finding the typical histological lesions on liver biopsy. These include mid-zone necrosis, fatty degeneration and intracellular hyaline necrosis (Councilman bodies).

TREATMENT

Treatment is supportive. Bed rest, analgesics, and maintenance of fluid and electrolyte balance are important.

PREVENTION AND CONTROL

Yellow fever is an internationally notifiable illness. It is easily prevented using either the 17-day chick embryo vaccine, which is more popular, or the Dakar vaccine. Eradication of the breeding places of the vectors will help in decreasing the prevalence of the disease.

Dengue

Dengue is a viral disease found mainly in Asia and Africa, although it has been reported from the USA as well. Six different antigenic varieties of the dengue virus are recognized and are all transmitted by the daytime-biting *Aedes aegypti*. Humans are infective during the first 3 days of the illness (viraemic stage). Mosquitoes become infective about 2 weeks after feeding on an infected individual, and remain so for the rest of their lives. The disease is usually endemic, but epidemics have been recorded. Immunity after the illness is partial.

CLINICAL FEATURES

The incubation period varies from 5 to 6 days. Two clinical forms are recognized.

Classic dengue fever is characterized by the abrupt onset of fever, malaise, headache, retrobulbar pain which worsens on eye movements, conjunctival suffusion and severe backache, which is a prominent symptom. Lymphadenopathy, petechiae on the soft palate and skin rashes may also occur. The rash is transient and morbilliform. It appears on the limbs and then spreads to involve the trunk. Desquamation occurs subsequently. Cough is uncommon. The fever subsides after 3–4 days, the temperature remains normal for a couple of days, and then the fever returns, together with the features already mentioned, but is milder. This biphasic or saddle-back pattern is considered characteristic. Severe fatigue, a feeling of being unwell and depression are common for several weeks after the fever has subsided.

Dengue haemorrhagic fever is a severe form of dengue fever and is believed to be the result of two sequential infections with different dengue serotypes. It is a disease of children and has been described almost exclusively in south-east Asia. The disease has a mild start, often with symptoms of an upper respiratory tract infection. This is then followed by the abrupt onset of shock and haemorrhage into the skin and ear, epistaxis, haematemesis and melaena. Serum complement levels are depressed and there is laboratory evidence of a consumptive coagulopathy.

DIAGNOSIS

Isolation of the dengue virus by tissue culture in sera obtained during the first few days of illness is diagnostic. Demonstrating rising antibody titres by neutralization (most specific), haemagglutination inhibition or complement-fixing antibodies in sequential serum samples is presumptive evidence of dengue virus infection.

TREATMENT

Treatment is symptomatic.

Rift Valley fever

Rift Valley fever is primarily an acute febrile illness of livestock, sheep, goats and camels. It is found in south and east Africa. The vector in east Africa is *Culex pipiens* and in south Africa, *Aedes caballus*. Following an incubation period of 3–6 days, the patient has an acute febrile illness which is difficult to distinguish clinically from other viral fevers. The temperature pattern is usually biphasic. The initial febrile illness lasts 2–4 days, and is followed by a remission and a second febrile episode. Complica-

tions are indicative of severe infection and include retinopathy, meningoencephalitis, haemorrhagic manifestations and hepatic necrosis. Mortality approaches 50% in severe forms of the illness. Treatment is symptomatic.

Japanese encephalitis

Japanese encephalitis is a mosquito-borne encephalitis caused by a flavivirus. It has been reported most frequently from the rice growing countries of south-east Asia and the Far East. *Culex tritaeniorhynchus* is the most important vector and feeds mainly on pigs as well as birds such as herons and sparrows. Humans are accidental hosts.

As with other viral infections, the clinical manifestations are variable. The onset is heralded by severe rigors. Fever, headache and malaise last from 1 to 6 days. Weight loss is prominent. In the acute encephalitic stage the fever is high (38–41°C), neck rigidity occurs and neurological signs such as altered consciousness, hemiparesis and convulsions develop. Mental deterioration occurs over a period of 3 to 4 days and culminates in coma. Mortality varies from 7 to 40% and is higher in children. Residual neurological defects such as deafness, emotional lability and hemiparesis occur in about 70% of patients who have had CNS involvement. Convalescence is prolonged. Treatment is symptomatic.

ORTHOMYXOVIRUSES

Influenza

Three types of influenza virus are recognized—A, B and C. The influenza A virus is a spherical or filamentous enveloped virus. Haemagglutinin, a surface glycopeptide, aids attachment of the virus to the wall of susceptible host cells at specific receptor sites. Cell penetration, probably by pinocytosis, and release of replicated viruses from the cell surface is effected by budding through the cell membrane or by the action of viral neuraminidase.

- *Influenza A* is generally responsible for pandemics and epidemics.
- *Influenza B* often causes smaller or localized outbreaks, e.g. in camps or schools.
- *Influenza C* rarely produces disease in humans.

Antigenic shift (major antigenic change within an influenza subtype) usually heralds the onset of a pandemic.

Sporadic cases of influenza and outbreaks amongst groups of people living in a confined environment are frequent. The incidence increases during the winter months, when crowding is common. Spread is mainly by droplet infection, but fomites and direct contact have also been implicated.

The clinical features, diagnosis, treatment, and prophylaxis of influenza are discussed on p. 576.

PARAMYXOVIRUSES

These are a heterogenous group of enveloped viruses of varying size which are responsible for parainfluenza, mumps, measles and respiratory infection.

Parainfluenza

Parainfluenza is caused by the parainfluenza viruses types I to IV, which have a world-wide distribution. Type IV has been identified only in the USA.

Parainfluenza is essentially a disease of children and presents with features similar to the common cold. When severe, a brassy cough with inspiratory stridor and features of laryngotracheobronchitis (croup) are present. Treatment is symptomatic. The role of steroids is controversial.

Measles (rubeola)

Measles is a highly communicable disease which occurs world-wide. With the introduction of aggressive immunization policies, the incidence of measles has fallen dramatically in the West, but it still remains one of the commonest childhood infections in the Third World, where it is associated with a high morbidity and mortality. It is spread by droplet infection.

CLINICAL FEATURES

The incubation period varies from 8 to 14 days. Two distinct phases of the disease can be recognized:
- The *infectious pre-eruptive and catarrhal stage*. This is the stage of viraemia and viral dissemination. Malaise, fever, rhinorrhoea, cough, conjunctival suffusion and the pathognomonic Koplik's spots are present during this stage. Koplik's spots are small, greyish, irregular lesions surrounded by an erythematous base and are found in greatest numbers on the mucous membrane opposite the second molar tooth. They occur a day or two before the onset of the rash.
- The *non-infectious eruptive or exanthematous stage*. This is characterized by the presence of a maculopapular rash (Table 1.32), which initially occurs on the face, chiefly the forehead, and then spreads rapidly to involve the rest of the body. At first the rash is discrete but later it may become confluent and patchy, especially on the face and neck. It fades in about a week and leaves behind a brownish discoloration with desquamation.

Although measles is a relatively mild disease in the healthy child, it carries a high mortality in the

Table 1.32 Some viral infections associated with a maculopapular rash.

Adenovirus infection
Arbovirus infection
Measles
Cytomegalovirus infection
Enterovirus infection
Hepatitis B virus
Infectious mononucleosis
Rubella
Rubeola

malnourished and in those who have other diseases. Complications are common in such individuals and include bacterial pneumonia, bronchitis, otitis media and gastroenteritis. Less commonly, myocarditis, hepatitis and encephalomyelitis may occur. The virus has also been implicated in the rare condition subacute sclerosing panencephalitis.

Maternal measles, unlike rubella, does not cause congenital fetal abnormalities. It is, however, associated with spontaneous abortions and premature delivery.

DIAGNOSIS

The clinical features are distinctive and hence serological tests, such as the haemagglutination inhibition test, are rarely used to confirm the diagnosis. The measles virus is difficult to culture.

TREATMENT

Treatment is symptomatic. Antibiotics are indicated only if secondary bacterial infection occurs.

PREVENTION

A previous attack of measles confers a high degree of immunity and second attacks are uncommon.

Human immunoglobulin 0.25 ml·kg^{-1} given within 5 days of exposure effectively aborts an attack of measles. It is indicated for previously unimmunized children below 3 years of age, during pregnancy, and in those with debilitating disease.

Active immunization involves a single dose of 0.5 ml live attenuated measles vaccine given subcutaneously. The measles vaccine has recently been adapted for administration as an aerosol.

Mumps

Mumps is the result of infection with an intermediate-sized paramyxovirus. It is spread by droplet infection, by direct contact or through fomites. Humans are the only known natural hosts. The peak period of infectivity is 2–3 days before the onset of the parotitis and for 3 days afterwards.

CLINICAL FEATURES

The incubation period averages 18 days. Although no age is exempt, it is primarily a disease of school-age children and young adults; it is uncommon before the age of 2 years. The prodromal symptoms are non-specific and include fever, malaise, headache and anorexia. This is followed by severe pain over the parotid glands, with either unilateral or bilateral parotid swelling. The enlarged parotid glands obscure the angle of the mandible and may elevate the ear lobe, which does not occur in cervical lymph node enlargement. Trismus due to pain is common at this stage. Submandibular gland involvement occurs less frequently.

COMPLICATIONS

Central nervous system involvement is the commonest extra-salivary gland manifestation of mumps. Clinical meningitis occurs in 5% of all infected patients, and 30% of patients with CNS involvement have no evidence of parotid gland involvement.

Epididymo-orchitis develops in about one-third of patients who develop mumps after puberty. Bilateral testicular involvement results in sterility in only a small percentage of these patients.

Pancreatitis, oophoritis, myocarditis, mastitis, hepatitis and polyarthritis may also occur.

DIAGNOSIS

The diagnosis of mumps is on the basis of the clinical features. In doubtful cases, serological demonstration of a fourfold rise in antibodies detected by complement fixation or indirect haemagglutination or neutralization tests on acute and convalescent sera is diagnostic.

TREATMENT

Treatment is symptomatic. Attention should be given to adequate nutrition and mouth care. Analgesics should be used to relieve pain. The role of steroids in the treatment of mumps orchitis is controversial.

PREVENTION

Live attenuated mumps virus vaccine given as a single 0.5 ml intramuscular dose can prevent the disease in children over the age of 1 year. This vaccine should not be used in children below this age as it interferes with transplacentally acquired maternal antibodies. Vaccination is contraindicated in immunosuppressed individuals, during pregnancy, or in those with severe febrile illnesses because the live attenuated vaccine may cause disease.

Respiratory syncytial virus infection

Respiratory syncytial virus is a paramyxovirus which causes many respiratory infections. It is a common cause of bronchiolitis in infants, which is complicated by pneumonia in approximately 10% of cases.

RHABDOVIRUSES

Rabies

This is a major problem in some countries and carries a high mortality.

The rabies virus is bullet-shaped and has spike-like structures arising from its surface containing glycoproteins which cause the host to produce neutralizing, haemagglutination inhibiting antibodies. The virus has a marked affinity for nervous tissue and the salivary glands. It exists in two major epidemiological settings:

- *Urban rabies*, which is most frequently transmitted to humans through rabid dogs and, less frequently, cats
- *Sylvan (wild) rabies*, which is maintained in the wild by a host of animal reservoirs such as foxes, skunks, jackals, mongooses and bats

With the exception of Australia, New Zealand and the Antarctic, human rabies has been reported from all other continents. Transmission is through the bite of an infected animal. However, only 50% of rabid bites result in clinical disease. Human-to-human transmission is rare. Rabid animals can also transmit the disease by licking abraded skin or mucosa. Rarely airborne droplet infection occurs.

Having entered the human body, the viruses replicate in the muscle cells near the entry wound. They penetrate the nerve endings and travel in the axoplasm to the spinal cord and brain. In the central nervous system the viruses again proliferate before they spread to the salivary glands, lungs, kidneys and other organs via the autonomic nerves.

CLINICAL FEATURES

The incubation period is variable and may range from a few weeks to several years; on average it is 1–3 months. In general, bites on the head, face and neck have a shorter incubation period than those elsewhere. In humans, two distinct clinical varieties of rabies are recognized:

- 'Furious rabies'—the classical variety
- 'Dumb rabies'—the paralytic variety

Furious rabies

The only characteristic feature in the prodromal period is the presence of pain and tingling at the site of the initial wound. Fever, malaise, myalgia, and headache are also present. About 10 days later marked anxiety and agitation or depressive features develop. Hallucinations, bizarre behaviour and paralysis may also occur. Hyperexcitability, the hallmark of this form of rabies, is precipitated by auditory or visual stimuli. Hydrophobia (fear of water) is present in 50% of patients and is due to severe pharyngeal spasms on attempting to eat or drink. Aerophobia (fear of air) is considered pathognomonic of rabies. Examination reveals hyperreflexia, spasticity, and evidence of sympathetic overactivity indicated by pupillary dilatation and diaphoresis.

The patient goes on to develop convulsions, respiratory paralysis and cardiac arrhythmias. Death usually occurs in 10–14 days.

Dumb rabies

Dumb rabies or paralytic rabies presents with a symmetrical ascending paralysis resembling the Guillain–Barré syndrome. This variety of rabies commonly occurs after bites from rabid bats.

It is unusual for patients to survive an attack of rabies; only a few cures have been documented.

DIAGNOSIS

The diagnosis of rabies is generally made clinically. Recently fluorescent antibody has been used to detect rabies antigen in corneal impressions or in salivary secretions; this is a useful test. The classical Negri bodies are detected at post mortem in 90% of all patients with rabies; these are eosinophilic, ovoid bodies, 2–10 nm in diameter, seen in greatest numbers in the cells of the hippocampus and the cerebellum.

TREATMENT

Once the disease is established, therapy is symptomatic. The patient should be nursed in a quiet, darkened room. Nutritional, respiratory and cardiovascular support may be necessary.

Drugs such as morphine, diazepam and chlorpromazine should be used liberally in patients who are excitable.

The wound should be carefully cleaned, adequately debrided and left open. Cauterization of the wound with one of the quaternary ammonium compounds such as cetrimide or 1% benzalkonium chloride should then be performed. Antirabies serum injected locally around the site of the wound may be helpful.

PREVENTION

The vaccine of choice is the human diploid cell strain vaccine (HDCSV).

Post-exposure prophylaxis

Five 1.0 ml doses of HDCSV should be given intramuscularly: the first dose is given on day 0 and is followed by injections on day 3, 7, 14 and 28. Duck embryo vaccine (DEV), a killed virus vaccine, is another safe alternative. Reactions to these vaccines are uncommon.

Pre-exposure prophylaxis

This is given to individuals with a high risk of contracting rabies, e.g. laboratory workers, animal handlers and veterinarians. HDCSV 1.0 ml intramuscularly on day 0, 7 and 21 should provide effective immunity. If DEV is used, two 1.0 ml subcutaneous injections 1 month apart, followed by a third dose at 6 months also offers adequate protection. Vaccines of nervous tissue origin are still used in some parts of the world. These, however, are associated with significant side-effects and are best avoided if HDCSV or DEV is available.

Vesicular stomatitis

Vesicular stomatitis is a viral disease of animals. In humans the virus produces a severe influenza-like infection. Sore throat and cervical or submandibular lymphadenopathy are usual. Raised vesicular lesions on the buccal mucosa are characteristic. Occasionally these vesicles may be seen on the fingers. The disease is self-limiting and rarely lasts more than 5 days.

RETROVIRUSES

Infection with human immunodeficiency virus (HIV)

HIV is the virus responsible for the acquired immunodeficiency syndrome (AIDS), which probably first became apparent in 1979 but was not fully appraised by clinicians and scientists until 1981. The syndrome is characterized by a profound defect in cell-mediated immunity resulting in opportunistic infections, particularly *Pneumocystis carinii* pneumonia, and otherwise uncommon malignancies such as Kaposi's sarcoma.

EPIDEMIOLOGY

AIDS is transmitted by sexual contact and blood products. These limited modes of transmission have resulted in the emergence of well-defined risk groups (Table 1.33). More than 70% of reported cases are in homosexual or bisexual men and 17% in

Table 1.33 Risk groups for acquired immunodeficiency syndrome (AIDS).

Homosexual or bisexual males

Intravenous drug users

Haemophiliacs or transfused patients

Female sexual partners of AIDS patients

Infants of mothers with AIDS

People from certain geographical locations, e.g. some parts of central Africa (Zaire, Chad, Rwanda)

intravenous drug abusers. Patients with haemophilia and those receiving blood transfusion constitute about 1% of the total reported cases.

The origins of AIDS are unknown. One theory suggests that the virus has been present in Central Africa for many years but was spread from Zaire to Haiti in the late 1960s and from there to the USA.

Epidemiological evidence in Africa suggests that AIDS is spread by heterosexual activity and in Zaire females are affected as frequently as males. This is different from the situation seen at present in the USA and Europe.

The incubation period appears to depend on the mode of transmission, varying from approximately 1 year following sexual contact to up to 4 years after transfusion of contaminated blood. Infants born to women with AIDS develop the disease within a few months.

CLINICAL FEATURES

A broad spectrum of disease is caused by HIV (Table 1.34). Immediately after infection the virus com-

Table 1.34 Summary of classification system for HIV infections.

Group I	Acute infection (transient symptoms with seroconversion)
Group II	Asymptomatic infection
Group III	Persistent generalized lymphadenopathy
Group IV	Other manifestations:
	(a) Chronic constitutional disease, e.g. lassitude, fever, weight loss
	(b) Neurological disease, e.g. dementia (subacute encephalitis), peripheral neuropathy, atypical aseptic meningitis
	(c) Specified secondary infections (see Table 1.35)
	(d) Specified secondary cancers, e.g. Kaposi's sarcoma, primary brain lymphoma, probably other carcinomas (anal canal, tongue)
	(e) Other conditions, e.g. diarrhoea

monly causes an acute febrile illness which might be mistaken for influenza or infectious mononucleosis. The individual may then remain symptom-free for months or several years, and then present with progressive weight loss, intermittent fever, generalized lymphadenopathy, chronic diarrhoea, one or more opportunistic infections (see Table 1.35), widespread Kaposi's sarcoma, and even a progressive encephalopathy.

It is still unclear as to what proportion of such patients will eventually go on to develop the complete syndrome of AIDS (group IV, Table 1.34).

The total number of reported cases of HIV infections is now well in excess of 30 000, with a current mortality rate of over 40%. The mortality for the full syndrome would appear to be almost 100%.

DIAGNOSIS

The diagnosis should be suspected in individuals from a high-risk group with all or some of the clinical features of AIDS. These patients should have no other obvious cause for immunodeficiency with or without opportunistic infection. The presence of the virus can now be confirmed by detecting the presence of antibody to HIV by ELISA. There are multiple immunological abnormalities in AIDS, the characteristic pattern being lymphopenia, with a quantitative and qualitative defect in the T_4 or Leu 3 inducer/helper subset of T cells resulting in a marked defect in cell-mediated immunity. In addition there are B cell abnormalities, with polyclonal activation of B cells and increased immunoglobulin secretion, causing hypergammaglobulinaemia.

TREATMENT

There is no definitive treatment which will eradicate HIV and the management of AIDS rests entirely on supportive care and active treatment of the complications, in particular the opportunistic infections.

Table 1.35 Organisms causing opportunistic infections in AIDS.

Pneumocystis carinii (causing pneumonia)

*Mycobacterium avium–intracellulare**

Cryptococcus neoformans meningitis*

*Mycobacterium tuberculosis**

*Candida**

Cytomegalovirus*

Herpes simplex virus*

Toxoplasma gondii (with CNS involvement)

Cryptosporidium

*Often with disseminated infection.

Pneumocystis carinii pneumonia occurs in approximately 60% of patients and is the commonest cause of death in AIDS. Treatment is with high-dose co-trimoxazole (see p. 597).

Cryptosporidiosis is an important cause of watery diarrhoea and extremely difficult to treat, although recent reports suggest that spiramycin may be helpful in some cases.

PREVENTION

'Safe sex', i.e. the use of condoms, and restricting the number of partners must be advised. All blood products should be screened for HIV.

ARENAVIRUSES

These are pleomorphic, round or oval viruses with diameters ranging from 50–300 nm. The virion surface has club-shaped projections, and the virus itself contains a variable number of characteristic electron-dense granules which represent host ribosomes. Infection with the prototype virus of this group produces lymphocytic choriomeningitis. Arenaviruses are also responsible for Argentinian and Bolivian haemorrhagic fevers and Lassa fever.

Lassa fever

This illness was first documented in the town of Lassa, Nigeria, in 1969 and is confined to sub-Saharan West Africa (Nigeria, Liberia and Sierra Leone). The multimammate rat, *Mastomys natalensis*, is known to be a reservoir. Humans are infected by ingesting foods contaminated by rat urine or saliva containing the virus. Direct inoculation and inhalation of this virus are also common modes of spread of this disease.

CLINICAL FEATURES

The incubation period varies from 1 to 24 days. The disease is insidious in onset and is characterized by fever, myalgia, severe backache, malaise and headache. A transient maculopapular rash may be present. Sore throat and lymphadenopathy occur in over 50% of patients. In severe cases epistaxis and gastrointestinal bleeding may occur, hence the classification of Lassa fever as a viral haemorrhagic fever. The fever usually lasts from 1 to 3 weeks and recovery within a month of the onset of illness is usual. However, death occurs in 15–20% of hospitalized patients, usually from irreversible hypovolaemic shock.

DIAGNOSIS

The diagnosis is established by serial serological tests (including the Lassa-specific IgM titre) or by culturing the virus from the throat, serum or urine.

TREATMENT

Treatment is supportive. Human convalescent serum has produced some clinical improvement, but its value has been questioned. Ribavirin, an antiviral drug, has been useful in preventing haemorrhagic manifestations in rhesus monkeys and dramatically reduces mortality in human infection.

In non-endemic countries, strict isolation procedures should be used, the patient ideally being nursed in a flexible film isolator or by medical and nursing staff wearing full protective clothing, including respirators or ventilated hoods. Prevention of spread of the virus is best achieved by treating patients in the endemic area where they contracted the disease, since a high proportion of the local population will be immune.

Lymphocytic choriomeningitis (LCM)

This infection is a zoonosis, the natural reservoir of the LCM virus being the house mouse. Infection is characterized by either:
- Non-nervous system illness, with fever, malaise, myalgia and headache
- A typical aseptic meningitis-type illness, with signs of meningism in addition to the above symptoms. Occasionally, a more severe form occurs, with encephalitis leading to disturbance of consciousness.

This illness is generally self-limiting and requires no specific treatment.

MARBURG VIRUS DISEASE AND EBOLA VIRUS DISEASE

These severe, haemorrhagic, febrile illnesses are discussed together because their clinical manifestations are similar. These diseases are named after Marburg in Germany and the Ebola river region in the Sudan and Zaire where these viruses were first isolated. The natural reservoir for these viruses has not been identified and the precise mode of spread from one individual to another has not been elucidated.

The illness is characterized by the acute onset of severe headache, severe myalgia and high fever, followed by prostration. On about the fifth day of illness a non-pruritic maculopapular rash develops on the face and then spreads to the rest of the body. Diarrhoea is profuse and is associated with abdominal cramps and vomiting. Haematemesis, melaena or haemoptysis may occur between the seventh and sixteenth day. Hepatosplenomegaly and facial oedema are usually present. In Ebola virus disease, chest pain and a dry cough are prominent symptoms.

Treatment is symptomatic. Convalescent human serum appears to decrease the severity of the attack.

Fungal infections

Morphologically, fungi can be grouped into two major categories:
● Yeasts, which reproduce by budding
● Moulds, which grow by branching and longitudinal extensions of hyphae

Dimorphic fungi are those which behave as yeasts in the host but as moulds in vitro, e.g. *Histoplasma* and *Sporothrix*. Despite the fact that fungi are ubiquitous, fungal infections are uncommon. Fungal infections are transmitted by inhalation of spores or by contact with the skin.

Diseases are usually divided into:
● Systemic
● Subcutaneous
● Superficial

Systemic mycoses are unusual, but opportunistic mycoses can cause disease in immunocompromised patients. Fungi do not produce endotoxin, but exotoxin, e.g. aflatoxin (p. 224), production has been documented in vitro. Fungi may also produce allergic disease (see p. 611).

In general, human fungal infections are indolent and respond poorly to treatment. Some fungi such as *Candida albicans* are human commensals.

Systemic fungal infections

Histoplasmosis

Histoplasmosis is caused by *Histoplasma capsulatum*, a non-encapsulated, dimorphic fungus. Spores can survive in moist soil for several years, particularly when enriched by bird and bat droppings. Histoplasmosis occurs world-wide and is commonly seen in Ohio and the Mississippi river valley. Transmission is mainly by inhalation of the spores.

CLINICAL FEATURES

Fig. 1.16 summarizes the pathogenesis, main clinical forms and sequelae of *Histoplasma* infection.

Primary pulmonary histoplasmosis is usually asymptomatic. The only evidence of infection is conversion of a histoplasmin skin test from negative to positive, and radiological features similar to those seen with the Ghon primary complex of tuberculosis (see p. 599). Calcification in the lungs, spleen and liver occurs in patients from areas of high endemicity. When symptomatic, primary pulmonary histoplasmosis generally presents as a mild influenza-like illness, with fever, chills, myalgia and cough. The systemic symptoms are pronounced in severe disease.

Complications such as atelectasis, secondary bacterial pneumonia, pleural effusions, erythema nodosum and erythema multiforme may also occur.

Chronic pulmonary histoplasmosis is clinically indistinguishable from pulmonary tuberculosis (see p. 601). It is usually seen in white males over the age of 50 years. Radiologically, pulmonary cavities, infiltrates and characteristic fibrous streaking from the periphery towards the hilum are seen.

Disseminated histoplasmosis resembles disseminated tuberculosis clinically. Fever, lymphadenopathy, hepatosplenomegaly, weight loss, leucopenia and thrombocytopenia are common. Rarely features of meningitis, hepatitis, Addison's disease, endocarditis and peritonitis may dominate the clinical picture.

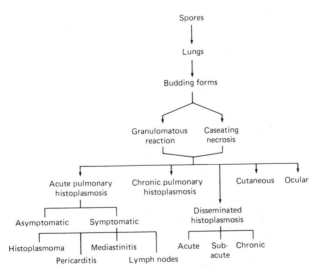

Fig. 1.16 A summary of the pathogenesis, main clinical forms and sequelae of *Histoplasma* infection.

DIAGNOSIS

Definitive diagnosis is possible only by culturing the fungi or by demonstrating them on histological sections. The histoplasmin skin test is usually positive.

Antibodies usually develop within 3 weeks of the onset of illness and are best detected by the complement fixation test. Titres of above 1:32 are suggestive of *Histoplasma* infection. Agar gel diffusion and latex agglutination antibody tests may also be helpful.

TREATMENT

Only severe acute pulmonary histoplasmosis, chronic histoplasmosis and acute disseminated histoplasmosis require therapy. Intravenous amphotericin 0.5–0.6 mg·kg^{-1} daily or 1.0–1.2 mg·kg^{-1} on alternate days for 10 weeks is the mainstay of therapy. Surgical excision of histoplasmomas (pulmonary granuloma due to *H. capsulatum*) or chronic cavitatory lung lesions and release of adhesions following mediastinitis may be required.

African histoplasmosis

African histoplasmosis is caused by *Histoplasma duboisii*, the spores of which are larger than that of *H. capsulatum*. Skin lesions, e.g. abscesses, nodules, lymph node involvement and lytic bone lesions are prominent. Pulmonary lesions do not occur. Treatment is similar to that for *H. capsulatum* infection.

Aspergillosis

Aspergillosis is caused by several dimorphic fungi of the Aspergillus species. Of these, *Aspergillus fumigatus* is the commonest cause of disease in humans, although *A. flavus* and *A. niger* have also been implicated as pathogens. These fungi are ubiquitous in the environment and are commonly found on decaying leaves and trees. Humans are infected by inhalation of the spores. Disease manifestation depends on the dose of the spores inhaled as well as the immune response of the host. Three major forms of the disease are recognized:

- *Bronchopulmonary allergic aspergillosis* (p. 608), with symptoms suggestive of bronchial asthma
- *Aspergilloma* (p. 609), sometimes referred to as a pulmonary mycetoma
- *Fulminant disease*, which occurs in immunosuppressed patients, presenting as acute pneumonia, meningitis or an intracerebral abscess, lytic bone lesions, and granulomatous lesions in the liver; less commonly endocarditis, paranasal *Aspergillus* granuloma or keratitis may occur

Urgent treatment with intravenous amphotericin is required. The diagnosis and treatment are described in more detail on p. 608.

Cryptococcosis

Cryptococcosis is caused by the yeast-like fungus, *Cryptococcus neoformans*. It has a world-wide distribution and appears to be spread by birds, especially pigeons, in their droppings. The spores gain entry into the body through the respiratory tract, where they elicit a granulomatous reaction. Pulmonary symptoms are, however, uncommon and meningitis, which is clinically indistinguishable from bacterial meningitis, is the usual mode of presentation.

Lung cavitation, hilar lymphadenopathy, pleural effusions and occasionally pulmonary fibrosis occur. Less commonly the skin and bones are involved.

DIAGNOSIS

This is established by demonstrating the organisms in appropriately stained tissue sections. A positive latex cryptococcal agglutinin test performed on the CSF is diagnostic of cryptococcosis.

TREATMENT

Amphotericin (0.3–0.5 mg·kg^{-1} daily i.v.), alone or in combination with flucytosine (100–200 mg·kg^{-1} daily), has reduced the mortality of this once always fatal condition. Therapy should be continued for 3 months if meningitis is present.

Coccidioidomycosis

Coccidioidomycosis is caused by the non-budding spherical form (spherule) of *Coccidioides immitis*. This is a soil saprophyte and is found in the southern United States, Central America and parts of South America.

Humans are infected by inhalation of the thick-walled barrel-shaped spores called arthrospores. Occasionally epidemics of coccidioidomycosis have been documented following dust storms.

CLINICAL FEATURES

The majority of patients are asymptomatic. Infection is detected by the conversion of a skin test using either coccidioidin (extract from a culture of mycelial growth of *C. immitis*) or spherulin (the soluble fraction from a culture of *C. immitis* spherules) from negative to positive.

Acute pulmonary coccidioidomycosis presents, after an incubation period of about 10 days, with fever, malaise, cough and expectoration. Erythema nodosum, erythema multiforme, phlyctenular conjunctivitis and, less commonly, pleural effusions may occur. Complete recovery is usual.

Pulmonary cavitation with haemoptysis, pulmonary fibrosis, meningitis, lytic bone lesions, hepatosplenomegaly, and skin ulcers and abscesses may occur in severe disease.

DIAGNOSIS

Because of the high infectivity of this fungus, and consequent risk to laboratory personnel, serological tests (rather than culture of the organism) are widely used for diagnosis. These include the highly specific latex agglutination and precipitin tests. A positive complement fixation test performed on the CSF is diagnostic of coccidioidomycosis meningitis.

TREATMENT

Mild pulmonary infections are self-limiting and require no treatment, but progressive and disseminated disease requires urgent therapy. Amphotericin is the drug of choice. Surgical excision of cavitatory pulmonary lesions or localized bone lesions may be necessary. For meningitis, intrathecal amphotericin may be required; the role of steroids remains controversial. Ketoconazole or miconazole may be of value.

Paracoccidioidomycosis

Paracoccidioidomycosis is caused by the dimorphous fungus *Paracoccidioides brasiliensis*. Paracoccidioidomycosis is confined to Central and South America. Males are affected more often than females. The commonest presentation is an indolent pulmonary infection characterized by fever, cough, weight loss and night sweats. Radiologically there may be evidence of consolidation, fibrosis, cavitation, and hilar or mediastinal lymphadenopathy. Unlike in tuberculosis, calcification is not prominent. Ulceration of mucocutaneous junctions is the second commonest form of presentation. Less commonly, disseminated paracoccidioidomycosis may occur as a rapidly progressive disease.

TREATMENT

Amphotericin is the mainstay of therapy. Ketoconazole orally (200–400 mg daily) may be an effective alternative. Sulphonamides may be useful in milder infections.

Blastomycosis

Blastomycosis is a systemic infection caused by the biphasic fungus *Blastomyces dermatitidis*. Although initially believed to be confined to certain parts of North America, it has recently been reported in Canada, Africa, Israel, Eastern Europe and Saudi Arabia.

CLINICAL FEATURES

Blastomycosis primarily involves the skin, where it presents as non-itchy papular lesions which later develop into ulcers with red verrucous margins. The ulcers are initially confined to the exposed parts of the body but later involve the unexposed parts as well. Atrophy and scarring may occur. Pulmonary involvement may present as a solitary lesion resembling a malignancy or give rise to radiological features similar to the primary complex of tuberculosis. Systemic symptoms such as fever, malaise, cough and weight loss are usually present. Bone lesions are common and present as painful swellings.

DIAGNOSIS

The diagnosis is confirmed by demonstrating the organism in histological sections or by culture. Serology is not useful because of the marked cross-reactivity of antibodies to *Blastomyces* with *Histoplasma*.

TREATMENT

The drug of choice is amphotericin.

Systemic phycomycosis

Systemic phycomycosis (systemic zygomycosis, mucormycosis) is rare and is caused by several fungi, including *Mucor*, *Rhizopus* and *Absidia*. It occurs in ill patients. The hallmark of the disease is vascular invasion with marked haemorrhagic necrosis.

Rhinocerebral mucormycosis is the commonest form. Nasal stuffiness, facial pain and oedema, and necrotic, black nasal turbinates are characteristic. Treatment is with amphotericin. This condition is invariably fatal if left untreated.

Candidiasis

Candidiasis is the most common fungal infection in humans and is caused by *Candida albicans*. *Candida* are small asexual fungi. All the species which are pathogenic to humans are normal oropharyngeal and gastrointestinal commensals. Candidiasis is found world-wide.

CLINICAL FEATURES

Practically any organ in the body can be invaded by *Candida*, but oral thrush (p. 155) is the commonest form. This is seen in the very young, in the elderly, following antibiotic therapy and in those who are immunosuppressed. Candidial oesophagitis may present with painful dysphagia.

Cutaneous candidiasis (p. 927) typically occurs in intertriginous areas. It is also an important cause of paronychia, balanitis and vaginitis.

Chronic mucocutaneous candidiasis is a rare manifestation, usually occurring in children, and is associated with a T-cell defect. It presents with hyperkeratotic plaque-like lesions on the skin, especially the face, and on the finger nails. It is associated with several endocrinopathies, including hypothyroidism and hypoparathyroidism. Less commonly dissemination of candidiasis may lead to a haematogenous spread, with meningitis, pulmonary involvement, endocarditis or osteomyelitis.

DIAGNOSIS

The fungi can be demonstrated in scrapings from infected lesions.

TREATMENT

This varies depending on the site and severity of infection. Oral lesions respond to nystatin, oral amphotericin or miconazole. For more severe systemic infections, parenteral therapy with amphotericin or ketoconazole, or oral therapy with flucytosine 50–75 mg·kg^{-1} daily for 2–3 weeks may be required.

Local fungal infections

Dermatophytosis

Dermatophytoses are chronic fungal infections of keratinous structures such as the skin, hair or nails (see p. 928). *Trichophyton*, *Microsporum* and *Epidermophyton* are traditionally referred to as dermatophytes, although other fungi such as *Candida* can also infect keratinous structures.

Sporotrichosis

Sporotrichosis is due to the saprophytic fungus *Sporothrix schenckii*, which is found world-wide. Infection usually follows cutaneous inoculation, at the site of which a reddish, non-tender, maculopapular lesion, referred to as 'plaque sporotrichosis', develops. Pulmonary involvement and disseminated disease rarely occur.

TREATMENT

Treatment with saturated potassium iodide (10–12 ml daily orally for adults) is curative in the cutaneous form. Amphotericin or miconazole is required for systemic infection.

Subcutaneous phycomycosis

Subcutaneous phycomycosis (zygomycosis) is caused by several filamentous fungi of the *Basidiobolus* genus. The disease usually remains confined to the subcutaneous tissues and muscle fascia. It presents as a brawny, woody infiltration involving the limbs, neck and trunk. Less commonly, the pharyngeal and orbital regions may be affected.

Treatment is with saturated potassium iodide solution given orally.

Chromomycosis

Chromomycosis (chromoblastomycosis) is caused by fungi of the genus *Philalophora* and *Cladosporium carrionii*. It presents initially as a small papule, usually at the site of a previous injury. This persists for several months before ulcerating. The lesion later becomes warty and encrusted and gradually spreads. Satellite lesions may be present. Itching is frequent. The drug of choice is flucytosine in combination with amphotericin in small doses.

Rhinosporidiosis

Rhinosporidiosis is caused by *Rhinosporidium seeberi*. This organism has not been cultured. Although recognized world-wide, it is seen mainly in South India and Sri Lanka. Mucosal lesions present as polyps which are friable and vascular; the nose, nasopharynx and soft palate are most frequently involved. Haematogenous dissemination may occur. Treatment is surgical excision and cautery.

Protozoal infections

Blood and tissue infections

Leishmaniasis

Three clinical entities caused by *Leishmania* have been described:
● Visceral leishmaniasis (kala-azar)
● Cutaneous leishmaniasis of the New World
● Cutaneous leishmaniasis of the Old World

The geographical distribution is shown in Fig. 1.17.

The life-cycle of the parasite involves two stages:
1 The *amastigote* (Leishman–Donovan body) occurs in vertebrate hosts such as humans, dogs or rodents. The parasites infect macrophages and reticuloendothelial cells and multiply until the cells rupture, releasing the organisms into the circulation. When the female sandfly (*Phlebotomus* or *Lutzomyia*) bites an infected host, it draws blood containing the amastigotes.
2 In the sandfly the parasites develop into the infective *promastigotes*, which move to the salivary glands in about 10 days.

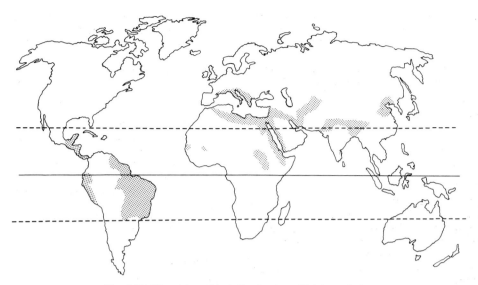

Fig. 1.17 The geographical distribution of leishmaniasis.

The cycle is completed by the sandfly biting another vertebrate.

The presentation in humans is dependent on the patient's cellular immunity as well as the parasite species.

In the *kala-azar syndrome* there is little or no immune response and the reticuloendothelial system is laden with amastigote-laden histiocytes. In subjects with an increased immune response, hepatic and lymph node granulomas are found and there are either no clinical symptoms or a localized lesion is seen.

Inapparent infection is common in endemic areas and is recognized by the high incidence of leishmanin-positive skin tests. There is usually no previous history of skin ulceration or systemic disease. Infection is eradicated by the immune system and the subject is left with permanent immunity to that species of *Leishmania*.

Visceral leishmaniasis (kala-azar)

Visceral leishmaniasis is caused by *L. donovani* and occurs in Asia, the Mediterranean, South America and Africa. Dogs, foxes, jackals and wild rodents can be reservoirs, but in India humans are the only known reservoir. Primary skin lesions (leishmaniomas) are usually small, but can be found at the site of the sandfly bite.

The disease usually affects young people. The incubation period may be months or years. The onset is abrupt or insidious. The patient feels remarkably well despite many symptoms and signs. Fever occurs and may exhibit a characteristic biphasic pattern. Cough is frequent and diarrhoea may occur. The skin is dry and rough and with time becomes pigmented. Splenic enlargement may be massive and hypersplenism is chiefly responsible for the pancytopenia seen. Epistaxis may occur due to thrombocytopenia. Hepatomegaly is less prominent than the splenomegaly. In African kala-azar, warty skin eruptions and lymphadenopathy also occur.

If left untreated, death occurs within 3 years in the majority of patients and is due to pulmonary or gastrointestinal superinfection, to which these patients are predisposed.

Infantile kala-azar is seen chiefly in the Mediterranean region and is a disease of children below the age of 5 years.

Post-kala-azar dermal leishmaniasis (PKDL) occurs 1–2 years after successful treatment for visceral leishmaniasis in a small proportion of patients in India and less often in Africa. It is characterized by macular, erythematous lesions and pale pink nodules on the face.

INVESTIGATION AND DIAGNOSIS

- The characteristic Leishman–Donovan bodies may be demonstrated in buffy coat preparations or in bone marrow smears or lymph node, liver or spleen aspirates.
- The organism can be cultured in the Nicolle–Novy–MacNeal culture medium.
- Complement-fixing antibodies may be detected by indirect immunofluorescence, ELISAs and haemagglutination.
- A formol gel test is positive due to hyperglobulinaemia.

An intradermal leishmanin skin test (a test of delayed hypersensitivity) is of no value in diagnosis since it is negative early in the course of the disease.

TREATMENT

Response to therapy varies. African kala-azar is relatively resistant to treatment and the duration of therapy is necessarily longer. Pentavalent antimony compounds are the drugs of choice. Sodium stibogluconate 10 mg·kg^{-1} in adults is often used. Treatment should be continued for 10 days in Indian kala-azar and 30 days in all other forms. Meglumine antimonate 50 mg·kg^{-1} daily for 10–30 days is a useful alternative.

Intercurrent pulmonary infections should be treated with appropriate antibiotics. Blood transfusions are rarely required.

Intravenous amphotericin or pentamidine (up to four courses of 3 mg·kg^{-1} daily for 10 days) may be required for patients whose initial response to therapy is poor. Pentamidine is ineffective in the treatment of PKDL.

PREVENTION

In endemic areas control of vectors plays an important part. Spraying with an effective insecticide should be carried out at regular intervals. There should also be an attempt to decrease the reservoir of infection by destroying infected animals and treating infected humans early.

Cutaneous leishmaniasis of the New World (American cutaneous leishmaniasis)

Four forms are recognized:

Chiclero's ulcer
This is caused by *L. mexicana* and is found in Mexico, Guatemala, Brazil, Venezuela and Panama. It occurs on the exposed parts of the body, and runs a benign course with spontaneous healing within 6 months. However, infection of the pinna (chiclero's ear) results in gross destruction of the external ear. A lesion at this site may persist for over 20 years.

Espundia (mucocutaneous leishmaniasis)
This is caused by *L. braziliensis* and is found in Brazil, Ecuador, Bolivia, Uruguay and northern Argentina. Initially painful, itchy nodules appear on the lower limbs, and then ulcerate. Lymphangitis is usual. Healing occurs spontaneously in 6 months.

Several years later secondary lesions develop at mucocutaneous junctions such as the nasopharynx. There is evidence of nasal obstruction, ulceration, septal perforation and destruction of the nasal cartilages. Death usually occurs from secondary bacterial infection or aspiration.

Diffuse cutaneous leishmaniasis
This is caused by *L. amazonensis* and is characterized by diffuse infiltration of the skin by Leishman–Donovan bodies. Visceral lesions are absent. Clinically this chronic condition resembles lepromatous leprosy, although it does not involve the nasal septum.

Uta
Uta is a similar disease to diffuse cutaneous leishmaniasis and is caused by *L. peruviana*. It occurs in cooler climates in the Andes. It produces single or multiple ulcers which usually heal spontaneously.

DIAGNOSIS

The diagnosis is established by demonstrating Leishman–Donovan bodies in spleen or bone marrow smears or histological sections of tissues. Parasites are scanty and hence a positive leishmanin skin test is useful.

TREATMENT

Chiclero's ulcer has been effectively treated with a single intramuscular injection of cycloguanil pamoate. Sodium stibogluconate in a dose similar to that used for kala-azar is effective for most other forms of cutaneous and mucocutaneous leishmaniasis. Amphotericin is usually required for severe infections. Reconstructive surgery of any deformity is an important part of therapy.

Cutaneous leishmaniasis of the Old World

This is a mild form of leishmaniasis caused by *L. tropica* or *L. aethiopica*. *L. tropica* is found in urban areas of the Mediterranean, USSR and India.

L. tropica minor causes a red pruritic papule which ulcerates (oriental sore) and heals by scarring. Leishmaniasis recidiva, which is characterized by features resembling lupus vulgaris, may complicate this form of cutaneous leishmaniasis.

L. tropica major usually results in multiple clusters of nodules which ulcerate. A marked inflammatory reaction is present. Regional lymphadenopathy and satellite lesions are common. Marked scarring occurs on healing.

L. aethiopica is found in the highlands of Ethiopia and Kenya. The cutaneous lesions have a tendency to become diffuse.

TREATMENT

Cutaneous lesions respond to application of direct heat (40°C). Pentavalent antimony compounds provide the mainstay of therapy. In patients with indolent lesions, levamisole has been used with some success.

TRYPANOSOMIASIS

Trypanosomes are protozoa which at some stage of their life-cycle have a flagellum. The development of the trypanosomes consists of several stages. They usually exist as trypomastigotes in vertebrate hosts such as humans, although some may also exist as amastigotes, e.g. *Trypanosoma cruzi*. Two main types of development of the parasite in its vector are recognized:

- *Anterior station development (salivaria)*, where the organism is transmitted through the bite of the insect (e.g. *T. brucei*)
- *Posterior station development (stercoraria)*, where transmission occurs by rubbing faecal matter from the insect into the bite wound or conjunctiva (e.g. *T. cruzi*)

African trypanosomiasis

African trypanosomiasis (sleeping sickness) follows the bite of the tsetse fly and is caused by *T. brucei*, which develops by anterior station. *T. brucei* is found in west and central Africa between the 20° north and 20° south parallels of latitude (Fig. 1.18). Two clinical forms are recognized (Table 1.36):

- *Gambian sleeping sickness*, which is found mainly in West Africa, including southern Sudan and Uganda
- *Rhodesian sleeping sickness*, which is found from Ethiopia in the north to Botswana in the south

Gambian sleeping sickness is caused by *T. b. gambiense* and transmitted to humans by the tsetse fly species *Glossina palpalis* and *G. tachinoides*. Humans are the only important reservoirs.

T. b. rhodesiense, the causative agent of Rhodesian sleeping sickness, is a zoonosis and is transmitted by *Glossina pallidipes*, *G. morsitans*, *G. swynnertoni*, and *G. palpalis*. Pigs are possible reservoirs of *T. b. rhodesiense*.

Tsetse flies are daylight biting and both males and females can be infected. Following the bite of a tsetse fly, metacyclic forms (the infective forms of trypomastigotes) are deposited into the sub-cutaneous tissue, where a marked perivascular reaction occurs. Lymphatics are then invaded, followed by spread to the lymph nodes. Invasion of the bloodstream occurs in 2 or 3 weeks, at which time the organisms reach all parts of the body, especially the CNS. In the CNS they elicit a marked perivascular mononuclear infiltration which results in leptomeningitis or encephalomyelitis. The presence of a toxin, although postulated, has not been demonstrated.

CLINICAL FEATURES

The incubation period is about 3 weeks. The clinical manifestations of Gambian and Rhodesian sleeping sickness are similar. Gambian sleeping sickness is a chronic illness with symptom-free periods, while Rhodesian sleeping sickness is an acute, more severe form, and death usually occurs within a year, often due to myocarditis. Features of CNS involvement are therefore less prominent in the Rhodesian form (Table 1.36).

Following a bite by an infected tsetse fly, a nodule appears at the site of the bite. This is referred to as a trypanosoma chancre and is seen more commonly in Rhodesian sleeping sickness and in Caucasians. Tachycardia and persistent headache are common.

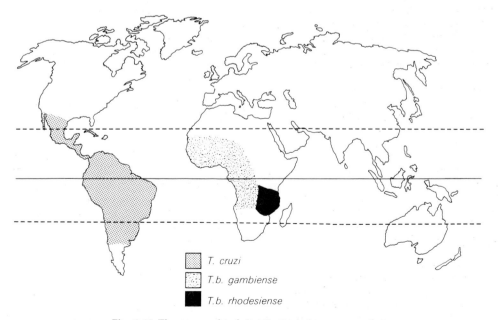

T. cruzi
T.b. gambiense
T.b. rhodesiense

Fig. 1.18 The geographical distribution of trypanosomiasis.

Table 1.36 Comparison between Gambian and Rhodesian sleeping sickness.

	Gambian	Rhodesian
Causative agent:	*Trypanosoma brucei gambiense*	*Trypanosoma brucei rhodesiense*
Main insect vector:	*Glossina palpalis*	*Glossina morsitans*
Transmission:	Anterior station	Anterior station
Reservoir:	Humans (pigs, goats, cattle, ? dogs)	Humans, wild animals (antelopes and hogs), cattle
Geographical distribution:	West Africa (Gambia to Congo), central Africa, scattered areas in east Africa	East Africa
Clinical features		
Duration:	Chronic	Acute
Severity:	Mild	Severe
Trypanosoma chancre:	Uncommon	Common
Fever:	Insidious and low grade	Acute and with large variations
Lymphadenopathy:	Prominent, especially posterior cervical group (Winterbottom's sign)	Less prominent
Hepatosplenomegaly:	Present	Present
CNS abnormalities:	Marked	Less marked
Other organs involved	Uncommon	Common
Treatment with melarsoprol:	Effective	Ineffective
Chemoprophylaxis:	Effective	Less effective

Spontaneous healing of the chancre is followed by haematogenous dissemination.

The lymph glands are discrete, non-tender and have a peculiar rubbery consistency. Splenomegaly and hepatomegaly may also occur. After a variable period of time, there is evidence of central nervous system involvement and features of a chronic meningoencephalomyelitis with behavioural changes. The patient loses interest in his surroundings, becomes apathetic, has a mask-like facies, and a tendency to fall asleep during the day and inability to sleep at night. The eyelids tend to droop, there is facial puffiness, the lower lips are swollen and hang loosely and the patient's attention span decreases. Later, tremor of the hands, areas of hyperaesthesia, especially over the ulnar nerve (Kerandel's sign), choreiform movements, seizures and finally coma develop. Myocarditis, hepatitis, petechiae and pleural effusions may occur, particularly in Rhodesian sleeping sickness.

Unusual manifestations
An erythematous, patchy, annular rash which fades in a week may be seen in the early stages of infection in Caucasians. Facial oedema, paraesthesiae, periosteitis, especially of the tibia resulting in hyperaesthesia, iridocyclitis and choroiditis may occur. Endocrine dysfunction may develop, manifesting as amenorrhoea or impotence.

DIAGNOSIS

The definitive diagnosis depends on demonstrating trypomastigotes in the peripheral blood, lymph node aspirates or CSF. If the organism is not easily demonstrated, concentration techniques should be utilized. IgM levels in the serum and CSF are markedly elevated.

TREATMENT

Therapy is usually effective if commenced before CNS symptoms develop.

Suramin, a polysulphated compound, is given intravenously; initially 0.1 g is given as a test dose to exclude an idiosyncratic reaction, followed by 1.0 g intravenously on the 1st, 3rd, 7th, 14th and 21st days. If proteinuria or haematuria develop, therapy should be discontinued. Pentamidine 3–4 $mg \cdot kg^{-1}$ intramuscularly on alternate days for 10 injections is an effective alternative. Rapid intravenous injection of pentamidine results in hypotension.

Although suramin and pentamidine have been found to be effective and should be used initially to control the fever, they do not cross the blood–brain barrier. It is currently believed that relapse or failure to respond to therapy will occur when CNS involvement occurs early in the disease. Hence drugs which penetrate the blood–brain barrier are being recommended as part of the initial treatment of trypanosomiasis. Melarsoprol, a trivalent arsenic, is used most widely for this purpose. Three to four consecutive injections of 2.0–3.6 mg·kg^{-1} body weight (up to a maximum of 250 mg per injection) are given intravenously. The course is usually repeated after an interval of 2 weeks. Major side-effects include an acute encephalitis-like condition and skin rashes.

A water-soluble analogue of melarsoprol, melarsonyl potassium, has also been found effective in Gambian but not in Rhodesian sleeping sickness.

Nitrofurazone 10 mg·kg^{-1} in divided doses three times daily for 10 days has also been found to be useful in cerebral trypanosomiasis. Peripheral neuritis and haemolytic anaemia may be troublesome side-effects in patients with glucose-6-phosphatase deficiency.

PREVENTION AND CONTROL

Elimination of the vector, the tsetse fly, by insecticides or by making environmental conditions unsuitable for its inhabitation would effectively eradicate trypanosomiasis. Both these approaches require formidable mobilization of manpower and money. Insect repellents should be used when visiting endemic areas.

A single intramuscular prophylactic injection of pentamidine 4 mg·kg^{-1} body weight (up to a maximum dose of 300 mg) gives effective protection against Gambian sleeping sickness, but is less effective against Rhodesian sleeping sickness.

African trypanosomiasis in children

In children the early manifestations and CNS symptoms overlap. Lymphadenopathy and neurological abnormalities may occur together. Seizures and choreiform movements are not uncommon. Treatment is as for the adult form.

American trypanosomiasis (Chagas' disease)

This is a zoonotic disease caused by *T. cruzi* which is transmitted by various reduviid insects. The principal vectors are *Triatoma infestans*, and *Rhodnius prolixus* (Latin America) and *Panstrongylus megistus* (Venezuela). Once infected, these insects remain infective for at least 2 years. Humans constitute the main reservoir, although domesticated and wild animals are also important reservoirs. Humans are infected when a bite is contaminated by the faeces of an infected insect or when infected faeces are rubbed into an abrasion or mucosal surface such as the conjunctiva. Less commonly the infection may spread via blood transfusions or transplacentally.

Chagas' disease is confined to South and Central America. Occasional cases have also been reported from southern Texas.

CLINICAL FEATURES

The incubation period varies from 1 to 3 weeks. Two clinically distinct presentations are recognized:

Acute Chagas' disease
Acute Chagas' disease predominantly affects children. An erythematous, indurated papule (chagoma) develops at the site of bite, and is associated with regional lymphadenopathy. This resolves spontaneously. If the portal of entry is the conjunctiva, unilateral periorbital and palpebral oedema (Romaña's sign), conjunctivitis and preauricular lymphadenopathy develop. Systemic findings such as fever, a transient morbilliform or urticarial rash, a peculiar gelatinous oedema of the face and trunk, tender lymphadenopathy and hepatosplenomegaly may be present. Death may occur in a small proportion of patients due to myocarditis or meningoencephalitis. More commonly the patient recovers completely in a few weeks.

Chronic Chagas' disease
Chronic Chagas' disease occurs in previously asymptomatic individuals. It is due to an autoimmune reaction mediated by cytotoxic T cells and antibodies against the endocardium, vascular tissue and striated muscle, together with myenteric plexus damage by amastigotes. The heart is invariably involved. The patient may complain of chest pain, dyspnoea or syncope. Cardiac abnormalities and arrhythmias are usual. Signs of right-sided cardiac failure may be present. Thromboembolic phenomena may occur.

With gastrointestinal involvement, megaoesophagus, leading to dysphagia and aspiration pneumonia, and megacolon, giving constipation and progressive abdominal distension, may occur. Dilatation of the biliary tree and of the bronchi have also been documented.

DIAGNOSIS

In acute Chagas' disease trypomastigotes may be demonstrated in peripheral blood. If parasites are not demonstrated in the blood, xenodiagnosis may be used: a parasite-free laboratory-reared vector feeds on a patient suspected to have the disease and 2–3 weeks later the intestinal contents of the vector are examined for parasites.

In chronic Chagas' disease complement fixation (Machado–Guerreiro reaction), indirect fluorescent antibody or haemagglutination tests may be used. Radiological assessment of gastrointestinal abnormalities is helpful.

TREATMENT

Nifurtimox, a nitrofurazone derivative, has been found to be useful in acute disease. The dose is 20 mg·kg^{-1} daily for children below the age of 2 and 8–10 mg·kg^{-1} daily for 3–4 months in older children and adults. Side-effects are few and include transient leucopenia, vomiting, sleeplessness and paraesthesiae. Benzimidazole is a useful alternative drug.

Over 80% of patients with the acute form of the disease and slightly more with the chronic form are cured of the infection.

PREVENTION AND CONTROL

No vaccine or chemoprophylactic agent is available. Prevention therefore involves the regular spraying of houses with benzene hexachloride in order to decrease the vector population.

TOXOPLASMOSIS

Toxoplasmosis is caused by *Toxoplasma gondii*, an obligate intracellular protozoa, which requires for completion of its life-cycle a definitive host, e.g. a cat, sheep or pig, and an intermediate host, e.g. a human. Infection of humans occurs either congenitally or by ingestion of foodstuffs contaminated by infected cat faeces or lamb or pork contaminated with *T. gondii* cysts. Toxoplasmosis is rare in the UK.

CLINICAL FEATURES

Five major clinical forms of toxoplasmosis are recognized:
1 *Asymptomatic lymphadenopathy*, the commonest mode of presentation
2 *Lymphadenopathy*, usually involving the cervical lymph nodes and associated with a febrile illness. This may clinically be indistinguishable from infectious mononucleosis but the Paul–Bunnell test is negative.
3 *Neurological abnormalities*, which include neck stiffness and headache, associated with sore throat and maculopapular rashes. The CSF is under pressure and the level of protein is elevated.
4 An *acute febrile illness*, with a maculopapular rash, hepatosplenomegaly and reactive lymphocytes in the peripheral blood. Uveitis, chorioretinitis, myocarditis and hepatitis may occur.

In the immunocompromised host, features present in the acute febrile and neurological forms are prominent.

5 *Congenital toxoplasmosis*, in which the symptoms and signs are indicative of CNS involvement. The characteristic 'syndrome of Savin', which comprises internal hydrocephalus, chorioretinitis, convulsions and cerebral calcification, may be seen. Tremors, nystagmus, micro-ophthalmia and pneumonitis are also present. The prognosis is usually poor, the survivors generally exhibiting mental retardation, epilepsy and spastic paraplegia.

DIAGNOSIS

Serological tests are the mainstay of diagnosis of acquired infection. The Sabin–Feldman dye test, a measure of IgG antibodies, has been widely used. Antibodies can also be detected by indirect fluorescence or indirect haemagglutination. Raised antibody levels are common in the general population and only a rising antibody titre is highly suggestive of toxoplasmosis. The IgM–immunofluorescent antibody (IgM–IFA) test is particularly useful for detecting acute infection since titres rise early and fall rapidly.

T. gondii can be isolated by injecting the peritoneum of mice with tissue extracts, e.g. bone marrow, body fluids or CSF when available, and examining the peritoneal fluid 6–10 days later for the organism.

TREATMENT

Most patients require no therapy as the disease is mild. Pyrimethamine (25–50 mg three times daily) and sulphadiazine (4–5 g daily) are used in combination for severe disease since they are synergistic. Therapy should be continued for at least 1 month. Since pyrimethamine is teratogenic, spiramycin is a useful alternative during pregnancy. Steroids are probably useful in ocular toxoplasmosis.

PREVENTION

Domestic cats that kill mice and birds are the chief source of infection and care should be taken in handling their faeces.

BABESIOSIS

This is a tick-borne disease, found chiefly in North America and Europe, and is occasionally transmitted to humans, especially those who are immunosuppressed. The causative organism is the plasmodium-like *Babesia microti*. The incubation period averages 10 days. In patients with normal splenic function, the symptoms are mild and usually comprise fever, nausea, myalgia, chills, vomiting and abdominal pain. Hepatosplenomegaly and mild to moderate haemolytic anaemia may also be present. In splenectomized individuals, systemic symptoms are more pronounced and haemolysis is associated with haemoglobinuria, jaundice and renal failure. Examination of a peripheral blood smear may reveal the characteristic plasmodium-like organisms.

TREATMENT

Treatment is mainly symptomatic. In severe cases pentamidine may be used but is effective only in reducing the numbers of but not eradicating the parasite. Chloroquine is reasonably effective.

MALARIA

Malaria affects more than 100 million people each year and has a mortality rate of 1%.

Endemic and epidemic malaria are found in all countries between the 40° south and 60° north lines of latitude (Fig. 1.19). Malaria is primarily a disease of hot, humid countries at altitudes less than 2200 metres above mean sea level, where conditions are ideal for prolific breeding of the mosquito vector, *Anopheles*. It is endemic in India, in parts of Africa and parts of South and Central America.

In humans, malaria is caused by four species of *Plasmodium*:

- *P. vivax* causes tertian malaria.
- *P. falciparum* causes malignant tertian malaria.
- *P. malariae* causes quartan malaria.
- *P. ovale* causes tertian malaria.

The four species are distinguishable from each other on examination of peripheral blood smears.

P. ovale has been reported predominantly from East and West Africa. *P. vivax* is the major species in temperate zones, whereas in the tropics all forms of malaria are seen. With present-day ease and speed of travel, sporadic cases of malaria are being increasingly recognized. Unfortunately, the initial impact of the WHO eradication programme lost its impetus in several countries in the early 1970s and malaria has once more become a major cause of morbidity and mortality in tropical and subtropical countries.

Humans, the intermediate hosts, are infected following the bite of an infected female *Anopheles* mosquito, the definitive host. The parasite can also be transmitted by blood transfusion, transplacentally, and, increasingly, between drug addicts who use improperly cleaned syringes.

The introduction of sporozoites, the infective form of the parasite, through the skin by the *Anopheles* mosquito heralds the commencement of the human cycle (Fig. 1.20). The following stages occur:

Pre-erythrocytic schizogony

During this phase clinical symptoms are absent and humans are not infective. Those sporozoites which are not removed by the body's defence mechanisms undergo development within the liver. A variable number of days later micromerozoites are liberated (primary attack). Other sporozoites (*P. vivax* and probably *P. ovale*) remain in a latent form in the liver as hypnozoites.

Erythrocytic schizogony

This is the phase when red blood cells (RBCs) become infected by the micromerozoites. In the RBCs they pass through several stages of development, namely trophozoites, schizonts and finally merozoites. These asexual parasitic forms are found in peripheral blood about 12 days after inoculation of the sporozoites in *P. vivax* infection and 9 days in *P. falciparum* infection. The different *Plasmodium* species differ in their ability to invade RBCs. *P. falciparum* is capable of invading all RBCs, especially young RBCs.

Fig. 1.19 The geographical distribution of malaria.

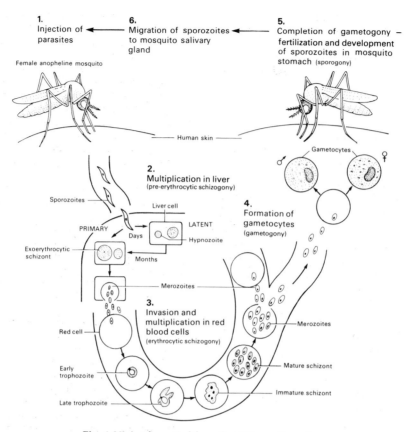

Fig. 1.20 A schematic life-cycle of *Plasmodium vivax*.

It therefore has the potential to produce the most severe form of malaria. *P. vivax* and *P. ovale* preferentially invade reticulocytes and young RBCs, whereas *P. malariae* invades senescent RBCs. Each cycle in the red cells terminates with rupture of the cell and release of merozoites into the circulation. This occurs every 48 h in *P. falciparum* infection, every 48–72 h in *P. vivax* and *P. ovale* infection, and approximately every 72 h in *P. malariae*.

Gametogony
The erythrocytic phase may continue for a considerable period of time before the stage of gametogony occurs. In this stage a few merozoites develop into the sexual form of the parasites known as gametocytes. Of these only the mature forms are found in peripheral blood. At this stage the patient is infective.

Exoerythrocytic schizogony
This fourth stage, which occurs in the liver, is found only with *P. vivax*, probably *P. ovale* and possibly *P. malariae* infections. It does not occur with *P. falciparum* infection and is believed to be responsible

for the relapses in *P. vivax* and *P. ovale* infections. The parasites in this phase are referred to as hypnozoites.

When an *Anopheles* mosquito ingests human blood containing gametocytes it marks the commencement of the sexual cycle in the mosquito. The external incubation period varies from 7 to 20 days.

IMMUNITY

This may be natural or acquired. Natural immunity is present in individuals of West African extraction, who are blood group Duffy-negative (FyFy) and therefore lack the specific receptor on the RBC surface to which the merozoites attach. They cannot develop *P. vivax* malaria. The presence of haemoglobin S, glucose-6-phosphatase deficiency, thalassaemia and pyridoxal kinase deficiency also offer resistance against *P. falciparum*. The presence of abnormal haemoglobins or altered red cell metabolism retards *P. falciparum* maturation and reduces the severity of the disease.

The spleen plays an important role in natural immunity since splenectomized individuals are highly susceptible to the malarial parasite.

Infants are protected by the transfer of maternal IgG antibodies across the placenta.

Partial immunity may be acquired following an attack of malaria, and is attributed to macrophage stimulation by T cells.

CLINICAL FEATURES

The incubation period varies:
- 10 to 14 days in *P. vivax*, *P. ovale* and *P. falciparum*
- 18 days to 6 weeks in *P. malariae* infection

Although individual variations in clinical presentation are noted, febrile paroxysms, anaemia, splenomegaly and hepatomegaly are usually present. Malarial febrile paroxysms typically have three stages:
1 The *'cold stage'* is characterized by marked vasoconstriction and lasts from 30 minutes to 1 h. The patient feels intensely cold and uncomfortable. There is marked shivering. The temperature rises rapidly, often to as high as 41°C.
2 The *'hot stage'* abruptly follows and lasts for 2–6 h. The patient feels intensely hot and uncomfortable. Delirium may be present.
3 The *'sweating stage'* then occurs, during which the bedclothes are drenched. The patient feels fatigued and exhausted but otherwise well and often sleeps. The fever is due to schizont rupture and the release of pyrogens.

Herpes labialis frequently occurs in established malaria. Anaemia is usually present and is largely a result of haemolysis.

Tertian malaria
Tertian malaria is caused by *P. vivax* and *P. ovale* and is so called because the fever recurs every third day. These species of *Plasmodium* give rise to a clinically mild infection. The presence of an exoerythrocytic stage is responsible for relapses and makes eradication of the organisms difficult.

Quartan malaria
Quartan malaria is caused by *P. malariae* and results in fever every fourth day. It is usually a mild disease, but tends to run a more chronic course. The nephrotic syndrome can complicate this type of malaria and may be fatal between the ages of 4 and 5 years. Because of its chronicity the patient develops a sallow complexion, marked muscle wasting, mild icterus and massive splenomegaly. Growth retardation may occur in children.

Falciparum malaria
Falciparum malaria (pernicious malaria) due to *P. falciparum* is potentially the most severe form of malaria, with high levels of parasitaemia. Infected RBCs develop peculiar knob-like surface projections which facilitate adhesion of these RBCs to the endothelium of blood vessels. The consequent vascular occlusion causes severe organ damage, chiefly in the kidneys, liver, brain and gastrointestinal tract. The prodrome tends to be severe. The fever follows no particular pattern. Splenomegaly tends to occur late and the characteristic cold, hot and sweating stages are not prominent. The following clinical forms of falciparum malaria are recognized and are likely to occur when more than 5% of RBCs are parasitized:
- *Cerebral malaria* is characterized by a marked elevation in body temperature, a rapid deterioration in consciousness, convulsions, coma and death.
- *Algid malaria* is characterized by the presence of severe vomiting, diarrhoea and peripheral circulatory collapse.
- *Septicaemic malaria* results in a high, continuous fever, vomiting and signs and symptoms mimicking typhoid fever. Pulmonary circulatory insufficiency may be present, with cough, haemoptysis and features of shock lung. The hepatorenal syndrome and spontaneous splenic rupture may also occur.
- *Blackwater fever*, so called because of the production of dark brown-black urine due to intravascular haemolysis, is seen only in falciparum malaria. It can be precipitated by very small amounts of quinine in quinine-sensitive cases. This is a rapidly progressive illness characterized by the abrupt onset of fever, marked haemolysis, haemoglobinuria, hyperbilirubinaemia, vomiting, circulatory collapse and acute renal failure. Malarial parasites cannot usually be detected in peripheral blood smears after the onset of intravascular haemolysis.

Tropical splenomegaly syndrome
Tropical splenomegaly syndrome is seen in areas where malaria is hyperendemic. It is uncommon before 10 years of age. Characteristic features are massive splenomegaly, marked elevation in serum IgM levels, and IgM aggregates (detected by immunofluorescence) in Kupffer's cells in the liver. The splenomegaly responds to antimalarial therapy. However, malarial parasites are not detected in the spleen or peripheral blood smears.

PREVALENCE

Several indices are used to measure the prevalence of malaria:
- The *spleen rate*, defined as the percentage of children between 2 and 10 years of age with splenomegaly, is used as a measure of the endemicity of malaria in a community.
- The *infant parasite rate*, defined as the percentage of infants below 1 year of age in whom malarial parasites are demonstrable in peripheral blood smears, is regarded as the most sensitive index of transmission of malaria to a locality.

INCIDENCE

The *annual parasite index* is a sensitive indication of the incidence of malaria in a community. It is calculated thus:

$$\frac{\text{Number of confirmed cases during 1 year}}{\text{Population under surveillance}} \times 1000$$

DIAGNOSIS

The parasite can be demonstrated in either thin or thick peripheral blood smears stained with Giemsa, Wright or Leishman stains. Two to three blood smears taken each day for three or four days and found to be negative are necessary before a patient is declared malaria-free.

Serological methods are not widely used but include indirect immunofluorescence, indirect haemagglutination and gel diffusion techniques.

Enzyme-linked immunosorbent assays (ELISA) are currently being evaluated for use in detecting malarial antigens.

TREATMENT

General

Analgesics and antipyretics such as aspirin and paracetamol are given as necessary. Intravenous fluids may be required to combat dehydration and shock.

Treatment of an acute attack:

The 4-aminoquinolines are the drugs of choice. Chloroquine-sensitive malaria is treated with chloroquine 600 mg of the base followed by 300 mg in 6 hours and then 150 mg twice daily for 3 days, or amodiaquine hydrochloride 600 mg of the base followed by 400–600 mg daily for 2 days up to a total maximum dose of 2400 mg.

Chloroquine-resistant malaria is treated with quinine sulphate 650 mg three times daily for 5 days given in combination with pyrimethamine 25 mg twice daily for 3 days and sulphadiazine 500 mg twice daily for 5 days. Alternatively, quinine sulphate may be followed by a single dose of sulfadoxine 1.5 g combined with pyrimethamine 75 mg (available as Fansidar).

If the patient is intolerant to oral therapy, for example due to vomiting, intravenous or intramuscular therapy can be given initially.

Drug side-effects. These drugs are potentially toxic. With quinine, tinnitus, haemolytic anaemia and drug fever may occur. Chloroquine may cause vomiting, abdominal pain, agranulocytosis or convulsions.

Eradication

P. falciparum. Chloroquine alone or in combination with either pyrimethamine 25 mg or primaquine 45 mg as a single dose effects a radical cure because there is no exoerythrocytic stage in falciparum malaria.

P. vivax, P. malariae and P. ovale. Primaquine, an 8-aminoquinoline, is essential for eliminating the exoerythrocytic cycle and effecting a radical cure. A course of one of the 4-aminoquinolines should be followed by primaquine 7.5 mg daily for 14 days. Alternatively 300 mg chloroquine combined with 45 mg primaquine once a week for 8 weeks is also effective.

Treatment of severe malaria (more than 1% of RBCs infected) or any of the pernicious forms of falciparum malaria constitutes a medical emergency. Therapy is initially with intravenous chloroquine 5 mg·kg^{-1} or quinine hydrochloride 10 mg·kg^{-1} with the dose being repeated every 8 h until oral therapy can be tolerated.

PREVENTION AND CONTROL (see Table 1.7)

Owing to changing patterns of resistance, advice about chemoprophylaxis should be sought prior to leaving for a malaria-endemic area. Chemoprophylaxis is essential for those visiting endemic areas; generally chloroquine 400–500 mg once a week or proguanil 100–200 mg daily is used. Prophylaxis should be continued for 6 weeks after leaving a high-risk area. If chloroquine resistance is suspected, prophylaxis should be pyrimethamine 12.5 mg with dapsone 100 mg once a week or pyrimethamine 25 mg with sulfadoxine 500 mg once a week, and should be continued for 6 weeks after leaving the endemic area.

Based on the 1979 WHO Expert Committee report on malaria, the following preventive measures have been suggested. Measures to be applied to the community include prevention of man–vector contact, destruction of adult mosquitoes and mosquito larvae, and active elimination of human infection by presumptive (i.e. treatment of all fevers in endemic areas with antimalarials) and radical treatment. Measures to be applied to individuals include use of mosquito repellents, chemoprophylaxis and chemotherapy where indicated.

PNEUMOCYSTIS CARINII INFECTION

Pneumocystis carinii is an important cause of interstitial pneumonia in the immunocompromised host. The taxonomy of *P. carinii* remains controversial: some authorities regard it as a protozoan whilst others prefer to leave it unclassified. The organism exists as a trophozoite, which is probably motile and reproduces by binary fission. After the trophozoite invades the lung parenchyma, its wall thickens and forms a cyst. On maturation, further division takes place to yield eight merozoites which, after cyst wall rupture, develop into trophozoites.

CLINICAL FEATURES

Infection is probably common in infancy but most infections in otherwise healthy infants remain undetected. Outbreaks in infant nurseries have been reported but are now less common. Infection in adults is associated with a major defect in cell-mediated immune mechanisms. Thus infection with *P. carinii* is one of the most common opportunistic infections in AIDS and an important cause of death in these patients. The illness presents as a severe pneumonia with progressive respiratory distress, a non-productive cough, tachypnoea, hypoxia and fever. Physical signs in the chest are minimal and may be absent. Chest radiographs generally show bilateral diffuse granular opacities spreading from the hilar region and initially sparing the periphery. These radiographic changes may develop late; they may be absent for 1 or 2 days even in a patient with severe dyspnoea.

DIAGNOSIS

Demonstration of the organism in lung tissue is essential to make a confident diagnosis of *Pneumocystis* infection. The organism cannot easily be isolated from sputum or aspirated pulmonary secretions. The currently favoured way to detect the organism is in lung tissue obtained by transbronchial biopsy during fibreoptic bronchoscopy or open lung biopsy. Needle aspiration of lung parenchyma has been used in the past but has a high complication rate (pneumothorax or haemorrhage) and is no longer in general use.

TREATMENT

High-dose co-trimoxazole (640 mg trimethoprim, 3.2 g sulphamethoxazole) 12-hourly, usually intravenously initially, is given for 2–4 weeks. There is some evidence that prophylactic co-trimoxazole is useful in protecting high-risk patients from *P. carinii* infection. Other drugs used to treat this infection include pentamidine, and a combination of pyrimethamine and sulfadoxine appears to be an effective prophylactic preparation.

Intestinal and genital infections

Amoebiasis

The most important human disease due to amoebae is amoebiasis, which is caused by *Entamoeba histolytica*. This intestinal pathogen can be differentiated from other enteric amoebae such as *Entamoeba hartmani*, *Entamoeba coli* and *Endolimax nana*, since *E. histolytica* is the only amoeba found in the intestine which phagocytoses red blood cells. It occurs worldwide, although much higher incidence rates are found in the tropics and subtropics. It can be found in active male homosexuals who carry the pathogen (usually strains of low virulence) and between whom it is spread by sexual contact.

LIFE-CYCLE AND PATHOGENESIS

The organism exists both as a motile trophozoite and as a cyst which can survive outside the body. Cysts are transmitted chiefly by ingestion of contaminated food or water or spread directly by person-to-person contact. Trophozoites emerge from the cyst in the small intestine and then pass on to the colon where they multiply (Fig. 1.21). Many individuals can carry the pathogen without obvious evidence of clinical disease (asymptomatic cyst passers). However, under certain conditions, *E. histolytica* trophozoites invade the colonic epithelium, probably with the aid of their own cytotoxins and proteolytic enzymes. The parasites continue to multiply and finally frank ulceration of the mucosa occurs. If penetration continues trophozoites may enter the portal vein, via which they reach the liver and cause hepatitis and intrahepatic abscesses. This invasive form of the disease is particularly serious and unless treated promptly is often fatal.

CLINICAL FEATURES

The incubation period is highly variable and may be as short as a few days or as long as several months or even a year. The presentation of amoebic colitis may be:

- Gradual onset with mild intermittent diarrhoea and abdominal discomfort, usually progressing to bloody diarrhoea with mucus. Systemic manifestations such as headache, nausea and anorexia are often present.

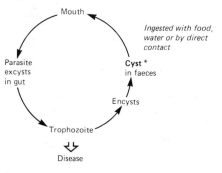

* Infective form for humans

Fig. 1.21 A schematic life-cycle of intestinal protozoa.

- Severe acute (amoebic) dysentery, closely resembling that due to *Shigella* (bacillary dysentery)
- A fulminating colitis

Typically, patients with amoebic colitis appear less unwell than those with bacillary dysentery, fever is low grade or absent, and dehydration is unusual.

COMPLICATIONS

Complications are unusual, but include:
- Progression of fulminant colitis to toxic dilatation of the colon with perforation and peritonitis
- Chronic infection leading to stricture formation
- Severe haemorrhage
- Development of a mass of fibrotic granulation tissue (amoeboma), most commonly in the caecum or rectosigmoid region. Amoebomas occur in 10% of patients and may bleed, cause obstruction, intussuscept and are sometimes mistaken for a carcinoma.
- Amoebic liver abscess, which often develops in the absence of a recent episode of colitis. Tender hepatomegaly, a high swinging fever and profound malaise are characteristic, although early in the course of the disease both symptoms and signs may be minimal. The clinical features are described in more detail on p. 244.

DIAGNOSIS

Serodiagnosis
The amoebic fluorescent antibody titre (FAT) is positive in at least 90% of patients with liver abscess or active colitis. Seropositivity is low in asymptomatic cyst passers.

Colonic disease
Direct examination of colonic exudate obtained at sigmoidoscopy or of freshly passed stool as a saline-wet mount is the most rapid and least expensive way of confirming amoebic infection. *E. histolytica* trophozoites must be distinguished from non-pathogenic amoebae and from polymorphonuclear leucocytes, with which they are sometimes confused. Cysts may also be present in the stool. Sigmoidoscopy and barium enema examination may show colonic ulceration but are rarely diagnostic.

Liver disease
Liver abscess should be suspected if the serum alkaline phosphatase is elevated, even when clinical signs are absent. Hepatic ultrasound scan should confirm the presence of an abscess, which may be either single or multiple. Pus from an amoebic abscess has a classic 'anchovy sauce' appearance and may contain trophozoites.

TREATMENT

Metronidazole 800 mg three times daily for 5 days is given in amoebic colitis and a more prolonged course for 10–14 days in liver abscess or other extraintestinal spread.

Alternative drugs include the newer nitroimidazole derivative, tinidazole or dehydroemetine. Diloxanide furoate is a luminal amoebicide and may be a helpful adjunct in clearing cysts.

Large, tense abscesses in the liver may require percutaneous drainage, using an ultrasound scan to accurately localize the abscess and to position the drainage needle.

CONTROL AND PREVENTION

This disease will be difficult to eradicate because of the substantial human reservoir of asymptomatic cases. There is no immediate hope of vaccine development, particularly as the same individual may experience several episodes of amoebic infection, indicating that only partial protective immunity develops after exposure to the pathogen. Improved standards of personal hygiene and water quality are important. Cysts are destroyed by boiling water for at least 10 minutes, but the effects of chlorination are variable.

Balantidiasis

Balantidium coli is the only ciliate which produces clinically significant infection in humans. It is found throughout the tropics, particularly in Central and South America, Iran, New Guinea and the Philippines. It is usually carried by pigs and infection is most common in those communities which live in close association with swine. Its life-cycle is identical to that of *Entamoeba histolytica*.

B. coli produces a dysenteric illness due to invasion of the distal ileal and colonic mucosa. The colitis may be acute and fulminant and if untreated may be fatal. Trophozoites rather than cysts are found in the stool. Treatment is with tetracycline, ampicillin or metronidazole.

Giardiasis

Giardia lamblia is a flagellate which is found worldwide. It causes small intestinal disease, with diarrhoea and malabsorption. Prevalence is high throughout the tropics. It is an important cause of traveller's diarrhoea, in certain parts of Europe, the USSR, and in some rural and mountainous areas of North America where large waterborne epidemics have been reported. Person-to-person spread is common in day nurseries, residential institutions and between male homosexuals. Like *Entamoeba histolytica*, the organism exists both as a trophozoite and a cyst, the latter being the form in which the protozoa is transmitted.

The organism colonizes and multiplies within the small intestine and may remain there without causing detriment to the host. Severe malabsorption may occur and is thought to be related to morphological damage to the small intestine; changes in villus architecture vary from mild partial villus atrophy to subtotal villus atrophy. Bacterial overgrowth has also been found in association with giardiasis and may contribute to fat malabsorption.

CLINICAL FEATURES

Many individuals excreting *Giardia* cysts have no symptoms and are therefore carriers. Others develop symptoms within 1 or 2 weeks of ingesting cysts. These include diarrhoea, often watery in the early stage of the illness, nausea, anorexia, abdominal discomfort and distension. Stools may then become paler, with the characteristic features of steatorrhoea. If the illness is prolonged, weight loss ensues which, even in previously healthy adults, can be marked.

DIAGNOSIS

Both cysts and trophozoites can be found in the stool, but negative stool examination does not exclude the diagnosis since the parasite may be excreted at irregular intervals. The parasite can also be seen in duodenal aspirates and in histological sections of jejunal mucosa. Raised IgG and, in acute infections, IgM antibodies are found.

TREATMENT

Metronidazole 2 g as a single dose on three successive days will cure the majority of infections, although sometimes a second or third course is necessary. *Giardia* is also sensitive to mepacrine. Preventive measures are similar to those outlined for *Entamoeba histolytica*.

Cryptosporidium

Cryptosporidium is a member of the sporozoa and has been known to be an animal pathogen for many years. The first human case was described in 1976 in an immunocompromised individual, but it is now known to also affect otherwise healthy subjects. The organism is found world-wide. It produces a devastating diarrhoeal illness in patients with immunodeficiency, particularly those with AIDS.

The parasite is able to reproduce both sexually and asexually and has a life-cycle in the intestine very similar to that of *Plasmodium*. The disease is spread by oocysts excreted in the faeces.

CLINICAL FEATURES

In healthy individuals cryptosporidiosis is a self-limiting illness lasting for 7–10 days. Acute watery diarrhoea is associated with fever and general malaise, but otherwise the disease follows a benign course. In the immunocompromised patient diarrhoea is followed by severe weight loss and general debility, contributing significantly to the downhill course of AIDS. As yet there is no effective treatment for this infection, although encouraging results have been reported with spiramycin.

Trichomoniasis

Trichomonas vaginalis is a flagellate which causes vaginitis and urethritis. The resulting vaginal discharge is profuse, greenish and malodorous and associated with vulval irritation. The organism also colonizes the male urethra where it may produce little or no effect or may alternatively cause frank urethritis. Infection is transmitted sexually. Motile trichomonads can be readily seen in wet preparations of urethral or vaginal discharge. Infection responds to metronidazole (2 g as a single oral dose) and it is advisable to also treat the patient's sexual partner.

Helminthic infections

Nematode (roundworm) infections

FILARIASIS

Several nematodes belonging to the superfamily Filarioidea are responsible for filariasis (Table 1.37). The adult worms are thread-like. Females are larger than males. The viviparous females give birth to larvae known as microfilariae. The microfilariae of various species can be easily differentiated from each other by the presence or absence of a sheath and the pattern of nuclear distribution in the tail. These nematodes require two hosts to complete their life-cycle.

Bancroftian and Malayan filariasis

Wuchereria bancrofti is found mainly in the tropics and subtropics, in northern Australia, Pacific islands, West and Central Africa, South America and India. *Brugia malayi* infection is less widespread than Bancroftian filariasis and is found in India, southern China, Malaysia, Indonesia and Borneo (Fig. 1.22).

Table 1.37 Habitat, vectors and major clinical manifestations of some nematodes of the superfamily Filarioidea.

Organism	Habitat of adult worms in humans	Vector	Clinical manifestations
Wuchereria bancrofti	Lymphatics, lymph nodes	*Culex, Aedes, Anopheles*	Fever, lymphangitis, elephantiasis of limbs, breasts and scrotum
Brugia malayi	Lymphatics	*Mansonia*	Fever, lymphangitis, elephantiasis (scrotal involvement is uncommon)
Loa loa	Subcutaneous tissue, subconjunctiva	*Chrysops*	'Calabar swellings', urticaria
Onchocerca volvulus	Subcutaneous tissue	*Simulium*	Subcutaneous nodules, elephantiasis, ocular lesions
Dipetalonema	Body cavities	*Culicoides*	Occasionally dermatitis

Humans are the definitive hosts and mosquitoes of various types are the intermediate hosts. Humans are the only known reservoirs of Bancroftian filariasis, whereas, in addition to humans, animals such as cats are reservoirs of Malayan filariasis. *Culex fatigans* is the main vector of Bancroftian filariasis. *Aedes* and *Anopheles* species have also been implicated. The major vector for Malayan filariasis is *Mansonia annulifera*.

Following the bite of an infected mosquito, the larvae penetrate the skin, enter the lymphatics and are carried to the regional lymph nodes. Here they grow and mature for up to 18 months. After fertilization the microfilariae produced are carried from the lymphatics into the blood; they do not produce any symptoms or signs. Adult worms produce lymphangitis, which is believed to be a hypersensitivity reaction. The lymphangitis is followed by fibrosis, a granulomatous reaction and later irreversible lymphatic blockade. Secondary bacterial infection may add considerably to the inflammatory response and resultant fibrosis.

CLINICAL FEATURES

Following an incubation period which averages 10–12 months, the patient presents with fever ranging from 39–41°C accompanied by lymphangitis, both of which usually subside in 3–5 days. Lymphangitis typically involves the lymphatics of the lower or upper limbs or of the abdomen. Involvement of the lymphatics of the epididymis, testis and spermatic cord occurs almost exclusively in Bancroftian filariasis. The involved superficial lymphatics appear as red streaks on the skin, and are tender and cord-like. The inflammation may subside either with treatment or spontaneously but there is a tendency for recurrences to occur. The inflammatory phase is usually followed by the obstructive phase, which is characterized by features of lymphatic blockade.

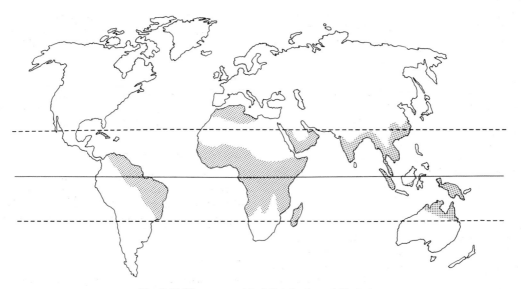

Fig. 1.22 The geographical distribution of filariasis.

Many sites may be affected but lower limb and scrotal oedema occur frequently. Long-standing obstruction produces thick, rough skin, which occasionally ulcerates. Less frequently chyluria, chylous ascites and pleural effusions occur. The obstructive phase may be punctuated by episodes of acute lymphangitis.

DIAGNOSIS

The clinical presentation is characteristic. Eosinophilia and the presence of microfilariae in thin or thick peripheral blood smears is diagnostic. Since *W. bancrofti* and *B. malayi* are released into the peripheral circulation at night, blood for examination should be taken between 9 p.m. and 1 a.m. If, despite repeated examination, microfilariae cannot be demonstrated in thick or thin blood smears, diethylcarbamazine 100 mg given as a single dose followed by blood removal 30 minutes later for examination may give a positive yield. Various parasite concentration techniques such as Knott's concentration or membrane filtration techniques have resulted in a higher positive yield. Serological tests are not specific.

TREATMENT

Diethylcarbamazine (DEC) 2–6 mg·kg^{-1} daily in three divided doses for 2–3 weeks is recommended. A second course after 6 weeks increases the cure rate. The WHO Expert Committee has recommended that a total of 72 mg·kg^{-1} be given for eradication of Bancroftian filariasis and 30–40 mg·kg^{-1} for Malayan filariasis. DEC is filaricidal. Following initiation of therapy, marked allergic reactions can occur and require concomitant administration of antihistamines or steroids.

Associated bacterial infections should be appropriately treated. Reconstructive surgery plays an important role in removing unsightly tissue.

PREVENTION AND CONTROL

Mass chemotherapy with DEC has been effective in decreasing the *microfilariae rate* (the percentage of individuals who have microfilariae in a unit volume of their blood in a given population) and the *microfilariae density* (the number of microfilariae per unit volume of blood in individual patients). Primary prophylaxis should be aimed at vector control and protection of humans from mosquitoes.

Tropical eosinophilia

Tropical eosinophilia has been attributed to microfilariae such as *Dirofilaria* and more recently to *W. bancrofti* and *B. malayi*. Two forms are recognized, one characterized by lymphadenopathy and splenomegaly, and the other by cough,

bronchospasm and an asthma-like picture (see p. 609).

Loiasis

Loiasis is caused by *Loa loa*. As in Bancroftian and Malayan filariasis, the microfilariae of *L. loa* do not produce any symptoms. Unlike in Bancroftian filariasis, the microfilariae are found in the peripheral circulation mainly during the day. The disease is confined to the hot, humid, swampy areas of West and Central Africa, in which environment the deerfly vectors *Chrysops silacea* and *Chrysops dimidiata* thrive. Following the bite of a female *Chrysops*, the microfilariae are introduced into the skin of the human host and tend to migrate in the subcutaneous tissues. They have a predilection for subconjunctival and periorbital tissues.

CLINICAL FEATURES

The main feature of loiasis is *Calabar swellings*, which are painless, localized, transient, hot, soft tissue swellings, often near joints. They persist for periods varying from a few hours to several weeks. They occur more commonly during the hotter months and may be preceded by numbness and tingling. They are produced by toxin released from the adult worm.

Urticaria, pruritus, lymphoedema, arthritis and chorioretinitis may occur.

A picture resembling meningoencephalitis, which occurs only during treatment, is thought to be an allergic reaction.

DIAGNOSIS

The worm can be seen in subcutaneous tissues or crossing the conjunctivae.

The characteristic microfilariae may be demonstrable in peripheral blood smears. Serological tests such as the complement fixation test are also useful.

TREATMENT

Diethylcarbamazine (DEC) 2–6 mg·kg^{-1} is effective against both adult worms and microfilariae. Treatment should be continued for 2–3 weeks.

PREVENTION AND CONTROL

Prevention is best effected by adequate personal protection. In addition, houses should be sprayed with dieldrin. Mass treatment of all the inhabitants of villages with DEC 2 mg·kg^{-1} daily for 3 days has reduced the incidence of this disease.

Onchocerciasis

Onchocerciasis is produced by the unsheathed, filarial worm, *Onchocerca volvulus*. The gravid female has a life-expectancy of 15 years. The microfilariae are found in the skin and subcutaneous tissue. Man is the only known definitive host and the day-biting female black fly of genus *Simulium* is the vector; the species involved are *S. damnosum* and *S. naevi* in Africa and *S. metallicum* in Venezuela. The disease is confined to west, central and east Africa, Central and South America, and southern parts of Saudi Arabia.

CLINICAL FEATURES

The incubation period averages 1 year. Initially a papular, reddish, itchy rash develops. With repeated infections, characteristic subcutaneous nodules of various sizes appear. Usually they number less than 10 and are unevenly distributed over the body. In chronic disease, lichenification, xeroderma, pseudoichthyosis and atrophy of the skin occur. The nodules may be associated with the development of genital elephantiasis, hydrocele and the so-called 'hanging groin', in which large folds of wrinkled and thickened skin develop in the groin.

Ocular lesions represent the most serious manifestation of this disease and are the cause of up to 15% of the blindness in some areas. Initially the patient complains of lacrimation, photophobia and a foreign body sensation in the eye. Conjunctivitis, iridocyclitis, chorioretinitis, secondary glaucoma and optic atrophy may occur. The eye lesions have been attributed to toxin production by the microfilariae and adult worms, mechanical irritation and hypersensitivity.

DIAGNOSIS

This is established by demonstrating microfilariae in snips of bloodless tissue obtained from the nodules and kept in saline for 30 minutes to 1 h before microscopic examination. The organism may also be identified in the anterior chamber of the eye by slit-lamp examination. Mazzotti's test is suggestive of the diagnosis and is positive if pruritus and a rash develop within a few hours of taking 50–100 mg of diethylcarbamazine (DEC) orally. Serological tests are not helpful in the indigenous population as the positivity rate is high. Eosinophilia occurs.

TREATMENT

In endemic areas not all people require treatment. The major indications for treatment are:
● The threat of eye damage
● Severe pruritus

DEC is the drug of choice. It is effective against the microfilarial form but not the adult worms. In order to prevent a marked hypersensitivity reaction, the initial dose is small; 50 mg is given on the first day, and then the dose is gradually increased over a period of 1 week to 12 mg·kg^{-1} daily for a further 3 weeks. Exacerbation of symptoms while on therapy is effectively controlled by antihistamines or steroids. Mebendazole may be useful but its efficacy has not been established with certainty. Suramin is effective against the adult form but should be used with care because of its toxicity; the dose is 0.1 g intravenously initially to test for hypersensitivity followed by 1.0 g intravenously once a week up to a maximum of 5 g.

PREVENTION AND CONTROL

Prevention and control is confined to personal protection and attempts at destroying the vector. Chemoprophylaxis has not been found to be practical or effective.

Dipetalonemiasis

Dipetalonema perstans and *D. streptocerca* can infect man. Their major importance lies in the fact that they may be confused with other more common microfilariae. They are transmitted by blood-sucking gnats of the genus *Culicoides*. In humans, *D. perstans* is considered to be non-pathogenic and inhabits mesenteric tissue, pleural and pericardial cavities. Occasionally it gives rise to fever, itchy erysipelas-like lesions and abdominal pain. As with other microfilariae, peripheral eosinophilia is common. *D. streptocerca* inhabits dermal collagen tissue and causes a papular, itchy rash which is occasionally hyperpigmented. Normally, no treatment is required. Diethylcarbamazine is effective against both species.

Mansonelliasis

Mansonella ozzardi is confined to tropical Central America and the Caribbean. In general, mansonelliasis is totally asymptomatic, although fever, lymphadenopathy and hydrocele may occur.

Dirofilariasis

Dirofilariasis is caused by *Dirofilaria immitis* and is transmitted to man by mosquitoes. Typically patients are asymptomatic; small round lesions (coin lesions) on pulmonary radiographs, haemoptysis and fever may rarely occur.

DRACUNCULIASIS

Dracunculiasis (guinea worm infection) results from infection with *Dracunculus medinensis*. It is found sporadically throughout the tropics but is common in certain parts of India, central, east and west Africa, Pakistan, the Middle East, parts of South America and the eastern regions of the USSR.

Humans are the definitive host and are infected by ingestion of water containing infected *Cyclops*. The larvae are liberated in the human stomach by the action of acid. These penetrate the intestinal wall, where the male dies after fertilizing the female. The gravid female then wanders in connective tissue for several months before emerging through the skin. On reaching the skin, it elicits an allergic reaction with blister formation and later protrusion of the worm associated with the discharge of motile larvae. The larvae are then taken up by *Cyclops*, which once again are infective to man.

CLINICAL FEATURES

A generalized reaction can occur which is associated with nausea, vomiting, generalized urticaria and diarrhoea. These symptoms abate with rupture of the blister. Secondary bacterial infection, especially with streptococci, is common and results in cellulitis and abscess formation. In Nigeria, tetanus is a frequent complication. If attempts at extraction of the worm result in damage to it, intense cellulitis may occur. Arthritis, synovitis, ankylosis of joints and epididymitis are rare sequelae.

DIAGNOSIS

Keeping the appropriate part of the body immersed in water may induce the worm to wriggle out. Fluorescent antibody tests may be useful. Radiography may reveal the presence of the worm.

TREATMENT

Gradual physical extraction of the worm by winding it carefully around a stick is the treatment of choice. It may take several days before the entire worm is extruded. Niridazole 25 mg·kg^{-1} body weight daily in three divided doses for 7–10 days has been found useful. Thiabendazole 25 mg·kg^{-1} body weight twice daily for 2 days is also effective in the relief of symptoms.

PREVENTION AND CONTROL

Prevention of this parasitosis is easily effected by chemically treating infected sources of water.

ANIMAL NEMATODES

Toxocariasis

Toxocariasis (visceral larva migrans) occurs worldwide and is caused by *Toxocara canis* or *T. cati*. The adult worm is found in the intestine of dogs and cats. The infective ova are passed in animal faeces and may be accidentally ingested by humans. The liberated larvae penetrate the intestinal wall and reach the liver and lung via the circulation. Epidemiologically, puppies are the most important natural hosts and the infection is most commonly seen in children between 1 and 4 years of age. Several viscera may be involved and the clinical manifestations are dependent on the organ involved and the intensity of infection. Eosinophilia is common. Urticaria and dermatitis may occur. With pulmonary involvement the presentation is that of bronchial asthma. Chest radiographs may reveal transient pulmonary infiltrates. Splenomegaly and hepatomegaly may occur. Rarely involvement of the myocardium and central nervous system may result in death. Eye involvement produces a retinoblastoma-like picture.

DIAGNOSIS

The presence of marked eosinophilia, hepatomegaly, and elevated IgG, IgM and IgE is suggestive, as is the identification of foreign body eosinophilic granulomas in histological sections. Recently detection of antibodies by enzyme-linked immunoassay has been found to be useful.

TREATMENT

Treatment is difficult to evaluate in view of the mild nature of the illness and the tendency for spontaneous cure. Diethylcarbamazine 2–6 mg·kg^{-1} daily in divided doses for 3 weeks or thiabendazole 25 mg·kg^{-1} twice daily for 5 days is probably effective.

Cutaneous larva migrans

Cutaneous larva migrans (creeping eruption) is a disease of the hot, humid areas of tropical and subtropical countries. It is caused by the dog and cat hookworms *Ancylostoma braziliense* and *A. caninum* and, occasionally, the human parasites *A. duodenale*, *Necator americanus* and *Strongyloides stercoralis*, the adult forms of which are found in the intestine of the host (see p. 87). The filariform larva emerges from the ova passed in the faeces and penetrates intact human skin. An itchy papule develops at the site of larval entry. Two to three days later a markedly itchy, erythematous, serpiginous skin lesion develops. This is due to the larva which slowly migrates at 1–2 mm per day. The skin over the lesion may vesiculate. Healing occurs by crusting. Although the lesions are more frequent on the lower limbs, any part of the body may be affected. Secondary bacterial infection may result in a mistaken diagnosis of pyoderma. The only systemic manifestations are transient pulmonary infiltrates and occasional breathlessness. Peripheral eosinophilia is seen.

TREATMENT

Thiabendazole applied locally as a 10% solution or given systemically (25 mg·kg^{-1} for 5 days) is effective.

Anisakiasis

Anisakiasis (herring worm disease) is caused by the larval stage of several species of *Anisakis*, and possibly of the related nematode *Phocanema*, which are found in abundance in herring, and dolphins, whales and other large sea mammals. The disease is prevalent in Japan and northern Europe where eating raw herring and other raw fish is considered a delicacy. In Japan the illness is characterized by an acute gastric syndrome which presents as epigastric pain, nausea and vomiting. Upper gastrointestinal endoscopy may reveal the presence of larvae in the gastric mucosa. In contrast, in Europe the small intestine is predominantly involved and the patient presents with colicky, generalized abdominal pain and fever. Eosinophilia is unusual.

Angiostrongyliasis

Angiostrongyliasis is a disease endemic to south-east Asia and the Pacific and is caused by the rat lungworm *Angiostrongylus cantonensis*, which gives rise to eosinophilic meningitis. Transmission to humans is by ingestion of infected crustaceans and molluscs. It is a self-limiting disease presenting with features of meningitis, and has a low mortality. Cranial nerve palsies may be present. Examination of the CSF reveals a leucocytosis characterized by the presence of a large number of eosinophils, usually more than 50 per mm^3.

A. costaricensis, a parasite of the cotton rat, causes an eosinophilic gastroenteritis, presenting with features suggestive of appendicitis. Intestinal obstruction and perforation may occur. The usefulness of thiabendazole needs to be evaluated.

Gnathostomiasis

Humans, the incidental hosts, are infected by ingesting meats, especially fish, contaminated by the third larval stage of *Gnathostoma spinigerum*. Abdominal pain, eosinophilic meningitis or radiculitis may occur. In the subcutaneous tissues the larvae elicit a marked inflammatory response associated with pruritus. Treatment is surgical removal of the worm. Prevention is by adequate cooking of fish, pork and chicken, and ensuring drinking water is of good quality.

Trichinosis

This is caused by the intestinal nematode, *Trichinella spiralis*. The larval form is found in rats, hares, pigs, dogs and cats. Although cases of trichinosis have been reported from all parts of the world, it is found predominantly in the USA and Europe. It is uncommon in India. Transmission to humans occurs when improperly cooked meats, contaminated with infective larvae, are eaten.

CLINICAL FEATURES

Vomiting, diarrhoea, abdominal pain and headache occur 24–72 h after ingestion of contaminated meat. The severity of the clinical manifestations depends on the number of infecting larvae.

The larvae mature into the adult form in the intestine, where they reproduce and discharge larvae into the circulation. When these larvae migrate into the bloodstream and striated muscles (a stage which lasts 10–21 days), periorbital oedema, conjunctivitis, photophobia, fever with chills, and muscle pain and spasm occur. An urticarial rash, diarrhoea, dyspnoea and pleurisy may also occur. Myocardial and central nervous system involvement is unusual and, if it occurs, may result in death. In the next stage of development, larvae encyst in striated muscle. During encystment symptoms gradually subside, although weakness, muscle pain and cramps may persist for several months.

DIAGNOSIS

A firm diagnosis can be made on the clinical presentation, marked peripheral eosinophilia, and an antibody titre greater than 1:5 detected by the bentonite floculation test. If necessary the diagnosis can be established by biopsying the deltoid or gastrocnemius muscle 3 weeks after the onset of illness and demonstrating the presence of the larvae.

TREATMENT

Analgesics, sedatives and bed rest are the mainstays of treatment. Steroids are indicated only in the presence of myocarditis, central nervous system involvement or marked allergic phenomena. Thiabendazole 25 mg·kg^{-1} body weight twice daily for 7 days is effective against intestinal worms and larvae.

INTESTINAL NEMATODE INFECTION
(Table 1.38)

Some adult nematodes live within the intestinal lumen. The disease is spread to man (Fig. 1.23):
- Passively by ingesting infective eggs, as occurs with *Ascaris lumbricoides* ('roundworm'), *Trichuris trichiura* (whipworm) and *Enterobius vermicularis* (threadworm)
- Actively by percutaneous spread of filariform larvae which penetrate the skin (hookworm and *Strongyloides*)

Table 1.38 Intestinal nematode (roundworm) infections.

Organism	Site	Clinical manifestations
Strongyloides stercoralis	Small intestine	Malabsorption
Hookworm: *Ancylostoma duodenale* and *Necator americanus*	Small intestine	Iron-deficiency anaemia
Capillaria philippinensis	Small intestine	Malabsorption
Ascaris lumbricoides ('roundworm')	Small intestine	? Undernutrition, intestinal obstruction
Trichuris trichiura (whipworm)	Large intestine	Usually nil, colitis, rectal prolapse
Enterobius vermicularis (threadworm)	Large intestine	Usually nil, pruritus ani

Ascaris deviates from the simplified life-cycle shown in Fig. 1.23 in that it invades the duodenum and enters the venous system, via which it reaches the lungs. The worm is eventually expectorated and swallowed, entering the intestine where it completes its maturation. *Strongyloides* is the only nematode that is able to complete its life-cycle in man; its rhabditiform larvae, which hatch in the intestine, are able to re-infect the host by penetrating the intestinal wall and entering the venous system.

Strongyloidiasis

Strongyloides stercoralis is found world-wide, but is particularly common in warm, wet regions such as parts of Central America and south-east Asia. Adult worms inhabit the crypts of the small intestine causing little damage, but in heavy infection worms are embedded in the mucosa and cause an inflammatory response with mucosal injury. The worms are passed in the stools and auto-infection is common.

CLINICAL FEATURES

After penetration of the skin by the filariform larvae, a local reaction occurs characterized by itching, erythema, oedema and urticaria. This subsides within 2 days. A week later migration of the adolescent worms causes irritation of the upper airways, producing cough and occasionally more severe respiratory symptoms. After about 3 weeks, intestinal colonization occurs, often leading to abdominal discomfort and intermittent diarrhoea and constipation. These symptoms can be mild and may pass unnoticed. However, in some individuals, heavy infection may lead to persistent diarrhoea, nausea, anorexia, and evidence of intestinal malabsorption, notably steatorrhoea. Hypoalbuminaemia and weight loss also occur. Disseminated strongyloidiasis is a very serious and often fatal condition and has been described in patients receiving corticosteroid or other immunosuppressive therapy or in those who are immunocompromised for other reasons.

Fig. 1.23 Schematic life-cycles of intestinal nematodes.

DIAGNOSIS

Motile rhabditiform larvae can be detected in fresh stool or in duodenal aspirate. Eosinophilia is common. In heavy infection, anaemia and biochemical evidence of malabsorption are found.

TREATMENT

Treatment consists of thiabendazole 1.5 g twice daily for 2 days. Therapy should be given for at least 5 days (often longer) in the hyperinfected patient with disseminated disease. As the mortality is high, treatment should include i.v. broad spectrum antibiotics as there is often an accompanying gram-negative septicaemia.

Hookworm infection

Hookworm is seen world-wide and affects approximately 25% of the world population. *Ancylostoma duodenale* is found in Europe, the Middle East and North Africa, whereas *Necator americanus* is found in the Western Hemisphere, sub-Saharan Africa, south-east Asia and the Far East.

Adult worms inhabit the small intestine and attach firmly to the intestinal mucosa by the teeth or cutting plates in their large buccal capsule. Blood loss is approximately 0.2 ml per day in *A. duodenale* infection (5- to 10-fold less with *N. americanus*); in heavy infection it has been estimated that up to 100 ml of blood is lost daily.

CLINICAL FEATURES

Local irritation at the site of larval entry in the skin is known as 'ground itch', but this rapidly disappears to be followed some 2 weeks later by mild and transitory pulmonary symptoms. Most patients are asymptomatic once the larvae have reached the small intestine. Some patients experience ulcer-like symptoms and those with heavy chronic infection eventually develop symptoms and signs of anaemia. Hookworm infection is the commonest cause of iron-deficiency anaemia world-wide.

DIAGNOSIS

Hookworm ova appear in the stool, the number of eggs present giving a guide to the severity of the infection. Early in the infection eosinophilia may be found in the peripheral blood. This is followed later by the appearance of iron-deficiency anaemia.

TREATMENT

Mebendazole 100 mg twice daily for 3 days is effective in both types of hookworm, although the infection may not be cleared with a single course of treatment.

Capillaria philippinensis infection

Capillaria philippinensis was first shown to produce human disease in 1964 when an epidemic was reported in the Philippines. It inhabits the small intestine. Transmission to humans is thought to be accomplished by ingestion of larva-infected fish.

Symptoms include epigastric or generalized abdominal pain, chronic diarrhoea and often severe debility. Untreated, the infection lasts 6–12 months and results in marked cachexia with a 20% mortality rate. Mebendazole and thiabendazole are effective treatment, but general supportive measures are important in chronic infection.

Ascaris lumbricoides ('roundworm') infection

Ascaris lumbricoides is a large worm which is found world-wide but is particularly common in poor rural communities where there is heavy faecal contamination of the immediate environment. Infection may be entirely asymptomatic, although heavy infections are associated with nausea, vomiting, abdominal discomfort and anorexia. Worms may obstruct the small intestine, the commonest site being at the ileocaecal valve. Worms occasionally invade the appendix, causing acute appendicitis, or the bile duct, resulting in biliary obstruction and suppurative cholangitis. The nutritional impact of *Ascaris* infection in children is controversial, although it is likely that heavy infection in malnourished children certainly compounds the situation, largely by competition for host nutrients.

DIAGNOSIS

Ascaris eggs may be identified in the stool and occasionally adult worms emerge from the mouth or the anus.

TREATMENT

Mebendazole 100 mg twice daily for 3 days or a single dose of piperazine (100 mg·kg^{-1}) or pyrantel pamoate (10 mg·kg^{-1}) is effective. Surgical intervention may be required for intestinal or biliary obstruction.

Trichuris trichiura (whipworm) infection

Trichuris trichiura is a common parasite and is found world-wide. Prevalence varies from 1 to 90%, being highest in poor communities with inadequate sanitation. Adult worms are most commonly found in the distal ileum and caecum, although in heavy infection no part of the colon is spared. The adult worm embeds its cephalic region into the intestinal mucosa, leaving the distal tail free within the lumen. Such invasion damages the intestinal mucosa and in heavy infection overt colonic and rectal ulceration may result, leading to significant blood and protein loss.

CLINICAL FEATURES

Most infections are asymptomatic and haematological or biochemical deficits do not occur provided nutritional intake is adequate. Heavy infection is associated with diarrhoea with blood and mucus, often associated with abdominal discomfort, tenesmus, anorexia and weight loss. Involvement of the appendix can cause appendicitis, and rectal prolapse has been reported in children.

DIAGNOSIS

Stool examination confirms the presence of typical barrel-shaped eggs. Proctosigmoidoscopy may reveal adult worms firmly attached to the rectal mucosa.

TREATMENT

Mebendazole (100 mg twice daily for 3 days) or a single dose of pyrantel pamoate (10 mg·kg^{-1}) is effective therapy.

Enterobius vermicularis (threadworm) infection

This parasite occurs world-wide but is more prevalent in temperate and cold climates. Children are most commonly infected, but it may affect whole families, inhabitants of residential institutions, and any group of people living in overcrowded circumstances. Adult worms reside largely in the colon, the female migrating to the anus to deposit embryonated eggs on the perianal and perineal areas. Superficial damage to the colonic mucosa occurs during heavy infection and secondary bacterial infection of these lesions may rarely result in submucosal abscesses.

CLINICAL FEATURES

Intense pruritus ani is usually the only symptom of threadworm infection. This is usually nocturnal and related to egg-laying in the perianal region by the female worms. Scratching results in dissemination of eggs and auto-infection. Infection has little significance while the parasite remains within the intestinal lumen, although on occasions migration occurs to the peritoneum and the viscera may be involved.

DIAGNOSIS

Diagnosis is best achieved by applying a piece of clear adhesive tape to the perianal region which may then be examined microscopically for the presence of adherent eggs. Adult worms may be observed leaving the anus by the child's parents.

TREATMENT

A single dose of mebendazole 100 mg followed by a second dose 2 weeks later is usually effective. Alternatives include pyrantel pamoate or piperazine.

Trematode (fluke) infections (Table 1.39)

BLOOD INFECTIONS

Schistosomiasis (bilharzia)

Three major species of schistosomes produce human disease. These have marked differences in geographical distribution (Fig. 1.24). Prevalence is dependent on the presence of a susceptible intermediate snail host and faecal contamination of water supplies. The size of snail populations varies with the season and availability of freshwater breeding grounds. An increase in the world prevalence of schistosomiasis is partly due to dam construction and irrigation programmes.

LIFE-CYCLE AND PATHOGENESIS

Human infection occurs after penetration of the skin or mucous membranes by cercariae, the infective

Table 1.39 Trematode (fluke) infection.

Organism	Location	Major disease site(s)
Schistosoma mansoni	Mesenteric veins	Liver, colon
Schistosoma japonicum	Mesenteric veins	Liver, colon, small intestine
Schistosoma haematobium	Pelvic veins, vesical plexus	Bladder, distal colon, rectum
Fasciola hepatica	Bile ducts	Bile ducts, liver
Clonorchis sinensis	Bile ducts	Bile ducts, liver
Fasciolopis buski	Small intestine	Small intestine
Paragonimus westermani	Lung	Lung

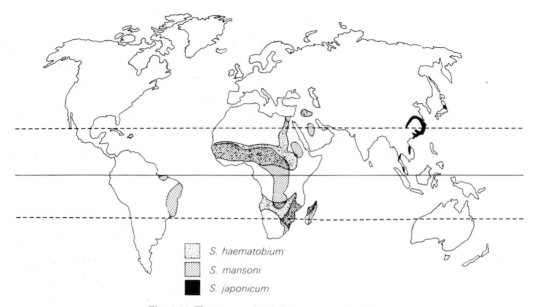

Fig. 1.24 The geographical distribution of *Schistosoma*.

form of the parasite which is liberated into fresh water by the specific intermediate snail host (Fig. 1.25). Cercariae penetrate unbroken skin and migrate as schistosomules through the venous circulation to the liver, where the adult worms mature. Eventually pairs of male and female worms migrate upstream along the portal vein to the mesenteric venules, until the calibre of the vessels halts their progress. They remain in this location for many years copulating continuously and producing enormous numbers of eggs. To complete the life-cycle, eggs must leave the body, either by penetrating the intestinal wall (*Schistosoma mansoni* and *S. japonicum*) or the bladder wall (*S. haematobium*) and returning to the environment via faeces or urine, respectively.

The larvae (miracidia) develop inside the eggs but do not hatch until they arrive in fresh water, when they search actively for the specific snail host to invade. Once inside the snail multiplication occurs, a single miracidium producing up to a 100 000 cercariae released at the rate of 5000 per day.

Eggs retained in host tissues, particularly the liver, urinary bladder and intestine, are responsible for the clinical manifestations of schistosomiasis. Egg antigens initiate both immediate and delayed type hypersensitivity reactions with granuloma formation. Humoral substances such as lymphokines, macrophage migration inhibitory factor and fibroblast stimulating factors are found at the site of these granulomas and presumably support the cell-

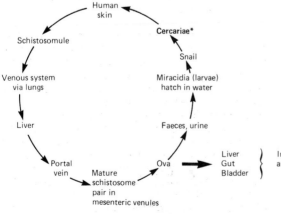

* Infective form for humans

Fig. 1.25 A schematic life-cycle of *Schistosoma*.

ular inflammatory response. Healing eventually occurs by fibrosis.

CLINICAL FEATURES

The first clinical sign of an acute infection is a local inflammatory response at the site of the invading cercariae known as 'swimmer's itch'. Within a week or more there is a generalized allergic response characterized by fever, urticaria, eosinophilia, myalgia and malaise. Nausea, vomiting and profuse diarrhoea are common, as are respiratory symptoms, particularly cough. Clinical findings at this time include generalized lymphadenopathy, hepato-splenomegaly and signs of patchy pneumonia. In Asia the acute disease is called Katayama fever. It is most pronounced in infection with *S. japonicum* and *S. mansoni*.

Chronic schistosomiasis varies in its clinical presentation depending on the type of schistosome involved.

S. mansoni and S. japonicum

S. mansoni is found predominantly in Africa, South America and the West Indies, whereas *S. japonicum* is common in China and other specific sites in south-east Asia.

S. mansoni predominantly affects the colon, where the presence of ova produce macroscopic lesions such as mucosal granularity, erythema and superficial ulceration. However, a particularly severe form of colonic disease is seen in Egyptians, with gross ulceration and polyp formation, particularly in the rectosigmoid; extensive polyposis results in significant blood and protein loss from the colon. Progressive fibrosis in the intestinal wall leads to rigidity and stricture formation, although intestinal obstruction is rare. A localized granulomatous reaction in the intestine (pseudotumour or bilharzioma) may be mistaken for a colonic cancer.

The development of granulomatous hepatitis, followed by progressive periportal fibrosis and portal hypertension, is signified by marked hepato-splenomegaly, often associated with oesophageal varices. In advanced cases death is due to the complications of portal hypertension, as hepatocellular function remains remarkably good.

S. japonicum affects the small intestine and proximal colon in addition to causing fibrotic liver disease. *S. japonicum* produces larger numbers of eggs than *S. mansoni*, which accounts for the more extensive pattern of disease and the frequency of ectopic deposition of ova, particularly in the lungs, spinal cord and brain. The latter may result in fits or hemiplegia.

Epithelial dysplasia in the colon has been reported in patients with chronic *S. japonicum* colitis, and it is now clear that this condition has premalignant potential in endemic areas.

S. haematobium

This is predominantly a urinary tract schistosome found predominantly in Egypt, east Africa and the Middle East. Chronic inflammation is found in the bladder, ureters and urethra, causing urinary frequency, dysuria and haematuria. Chronic infection leads to obstructive uropathy, chronic pyelonephritis and renal failure, and contraction of the bladder. Epidemiological studies confirm an association between bladder carcinoma and this infection. The internal genitalia may be involved and rectal inflammation and ulceration may be found in up to 70% of patients.

DIAGNOSIS

In endemic areas a confident diagnosis can often be obtained on clinical grounds. Confirmation is achieved by detecting the characteristic eggs in the stools, the urine or in a rectal biopsy. Different species of *Schistosoma* can be distinguished not only by the clinical pattern but also by egg morphology.

A plain abdominal radiograph may reveal intramural calcification in the wall of the bladder or the colon. Barium contrast studies of the colon show spiculating mucosal ulceration, polyposis, strictures, and possibly a mass lesion which could either be a bilharzioma or, in the case of *S. japonicum* infection, a carcinoma.

Intravenous urography may confirm an obstructive uropathy and demonstrate bladder contraction.

Immunodiagnostic tests are available, the most sensitive of which detect antibodies against a gut-associated polysaccharide antigen by either ELISA or by indirect immunofluorescence.

TREATMENT

The two major objectives of treatment of schistosomiasis are:
● Reduction in egg production
● Prevention or reduction of tissue damage by eggs already in situ

In endemic and hyperendemic areas, curative therapy is usually inappropriate since reinfection occurs rapidly, whereas infected individuals who are no longer exposed to the parasite can be effectively treated. Suppressive non-curative chemotherapeutic approaches have been used in mass treatment programmes in Egypt with good clinical improvement following a reduction in the 'worm burden'. All antischistosomal drugs have the same effect: they cause worms to leave the mesenteric and vesical veins and to enter the liver and lungs where they are eventually destroyed by host tissue responses.

Praziquantel is active against all species of schistosome and is probably the drug of choice as it is well tolerated and relatively free from serious side-effects. A single dose (40 mg·kg^{-1}) cures more than 90% of patients with *S. haematobium*, with slightly lower rates against *S. mansoni*. *S. japonicum* is best treated with a total dose of 60 mg·kg^{-1} given in divided doses over 1 or 2 days.

Oxamniquine is active against *S. mansoni* and metriphonate against *S. haematobium*. Niridazole is now used much less commonly, but, in addition to its activity against *S. haematobium*, it causes dramatic regression of colonic polyps.

Colonoscopic polypectomy can control the number of colonic polyps, but surgery may be required to relieve obstructive uropathy and for inflammatory masses in the central nervous system.

LIVER AND BILIARY TRACT INFECTIONS

Fascioliasis

Fasciola hepatica infects sheep, goats and cattle, in which it produces liver disease, and is only accidentally transmitted to man via consumption of wild watercress grown on the grazing land of infected animals. The disease is found world-wide, including the United Kingdom. Animals excrete eggs in their faeces from which ciliated miracidia emerge. These enter the freshwater snail (the intermediate host) in which larval development takes place. Eventually cercaria are released and these encyst on aquatic or surface vegetation.

After ingestion by a mammalian host the parasites excyst, migrate through the intestinal wall and penetrate the liver capsule after traversing the peritoneal cavity. Immature flukes reach the bile duct by passing through liver parenchyma and after maturation begin to produce eggs. Adult flukes remain within the biliary tract for many years.

CLINICAL FEATURES

Early symptoms of intermittent fever, malaise, weight loss, right upper quadrant pain and urticaria relate to migration of flukes through the liver and generally occur 2–3 months after infection.

A second phase of the illness relates to the presence of flukes in the biliary tract, where they can cause obstructive jaundice and cholangitis, although infection may remain asymptomatic. Flukes have been found in many ectopic sites, including lung, brain and skin.

DIAGNOSIS

Eosinophilia is common in the early phase of the illness and is often associated with liver function test abnormalities and a positive complement fixation test. Ova are not found in the stool until the second phase of the illness when the mature flukes are established in the biliary tract. However, in up to 30% of cases, stools remain negative; the diagnosis can then be confirmed either by identifying ova in duodenal aspirate or by serological tests. Treatment is with bithionol 30–50 mg·kg^{-1} for 10–15 doses given either daily or on alternate days.

Clonorchiasis

Clonorchis sinensis is a common fluke of the dog, cat and pig affecting millions of animals in the Far East, particularly Indochina, Japan, Korea, Hong Kong and Vietnam. A related fluke, *Opisthorchis felineus*, also affects foxes and is found predominantly in India, the Philippines, Korea and Japan. The lifecycle of both these flukes are similar to that of *Fasciola hepatica*, except that freshwater fish become infected by the cercaria and thereby function as a second intermediate host. Human infection occurs by ingestion of infected, raw fish.

CLINICAL FEATURES

Infected individuals may remain symptom-free, although prolonged exposure with heavy infection results in recurrent obstructive jaundice, suppurative cholangitis, liver abscess and cholangiocarcinoma.

DIAGNOSIS

The diagnosis is made on microscopic examination of faeces or duodenal aspirate.

TREATMENT

Praziquantel 25 mg·kg^{-1} as a single dose is the treatment of choice.

INTESTINAL INFECTIONS

Fasciolopsiasis

Fasciolopsis buski causes intestinal infection in man and pigs. There are two intermediate hosts—freshwater snails and water plants. Human infection is initiated by oral contact with contaminated water plants. These large flukes, which are several centimetres in length, are common in China, Vietnam, Thailand and Taiwan.

Mucosal ulceration and inflammation are apparent at the site of attachment in the intestine; abscess formation, haemorrhage and occasionally bowel obstruction may result. The symptoms are usually non-specific. Heavy infection in children may simulate or precipitate protein–energy malnutrition. Anaemia and eosinophilia are common.

DIAGNOSIS

The diagnosis may be simple if the patient is vomiting or passing flukes per rectum, but may be confirmed by identifying ova in the stools.

TREATMENT

Treatment is with tetrachloroethylene 0.12 ml·kg^{-1} as a single dose (maximum dose of 5 ml) or dichlorophen 100 mg·kg^{-1} as a single dose (which may be repeated 1 week later).

LUNG INFECTIONS

Paragonimiasis

Paragonimus westermani is found most commonly in the Far East, particularly in Korea. Adult worms reside in necrotic capsulated areas in the lung parenchyma and produce ova which are either coughed up in the sputum or swallowed and excreted in the faeces. On reaching fresh water the first larval stage, the miracidium, emerges and within 24 h must find its first intermediate host, the snail. Freshwater crabs or crayfish, the second intermediate hosts, become infected either by eating the digestive glands of the snails or are penetrated directly by the second larval stage, the cercaria. Humans are infected by eating raw freshwater crabs or crayfish. The parasite migrates through the wall of the small intestine into the peritoneal cavity and finally reaches the lungs by penetrating the diaphragm.

CLINICAL FEATURES

Chronic cough with blood-stained or reddish-brown sputum is the usual presentation (hence 'endemic haemoptysis'). Up to one-quarter of patients, however, may be totally asymptomatic. Pleuritic chest pain, pleural effusion and empyema also occur.

Flukes may migrate to ectopic foci such as the abdomen and pelvis, retroperitoneum, scrotum, kidney and mediastinum. CNS involvement results in epilepsy, hemiplegia and visual disturbances.

DIAGNOSIS

Ova may be found in the sputum or faeces. Ectopic flukes may be detected by aspiration or biopsy. Radiological abnormalities are particularly common in the mid-zones of the lungs, usually cavities within an area of consolidation.

TREATMENT

Treatment is with praziquantel or bithionol.

PREVENTION

Human infection can be avoided by not eating raw crab or crayfish.

Cestode (tapeworm) infections

Tapeworms belong to the subclass Cestoda. These are flat worms measuring from a few millimetres (*Echinococcus granulosus*) to several metres in length (*Taenia saginata*). Structurally they consist of a head which is adorned with suckers and hooks (*Taenia solium*) or suckers alone (*T. saginata*). The head is attached via a short slender neck to several segments or proglottids which form a chain-like structure or strobila. The terminal proglottid is the most mature. The entire worm is covered with a continuous elastic cuticle. Tapeworms are devoid of a gastrointestinal tract or vascular system; nutrients are absorbed directly through the cuticle. They are hermaphrodites and cross-fertilization between proglottids is frequent.

Adults live in the intestinal tract of vertebrates, whereas the larvae (oncospheres) exist in the tissues of vertebrates and invertebrates. Infection is transmitted to humans by ingestion of meats infected with larval forms. Four tapeworms commonly infect humans: *T. saginata*, *T. solium*, *Diphyllobothrium latum* and *Hymenolepis nana*.

Taenia saginata (beef tapeworm) infection

T. saginata measures up to 10 m in length, inhabits the upper jejunum, and is prevalent in humans in all beef-eating countries. The majority of patients are asymptomatic. Symptoms are mild, with vague epigastric and abdominal pain, and occasional diarrhoea and vomiting. Weight loss is unusual. Rarely appendicitis and pancreatitis due to obstruction of the appendix and pancreatic ducts, respectively, by the adult worms may occur. The commonest symptom is the presence of proglottids in the faeces, bed or underclothing.

DIAGNOSIS

The presence of proglottids, which are visible macroscopically, or the eggs, which are seen microscopically, in the faeces or perianal region is diagnostic. A higher positive yield is obtained by examining perianal clear adhesive tape swabs for ova, in which case the scolex (the head) or proglottids are required to establish the species.

TREATMENT

Praziquantel 10 mg·kg^{-1} as a single dose is probably the treatment of choice. Niclosamide 2 g as a single chewed dose is also effective.

PREVENTION

Prevention is easily effected by careful inspection of beef for cysticerci (encysted larval forms). Refrigeration of beef at −10°C for 5 days or cooking it at 57°C for a few minutes destroys the cysticerci.

Taenia solium infection and cysticercosis

Taenia solium (the pork tapeworm) measures up to 6 m in length. It has a world-wide distribution, but is seen most frequently in eastern Europe, south-east Asia and Africa. In the adult form it lives in the human upper jejunum. The clinical features are similar to those caused by *T. saginata*.

Treatment is similar to that for *T. saginata*. However, because release of ova can occur during treatment and, theoretically, these could be carried back into the stomach, releasing the intermediate larval stage, treatment for *T. solium* should be followed by a saline purge.

Human cysticercosis

Cysticercosis occurs after autoinfection or hetero-infection by eggs of *T. solium* and invasion of tissues by the intermediate larval form, *Cysticercus cellulosae* (Fig. 1.26). Cysticercosis is most commonly seen in parts of Asia, Africa and South America. Cysticerci may develop in any tissue in the body. Most commonly, however, three clinical forms are recognized:

- *Cerebral cysticercosis* may present as various forms of epilepsy, as a space-occupying lesion or as focal neurological deficits including hemiplegia and behavioural changes.
- *Ocular cysticercosis* may present as retinitis, uveitis, conjunctivitis or choroidal atrophy. Blindness may ensue.
- *Subcutaneous cysticercosis* presents as small, pea-sized, hard nodules in the subcutaneous tissue.

The diagnosis is established by biopsying a subcutaneous nodule and demonstrating the characteristic translucent membrane. Radiography may demonstrate calcified degenerating cysticerci. Indirect haemagglutination tests are useful.

Treatment involves surgical excision of the cysticerci. Mebendazole has recently been shown to be active against both the adult and larval stages, but its efficacy needs to be further evaluated. Praziquantel is also effective and may be the drug of choice for cerebral cysticercosis.

Diphyllobothrium latum infection

Diphyllobothriasis is particularly prevalent in Scandinavian countries, the Baltic region, Japan and the lake region of Switzerland. Infection in humans, the definitive host, results from ingestion of fish which contain the infective plerocercoid form. The adult tapeworm measures several metres in length. The proglottids differ from those of *Taenia* in that they are more wide than long. The adult worm usually attaches itself to the jejunum.

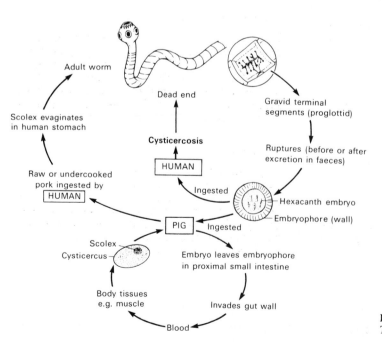

Fig. 1.26 A schematic life-cycle of *Taenia solium*.

The clinical features are usually mild and consist of vague abdominal discomfort, anorexia, nausea and vomiting. Megaloblastic anaemia, due to competitive utilization of ingested vitamin B_{12} by the parasite, may occur in a small percentage of patients. Rarely intestinal obstruction occurs.

Treatment is similar to that described for *T. saginata*. Vitamin B_{12} should be administered where indicated.

Hydatid disease

Hydatid disease occurs when humans ingest the hexacanth embryos of the dog tapeworm, *Echinococcus granulosus* or of *E. multilocularis*.

Human infection with *E. granulosus* frequently occurs in early childhood by direct contact with infected dogs, or by eating uncooked, improperly washed vegetables contaminated with infected canine faeces. In the duodenum the hexacanth embryos hatch, penetrate the intestinal wall, enter the portal system and are then carried to the liver. Further dissemination of embryos to the lung and to almost every organ in the body may occur, where they form hydatid cysts (Fig. 1.27). The disease is seen in all parts of the world, particularly in those countries where sheep- and cattle-raising constitutes an important means of livelihood. These animals perpetuate the life-cycle of the parasite.

Symptoms largely depend upon the site of the unilocular hydatid cyst. The liver is the commonest site for cyst formation (60%), followed by the lung (20%), kidneys (3%) and brain (1%). In the liver the majority of cysts are situated in the right lobe. The symptoms are those of a slowly growing benign tumour. Pressure on the bile ducts may cause obstructive jaundice. Rupture into the abdominal cavity, pleural cavity or biliary tree may occur. In the

latter instance intermittent jaundice, abdominal pain and fever associated with eosinophilia result. A cyst rupturing into a bronchus may result in its expectoration and spontaneous cure, but if secondary infection supervenes a chronic pulmonary abscess will form. Haemoptysis, dyspnoea and chest pain may lead to a mistaken diagnosis of malignancy. Focal seizures may occur if cysts are present in the brain. Renal involvement produces lumbar pain and haematuria. Calcification of the cyst occurs in about 40% of cases.

The alveolar hydatid cyst caused by *E. multilocularis* results from its larval stage. *E. multilocularis* is seen in parts of Canada, the USSR, and Alaska. Foxes and small rodents constitute the intermediate hosts; humans are accidental hosts. The majority of the lesions are in the liver and metastasis may occur.

The diagnosis and treatment of hydatid disease are described on p. 245.

Hymenolepis nana infection

Hymenolepis nana (dwarf tapeworm) is a short worm measuring about 20 mm in length. Humans, rats and mice constitute the definitive hosts. Infection of humans is caused by ingestion of the eggs. The adult worm inhabits the small intestine. No intermediate host is required.

Most patients remain asymptomatic. The diagnosis is established by identifying the ova in faeces.

Treatment is with praziquantel 20 mg·kg^{-1} as a single dose, niclosamide 2 g daily for 7 days, or paromomycin 45 mg·kg^{-1} for 7 days.

Sparganosis

Sparganosis results when the plerocercoid larva (sparganum) of various diphyllobothriid tapeworms, including *Diphyllobothrium mansoni*, are ingested by humans, the second intermediate host. They give rise to painful subcutaneous swellings which on excision reveal the presence of a mass of worms. Treatment is surgical excision.

Dipylidiasis

Dogs, cats and wild carnivora are the definitive hosts for *Dipylidium caninum*. Ingestion of fleas containing the infective larval form causes human infection. Children are usually affected. Symptoms are uncommon and diagnosis is established by identifying the characteristic orange-brown proglottids in the faeces. Treatment is as for *T. saginata*.

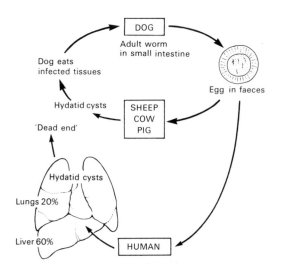

Fig. 1.27 A schematic life-cycle of *Echinococcus granulosus*.

Further reading

Bannister B (1983) *Infectious Diseases*. London: Baillière Tindall.

Braude AI (1985) *Infectious Diseases and Medical Microbiology*, 2nd edn. Philadelphia: WB Saunders.

Mandel GL, Douglas RG & Bennett JE (1985) *Principles and Practice of Infectious Diseases*, 2nd edn. New York: John Wiley.

Manson-Bahr PEC & Bell D (1987) *Manson's Tropical Diseases*, 19th edn. London: Baillière Tindall.

Youmans GP, Paterson PY & Sommers HM (eds) (1985) *The Biologic and Clinical Basis of Infectious Diseases*, 3rd edn. Philadelphia: WB Saunders.

2

The Basics of Genetics, Molecular Biology and Immunology

- Unifactorial genetic disorders are usually due to single gene defects, e.g. Huntington's chorea.
- In multifactorial disorders many genes may be involved (polygenic), e.g. congenital dislocation of the hip.

A glossary of terms commonly used in genetics can be found on p. 125.

MOLECULAR BASIS OF GENETICS

DNA (deoxyribonucleic acid)

Genetic information is stored in the form of double-stranded DNA. Each strand of DNA is made up of a deoxyribose phosphate backbone and a series of purine [adenine (A) and guanine (G)] and pyrimidine [thymine (T) and cytosine (C)] bases. The two strands of DNA are held together by hydrogen bonds between the bases. As T always pairs with A, and G with C there are only four possible pairs of nucleotides—TA, AT, GC and CG. The nucleus of each diploid cell contains 6×10^9 base pairs worth of DNA and of this 5×10^6 are likely to be transcriptionally active.

The sequence of nucleotides contains the information which determines the sequence of amino acids in a newly formed polypeptide chain and hence its composition and primary structure.

RNA (ribonucleic acid)

RNA is found mainly in the nucleolus and cytoplasm and is similar in stucture to DNA, except that thymine is replaced by uracil (U).

Amino acids

Three adjacent nucleotides (a codon) code for a particular amino acid on messenger RNA (see below). There are only 20 common amino acids, but 64 possible codon combinations. Some of these other codons are used as signals for 'initiating' or 'terminating' polypeptide chain synthesis.

This chapter describes the essential facts required for an understanding of genetics, molecular biology and immunology. The first half is concerned with genes, inheritance and the human leucocyte antigens, whilst the latter half of the chapter describes the basic immunological reactions.

The broad mechanisms of the pathogenesis of diseases are discussed here, but details of the abnormalities found within each disease state are discussed with the clinical findings elsewhere in this book.

Genetics and molecular biology

Introduction

The nucleus of every cell in the body contains DNA. This is the chemical basis of the genes which specify the construction of each and every protein in the body and thus control the normal variations in physical characteristics such as height. Genes also have an effect on the susceptibility of an individual to disease.

The analysis of the detailed structure and function of genes has been made possible by the application of recombinant DNA technology to genetics. This has helped in the understanding of the inheritance of diseases caused by the alteration or mutation of a single gene, but the problems of unravelling the simultaneous effects of several different genes are still immense.

Human diseases may be due to entirely genetic or environmental causes (unifactorial) or to a combination of both factors (multifactorial):

Genes

A gene is a portion of DNA which codes for a single polypeptide sequence (called a cistron). There are two main types:

- *Structural genes*, which are responsible for synthesis of specific proteins, e.g. enzymes, haemoglobin and collagen
- *Control genes*, which are thought to modify the action of structural genes

Structural genes consist of lengths of DNA which contain sufficient nucleotide triplets to code for the appropriate number of amino acids in the polypeptide chains of a particular protein. However, these coding sequences (called exons) are interrupted by intervening sequences (IVS) which are non-coding (called introns) at various positions (see below).

Transcription

Genetic information is carried from the nucleus to the cytoplasm by a form of RNA called messenger RNA (mRNA) which acts as a template for protein synthesis.

Each base in the mRNA molecule is lined up opposite to the corresponding base in the DNA—C to G, G to C, T to A and A to U (instead of T) (see Fig. 2.1).

This initial mRNA is a complete transcription of one strand of DNA and therefore contains both introns and exons. Before leaving the nucleus, the introns are excised and the exons spliced together. The mRNA migrates out of the nucleus into the cytoplasm. Polysomes (groups of ribosomes) become attached to the mRNA; these will carry the growing peptide chain. This definitive mRNA now has the exact coding sequence for the order of amino acids in a polypeptide chain. It also contains specific 'start' (e.g. AUG) and 'stop' (e.g. UAA) codons, which determine the points of initiation and termination of peptide chain synthesis.

The cytoplasm contains another form of RNA called transfer RNA (tRNA). Each molecule of tRNA is specific for one amino acid and has three unpaired nucleotide bases (the anti-codon) that correspond to the appropriate codons of the mRNA (see Fig. 2.2).

The mRNA therefore can act as a template—a particular codon in the mRNA is related through the tRNA to specific amino acids. The ribosome moves along the mRNA like a 'zipper', linking the assembled amino acids to form a polypeptide chain (protein synthesis).

The regulation of protein synthesis is extremely complex and not entirely understood. The rates of transcription and protein production are thought to be regulated by sequences in the 'flanking' regions at each end of the genes. The NC (non-coding) region directs the production of mRNA regions which are not translated into a protein product.

Changes in DNA (mutations)

Changes in DNA are random and can be inherited.

Substitution

This is the simplest type of change and involves the substitution of one base or one triplet for another. For example, the triplet AAA, which codes for phenylalanine, may become AGA, which codes for serine.

Whether a substitution produces a clinical disorder or not depends on whether it results in a change in a critical part of the protein molecule produced. Fortunately, many substitutions have no effect on the function or stability of the proteins produced as several triplets code for the same amino acid. However, in others the effects may be severe; for example, in sickle cell disease a change in the DNA results in the substitution of valine for glutamic acid and the production of HbS rather than HbA. Over 300 variants of haemoglobin have been described, as single amino acid changes can alter the electrophoretic mobility of the haemoglobin molecule. Many others, however, remain undetected as some substitutions do not alter the protein sufficiently to change the electrophoretic mobility.

Other examples include glucose-6-phosphate deficiency in Negroes, which is known to result from the production of an enzyme variant with a single amino acid mutation. DNA substitution is also seen in a rare form of diabetes in which a change in a single amino acid prevents the normal cleavage of pro-insulin to insulin.

Insertion or deletion

Insertion or deletion of one or more bases is a more serious change, as it results in the alteration of the rest of the following sequence. For example, if the original code was:

TAA GGA GAG TTT

and the third nucleotide (A) is deleted, the sequence becomes:

TAG GAG AGT TT...

Deletions of part or all of the structural gene cause changes in amino acid sequences. This type of change is responsible for some forms of thalassaemia or growth hormone deficiency.

DNA
(single strand, coiled)

| A | C | G | A | A | G |
| U | G | C | U | U | C |

mRNA

Fig. 2.1 Transcription. One strand of DNA forms a template for the synthesis of messenger RNA (mRNA).

Fig. 2.2 Genetic control of protein synthesis. NC = non-coding; mRNA = messenger RNA; AUG = 'start' coding sequences; UAA = 'stop' coding sequence. From Weatherall D (1985) The new genetics with reference to inborn errors of metabolism. *Medicine International* 14: 585–589. With permission.

Normal chain termination occurs when the ribosomes on the mRNA reach one of the chain termination codons (e.g. UAA, UAG or UGA). Mutations can involve these termination codons. For example, premature termination may occur when a coding sequence for 'termination' of a polypeptide chain is produced by a mutation. Alternatively, a chain may not terminate correctly when instead of the sequence reading 'stop' it allows the insertion of another amino acid. Haemoglobin Constant Spring—a haemoglobin variant—is formed when, instead of the 'stop' sequence, there is a single base change allowing the insertion of an amino acid.

Other types of mutations include gene fusion and gene inversions.

ANALYSIS AND ISOLATION OF GENES

Recombinant DNA technology and gene mapping have now made it possible to analyse human genes and their mRNAs and define defects at a molecular level in some genetic disorders. These techniques, which include both biochemical and bacteriological steps, involve:

- The isolation of a human gene from most cells
- Its incorporation into a vector, e.g. a plasmid, bacteriophage or cosmid (see below) (recombinant step)
- The introduction of the vector into an organism, e.g. a bacterium
- The production of multiple 'copies' of the gene (cloning)
- Subsequent selection and harvesting

Amino acid sequencing techniques for DNA permit positive identification of the gene under study.

Recombinant DNA technology

Molecular hybridization
A fundamental property of strands of DNA is that when the two strands are separated, for example by heating, they will always re-associate and stick together again because of their complementary base sequences. The presence and position of a particular

gene can therefore be identified using a gene 'probe' consisting of DNA with a base sequence that is complementary to that of the gene. A probe can be made in the following way:

- The enzyme reverse transcriptase, isolated from certain RNA tumour viruses, can be used to synthesize DNA (complementary DNA or cDNA) when mixed with any purified mRNA isolated from mammalian cells.
- This is folowed by cloning (i.e. by selectively purifying and amplifying) bacteria containing this DNA (see below).

By incorporating radioactive isotopes, usually phosphorus-32, into the nucleotides the synthesized DNA probe is made radio-active and then can be used as a 'hybridization' probe to look for similar sequences in genomic DNA or cellular RNA. As cDNAs can hybridize in a highly specific manner to appropriate DNAs or RNAs, it is possible to test for the presence of and quantify these RNA or DNA sequences. In this way a genetic disorder may be discovered to be associated with the absence of a particular structure, e.g. one form of thalassaemia has been demonstrated to be due to a gene deletion.

With this technique it is possible to clone a chosen DNA or cDNA sequence. Foreign DNA is inserted into a vector, e.g. a bacterial plasmid, a viral vector or a cosmid. Plasmids are extremely simple organelles which live and replicate in the cytoplasm of bacteria. They consist of a circular ring of DNA which can be cleaved by a specific restriction endonuclease to produce a linear structure. Viral vectors are mostly derived from the bacteriophage lambda. They work in the same way as plasmids but form plaques by killing. A cosmid vector is a plasmid into which the phage lambda *cos* gene has been inserted. This enables larger amounts of DNA to be packaged in vitro into the phage head.

Restriction endonucleases are bacterial enzymes which cleave DNA at a number of specific sites. For example, the DNA of the microorganism *Escherichia coli* RY 13 is cleaved by the restriction enzyme Eco R1 at the points indicated below:

5' GAATTC 3'

3' CTTAAG 5'

The DNA for insertion into a vector is broken up by using restriction enzymes and is mixed with the plasmids and joined by a ligase. Some plasmids in the mixture now incorporate the foreign DNA and reform into circular structures (see Fig. 2.3). These reformed plasmids and some suitable bacteria are then mixed together and a small proportion of the plasmids will enter the bacterial cytoplasm. These bacteria can be selected out by different techniques;

Fig. 2.3 Recombinant DNA technique, showing the construction of a bacterial plasmid to contain foreign DNA.

for example, the plasmid may confer antibiotic resistance to the bacteria and this can be detected on culture. Using the technique of hybridization, bacterial colonies can be screened to search for the particular clone which contains the inserted DNA. If one is found it can be grown in large quantities to produce the required DNA.

There are now gene libraries and banks of cloned DNA fragments with known sequences growing in suitable hosts such as *E. coli*. This allows easy identification of individual genes for given amino acid sequences and the manufacture of probes for gene mapping. For example, using this technique the gene defect in sickle cell disease has been shown to be a mutation of GAG (glutamic acid) to GTG (valine).

Gene mapping (see Fig. 2.4)
DNA fragments produced by restriction endonucleases are separated by electrophoresis in agarose gel. A nitrocellulose filter is placed on top of the gel and the DNA is sucked from the gel onto the filter, to which it sticks very firmly. This process is called 'Southern blotting'. The filter is then exposed to a radioactively labelled cDNA probe which has a complementary sequence of bases to the gene that is being sought and so will hybridize to it. The position of the fragments of DNA containing the gene is then determined by autoradiography. By using different enzymes for cleavage it is possible to build up restriction enzyme maps of appropriate areas of the genome.

A similar technique using RNA fragments is known as Northern blotting, and one using virus polypeptides which can then be reacted with specific antibody is called Western blotting.

The chromosomal localization of genes is usually performed by using rodent/human cell hybrids or by in situ hybridization techniques.

When the loci occupied by the genes are very close together on the same chromosomes, the genes tend to be inherited together and are said to be 'linked'. The closer the loci are to each other, the less likely they are to be separated during the 'crossing over' process.

Fig. 2.4 Gene mapping, showing the technique for identifying a particular gene. From Weatherall D (1985). The new genetics with reference to inborn errors of metabolism. *Medicine International* 14: 585–589. With permission.

So far over 100 genetic loci have been mapped on the human X chromosome, and about 500 on autosomal chromosomes.

Table 2.1 shows some of the diseases that are controlled by genes on various chromosomes.

APPLICATIONS OF MOLECULAR GENETICS

The use of molecular biological techniques in genetics will undoubtedly have a large impact on the investigation, diagnosis, treatment and control of genetic disorders. Some of its applications include:

● The investigation of gene structure, function and mapping, e.g. immunoglobulin genes, globin genes
● The control of genetic disease, e.g. prenatal diagnosis, carrier detection
● The diagnosis of genetic disorders, e.g. sickle cell disease, Huntington's chorea
● The biosynthesis of substances, e.g. insulin, growth hormone, vaccines
● The future treatment of genetic disease by the insertion of cloned normal genes and deletion of abnormal genes

Very careful control and supervision of gene manipulation will, however, be necessary because of its potential hazards and ethical implications.

ONCOGENES

Oncogenes are genes present in normal cells but which become altered in structure or expression in cancer cells. The initial studies that led to their discovery were on RNA tumour viruses such as human T cell leukaemia virus. An oncogenic virus that infects a cell converts its RNA genome into DNA using the enzyme reverse transcriptase (i.e. it is a retrovirus). The DNA becomes integrated into the host's chromosomal DNA and the subsequent proteins produced are then copies of the virus protein. The new DNA also controls the malignant transformation of the cell. Genes have now been found in non-infected cells with very similar structures to the DNA produced by oncogenic viruses. They are present in normal cells of all vertebrate species and they are very highly conserved in evolution, suggesting that they have obvious survival value. Over 30 of these oncogenes have now been identified, mole-

Table 2.1 Some examples of diseases or factors controlled by genes on particular chromosomes.

Chromosome	Factor or disease
Chromosome 1	6-Phosphogluconate dehydrogenase Rhesus blood group Elliptocytosis Amylase (salivary and pancreatic) Duffy blood group
Chromosome 6	Major histocompatibility complex (HLA) Properdin factor B Complement 4 Haemochromatosis
Chromosome 9	ABO blood groups Adenylate kinase
Chromosome 11	Structure of beta, gamma and delta haemoglobin chains Insulin-dependent diabetes
Chromosome 12	Phenylketonuria
Chromosome 16	Structure of alpha haemoglobin chain
Chromosome 19	Familial hypercholesterolaemia
Chromosome 21	Phosphofructokinase (liver type)
Chromosome 22	Beta-galactosidase 2 Alpha-galactosidase B (*N*-acetyl-alpha-D-galactosaminidase)

cularly cloned and sequenced. Activation of oncogenes has obvious implications in the development of cancer. This may occur, for example, due to chromosome abnormalities such as:

- The Philadelphia chromosome (see p. 103). The oncogene c-*abl* is situated near the breakpoint on chromosome 9. On translocation c-*abl* fuses at the breakpoint cluster region (*bcr*) of chromosome 22 to form a chimaeric gene *bcr-abl*. On transcription a new protein results and this is analogous to a viral oncogene (v-*abl*) associated with a murine leukaemia virus. Thus the juxtaposition of c-*abl* and *bcr* may be critical for the development of chronic granulocytic leukaemia.
- Burkitt's lymphoma. A translocation involving chromosomes 8 and 14 occurs. The breakpoint in chromosome 8 is the c-*myc* region which is inserted with the Ig heavy chain region of chromosome 14.

Proteins produced by three oncogenic products have been shown to be involved in growth control:

- The product of c-*sis* gene, b 28^{c-sis}, has the same amino acid structure to a platelet derived growth factor, a protein known to increase cellular activity.
- The product of c-*erbB* has the same structure as the epidermal growth factor receptor. This factor activates protein kinases within cells, increasing their growth.
- The product of c-*myc* is involved in cell cycle control.

Alteration in the structure or control of these genes could be important in the control of cell growth and the development of malignant potential. Monoclonal antibodies to oncogenic proteins are being developed so that assays of oncogenes in normal and abnormal cells can be made. DNA hybridization techniques have already shown vast increases of certain genes in tumour tissues, e.g. N-*myc* in neuroblastoma, and H-*ras* mRNA in colonic carcinoma, colonic polyps and breast cancer.

CHROMOSOMES

Chromosomes are only visible in a cell when it is undergoing mitotic division. Every nucleated cell in the body, except the gametes, has 46 chromosomes. Each chromosome contains one molecule of double-stranded DNA. Two chromosomes determine the sex of the individual and are known as sex chromosomes; the remaining 44 are called autosomes.

During division, a chromosome consists of two identical chromatids joined together at a centromere (Fig. 2.5). They are classified according to their size and the site of the centromere. The centromere can be at three locations:

- Metacentric (central)

Fig. 2.5 A schematic diagram showing the structure of a chromosome with the sites at which it can split. The nomenclature for describing loci on chromosomes is as follows:

  Number of chromosome or X or Y + short arm (p) or long arm (q)

The region or subregion is defined by bands stained with quinacrine or giemsa.

- Submetacentric (nearer one end than the other)
- Acrocentric (at one extreme end)

The chromosomes in the nucleus are arranged in pairs. The two members of each pair of autosomes (one derived from each parent) resemble one another and are said to be homologous. However, the sex chromosomes differ—in the female the sex chromosomes are homologous (XX), but in the male pair they are not (XY).

During cell division (mitosis), each chromosome divides into two so that each daughter nucleus has the same number of chromosomes as its parent cell. During gametogenesis, however, the number of chromosomes is halved by meiosis, so that after conception the number of chromosomes remains the same and is not doubled. In the female each ovum contains one or other X chromosome, but in the male the sperm bears either an X or a Y chromosome.

Chromosomal abnormalities
Chromosomal abnormalities are much commoner than generally appreciated. In a study of spontaneous abortions, half were due to chromosomal abnormalities, as compared with an incidence of only four to six abnormalities per 1000 live births.

Specific chromosomal abnormalities can lead to well-recognized and disabling clinical syndromes. The incidence of such abnormalities is divided equally between abnormalities in the autosomes and abnormalities in the sex chromosomes. Abnormalities may occur in either the number or the structure of the chromosomes.

Abnormal chromosome numbers (non-disjunction)
This is an abnormality of nuclear division, with failure of chromosomes or chromatids to separate either in meiosis or mitosis. If it occurs during meiosis it can lead to an ovum or sperm having either an extra chromosome which, if involved in conception, produces a fetus with an extra chromosome (i.e. three instead of two of one type—called trisomy) or only one (monosomy). Fetuses with the latter defect are usually non-viable. Non-disjunction can occur with autosomes or sex chromosomes.

Occasionally non-disjunction can occur during mitosis shortly after two gametes have united. It will then result in the formation of two cell lines, each with a different chromosome complement. This occurs more often with the sex chromosome, and is called 'mosaicism'.

Abnormal chromosome structure
The following changes can occur:
● *Translocation.* This occurs when two homologous chromosomes lying together break simultaneously and a portion of one joins up with a portion of the other. Here the cell still has 46 chromosomes, but the structure of two of them has been rearranged. The carrier of this balanced reciprocal translocation is healthy, but if at meiosis the homologous pair separate and a child gets one normal and one abnormal chromosome, i.e. an unbalanced translocation, development may be disturbed.

Philadelphia chromosome (Ph') is a chromosome 22 with a shortened long arm due to a reciprocal translocation with the tip of the long arm of chromosome 9 (see Fig. 2.6). Usually the Ph' chromosome is associated with chronic granulocytic leukaemia (see Fig. 7.11, p. 314), but all Ph' chromosomes are not identical as the breakpoint may be different. Recent evidence suggests that the material translocated from chromosome 9 to 22 contains the cellular oncogene *c-abl* (see p. 102.
● *Deletion.* This is a loss of a section of chromosome together with the genes contained in it; for example, in the cri du chat syndrome there is a deletion of the short arm of chromosome 5.
● *Inversion.* This is an end-to-end reversal of a segment within a chromosome, e.g. abcdefgh becomes abcdhgfe.
● *Duplication.* This is where part of the chromosome is duplicated, e.g. abcdef becomes abcabcdef.

Fig. 2.6 The Philadelphia chromosome (Ph'). The long arm (q) of chromosome 22 has been shortened by the reciprocal translocation with chromosome 9.

● *Ringed chromosomes.* These occur when two ends of a chromosome have been deleted and the broken 'sticky' ends fuse together.
● *Isochromosomes.* These occur when the centromere divides horizontally instead of longitudinally, forming chromosomes with two short or two long arms (see Fig. 2.5).

Abnormalities of chromosome number or structure can be seen in both autosomes and sex chromosomes; some of the resulting syndromes are shown in Table 2.2. Many individuals have an extra sex chromosome which remains unrecognized. However, since this abnormality is associated with an increased incidence of mental retardation and psychiatric problems, a disproportionate number of such individuals are seen in psychiatric and mental institutions.

Chromosome studies

Chromosomes can only be seen in actively dividing cells. Lymphocytes from the peripheral blood are therefore stimulated by phytohaemogglutanin for these studies. Alternatively, skin cells can be used. Culture and preparation takes about three days for lymphocytes and much longer with skin cells. On staining, for example with the Giemsa stain, the chromosomes show a distinctive pattern of light and dark bands, enabling each chromosome to be identified.

Table 2.2 Chromosomal abnormalities.

Syndrome	Chromosome defect	Total number of chromosomes	Incidence and risks	Clinical features	Mortality
AUTOSOMAL ABNORMALITIES					
Down's syndrome	Trisomy of chromosome 21 (95%) Mosaicism Translocation } (5%)	47	1:800 (Risk with 20–29 year old mother = 1:1000; >45 year old mother = 1:30)	Flat facies, slanting eyes, epicanthic folds, small ears, simian crease, short, hypotonia, variable mental retardation, congenital heart disease (up to 50%)	High in first year, but some survive to adulthood
Patau's syndrome	Trisomy of chromosome 13	47	1:8000	Low-set ears, cleft lip and palate, micro-ophthalmia, mental retardation	Rarely survive for more than a few weeks
Edwards' syndrome	Trisomy of chromosome 18	47	1:5000	Low-set ears, micrognathia, rocker-bottom feet, mental retardation	Rarely survive for more than a few weeks
SEX CHROMOSOME ABNORMALITIES					
Female					
Turner's syndrome	Monosomy of X chromosome	45	1:2500	Infantilism, primary amenorrhoea, short stature, webbed neck, cubitus valgus, normal IQ	
Triple X syndrome	XXX	47	1:800	No distinctive somatic features, mental retardation	
Others	XXXX XXXXX	48 49 }	Rare	Amenorrhoea, infertility, mental retardation	
Male					
Klinefelter's syndrome	XXY (or XXYY)	47	1:800 (more in sons of older mothers)	Decreased crown–pubis: pubis–heel ratio, eunuchoid, testicular atrophy, infertility, gynaecomastia, mental retardation (20%; related to number of X chromosomes)	
Double Y syndrome	XYY	47	1:800	Tall, fertile, minor mental and psychiatric illness, high incidence in tall criminals	
Others	XXXY XXXXY	48 49		Mental retardation, testicular atrophy	

Indications

Chromosome studies may be performed for various reasons at the following times:

- Antenatally:
  - (a) Sexing of fetus in X-linked disorders
  - (b) Diagnosis of autosomal trisomy
- In the neonate:
  - (a) Malformations
  - (b) Suspicion of trisomy
  - (c) Ambiguous genitalia
- In the adolescent:
  - (a) Primary amenorrhoea
- In the adult:
  - (a) Screening of patients with a child with a chromosomal abnormality for further genetic counselling
  - (b) Infertility or recurrent abortion

For families at risk of genetic disease an intrauterine diagnosis is important; the methods available for prenatal diagnosis are shown in Table 2.3.

Amniocentesis is a widely available technique in the UK. Pregnancies can be screened and abortion offered if abnormalities are found.

Nuclear sexing

Methods for preparing complete karyotypes are now available. Sex chromosomes can also be studied by looking for 'Barr bodies' in buccal smears. These Barr bodies, which are also known as sex chromatin bodies, represent genetically inactive X chromosomes in the female nuclei and appear as a distinctive mass of nuclear chromatin near the nuclear membrane. The Lyon hypothesis states that in cells with more than one X chromosome there is random inacti-

Table 2.3 Methods available for prenatal diagnosis.

Method	Comments
Amniocentesis	(See Box)
Ultrasonography	Used for suspected neural-tube defects or skeletal abnormalities
Fetoscopy	Available in specialized centres to detect specific malformations
Fetal blood sampling	Samples used for recombinant DNA techniques to diagnose, for example, haemoglobinopathies
Trophoblast biopsy at 8–10 weeks	Being developed, and is replacing fetal blood sampling for DNA techniques. The incidence of fetal loss using this technique is uncertain

vation of all but one of the X chromosomes, with the formation of Barr bodies. Once this chance selection is made, it is passed on to all the descendants of these cells. Therefore, a normal female (XX) has one Barr body, a female with Turner's syndrome (XO) has

---

Amniocentesis

- This is performed at 14–17 weeks' gestation.
- Ultrasound is used to localize placenta and to detect the presence of twins.
- Sterile precautions are used during aspiration of approximately 20 ml of amniotic fluid via the transabdominal route.
- The specimen is centrifuged:
  (a) The *supernatant* is used for chemical analysis to detect defects such as the adrenogenital syndrome.
  (b) The *cell deposit* can be cultured and used for cytogenetics (or chromosomal analysis) or enzyme studies for the detection of inborn errors of metabolism such as Tay–Sachs disease.

Indications
Amniocentesis should be offered if the following are suspected:
- Chromosomal abnormality—*all* mothers over 35 years, or those with a previous child with a chromosome abnormality
- X-linked disorders (for fetal sexing)
- Inborn errors of metabolism (family history)
- Neural tube defects—couples who have had a previous baby with a neural tube defect, e.g. spina bifida, or if one parent is affected, and women who have an unexplained raised alpha-fetoprotein level on routine screening of maternal serum

---

none, whilst a male with Klinefelter's syndrome (XXY) will have one Barr body.

A buccal smear is prepared by scraping the inside of the cheek with a spatula and spread on to a slide. After staining it is examined for the presence of Barr bodies, which are usually seen in 30–60% of nuclei of normal females.

In another technique using stained smears of peripheral blood from females, the polymorphonuclear leucocytes show a small accessory nuclear lobule (a drumstick) projecting from the nuclear lobes. However, the number of drumsticks is not related to the number of X chromosomes, unlike the number of Barr bodies.

The counterpart of these studies in males is the F body (or Y chromatin), which is a fluorescent spot on the interphase nuclei of cells when stained with quinacrine. This test can be performed on buccal smears.

INHERITANCE

Unifactorial inheritance

Monogenetic disorders can be inherited as dominant, recessive or sex-linked characteristics. As chromosomes are present in duplicate, nearly all the genes are represented twice. If both the *alleles* (i.e. genes at a given locus) are the same, the subject is said to be *homozygous* for that gene. Alternatively, if there are two different genes at the same locus, the individual is said to be *heterozygous*.

A harmful mutation of one allele (i.e. heterozygous) will usually cause no harm if the other is normal. However, if both alleles are affected (i.e. homozygous), the mutation will be expressed as disease. The conditions produced are known as *recessive* disorders.

Alternatively, at the same loci, a single normal gene may not be adequate for the normal functioning of the individual. In this situation a single harmful mutation in one allele will manifest itself as disease; this is known as a *dominant* disorder.

Table 2.4 gives a list of inherited diseases. Some diseases show a racial or geographical prevalence. Thalassaemia is seen mainly in Greeks, south-east Asians and Italians, porphyria variegata occurs more frequently in the South African white population, and Tay–Sachs disease particularly occurs in Ashkenazi Jews.

Inheritance occurs according to simple Mendelian laws, making predictions of disease in offspring and therefore genetic counselling more straightforward. Disorders are usually due to defects of a single gene. Over 16 000 single gene defects are known to exist; of these approximately 900 are inherited in an autosomal dominant manner, 600 in an autosomal recessive manner and over 100 are X-linked.

Table 2.4 Some examples of inherited disorders.

Autosomal dominant
Achondroplasia
Crigler–Najjar syndrome type II
Dystrophia myotonica
Hereditary spherocytosis
Huntington's chorea
Hyperlipoproteinaemia type IIa
Marfan's syndrome
Neurofibromatosis
Osteogenesis imperfecta
Adult polycystic kidney disease
Familial adenomatous polyposis
Acute intermittent porphyria
Rotor's syndrome
Tuberous sclerosis
von Willebrand's disease (classical)

Autosomal recessive
Albinism
Ataxia telangiectasia
Crigler–Najjar syndrome type I
Cystic fibrosis
Dubin–Johnson syndrome
Fanconi syndrome
Friedreich's ataxia
Galactosaemia
Gaucher's disease
Glycogen storage disease
Hurler's syndrome
Phenylketonuria
Infantile polycystic kidney disease
Sickle cell anaemia
Tay–Sachs disease
Beta-thalassaemia
Wilson's disease

X-linked recessive
Christmas disease
Duchenne muscular dystrophy
Glucose-6-phosphate dehydrogenase deficiency
Haemophilia A
Hunter's syndrome
Nephrogenic diabetes insipidus
Menkes' syndrome
Wiskott–Aldrich syndrome

Some conditions, e.g. Ehlers–Danlos syndrome, can
have a variable inheritance.

Fig. 2.7 Different modes of inheritance. (a) Autosomal
dominant. (b) Autosomal recessive. (c) X-linked recessive.
(d) X-linked dominant.

Autosomal dominant disorders (see Fig. 2.7a)
A dominant gene can be manifested in the heterozygote form and is transmitted by an affected person
to half of his offspring. These disorders generally
produce less severe abnormalities and have a greater
variability than recessive disorders. Incomplete
penetrance is said to occur if some patients have the
dominant gene but in whom it does not manifest
itself clinically. This gives the appearance of the gene
having 'skipped' a generation when in fact it is still
present.

If the disease is very severe, affected individuals
may not survive to have children or are infertile and

therefore the condition becomes extinct in a family.
New cases appearing in a previously unaffected
family are usually a result of a new mutation, ille-
gitimacy or of one parent being minimally affected
and therefore not having been diagnosed
previously.

Other autosomal dominant traits are extremely
variable in severity, i.e. the degree to which the effect
of the gene is expressed (*variable expression*). For
example, in conditions like polydactyly patients may
have abnormalities of either all four extremities, or
only three, two or one, or the hands and feet may
even appear normal.

The overall incidence of autosomal dominant
disorders is 7 per 1000 live births.

Autosomal recessive disorders (see Fig. 2.7b)
These disorders are only present where an
individual is homozygous for that gene. Heterozygotes are usually unaffected but may be detected
by testing and are said to be *carriers*.

Recessive conditions are rare as it is unlikely that
an affected (i.e. homozygous) or heterozygous person will marry someone who is homozygous or
heterozygous for the same mutant gene. When carriers marry the offspring will have:

- A 1 in 4 chance of being homozygous and affected
- A 1 in 2 chance of being a carrier
- A 1 in 4 chance of being genetically normal

Recessive traits cannot usually be traced from one generation to the next. However, there is a 1 in 8 chance of first cousins carrying the same recessive gene. Although the offspring of marriages of first cousins have an increased perinatal mortality and an increased frequency of congenital abnormalities, the actual risks for producing an abnormal child are probably only slightly higher than in the general population.

The clinical features of autosomal recessive disorders are usually severe; patients often present in the first few years of life and have a high mortality.

Many inborn errors of metabolism are recessive diseases. The commonest recessive disease in the UK is cystic fibrosis, with 1 in 22 of the population being a carrier. Cystic fibrosis affects 1 in every 2000 live births.

The overall incidence of autosomal recessive disorders is about 2.5 per 1000 live births in the UK. World-wide, diseases such as thalassaemia and sickle cell disease are very common: the frequency of these diseases may be as high as 20 per 1000 births in some populations.

Sex-linked disorders
Genes carried on the X chromosome are said to be X-linked and can be dominant or recessive in the same way as autosomal genes.

Genes carried on the Y chromosomes are said to be Y-linked and only males can be affected. However, there are no known examples of Y-linked single gene disorders, with the possible exception of hairy ears and azoospermia (spermatogenesis may be controlled by part of the long arm of the Y chromosome).

X-linked recessive disorders (see Fig. 2.7c). In the male, X-linked recessive genes are always manifested as there is no normal gene on an additional X chromosome (as there is in the female) to oppose the action of the abnormal gene. In the female, X-linked recessive genes are only manifested when the gene is homozygous. These conditions therefore usually affect males. They are transmitted by healthy female carriers or affected males if they survive to reproduce.

The best known example of an X-linked recessive disorder is haemophilia. Half the female offspring of a carrier female (married to a normal man) will be carriers and half will be normal; half the male offspring will have haemophilia and half will not. The male offspring of a male with haemophilia will not have the disease as long as his wife is not a carrier, but all the female offspring will be carriers. Very rarely a female will have haemophilia, either because she is homozygous or due to the effect of Lyonization, which is a random process.

Other examples are shown in Table 2.4.

X-linked dominant disorders (see Fig. 2.7d). These are rare. Vitamin D resistant rickets is the best example. Females who are heterozygous for the mutant gene

Table 2.5 Some conditions that may have a polygenic inheritance.

Hypertension
Peptic ulceration
Rheumatoid arthritis
Diabetes mellitus
Epilepsy
Ischaemic heart disease
Congenital dislocation of the hip
Cleft palate
Pyloric stenosis
Congenital heart disease
Neural tube defects

and males with the gene on their single X chromosome will manifest the disease. Half the male or female offspring of an affected mother and all the female offspring of an affected man will have the disease. Affected males tend to have the disease more severely than the heterozygous female.

Sex-limited inheritance
Occasionally a gene can be carried on an autosome but manifests itself only in one sex. For example, frontal baldness is an autosomal dominant disorder in males but behaves as a recessive disorder in females.

Multifactorial inheritance

Characteristics resulting from a combination of genetic and environmental factors are said to be multifactorial; those involving multiple genes can also be said to be polygenic. Measurements of most biological factors, e.g. height, show a variation between individuals in a population and a unimodal, symmetrical (gaussian) frequency distribution curve can be drawn. This variability is due to variation in the genetic factors, the environmental factors or both. Environmental factors may play an important part in determining some characteristics, such as weight, whilst other characteristics such as intelligence or height may be largely genetically determined. The genetic component is thought to be due to the additive effects of a number of alleles at a number of loci (polygenic), many of which can be individually identified using molecular biological techniques. One such condition which has been studied is congenital pyloric stenosis. This is commoner in boys but if it occurs in girls the latter have a larger number of affected relatives. This difference suggests that a larger number of the relevant genes are required to produce the disease in girls than in boys.

Other conditions that may have a polygenic inheritance are shown in Table 2.5.

Population genetics

The genetic constitution of a population depends on many factors. The Hardy–Weinberg equilibrium is a concept, based on a mathematical equation, which describes the outcome of random mating within populations. It states that 'in the absence of mutation, non-random mating, selection and genetic drift, the genetic constitution of the population remains the same from one generation to the next'.

This genetic principle has clinical significance in terms of the number of abnormal genes in the total gene pool of a population. The Hardy–Weinberg equation states that:

$$p^2 + 2pq + q^2 = 1$$

where p is the frequency of the normal gene in the population, q is the frequency of the abnormal gene, p^2 is the frequency of the normal homozygote, q^2 is the frequency of the affected abnormal homozygote, $2pq$ is the carrier frequency, and $p + q = 1$.

This equation can be used, for example, to find the frequency of heterozygous carriers in cystic fibrosis:

The incidence of cystic fibrosis is 1 in 2000 live births. Thus, $q^2 = 1/2000$,

$$q = \sqrt{(1/2000)} = 1/44,$$
$$\text{and } p = 1 - q = 43/44$$

The carrier frequency is represented by $2pq$, i.e. $2 \times 43/44 \times 1/44 = 1/22$

Thus 1 in every 22 persons in the population is a heterozygous carrier for cystic fibrosis

Genetic counselling

People with a history of a congenital abnormality in a member of their family often seek advice about the risks of producing abnormal offspring. In any pregnancy the risk of a serious developmental abnormality is approximately 1 in 30 pregnancies and it has been suggested that 15% of paediatric inpatients have a multifactorial disorder with a predominantly genetic element. In advising patients, it is important to take a very full family history and to establish an accurate diagnosis of the condition which has occurred.

Precise genetic counselling can only be given if there is:
- A single gene defect inherited along Mendelian lines with a high penetrance and expressivity
- A chromosomal disorder (see p. 104)

In many common conditions only an empirical assessment of risk can be given. This should be explained carefully and patiently to the individuals seeking advice and the risks should be put in perspective. However, although the physician can help, the ultimate decision about whether to have children should always be left to the couple. If possible, it is advisable to send couples to the nearest genetic clinic unless the diagnosis and type of inheritance is straightforward. Prenatal diagnosis must be undertaken.

HUMAN LEUCOCYTE ANTIGENS (HLA)

The HLA system consists of a series of closely linked genetic loci situated in the major histocompatibility complex (MHC) on the short arm of chromosome 6. Fig. 2.8 shows the classification of these antigens. The class I or A, B and C series of genes are expressed on all nucleated cells, whereas the class II series of genes are expressed predominantly on B lymphocytes. A feature of these loci is that they are highly polymorphic, i.e. a large number of different alleles occur; more than 20 HLA-A, 40 HLA-B, 10 HLA-C, 15 HLA-DR and 3 HLA-DQ antigens have been identified so far. The class III series of genes express complement.

Genetic linkage

The genes at a given locus are inherited as co-dominants, so that each individual expresses both alleles, one transmitted from the mother and the other from the father. Because of the close linkage between the loci, all the genes in the MHC tend to be inherited together. The term 'haplotype' is used to indicate the particular set of HLA genes an individual carries on each chromosome 6.

Fig. 2.8 Human leucocyte antigens (HLA). A schematic diagram of the short arm of chromosome 6 showing the position of different HLA antigen classes.

'Crossing over' can occur within the HLA region. However, certain alleles occur more frequently in the same haplotype than expected by chance and this is known as linkage disequilibrium; for example, the haplotype A1 B8 occurs more frequently than would be expected from the individual gene frequencies of A1 or B8.

There is a wide inter-racial variation in HLA antigens; for example, the HLA haplotype A1 B8 is found mainly in caucasians, while the antigen B42 is seen only in blacks.

Products of the HLA genes

The HLA genes code for cell surface glycoproteins that extend from the plasma membrane to the cytoplasm and are known as class I and class II molecules. These glycoproteins consist of two chains of unequal size (alpha and beta chains), and are antigenic.

Class I molecules consist of a 45 kilodalton alpha chain, which extends through the membrane into the cytoplasm, and is encoded by the HLA genes, and a beta-2-microglobulin, which is encoded by chromosome 15. HLA-A, -B and -C antigens can be distinguished serologically by the microlymphocytotoxic test. Lymphocytes from the peripheral blood are incubated with a range of antibodies of known specificity (obtained from parous women or immunized individuals) in the presence of complement and trypan blue dye (which penetrates and stains cells with a damaged cell membrane). If the antibody does not react with the antigen, the lymphocytes survive and exclude the dye; in a positive reaction the dye enters the dead cells, indicating the presence of the specific antigen on that cell.

Class II molecules consist of an alpha (31–33 kilodaltons) and a beta chain (27–29 kilodaltons), both of which are encoded in the HLA region. They are important in presenting antigens to certain subpopulations of T cells. HLA-D antigens are recognized by the mixed lymphocyte culture (MLC) technique, which requires a panel of different HLA-D homozygous standard typing cells. The homozygous typing cell (HTC) is treated with mitomycin or irradiation to prevent it from dividing when it is cultured with the test responder lymphocytes. The latter will not proliferate (measured by incorporation of tritiated thymidine) if it possesses the same D antigen as the HTC, but it will proliferate if it lacks this antigen. The DR (D-related) antigens are very closely related to D antigens and are also detected on B cells (B cell allo-antigens) using a cytotoxic antibody test. These antigens probably are the counterpart of the 'immune-associated' (Ia) antigens on the surface of B cells and macrophages in the mouse.

Immunoregulatory function of HLA molecules

In the mouse, the *Ir* gene controls the magnitude of the immune response by helping T cell recognition of the macrophage-bound antigen. Thus T cells use HLA antigens as recognition molecules (see Fig. 2.9). Helper T (T$_H$) cells (identified by monoclonal antibody CD4) usually use class II antigens, whilst cytotoxic T cells (identified with monoclonal antibody CD8) generally use class I antigens. Thus:

- T$_H$ cells only cooperate with B cells if they share the same Ia (HLA-DR) antigens.
- Macrophages presenting an antigen to a T$_H$ cell must also share the same Ia (DR) antigen in order to stimulate it.
- Cytotoxic T cells also require the same class I HLA molecules to be present on the target cell for cytotoxicity. For example, cytotoxic lymphocytes lyse target cells which have been infected with the

Fig. 2.9 T cell recognition of macrophage-bound antigen via the HLA glycoprotein. From Batchelor JR (1984) Genetic role in autoimmunity. *Triangle* (Sandoz Journal of Medical Science) **23** (3/4): 77–83. Copyright Sandoz Ltd, Basle, Switzerland. With permission.

specific virus and carry one or more of the same class I antigens, but do not lyse target cells infected with a different virus and/or which do not share the same class I antigens.

Transplantation requirements
Tissue typing for organ grafting requires HLA typing for A, B, C and DR antigens. The match should be as close as possible as this increases graft survival. Requirements for matching in bone marrow transplantation are much more stringent, as the rejection process can be either host-versus-graft or graft-versus-host (see p. 274).

Genetic markers and disease associations
The susceptibility to certain diseases appears to be associated with certain HLA alleles (see Table 2.6). In some disorders more than one allele is required to produce the disease; for example, the highest relative risk for developing type I diabetes mellitus is the presence of both DR3 and DR4.

Coeliac disease was originally thought to be associated with HLA-DR3 and -DR7, but it has now been shown that the association is much stronger with -DQW2, which is in linkage disequilibrium with

Table 2.6 HLA associations with some clinical disorders.

HLA	Associated diseases
B8, DR3	Myasthenia gravis Thyrotoxicosis Primary Addison's disease Dermatitis herpetiformis Sjögren's syndrome Chronic active hepatitis (HbsAg negative) Systemic lupus erythematosus
B27	Ankylosing spondylitis Reiter's syndrome 'Reactive' arthritis Psoriatic arthritis Acute anterior uveitis
B8, DR3, DR7, DQW2	Coeliac disease
DR4, DR3, (B8, 15(62), 18)	Diabetes mellitus type I
DR4	Rheumatoid arthritis
A3, B14	Haemochromatosis
CW6 (B13, 17)	Psoriasis
DR2	Multiple sclerosis Narcolepsy (100% association)
B5	Behçet's syndrome

DR3-positive patients have a higher titre of autoantibodies and antibodies against viruses and other antigens. DR2-positive patients have a lower titre of antibodies and low risks for diabetes mellitus type I and myasthenia gravis.

-DR3 and -DR7. Nevertheless, no disease shows an absolute correlation with any one or more HLA allele. The likely explanation is that these genes are not disease susceptible genes per se but are in linkage disequilibrium with the as yet unidentified responsible gene.

HLA alleles and adverse drug reactions
Associations between HLA antigens and adverse drug reations are becoming increasingly recognized. For example HLA-DRW4 is present in 75% of patients with systemic lupus erythematosus (SLE) due to hydralazine compared with 25% of idiopathic SLE patients and slow acetylators who did not develop SLE on hydralazine.

Immune mechanisms in health and disease

Introduction

The exposure of an individual to foreign substances elicits an immune reaction. The results of this response are to:
- Eliminate the foreign material
- Confer protection against future contact with the antigen

Immune responses conferring protection against disease can be induced by direct infection or by artificial exposure of the individual to inactive forms of the infectious organism, i.e. immunization.

From as early as 1500 BC, attempts were made to prevent infection by immunization, but it was not until the studies of Edward Jenner in 1796 and Louis Pasteur in 1847 that the advantages of immunization were appreciated. By the end of the nineteenth century, vaccination was possible against many of the great killers of the day, including smallpox, anthrax and diphtheria.

Metchnikoff, from his studies on leucocytes carried out between 1882 and 1887, proposed a cellular mechanism of immunity which involved the destruction of invading microorganisms by phagocytosis. Cellular defence was felt to play a primary role in the immune response until the work of Bordet and Ehrlich in the 1890s. From their studies on red cell agglutination by cholera bacteria, they were able to show that the destruction of these organisms was dependent on two factors, one of which was heat stable and specific, which they called a sensitizer, and the other which was thermolabile and non-specific, which they called alexin. These two factors, now known as antibody and complement respectively, formed the basis for their theory of humoral immunity. In the end both the cellular and the humoral theories became accepted when it was established that humoral factors originated from lymphoid cells.

A glossary of terms commonly used in immunology can be found on p. 127.

Lymphoid tissue

Lymphoid organs appear early in gestation. The thymus appears first, producing cells at 8 weeks which become immunocompetent by 11 weeks. The total population of the lymphoid tissue is completed by 16 weeks of gestation.

Lymphocytes are distributed in all organs, tissues and interstitial fluids except the brain. Many lymphocytes constitute a 'circulating pool' and are constantly entering and leaving the blood and lymph. Other lymphocytes are concentrated in certain areas and constitute lymphoid organs. Lymphoid tissues in man (see Fig. 2.10) are the bone marrow, spleen, thymus, lymph nodes and mucosally associated lymphoid tissue (MALT). MALT is present in:

- The gut
- The pharynx
- The bronchi
- Breast tissue
- The genitourinary system
- The salivary and lacrimal glands

The resting lymphoid tissue consists of three areas:

- The cortex, which contains B lymphocytes
- The paracortex, which contains T lymphocytes
- The medulla, which contains connective tissue

Following antigenic stimulation the following changes result:

- The cortex contains actively dividing cells.
- The paracortex contains blast-like cells and 'germinal centres' containing actively dividing cells.
- The medulla is packed with plasma cells secreting antibodies; each plasma cell lives for a few days.

THE IMMUNE RESPONSE

The immune response has two limbs:

- The afferent limb is concerned with the recognition of the antigen, the processing of this antigen, and the induction of the immune response.
- The efferent limb, activated by contact with the antigen, sets in motion a series of cellular and humoral mechanisms against the antigen.

This series of events involves cooperation between lymphocytes and phagocytic cells and the release of many soluble factors (see below).

Cells participating in the immune response

All cells involved in the immune response are derived from a common stem cell in the marrow (see p. 260). This gives rise to the lymphoid progenitor cells, which then produce lymphocytes, or the myeloid progenitor, which then produces macrophages, monocytes, eosinophils, neutrophils and mast cells.

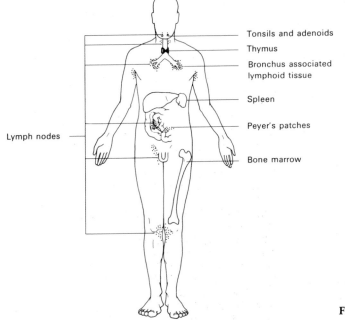

Tonsils and adenoids

Thymus

Bronchus associated lymphoid tissue

Spleen

Peyer's patches

Bone marrow

Lymph nodes

Fig. 2.10 The lymphoid system.

Lymphocytes
Lymphocytes account for up to 45% of the circulating blood leucocytes. They are divided into:
- T lymphocytes (70% of total lymphocytes)
- B lymphocytes (20% of total)
- 'Null' cells (10% of total)

T cells are mainly involved with cell-mediated immunity, whilst B cells are involved in humoral immunity. Immunological memory is carried by long-living T and B cells.

T lymphocytes. These cells migrate from the bone marrow to the thymus where they are processed by the thymic epithelial cell hormone, which transforms them into immunocompetent cells. They are activated to form 'blast' cells by specific antigens as well as non-specific mitogens such as phytohaemagglutinin (PHA); the latter can be demonstrated in vitro. This activation involves macrophages, which process and present the antigen to the lymphocytes (see Fig. 2.9).

T lymphocytes are divided into subsets depending on their role in the immune response, either regulating antibody production or taking part in delayed hypersensitivity reactions:
- T helper (T_H)
- T suppressor (T_S)
- T cytotoxic (T_C)
- T delayed hypersensitivity (T_D)

The following factors are important in T cell function:
- T_H and B cell interaction is essential for an optimal humoral response to most antigens.
- T cell mediated immunity can be transferred by giving T cells to a genetically compatible individual.
- Transfer factor, a soluble extract of T cells, can transfer some T cell functions.
- T cell interaction with antigen releases non-specific factors called *lymphokines* and *interleukin*, which amplify the immunological response (see p. 121).
- T lymphocytes live for months or years.

B lymphocytes. These are derived from the bone marrow, are thought to be processed in the fetal liver and spleen and the adult bone marrow (in mammals), and live for days or weeks. They are transformed into antibody-producing plasma cells. Antibody synthesis is inhibited by T_S cells.

T and B lymphocytes also differ in their surface receptors and markers (Table 2.7).

'Null' cells. These are lymphocytes that do not possess the phenotype surface markers of either T or B cells. They originate in the bone marrow. Some may be identical to 'killer' (K) cells, which have cytotoxic properties against target cells coated with antibody, and some may be 'natural killer' (NK) cells, which are thought to lyse certain tumour cells.

Table 2.7 Receptors and surface antigens present on T and B lymphocytes.

| | Lymphocytes | | |
	T	B	Comments
Receptors			
Complement			
C3b	−	+	
C4b	−	+	
Immunoglobulin	−	+	Receptors mainly for IgM but also for IgA, IgG and IgE
			Most are of low affinity, but 10% have high affinity receptors for IgG. It has been suggested these are 'null' cells
Sheep erythrocyte (E receptor)	+	−	Present on 60–65% of all circulating T lymphocytes
Surface antigens/markers			
1a	+	−	Present on circulating lymphocytes and involved in cell–cell cooperation
Immunoglobulin	−	+	
CD3 (T3)	+	−	Expressed on all circulating T lymphocytes (and immature T cells)
CD4 (T4)	+	−	Expressed on T helper/inducer cells Present on 55–65% of circulating T cells
CD5 (T5)	+	−	Expressed on T suppressor cells
CD8 (T8)	+	−	Present on 20–30% of circulating T cells Expressed on T cytotoxic cells/suppressor cells

Mononuclear phagocytes

Mononuclear phagocytes originate from bone marrow promonocytes. They are present as tissue macrophages and blood monocytes, which constitute approximately 5% of the total number of leucocytes. Mononuclear phagocytes bear surface receptors for IgG and IgE, and C3 and C5.

The primary activities of mononuclear phagocytes are:
- The engulfment and digestion of cell debris and foreign material. This is important in non-specific immunity.
- The presentation of partially degraded antigen–antibody complexes or free antigen to T and B lymphocytes. This is important in humoral immunity.

Neutrophils

Polymorphonuclear granulocytes (neutrophils) originate from bone marrow derived myeloid cells and circulate in the bloodstream. Neutrophils live for 6–20 h and constitute approximately 60% of the total number of leucocytes. They bear surface receptors for IgA, IgG and complement components.

Neutrophils play a primary role in non-specific immunity by engulfing and digesting microorganisms; their absence usually proves fatal.

Mast cells and basophils

Mast cells are present in the skin and mucosal surfaces, and basophils circulate in the blood, where they constitute 0.5–2% of the circulating leucocytes. Although direct proof of a common origin is lacking for these cells, they are normally grouped together due to their similar mediator content and mechanisms of activation.

Both mast cells and basophils are involved in immediate hypersensitivity reactions, when they release mediators following allergen binding to IgE on their surface (see Fig. 2.16, p. 119). They also bear receptors for complement components.

The number of basophils in the circulation is small, but may show an increase in allergic disease states. They are also seen in the secretions of patients with allergic rhinitis.

Eosinophils

Eosinophil granulocytes originate from myeloid precursors in the bone marrow and circulate in the bloodstream, where they constitute 2–5% of the total number of leucocytes, although they may account for up to 20% in individuals with immediate hypersensitivity diseases or helminth infestation (see below). They live for 6–20 h and bear receptors on their surface for IgG and complement components.

The primary activities of eosinophils are:
- The engulfment and/or digestion of antigen–antibody complexes. This is important in the immune response against helminth infestation.
- The release of enzymes that are able to inactivate biologically active substances such as histamine. This is important in type I hypersensitivity reactions.

Types of immune response

The ability of a substance to induce an immune response is termed its antigenicity and is determined by the size, foreignness and complexity of the material. The type of immune response will depend on the antigen and the immunological maturity of the immune system. It can take the form of antibody production, immune tolerance or a cell-mediated response (see p. 6).

Humoral response

Antibody production

Lymphocytes and cells of the monocyte–macrophage series play a central role in antibody production:
- Macrophages, present on mucosal surfaces and in tissues, trap the antigen and partially degrade it.
- This degraded antigen, fixed on or near the cell surface in conjunction with cell antigens, is transported and presented to T and B lymphocytes.
- Receptive T and B lymphocytes undergo 'blast formation', producing a clone (a family of cells).

Prior to antigen exposure, a few specific lymphocytes arise by random mutation. Antigen exposure, however, produces 'memory' T and B cells which rapidly generate antibody on a second exposure.

Proliferation of T and B lymphocytes produces:
- Plasma cells from B lymphocytes, which synthesize antibody
- T helper cells, which cooperate with plasma cells in the synthesis of certain antibodies
- T suppressor cells, which regulate antibody synthesis

The synthesis of antibody can be stimulated in two ways (Fig. 2.11):
- Free antigen becomes bound to the surface antigen receptor (immunoglobulin) of plasma cells. This is the method by which antibody production against thymus (T) independent antigens, such as *Escherichia coli* and pneumococcal polysaccharides, is stimulated.
- T helper cells present the antigen to the plasma cells. This is the method by which antibody production against T dependent antigens, such as serum proteins and erythrocytes, is stimulated (Fig. 2.11).

The interactions between macrophages, T lymphocytes and B lymphocytes (as shown in Fig. 2.11) occur primarily within lymphoid tissue.

The class of antibody produced depends on the

Fig. 2.11 T cell and non T cell dependent antibody production. The macrophage presents an antigen to the T or B lymphocytes, which undergo blast formation. Further differentiation leads to the formation of T helper and suppressor cells and plasma cells. Further cooperation between T helper cells and plasma cells leads to the production of antibodies, except with certain antigens (see text), when T cell cooperation is not required.

type of humoral response mounted: a primary response chiefly leads to the production of immunoglobulin M (IgM), whereas a secondary response leads to IgG production.

Immunoglobulins
These are a group of glycoproteins present in the serum and tissue fluids. All antibodies to date have been shown to be immunoglobulins, but it is not yet clear whether all immunoglobulins are antibodies.

Immunoglobulins consist of two types of polypeptide chain, heavy and light, which are linked together by disulphide bonds (Fig. 2.12).

Light chains are of two types: kappa and lambda. Heavy chains are of five types, which are determined by isotypic variation. The type of heavy chain present determines the antibody class:

- Alpha (α)—IgA
- Delta (δ)—IgD
- Epsilon (ε)—IgE
- Gamma (γ)—IgG
- Mu (μ)—IgM

Immunoglobulins all have the same basic subunit structure (Fig. 2.12) and each antibody consists of only one type of light and one type of heavy chain.

Papain splits immunoglobulins into two regions:
- A fragment with which antibody combines (Fab). This is divided into a variable (V) and constant homology (CH) region or domain. The variable region is unique for each antibody due to idiotypic variation.
- A constant region fragment (Fc) codes for α, δ, ε, γ and μ chains and determines the class of immunoglobulin. It contains two CH domains (CH2 and CH3) in IgA, IgD and IgG, and an additional one (CH4) in IgM and IgE as these have larger heavy chains. The constant region determines the cytophilic activities of immunoglobulin.

Immunoglobulins vary both in structure (Fig. 2.13) and in their physicochemical properties (Table 2.8).

Complement

Complement is a series of nine plasma proteins which become bound to antigen–antibody complexes in a specific sequence (cascade). Binding, or fixation, of complement results in either the lysis or engulfment by phagocytes of the antigen, and can occur by two major routes—the classical and the alternative pathways.

Fig. 2.12 Basic subunit structure of immunoglobulins.

IgM   IgE, IgD, IgA   Secretory IgA

--- Disulphide bonds
~~~ J-chain
|||| Secretory piece

Fig. 2.13 Structure of the different classes of immunoglobulins.

Table 2.8 Properties of immunoglobulins (Ig).

	IgA	sIgA*	IgD	IgE	IgG	IgM
Molecular weight (kilodaltons)	160	400	185	200	150	900
Proportion of Ig pool	10%	—	1%	Trace	70–75%	10%
Number of subclasses	2 (IgA$_1$, IgA$_2$)	2 (IgA$_1$, IgA$_2$)	1	1	4 (IgG$_1$, IgG$_2$, IgG$_3$, IgG$_4$)	1
Number of basic subunits	1	2	1	1	1	5
J chain†	−	+	−	−	−	+
Secretory piece‡	−	+	−	−	−	−§
Able to cross placenta	−	−	−	−	+	−
Able to fix complement	±	+	−	−	+	+
Cytophilic binding						
Mast cells/basophils	−	−	−	+	−	−
Macrophages/monocytes	−	−	−	?+	+	−
Neutrophils	+	+	−	−	+	−
Lymphocytes	+	+	−	+	+	+
Eosinophils	−	−	−	?	+	−

* Secretory IgA
† Joining chain – links immunoglobulin sub-units together
‡ Allows immunoglobulins to resist proteolysis; molecular weight = 60 kilodaltons
§ Present on secretory IgM

The classical pathway (Fig. 2.14)
- The classical pathway is triggered by two molecules of IgG or one molecule of IgM bound to antigenic material.
- The Fc sites of the antibodies produce a binding site for the first component of complement (C1).
- C1 binds to the complex in the presence of calcium and undergoes a structural transformation to become an esterase, C1a.
- C4 and C2 become bound to the complex in the

presence of magnesium ions. C1a activates the C4, 2 complex to form C3 convertase.
- The binding of C3 to the complex causes the particles which are being coated to agglutinate (immune adherence). C3 convertase splits C3 into C3a (anaphylatoxin I), which is released, and C3b, which remains bound to the complex.
- C5, C6 and C7 become bound to the complex, with the liberation of C5a (anaphylatoxin II). Some C5, 6, 7 complexes are free and can mediate

Fig. 2.14 The classical pathway of complement activation.

'bystander lysis' by attaching themselves to nearby cells.
● C8 causes cells to become 'leaky' and C9 lyses the antigenic material.

Several biologically active molecules are produced during the complement cascade:
● C3a (anaphylatoxin I) is chemotactic for neutrophils and liberates histamine from mast cells. Receptors for this complement component are present on monocytes, neutrophils, mast cells, basophils and eosinophils.
● C3b enhances engulfment of antigenic particles by phagocytes. Receptors for this complement component are present on neutrophils and eosinophils.
● C5a (anaphylatoxin II) is chemotactic for neutrophils and monocytes and also liberates histamine from mast cells. Receptors for this complement component are present on monocytes, neutrophils, mast cells, basophils and eosinophils.
● The C5,6,7 complex is chemotactic for neutrophils.

The alternative pathway (Fig. 2.15)
● The alternative pathway can be triggered by IgA, IgE, cobra venom and bacterial endotoxins. It is initiated by particle-bound C3b.
● Factor B is an 80 000 dalton protein that is bound to C3b in the presence of magnesium ions.

● Factor D is a 25 000 dalton plasma serine esterase that cleaves the C3b–factor B (3bB) complex into two fragments. The larger fragment (3bBb) remains bound and acts as a C3 convertase.
● Properdin is a 220 000 dalton protein that stabilizes the 3bBb complex.
● C3bBb acting as a C3 convertase produces a positive feedback loop that enhances the rate at which complement is fixed.
● C5, C6, C7, C8 and C9 bind as in the classical pathway, with the liberation of C5a.

Modulation of the complement cascade is achieved by several factors such as:
● C1 esterase inhibitor
● Anaphylatoxin inactivator (attacks C3a and C5a)
● C3b inactivator

Derangement of these factors leads to diseases (see below).

Immune tolerance and autoimmunity

When cells from the immune system of an animal which has not reached immunological maturity are exposed to antigenic material they are unable to produce antibodies against it. This state of specific unreactivity, which can also be acquired in adults, is termed 'immunological tolerance'.

Immunological tolerance to the body's own tissues is thought to be acquired during fetal life;

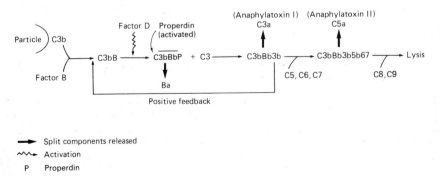

Fig. 2.15 The alternative pathway of complement activation.

therefore the body does not mount significant antibodies against its own tissues. Nevertheless, some clones of cells which can produce 'autoantibody' ('forbidden clones') are thought to be produced throughout life and are either:

- Suppressed by large amounts of 'self' antigen
- Suppressed by antigen-specific T suppressor cells

Autoimmune disease states are thought to arise when this system for mopping up forbidden clones breaks down. 'Autoantibodies' are produced to a wide variety of antigens in autoimmune disease. These antibodies may be organ-specific, e.g. intrinsic factor antibodies in pernicious anaemia, thyroid antibodies in Hashimoto's disease, or non-organ specific, e.g. antinuclear factor in systemic lupus erythematosus.

These and other autoimmune diseases are discussed in the relevant chapters.

ABNORMALITIES OF THE IMMUNE RESPONSE

Immunodeficiency diseases

Some individuals are unable to produce an immune response to antigenic material and are termed immunodeficient. Immunodeficiency may be inherited or may occur as a result of infection or drug therapy. It includes defects in antibody production, complement fixation, and lymphocyte and phagocyte functioning.

Antibody deficiency syndromes
Table 2.9 shows syndromes associated with defective antibody production.

Complement deficiencies
Deficiencies of the following can occur:

- C1 esterase inhibitor, causing hereditary angioedema (see p. 915) (the deficiency is inherited in an autosomal dominant manner)
- C1q, leading to persistent skin lesions (discoid lupus erythematosus)
- C1q, C1r, C4 or C2, causing an increased tendency to immune complex vasculitis
- C3 or C3b inhibitor, leads to exhaustion of the alternative pathway and is associated with Klinefelter's syndrome
- C5, C6, C7 or C8, caused by a genetic defect and leading to recurrent infections with *Neisseria*

Immunodeficiency diseases involving defective T lymphocyte functions
In these diseases, cell-mediated immunity is impaired in all cases. They include:

- *Thymic aplasia*, either with hypoparathyroidism (DiGeorge's syndrome) or with normal parathyroids (Nezelof syndrome). Antibody production is normal but patients usually die in infancy. Fungal infections are common (see p. 67).
- *Purine nucleoside phosphorylase deficiency*. Antibody production is normal but some patients also have abnormal red blood cells.
- *Ataxia telangiectasia*. This is inherited as an autosomal recessive and is associated with selective IgA deficiency, cerebellar ataxia and oculocutaneous telangiectasia. Onset is early and children die in the second decade due to infections.
- *Wiskott–Aldrich syndrome*. This is an X-linked recessive defect thought to involve faulty presentation of antigen by macrophages. Males present with thrombocytopenia, eczema and recurrent infections. The immunoglobulins are normal but no antibody is produced against polysaccharide antigens.
- *Bloom's syndrome*. Immunoglobulin levels are reduced, with sometimes only IgA being affected. Lymphomas are seen.
- *Severe combined immunodeficiency (SCID)*. This presents in the first few months of life and has a variable inheritance. No specific antibodies are produced and low numbers of T and B lymphocytes are seen. Death is usual before the age of 2 years. It can occur in association with other diseases, e.g. short-limbed dwarfism.

Immunodeficiency diseases involving defective phagocyte functions
Patients suffer from repeated infections, mainly involving the skin. Diseases include:

- *Job's syndrome*. High levels of serum IgE and defective neutrophil chemotaxis are seen.
- *Chronic granulomatous disease (CGD)*. This is a sex-linked disease in which chemotaxis is normal but intracellular killing of catalase-positive organisms in polymorphonuclear leucocytes and macrophages is impaired.
- *Chédiak–Higashi syndrome*. Neutrophil lysosomal formation is affected, leading to impaired killing. It is associated with oculocutaneous albinism, and staphylococcal and candidal infections are common.
- *Myeloperoxidase deficiency*. This is an autosomally recessive-linked disease producing reduced levels of myeloperoxidase enzyme in neutrophils and monocytes. Systemic candidiasis is common.

Hypersensitivity reactions

Immunological priming can lead, on further exposure to antigen, to either secondary boosting of the immune response or to an excessive damaging reaction termed hypersensitivity. Six types of hypersensitivity have been described (Fig. 2.16 and Table 2.10): types I, II, III and V are mediated by antibody and types IV and VI by cellular mechanisms. In practice, these reactions may not necessarily occur

Table 2.9 Immunodeficiency syndromes associated with defective antibody production.

Syndrome	Antibodies/immunoglobulins	Circulating B lymphocytes	Circulating T lymphocytes	Comments
X-linked 'agamma-globulinaemia'	Small amounts of IgG and IgM	Absent	Immature	Familial. Sometimes only male offspring and siblings affected
Transient hypogamma-globulinaemia in childhood	Produced against potent antigens, e.g. tetanus toxoid, only	Normal	Low numbers of T helper cells	Recurrent infections
Late onset primary hypogammaglobulinaemia	Low levels, especially of IgA	Normal, produce mainly IgM	Fail to differentiate. Some patients have increased numbers of T suppressor cells	Recurrent respiratory tract infections, especially *H. influenzae*. Also gut infections, haematological abnormalities and arthritis
Functional antibody deficiency	Impaired response to antigens such as tetanus toxoid	Normal	Normal	Mechanisms unknown. May follow chronic infection or smoking
Thymoma and hypogamma-globulinaemia	Low IgA. Moderate hypogammaglobulinaemia	Absent (also precursors)	Normal	Patients usually 40–70 years of age at presentation
Low IgG and IgA with hyper-IgM	Low levels of IgG and IgA, high levels of IgM			
IgA deficiency	IgG and IgM normal. IgM and IgD found in secretions	Normal	Normal	
IgG subclass deficiencies	IgM and IgA normal. Sometimes IgG normal, except for one subclass			Sometimes familial
IgM deficiency	Normal	Normal	T helper cell defect	Rare. Usually other immunoglobulins involved

Fig. 2.16 Hypersensitivity reactions. (a) Type I: immediate anaphylactic hypersensitivity. (b) Type II: membrane damage/cytolytic hypersensitivity. (c) Type III: immune complex hypersensitivity. (d) Type IV: delayed hypersensitivity. (e) Type V: stimulatory hypersensitivity. (f) Type VI: antibody-dependent cell-mediated cytotoxicity (ADCC). MAF = macrophage-activating factor.

singly. For example, types II–VI may be involved in producing autoimmune diseases.

Type I reaction (reaginic/anaphylactic/immediate hypersensitivity reaction)
This is an allergic reaction produced within 30 min of exposure to a specific allergen. Allergens, e.g. house dust, pollens, animal danders or moulds, only elicit reactions in certain genetically predisposed individuals, who are said to be atopic (see p. 586). Atopy is diagnosed on skin prick testing (see Fig. 12.16, p. 570), when a reaction is elicited by sensitizing allergens. Allergic reactions were first described by Prausnitz and Küstner in 1921, who showed that the passive transfer of a serum factor (reagin) from an allergic person to the skin of a normal person could produce a reaction in the latter in response to the allergen. Küstner was allergic to fish. His serum was injected into the skin of Prausnitz, who was not allergic to fish. When fish antigen was injected into the sensitized site, an immediate wheal and flare reaction occurred.

Type I reactions occur as follows:
- The allergen stimulates B cells to produce specific IgE, with the aid of T helper cells.
- This IgE, which is allergen-specific, binds to mast cells via their Fc receptors.
- On subsequent exposure to the allergen, the allergen cross-links the surface-bound IgE on the sensitized mast cell.

- This triggers the mast cell to degranulate and release mediators, producing the type I hypersensitivity reaction.

Type II reactions (cytotoxic/membrane reactions)
In this type of reaction, antibodies of the IgG or IgM class are directed against cell surface or tissue antigens. These antibodies interact via their Fc regions and fix complement as well as the effector cell. Thus antibodies are produced against antigens on the patient's own cells and can lead to the development of autoimmune diseases, e.g. autoimmune haemolytic anaemia.

Antibodies can also 'block' a receptor site, preventing its normal function: for example, in insulin-resistant diabetes antibodies react with the insulin receptors. In this particular type of reaction complement is not involved.

In certain conditions, IgG autoantibodies are present but it is not clear whether they are involved in the pathogenesis of the disease, e.g. intrinsic factor antibodies are found in pernicious anaemia.

Type III reactions (immune complex mediated hypersensitivity reactions)
Antibodies (IgG or IgM) can complex with antigen to form immune complexes. These are usually removed by the reticuloendothelial system, but a hypersensitivity reaction can sometimes occur when these complexes are deposited in the tissues. Complement

Table 2.10 Summary of hypersensitivity reactions.

	I (immediate)	II (cytotoxic)	III (immune complex)	IV (delayed)	V (stimulating)	VI (antibody-dependent cell-mediated cytotoxicity)*
Antigens	Dust, pollens, moulds, mites, drugs, food and parasites	Cell surface or tissue bound	Exogenous (bacteria, fungi, parasites) Autoantigens	Cell/tissue bound	Cell surface	Antibody complexed on cell surface of target cells
Mediators	IgE and mast cells	IgG, IgM and complement	IgG, IgM, IgA and complement	T_D, T_C activated macrophages and lymphokines	IgG	K cells
Diagnostic tests	Skin prick tests—wheal and flare RAST	Coombs' test Indirect immunofluorescence (antibodies) Red cell agglutination Precipitating antibodies	Skin test—oedema, erythema (Arthus reaction) Immune complexes	Skin test—erythema induration (e.g. tuberculin test)	Indirect immunofluorescence	As for type II
Time taken for reaction to develop	15-30 min	Rapid	4-12 h	12-48 h	Variable	Variable
Histology	Oedema, vasodilatation, mast cell degranulation, eosinophils	Damage to target cells	Acute inflammatory reaction, neutrophils, vasculitis	Perivascular inflammation, mononuclear cells, fibrin Caseation and necrosis in TB	Hypertrophy	Damage to target cells
Diseases and conditions produced	Asthma (extrinsic) Eczema (atopic) Urticaria Allergic rhinitis Anaphylaxis	Autoimmune haemolytic anaemia Transfusion reactions Haemolytic disease of newborn Goodpasture's syndrome Addisonian pernicious anaemia Myasthenia gravis	Autoimmune e.g. SLE, glomerulonephritis, rheumatoid arthritis Low-grade persistent infections, e.g. viral hepatitis Disease caused by environmental antigens, e.g. farmer's lung	Pulmonary TB Contact dermatitis Graft-versus-host disease Insect bites Leprosy	Neonatal hyperthyroidism Graves' disease	Autoimmune tumour rejection Defence against helminthic infection
Treatment	Antigen avoidance Antihistamines Corticosteroids (usually local) Sodium cromoglycate	Exchange transfusion Plasmapheresis	Corticosteroids Immunosuppressives Plasmapheresis	Immunosuppressives Corticosteroids	Treatment of individual disease	Treat symptomatically

* Type VI hypersensitivity may also be classified with type II reactions.

is activated and this results in an inflammatory reaction leading to cellular damage.

Immune complexes can be:

● *Soluble.* These are formed when the antigen is in excess and can be produced, for example, by injecting large amounts of heterogenic serum into the circulation, leading to 'serum sickness'.

● *Insoluble.* These precipitates are formed when the concentrations of antibody and antigen are equivalent or when there is an excess of antibody. The size of the complexes determines the site at which they are deposited. An intradermal injection of antigen in a patient with a high circulating level of antibody will produce a red, oedematous area at the site of the injection within 4–12 h. This is called the 'Arthus reaction'. Examples of conditions in which insoluble complexes are formed include pulmonary aspergillosis (when the complexes are deposited in bronchial walls) and erythema nodosum (when the complexes are deposited in the vessels).

Tissue damage occurs as follows:

● Complement fixation leads to generation of C3a and C5a.
● C3a and C5a have chemotactic properties and cause release of vasoactive amines from mast cells and basophils.
● Vascular permeability is thus increased and polymorphonuclear leucocytes are sequestered.
● Lysosomal enzymes are released and cause tissue damage.
● Complexes also interact with platelets through their Fc receptors, causing them to aggregate and microthrombi to form.

The diseases produced by immune complex deposition can be divided according to the type of antigen:

● Autoimmune diseases, e.g. systemic lupus erythematosus, are caused by the production of an antibody to a *self-antigen*, which leads to immune complex formation and deposition.
● Low-grade persistent infection with a *microbial antigen* with a weak antibody response leads to chronic immune complex formation, e.g. in viral hepatitis B or staphylococcal infective endocarditis.
● Repeated inhalation of an *environmental antigen*, e.g. moulds or an animal antigen, can produce an extrinsic allergic alveolitis, e.g. farmer's lung disease. The antibodies are IgG rather than IgE.

Type IV reactions (cell-mediated/delayed hypersensitivity reactions)
These reactions take more than 12 h to develop and can be produced in several ways (see below). Type IV reactions can be transferred from one animal to another by certain types of lymphocytes but not by serum.

The reaction is mediated by:

● T delayed hypersensitivity cells (T_D) that have become sensitized to a particular antigen previously; these release lymphokines and interleukins
● T cytotoxic cells (T_C), which directly damage infected target cells, e.g. virus-infected cells, allogenic cells or host cells in graft-versus-host disease.

Lymphokines have several activities (see Fig. 12.29, p. 589), including:

● The production of macrophage activation factor (MAF) and migration inhibition factor (MIF), which increase the ability of macrophages to kill
● The production of chemotactic factors. Lymphokines attract macrophages, neutrophils, eosinophils and basophils.
● The inhibition of leucocyte migration
● The production of mitogenic factor, which causes mitosis in uncommitted lymphocytes
● They prevent viral replication by the production of interferon by the lymphocytes.
● The production of skin reactive factor, which causes cellular exudation

Interleukins are specific lymphokines which pass signals between cells of the immune system and affect antibody production.

● *Interleukin-1 (IL-1)* is produced by macrophages that have been stimulated with MAF. It used to be called leucocyte activating factor (LAF). It causes T helper cells to differentiate, and these cells then secrete another lymphokine called interleukin-2.
● *Interleukin-2 (IL-2)* comprises T cell growth factor (TCGF), which allows clonal expansion of specific T helper and cytotoxic cells, and T cell replacing factor, which allows B lymphocytes to differentiate into plasma cells.
● *Interleukin-3 (IL-3)* is released by lymphocytes and promotes the differentiation of and/or amplification of T helper cells.

Cell recruitment in type IV reactions is initially neutrophil in nature (within a few hours) and is followed by lymphocyte and macrophage infiltration (24–48 h).

Type IV reactions are seen in association with viral infections, tuberculosis and brucellosis. They have also been implicated in autoimmune diseases such as Hashimoto's thyroiditis and homograft rejection.

Type V reaction (stimulating antibody reaction)
Antibodies of the IgG class directed against cell surface antigens can 'stimulate' some cells instead of killing them. They may be important in the pathogenesis of neonatal hyperthyroidism, as IgG

stimulating antibodies directed against thyroid cells would be capable of crossing the placenta.

Type VI reaction (antibody-dependent cell-mediated cytotoxicity; ADCC)

Killer lymphocytes (K cells) can lyse target cells coated with antibody. They are 'activated' by antigen–antibody complexes. The K cells interact with the Fc region of cell-bound antibody, and destroy the target cells by the release of proteolytic enzymes.

Type VI reactions are involved in autoimmune diseases, tumour rejection and defence against helminthic parasites.

RESISTANCE TO INFECTION

Innate immunity

Mechanical barriers
Skin. Entry to the skin is prevented by:
- The upper, hard keratinized layer of epidermis
- Antimicrobial substances, i.e. lactic and fatty acids present in sweat

Mucosal surfaces. Protection of mucosal surfaces is achieved by:
- Mucus. This forms an adhesive blanket that traps foreign material. It is secreted by the ciliated layer of respiratory mucosal cells and is eliminated from the respiratory tract by coughing, sneezing and swallowing, and by defecation from the gastrointestinal tract.
- Bacterial competition. The gut flora prevents colonization by pathogenic bacteria by competing for nutrients. The gut also secretes antibacterial substances.
- The flushing action of tears, urine and saliva
- Antimicrobial substances present in secretions. For example, lysozyme, a proteolytic enzyme which destroys bacterial cell walls, is present in nasal secretions, saliva and tears.

Systemic immunity
Humoral mechanisms. These include:
- Interferon. This prevents viral replication and infection by a second virus. It is synthesized by infected cells.
- Lysozyme
- 'Natural' antibody. This is found in the absence of specific antigen, probably due to contact with organisms possessing related antigens. It is chiefly of the IgM class and fixes complement. Examples include antibodies active against typhoid endotoxin and *Streptococcus viridans*.
- C-reactive protein. The blood level is raised in any acute infection, e.g. pneumonia, or in an inflam-

matory reaction. C-reactive protein attaches to, for example, the *Pneumococcus* antigen and binds complement, opsonizing or lysing the bacteria.

Cellular mechanisms. Opsonized particles are engulfed and digested by neutrophil and mononuclear phagocytes.

Acquired immunity

Humoral defences
These are involved in immune responses against bacteria and extracellular viruses and include:
- Opsonization and phagocytosis. These mechanisms provide an efficient clearance mechanism in patients with a normal immune system. IgG, IgM and IgA are involved. Failure of this mechanism results in recurrent infections, as seen in patients with immunodeficiency diseases.
- Complement fixation and lysis
- Prevention of adherence of microorganisms at mucosal surfaces by specific secretory IgA. Some organisms, e.g. *Neisseria meningitidis*, overcome this by producing an IgA protease.

Cell-mediated defences
These are involved in immunity against intracellular viruses, parasites, and bacteria resistant to phagocytosis.

Viruses. The following occur (see Fig. 2.17):
- Interferon is released by T lymphocytes and macrophages.
- T cytotoxic cells kill infected cells and halt viral spread if it has not been transferred to another cell.
- Activated macrophages (activated by MAF released by sensitized T cells) break intracellular bridges, preventing viral spread.

Protozoa and bacteria resistant to phagocytosis. Activated macrophages (activated by MAF from sensitized T cells) can eliminate protozoa and organisms which normally survive phagocytosis such as *Leishmania braziliensis*, *Toxoplasma gondii*, *Mycobacterium leprae* and *tuberculosis*, and *Listeria monocytogenes* (see Fig. 2.18).

Helminths. Antibodies can kill helminths, e.g. *Schistosoma mansoni*, by mechanisms involving antibody-dependent cytotoxicity. Cytotoxic cells, e.g. eosinophils or macrophages, adhere to worms via the Fc and C3 receptors in the presence of antibodies. Eosinophils bind to the opsonized helminth and destroy it by releasing eosinophil cationic protein and major basic protein.

Fig. 2.17 Cell-mediated immunity against viruses (see text). MAF = macrophage-activation factor; MIF = macrophage-inhibition factor.

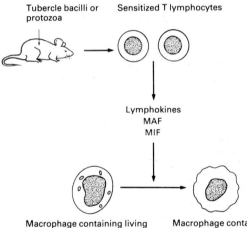

Macrophage containing living tubercle bacilli or protozoa   Macrophage containing no surviving organisms

Fig. 2.18 Cell-mediated immunity against bacterial and protozoal infections. Many bacteria and protozoa can survive within phagocytic cells (macrophages). These cells may be activated by products (lymphokines) from specifically sensitized T lymphocytes, causing release of intracellular lysosomal enzymes and destruction of the infecting agents. MAF = macrophage-activation factor; MIF = macrophage-inhibition factor.

INVESTIGATIONS

Measurement of immunoglobulins and other proteins

Immunoprecipitation
Immune precipitates are formed when antigen and antibody are combined in proportions of near equivalence. This technique is used for estimation of the concentration of many proteins.

In the single radial immunodiffusion test, an antiserum specific for the heavy chain of the immunoglobulin to be measured, is mixed with melted agar and poured on to a plate. When set, holes are cut and the patient's serum as well as a series of control immunoglobulins to form a standard curve are placed in the well. The diameter of precipitate produced is measured and read off the standard curve to give the actual concentration.

Immunoelectrophoresis
This involves separation of antigens present in, for example, serum by placing an electric charge across it on an agar plate. Positively charged proteins move to the negative electrode and vice versa. A longitudinal trough is then cut in the agar parallel to the direction of the current and filled with antibody. The antibody diffuses into the agar, and arcs of precipitates form where antigen and antibody meet. The plates can then be stained. Serum protein electrophoresis will screen for paraproteins (monoclonal bands).

In counter-current electrophoresis the pH of the gel is chosen so that the antibody is positively charged and the antigen negatively charged. On passing a current, the antigen and antibody move towards each other and precipitate; this increases the sensitivity of the test. In rocket electrophoresis antigens are electrophoresed into an antibody-containing gel.

For the measurement of cryoglobulin (i.e. immunoglobulins that form precipitates in the cold), a fresh specimen of blood should be taken in a warm syringe and allowed to clot at 37°C. The serum should then be left at 4°C for 48 h to precipitate the cryoglobulin. The precipitate redissolves on warming back to 37°C, at which temperature the tests are then performed.

Bence Jones proteins (free monoclonal light chains) are detected in concentrated urine on cellulose acetate electrophoresis, when an M band is seen. The presence of monoclonal free kappa or lambda light chains can be confirmed using immunoelectrophoresis.

Radioimmunoassay (RIA), enzyme-linked immunoabsorbent assay (ELISA) and the radioallergosorbent test (RAST)
These are extremely sensitive methods of detecting antigens and antibodies in low concentrations.

RIA. This is described on p. 684.

ELISA. This method is like RIA but the ligand used not only detects the antibody but is also coupled to an enzyme, e.g. peroxidase which can be visualized by adding chromogen. Chromogen is colourless but becomes coloured when the enzyme portion of the ligand acts on it. The coloured end-product, i.e. the amount of antibody, is measured by optical density scanning of the plate.

RAST. This test measures IgE to a specific antigen. It is like RIA but the allergen (antigen) is bound to a tiny cellulose disc rather than a large plastic plate, thus increasing the ability of the test to detect tiny amounts of IgE in the serum. The ligand used is labelled anti-IgE antibody.

Antibodies that can be detected include intrinsic factor antibody, double-stranded DNA antibody, glomerular basement membrane antibody, acetylcholine receptor antibody and platelet antibody. Specific IgE antibodies to inhalants or food can also be measured.

Autoantibodies
These can be detected by haemagglutination, indirect immunofluorescence or counter-current immunoelectrophoresis.

Haemagglutination. This depends on the ability of the antibody to cross-link surface antigens on red blood cells. The antibody is serially diluted in wells with saline; positive and negative controls are also used. A red cell suspension is added to each well. If no antibody is present the cells settle to form a pellet; if antibody is present, it agglutinates the red cells to form a hazy red appearance.

This test is used to detect rheumatoid factor, thyroglobulin antibody, thyroid microsomal antibody and erythrocyte autoantibodies (Coombs' test; see p. 285).

Indirect immunofluorescence. This detects autoantibodies and antibodies to tissues and cellular antigens. Sections of frozen animal tissues (e.g. liver, kidney, stomach or thyroid) are cut at −20°C on a cryostat. The sections are incubated with the patient's serum, washed and then incubated with a second antibody with a fluorescein tag. The latter reacts with any antibody in the patient's serum which has combined with antigens in the substrate and can be visualized using fluorescent microscopy.

This test is used to detect nuclear, smooth muscle, mitochondrial, reticulin, DNA, gastric parietal cells, thyroid microsomal, adrenal, pancreatic islet cell, salivary gland, skeletal muscle, cardiac muscle and skin antibodies.

Counter-current immunoelectrophoresis. This is used for detecting autoantibodies against 'extractable nuclear antigens'.

Skin tests for antigens and allergens

Prick tests
Prick tests for type I IgE-mediated reactions to allergens are described on p. 570.

Intradermal tests
These are used to demonstrate the Arthus reaction (appearing after 6–24 h) to fungal antigens (e.g. *Aspergillus*) or bird proteins. Delayed hypersensitivity can also be demonstrated, e.g. using tuberculin in the Mantoux test (p. 602). Immune deficiency can be assessed by testing with a panel of common antigens such as *Candida albicans*, streptokinase–streptodornase or mumps virus. Ninety-five per cent of normal adults respond to at least one of these antigens. Children not exposed to these antigens can be tested by sensitization followed by a challenge with dinitrochlorobenzene (DNCB).

Patch tests (see p. 907)
These demonstrate delayed hypersensitivity to a variety of sensitizing antigens in contact dermatitis, e.g. ointments, rubber extracts or metallic ions.

Detection of immune complexes

Immune complexes can be detected by looking for evidence of complex deposition in tissues using direct immunofluorescence or by measuring complexes in the blood or in body fluids. There are many methods based on either the physical properties (e.g. morphology and size) or biological properties of the immune complexes. The latter include complement binding (e.g. the C1q binding assay) or cell binding to either Fc receptors (e.g. platelet aggregation) or to Fc and C3b receptors (e.g. Raji cell assay).

All methods detect aggregated immunoglobulin and therefore immune complexes are sometimes difficult to distinguish from non-specifically aggregated immunoglobulins. These tests are not routinely performed and are not essential for the diagnosis of diseases thought to be mediated by immune complexes.

Lymphocyte separation

Lymphocytes can be separated from other blood constituents by using their different densities. Diluted defibrinated whole blood is layered on top of Ficoll Isopaque and centrifuged. The lymphocytes settle at the plasma–Ficoll interface, whilst other blood constituents fall to the bottom.

Human T lymphocytes have receptors for sheep red cells and form rosettes when mixed together. They can be separated from non-rosetting B cells by using Ficoll gradients as above.

Lymphocyte subpopulations can also be separated on antibody-sensitized plates where antigen-positive cells will bind to the plate and antigen-negative cells are washed off. Thus T cells can be separated from B cells by using anti-Ig which binds B cells or T_H from T_S by using the appropriate antibody.

Monoclonal antisera can distinguish and quantitate helper T cells, which stain with horse-radish peroxidase linked CD4, from suppressor/cytotoxic T cells, which stain with linked CD8 (OKT8).

B lymphocytes have surface immunoglobulins which can be identified by direct immuno-fluorescence using fluorescein-conjugated antisera to human immunoglobulin. They can then be counted with a fluorescent microscope or by using a fluorescent activated cell sorter (FACS).

In vitro tests of cell-mediated immunity

Lymphocyte transformation test
When sensitized lymphocytes are cultured with the appropriate antigen they undergo blast transformation and DNA is synthesized. This can be measured by adding tritiated thymidine 16 h before the cells are harvested. Thymidine is taken up by the cells and incorporated into DNA. The radioactivity of the cells is measured; a high count indicates lymphocyte transformation and thus sensitivity to the antigen.

Macrophage migration inhibition test
Lymphocytes produce lymphokines when exposed to a sensitizing antigen. One of these lymphokines is the macrophage migration inhibition factor (MIF). Macrophages and lymphocytes are packed into capillary tubes and cultured in media with and without antigen. If migration of the cells out of the capillary tubes is inhibited it suggests that the lymphocytes are sensitive to the antigen and are producing MIF.

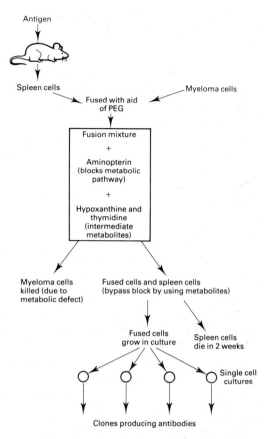

Fig. 2.19 Monoclonal antibody production. PEG = polyethylene glycol.

Monoclonal antibody production

This involves the production of a cell which can generate a single specific antibody (Fig. 2.19).

Glossary

TERMS COMMONLY USED IN GENETICS

Acrocentric—used to describe a chromosome in which the centromere lies close to one end, producing one long and one short arm

Allele (allelomorph)—alternative form of a gene occupying the same locus on a particular chromosome

Aneuploid—used to describe cells with a chromosomal number which is not the exact multiple of the normal haploid number

Autosome—any chromosome that is not a sex chromosome; there are 22 pairs of autosomes in humans

Centromere—the point at which two chromatids of a chromosome are joined and also where the spindle fibres become attached during mitosis and meiosis

Character (trait)—an observable phenotypic feature of an individual

Chromatid—one of the two strands, held together by the centromere, which make up the chromosome as seen during cell division

Chromosomal aberration—an abnormality in the number or structure of a chromosome

Chromosome—a thread-like body containing DNA and protein, situated in the nucleus, and carrying genetic information

Cistron—the smallest unit of genetic material which is responsible for the synthesis of a specific polypeptide; also known as a gene

Clone—cells having the same genetic constitution and derived from a single cell by repeated mitoses

Codon—three adjacent nucleotides in a nucleic acid which code for one amino acid

Concordance—the occurrence of the same trait in both members of a pair of twins

Deletion—loss of a part of a chromosome

Diploid—used to describe cells containing two sets of chromosomes

Dominant—used to describe a trait expressed in individuals who are heterozygous for a particular gene

Expressivity—the degree to which the effect of a gene is expressed

Gene—part of a DNA molecule which directs the synthesis of a specific polypeptide chain; it consists of many codons

Gene pool—the total genetic information contained in all the genes in a breeding population at a given time

Genetic marker—a genetically controlled phenotypic feature used in inheritance studies

Genetics—the science of heredity and variation

Genome—the total amount of genetic material in the cell

Genotype—the genetic constitution of an individual

Haploid—used to describe cells containing one set of chromosomes

Heterozygote—an individual possessing two different alleles at the corresponding loci on a pair of homologous chromosomes

Homozygote—an individual possessing identical alleles at the corresponding loci on a pair of homologous chromosomes

Hybrid—the progeny of a cross between two genetically different organisms

Hybridization—the pairing of complementary DNA or RNA strands to give DNA–DNA or DNA–RNA strands; for example, it is used to search for particular DNA fragments after Southern blotting

Karotype—the number, size and shape of the chromosomes in a cell

Linkage disequilibrium—the association of particular alleles at two linked loci more frequently than expected by chance

Locus—the site of a gene on a chromosome

Monosomy—loss of one chromosome of a homologous pair, resulting in 45 chromosomes

Non-disjunction—failure of a chromosome pair to separate during cell division, resulting in both chromosomes passing to the same daughter cell

Nucleotide—the basic unit of nucleic acids, which is made up of a pyrimidine or purine base, a pentose sugar and a phosphate group

Penetrance—the proportion of individuals with a particular genotype who also have the corresponding phenotype; full penetrance occurs when a dominant trait is always seen in an individual with one such allele, or when a recessive trait is seen in all individuals possessing two such alleles

Phenotype—the appearance of an individual resulting from the effects of both environment and genes

Recessive—used to describe a trait expressed in individuals who are homozygous for a particular gene but not seen in the heterozygote

Sex linkage—genes carried on the sex chromosomes

Transcription—the process by which genetic information is transmitted from the DNA in the chromosomes to messenger RNA

Translation—the process by which genetic information from messenger RNA is 'translated' into protein synthesis

Translocation—the transfer of a piece of one chromosome to another non-homologous chromosome

Trisomy—representation of a chromosome three times rather than twice, giving a total of 47 chromosomes

TERMS COMMONLY USED IN IMMUNOLOGY

Allergen—an antigen provoking an allergic response; the term usually restricted to antigens such as grass pollen involved in type I hypersensitivity

Allergy—*see* Immune response

Allotype—genetically determined epitopes which vary between different members of the same species, e.g. blood group antigens

Antibody—an immunoglobulin capable of binding to an antigen via specific areas of the protein termed combining sites

Antigen—a substance which produces an immune response when introduced into a vertebrate animal

Atopy—genetically determined tendency to develop immediate hypersensitivity/allergic reactions to common allergens involving the production of immunoglobulin E

Complement—a serum enzyme cascade usually activated by antibody–antigen complexes; the enzymes released are capable of lysing red cells, nucleated cells and bacteria to which antibody is attached

Cell cooperation—cell interaction which is either between T and B lymphocytes, which leads to antibody production, or between T lymphocytes, which regulates humoral immunity

Cell-mediated immunity—specific immunity which is dependent on T lymphocytes

Epitope—an antigenic determinant of known molecular structure present on complex antigens

Graft-versus-host reaction—the response of a graft containing immunologically functional cells against its non-identical host or recipient

Idiotype—the unique determinant present in the antigen combining site of an antibody

Immune response—the development of a state of altered reactivity following exposure to an antigen; it may be cell-mediated, humoral or both

Immunoglobulin—a glycoprotein composed of heavy and light polypeptide chains; the class to which immunoglobulins belong is determined by the type of heavy chain

Immunological tolerance—the development of a specific unresponsiveness to a particular antigen which, in other circumstances, is capable of inducing an immune reaction

Isotype—antigenic variation common to all members of the same species, e.g. differences in the immunoglobulin chains and classes

Monoclonal antibody—an antibody produced by a single clone (family) of cells

Opsonization—the coating of, e.g. microorganisms, with either antibody or antibody and complement; it facilitates phagocytosis of the particles

Paratope—the part of an antibody that combines with the epitope of an antigen

Phagocytosis—the process of engulfment of particles, e.g. microorganisms, by cells

Syngeneic (isogeneic)—used to describe cells or tissues transferred between genetically identical individuals (e.g. identical twins)

Vaccine—material containing antigens. May be:
- Inactivated (contains organisms incapable of replication, e.g. whooping cough vaccines)
- Live (actual pathogen given by unusual route, e.g. contagious bovine pleuropneumonia vaccine)
- Attenuated (live vaccine containing organisms treated to lose their virulence, e.g. polio and BCG vaccines)
- Heterologous (protects against organisms not present in the vaccine by cross-reaction, e.g. cowpox vaccine protects against smallpox)

Xenogeneic (heterogeneic)—used to describe cells or tissues transferred between different species

Further reading

Emery AEH (1983) *Elements of Medical Genetics*, 6th edn. Edinburgh: Churchill Livingstone.

Galton DJ (1985) *Molecular Genetics of Common Metabolic Disease*. London: Edward Arnold.

Harper PS (1984) *Classical Genetic Counselling*. Bristol: John Wright.

Holborrow EJ & Reeves WG (1983) *Immunology in Medicine* London: Grune and Stratton.

McKusick VA (1983) *Mendelian Inheritance in Man*, 6th edn. Baltimore: Johns Hopkins University Press.

Roitt I, Brostoff J & Male D (1985) *Immunology*. London: Gower Medical/Churchill Livingstone.

Weatherall DJ (1986) *The New Genetics in Clinical Practice*, 2nd edn. Oxford: Oxford University Press.

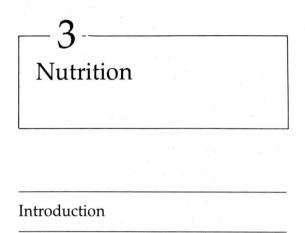

3
Nutrition

Introduction

In the Western World, excess food is available and the commonest nutritional problem is obesity. In the Third World, a lack of food supply and poor utilization of the available food results in protein–energy malnutrition.

Diet and disease can be interrelated in many ways. First, diet can be a causative factor in the development of certain diseases. Excess energy intake, particularly when high in animal (saturated) fat content, is thought to be responsible for a number of diseases including ischaemic heart disease and diabetes. The importance of the relationship between nutrition and cancer has been realized in recent years, largely due to epidemiological studies. There is evidence that vitamin A deficiency may be associated with certain tumours, and a high fat intake is also thought to be of importance in producing cancer. Numerous carcinogens, either intentionally added to food, e.g. nitrates for preserving foods, or accidental contaminants, e.g. moulds producing aflatoxin and fungi, may also be involved in the development of cancer.

Second, special diets are necessary to control certain disease states, e.g. a low sodium diet can be used in renal and liver disease and a gluten-free diet in coeliac disease.

Finally, the proportion of processed foods eaten may affect the development of disease. A number of processed convenience foods have a high sugar and high fat content and therefore predispose to obesity and dental caries. They also have a low fibre content, and dietary fibre is possibly important in the prevention of a number of diseases (see p. 130).

A link between diet and disease is also present when industrial pollution of food supplies occurs, e.g. with insecticides, herbicides or preservatives.

The overall role of the doctor is not only to advise the patient to take a balanced diet, but also to help him avoid any 'food fadism' which can easily develop as a result of extensive advertisements based on commercial interests rather than concerns about health.

Water and electrolyte balance
Water and electrolyte balance is dealt with fully in Chapter 10. Approximately 1 l of water per day is required in the diet to balance insensible losses, but much more is usually drunk, the kidneys being able to excrete large quantities.

Energy balance
Food is necessary to provide the body with energy (Fig. 3.1). The oxidation of carbohydrate, fat and protein eventually leads to the generation of high-energy bonds in adenotriphosphate (ATP), which is then used for all energy requirements. In addition to providing energy, some of these oxidative products are utilized to generate the carbohydrates, fats and proteins of which the body is composed.

Table 3.1 shows the normal energy requirements in man. These increase with exercise, fever and trauma. In the basal state, energy demands for muscle are 30% of the total energy required, abdominal organs 25%, brain 20% and heart 10%. The increase in muscle energy requirements during exercise is 10-fold.

The normal body composition of a 70 kg man is shown in Table 3.2. Energy is derived from various stores. The fat content of the body is extremely variable; it may be increased twofold in an obese subject. One-third of protein (e.g. in bone) is unavailable as an energy source, muscle being the main available protein source. Muscle contains three times its own weight of water and protein breakdown provides only 4 kcal (17 kJ) of energy per gram. This compares with fat which is anhydrous and provides 9 kcal (37 kJ) of energy per gram. Adipose tissue is therefore an efficient way of storing energy and is the only major source of fuel available, apart from muscle protein, in the long-term fasting state. Fat is broken down into free fatty acids and

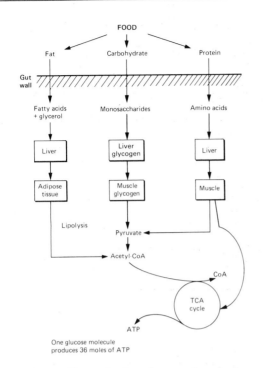

Fig. 3.1 The production of energy from food.

Table 3.1 Approximate energy expenditure of a normal adult.

	kcal	kJ
Male		
Rest	500	2100
Light work	1000	4200
Heavy work	2500	10500
Female		
Rest	420	1760
Light work	840	3520
Heavy work	1500	6300

Table 3.2 Normal composition of a 70 kg man.

	kg	Per cent of body weight
Water	42	60
Fat	13	18
Protein	11	16
Carbohydrate	0.5	0.7
Minerals	3.5	5.2

ketone bodies, and protein into amino acids, prior to oxidation to provide energy. Carbohydrate stores are small, consisting of glycogen in the liver and a small amount of circulating glucose.

The average daily energy intake of a 70 kg man is 2700 kcal (approximately 12 000 kJ). These calories are normally provided as approximately:

- 320 kcal (1360 kJ) of protein (80 g)
- 1200 kcal (4800 kJ) of carbohydrate (300 g)
- 1125 kcal (4625 kJ) of fat (125 g)

Recent recommendations from the Health Education Council in the UK suggest a decrease in the fat content of the diet and an increase in complex carbohydrates, with the protein content remaining much the same.

The basal metabolic rate decreases with age by up to 10% per decade. Activity increases energy demands—50% in moderate exercise and 100% or more in severe exercise (Table 3.1). Growth, pregnancy and lactation all increase the daily requirement of energy.

Protein

The recommended daily intake of protein is 0.8 g per kg per day, with protein representing at least 10% of the total energy intake. Most people eat more than this, consuming 80–100 g of protein per day. The total amount of nitrogen excreted in the urine represents the balance between protein breakdown and synthesis. In order to maintain nitrogen balance, at least 40–50 g of protein are needed. The amount of protein required to maintain nitrogen balance in a particular individual can be calculated from the amount of nitrogen excreted in the urine using the following equation:

Urinary nitrogen $\times$ 6.25 = g of protein required

Protein contains many amino acids of which at least eight (probably nine) are essential amino acids necessary for protein synthesis and for maintenance of nitrogen balance. The biological value of a protein is defined as the amount of absorbed protein retained by the body, and this primarily depends on the essential amino acids present. Egg and milk have high biological values, whereas plant proteins have low biological values as at least one essential amino acid is missing. Adequate energy is required in addition to protein for the normal diet, otherwise protein will be directed towards oxidative pathways and eventually gluconeogenesis for energy.

Fat

The average fat intake per day varies from 90 to 180 g. It has recently been suggested that the average total fat intake be reduced from 128 g (38% of total energy) to 115 g (34% of total energy). Dietary fat is chiefly in the form of triglycerides. Forty per cent of dietary fat is saturated, but gradually more vegetable oils containing polyunsaturated fats are being introduced into the diet.

Currently the ratio of polyunsaturated to saturated fatty acids in the Western diet is 0.3. Studies, largely epidemiological, suggest that an increase in polyunsaturated fatty acids will decrease the incidence of ischaemic heart disease. However, the advisability of any increase in polyunsaturated fats is still questionable, remembering that it cannot be achieved without a substantial change from meat and dairy products to vegetable fats. A reasonable compromise would be to try to bring the ratio of saturated to polyunsaturated fats nearer to 1.0, which would at least probably do no harm. Recently a reduction in the proportion of saturated fatty acids to 15% of the total energy intake has been recommended.

Essential fatty acids

Only linoleic acid, from which arachidonic acid is derived, is an essential fatty acid. Essential fatty acid deficiency may accompany protein–energy malnutrition, but it has only been clearly defined as a clinical entity in patients on long-term parenteral nutrition given glucose and protein and no fat.

Carbohydrate

Carbohydrate intake comprises the polysaccharide starch, some disaccharides (mainly sucrose) and a small amount of lactose. Carbohydrates are cheap compared with other foodstuffs; a great deal is therefore eaten, usually more than required.

Dietary fibre, which is largely non-starch polysaccharide, is removed in the processing of food, leaving highly refined carbohydrate such as sucrose.

The principal classes of dietary fibre are cellulose, hemicelluloses, lignins, pectins and gums, all of which are not digested by gut enzymes. However, fibre is partly broken down in the GI tract, mainly by colonic bacteria, producing gas and volatile fatty acids.

All plant food, when unprocessed, contains fibre, so that all unprocessed food eaten will increase the fibre content of the diet. Bran, the fibre from wheat, is an easy way of adding additional fibre to the diet. It increases faecal bulk and is helpful in the treatment of constipation. Dietary fibre deficiency is now accepted as an entity by many workers in the UK and it is suggested that the total dietary fibre be increased to 25–30 g per day. This could be achieved by increased consumption of bread, potatoes, fruit and vegetables, with a reduction in sugar intake.

Wholemeal food, that is food with fibre still present, is thought to prevent a number of chronic conditions, e.g. diverticular disease, but this has not been proved. Refined carbohydrate, with little or no fibre, is less filling and can be eaten in larger quantities. This contributes to obesity.

Recently, pectins and gums have been added to food to slow down monosaccharide absorption, particularly in diabetes.

Protein–energy malnutrition (PEM) as seen in developed countries

Starvation is unusual in developed countries, although some degree of undernourishment is seen in very poor areas. Most nutritional problems occurring in the population at large are due to eating wrong combinations of food, e.g. excess of refined carbohydrate or diets low in fresh vegetables.

Common causes of protein–energy malnutrition
With the exception of thyrotoxicosis where there are increased energy demands, loss of weight leading to malnutrition is almost always due to a poor dietary intake. Table 3.3 gives a list of conditions in which malnutrition is commonly seen. Surgical complications, with sepsis, are the commonest cause in most hospitals. All are associated with a decreased appetite. Malabsorption is sometimes thought to be a cause of weight loss, but failure to absorb nutrient is

Table 3.3 Common conditions associated with protein–energy malnutrition (PEM).

Sepsis

Surgery, particularly of gastrointestinal tract, with complications

Gastrointestinal disease, particularly involving small bowel

Psychological—anorexia nervosa

Malignancy

Metabolic disease—renal failure

Any very ill patient

never so great that it cannot be overcome by increased intake (see p. 175).

Pathophysiology of starvation (Fig. 3.2)
In the first 24 h following low dietary intake the body relies on the breakdown of hepatic glycogen to glucose for energy. Hepatic glycogen stores are small and therefore gluconeogenesis is soon necessary to maintain glucose levels. Gluconeogenesis takes place mainly from lactate, glycerol and amino acids. All endogenous proteins can be utilized to provide amino acids for gluconeogenesis and loss of muscle bulk eventually occurs.

Lipolysis, the breakdown of the body's fat stores, also occurs. It is inhibited by insulin, but the level of this hormone falls off as starvation continues. Gradually a decrease in metabolic rate and total body energy expenditure occurs. Central nervous metabolism changes from glucose as a substrate to ketone bodies (derived from fatty acid oxidation in the liver), which now become the main source of energy. Gluconeogenesis in the liver decreases with a consequent reduction of protein breakdown, both being inhibited directly by ketone bodies. Most of the energy at this stage comes from adipose tissue, with some gluconeogenesis from amino acids, particularly glutamine, occurring in the kidney. Any form of

trauma or surgery will increase catabolism, and muscle breakdown can be massive.

Regulation of metabolism
The unavailability of the various substrates in starvation produces dramatic changes in hormone levels, these hormones being the main factors in controlling intracellular metabolism.

In the fed state, insulin/glucagon ratios are high. Insulin promotes synthesis of glycogen, protein and fat, and inhibits lipolysis and gluconeogenesis.

In the fasted state, the insulin/glucagon ratios are low. Glucagon acts mainly on the liver and has no action on muscle. It increases glycogenolysis and gluconeogenesis, as well as increasing ketone body production from fatty acids. It also stimulates lipolysis in adipose tissue. Catecholamines have a similar action to glucagon but also affect muscle metabolism. These agents both act via cyclic AMP to stimulate lipolysis, producing free fatty acids which can then act as a major source of energy.

CLINICAL FEATURES

Patients are sometimes seen with loss of weight or malnutrition (failure to thrive in children) as the primary symptom. Mostly, however, malnourish-

Fig. 3.2 Metabolism in the fed and the fasted state. (a) The fed state. (b) The fasted state. FFA = free fatty acids.

ment is only seen as an accompaniment of some other disease process, e.g. malignancy. A careful history may indicate the cause of the weight loss, but if nothing obvious is found hyperthyroidism must be considered.

Anorexia nervosa commonly occurs in young adolescent females (see p. 896).

Severe malnutrition is mainly seen with advanced organic disease or after surgical procedures followed by complications. PEM leads to a depression of the immunological defence mechanism, leading to decreased resistance to infection (see p. 7).

Patients who have lost more than 10% of their body weight (unless dieting) suffer from malnutrition. Indicators of malnutrition are given in Table 3.4. The clinician can, however, usually decide whether the patient is malnourished by the patient's general appearance. Retrospective dietary evaluation is unfortunately not helpful because of the degree of error in the patient's recollection of his intake.

It is important to establish the cause of the malnutrition, as the treatment often depends on the underlying disease.

TREATMENT

When malnutrition is obvious and the underlying disease cannot be corrected at once, some form of nutritional support is necessary. Nutrition should always be given enterally if the GI tract is functioning adequately. This can most easily be done by encouraging the patient to eat more often and by giving a high-calorie supplement. If this is not possible, a liquified diet may be given intragastrically via a fine-bore tube.

If both of these measures fail, parenteral nutrition is given. Details of nutritional support are given on p. 142.

Table 3.4 Hallmarks of protein–energy malnutrition.

	Males	Females
Weight loss	>10%	
Triceps skinfold thickness*	<10 mm	<13 mm
Arm muscle circumference*	<23 cm	<22 cm
Serum albumin	<35 g·l^{-1}	
Serum transferrin	<1.5 g·l^{-1}	
Lymphocyte count	<1.5 × 10^9/l	
Cell-mediated immunity	Negative *Candida* skin test	

* Values obtained in the UK.

Protein–energy malnutrition in Third World countries

In many areas of the world many people border on malnutrition. If events such as drought, war or changes in political climate occur in addition, millions suffer from starvation. Although the basic condition of PEM is the same in all parts of the world from whatever cause, malnutrition due to long periods of near total starvation produces unique clinical appearances virtually never seen in the Western World (Table 3.5).

The term PEM covers all the clinical conditions seen in adults and children (Table 3.6). It is possible to make a clinical distinction between marasmus and kwashiorkor, but this means very little. The protein content of food has been shown to be the same in both groups and the aetiology of each type is complex. All patients who have a deficiency in protein intake also have deficiencies of total calorie intake and of other, often unspecified, nutrients. It is therefore not possible to be sure which is the most important feature causing any one clinical picture. In addition, infection, diarrhoea and protein loss can affect the clinical picture.

Table 3.5 Clinical features of protein–energy malnutrition in Third World countries.

Failure of growth
Apathy, anorexia
Diarrhoea
Hepatomegaly
Muscle wasting
Oedema
Signs of multiple vitamin and mineral deficiency, e.g. corneal keratinization (blindness)
Anaemia
Hair thinning
Angular stomatitis and sore tongue
Skin changes (changes in pigmentation, dryness)

Table 3.6 Wellcome classification of protein–energy malnutrition.

Weight (per cent of standard for age)	Oedema	
	Present	Absent
60–80%	Kwashiorkor	Undernutrition
<60%	Marasmic kwashiorkor	Marasmus

CLINICAL FEATURES

PEM occurs chiefly in children under 5 years of age, but no age is spared; the clinical manifestations in adults are not so severe. Children show failure of growth, often present from the moment of weaning. Oedema is present in kwashiorkor and this hides muscle wasting. The child is usually apathetic, miserable and suffers from anorexia (Fig. 3.3). Diarrhoea is always present, and hepatomegaly due to fatty infiltration is often found. Hyper- or hypopigmentation may be present, with skin atrophy and eventually ulceration, particularly of the legs, perineum and buttocks. Hair is very thin and changes colour to red and eventually blond, and nails fail to grow. All tissues and organs malfunction in PEM, but most will recover if nutrition is available and the patient is not in the extreme state.

Signs of infection must be looked for carefully as malnutrition depresses normal responses to infection (see p. 7). Specific nutritional deficiencies of vitamins and trace elements also occur and these produce specific signs (see p. 134).

INVESTIGATION

Investigation is not always practicable. Anaemia due to folate, iron and copper deficiency is often present, but the haematocrit may be high due to dehydration. Electrolyte disturbances are common. Blood should be examined for malarial parasites and the stools for pathogens. Tuberculosis is common and is easily missed if a chest x-ray is not performed.

TREATMENT

Treatment must involve the provision of protein and energy supplements and the control of infection.

The severely ill child will require resuscitation, but intravenous therapy should be avoided if possible because of the danger of fluid overload.

Fig. 3.3 A malnourished child.

Feeding needs to be carefully planned and during the initial treatment of the acute case only enough energy and protein is given to maintain a steady state. Large increases in energy lead to heart failure, circulatory collapse and death. A child requires approximately 100 kcal·kg^{-1} (450 kJ·kg^{-1}) daily, which is provided by 0.6 g·kg^{-1} of protein. This is often given as milk with additional water, flour, maize or whatever is available locally. Sugar mixed with dried skimmed milk and small amounts of cotton seed oil (DISCO) is frequently used. Attempts should be made to give the feeds as slowly and as often as possible, although anorexia is often a problem and can be exacerbated by excess feeding. If necessary, fluids and food should be given by nasogastric tube. The child is then gradually weaned to liquids and then solids by mouth.

Hypothermia and hypoglycaemia occur in severely ill children, often with an accompanying infection, and need to be treated urgently. Because of the cold temperatures at night, blankets and sometimes additional heat are necessary. Gradually, as the child improves, more energy can be given and during rehabilitation maximum weight gain is achieved in the shortest time by extra calories ('catch-up weight gain'). The children who have been severely ill need constant attention right through the convalescent period as often home conditions are poor and feeds are refused.

Supplements of vitamins (A, D, B, and C) should always be given, together with folic acid and iron. Many children are deficient in minerals such as zinc, copper and selenium, and supplements should be given if deficiency is suspected (see p. 139).

Diarrhoea can lead to potassium deficiency, and glucose electrolyte mixtures (such as the WHO formulation—p. 30) are sometimes necessary. Diarrhoea is often due to bacterial or protozoal overgrowth and metronidazole is very effective and is often given routinely. Parasites are also common and, as facilities for stool examination are usually not available, mebendazole 100 mg twice daily for 3 days should be given. In high-risk areas, antimalarial therapy is given.

Adults do not usually suffer such severe malnutrition, but the same principles of treatment should be followed.

PROGNOSIS

Children with extreme malnutrition have a mortality of over 50%. By careful management this can be significantly reduced to 1–2%. This will depend on the availability of facilities.

Brain development takes place in the first years of life, a time when severe PEM frequently occurs. There is evidence that intellectual impairment and behavioural abnormalities occur in severely affected children. Physical growth is also impaired. Probably both of these effects can be alleviated if it is possible to maintain a high standard of living with a good diet and freedom from infection over a long period.

PREVENTION

Prevention of PEM depends not only on adequate nutrients being available, but also on education of both governments and individuals of the importance of good nutrition. Short-term programmes are useful for acute shortages of food, but long-term programmes involving improved agriculture are equally important.

Bad feeding practices and infections are more important than actual shortage of food in many areas of the world. However, good surveillance is necessary to avoid periods of famine.

Food supplements (and additional vitamins) should be given to 'at risk' groups by adding high energy food, e.g. milk powder, meat concentrates, to the diet. Pregnancy and lactation are times of high energy requirement and supplements have been shown to be beneficial.

Finally, generally good health care with treatment of infections is particularly beneficial in alleviating severe PEM.

Vitamins (Table 3.7)

Deficiencies due to inadequate intake are commonly seen in Third World countries and are always present with protein–energy malnutrition. In the Western World, deficiency of vitamins is rare except in the specific groups shown in Table 3.8. The widespread use of vitamins as 'tonics' is unnecessary and should be discouraged. Toxicity from excess fat-soluble vitamins is occasionally seen.

FAT-SOLUBLE VITAMINS

Vitamin A

Vitamin A (retinol) is found in dairy products, liver and fish, but is also synthesized in the intestinal wall from β-carotene found in vegetables.

Vitamin A deficiency
Since vitamin A is absorbed in a similar way to all lipids (see p. 172), deficiency can be seen in all

Table 3.8 Some causes of vitamin deficiency in the Western World.

> *Decreased intake*
> Alcoholics—chiefly B vitamins, e.g. thiamine
> Small bowel disease—chiefly folic acid, occasionally fat-soluble vitamins
> Vegans—vitamin D (if no exposure to sunlight), vitamin B_{12}
> Elderly with poor diet—chiefly vitamin D (if no exposure to sunlight), folic acid
> Anorexia from any other cause—chiefly folate
>
> *Decreased absorption*
> Ileal disease/resection—only vitamin B_{12}
> Liver and biliary tract disease—fat–soluble vitamins
>
> *Miscellaneous*
> Long–term enteral or parenteral nutrition—usually vitamin supplements are given
> Renal disease—vitamin D
> Drug antagonists, e.g. methotrexate interfering with folate metabolism

Table 3.7 Fat-soluble and water-soluble vitamins.

Vitamin	Daily requirement	Major clinical features of deficiency
Fat-soluble		
A (retinol)	750 µg	Xerophthalmia, night blindness, keratomalacia, follicular hyperkeratosis
D (cholecalciferol)	2.5–10 µg and sunlight	Rickets, osteomalacia
K	50–150 µg	Coagulation defects
E (α–tocopherol)	10–30 mg	Neurological disorders, e.g. ataxia
Water-soluble		
B_1 (thiamine)	1 mg	Beriberi; Wernicke–Korsakoff syndrome
B_2 (riboflavin)	1–2 mg	Angular stomatitis
Niacin	15–20 equivalents (see text)	Pellagra
B_6 (pyridoxine)	2 mg	Peripheral neuropathy
Pantothenic acid	? 5–10 mg	? No deficiency
Biotin	0.4 mg	Dermatitis
B_{12} (cobalamin)	5 µg	Megaloblastic anaemia; neurological disorders
Folic acid	300 µg	Megaloblastic anaemia
C (ascorbic acid)	30 mg	Scurvy

chronic conditions where there is fat malabsorption. Nevertheless, the clinical features of vitamin A deficiency are rare in most of these malabsorptive conditions. They are normally only seen associated with severe protein–energy malnutrition and other multiple deficiencies in Third World countries. As a result of multiple deficiencies being present, it is not always clear which nutrient deficiency is responsible for any one clinical syndrome.

Clinical features. The clinical features of vitamin A deficiency are impaired dark adaptation followed by night blindness. Later, dryness of the conjunctiva and the cornea (xerophthalmia) occurs as a result of keratinization. Bitot's spots—white plaques of keratinized epithelial cells—are found on the conjunctiva of young children with vitamin A deficiency. These spots can, however, be seen without vitamin A deficiency, possibly due to exposure. Corneal ulceration and dissolution keratomalacia eventually occur; superimposed infection is a frequent accompaniment. Both may lead to blindness. Vitamin A deficiency is a common cause of blindness in Third World countries, affecting 250 000 children per year. Follicular hyperkeratosis, in which there is thickening and dryness of the skin, is also seen with vitamin A deficiency. It is also sometimes seen without vitamin A deficiency.

Diagnosis. In parts of the world where the deficiency is common, diagnosis is made on the basis of the clinical features and deficiency should always be suspected if any degree of malnutrition is present. Blood levels of vitamin A will usually be low, but the best guide to the diagnosis is a response to replacement therapy.

Treatment. Retinol palmitate 30 mg orally (100 000 iu) should be given on two successive days. In the presence of vomiting and diarrhoea, vitamin A 30 mg i.m. is given. Associated malnutrition must be treated, and superadded bacterial infection should be treated with antibiotics. Referral for specialist ophthalmic treatment is necessary in severe cases.

Prevention. Recommended daily intakes of vitamin A are 750 µg for adults and approximately 500 µg for children, depending on age. Lactating women require 1200 µg. Most Western diets contain enough dairy products and green vegetables, but vitamin A is added to foodstuffs in some countries. Vitamin A is not destroyed by cooking. Education of the population is important; in particular, pregnant women and children should be encouraged to eat green vegetables.

Vitamin D

Vitamin D is produced in the skin as cholecalciferol (vitamin D_3) by photoactivation of 7-dehydro-cholesterol. This, rather than dietary vitamin D, is the chief source of vitamin D metabolites in man. Cholecalciferol is firstly hydrolysed in the liver to 25-hydroxycholecalciferol and then by the kidney to 1,25-dihydroxycholecalciferol, which is the active molecule. A small amount of physiologically active 24,25-dihydroxycholecalciferol is also produced. The metabolism and actions of vitamin D are shown in Fig. 3.4 and its role with parathormone in regulating calcium metabolism is discussed on p. 733.

Vitamin D is only found in small amounts in natural foods and hence poor nutrition is only of small importance in producing vitamin D deficiency. Conversely, vitamin D can easily be added to food, e.g. margarine.

Vitamin D deficiency

Clinical features. Vitamin D deficiency produces growth failure and rickets in children and osteomalacia in adults (see p. 734). Osteomalacia is common in the elderly population who are immobile and do not go out of their homes. It is also seen frequently in Asians in the UK; Asian women and children are often completely covered by clothes and thus their skin is not exposed to sunlight. This is exacerbated by the fact that many are vegans, who take no animal products, and therefore do not benefit from the small amounts of dietary vitamin D found in dairy products.

Vitamin D stores are decreased, like other fat-soluble vitamins, when there is fat malabsorption.

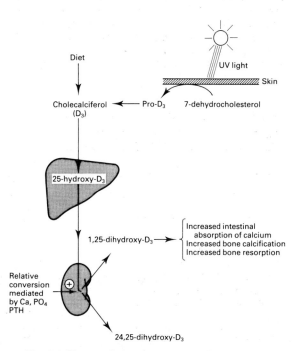

Fig. 3.4 The metabolism and actions of vitamin D.

Diagnosis. Vitamin D deficiency is often subclinical and diagnosis is made on the basis of a raised serum alkaline phosphatase due to increased bone turnover. Bone x-rays show osteomalacia. A low serum level of 1,25-dihydroxycholecalciferol reflects the deficiency, but this test is not readily available at present.

Treatment. The simplest treatments are exposure to sunlight and oral vitamin D supplements. Vitamin D 1 mg (40 000 units) daily should be given as a supplement to patients with chronic fat malabsorption. Larger amounts, e.g. 5 mg, are given in hypocalcaemia. 1α-Hydroxycholecalciferol (1 μg daily) is the usual treatment for vitamin D deficiency in renal disease and other conditions. 1α,25-Dihydroxycholecalciferol is now also available.

All patients receiving pharmacological doses of vitamin D should have their serum calcium measured regularly. Hypervitaminosis D presents with nausea and vomiting and other features of hypercalcaemia.

Vitamin K

Vitamin K is present in many plant foods as phylloquinone (vitamin K_1). Intestinal bacteria can synthesize menaquinone (vitamin K_2), but this is only of minimal importance overall. Synthesized vitamin K or that derived from the diet (leafy vegetables) is absorbed in a similar manner to other fat-soluble substances and therefore deficiency occurs with malabsorption of fat. Deficiency is most commonly seen in biliary obstruction, when no bile salts are available to facilitate absorption. Antibacterial drugs also interfere with bacterial synthesis of vitamin K.

Vitamin K is a co-factor necessary for the synthesis of clotting factors (see p. 215). Vitamin K deficiency is inferred if the prothrombin time is prolonged and no other cause is found. Treatment is by vitamin K injection (Phytomenadione 10 mg i.m.), but this will be ineffective if the prothrombin time is prolonged because of liver disease rather than vitamin K malabsorption. Phytomenadione (1 mg) is given to all newborn babies.

Vitamin E

α-Tocopherol (vitamin E) occurs mainly in vegetable oils, but is also found in fish. Its role in human nutrition is uncertain, but severe deficiency leads to anaemia, haemolysis and muscle disorders as well as central nervous lesions. Deficiency is only seen in patients who are virtually unable to absorb any fat or fat-soluble vitamins, e.g. in biliary atresia. In children with abetalipoproteinaemia the severe neurological deficit (gross ataxia) can be prevented by vitamin E injection.

WATER-SOLUBLE VITAMINS

These are non-toxic, relatively cheap and can therefore always be given in excess if a deficiency is possible. The daily requirements of water-soluble vitamins are given in Table 3.7.

Thiamine

Thiamine is a co-factor of many enzyme reactions, particularly in the glycolytic pathway. Body stores are small and signs of deficiency will quickly develop with an inadequate intake. Thiamine is found in many foodstuffs and deficiency is only seen:

● As beriberi, where the only food consumed is polished rice
● In chronic alcoholics who are consuming virtually no food at all

Beriberi
This is now confined to the poorest areas of Asia. It can be prevented by eating undermilled or parboiled rice, or by fortification of rice with thiamine. Probably the most important factor in the reduction of beriberi is the general increase in overall food consumption so that the staple diet is varied and contains legumes and pulses, which contain a large amount of thiamine. There are two main clinical types of beriberi:

● *Dry beriberi* usually presents insidiously with a symmetrical polyneuropathy. The initial symptoms are heaviness and stiffness of the legs, followed by weakness, numbness, and pins and needles. The ankle jerk reflexes are lost and eventually all the signs of polyneuropathy which may involve the trunk and arms, are found (see p. 857). Cerebral involvement occurs, producing the picture of the Wernicke–Korsakoff syndrome (p. 859). In endemic areas mild symptoms and signs may be present for years without unduly affecting the patient.
● In *wet beriberi* oedema occurs. Initially this is of the legs, but it can extend to involve the whole body, with ascites and pleural effusions. The peripheral oedema may mask the accompanying features of dry beriberi.

In thiamine deficiency, glucose is inadequately metabolized and lactate and pyruvate accumulate, producing peripheral vasodilatation and eventually oedema. The heart muscle is also affected and heart failure occurs, causing a further increase in the oedema. Initially there are warm extremities, a full, fast, bounding pulse and a raised venous pressure ('high output state'), but eventually heart failure advances and a poor cardiac output ensues. The electrocardiogram may show conduction defects.

Infantile beriberi occurs, usually acutely, in breast-fed babies at approximately 3 months old. The mothers may show no signs of thiamine deficiency, but presumably their body stores must be virtually nil. The infant becomes anorexic, develops oedema and has some degree of aphonia. Tachycardia and tachypnoea develop and, unless treatment is instituted, death occurs quickly.

Diagnosis. In endemic areas the diagnosis of beriberi should always be suspected and if in doubt treatment with thiamine instituted. A rapid improvement in the heart failure after thiamine (50 mg i.m.) is diagnostic. Other causes of oedema must be considered, e.g. renal or liver disease, and the polyneuropathy is indistinguishable from that due to other causes. The diagnosis is confirmed by measurement of transketolase activity in red cells. This enzyme is dependent on thiamine pyrophosphate (TPP). The assay is performed with and without added TPP; an increase in activity of 30% with TPP indicates deficiency.

Treatment. Thiamine 50 mg i.m. is given for 3 days, followed by 20 mg of thiamine daily by mouth. The response in wet beriberi occurs in hours, giving dramatic improvement, but in dry beriberi improvement is often slow to occur. In most cases all the B vitamins are given because of multiple deficiency. Infantile beriberi is treated by giving thiamine to the mother, which is then passed on to the infant via the breast milk.

Thiamine deficiency in chronic alcoholics
In the Western hemisphere chronic alcoholics are the only group to suffer from thiamine deficiency. Rarely they develop wet beriberi, which must be distinguished from alcoholic cardiomyopathy. More usually, however, thiamine deficiency presents with polyneuropathy or with the Wernicke–Korsakoff syndrome. This syndrome, which consists of dementia, ataxia, varying ophthalmoplegia and nystagmus (see p. 859), presents acutely and should be suspected in all chronic alcoholics. If treated promptly, it is reversible, but if left it becomes irreversible; it is a major cause of chronic dementia in the USA.

Treatment is with thiamine 50–100 mg i.m. or i.v., often given in combination with other vitamin B complex vitamins.

Riboflavin

Riboflavin is widely distributed through all plant and animal cells. Good sources are dairy products, offal and leafy vegetables. Riboflavin is not destroyed appreciably by cooking, but is destroyed by sunlight. Riboflavin is a flavoprotein which is a co-factor for many oxidative reactions in the cell.

The characteristic features of riboflavin deficiency are:

- Angular stomatitis or cheilosis (fissuring at the corners of the mouth); this lesion can also occur with other vitamin deficiencies as well as from other non-specific causes
- A red, inflamed tongue
- Seborrhoeic dermatitis, particularly involving the face (around the nose) and the scrotum or vulva
- Rarely, neurological damage and vascularization of the cornea

All of these changes often also accompany pellagra—see below.

The diagnosis is made on the basis of the clinical features, although riboflavin can be measured in blood and urine. There is always a good response to riboflavin therapy (10 mg daily), but usually the whole vitamin B complex is given because of other accompanying deficiencies.

Niacin

This is the generic name for the two chemical forms nicotinic acid and nicotinamide, the latter being found in the two pyridine nucleotides nicotinamide adenine dinucleotide (NAD) and nicotinamide adenine dinucleotide phosphate (NADP). Both act as hydrogen acceptors in many oxidative reactions and in their reduced forms (NADH and NADPH) act as hydrogen donors in reductive reactions. Many oxidative steps in the production of energy require the nucleotide NAD, and NADP is equally important in the hexose monophosphate shunt for the generation of NADPH, which is necessary for fatty acid synthesis.

Niacin is found in many foodstuffs, including plants, meat (particularly offal) and fish. Niacin is lost by removing bran from cereals, but is added to processed cereals and white bread in many countries.

Niacin can be synthesized in humans from tryptophan, 60 mg of tryptophan being converted to 1 mg of niacin (Fig. 3.5). The amount of niacin in food is given as the niacin equivalent, which is equal to the amount of niacin plus one-sixtieth of the tryptophan content.

Pellagra
This is nowadays almost always only found in areas where the main constituent of the diet is maize. It has occurred world-wide, including India, Asia, the southern states of the USA and South America. It is now rarely seen apart from in southern Africa in Bantu homelands and in India. Maize contains niacin in the form of niacytin, which is biologically unavailable, and has a low content of tryptophan. Many of the features of pellagra can be explained purely by niacin deficiency; some, however, are probably due to multiple deficiencies, including proteins and other vitamins.

The clinical features are of dermatitis, diarrhoea and dementia. Although this is an easily remem-

Fig. 3.5 The oxidative pathway of tryptophan metabolism.

bered triad, not all are always present and the mental changes are not a true dementia.

Dermatitis. Initially there is a redness of the skin in the areas exposed to sunlight. This is followed by cracks in the skin, with occasional ulceration. Chronic thickening, dryness and pigmentation develop. Casal's necklace or collar is the term given to the skin lesion around the neck, which is confined to this area by the clothes worn.

Diarrhoea. This is often a feature, but constipation is occasionally seen. Other GI manifestations include a painful red raw tongue, glossitis and angular stomatitis. Recurring mouth infections occur.

Dementia. This occurs in chronic disease. In milder cases there are symptoms of depression, apathy and sometimes thought disorders. Hallucinations and acute psychosis are seen with more severe cases.

Pellagra may also occur in:
- Isoniazid therapy, as this can lead to a deficiency of vitamin B_6, which is needed for the synthesis of nicotinamide from tryptophan; vitamin B_6 is now given concomitantly with isoniazid
- Hartnup disease, a rare inborn error whereby basic amino acids including tryptophan are not absorbed by the gut and there is also loss of this amino acid in the urine
- Generalized malabsorption (rare)

- Chronic alcoholics who do not eat
- Very low protein diets given for renal disease or taken as a food fad
- Carcinoid syndrome and phaeochromocytoma, in which tryptophan metabolism is diverted away from the formation of nicotinamide to form amines

Diagnosis. In endemic areas this is based on the clinical features, remembering that other vitamin deficiencies can produce similar changes, e.g. angular stomatitis. Nicotinamide (approximately 300 mg daily by mouth) with a maintenance dose of 50 mg daily is given. Mostly, however, vitamin B complex is given, as other deficiencies are often present.

An increase in the protein content of the diet and treatment of malnutrition and other vitamin deficiencies is essential.

Vitamin B_6

Vitamin B_6 exists as pyridoxine, pyridoxal and pyridoxamine, and is found in plant and animal foodstuffs. Pyridoxal phosphate is involved in the metabolism of amino acids. Dietary deficiency is extremely rare, but has been described in coeliac disease and after the administration of drugs antagonistic to B_6, e.g. isoniazid, hydralazine and penicillamine. The peripheral neuropathy occurring after isoniazid usually responds to vitamin B_6.

Sideroblastic anaemia occasionally responds to vitamin B$_6$ (see p. 267).

Biotin

Biotin is involved in a number of carboxylase reactions. It occurs in many foodstuffs and the dietary requirement is small. Deficiency is extremely rare and is confined to a few people who consume raw eggs, which contain an antagonist (avidin) to biotin. It causes a dermatitis which responds to biotin replacements.

Pantothenic acid

Pantothenic acid is necessary for a number of metabolic reactions, including fatty acid synthesis. It is widely distributed in all foods and deficiency in humans has not been described.

Vitamin C

Ascorbic acid is a simple sugar and a powerful reducing agent, its main role being to control the redox potential within cells. It is involved in the hydroxylation of proline to hydroxyproline, which is necessary for the formation of collagen. The failure of this biochemical pathway in vitamin C deficiency accounts for virtually all of the clinical effects found.

Man, along with a few other animals (e.g. primates and the guinea-pig), is unusual in not being able to synthesize ascorbic acid from glucose.

Vitamin C is present in all animals and plants, fresh fruit and vegetables being the best sources. Unfortunately, ascorbic acid is easily leached out of vegetables when they are placed in water and it is also oxidized during cooking. Potatoes are a good source as many people eat a lot but, as with other vegetables, vitamin C is lost during storage.

Vitamin C deficiency is mainly seen in infants fed boiled milk and elderly and single people who cannot be bothered to eat vegetables. In the UK it is also seen in Asians eating only rice and chapattis and in food fadists.

Scurvy

In adults the early symptoms may be non-specific, with weakness and muscle pain. Other features are shown in Table 3.9. In infantile scurvy there is irritability, painful legs, anaemia, and characteristic subperiosteal haemorrhages, particularly into the ends of long bones.

Diagnosis. The anaemia is usually hypochromic but occasionally a normochromic or megaloblastic anaemia is seen. The type of anaemia depends on whether iron deficiency (due to decreased absorption and loss due to haemorrhage) or folate deficiency (folate is largely found in green vegetables) is present.

Table 3.9 Clinical features of vitamin C deficiency.

Keratosis of hair follicles with 'corkscrew hair'
Perifollicular haemorrhages
Swollen, spongy gums with bleeding and superadded infection; loosening of teeth
Spontaneous bruising
Spontaneous haemorrhage
Anaemia
Failure of wound healing

Plasma ascorbic acid is very low in obvious deficiency and a vitamin C level of less than 0.1 μg·dl^{-1} in the leucocyte-platelet layer (buffy coat) of centrifuged blood indicates deficiency.

Treatment. Ascorbic acid should be given in doses of up to 1 g a day initially and patients should be encouraged to eat fresh fruit and vegetables.

Prevention. Orange juice should be given to bottle-fed infants. The intake of breast-fed infants depends on the mother's diet.

In the elderly, eating adequate fruit and vegetables is the best way to avoid scurvy. Careful surveillance of the elderly, particularly those who live alone, is necessary. Ascorbic acid supplements should only be necessary occasionally.

Ascorbic acid in high dosage has been suggested as a treatment of cancer and the common cold. There is some scientific support for its value; however, clinical trials in the common cold have shown that it is of no help.

Vitamin B$_{12}$ and folate

These are dealt with on p. 268 and in Table 3.7.

Minerals

A number of minerals have been shown to be essential in animals and an increasing number of deficiency syndromes are becoming recognized in humans. Long-term total parenteral nutrition allowed trace element deficiency to be studied in controlled conditions; now trace elements are always added to long-term parenteral nutrition regimens. It is highly probable (but difficult to study because of multiple deficiencies) that trace element deficiency is also an important accompaniment of all protein–energy malnutrition states.

Apart from poor dietary intake, trace element

deficiency can occur as a result of generalized or specific malabsorption. The role of excess loss, e.g. with severe diarrhoea, is less clear.

A number of the more important elements are discussed below.

Copper

Deficiency
Menkes' kinky hair syndrome is a rare condition due to malabsorption of copper. Infants with this sex-linked abnormality develop growth failure, mental retardation, bone lesions and brittle hair. Anaemia and neutropenia also occur. This condition, which serves as a model for copper deficiency, supports the idea that some of the clinical features seen in protein–energy malnutrition are due to copper deficiency. Breast and cow's milk are low in copper and supplementation is occasionally necessary when first treating PEM.

Toxicity
Copper toxicity occurs in Wilson's disease—see p. 240.

Zinc

Acrodermatitis enteropathica
This inherited disorder is due to malabsorption of zinc. Infants develop growth retardation, severe diarrhoea, hair loss and associated *Candida* and bacterial infection. Zinc supplement results in a complete cure.

This condition provides a model for zinc deficiency, which may play a role in protein–energy malnutrition.

Zinc levels have also been shown to be low in a number of conditions associated with malabsorption, skin disease and diarrhoea.

Fluorine

In areas where the level of fluorine is less than one part per million, dental caries is more prevalent. Fluoridation of the water seems to reduce this.

Excessive fluorine intake can result in fluorosis, in which there is infiltration of the enamel of the teeth with fluorine, producing pitting and discoloration.

Calcium (see p. 733)

This is found in many foods but particularly in milk. Its absorption from the GI tract is vitamin D-dependent. Ninety-nine per cent of body calcium is in the skeleton. Increased calcium is required in pregnancy and lactation when dietary intake must be increased. Calcium deficiency is usually due to vitamin D deficiency.

Table 3.10 Other trace elements (see text).

Element	Deficiency
Cadmium	?
Chromium	Glucose intolerance
Cobalt	Anaemia
Manganese	Growth retardation, skeletal abnormalities, glucose intolerance
Molybdenum	? Animals only
Nickel	? Animals only
Selenium	Growth retardation

Phosphate

Phosphates are present in all natural foods and dietary deficiency has not been described. Patients taking large amounts of aluminium hydroxide can, however, develop phosphate deficiency due to binding in the gut lumen. It can also be seen in total parenteral nutrition. Symptoms include anorexia, weakness and osteoporosis.

Other trace elements which have been found to be necessary are shown in Table 3.10.

Obesity

Some degree of obesity is almost invariable in the Western World and almost all people develop some obesity as they get older. Obesity implies the excess storage of fat and this can most easily be detected by looking at the undressed patient.

Tables of desirable weights for a given height can be found in the Appendices, 10% greater than the ideal weight being described as overweight, 20% or more than the ideal weight as morbid obesity.

Causes of obesity
There are a few unusual causes (Table 3.11), but most

Table 3.11 Unusual causes of obesity.

Genetic syndromes associated with hypogonadism, e.g. Prader–Willi syndrome, Laurence–Moon–Biedl syndrome
Hypothyroidism
Cushing's syndrome
Stein–Leventhal syndrome
Drug-induced, e.g. corticosteroids
Hypothalamic damage, e.g. due to trauma, tumour

patients suffer from simple obesity. Hormonal imbalance is often incriminated in women, e.g. post-menopause or taking contraceptive pills, but most weight gain in such cases is usually small and due to water retention.

Simple obesity

Not all obese people eat more than the average, but all obviously eat more than they need.

Suggested mechanisms
Genetic and environmental factors. These are difficult to separate, but obese children mostly have obese parents (usually the mother). The relative importance of genetic make-up compared with the importance of food eating patterns is complex. It has been suggested that body size is determined in the first few months of life, but not all obese children become obese adults. On the other hand, obese teenagers often remain obese.

Food intake. Many factors related to the home environment, e.g. finance and the availability of sweets and snacks, will affect food intake. Some patients eat more during periods of heavy exercise or during pregnancy and are unable to get back to their former eating habits. The increase in obesity in social class 5 can usually be related to the type of food consumed, i.e. food containing sugar and fat. The underlying mechanisms for controlling satiety are ill understood; psychological factors and how food is presented may override complex biochemical interactions.

Exercise. Any physical exercise, however small, increases energy requirements. For example, the energy expended on walking at 3 miles per hour is 3.7 kcal·min^{-1} (15.5 kJ·min^{-1}). Increased body fat develops insidiously over the years, often due to small discrepancies in energy balance, and therefore any decrease in physical activity is important. The obese person usually takes less physical exercise than the non-obese, and obesity itself can impair physical activity.

Thermogenesis. Brown adipose tissue in animals, when stimulated by cold or food, dissipates the energy derived from ingested food as heat. This can be a major component of overall energy expenditure and it has been suggested that this may also apply to man, so that excess intake in normal subjects is dissipated as heat. A defect in thermogenesis would explain why some obese patients require a very low calorie intake to maintain any weight loss achieved and gain weight easily after only small calorie increases. Overall, this mechanism probably does not play a major role.

CLINICAL FEATURES

Most patients recognize their own problem, although often they are unaware of the main foods that cause obesity. Many symptoms are related to psychological problems, e.g. in women who cannot find fashionable clothes to wear. Social pressures are also important.

The degree of obesity is assessed by comparison with tables of ideal weight for height (see Appendices) and also by measuring skinfold thickness. This should be measured over the middle of the triceps muscle; normal values are 20 mm in a man and 30 mm in a woman.

Table 3.12 shows the conditions and complications that are associated with obesity. The relationship between cardiovascular disease (hypertension or ischaemic heart disease), hyperlipidaemia, smoking, physical exercise and obesity is complex. Difficulties arise in interpreting mortality figures because of the number of factors involved. Many studies of obesity do not, for instance, differentiate between smokers and non-smokers or between the types of physical exercise that are taken. Many do not take into account the cuff-size artefact in the measurement of blood pressure; an artefact will occur if a large cuff is not used in patients with a large arm. Nevertheless, obesity almost certainly plays a part in all of these diseases and should be treated. The only exception is that stopping smoking, even if accompanied by weight gain, is more important than any of the other factors.

Table 3.12 Conditions and complications associated with obesity.

Psychological
Osteoarthritis
Varicose veins
Hiatus hernia
Gallstones
Postoperative problems
Back strain
Accident proneness
Hypertension
Breathlessness
Ischaemic heart disease
Stroke
Diabetes mellitus
Hyperlipidaemia
Menstrual abnormalities

TREATMENT

This largely depends on a reduction in calorie intake. The commonest diets allow an intake of approximately 1000 kcal (4200 kJ) per day, although this may need to be nearer 1500 kcal (6300 kJ) per day for someone engaged in physical work. A diet which is too low in total calories will usually result in the patient cheating and only keeping to the diet for short periods.

Patients must realize that prolonged dieting is necessary for large amounts of fat to be lost. Furthermore, a permanent change in eating habits is required to maintain the new low weight. It is relatively easy for most patients to lose the first few kilograms, but long-term success in moderate obesity is poor, with an overall success rate of no more than 10–20%.

The aim of any dietary regimen is to lose approximately 1 kg per week, which corresponds to a loss of 7700 kcal (3200 kJ) from adipose tissue. Weight loss will be greater initially due to accompanying protein and glycogen breakdown and consequent water loss. After three to four weeks, weight loss may be very small, as only adipose tissue is broken down and there is no accompanying water loss.

Patients must understand the principles of energy intake and expenditure, and the best results are obtained in educated, well-motivated patients. Constant supervision, either by a doctor, close relatives or through slimming societies (e.g. Weight Watchers) helps to encourage compliance.

An increase in exercise will increase energy expenditure and should be encouraged, as long as there is no contraindication such as cardiovascular disease. Weight cannot be lost by exercise alone. Nevertheless, a 15-minute brisk daily walk will use the energy contained in a small slice of bread and butter.

The diet should contain adequate amounts of each nutrient; a diet of 1000 kcal (4200 kJ) per day should be made up of approximately 100 g of carbohydrate, 50 g of protein and 40 g of fat. The carbohydrate should be in the form of complex carbohydrates such as vegetables and fruit rather than simple sugars. Alcohol contains 7 kcal·g^{-1} and should be discouraged. It can be substituted for other foods in the diet but it often reduces the willpower. With a varied diet, vitamins and minerals will be adequate and supplements are not necessary. A balanced diet, attractively presented, is of much greater value and safer than any of the slimming regimens often advertised in women's magazines.

Drug therapy

Drugs can be used as an adjunct to the dietary regimen but they do not substitute for strict dieting. Amphetamine is addictive, although some less stimulating derivatives are now available which produce anorexia. However, their use should be discouraged as they cause dependency and psychotic states. The most commonly used drugs are diethylproprion (75 mg daily) and fenfluramine. The latter differs in that it acts on the serotoninergic system rather than the catecholaminogenic pathway which is affected by the amphetamine derivatives. It can be given in doses up to 100 mg daily but side-effects are frequent. None of the drugs should be given long-term; they should be withdrawn slowly.

Surgical treatment

Operations involving bypass of parts of the small intestine have fallen out of favour because of their side-effects and cannot now be recommended. Jejunoileal bypass was the commonest operation and involved the anastomosis of approximately 18 cm of jejunum to the terminal 18 cm of the ileum. Complications are chiefly those of intestinal resection (see p. 181). A fatty liver often occurs and in a few patients cirrhosis is seen.

Two operations are still performed in cases of severe morbid obesity:
- *Wiring the jaws* to prevent eating and allow liquid feeds only. This can be used as a temporary measure, but good dental hygiene is essential. Weight gain usually occurs after the wires have been removed.
- *Gastric plication*, in which a small gastric pouch is created by stapling across the wall of the stomach. Good results are claimed without the side-effects of bypass operations.

MORBIDITY AND MORTALITY

There is an increase in death in obesity, mainly from diabetes, coronary heart disease and cerebrovascular disease. The greater the obesity the higher the morbidity and mortality figures. For example, men who are 10% overweight have a 13% increased risk of death, whilst the increase in mortality for those 20% overweight is 25%. The rise is less in women. Weight reduction reduces this mortality and therefore should be strongly encouraged.

Nutrition in the hospital patient

Over the past 10 to 15 years it has been realized that many patients are suffering from malnutrition on admission to hospital. This may then be made worse by the patient being unable to eat whilst in hospital, due either to the symptoms of the disease or to the treatment, e.g. surgery of the GI tract.

Malnutrition has been dealt with earlier (p. 130); here the forms of nutritional supplements that are available are discussed.

Principles

Some form of nutritional supplementation is needed in those patients who cannot eat, will not eat or cannot eat enough. This can be given as:
- enteral nutrition
- parenteral nutrition

If the gastrointestinal tract is functioning normally, enteral nutrition should always be used rather than parenteral nutrition. Feeds can be given either by mouth, via a fine-bore nasogastric tube or, very occasionally, via a jejunostomy.

Enteral feeding

The methods of providing nutritional support enterally are shown in Table 3.13.

Initially, oral feeding should be attempted, but in ill patients anorexia is a major problem and often oral feeding is not well tolerated. It is in these patients that feeding via a nasogastric tube is particularly useful.

Diet formulation

Patients with normal gastrointestinal function should be given diets containing whole protein as the nitrogen source, with triglycerides and carbo-hydrates (as glucose polymers) as the energy source. The composition of an ideal standard enteric diet is shown in Table 3.14.

In patients with impaired gastrointestinal function, nutrients can be given in a predigested form, although this is only indicated in very occasional

Table 3.13 Methods of providing enteral nutrition.

Route	Food
Oral	Liquidized food

Nasogastric tube	Enteral diet:
	    Whole protein liquid feed
	    Elemental diet
	    Glucose polymer

Gastrostomy Jejunostomy	Enteral diet

Table 3.14 Standard enteric diet (2000–3000 kcal, approximately 12 000 kJ).

Energy
    Carbohydrate as glucose polymers (70%)
    Fat as triglycerides (30%)

Nitrogen
    Whole protein (9–15 g)
    Ratio of energy to nitrogen (kcal:g) = 150:1

Osmolality = 285–300 mosmol·kg^{-1}
Additional electrolytes, vitamins and trace elements

patients. The carbohydrate source is still given in the form of glucose polymers, but when fat digestion is impaired, triglycerides should contain medium-chain fatty acids which can be absorbed in the absence of luminal hydrolysis. The nitrogen source can contain partial enzyme hydrolysates of whole protein or mixtures of amino acids rather than whole protein.

In most patients these feeds should be given via a narrow-bore nasogastric tube. The tube is passed into the stomach under radiographic control. The aim of the regimen is to achieve a positive nitrogen balance, which can usually be obtained by giving 3–5 g of nitrogen in excess of output. Nitrogen loss can be calculated in grams per 24 hours, this being equal to the urinary urea (mmol per 24 hours) × 0.028 + 2, the 2 representing non-urinary nitrogen excretion.

The success of enteral feeding depends on careful supervision of the patient. Complications include:
- Those related to the tubes, e.g. oesophagitis
- Gastrointestinal side-effects, the most common being diarrhoea
- Metabolic complications, including hypergly-caemia and low levels of potassium, magnesium, calcium and phosphate

Any patient requiring long-term therapy will need vitamin and essential trace metal supplements.

Parenteral nutrition

This is only used for the malnourished patient when the enteral route is unavailable. Parenteral nutrition is much more complicated and potentially more dangerous than enteral nutrition. It should therefore not be used unless absolutely necessary. It is seldom necessary for periods of less than 14 days.

Catheter placement

A silicon catheter is placed into a central vein, usually using the infraclavicular approach to the subclavian vein. The skin entry site should be dressed carefully and not disturbed unless there is a suggestion of catheter-related sepsis.

Complications of catheter placement include central vein thrombosis, pneumothorax and embolism, but the major problem is catheter-related sepsis. Organisms, mainly staphylococci, enter along the side of the catheter, leading to septicaemia. Sepsis can be prevented by careful and sterile placement of the catheter, by not removing the dressing over the catheter entry site, and by not giving other substances (e.g. blood products, antibiotics) via the central vein catheter.

Sepsis should be suspected if the patient develops fever and leucocytosis. In two-thirds of cases, organisms can be grown from the catheter tip. Treatment involves removal of the catheter and appropriate systemic antibiotics.

Catheter placement for parenteral nutrition

This should be performed only by experienced clinicians under aseptic conditions in an operating theatre.

- The patient is placed supine with 5° of head down tilt to avoid air embolism.
- The skin below the midpoint of the left clavicle is infiltrated with 1–2% lignocaine and a 1 cm skin incision made.
- A 20-gauge needle on a syringe is inserted beneath the clavicle and first rib and angled towards the tip of finger held in the suprasternal notch.
- When blood is aspirated freely, the needle is used as a guide to insert the cannula through the skin incision and into the subclavian vein.
- The catheter is advanced 20–30 cm so that its tip lies in the distal part of the superior vena cava.
- A skin tunnel is created under local anaesthetic using an introducer inserted through a point about 10 cm below and medial to the incision and passed upwards to the incision.
- The proximal end of the catheter (with hub removed) is passed backwards through the introducer to emerge 10 cm below the clavicle, where it is sutured to the chest wall.
- The original infraclavicular entry incision is now sutured.

Nutrition

With parenteral nutrition it is possible to provide sufficient nitrogen for protein synthesis and calories to meet energy requirements. Electrolytes, vitamins and trace elements are also necessary. All of these substances are infused simultaneously.

Nitrogen source. Synthetic L-amino acid solutions are used, which contain between 9 and 17 g of nitrogen per litre. Most patients require at least 14 g of nitrogen per day.

Energy source. This is mainly provided by glucose as a 20% solution, with additional calories provided by a fat emulsion. Fat infusions provide a greater number of calories in a smaller volume than can be provided by carbohydrate. They are not hypertonic and they also prevent essential fatty acid deficiency.

Essential fatty acid deficiency has been reported in long-term parenteral nutritional regimens without fat emulsions. It causes a scaly skin, hair loss and a delay in healing.

The calorie to nitrogen ratio in parenteral nutrition should be approximately 150 to 1.

Electrolytes and trace elements (Table 3.15). The electrolyte status should be monitored on a daily basis and electrolyte solutions given as appropriate. Water-soluble vitamins can be given daily but fat-soluble vitamins should be given weekly as overdose can

Table 3.15 Daily dietary electrolytes and trace elements required for long-term maintenance.

Na^+	70–220 mmol
K^+	60–120 mmol
Mg^{2+}	5–20 mmol
Ca^{2+}	5–10 mmol
Zn^{2+}	50 μmol
Mn^{2+}	7 μmol
Fe^{3+}	70 μmol
Cu^{2+}	8 μmol
Cl^-	70–220 μmol
PO_4^{3-}	20–40 mmol
F^-	50 μmol
I^-	>1 μmol

occur. A trace metal solution is available for patients on long-term parenteral nutrition, but if the patient requires blood transfusions trace metal supplements are not needed.

Most hospitals now administer parenteral nutrition using 3 l bags pre-mixed under sterile conditions by the pharmacy. A standard parenteral nutrition regimen is given in the Appendices.

Complications
- Metabolic, e.g. hyperglycaemia—insulin therapy may be necessary
- Electrolyte disturbances
- Hypercalcaemia
- Liver dysfunction

Monitoring of patients on parenteral nutrition
Essential monitoring includes daily plasma electrolytes and weekly assessments of nutritional status (weight and skinfold thickness). Nitrogen balance should also be measured on a weekly basis.

Home parenteral nutrition is occasionally required for patients with virtually no small bowel.

Food allergy and food intolerance

Some patients have allergic reactions to particular foods, e.g. urticaria, vomiting or diarrhoea after eating strawberries or shellfish. Vague, non-specific symptoms such as headaches, panic attacks, palpitations and anxiety, although related to food ingestion, may not be due to an allergic reaction and often have a psychological basis. Unfortunately, as symptoms are usually subjective, differentiating between true food allergy and psychiatric ill-health is often difficult.

Definition

Food intolerance may be due to pharmacological, idiosyncratic or allergic mechanisms (Fig. 3.6):
- Pharmacological reactions to a constituent of food, e.g. the histamine in mackerel or canned food, or the tyramine in cheeses
- Reactions to chemical mediators released by food, e.g. histamine may be released by tomatoes or strawberries
- Reactions to toxic chemicals found in food, e.g. the food additive tartrazine
- Irritation of the GI tract by foods containing spices
- Reactions due to an enzyme deficiency, e.g. milk-induced diarrhoea in alactasia, or fava bean-induced haemolytic anaemia in glucose-6-phosphate dehydrogenase deficiency

Food allergy. This term should be restricted to patients with an immunological hypersensitivity reaction mediated by IgE.

Mechanisms

The exact mechanism of the causation of food allergy is unclear. Antigenic food proteins are absorbed across healthy gastrointestinal mucosa and, although small in amount, they are sufficient to immunize and lead to the production of antibodies. This is a normal reaction to the ingestion of foreign material and does not usually lead to symptoms. In some patients inappropriate allergic reactions to food may lead to local gastrointestinal or distant systemic symptoms.

Excess antigen absorption across an intact gastrointestinal mucosa is prevented by several mechanisms (see p. 173). When an infant first eats a food, a small amount of the antigen appears in the blood and an antibody (usually IgE) is produced. On subsequent ingestion of the antigen, very little enters the blood due to the protective response (immune exclusion). Ingestion of an antigen also induces partial immunological tolerance to subsequent parenteral contact with the antigen.

The type of antigen absorbed is important. Some foods, e.g. egg, milk, fish and wheat, have a very strong tendency to sensitize, while others are fairly innocuous. Cross-sensitization between related vegetables, e.g. soy bean and peas, also occurs.

However, the nature of the actual allergen in any particular food is still uncertain.

Genetic predisposition may be important, as there appears to be a familial tendency to certain food allergies. In coeliac disease (see p. 178), where the lesion is produced by gluten ingestion, there is an increase in the incidence of HLA-B8, DR3. Atopic patients with eczema may also have an increase in the incidence of HLA-B8. Environmental factors may also play a part, as concordance of atopic allergic disease in monozygotic twins is not total.

CLINICAL FEATURES

It must be emphasized that of all the many disorders thought to be due to food allergy, most patients have a food fad or a psychiatric problem rather than a true allergy. These psychiatric disorders may vary from simple avoidance of a food as an attention-seeking ploy to anorexia nervosa associated with extreme weight loss (p. 896).

Symptoms of allergy may be immediate or delayed:
- *Immediate symptoms* start within a few hours of ingestion of the particular food, with swelling of the lips or tongue, vomiting, rhinorrhoea, urticaria, eczema, asthma or migraine. These reactions are usually thought to be mediated by IgE.
- *Delayed symptoms* are much more difficult to delineate. They may develop hours or even days after the ingestion of food and a causal relationship between the ingestion of the food and the symptoms is often difficult to prove.

Multiple vague symptoms, e.g. tiredness or malaise, are unlikely to be due to food allergy or intolerance and probably have a psychiatric basis.

Migraine, arthritis, behaviour and affective disorders, the irritable bowel syndrome and Crohn's disease have all been suggested to be due to food allergy. However, the results of double-blind studies, in which foods are administered in unmarked capsules, have usually been negative. Nevertheless, cases of immediate food-induced rhinitis and asthma are well recognized, migraine attacks can be provoked by certain foods in some people, and some cases of urticaria have been shown to be due to certain foods.

INVESTIGATION AND DIAGNOSIS

There are no reliable laboratory tests for food allergy. A careful history may help to delineate the causative agent, particularly if the effects are immediate. Delayed reactions are more difficult to diagnose, as laboratory testing is usually negative. Laboratory tests include:
- Skin-prick testing with allergens—positive results correlate poorly with clinical symptoms
- Serum IgE—this may be raised in an allergic

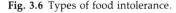

Fig. 3.6 Types of food intolerance.

response (particularly if it is an immediate reaction)

- Radioallergosorbent tests (RASTs) for specific antigen IgE—these may occasionally demonstrate circulating antibody levels to specific foods, but the correlation with symptoms is poor
- Measurement of circulating immune complexes, leucocyte histamine release tests, organ culture tests, etc.—these have all been performed in various conditions but at the moment are research tools only. Humoral antibodies against various foods are seen in normal individuals but may be helpful in assessing treatment in patients if antibody titres fall
- 'Fringe' techniques such as hair analysis—although widely advertised, these are valueless and possibly fraudulent
- Diagnostic exclusion diets—these diets are time-consuming and cumbersome and range from being very simple to extremely tedious. A basic exclusion diet usually excludes colourings, preservatives, milk, eggs, dairy products, fish and nuts. It empirically contains one meat, one vegetable and spring water. Patients are asked to introduce excluded foods one at a time at intervals of two to seven days; if symptoms do not occur the food involved is unlikely to be the cause of the symptoms
- Dietary challenge—this can take various forms. The patients may be 'challenged' with the food under test sublingually, by inhalation, by intragastric or intraduodenal instillation, or by dietary introduction using capsules containing the particular food or a placebo

MANAGEMENT

- Isolated reactions to particular foods, e.g. strawberries or shellfish, are best managed by simple avoidance. This is usually not a clinical problem as the patient has already learnt to avoid the suspected food.
- Multiple intolerance, if truly suspected, can be managed by a rigorous therapeutic exclusion diet. However, great care must be taken to ensure the diet is nutritionally adequate.
- Desensitization therapy using injections or oral or nasal administration has been used for immediate reactions, but with little success.
- Treatment of asthma, rhinitis, eczema or migraine is by avoidance of the particular food which the patient has recognized as causing the symptoms.
- In allergic diseases where the antigen is known, e.g. cow's milk protein intolerance in children and coeliac disease, patients should be treated with a milk-free or gluten-free diet, respectively.
- There is no specific drug therapy. Oral *sodium cromoglycate* has been tried and may have some value as an adjunct to a special diet. *Anti-histamines*, e.g. terfenadine, brompheniramine, have been tried with some success, and *prostaglandin synthetase inhibitors*, e.g. aspirin, and other non-steroidal anti-inflammatory drugs may be of some use.
- Most patients only require reassurance. Others may need psychiatric help.

Alcohol

Alcohol is a popular 'nutrient' consumed in large quantities all over the world.

Ethanol (ethyl alcohol) is metabolized chiefly in the liver, eventually to carbon dioxide and water, by the following mechanisms:

- Alcohol dehydrogenase, a mitochondrial enzyme, catalyses the oxidation of alcohol to acetaldehyde, which is then further metabolized in the Krebs cycle.
- Mixed function oxidases localized in the endoplasmic reticulum can also metabolize alcohol. These enzymes are inducible, which explains why people who often drink alcohol can metabolize alcohol at a faster rate than non-drinkers.

Ethanol itself produces $7 \ kcal \cdot g^{-1}$, but many alcoholic drinks also contain sugar, which increases their calorific value. For example, 1 pint of beer provides 250 kcal. Therefore the heavy drinker will be unable to lose weight if he or she continues to drink.

Effects of excess alcohol consumption

Excess consumption of alcohol leads to two major problems, both of which can be present in the same patient:

- Alcohol dependence syndrome—see p. 892
- Physical damage to various tissues

Each unit of alcohol, e.g. half a pint of beer, one single spirit, one small glass of wine, contains 8 g of ethanol (Fig. 3.7). All the long-term effects of excess alcohol consumption are due to excess ethanol irrespective of the type of alcoholic beverage, i.e. beer and spirits are no different in their long-term effects.

Short-term effects, such as hangovers, depend on additional substances, particularly other alcohols such as isoamyl alcohol, which are known as congeners. Brandy and bourbon contain the highest percentage of congeners.

The amount of alcohol which produces damage varies and not everyone who drinks to excess will get physical damage. For example, only 20% of people who drink heavily develop cirrhosis of the liver.

The effect of alcohol on different organs of the

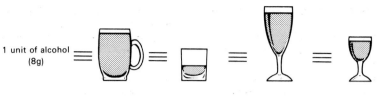

1 unit of alcohol (8g) = ½ pint of beer = 1 single measure (⅙ gill spirit) = 1 glass of wine = 1 glass of sherry

Fig. 3.7 Measures of alcohol.

body is not the same; in some patients the liver is affected, in others the brain or muscle. The differences may be genetically determined.

In general the effects of a given intake of alcohol seem to be worse in women. The following figures are for men and should be reduced by 50% for women.

For liver disease:
- 160 g ethanol per day (20 single drinks) carries a high risk
- 80 g ethanol per day (10 single drinks) carries a medium risk
- 40 g ethanol per day (4 single drinks) carries little risk

Heavy *persistent* drinkers for many years are at greater risk than heavy *sporadic* drinkers.

Susceptibility to damage to different organs is variable and the above figures are only a guide.

Alcohol consumption in pregnancy
Women are advised not to drink alcohol at all during pregnancy, as even small amounts of alcohol consumed can lead to 'small babies'.

The fetal alcohol syndrome is characterized by mental retardation, dysmorphic features and growth impairment; it occurs in fetuses of alcohol-dependent women.

A summary of the physical effects of alcohol is given in Table 3.16. Details of these diseases are discussed in the relevant chapters. The effects of alcohol withdrawal are discussed on p. 893.

Table 3.16 Physical effects of excess alcohol consumption.

Central nervous system (see Table 18.55)
Epilepsy
Wernicke–Korsakoff syndrome
Polyneuropathy
Muscles
Acute or chronic myopathy
Cardiovascular system
Cardiomyopathy
Beriberi heart disease
Cardiac arrhythmias
Metabolism
Hyperuricaemia (gout)
Hyperlipidaemia
Hypoglycaemia
Endocrine system
Pseudo-Cushing's syndrome
Respiratory system
Chest infections
Gastrointestinal system
Acute gastritis
Carcinoma of oesophagus and rectum
Pancreatic disease
Liver disease
Haemopoiesis
Macrocytosis (due to direct toxic effect on bone marrow, or folate deficiency)
Thrombocytopenia
Leucopenia
Bone
Osteoporosis
Osteomalacia

Guide to sensible drinking

- Daily maximum:
  6 units for men
  4 units for women
  To help achieve this:
  Use a standard measure
  Do not drink during the day
- Have alcohol-free days each week
- Remember:
  Health can be damaged without being 'drunk'
  Regular heavy intake is more harmful than occasional binges
  Do not drink to 'drown your problems'
- Drinking and driving *limit* is 800 mg·l^{-1} of blood (in the UK)
  1 unit of alcohol is eliminated per hour, therefore spread drinking time
  Food decreases absorption and therefore results in a lower blood alcohol level
  4–5 units are sufficient to put the blood alcohol level over the legal driving limit in a 70 kg man (less in a lighter person)

Further reading

Davidson S, Passmore R, Brock JF & Truswell AS (1979) *Human Nutrition and Dietetics*, 7th edn. Edinburgh: Churchill Livingstone.

Fairclough PD & Clark ML (1980) Alcohol-related diseases of the gastrointestinal tract. In Clark PMS & Krieta LJ (eds) *Medical Consequences of Alcohol Abuse*, pp 87–97. Chichester: Ellis Harwood.

Silk DBA (1983) *Nutritional Support in Hospital Practice*. Oxford: Blackwell Scientific.

4

Gastroenterology

Introduction

Gastrointestinal disease is a major cause of ill-health world-wide. In underdeveloped countries infection and malnutrition are common. For example, over a billion people are infested with roundworms and hookworms, and amoebiasis affects over 10% of the world population. Poor hygiene and malnutrition allows the spread of infective organisms and many infections could be prevented by improved sanitation and education.

The developed countries are also affected, as refined diets and food additives may well be causative in such diseases as diverticular disease and cancer. Despite the advances in both diagnosis (e.g. endoscopy and imaging techniques) and treatment (e.g. H_2-receptor antagonists), gastrointestinal diseases still represent over 15% of the general practitioner's work-load. Much of this load is due to non-organic disorders, which are also becoming a world-wide problem.

Common symptoms (Table 4.1)

Dysphagia

Dysphagia is difficulty in swallowing.

Heartburn

Heartburn is a retrosternal or epigastric burning sensation which spreads upwards to the throat.

Dyspepsia and indigestion

These are terms often used by lay people to describe any symptom, e.g. nausea, heartburn, acidity, pain or distension, that occurs as a result of eating or drinking. They may also be used to describe an inability to digest food. Careful questioning is required to elicit the exact nature of the patient's complaint. 'Indigestion' is common; 80% of the general population will have had indigestion at some time.

Flatulence

Flatulence is the term used to describe excessive wind. It indicates either belching, abdominal distension (see below) or the passage of flatus per rectum. Excessive belching is not usually associated with

Table 4.1 Common gastrointestinal symptoms.

Dysphagia
Heartburn
Dyspepsia/indigestion
Flatulence ('wind')
Vomiting
Diarrhoea/steatorrhoea
Constipation
Abdominal discomfort/pain
Abdominal distension
Anorexia and weight loss
Rectal bleeding

organic disease and is a common functional disorder. It is due to air swallowing (aerophagy), which many people do subconsciously. Some of the swallowed air is passed into the intestines, where most is absorbed. Intestinal bacterial breakdown of food, particularly high-fibre legumes, also produces a small amount of gas. Flatus consists of nitrogen, carbon dioxide, hydrogen and methane. On average, flatus is passed 10 to 20 times per day.

Hiccups

Hiccups are due to involuntary diaphragmatic contractions and are extremely common. Rarely, they become continuous, when treatment with chlorpromazine 50 mg three times daily or diazepam 5 mg three times daily may be effective.

Vomiting

The causes are shown in Table 4.2. There are three stages:
- Nausea—a feeling of wanting to vomit
- Retching—a strong involuntary effort to vomit
- Vomiting—the expulsion of gastric contents through the mouth

Nausea occurs first and is usually associated with decreased gastric motility. This is followed by *retching*, where the glottis remains closed and there is contraction of the diaphragm and the abdominal muscles. Finally, there is a relaxation of the cardia and sustained contraction of the abdominal muscles, which leads to *vomiting*. Vomiting may occur without nausea, particularly in pyloric stenosis. Most gastrointestinal conditions can cause vomiting, but

Table 4.2 Causes of vomiting.

| Any gastrointestinal disease |
| Acute infections, e.g. |
| influenza |
| pertussis |
| Central nervous disease, e.g. |
| raised intracranial pressure |
| meningitis |
| vestibular disturbances |
| migraine |
| Metabolic causes, e.g. |
| uraemia |
| diabetic ketoacidosis |
| hypercalcaemia |
| Drugs, e.g. |
| digitalis toxicity |
| opiates |
| cytotoxics |
| Reflex, e.g. |
| severe pain—myocardial infarction |
| Psychogenic |
| Pregnancy |
| Alcoholic excess |

chronic vomiting with no other abdominal symptoms is not usually due to gastrointestinal disease.

The vomiting centre is located in the medulla oblongata and can be stimulated in many ways, e.g. by drugs and various metabolic conditions. Chronic and recurrent vomiting in women is frequently due to psychological causes.

Diarrhoea

Diarrhoea is extremely common; a single episode is usually due to dietary indiscretion. It is important to establish what the patient means by this symptom. True diarrhoea implies the passing of increased amounts (>300 g) of loose stool and is different from the frequent passage of small amounts of stool which is commonly seen in functional bowel disease. The consistency of the stools is important; watery stools of large volume are always due to an organic cause. Bloody diarrhoea usually implies colonic disease.

Diarrhoea can be either acute or chronic. If acute, infective causes must be looked for.

Steatorrhoea

Steatorrhoea is the passage of pale, bulky stools, which contain fat, sometimes float in the lavatory pan and are difficult to flush away. These stools float because of the increased air content. Normally people with steatorrhoea complain of diarrhoea, but occasionally they may pass only one motion per day.

Constipation

This is difficult to define in terms of frequency of bowel action because there is considerable individual and geographical variation. Patients usually consider themselves constipated if their bowels are not opened on most days. The difficult passage of hard stools is also regarded as constipation, irrespective of stool frequency.

Abdominal pain

Severe acute abdominal pain can be due to a large number of gastrointestinal conditions, and normally presents as an emergency. An 'acute abdomen' can occasionally be due to referred pain from the chest, as in pneumonia, or to metabolic causes, such as diabetic ketoacidosis.

In patients with abdominal pain the following should be ascertained:
- The site, intensity, character and periodicity of the pain
- The aggravating and relieving factors
- Associated symptoms, including non-gastrointestinal symptoms

Upper abdominal pain
Epigastric pain. This can be due to many upper and lower gastrointestinal disorders. It is often a dull ache, but can be severe and sharp. Its relationship to food intake should be ascertained. It is a common feature of peptic ulcer disease.

Biliary colic. This describes pain either in the epigastrium or in the right hypochondrium and is usually due to gallstones in the common bile duct. It generally fluctuates in intensity, but it can be constant; it is not usually colicky. The pain usually lasts from 30 minutes to several hours. It may radiate to the back or to the right shoulder. The patient may vomit and be in great distress because of the pain. Commonly, when the episode of pain is over, the patient is well until the next episode.

Right hypochondrial pain. Hepatic congestion, e.g. in hepatitis, and sometimes peptic ulcer can present with pain in the right hypochondrium. Chronic, often persistent, pain in the right hypochondrium is a frequent symptom in healthy females suffering from functional bowel disease. This chronic pain is not due to gallbladder disease.

Lower abdominal pain
Pain in the lower abdomen is usually colonic in origin. It is most commonly associated with functional bowel disease (see p. 198). Persistent pain in the right iliac fossa over a long period is not due to appendicitis.

Proctalgia
Proctalgia is a severe pain deep in the rectum which comes on suddenly but lasts only for a short time. It is not due to organic disease.

Tenesmus
This is the painful passage of stools per rectum.

Abdominal distension

This is a feeling of a distended abdomen, often erroneously attributed to wind. It is commonly associated with the passing of flatus and, in the absence of physical signs, is due to functional bowel disease.

Weight loss

This is due to anorexia (loss of appetite) and is a frequent accompaniment of all gastrointestinal disease. Anorexia is also common in systemic disease and may be seen in psychiatric disorders, particularly anorexia nervosa (see p. 896). Anorexia often accompanies carcinoma, but it is a late symptom and not of diagnostic help. Weight loss with a normal or increased dietary intake occurs with hyperthyroidism. Malabsorption is never so severe as to cause weight loss without anorexia.

Rectal bleeding

This is the loss of red blood per rectum and is usually due to haemorrhoids.

Clinical examination

A general examination is performed, with particular emphasis on the examination of all lymph nodes and noting the presence of anaemia or jaundice. Detailed examination of the gastrointestinal tract starts with the mouth and tongue, and is followed by:

Examination of the abdomen (Acute abdomen, see p. 199; Liver disease, see p. 219)

Inspection
A normal abdomen is shown in Fig. 4.1; Fig. 4.2 shows a normal CT scan at T12.

Evidence of any abdominal distension, which may be due to flatus, fat, fetus, fluid, or faeces, must be looked for. Lordosis may give the appearance of a distended abdomen; it is a common feature of the 'abdominal distension' seen in functional bowel disease.

Fig. 4.1 Diagram showing (a) the regions of the abdomen, and (b) organs sometimes palpable in thin subjects (percentage given).

Fig. 4.2 CT scan of a normal abdomen at the level of T12. 1 = aorta; 2 = portal vein; 3 = inferior vena cava; 4 = tail of pancreas; 5 = liver; 6 = caudate lobe of liver; 7 = stomach containing air; 8 = right kidney; 9 = left kidney; 10 = spleen.

Palpation

The abdominal organs may be felt in some normal subjects (see Fig. 4.1), but this is not common and such organs are usually only just palpable.

Any palpable mass is carefully felt to decide which organs are involved and also to evaluate its size, shape and consistency and whether it moves with respiration.

The hernial orifices should always be examined. A strangulated hernia can cause intestinal obstruction.

A succussion splash suggests pyloric stenosis if the patient has not drunk for two to three hours; the splash of fluid in the stomach can be heard with a stethoscope laid on the abdomen when the patient is moved.

Percussion

This is performed in the usual way to detect the area of dullness caused by the liver and spleen, and possibly bladder enlargement. The presence of fluid in the abdomen, i.e. ascites, is detected by shifting dullness. The percussion note changes from resonance to dullness when the patient is moved from one side to the other. It is a good physical sign if performed carefully, but 1–2 l of fluid must be present to elicit it. A large ovarian cyst can sometimes produce an enlarged abdomen, but the dullness is more centrally placed than in ascites. A fluid thrill is a poor discriminating sign and should not be used.

Auscultation

Apart from in the evaluation of the acute abdomen, auscultation is not of great value in gastrointestinal disease. Abdominal bruits are often present in normal subjects, but these are not clinically significant.

Intestinal sounds do not help in diagnosis.

Examination of the rectum and sigmoid

Digital examination of the rectum should be performed in most patients with gastrointestinal symptoms and in all patients with a change in bowel habit. The anus should be inspected for anal tags, external haemorrhoids, fissures or fistulas. In males, the prostate projects into the rectum anteriorly and its size and consistency should be noted. In women the cervix or uterus may be felt anteriorly.

Sigmoidoscopy should be part of the routine examination in all cases of diarrhoea and in patients with lower abdominal symptoms such as a change in bowel habit or bleeding. *Proctoscopy* is performed in all patients with a history of bright red blood per rectum; the narrow sigmoidoscope does not distend the lumen and haemorrhoids can be missed.

Sigmoidoscopy

- The technique is easy to learn, provides valuable information and is safe in competent hands.
- The patient is placed in the left lateral position with the knees drawn up and buttocks over the edge of the couch.
- No bowel preparation is usually required.
- Rectal examination is performed initially.
- The sigmoidoscope is pointed towards the symphysis pubis and passed into the anus. The obturator is removed and the instrument passed under direct vision to the rectosigmoidal junction and beyond if possible (using air insufflation).
- The mucosa of the anus and rectum is inspected. The normal mucosa is shiny, superficial vessels can be seen, and no contact bleeding should occur.
- Biopsies can be taken from any lesion seen or from apparently normal-looking mucosa which may show histological evidence of inflammation.
- The technique is relatively painless. In the irritable bowel syndrome, the patient's pain is often reproduced by air insufflation.

Proctoscopy

- The proctoscope is passed into the anus directed towards the symphysis pubis; the obturator is removed.
- The patient strains down as the proctoscope is withdrawn. Haemorrhoids are seen as purplish veins in the left lateral, right posterior or right anterior positions.
- Fissures may also be seen.

Flexible fibre sigmoidoscopy

The rigid sigmoidoscope only allows inspection of the lower 20–25 cm of the bowel, but a 70 cm flexible fibreoptic sigmoidoscope allows much more bowel to be visualized. It also can be readily used in the outpatient department after minimal bowel preparation (a disposable enema). Seventy per cent of colonic neoplasms occur within the range of the flexible sigmoidoscope.

Inspection of stools
This is not often performed nowadays. Nevertheless it can be important to confirm the patient's symptoms, e.g. of passing blood or steatorrhoea. The shape and size may be helpful, e.g. rabbity stools in the irritable bowel syndrome. Stool charts for recording frequency and volume of defecation are useful in inpatients to follow the progress of their disease.

Clinical investigation

Many techniques are now available for the investigation of the gastrointestinal tract, the most important being radiology and endoscopy.

Plain x-rays

Plain x-rays of the abdomen are chiefly used in the investigation of the acute abdomen (see p. 199). Areas of calcification can be seen in chronic pancreatitis (see p. 257). Routine abdominal x-rays are of little use in the management of most gastrointestinal disease.

Barium contrast studies

Barium swallow
The oesophagus is visualized as barium is swallowed in the upright and prone positions. Motility abnormalities as well as anatomical lesions can then be observed. Reflux of barium from the stomach into the oesophagus is demonstrated with the patient tipped head down, but minimal reflux under these conditions may well have no clinical significance. Swallowing bread with barium (to add bulk) is sometimes useful in the investigation of undiagnosed dysphagia.

Barium meal
This is performed to examine the stomach and duodenum. A small amount of barium is given together with effervescent granules or tablets to produce carbon dioxide, so that a double contrast between air and barium is obtained. This technique has a high accuracy rate when performed carefully. Single-contrast studies are not usually recommended.

Small bowel follow-through
This is used to examine the small bowel. Barium is swallowed and allowed to pass into the small intestine through the jejunum and into the ileum. This technique is the only way of demonstrating the gross anatomy of the small intestine. It is particularly important to study the terminal ileum using fluoroscopy and to obtain films of the area.

Small bowel enema
A tube is passed through the duodenum and a large volume of dilute barium introduced. This technique is useful for visualizing suspicious areas seen on the follow-through, particularly strictures.

Barium enema
Barium and air are insufflated into the rectum via a retained catheter. A double-contrast view is then obtained of the whole colon, often with views of the terminal ileum as well. The patient must be prepared well with laxatives and wash-outs so that the colon is empty. This technique does not examine the lowest part of the rectum, and rectal examination and sigmoidoscopy should precede this examination.

Barium contrast studies

- Upper GI series patients are fasted overnight.
- Barium enema patients are given a low-fibre diet for three days and laxatives 24 h before the procedure. Washouts are performed immediately before the examination to ensure the colon is empty.
- The radiologist should be given correct clinical information so that he can concentrate on the particular areas under suspicion.
- The radiologist screens the patient so that any suspicious area can be re-examined immediately.
- X-rays should be reviewed by the clinician and the radiologist.

Computed tomography (CT) and ultrasound

These techniques are mainly used in the investigation of the liver and biliary tract, pancreas and retroperitoneal areas (see p. 216).

Endoscopy

A series of fibreoptic instruments have been developed to obtain a good view of the mucosal surface of the GI tract. The oesophagus, stomach and duodenum can be examined with a gastroscope, and the rectum, sigmoid and all parts of the colon and terminal ileum with a colonoscope. Biopsies can be taken from any area using forceps passed down through the instrument. Oesophagoscopy is of particular value in oesophageal disease and for the detection of varices. Colonoscopy allows good visualization of the whole colon with the advantage that biopsies can be obtained. The relative advantages and disadvantages of gastroscopy and barium studies in the investigation of dyspepsia are shown in Table 4.3. The choice, however, depends on local availability and expertise, but generally a barium meal is the first investigation performed.

Table 4.3 Gastroscopy versus double-contrast barium studies in the investigation of dyspepsia.

	Gastroscopy	Barium studies
Advantages	Slightly more accurate	Permanent record
	Mucosa visualized directly	Time to study and review results
	Biopsies obtainable	Accurate for the detection of extrinsic lesions
	No radiation	
	Better for post-operative stomachs	Good for the detection of hiatus hernia
	Treatment can be instituted, e.g. removal of a foreign body	
Disadvantages	Sedation may be necessary	Radiation
	Time-consuming for physician	Tissue diagnosis unavailable
	Less comfortable	
	Slightly more expensive	
	Associated with a small mortality	

Upper GI endoscopy

- The patient is fasted overnight and the procedure carried out as an outpatient.
- Sedation may be given intravenously.
- The instrument is passed into the pharynx with the patient swallowing. It is then passed under direct vision through the oesophagus into the stomach and duodenum.
- The forward-viewing instrument is used for visualization of the oesophagus, stomach and duodenal cap.
- The side-viewing instrument is needed to visualize certain areas, e.g. the ampulla of Vater.

Colonoscopy

Patient preparation:
- Two days before procedure—low-residue diet started
- One day before procedure—clear fluids only
- Afternoon prior to procedure—71 ml extract of senna with one pint of water given
- Three hours later—one sachet of sodium picosulphate with one pint of water given
- Day of procedure—one sachet of sodium picosulphate with one pint of water given

Alternative preparation consists of giving large volumes of balanced electrolyte solution by mouth on the day of the test.

The instrument is passed under direct supervision and manoeuvred around to the caecum.

Endoscopic retrograde cholangiopancreatography (ERCP)

This technique has proved very useful in the investigation of pancreatic and biliary tract disease; it is discussed on p. 217.

Radionuclide imaging

Radionuclides are being increasingly used for imaging of the liver and biliary tract (see p. 217). Other uses include demonstration of oesophageal reflux and gastric emptying (using technetium-99m sulphur colloid), Meckel's diverticulum (using [^{99m} Tc] pertechnetate, which has an affinity for gastric mucosa) and inflammatory lesions in inflammatory bowel disease (using indium-111 labelled white cells). All of these techniques require constant evaluation if they are to produce reliable and reproducible results.

The mouth

Mastication of the food takes place in the mouth. The food then passes into the pharynx. Problems in the mouth are extremely common and although they may be trivial they can produce severe symptoms. Poor dental hygiene is often a factor.

Stomatitis

Viral
Herpes simplex virus type 1 causes an acute stomatitis and recurrent herpes labialis (cold sore) (see p. 67).

Hand, foot and mouth disease due to coxsackie A virus produces mouth vesicles, usually in children. No treatment is required.

Herpes zoster involving the fifth cranial nerve can produce unilateral vesicular lesions (see p. 838).

Glandular fever due to the Epstein–Barr virus is associated with palatal petechiae with acute tonsillitis and pharyngitis (see p. 53).

Bacterial
Bacterial stomatitis is not common in Western countries, except as an accompaniment to a sore throat due to *Streptococcus*.

Vincent's stomatitis occurs in the malnourished patient with poor dentition. The sloughing ulceration involves primarily the gums but the whole oral cavity may be affected. The specific causative organisms are not known, but it is likely that a number of organisms are responsible. Anaerobic commensals found in normal subjects are present in large numbers in this infectious condition. Treatment is with metronidazole (200 mg three times a day for 4 days) with accompanying good mouth and dental hygiene.

Tuberculosis involving the mouth is very rare, and presents as a painful shallow ulcer.

Syphilitic infection due to *Treponema pallidum* is also rare. Primary syphilis produces a chancre; secondary syphilis produces a snail track ulcer.

Fungal

Fungal infection of the mouth is usually due to *Candida albicans* and in adults it is seen only in the severely ill or immunocompromised patient or after broad-spectrum antibiotics. White colonies, often coalescing to form a membrane, are seen. The lower pharynx and oesophagus can be involved, producing dysphagia. Treatment, which often needs to be prolonged, is with nystatin pastilles held in the mouth or with miconazole oral gel.

Angular stomatitis and the stomatitis associated with dentures can sometimes be due to *Candida*.

Non-infective

Recurrent aphthous ulceration is very common. The ulcers are superficial and are surrounded by erythema. They are very painful. They are usually small, multiple and recur frequently. They start in adolescence and often seem to resolve spontaneously as the patient gets older. The aetiology is unknown. They are sometimes associated with GI disease, notably Crohn's disease, ulcerative colitis and coeliac disease. *Granulomatous ulcers* can also occur in Crohn's disease. *Behçet's disease* presents with deep oral and genital ulceration. Hydrocortisone pellets may help all these conditions and symptomatic treatment with local anaesthetics relieves the pain. However, the efficacy of treatment for this condition has not been proved.

Stomatitis can occur with ill-fitting dentures or with a number of *vitamin deficiences*, including deficiencies of niacin, riboflavin, folate and B_{12}. Angular stomatitis and glossitis frequently occur together.

Stomatitis is frequently seen in *blood dyscrasias*, particularly acute leukaemia. A blue line on the gums is seen with *lead poisoning*.

Diseases of the tongue

A pale smooth tongue can be seen in iron deficiency. A sore tongue may result from glossitis associated with stomatitis, the various causes of which are described above.

The term 'geographical tongue' describes a migrating glossitis exclusively affecting the dorsum of the tongue. This condition has no clinical significance and the patient should be reassured.

Many patients who complain of a sore tongue do not have an obvious abnormality. Very occasionally this can be due to B_{12} or folate deficiency, but mostly there is no organic cause and the symptoms are psychological in origin. A bad taste in the mouth and

offensive breath (halitosis), particularly if only noticed by the patient, are also usually psychogenic symptoms. Rarely, patients with pyloric stenosis have halitosis.

Leukoplakia

Leukoplakia consists of white patches that cannot be removed. Any part of the mouth can be involved, particularly the tongue. Often no cause can be found, but leukoplakia can be due to viral infections or smoking. Five per cent of cases become malignant.

Squamous carcinoma

This may be related to excess smoking and alcohol consumption. It may present as a swelling or ulcer on any part of the mouth and tongue. Biopsy of any long-standing ulcer should always be performed. Treatment is with surgery and radiotherapy.

Lichen planus (see p. 911)

This can occur in all parts of the mouth and tongue, and produces white striae with small papules.

Bullous pemphigus (see p. 919)

This involves the mouth in all cases at some time. Painful blisters or bullae form and then burst, producing shallow ulcers.

The salivary glands

Xerostomia

Xerostomia means dryness of the mouth. Causes include:
- Psychogenic—anxiety
- Pyrexia
- Drugs—anticholinergics, antihistamines, tricyclic antidepressants and diuretics
- Sjögren's syndrome (see p. 335)
- Diabetic ketoacidosis and dehydration

The sensation of excess salivation (ptyalism) is chiefly psychogenic. It occurs before vomiting and with lesions of the mouth.

Bacterial and viral infections

These can affect any of the salivary glands, the commonest condition being acute parotitis due to the mumps virus. Acute parotitis due to an ascending infection with staphylococci or streptococci occurs often in elderly patients with dehydration and poor oral hygiene. Parotitis is also seen in alcoholics.

Sarcoidosis

This can produce parotid gland enlargement. When combined with lacrimal gland enlargement it is known as Mikulicz's syndrome.

Salivary duct obstruction due to calculus

Obstruction due to calculus usually involves the submandibular gland. There is painful swelling of the gland after eating. The stones can sometimes be felt in the floor of the mouth and their removal is usually followed by complete relief of symptoms.

Tumours

Salivary gland tumours are usually of a mixed type. They may involve any of the salivary glands, but usually affect the parotid. The gland becomes swollen but not tender and treatment is by removal, although local recurrences occur.

The pharynx and oesophagus

Structure

The oesophagus is a muscular tube, approximately 25 cm long, connecting the pharynx to the stomach. The muscle coat has two layers—an outer longitudinal layer and an inner circular layer of fibres. In the upper portion both muscle layers are striated. They gradually change to smooth muscle in the lower oesophagus, where they are continuous with the muscle layer of the stomach. The oesophagus is lined by stratified squamous epithelium, except near the gastro-oesophageal junction where columnar epithelium is found.

Function

The oesophagus is separated from the pharynx by the *upper oesophageal sphincter* which is normally closed by the continuous contraction of cricopharyngeus muscle. The *lower oesophageal sphincter (LOS)* consists of an area of the distal end of the oesophagus which has a high resting tone and which is largely responsible for the prevention of reflux. The reduction in tone and relaxation that occurs with swallowing is under the control of nervous (vagal) and hormonal mechanisms.

During swallowing the bolus of food is moved from the mouth to the pharynx voluntarily. Immediately, the upper sphincter relaxes and food enters the oesophagus. A primary peristaltic wave starts in the pharynx at the onset of swallowing and sweeps down the whole oesophagus. Secondary peristalsis occurs locally in response to direct stimulation (e.g. distension by the bolus) and helps to clear food residue from the oesophagus. Non-peristaltic, non-propulsive tertiary waves are frequent in the elderly. The LOS relaxes when swallowing is initiated, before the arrival of the peristaltic wave.

Symptoms of oesophageal disorders

Major oesophageal symptoms are:
● Dysphagia
● Heartburn
● Painful swallowing

Dysphagia
This is either due to a local lesion or is part of a generalized disease. Patients will complain of something sticking in their throat or chest during swallowing or immediately afterwards. It is always a serious symptom and the cause must be found. The causes are shown in Table 4.4. Globus hystericus is the name given to apparent dysphagia—the sensation of a 'lump in the throat' in patients who do not have true dysphagia and can therefore swallow. It has no organic cause and the treatment is reassurance.

Heartburn
Heartburn is a common symptom of acid reflux. The pain can spread to the neck, across the chest, and can be difficult to distinguish from the pain of ischaemic heart disease. It occurs at night when the patient lies flat or after bending or stooping. Hot drinks and alcohol often precipitate the pain.

Table 4.4 Causes of dysphagia.

Disease of mouth and tongue, e.g. septic throat
Neuromuscular disorders
Pharyngeal disorders
Bulbar palsy
Myasthenia gravis
Oesophageal motility disorders
Achalasia
Scleroderma
Diffuse oesophageal spasm
Presbyoesophagus
Diabetes
Chagas' disease
Extrinsic pressure
Mediastinal glands
Goitre
Enlarged left atrium
Intrinsic lesion
Foreign body
Stricture
Benign—peptic, corrosive
Malignant—carcinoma
Lower oesophageal rings
Oesophageal web
Pharyngeal pouch

Painful swallowing

Painful swallowing without real difficulty is occasionally seen in candidiasis (particularly in the immunosuppressed patient), herpes simplex, and following ingestion of tablets such as emepronium and potassium (slow release) which produce local ulceration if they lodge in the gullet when swallowed lying down and without water.

Signs of oesophageal disorders

There are very few signs associated with oesophageal disease, the main one being of weight loss as a consequence of dysphagia.

Investigation of oesophageal disorders

Investigation of oesophageal disorders mainly involves barium contrast studies and oesophagoscopy. Occasionally manometry and acid perfusion studies may be necessary; these are described later in this chapter.

MOTILITY DISORDERS

Achalasia

DEFINITION

This is a disease of unknown aetiology that is characterized by aperistalsis in the body of the oesophagus and failure of relaxation of the lower oesophageal sphincter on initiation of swallowing.

PATHOLOGY

Degenerative lesions are found in the vagus as well as a decrease in ganglionic cells in the nerve plexus of the oesophageal wall.

CLINICAL FEATURES

The disease can present at any age but is rare in childhood. The incidence is about 1 per 100 000 per year. Patients usually have a long history of intermittent dysphagia for both liquids and solids. Regurgitation of food from the dilated oesophagus may be induced by the patient or may occur spontaneously, particularly at night, and aspiration pneumonia may result. Occasionally food gets stuck, but patients often learn to overcome this by drinking large quantities, thereby increasing the head of pressure in the oesophagus and forcing the food through. Severe retrosternal chest pain occurs particularly in younger patients with vigorous non-peristaltic contraction of the oesophagus. The dysphagia in these patients can be mild and the pain misdiagnosed as cardiac in origin. Weight loss is usually not marked.

INVESTIGATION

A *chest x-ray* may show a dilated oesophagus with occasionally a fluid level behind the heart. The fundal gas shadow is not present.

A *barium swallow* will show dilatation of the oesophagus, lack of peristalsis and often synchronous contractions. The lower end gradually narrows (beak deformity); this appearance is due to failure of the sphincter to relax.

Oesophagoscopy is necessary to exclude a carcinoma at the lower end of the oesophagus, which can produce a similar x-ray appearance. When there is marked dilatation, extensive cleansing is necessary to remove food debris in order to obtain a clear view. In achalasia the oesophagoscope easily flops through the apparent narrowing without resistance.

Manometry may be used to measure oesophageal motility but is not routinely performed. It can confirm the aperistalsis of the oesophagus as well as the failure of relaxation of the lower oesophageal sphincter.

Chagas' disease (American trypanosomiasis, see p. 73) damages the neural plexus of the gut and produces a similar clinical picture.

TREATMENT

The lower oesophageal sphincter is dilated forcibly using a pneumatic bag (passed under x-ray control) so as to weaken the sphincter. This is successful in 80% of cases. Forced dilatation is quicker to perform than surgical division of the muscle at the lower end of the oesophagus (cardiomyotomy or Heller's operation), which is now mainly used in patients whose symptoms have not improved after many dilatations. Reflux oesophagitis complicates both procedures and the aperistalsis of the oesophagus remains.

COMPLICATIONS

There is an increased incidence of 5–10% of carcinoma of the oesophagus in both treated and untreated cases. Recurrent pneumonia may occur due to aspiration of oesophageal contents.

Systemic sclerosis

In 90% or more of patients with this disease there is oesophageal involvement, with diminished peristalsis detected manometrically or by barium swallow. This is due to replacement of the smooth muscle layers by fibrous tissue. The lower oesophageal sphincter pressure is also decreased, allowing reflux; mucosal damage may occur as a consequence. Strictures may develop. Initially there are no symptoms, but dysphagia and heartburn occur as the oesophagus becomes severely involved.

Similar findings may be found in other connective tissue disorders, particularly if Raynaud's phenomenon is present. Treatment is as for reflux (see p. 159) and stricture formation (see below).

Diffuse oesophageal spasm

This is a severe form of abnormal oesophageal motility which can sometimes produce retrosternal chest pain and dysphagia. Swallowing is accompanied by bizarre and marked contractions of the oesophagus without progression of the waves. On barium swallow the appearance may be of a 'cork screw'. However, asymptomatic abnormalities of oesophageal motility are not infrequent, particularly in patients over the age of 60 years (presbyoesophagus). Care must therefore be taken that the symptoms and the x-ray findings of oesophageal spasm are not falsely attributed.

TREATMENT

True oesophageal spasm producing severe symptoms is rare and treatment is often unhelpful. Antispasmodics, nitrates, or calcium channel blockers such as sublingual nifedipine 10 mg three times daily may be tried.

Miscellaneous motility disorders

Abnormalities of motility, which are mostly asymptomatic but occasionally produce dysphagia, are found in diabetes mellitus, myotonica dystrophica and myasthenia gravis, as well as any neurological disorder involving the brain stem.

OTHER OESOPHAGEAL DISORDERS

Oesophageal diverticulum

This is a pouch lined with epithelium which can produce dysphagia and regurgitation. It is usually asymptomatic and often detected accidentally on a barium swallow performed for other reasons.
Diverticula can occur:
- Immediately above the upper oesophageal sphincter (pharyngeal pouch). If large it may cause dysphagia as well as spillage of contents into the trachea
- Near the middle of the oesophagus (traction diverticulum produced by extrinsic inflammation)
- Just above the lower oesophageal sphincter (epiphrenic diverticulum)

Only when symptoms are severe should surgery be undertaken.

Rings and webs

A number of rings and webs have been described throughout the oesophagus.

Lower oesophageal or Schatzki ring

This is a narrowing of the lower end of the oesophagus due to a ridge of mucosa or a fibrous membrane. The ring may be asymptomatic, but it can very occasionally produce dysphagia after swallowing a large bolus of bread or meat. The narrowing or ring is seen on a barium swallow, with the oesophagus well distended with barium.

The treatment is reassurance and dietary advice.

Upper oesophageal web

In this condition atrophy of the squamous epithelium in the postcricoid region occurs near the upper oesophageal sphincter, with formation of a web. The web may be asymptomatic or may produce dysphagia. In the Plummer–Vinson syndrome (Paterson Brown Kelly syndrome) this web is associated with iron-deficiency anaemia, glossitis and angular stomatitis. This rare syndrome affects mainly women, and its aetiology is not understood. At oesophagoscopy the web may be difficult to see. Dilatation of the web is rarely necessary. Iron is given for the iron deficiency.

Benign oesophageal stricture

Peptic stricture secondary to reflux is the commonest cause of benign strictures. They also occur after the ingestion of corrosives, after radiotherapy, after sclerotherapy of varices and following prolonged nasogastric intubation. All strictures give rise to dysphagia. They are usually treated by dilatation, but occasionally surgery is necessary.

Oesophageal candidiasis

Infection with the fungus Candida is becoming increasingly recognized as a cause of painful dysphagia, particularly in immunosuppressed or debilitated patients. Oral candidiasis is not invariably present. The barium swallow shows ulceration, which on oesophagoscopy appears as white plaques on top of a friable mucosa. The diagnosis can be confirmed by examining a direct smear taken at endoscopy. Treatment is with nystatin or amphotericin. Most patients on large doses of immunosuppressive agents are treated prophylactically.

Mallory–Weiss syndrome

This is described on p. 170.

Carcinoma of the oesophagus

This is discussed on p. 202.

Hiatus hernia and reflux oesophagitis

These will be considered together, as a sliding hiatus hernia on its own does not produce symptoms. The symptoms occur because of the presence of the associated reflux. With a sliding hiatus hernia, the gastro-oesophageal junction 'slides' through the hiatus so that it lies above the diaphragm. With a para-oesophageal or rolling hernia, a small part of the stomach rolls up through the hernia alongside the oesophagus (Fig. 4.3); the sphincter still remains below the diaphragm and remains competent. Occasionally a rolling para-oesophageal hernia will produce pain and need surgical treatment.

Fig. 4.3 Diagrammatic representation of the two types of hiatus hernia.

Reflux occurs because of failure of the antireflux mechanism, and commonly, but not necessarily, it accompanies a hiatus hernia. The antireflux mechanism includes the local anatomical arrangement of the gastro-oesophageal junction below the diaphragm and, more importantly, the tone of the lower oesophageal sphincter. In the majority of patients with reflux, sphincter pressure will be low. Reflux, however, commonly occurs sporadically in normal subjects several times a day. Presumably the transient nature of the reflux with rapid clearance by secondary peristalsis prevents inflammation in normal subjects. If, however, reflux is persistent and prolonged and clearance is poor, inflammation may result. Causes of increased reflux are shown in Table 4.5.

Table 4.5 Causes of increased oesophageal reflux.

Pregnancy or obesity
Fat, chocolate or coffee ingestion
Smoking
Anticholinergic drugs
Systemic sclerosis
After treatment for achalasia

CLINICAL FEATURES

Heartburn is the major feature of reflux oesophagitis. The burning is aggravated by bending, stooping or lying down and may be relieved by antacids. The patient may complain of pain on drinking hot liquids or alcohol. The correlation between heartburn and oesophagitis is poor. Some patients have little oesophagitis but severe heartburn; others have severe oesophagitis without symptoms and present with an iron-deficiency anaemia due to blood loss. Regurgitation of food into the mouth also occurs, particularly when lying flat. Aspiration into the lungs, producing pneumonia, is unusual without an accompanying stricture, but cough and nocturnal asthma from regurgitation and aspiration can occur.

INVESTIGATION

Barium swallow is still the most widely used investigation. Hiatus hernia occurs in approximately 30% of people of 50 years of age and by itself is of no diagnostic significance. Evidence of free reflux of barium must be demonstrated. Even here care must be taken not to over-interpret small amounts of reflux. Reflux can also be demonstrated with radio-labelled technetium or by using a pH probe. No single test is perfect and often a combination of tests is required.

Oesophagoscopy may show the presence of a red friable mucosa with linear ulceration. A Bernstein test may be helpful in investigating retrosternal chest pain; acid (or bicarbonate as a control) is infused into the oesophagus to try to reproduce the pain.

TREATMENT

Many patients can be treated successfully with antacids, a reduction in obesity, and raising the head end of the bed at night. Unfortunately, compliance with the latter two treatments is poor. Treatment with H_2-receptor antagonists such as cimetidine (400 mg two times daily) or ranitidine (150 mg two times daily) is frequently used. Proprietary antacids containing alginates (10 ml three times daily) may help. Unfortunately, even with these agents it is difficult to keep a neutral pH in the oesophagus.

Surgery is rarely needed and should never be performed for a hiatus hernia alone. The properly selected case with severe reflux and oesophagitis responds well to surgery. Repair of the hernia and some sort of additional antireflux surgery, e.g. Nissen fundoplication, is required.

COMPLICATIONS

The major complication of reflux is peptic stricture, which usually occurs in patients over the age of 60. The symptoms are those of intermittent dysphagia over a long period. Treatment is by dilatation and management of the reflux either medically or surgically. There is no increased incidence of carcinoma in hiatus hernia per se (but see Barrett's oesophagus, p. 202). Anaemia and occasionally frank haemorrhage may occur with oesophagitis. Recurrent aspiration pneumonia can occur when stricture formation is present.

The stomach and duodenum

Structure

The *stomach*, which varies considerably in size, is divided into the upper portion—the fundus, the mid region or body, and the antrum, which extends into the pyloric region. These areas are shown in Fig. 4.4.

There are two sphincters—the gastro-oesophageal sphincter and the pyloric sphincter, which is largely made up of a thickening of the circular muscle layer. The muscle wall of the stomach has three layers—an outer longitudinal, an inner circular, and an innermost oblique layer of smooth muscle.

The *duodenum* has outer longitudinal and inner smooth muscle layers. It is C-shaped and the pancreas sits in the concavity. It terminates in the jejunum at the duodenojejunal flexure.

The mucosal lining of the stomach, particularly in the greater curvature, is thrown into thick folds or rugae. The upper two-thirds of the stomach contain parietal cells, which secrete hydrochloric acid, and chief cells, which secrete pepsinogen. The junction between the body and the antrum of the stomach can often be seen macroscopically, but can be confirmed by measuring surface pH. The antrum contains only mucus-secreting cells and G cells, which secrete gastrin. There are two major forms of gastrin—G17 and G34, depending on the number of amino acid residues. G17 is the major form found in the antrum.

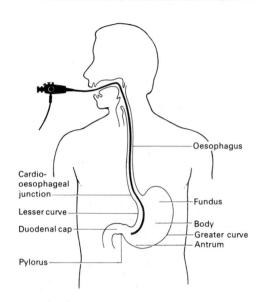

Fig. 4.4 Areas of the stomach as visualized through a gastroscope.

The duodenal mucosa contains Brunner's glands, which secrete alkaline mucus. This, along with the pancreatic and biliary secretions, helps to neutralize the acid secretion from the stomach when it reaches the duodenum.

Function

Acid secretion

The factors controlling acid secretion are shown in Fig. 4.5. Secretion is under neural and hormonal control. Both stimulate acid secretion through the release of histamine which acts directly on the parietal cells.

Fig. 4.5 Phases of and factors controlling acid secretion.

Other major gastric functions
- Reservoir for food
- Absorption (of only minimal importance)
- Emulsification of fat and mixing of gastric contents
- Secretion of intrinsic factor

Gastric emptying depends on many factors. There are osmoreceptors in the duodenal mucosa which control gastric emptying by local reflexes and the release of gut hormones. In particular, intra-duodenal fat delays gastric emptying by negative feedback through duodenal receptors.

GASTRITIS

This can be divided into acute and chronic. Unfortunately there is no universally accepted classification of this condition because there is a poor correlation between clinical, pathological and endoscopic findings. Some degree of gastritis can always be found if the stomach is examined by careful histological means, but these small areas of gastritis seem to have no significance.

Acute gastritis, acute ulceration and erosions

In *acute gastritis* there is acute inflammation of the gastric mucosa with destruction of the superficial epithelial cells.

In *mucosal erosion* there is destruction of small zones of the mucosa, but healing is complete and there is no subsequent fibrosis. Multiple small erosions, often with an oedematous mucosa, are known as acute erosive gastritis.

In *acute gastric ulceration* there is more extensive mucosal necrosis, and healing occurs with mucosal regeneration and the possibility of minimal fibrosis.

The aetiology is often obscure but gastritis can be produced by drugs such as aspirin and alcohol. Aspirin is thought to damage the mucosal barrier by allowing acid to diffuse into the gastric mucosa, where it causes the release of histamine, producing acute inflammation.

Acute ulcers are also seen after severe stress (stress ulcer) and secondary to burns (Curling ulcer), trauma, shock, renal or liver disease. The underlying mechanism for these ulcers is unknown but may be related to an alteration in blood flow.

CLINICAL FEATURES

The correlation between the pathological changes and symptoms is poor, but many patients wth acute gastritis will suffer from epigastric pain, indigestion and vomiting, usually for less than 24 hours. GI haemorrhage can occur (see p. 168).

DIAGNOSIS

In many patients the diagnosis is obvious (e.g. indigestion after a party), but endoscopy may be performed to confirm the presence of acute ulcers or erosions, particularly in patients admitted with GI haemorrhage.

TREATMENT

No specific therapy is required apart from removal of the offending cause. There is no evidence that acute gastritis will eventually lead to chronic gastritis or peptic ulceration.

Chronic gastritis

This occurs frequently, particularly in the elderly. Recently a new bacterium *Campylobacter pyloridis* has been implicated in the pathogenesis of non-autoimmune gastroduodenitis. Chronic gastritis is divided histologically into three categories.

Chronic superficial gastritis
Chronic superficial gastritis consists of an infiltration of lymphocytes and plasma cells into the superficial mucosa. The deeper mucosa is unaffected.

Atrophic gastritis
In atrophic gastritis there is more extensive inflammation of the mucosa, with loss of the parietal and chief cells in the deeper specialized parts of the glands. There is also intestinal metaplasia. This condition may be patchy or involve most of the body of the stomach.

Gastric atrophy
In gastric atrophy there is a decrease in mucosal thickness with almost complete loss of specialized glandular tissue. Intestinal metaplasia is virtually complete. Cellular infiltration is minimal.

Severe gastric atrophy occurs in less than 5% of the population. The causes are multiple, but seem to include cigarette smoking but probably not alcohol, which only causes an acute gastritis. Following a gastrectomy, most patients will have some degree of chronic gastritis due to biliary reflux.

There is a strong association between chronic gastritis and autoimmune diseases such as thyroid disease, diabetes mellitus and Addison's disease.

In *pernicious anaemia* there is always gastric atrophy with a lack of acid and intrinsic factor. Serum gastrin levels are high as a result of the anacidity. Circulating parietal cell antibodies are present in 50% of patients with atrophic gastritis and in 90% of patients with pernicious anaemia. Intrinsic factor antibodies are only present in one-third of patients with pernicious anaemia. Two types of intrinsic factor antibodies are found—blocking antibody, which prevents formation of the intrinsic factor/B_{12} complex, and a binding antibody, which binds this complex. The role of these antibodies in the pathogenesis is unclear.

Chronic gastritis is asymptomatic and requires no treatment. It is found incidentally at endoscopy or barium meal examination of the stomach (absence of mucosal folds). Accompanying pernicious anaemia is investigated and treated (see p. 269).

MENETRIER'S DISEASE

Menetrier's disease is a rare condition in which there is thickening and enlargement of the gastric mucosal folds. Histologically there is hyperplasia of the mucin-producing cells with glandular proliferation and loss of the parietal and chief cells.

The patient may complain of epigastric pain and occasionally peripheral oedema may occur due to hypoalbuminaemia resulting from protein loss through the gastric mucosa. Symptomatic treatment is all that is required for this condition. It is possibly premalignant.

DUODENITIS

Duodenitis is a condition frequently seen at endoscopy. The duodenal mucosa appears inflamed, haemorrhagic and friable. Occasionally small breaks in the mucosa are seen, i.e. erosions. Microscopically there is chronic inflammation.

The condition can occur in asymptomatic individuals and its relationship to symptoms is unknown. There is as yet no evidence that even severe inflammation will progress to frank chronic duodenal ulcer disease. Treatment is not necessary for the inflammation per se.

CHRONIC PEPTIC ULCER

This is an ulcer of the mucosa in or adjacent to an acid-bearing area. Most ulcers occur in the stomach or proximal duodenum, but they can occur in the oesophagus (with oesophageal reflux), in the jejunum in the Zollinger–Ellison syndrome or after a gastroenterostomy, and finally in a Meckel's diverticulum which contains ectopic gastric mucosa.

AETIOLOGY

The aetiology is unknown. Possible mechanisms include:

Gastric ulcer
Most patients with gastric ulcers have normal or low acid outputs and thus other factors are also responsible for the ulceration. These other factors include:

- Alteration in mucus production
- Biliary reflux
- Chronic gastritis, possibly produced by gastric stasis
- Mucosal ischaemia

Thirty per cent of gastric ulcers, mainly prepyloric ulcers, are associated with high acid output and duodenal ulcer disease.

Duodenal ulcer
Most patients with duodenal ulcer secrete excess acid and pepsinogen. Changes in mucosal resistance are thought to be less important. Bacteria (*Campylobacter* and spirochaetes) have been found in ulcers and it is suggested that they might play a role in pathogenesis.

Epidemiological factors. Duodenal ulceration is common; 15% of the population will suffer from a duodenal ulcer at some time. They are two to three times commoner than gastric ulcers. Duodenal ulcers are commoner in men than women (4:1) and both gastric and duodenal ulcers are more common in elderly people. There is considerable geographical variation. Duodenal ulcer is commoner in north England and Scotland than in other parts of the UK. South India has a higher incidence of duodenal ulcer than north India while south Nigeria has more patients with duodenal ulcer than north Nigeria. Both types of peptic ulcer are common in Australians.

Other aetiological factors of peptic ulcer are shown in Table 4.6. Peptic ulceration is also seen in hyperparathyroidism (since calcium stimulates acid secretion), the Zollinger–Ellison syndrome and in patients with renal transplants.

PATHOLOGY

Gastric ulcer can occur in any part of the stomach, but is most commonly found on the lesser curve.

Table 4.6 Some factors involved or thought to be involved in the causation of peptic ulceration.

Factors	Relationship
Diet	Weak
Alcohol	None
Anti-inflammatory drugs	Weak (but strong for aspirin for gastric ulcer in Australian women)
Steroid drugs	None
Smoking	Fair for duodenal ulcer
Psychological factors	Weak
Genetic factors	Strong for patients who do not secrete blood group O antigens into gastric secretions
Family history	Strong

Most duodenal ulcers are found in the duodenal cap. Histologically there is a break in the superficial epithelium with an increase in inflammatory cells and a necrotic ulcer base. The ulcer heals with fibrosis.

CLINICAL FEATURES

Symptoms

Epigastric pain or discomfort is the major feature of ulcer disease. The patient who points directly to the epigastrium as the site of the pain is most likely to have an ulcer. The pain of a duodenal ulcer classically occurs at night. In both types of ulcer, pain is helped by antacids. The relationship of the pain to food is variable and on the whole is not helpful in diagnosis. However, patients with a duodenal ulcer may complain of pains when they are hungry.

Nausea may accompany the pain, but vomiting is not frequent and when it occurs it may relieve the pain. Other symptoms include heartburn and flatulence, which are due to acid regurgitation. Anorexia and weight loss may occur, particularly with gastric ulcers.

The symptoms of a duodenal ulcer are periodic, with spontaneous relapses and remissions. Sixty per cent of patients will have a recurrence of symptoms within one year of the first episode. The natural history appears to be for the disease to remit over many years. Fifty per cent of patients with a gastric ulcer will have a recurrence within 2 years. If the patient complains of persistent and severe pain, complications such as penetration into other organs should be considered. Back pain may suggest a penetrating posterior duodenal ulcer.

Signs

The only signs are those of epigastric tenderness, but this is a poor discriminating sign. Tenderness does not necessarily imply disease and is frequently found in non-ulcer dyspepsia.

INVESTIGATION

- *Blood tests* are unhelpful.
- A *barium meal* using a double-contrast technique is still the most important test in diagnosis. A gastric ulcer is shown in Fig. 4.6 and a duodenal ulcer in Fig. 4.7.
- *Endoscopy* can be used as an alternative to a barium meal. It is slightly more accurate for both gastric and duodenal ulcers, but there is little to choose between the two techniques when both are performed competently. Endoscopy has the advantage that biopsies can be obtained from gastric ulcers, but even multiple biopsies do not exclude malignancy. The choice is dependent on local availability and expertise.
- *Gastric function tests.* Secretions from the stomach are collected via a nasogastric tube before (basal secretion) and following stimulation by an injection of pentagastrin. This is a synthetic peptide containing the terminal five peptides of gastrin. The acid status is not useful for the routine case of ulceration because of the overlap with normal values (see Fig. 4.8). The main use of this test is in the Zollinger–Ellison syndrome.
- *Serum gastrin.* Serum gastrin can be measured by radioimmunoassay, which measures the G17 form (see p. 160). Gastrin levels should always be assayed in patients with recurrent ulceration following surgery because of the possibility of the Zollinger–Ellison syndrome.

How to investigate epigastric pain

Patient under 35 years:
- Gastric or duodenal lesion unlikely
- No investigation—treat symptomatically initially

Patient over 35 years:
- Duodenal ulcer, gastric ulcer and gastric carcinoma are all possible
- Double-contrast barium meal is therefore performed
- If x-rays are negative after review, the diagnosis is non-ulcer dyspepsia (90% correct)
- Endoscopy for doubtful cases

TREATMENT

Duodenal ulcer

The treatment of duodenal ulcers has changed radically in the last few years since the introduction of *H₂-receptor antagonists* (Fig. 4.9). These agents have a molecular structure which fits the H_2 receptors on the parietal cells. They can reduce acid secretion by 60% over a 24-h period. Prior to their introduction, the treatment of duodenal ulceration was divided into symptomatic therapy, i.e. antacids, and therapy designed to heal the ulcer. Recently, however, it has been recognized that the symptoms of duodenal ulcer fluctuate and do not correlate with the degree of ulcer healing. Duodenal ulcer patients are now therefore advised to take either cimetidine or ranitidine for 3–4 weeks while they have severe symptoms, restarting as soon as their symptoms return. Some patients will require virtually continuous therapy, usually on a once-a-day basis. The H_2-receptor antagonists are remarkably free of side-effects, but confusion in the elderly, gynaecomastia and loss of libido have been described.

Any mild episodes of discomfort and indigestion can usually be managed by *antacids*. The chief antacids are magnesium trisilicate and aluminium hydroxide; the former often causes diarrhoea while the latter causes constipation. There is no place for the more complex antacid mixtures which have no increased buffering capacity and are expensive. Other side-effects of antacids at normal dosages ⹂re not a major problem, but many antacids contain

(a)

Fig. 4.6 Double contrast barium meal showing a gastric ulcer (arrow) on the lesser curve. The benign nature of the ulcer is demonstrated by a round niche within the wall of the stomach (a), with mucosal folds radiating to it (b).

(b)

Fig. 4.7 Barium meal showing a large chronic duodenal ulcer (arrow) on the anterior wall of the cap.

sodium which may exacerbate fluid retention. Aluminium hydroxide has less sodium than other antacids.

There are a number of other drugs available and some of these have been shown in clinical trials to be effective for both symptomatic relief and for ulcer healing (Table 4.7). However, their popularity has decreased since the introduction of H_2-receptor antagonists. The more traditional methods of healing duodenal ulcers with either bed rest or diet are now never used, but stopping smoking should always be strongly encouraged as smoking slows healing.

The effectiveness of treatment should be assessed symptomatically. There is no need for follow-up x-rays or endoscopy. If the patient fails to respond, the diagnosis should be reviewed. Duodenal ulcers are common and care must be taken not to falsely attribute abdominal symptoms to the finding of an ulcer.

Gastric ulcer
The treatment of a gastric ulcer differs in approach from that of a duodenal ulcer in that most physicians like to check that a gastric ulcer has completely

Fig. 4.8 Acid output in different conditions. DU = duodenal ulcer; GU = gastric ulcer.

Fig. 4.9 The chemical formulae of H_2-receptor antagonists. Note the similarity to histamine.

Table 4.7 Drugs other than H_2-receptor antagonists and antacids used in the treatment of peptic ulceration.

Drugs	Mechanism	Use	Daily dose	Side-effects
Anticholinergics				
Poldine methyl-sulphate	Reduce acid secretion	Occasionally in DU	2 mg × 3	Dry mouth; raised intraocular pressure
Propanthelene bromide			15 mg × 3	Blurred vision; urinary retention
Pirenzepine		Under study	50 mg × 2	More selective action, therefore fewer side-effects
Bismuth				
Tripotassium dicitrato-bismuthate	Forms protective coating on ulcer	GU and DU; reduces relapses	15 ml diluted in 15 ml water × 4 *or* 120 mg tablets × 4 (more palatable)	Unpleasant taste; black tongue, teeth and stools
Sucralfate				
Aluminium salt of sucrose octasulphate	Adherence to mucosa	GU and DU	1g × 4	Constipation
Liquorice derivatives				
Carbenoxolone	Effects mucosal resistance	GU	100 mg × 3	Sodium retention with oedema; hypokalaemia; hypertension; requires caution in elderly
Deglycyrrhizinized liquorice	? Effect on mucosal resistance	GU and DU	2 tablets × 3	Diarrhoea
Others				
Prostaglandin E_2	Cytoprotection, plus decreases acid	DU and GU	Under study	Under study

NB The main drugs used for peptic ulceration are H_2-receptor antagonists.
DU = duodenal ulcer; GU = gastric ulcer.

healed and thus follow-up x-rays or endoscopy are necessary. These differences in management are because:
- There is a better relationship between symptoms and the presence of an ulcer than for duodenal ulcer; nevertheless, asymptomatic gastric ulcers can occur.
- There is a risk that the ulcer may be malignant (see p. 203).

H_2-receptor antagonists are the most common agents used for treatment; follow-up with x-ray or endoscopy at 6 weeks is required. Failure to heal (or to achieve more than a 60% reduction in size) raises the question of malignancy and further endoscopy followed by surgery should be considered.

H_2-receptor antagonists are not so successful in the treatment of gastric ulcer as they are for duodenal ulcer but, because of their relative lack of side-effects, are still the drugs of first choice. Table 4.7 shows the other drugs that are sometimes used.

Once again, smoking should be strongly discouraged, but bedrest is now an outmoded form of therapy. Dietary changes are unnecessary and there is no reason to avoid spicy foods, coffee or alcohol unless they exacerbate symptoms. Antacids may be necessary to help with symptomatic relief.

Surgical management
The main indications for surgery are:
- All peptic ulcers:
  (a) Failure of medical treatment; operations in this group are decreasing since the introduction of H_2-receptor antagonists
  (b) Complications, including recurrent haemorrhage, perforation and outflow obstruction
- Gastric ulcers:
  (a) Failure to heal
  (b) Possibility of malignancy

Two types of operation are performed:
- Partial gastrectomy
- Vagotomy

Partial gastrectomy. The principle in both of the two types of gastrectomy performed for peptic ulcer disease is to remove the antral area which secretes gastrin, since this in turn stimulates acid production.

- *Billroth I partial gastrectomy* is now the commonest

operation for patients with a gastric ulcer. The lower part of the stomach is removed and the stomach remnant is connected to the duodenum.

- *Billroth II (Polya gastrectomy)* is now rarely performed, except for duodenal ulceration following a vagotomy. The stomach remnant is connected to the first loop of jejunum (a gastroenterostomy) and the duodenum is closed.

Vagotomy with or without drainage. A number of different types of operations have been performed over the years:

- Truncal vagotomy plus gastroenterostomy/ pyloroplasty
- Selective vagotomy (preserving the hepatic and coeliac branch of the vagus) plus gastroenterostomy/pyloroplasty.
- Highly selective vagotomy or proximal gastric vagotomy, in which only the nerves supplying the parietal cells are transected, and therefore no drainage is required. This is now the commonest operation for duodenal ulcer.

Some advantages and disadvantages of these operations are shown in Table 4.8.

Complications of surgery. The main complication is recurrent ulcer. This can occur in the stomach, duodenum or jejunum, often at the stoma. The symptoms are similar to those seen in the unoperated stomach, with pain being invariably present, although patients may present with haemorrhage. Because of the deformity of the stomach, investigation by endoscopy is preferred to x-ray examination. Treatment is either medical, using an H_2-receptor antagonist (usually long-term) or surgical. Consideration should be given to the possibility of the Zollinger–Ellison syndrome (see p. 208).

The following complications are all becoming less of a clinical problem as fewer and more conservative operations are being performed.

- *Dumping.* This is the term used to describe a number of upper abdominal symptoms, e.g. nausea and distension associated with sweating, faintness and palpitations, that occur in patients following gastrectomy or gastroenterostomy. It is due to 'dumping' of food into the jejunum, which is followed by rapid fluid dilution of the high osmotic load. A number of patients have mild symptoms of dumping but learn to cope with them. It is rare for it to be a clinical problem and if it is, the symptoms will have a functional element. Treatment should be reassurance and symptomatic therapy. Further operations are rarely needed.
- *Diarrhoea.* This is chiefly seen after vagotomy. It is not usually a problem, as many patients are happy with their increased stool looseness. Urgency or recurrent severe episodes occur in 1% and can be a major problem. Treatment consists of antidiarrhoeals such as codeine phosphate, but is not entirely satisfactory. Cholestyramine—a resin which binds bile salts—helps in some cases. Very occasionally the diarrhoea or steatorrhoea can be due to bacterial overgrowth in the blind loop of a Polya gastrectomy (see p. 181).
- *Vomiting (afferent loop syndrome/bilious vomiting).* The incidence of vomiting has decreased with the more conservative operations. Vomiting occurs because food gets trapped due to the altered anatomy. Treatment is symptomatic, except on the rare ocasions when reconstructive surgery is required.
- *Nutritional complications.* Anaemia is most commonly due to iron deficiency due to poor absorption. Treatment is with oral iron which may be needed long-term. Megaloblastic anaemia is uncommon but can be due to either folate defi-

Table 4.8 Advantages and disadvantages of operations for peptic ulceration.

Operation	Advantages	Disadvantages	Current usage
Partial gastrectomy	Low recurrence (< 1%) Diarrhoea < 1%	Increased operative mortality Increased complications, particularly metabolic Dumping 5% gastric 'cripple' Possible long-term malignancy	Gastric ulcer
Vagotomy	Decreased operative mortality Decreased metabolic complications	Higher recurrence (10%) Diarrhoea > 20%	Duodenal ulcer
Proximal gastric vagotomy	Little diarrhoea (only 2%) No drainage procedure necessary	Higher recurrence rate (5–10%) Needs experienced surgeon	Duodenal ulcer

ciency (due to poor intake) or B$_{12}$ deficiency (due to long-term atrophic gastritis resulting in intrinsic factor deficiency). Osteomalacia is an uncommon late complication (see p. 734). Patients often fail to gain weight due to anorexia after gastric surgery and a few suffer from severe protein–energy malnutrition as a result.

COMPLICATIONS OF PEPTIC ULCER

Haemorrhage
This is dealt with below.

Perforation (see also p. 199)
The frequency of perforation of a peptic ulcer is decreasing; this is partly attributed to the introduction of H$_2$-receptor antagonists. Duodenal ulcers perforate more commonly than gastric ulcers, usually into the peritoneal cavity. Perforation into the lesser sac may occur.

Management of perforation. Detailed management is described on p. 199. Surgery is performed to close the perforation and drain the abdomen. Conservative management using nasogastric suction, intravenous fluids and antibiotics is occasionally used in elderly and very sick patients.

Perforation of peptic ulcer

Look for:
- Other acute gastrointestinal conditions, e.g. cholecystitis, pancreatitis (check serum amylase)
- Non GI conditions, e.g. myocardial infarction
- Silent perforations in the elderly or patients on steroids

Remember:
- There *is* harm in leaving an undiagnosed perforation.
- There is no real harm in operating even if the perforation has occurred at a different site than expected clinically.
- Avoid laparotomy if pancreatitis is diagnosed.

Pyloric stenosis or obstruction
This is more accurately called gastric outflow obstruction as the obstruction may be prepyloric or in the duodenum. The obstruction occurs either because of an acute ulcer with surrounding oedema or because the healing of an ulcer has been followed by scarring. Occasionally the obstruction is due to a gastric malignancy.

The main symptom of this condition is vomiting, usually without pain as the characteristic ulcer pain has abated due to healing. Vomiting is projectile and huge in volume, and the vomitus contains particles of old food. On examination of the abdomen the patient may have a succussion splash.

Severe or persistent vomiting causes loss of acid from the stomach and a metabolic alkalosis occurs (see p. 446).

The diagnosis is made by barium meal examination, but can be suspected when large quantities of fluid are removed by gastric intubation in the fasting state. Fluid and electrolyte replacement is necessary, together with the regular removal of gastric contents via a nasogastric tube. In some patients with oedema rather than scarring the symptoms will settle with this conservative management. However, most patients require surgery. Postoperative gastric stasis can be a problem, particularly if a vagotomy has been performed, even when accompanied by drainage.

Acute and chronic gastrointestinal bleeding

This section should be read in conjunction with the descriptions of the specific conditions mentioned.

Acute upper gastrointestinal bleeding

Haematemesis is the vomiting of blood. Melaena is the passage of black tarry stools; the black colour is due to altered blood—50 ml or more are required to produce this. Melaena can occur with bleeding from any lesion from areas proximal to and including the caecum. Following a massive bleed from the upper GI tract, unaltered blood (due to rapid transit) can appear per rectum, but this is rare.

AETIOLOGY

Chronic peptic ulceration still accounts for approximately half of all cases of upper GI haemorrhage. This and other causes are shown in Fig. 4.10. The relative incidences of these causes vary depending on the patient population. Aspirin and other non-steroidal anti-inflammatory drugs can undoubtedly produce gastric lesions and probably are the cause of some GI bleeds from acute ulcers. There is doubt, however, whether these agents make chronic ulcers more likely to bleed. Corticosteroids in the usual therapeutic doses probably have no influence on GI haemorrhage.

IMMEDIATE MANAGEMENT

All cases with a recent GI bleed (i.e. within 48 h) should be admitted to hospital. In many no further immediate treatment is required as the patient's cardiovascular system can compensate for the blood loss.

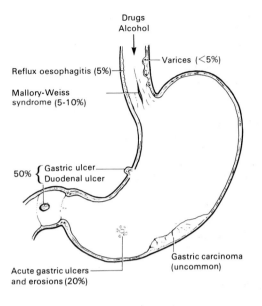

Drugs
Alcohol

Varices (<5%)

Reflux oesophagitis (5%)

Mallory-Weiss
syndrome (5-10%)

50% { Gastric ulcer
      Duodenal ulcer

Acute gastric ulcers
and erosions (20%)

Gastric carcinoma
(uncommon)

Other uncommon causes:

Hereditary telangiectasia (Osler-Weber-Rendu syndrome)
Pseudoxanthoma elasticum
Blood dyscrasias

Fig. 4.10 Causes of upper gastrointestinal haemorrhage. The approximate frequency is also given.

Factors affecting management
- Age (see below)
- The amount of blood lost, which may give some guide to the severity
- Continuing visible blood loss
- Signs of chronic liver disease on examination, as the bleeding is often severe and recurrent if it is from varices; liver failure can develop
- Presence of the classical clinical features of shock (i.e. pallor, cold nose, tachycardia and low blood pressure); remember that the peripheral constriction that occurs may keep the blood pressure falsely high

Urgent resuscitation is required in patients with large bleeds and the clinical signs of shock. Details of the management of shock are given in Chapter 13. The major principle is to restore the blood volume back to normal and this can only be satisfactorily achieved by transfusion of whole blood. It may be necessary in a severely shocked patient or in a patient with blood compatibility problems to give a blood substitute initially.

The rate of blood transfusion must be monitored carefully to avoid over-transfusion and consequent heart failure. The pulse rate and venous pressure are the best guides to transfusion rates.

Anaemia does not develop immediately as haemodilution has not taken place and therefore the haemoglobin level is a poor indicator of the need to transfuse. If the level is low (less than $10 \text{ g} \cdot \text{dl}^{-1}$) and the patient has either bled recently or is actively bleeding, transfusion may be necessary.

In most patients the bleeding stops, albeit temporarily, so that further assessment can be made.

Important factors in reassessment
- Age—below the age of 60 mortality from GI bleeding is small. Above the age of 80 the mortality is greater than 25%
- Recurrent haemorrhage—these patients have an increased mortality
- Most rebleeds occur within 48 h
- Melaena is usually less hazardous than haematemesis

Taking these factors into account, a decision can be made on future management. In addition, the cause of the haemorrhage should be looked for. The diagnosis may be obvious from the history, e.g. a long history of indigestion or, more significantly, previous haemorrhage from an ulcer. A history of aspirin or non-steroidal anti-inflammatory drug ingestion may suggest acute ulceration.

Signs of chronic liver disease, particularly with splenomegaly, suggest bleeding from oesophageal varices. The source of haemorrhage in most patients with chronic liver disease is their varices, but occasionally they may bleed from an accompanying peptic ulcer. The absence of splenomegaly does not rule out oesophageal varices.

After a careful history and examination, investigations should then be arranged within 12–24 h of admission. Endoscopy is now the preferred investigation in most centres, and the cause of the haemorrhage is found in 80% or more of cases. If stigmata of a recent bleed are seen, i.e. a visible vessel or adherent clot, the patient is more likely to re-bleed.

TREATMENT

Most conditions require no specific therapy after resuscitation. There is little evidence that H_2-receptor antagonists affect the mortality rate of GI haemorrhage but these agents are usually given to patients with ulcers because of their longer-term benefits. It may be necessary to operate if the bleeding is persistent, recurrent or if it cannot be controlled. Surgery should be avoided, if at all possible, in patients with acute gastric ulceration.

Specific conditions
Chronic gastric ulcer. These patients often require surgery after initial resuscitation as they are likely to rebleed.

Chronic duodenal ulcer. Since the advent of H_2-receptor antagonists, surgery has usually been avoided. When the patient is over his acute episode of haemorrhage, indications for surgery are the same as if the patient had not bled.

Gastric carcinoma. Most patients do not have large bleeds with this condition, but surgery may be performed for the lesion per se.

Oesophageal varices. These are discussed on p. 233.

Mallory–Weiss tear syndrome. This is a linear mucosal tear occurring at the oesophagogastric junction and produced by a sudden increase in intra-abdominal pressure. It occurs often after a bout of coughing or retching and is classically seen in the alcoholic. There may, however, be no antecedent history of retching. The haemorrhage may be large but most patients stop spontaneously. Rarely, surgery with oversewing of the tear will be required.

PROGNOSIS

The mortality of GI haemorrhage has not changed over the years despite many changes in management (see above). Early surgery has not so far reduced the mortality, partly because of the difficulty in recognizing the patient who will re-bleed.

Acute lower gastrointestinal bleeding

Massive bleeding from the lower GI tract is rare. On the other hand, small bleeds from haemorrhoids occur very commonly. Massive bleeding is usually due to diverticular disease or ischaemic colitis and may require urgent resuscitation. Surgery is rarely required as bleeding usually stops spontaneously. The causes of lower gastrointestinal bleeding are shown in Fig. 4.11.

MANAGEMENT

1 Resuscitation when required
2 Make diagnosis:
   ● Rectal examination, e.g. carcinoma
   ● Proctoscopy, e.g. haemorrhoids
   ● Sigmoidoscopy, e.g. inflammatory bowel disease
   ● Barium enema—any mucosal lesion
   ● Colonoscopy—diagnosis and removal of polyps
   ● Angiography—vascular abnormality, e.g. angiodysplasia
3 Treatment: individual lesions are treated as appropriate

Chronic gastrointestinal bleeding

Patients with chronic bleeding usually present with iron-deficiency anaemia (see Chapter 6).

Chronic blood loss producing anaemia in all men and all women after the menopause is always due to bleeding from the GI tract, so tests are not required to show this. Occult blood tests are not necessary.

Measurement of faecal occult blood

This is frequently performed *unnecessarily*. It is *only* of value in:
● Premenopausal women: if a history of menorrhagia is uncertain and the cause of iron deficiency is unclear
● As a mass population screening test for large bowel malignancy
   Advantages: cheap and easy to perform
   Disadvantages: high false-positive rate, leading to unnecessary investigations

---

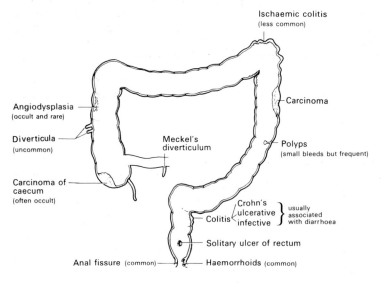

Ischaemic colitis (less common)

Angiodysplasia (occult and rare)

Diverticula (uncommon)

Meckel's diverticulum

Carcinoma of caecum (often occult)

Carcinoma

Polyps (small bleeds but frequent)

Crohn's
Colitis ⟨ ulcerative ⟩ usually associated with diarrhoea
infective

Solitary ulcer of rectum

Anal fissure (common)

Haemorrhoids (common)

Fig. 4.11 Causes of lower gastrointestinal bleeding. The sites shown are illustrative—many of the lesions can be seen in other parts of the colon.

DIAGNOSIS

Chronic blood loss can occur with any lesion of the GI tract that produces acute bleeding (see Fig. 4.10). In addition a Meckel's diverticulum and carcinoma of the caecum may present with an iron-deficiency anaemia. It should be remembered that, world-wide, hookworm is the commonest cause of chronic GI blood loss.

Careful history and examination may indicate the most likely site of the bleeding, but if no clue is available it is usual to investigate the lower bowel first with either a barium enema or colonoscopy. There is little to choose between these two techniques if both are performed well. The importance of having a clean, well-prepared bowel for both techniques cannot be overemphasized. The advantage of colonoscopy is that if a polyp is found it can be removed immediately.

If no lesion is found in the lower GI tract, the upper GI tract and small bowel are investigated. If these investigations are also negative, angiography may show up the site of bleeding, particularly when acute bleeding is occurring. Occasionally intravenous technetium-labelled colloid may be used to demonstrate the bleeding site in a Meckel's diverticulum.

The small intestine

Structure

The small intestine extends from the duodenum to the ileum. Its surface area is enormously increased by mucosal folds. In addition, the mucosa has numerous finger-like projections called villi, the surface area of which is further increased by microvilli (see Fig. 4.12). Each villus consists of a core containing blood vessels, lacteals (lymphatics) and cells and is covered by epithelial columnar cells which are absorptive. Opening into the lumen between the villi are the crypts of Lieberkühn.

The epithelial cells are formed at the bottom of these crypts and migrate to the tops of the villi, from where they are shed. This process takes three to four days. On its luminal side the epithelial cell has a brush border of microvilli which is covered by the glycocalyx. The lamina propria contains plasma cells, lymphocytes, macrophages, eosinophils and mast cells. Scattered throughout the gut are peptide-secreting cells.

Function (Table 4.9)

The small intestine is concerned with the digestion and absorption of nutrients, salt and water. It prod-

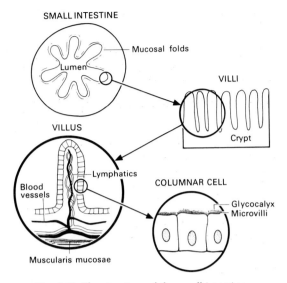

Fig. 4.12 The structure of the small intestine.

uces many enzymes and hormones in order to carry out these processes. It also has local defence mechanisms to prevent antigens from entering the body.

General principles of absorption
Simple diffusion. This process requires no energy and takes place if there is a concentration gradient from the intestinal lumen (high concentration) to the bloodstream (low concentration).

Active transport. This requires energy and can work against a concentration gradient. A carrier protein is required and the process is sodium dependent. For example, glucose enters the enterocyte on the luminal side via a sodium-dependent carrier molecule and leaves on the serosal side via a sodium-independent carrier which is found in the basolateral membrane. A gradient is maintained across the membrane by an energy-dependent sodium pump (Na^+–K^+ ATPase) which keeps the intracellular sodium concentration low.

Facilitated diffusion. This is an energy-independent carrier-mediated transport system which allows a faster absorption rate than simple diffusion, e.g. fructose absorption.

Table 4.9 Functions of the small intestine.

Absorption
Defence against antigen entry
Structural
Immunological
Hormone production
Motility—transit of nutrients

Absorption in the small intestine

Carbohydrate. Dietary carbohydrate consists mainly of starch with some sucrose and a small amount of lactose. Starch is a polysaccharide made up of numerous glucose units. Its hydrolysis begins in the mouth by salivary amylase. The majority of hydrolysis takes place in the upper intestinal lumen by pancreatic amylase. This hydrolysis is limited by the fact that amylases have no specificity for some glucose/glucose branching links.

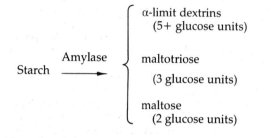

These breakdown products, together with sucrose and lactose, are hydrolysed on the brush border membrane by their appropriate oligo- and disaccharidases to form the monosaccharides glucose, galactose and fructose. These monosaccharides are transported into the cells, largely by sodium-dependent active transport systems.

Protein. Dietary and endogenous proteins (desquamated cells, intestinal secretions) are mainly digested by pancreatic enzymes prior to absorption. These proteolytic enzymes are secreted as proenzymes and transformed to active enzymes in the lumen. The presence of protein in the lumen stimulates the release of enterokinase which activates trypsinogen to trypsin, and this in turn activates the other proenzymes, chymotrypsin and elastase. These enzymes break down protein into oligopeptides. Some di- and tripeptides are absorbed intact by a carrier-mediated process, whilst the remainder are broken down into free amino acids prior to absorption in a similar way to disaccharides. These amino acids are transported into the cell by a number of different carrier systems.

Fat (Fig. 4.13). Dietary fat mainly consists of triglycerides with some cholesterol and fat-soluble vitamins. Emulsification of fat occurs in the stomach and is followed by hydrolysis of triglycerides in the duodenum by pancreatic lipase to yield fatty acids and monoglycerides.

Bile enters the duodenum following gallbladder contraction. Bile contains phospholipids and bile salts, both of which are partially water-soluble and act as detergents. They aggregate together to form micelles with their hydrophilic ends on the outside. Trapped in the hydrophobic centre of this micelle are

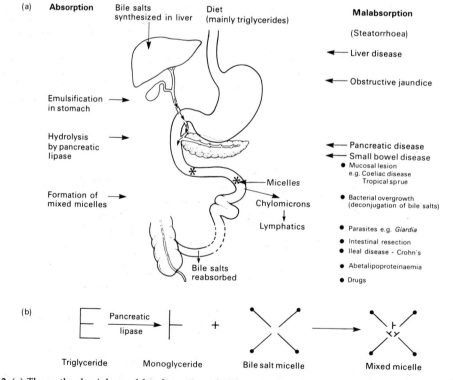

Fig. 4.13 (a) The pathophysiology of fat absorption. (b) Diagram showing the formation of mixed micelles.

the monoglycerides, fatty acids and cholesterol; these are then transported to the intestinal cell membrane. At the cell membrane the lipid contents of the micelle are absorbed, while the bile salts remain in the lumen. Inside the cell the monoglycerides and fatty acids are re-esterified to triglycerides. The triglycerides and other fat-soluble molecules (e.g. cholesterol, phospholipids) are then incorporated into chylomicrons to be transported into the lymph.

Medium-chain triglycerides (which contain fatty acids of chain length 6–12) as well as a small amount of long-chain fatty acid are transported via the portal vein.

Bile salts are not absorbed in the jejunum so that the intraluminal concentration in the upper gut is high. They pass down the intestine to be absorbed in the terminal ileum and are transported back to the liver. This enterohepatic circulation prevents excess loss of bile salts (see p. 213).

The pathophysiology of fat absorption is shown in Fig. 4.13. Interference with absorption can occur at all stages, as indicated, giving rise to steatorrhoea.

Water and electrolytes. A large amount of water and electrolytes, partly dietary but mainly from intestinal secretions, are absorbed coupled with monosaccharides and amino acids in the upper jejunum. Some water and electrolytes are absorbed in the ileum and right side of the colon, where active sodium transport occurs, but is not coupled to solute absorption. Intestinal secretion also takes place and abnormalities of this mechanism cause secretory diarrhoea (see p. 195).

Water-soluble vitamins, essential metals and trace elements. These all have to be absorbed in the small intestine. It must be remembered that vitamin B_{12} (see p. 268) is the only substance other than bile salts that is specifically absorbed in the terminal ileum

alone and malabsorption of both these substances will always occur following ileal resection.

Calcium. See p. 733.

Iron. See p. 264.

Defence against antigens
Structure and immunology. The normal intestinal mucosa forms an intrinsic barrier to the absorption of many antigens such as bacteria, viruses or dietary proteins. It is therefore not surprising that the GI tract acts as an important lymphoid organ. Lymphoid tissue is present either as lymphoid cells scattered throughout the gut mucosa or as lymphoid aggregates, e.g. the tonsils and Peyer's patches (see Fig. 4.14).

A specialized epithelial cell above these Peyer's patches called the M or microfold cell allows antigens to pass through the mucosa. The lymphocytes lying below the epithelium are stimulated by these antigens and pass to the local mesenteric lymph nodes and then, via the thoracic duct, to the circulation. Eventually these sensitized lymphocytes 'home' back again to the intestinal mucosa. Here they become immunoglobulin-producing plasma cells. The major immunoglobulin produced is monomeric IgA.

IgA is secreted into the gut lumen through the epithelial cell layer, where two molecules of IgA are joined together with a J chain. This dimeric IgA then has a 'secretor piece' attached to it. This is a glycoprotein which helps to protect the dimeric IgA from proteolysis by intestinal luminal enzymes (see Fig. 2.13, p. 115).

The function of dimeric IgA is to reduce antigen absorption and to prevent bacteria entering the wall by reducing their adherence to the mucosa. It thus acts as an 'antiseptic paint'. The GALT can also

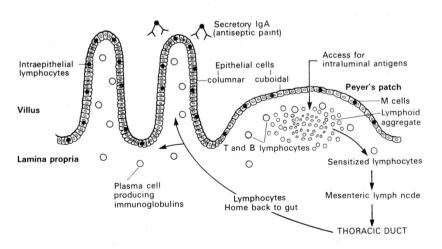

Fig. 4.14 Small intestinal mucosa with a Peyer's patch, showing the gut associated lymphoid tissue (GALT).

mount a local immune response to an antigen, independent of any circulating antibody. This local antibody production can either protect the host or can produce a hypersensitivity reaction resulting in damage to the mucosa, e.g. cow's milk protein intolerance in children.

Hormone production
The hormone-producing cells of the gut are scattered diffusely throughout its length and also occur in the pancreas. The cells that synthesize these hormones are derived from neural ectoderm and are known as APUD (amine precursor uptake and decarboxylation) cells. Many of these hormones have very similar structures. Although they can be detected by radioimmunoassay in the circulation, their action is often local.

Table 4.10 shows some gut hormones and their possible physiological actions. Many are also found in other tissues, particularly the brain. A number do not act as true hormones but act as neurotransmitters or have local effects on adjacent cells only (paracrine effects).

The exact physiological role of these peptides is still being evaluated. Their importance clinically is that they may be secreted in excess, particularly in endocrine tumours of the pancreas (see p. 207).

Gut motility
This is a complex process. Following a meal, food is propelled down the gut by a series of peristaltic contractions. In addition there are weaker contractions which enable the food to be mixed with the biliary and pancreatic secretions. Peristalsis is initiated by an electrical pacemaker in the lower part of the stomach and duodenum.

Table 4.10 Gut hormones.

Hormone	Possible physiological action	Main gut localization
Gastrin	Stimulates acid secretion Stimulates growth of mucosa	Gastric antrum
Secretin	Stimulates pancreatic secretion (bicarbonate and water)	Duodenum
Cholecystokinin (CCK)	Stimulates gallbladder contraction Stimulates pancreatic enzyme secretion Stimulates gut motility	Upper small gut
Pancreatic polypeptide (PP)	Unclear	Pancreas
Gastric inhibitory peptide (GIP)	Increases insulin secretion	Upper small gut
Somatostatin	Inhibits release of and antagonizes many hormones	Stomach, pancreas and intestine
Motilin	Increases gut contraction	Upper small gut
Neurotensin	Unclear; possible effect on gastric emptying	Ileum
Enteroglucagon	Unclear	Ileum and colon
Substance P	Unclear	Duodenum and colon
Bombesin	Unclear	Stomach and duodenum
Endorphins	Neurotransmitters	Whole gut
Vasoactive intestinal peptide (VIP)	Neurotransmitter; stimulates intestinal secretion	Whole gut
Peptide histidine isoleucine (PHI)	As for VIP	Whole gut

In the fasting state, a wave passes from the stomach to the colon; this is called the 'intestinal housekeeper' or migrating myoelectric complex (MMC). It is associated with a coincidental increase in biliary and pancreatic flow and ensures that the gut is emptied, especially of any bacterial content.

Presenting features of small bowel disease

Regardless of the cause, the common presenting features of small bowel disease are:
- Diarrhoea/steatorrhoea
- Abdominal pain or discomfort
- Weight loss
- Nutritional deficiencies

Diarrhoea and steatorrhoea

This is a common feature of small bowel disease, but approximately 10–20% of patients will have no diarrhoea or any other gastrointestinal symptoms.

Abdominal pain and discomfort

Abdominal distension can cause discomfort and flatulence. The pain has no specific character or periodicity and is not usually severe.

Weight loss

Weight loss is due to the anorexia which invariably accompanies small bowel disease. Although malabsorption occurs, the amount is small relative to intake.

Nutritional deficiencies

Deficiencies of iron, B_{12}, folate or all of these, leading to anaemia, are the only common deficiencies. Occasionally malabsorption of other vitamins or minerals occurs, causing bruising (vitamin K deficiency), tetany (calcium deficiency), osteomalacia (vitamin D deficiency), or stomatitis, sore tongue and aphthous ulceration (multiple vitamin deficiencies).

Ankle oedema may be seen and is partly nutritional and partly due to intestinal loss of albumin.

Physical signs of small bowel disease

These are few and non-specific. If present they are associated with anaemia and the nutritional deficiencies described above.

Abdominal examination is often normal, but sometimes distension and, rarely, hepatomegaly or an abdominal mass are found. In the severely ill patient gross malnutrition with muscle wasting is seen. A neuropathy, not always due to B_{12} deficiency, can be present.

Investigation of small bowel disease (Fig. 4.15)

Blood tests

The following are usually performed in all cases of suspected small bowel disease:
- *Full blood count and film.* Anaemia can be microcytic (low mean corpuscular volume [MCV]) or

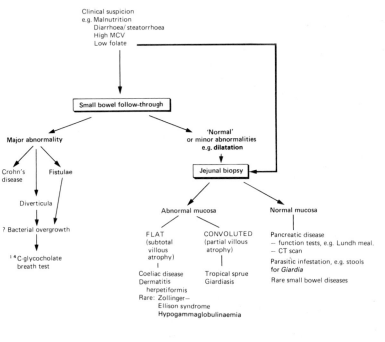

Fig. 4.15 Flow diagram for the investigation of patients with suspected small bowel disease.

macrocytic (high MCV). The blood film may also show other abnormal cells, e.g. Howell–Jolly bodies, which are seen in splenic atrophy associated with coeliac disease. *Serum iron and total iron-binding capacity* or *serum ferritin* are then performed if the MCV is low. *Serum B_{12}, serum folate and red cell folate* are performed if the MCV is high. However, with mixed deficiencies, the MCV may be normal.

- *Serum albumin.* This gives an indication of nutritional status.
- *Serum calcium and alkaline phosphatase.* These may indicate the presence of osteomalacia.
- *Red cell folate.* An accurately performed red cell folate using a microbiological assay is a good indicator of the presence of small bowel disease. Red cell folate is frequently low in both coeliac disease and Crohn's disease, which are also the two commonest causes of small bowel disease.

The following non-specific tests of malabsorption are being performed less often and are not always necessary. If the clinical suspicion of malabsorption is high, a definitive test should be performed next.

Non-specific function tests
Fat malabsorption. The fat content of stools is measured using a three-day collection of faeces with the patient on a diet containing 100 g of fat daily. Normal faecal fat excretion is less than 17 mmol (6 g) per day.

To avoid faecal collections, fat absorption can also be measured using breath analysis. Following oral administration of a radiolabelled fat load, the amount of $^{14}CO_2$ in the expired breath gives an indication of the amount of fat malabsorption. Comparison between a labelled triglyceride (^{14}C-Triolein) and a labelled fatty acid (tritiated oleic acid) is used to diagnose pancreatic disease, when fatty acid absorption will be normal.

D-*Xylose tolerance test.* Xylose is a synthetic sugar which is absorbed from the proximal small intestine. The urinary xylose excretion and the blood xylose level following an oral dose reflect its absorption. This test tends to produce many false-positives and should not be used when definitive tests are available.

Lactose tolerance test. This involves the oral ingestion of 50 g of lactose and the measurement of blood glucose. The test is of little use in adults as lactose intolerance is not a clinical problem as these patients avoid milk by choice. There is a high incidence of lactase deficiency in many parts of the world, e.g. the Mediterranean countries, and parts of Africa and Asia. It should be remembered that a glass of milk only contains approximately 11 g of lactose.

A glucose tolerance test should not be performed as

it is influenced by many factors other than absorption.

Definitive tests
Small bowel follow-through (see p. 153). This detects gross anatomical defects such as diverticula, strictures and Crohn's disease. Dilatation of the folds and a changed fold pattern may suggest malabsorption, but as these are not specific findings the diagnosis should not be based on these alone. Gross dilatation is seen in pseudo-obstruction.

Jejunal biopsy. This is used to assess the microanatomy of the small bowel. Specimens can be obtained using a Crosby–Kugler capsule (Fig. 4.16) or via an endoscope passed into the distal duodenum. The histological appearances will be described in the sections on individual diseases.

A smear of the jejunal juice or a mucosal impression can also be made and is helpful in the diagnosis of *Giardia lamblia* (see p. 80).

Jejunal biopsy

- The patient is fasted overnight.
- A Crosby–Kugler capsule is swallowed, guided through the pylorus with screening, and then allowed to pass to just beyond the duodeno-jejunal junction.
- A small piece of mucosa is sucked into the capsule; additional suction triggers the knife to remove a mucosal specimen.
- The capsule is immediately withdrawn.
- The specimen is examined immediately under a dissecting microscope.
- The specimen is then placed in 10% formalin for histological examination.

Complications
- Inability to swallow the capsule
- Haemorrhage or perforation (rare)

Other useful tests in specific diseases
^{14}*C-Glycocholic acid breath test* (Fig. 4.17). This is performed to look for bacterial overgrowth (see below). The patient is given ^{14}C-labelled bile salts by mouth. Bacteria deconjugate the bile salts, releasing ^{14}C-glycine, which is metabolized and appears in the breath as $^{14}CO_2$. This radioactivity in the breath can easily be measured. An early rise indicates either bacterial overgrowth in the upper small intestine or rapid transit to the colon where, of course, bacteria are normally present.

Direct intubation. Aspiration of intestinal juices is another method by which bacterial contamination can be detected. Bacterial counts are performed on aerobic and anaerobic cultures. Chromatography of bile salts can also be performed on the aspirate to detect evidence of deconjugation.

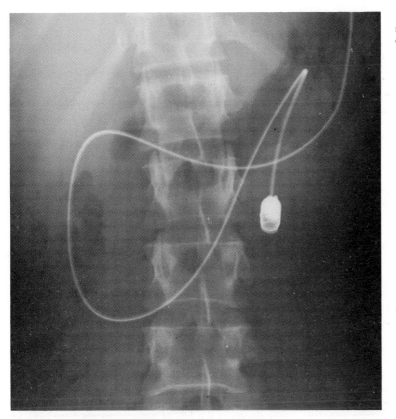

Fig. 4.16 A plain abdominal x-ray showing a Crosby capsule in the duodenojejunal flexure.

Fig. 4.17 The ^{14}C-glycocholic acid breath test. (a) The apparatus. (b) The amount of $^{14}CO_2$ expired in the breath after an oral dose of ^{14}C-glycocholic acid in a normal subject and in a patient with diverticula of the small intestine.

Hydrogen breath test. This can also be used to detect bacterial overgrowth. Oral lactulose is degraded by bacteria, with the production of hydrogen. An early rise in the breath hydrogen will indicate bacterial break down of lactulose in the small intestine or rapid transit of the lactulose to the large intestine.

Schilling test. This is performed to look for vitamin B_{12} malabsorption. It is described in detail on p. 270. In gastrointestinal disease it is used to detect:
- Pernicious anaemia
- Ileal disease (when vitamin B_{12} is given with intrinsic factor)
- Bacterial overgrowth (measurement of vitamin B_{12} plus intrinsic factor absorption is repeated after antibiotics)

Pancreatic tests (see p. 254). These may be required for the differential diagnosis of steatorrhoea.

Other blood tests. Serum immunoglobulins may be measured to exclude immune deficiencies. Auto-antibodies to reticulin or gliadin may be measured in suspected coeliac disease but are unhelpful in clinical practice in adult patients. Hormones, e.g. vasoactive intestinal peptide (VIP), may be measured in high-volume secretory diarrhoeas.

Test for protein-losing enteropathy. Intravenous radio-active chromic chloride is used to label circulating albumin. In excess gastrointestinal protein loss, the faeces will contain radioactivity. This test is rarely required unless a low serum albumin is a major clinical feature.

Intestinal permeability tests. These tests can be used for the detection of small bowel disease but are not in general use. They are based on the fact that the abnormal intestinal mucosa is permeable to large molecules such as lactulose and cellobiose. An oral load of these sugars is given and the sugars are then measured in the urine. Recently, radiolabelled sodium-EDTA has been used in a similar way and is said to be a more accurate investigation.

MALABSORPTION

In many small bowel diseases, malabsorption of specific substances occurs, but these deficiencies do not dominate the clinical picture. An example is Crohn's disease, in which malabsorption of vitamin B_{12} can be demonstrated, but this is not usually a problem and diarrhoea and general ill-health are the major features. Steatorrhoea—malabsorption of fat—is discussed on p. 172.

The major disorders of the small intestine that cause malabsorption are shown in Table 4.11.

Table 4.11 Disorders of the small intestine causing malabsorption.

Coeliac disease
Dermatitis herpetiformis
Tropical sprue
Bacterial overgrowth
Intestinal resection
Whipple's disease
Radiation enteritis
Parasite infestation, e.g. *Giardia lamblia*

Coeliac disease (gluten-sensitive enteropathy)

Coeliac disease is a condition in which there is an abnormal jejunal mucosa which improves morphologically when the patient is treated with a gluten-free diet and relapses when gluten is reintroduced. Gluten is contained in the cereals wheat, rye, barley and possibly oats.

Dermatitis herpetiformis is a skin disorder which is associated with a gluten-sensitive enteropathy (see below).

INCIDENCE

Coeliac disease is common in Europe, with an incidence in the UK of approximately 1 in 2000. In Ireland, however, it is 1 in 300. It occurs throughout the world, but is rare in the black African.

INHERITANCE

There is an increased incidence of coeliac disease in the families of patients, with 10–15% of the siblings being affected.

Eighty per cent of patients with coeliac disease have the genetic markers HLA-B8 and -DR3, compared with 25% in the control population. Coeliac disease is primarily associated with DR3 and the association with B8 is due to linkage disequilibrium of B8 with DR3. The finding that not all patients with coeliac disease have B8 and DR3, as well as the fact that there is a lack of complete concordance amongst identical twins, suggests an additional locus. It is possible that the additional locus is the immunoglobulin heavy chain allotype. Recently a class 2 antigen, DQW2, has been found in over 90% of patients with coeliac disease.

AETIOLOGY

Gluten obtained from wheat flour can be further fractionated into different peptides, one of which is alpha gliadin. It is this fraction that is injurious to the intestinal mucosa of patients with coeliac disease. How and why the damage occurs is still not understood. Initially it was suggested that there may be a deficiency of an intestinal peptidase, but the more popular view is that the damage is due to an abnormal immunological reaction to gluten. The association of coeliac disease with a particular HLA type which may be adjacent to an immune response locus makes an immunogenetic mechanism likely.

PATHOLOGY

The mucosa of the proximal small bowel is predominantly affected, the mucosal damage decreasing in severity towards the ileum as the gluten is digested into smaller non-toxic fragments.

Under the dissecting microscope (× 40) there is an absence of villi, making the mucosal surface flat. Histological examination shows that the crypts are elongated, with chronic inflammatory cells in the lamina propria (see Fig. 4.18). The lesion is described as *subtotal villous atrophy*, although true atrophy of the mucosa is not present because crypt hypertrophy compensates for villous loss and the total mucosal thickness is normal.

The surface cells become cuboidal. There is an increase in the intraepithelial lymphocytes, but this change is not specific for coeliac disease. In the lamina propria there is an increase in lymphocytes as well as plasma cells containing IgM.

CLINICAL FEATURES

Coeliac disease can present at any age. In infancy it appears after weaning onto gluten-containing foods. The peak incidence in adults is in the third and fourth decade, with a female preponderance. The symptoms are very variable and often non-specific, e.g.

(a)

(b)

(c)

(d)

Fig. 4.18 *(a) and (b)* The dissecting microscopic appearances of (a) normal mucosa and (b) abnormal mucosa from a patient with coeliac disease. *(c) and (d)* The histological appearances of (c) normal mucosa and (d) abnormal mucosa from a patient with coeliac disease.

tiredness and malaise. Common GI symptoms include diarrhoea or steatorrhoea, abdominal discomfort or pain and weight loss.

Mouth ulcers and angular stomatitis are frequent and can be intermittent. Rare complications include tetany, osteomalacia, neurological symptoms such as paraesthesia, muscle weakness or peripheral neuropathy, or gross malnutrition with peripheral oedema.

There is an increased incidence of atopy and autoimmune disease, including thyroid disease, insulin-dependent diabetes, inflammatory bowel disease, chronic liver disease, and fibrosing and allergic alveolitis.

Physical signs are usually few and non-specific and are related to anaemia and malnutrition.

INVESTIGATION

- *Jejunal biopsy.* The mucosal appearance of a jejunal biopsy specimen is diagnostic and this investigation should always be performed in suspected cases. Other causes of a flat mucosa in adults are rare and are shown in Fig. 4.15.
- *Haematology.* A mild or moderate anaemia is present in 50% of cases. Folate deficiency is almost invariably present in coeliac disease, giving rise in most instances to a high MCV. B_{12} deficiency is rare, but iron deficiency due to malabsorption of iron and increased loss of desquamated cells is common. A blood film may therefore show micro- and macrocytes as well as hypersegmented polymorphonuclear leucocytes and Howell–Jolly bodies (due to splenic atrophy).
- Antireticulin antibodies and antigliadin antibodies (IgA) are found in the serum of the majority of cases.
- Absorption tests are often abnormal (see p. 176), but are seldom performed.
- A small bowel follow-through may show dilatation of the small bowel with a change in fold pattern; folds become thicker and in the severer forms total effacement is seen.
- In the severely ill patient other biochemical abnormalities are seen, e.g. hypoalbuminaemia.

TREATMENT AND MANAGEMENT

A gluten-free diet usually produces a rapid clinical and morphological improvement. Replacement haematinics are given initially to replace body stores. The usual cause for failure to respond to the diet is poor compliance. A gluten challenge, i.e. reintroduction of gluten with evidence of jejunal morphological change, confirms the diagnosis. In the straightforward cases this is not necessary, although transient gluten intolerance has been described in early childhood.

Many patients do not keep to a strict diet but nevertheless maintain good health. The long-term effects of this low gluten intake are uncertain.

COMPLICATIONS

A few patients do not improve on a strict diet (unresponsive coeliac disease). Often no cause for this is found, but intestinal lymphoma or carcinoma are sometimes found. The incidence of small intestinal lymphoma is increased in coeliac disease. Carcinoma of the small bowel and oesophagus as well as extra-gastrointestinal cancers are also seen. Malignancy seems to be unrelated to the duration of the disease or its treatment.

Dermatitis herpetiformis (see p. 920)

This is an uncommon subepidermal blistering eruption of the skin associated with a gluten-sensitive enteropathy. Rarely there may be gross malabsorption, but usually the jejunal morphological abnormalities are not as severe as in coeliac disease. The inheritance and immunological abnormalities are the same as for coeliac disease. The skin condition responds to dapsone, but both the gut and the skin will improve on a gluten-free diet. On this diet the need for dapsone is reduced.

Tropical sprue

This is a condition presenting with malabsorption which occurs in residents of or visitors to a tropical area where the disease is endemic.

Malabsorption of a mild degree, sometimes following an enteric infection, is quite common and is usually asymptomatic. The term *tropical sprue* is reserved for severe malabsorption (of two or more substances) which is usually accompanied by severe diarrhoea and malnutrition. Tropical sprue is endemic in most of Asia, some Caribbean islands, Puerto Rico and parts of South America. Epidemics occur, lasting up to two years, and in some areas repeated epidemics occur at varying intervals of up to ten years.

AETIOLOGY

The aetiology is unknown but is likely to be infective because the disease occurs in epidemics and patients improve on antibiotics. A number of agents have been suggested, but none has been shown to be unequivocally responsible. Different agents could be involved in different parts of the world.

CLINICAL FEATURES

These vary in intensity and consist of diarrhoea, anorexia, abdominal distension and weight loss. The onset is sometimes acute and occurs either a few days or many years after being in the tropics. Epidemics can break out in villages, affecting thousands of people at the same time. The onset can also be insidious, with chronic diarrhoea and evidence of nutritional deficiency.

The clinical features of tropical sprue vary in different parts of the world, particularly as different criteria are used for diagnosis.

DIAGNOSIS

- Acute infective causes of diarrhoea must be excluded (see p. 197), particularly *Giardia* which can produce a syndrome very similar to tropical sprue.
- Malabsorption should be demonstrated, particularly fat and B_{12} malabsorption.
- The jejunal mucosa is abnormal, showing some villus atrophy (partial villus atrophy). In most cases the lesion is less severe than that found in coeliac disease, although it affects the whole small bowel. Mild changes can be seen in asymptomatic individuals in the tropics, so jejunal mucosal changes must be interpreted carefully.

TREATMENT

Many patients improve when they leave the sprue area and take folic acid (5 mg daily). Most patients also require an antibiotic (usually tetracycline 1 g daily) to ensure a complete recovery; it may be necessary to give this for up to six months.

The severely ill patient requires resuscitation with fluids and electrolytes for dehydration; any nutritional deficiencies should be corrected. Vitamin B_{12} is also given to all acute cases.

Bacterial overgrowth

The upper part of the small intestine is almost sterile, containing only a few organisms derived from the mouth. Gastric acid kills most organisms and intestinal motility keeps the jejunum empty. The normal terminal ileum contains faecal-type organisms, mainly *Escherichia coli* and anaerobes.

Bacterial overgrowth is normally only found associated with a structural abnormality of the small intestine, although it can occur alone in the elderly.

Aspiration of the upper jejunum will reveal the presence of *E. coli* and/or *Bacteroides*, both in concentrations greater than 10^6 per ml as part of a mixed flora. These bacteria are capable of deconjugating and dehydroxylating bile salts, so that unconjugated and dehydroxylated bile salts can be detected in aspirates by chromatography. Steatorrhoea (see p. 172) occurs as a result of conjugated bile salt deficiency.

The bacteria are able to metabolize B_{12} and interfere with its binding to intrinsic factor, thereby leading to B_{12} deficiency; this can be demonstrated using the Schilling test. Conversely some bacteria produce folic acid.

Bacterial overgrowth has only minimal effects on other substances absorbed from the small intestine. The clinical features are chiefly diarrhoea, steatorrhoea and vitamin B_{12} deficiency, although this is not so severe as to produce a neurological deficit.

Although bacterial overgrowth may be responsible for the presenting symptoms, it must be remembered that many of the symptoms may be due to the underlying small bowel pathology.

TREATMENT

If possible, the underlying lesion should be corrected, e.g. a stricture should be resected. With multiple diverticula, grossly dilated bowel, or in Crohn's disease, this may not be possible and courses of antibiotics are necessary.

Intestinal resection (Fig. 4.19)

Intestinal resection is usually well tolerated, but massive resection is followed by the short gut syndrome. The effects of resection depend on the extent and the areas involved.

Extent

Because the gut is long, a 30–50% resection can usually be tolerated without undue problems.

Site of resection

The ileum has specific receptors for the absorption of bile salts and vitamin B_{12}, so that relatively small resections will lead to malabsorption of these substances. Removal of the ileocaecal valve increases the incidence of diarrhoea. In ileal resection:

- Bile salts and fatty acids enter the colon and interfere with water and electrolyte absorption, causing diarrhoea.
- Increased bile salt synthesis can compensate for loss of approximately one-third of the bile salts in the faeces. Greater loss than this results in decreased micellar formation and steatorrhoea, and lithogenic bile and gallstone formation.
- Increased oxalate absorption is caused by the presence of bile salts in the colon. This gives rise to renal oxalate stones.
- There is a low serum B_{12} and macrocytosis.

However, in jejunal resection the ileum can take over jejunal absorptive function. Jejunal resection may lead to gastric hypersecretion with high gastrin levels; the exact mechanism of this is unclear.

Intestinal adaptation takes place, with an increase in the absorption per unit length of bowel. Patients with massive resection often require parenteral nutrition initially, but with adaptation most will eventually recover, although continuing to have diarrhoea and having little functional reserve should

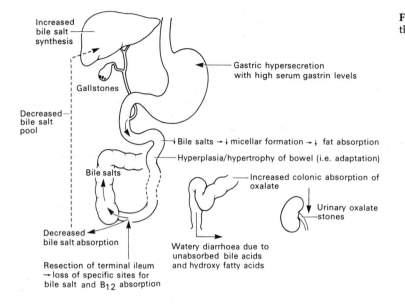

Fig. 4.19 The effects of resection of the distal small bowel.

another GI problem occur. A low-fat diet is often required.

Whipple's disease

In this rare disease there is a diffuse infiltration of the small intestinal mucosa. Histologically the villi are stunted and dilated by periodic acid–Schiff (PAS)-positive macrophages. On electron microscopy, bacilli of unknown type can be seen surrounding the macrophages. The disorder is a systemic one producing not only malabsorption but also arthritis, general signs of ill-health, and occasionally signs of heart, lung and brain involvement.

A dramatic improvement occurs with antibiotic therapy, which should include an antibiotic that crosses the blood/brain barrier, e.g. chloramphenicol.

Radiation enteritis

Radiation of more than 50 Gy will damage the intestine. The ileum and rectum are the areas most often involved as pelvic irradiation is the common cause. There may be acute signs of diarrhoea and abdominal pain at the time of the irradiation, but chronic symptoms develop after approximately one year.

Rectal damage produces a radiation proctitis with diarrhoea, with or without blood and tenesmus. Treatment is symptomatic; local steroids sometimes help.

Radiation enteritis produces muscle fibre atrophy, ulcerative changes due to ischaemia, and obstruction due to strictures produced by radiation-induced fibrosis. The symptoms are often that of

obstruction, which is usually partial but eventually may be complete. Malabsorption due to mucosal damage as well as bacterial overgrowth in dilated segments can occur. Treatment is symptomatic. Surgery should be avoided if at all possible, being reserved for life-threatening situations such as complete obstruction or occasionally perforation.

Parasite infestation

Giardia lamblia (see p. 80) not only produces diarrhoea but can produce malabsorption with steatorrhoea. Minor changes are seen in the jejunal mucosa and the organism can be found in the jejunal fluid or mucosa.

Cryptosporidiosis (see p. 81) can also produce malabsorption.

Other causes of malabsorption

- *Drugs* which bind bile salts, e.g. cholestyramine, and some antibiotics, e.g. neomycin, produce steatorrhoea.
- Diarrhoea, rarely with steatorrhoea, occurs in *thyrotoxicosis* due to increased gastric emptying and motility. Steatorrhoea occurs in the *Zollinger–Ellison* syndrome (p. 208).
- *Intestinal lymphangiectasia* produces diarrhoea and rarely steatorrhoea.
- *Lymphoma* which has infiltrated the small bowel mucosa causes malabsorption.
- In some patients with *diabetes mellitus*, diarrhoea, malabsorption and steatorrhoea, partly due to bacterial overgrowth from stasis, occur.
- *Hypogammaglobulinaemia*, which is seen in many conditions including lymphoid nodular hyper-

plasia, causes steatorrhoea due either to an abnormal jejunal mucosa or to secondary infestation with *Giardia lamblia*.

MISCELLANEOUS INTESTINAL DISORDERS

Protein-losing enteropathy

Protein-losing enteropathy is seen in many gastrointestinal and systemic conditions. Increased protein loss across an abnormal mucosa causes hypoalbuminaemia. Causes include inflammatory or ulcerative lesions, e.g. Crohn's disease, tumours, Menetrier's disease, coeliac disease and lymphatic disorders, e.g. lymphangiectasia. Usually it forms a minor part of the generalized disorder, but occasionally hepatic synthesis of albumin cannot compensate for the hypoalbuminaemia, and the peripheral oedema produced may dominate the clinical picture. The investigations are described on p. 178 and treatment is that of the underlying disorder.

Meckel's diverticulum

This is the commonest congenital abnormality of the GI tract, affecting 2–3% of the population. The diverticulum projects from the wall of the ileum approximately 60 cm from the ileocaecal valve. It is usually symptomless, but 50% contain gastric mucosa which secretes hydrochloric acid. Peptic ulcers can occur and may bleed (see p. 170) or perforate.

Acute inflammation of the diverticulum also occurs, and is indistinguishable clinically from acute appendicitis. Obstruction from an associated band rarely occurs. Treatment is surgical removal.

Tuberculosis

Tuberculosis (TB) can affect the intestine as well as the peritoneum (see p. 202).

Intestinal tuberculosis is due to reactivation of primary disease caused by *M. tuberculosis*. There is usually evidence of pulmonary tuberculosis on x-ray. Bovine TB occurs in areas where milk is unpasteurized.

The ileocaecal area is most commonly affected; the bowel is thickened with fibrosis and is similar in appearance to the bowel in Crohn's disease. The colon and rarely other parts of the gastrointestinal tract can also be involved.

CLINICAL FEATURES

These are chiefly diarrhoea and abdominal pain with generalized systemic manifestations, including anorexia and weight loss. Intestinal obstruction may develop.

On examination, a mass may be palpable and 50% have clinical evidence of pulmonary tuberculosis; this is an important aid to the diagnosis.

DIAGNOSIS

In the Western hemisphere TB must be differentiated from Crohn's disease and should always be considered as a possible diagnosis in Asian immigrants. Histological verification and culture of tissue is essential. Specimens can be obtained by colonoscopy, but often laparotomy is required.

TREATMENT

Drug treatment is similar to pulmonary TB, i.e. rifampicin, isoniazid and pyrazinamide (see p. 602).

Amyloid (see p. 323)

In systemic amyloidosis there is usually a diffuse involvement which may affect any part of the GI tract. Occasionally amyloid deposits occur as polypoid lesions. The symptoms depend on the site of involvement; amyloidosis in the small intestine gives rise to diarrhoea.

Connective tissue disorders

Systemic sclerosis (see p. 342) most commonly affects the oesophagus (see p. 157), although the small bowel and colon are often found to be involved if the appropriate radiological studies are performed. Frequently there are no symptoms of this involvement, but diarrhoea and steatorrhoea can occur. This is usually due to bacterial overgrowth of the small bowel as a result of reduced motility, dilatation and the presence of diverticula.

In *rheumatoid arthritis* (p. 336) and *systemic lupus erythematosus* (p. 342), gastrointestinal symptoms may occur but rarely predominate.

Chronic intestinal ischaemia

This is due to atheromatous occlusion of mesenteric vessels in the elderly, although such occlusion often does not produce clinical effects because of the collateral circulation. The characteristic symptom is abdominal pain occurring after food. This may be followed by acute mesenteric vascular occlusion (see p. 201). Loud bruits may be heard, but as these are heard in normal subjects they are of doubtful significance. The diagnosis is made using angiography.

The term 'coeliac axis compression syndrome' has been used in young patients with chronic abdominal pain, bruits and minor angiographic changes. Despite its plausible title, it is not an organic syndrome. Its suggested existence results from the false correlation of pain and bruits.

Eosinophilic gastroenteritis

This is a condition of unknown aetiology in which there may be eosinophilic infiltration and oedema of any part of the gastrointestinal mucosa. It usually involves the gastric antrum and proximal small intestine. Three main types are described depending on the different layer of the gut wall involved, i.e. submucosal, muscle or serosal layers.

The condition may occur at any age, but mainly in the third decade. Males are affected twice as often as females. The clinical presentation depends on the site of involvement. Abdominal pain, nausea and vomiting occur. An increased number of eosinophils in the blood is present in only 20% of patients. Radiology or endoscopy will demonstrate the lesion. Treatment is usually with steroids.

In some adults the condition appears to be allergic (allergic gastroenteritis) and is associated with peripheral eosinophilia and high levels of blood and tissue IgE.

Intestinal lymphangiectasia

Dilatation of the lymphatics may be primary or secondary to lymphatic obstruction, such as that occurring in malignancy or constrictive pericarditis. In the rare primary form it may be detected incidently as dilated lacteals on a jejunal biopsy or it can produce steatorrhoea of varying degrees. Hypoproteinaemia with ankle oedema is the main feature.

Abetalipoproteinaemia

In this rare condition there is failure of apoprotein synthesis in the intestinal cell so that chylomicrons are not formed. This leads to fat accumulation in the intestinal cells, giving a typical appearance on jejunal biopsy. Clinical features include acanthocytosis (spiky red cells due to membrane abnormalities), retinopathy, and mental and neurological abnormalities. The latter can be prevented by vitamin E injections.

Inflammatory bowel disease

Two major forms of *non-specific* inflammatory bowel disease are recognized: Crohn's disease, which can affect any part of the GI tract, and ulcerative colitis, which affects only the large bowel.

There is overlap between these two conditions in their clinical features, and histological and radiological abnormalities; in 10% of cases of colitis a definitive diagnosis of either ulcerative colitis or Crohn's disease is not possible. Currently, it is necessary to distinguish between these two conditions because of certain differences in their management. However, it is possible that these conditions represent two aspects of the same disease.

EPIDEMIOLOGY AND AETIOLOGY

Both diseases can occur at any age, including young children and the elderly. The peak incidence is between 20 and 40 years of age. Both sexes are equally affected.

The incidence of Crohn's disease varies from country to country but is approximately 3–7 per 100 000, with a prevalence of about 40 per 100 000 population, in the UK. Ulcerative colitis is commoner, with an incidence of 6–15 per 100 000 and a prevalence of approximately 80 per 100 000. Crohn's disease was on the increase but recently there seems to be a decline in incidence. The incidence of ulcerative colitis seems constant.

Both conditions have a world-wide distribution but are more common in the Western world. The incidence is lower in the non-white races. Jews are more prone to inflammatory bowel disease than non-Jews world-wide. These differences as well as other geographical clustering suggests an environmental and genetic cause. Ulcerative colitis and Crohn's disease are both seen more commonly amongst the relatives of patients than in the general population and there is a tendency for twins to both be affected. No overall association has been found with HLA markers, but there is, however, an association with HLA-B27, inflammatory bowel disease and ankylosing spondylitis.

The aetiology of both conditions is unknown. In Crohn's disease the most attractive hypothesis is a transmissible agent, but no bacterium, virus or parasite has been definitely identified.

Granulomas are characteristic of Crohn's disease, but are also seen in tuberculosis and sarcoidosis. This suggests a common pathogenesis between these diseases but no link has been found. There are many immunological abnormalities in Crohn's disease but these appear to be secondary to the disease process and may not be involved in the pathogenesis. There is also an increase in the incidence of atopy.

PATHOLOGY

Crohn's disease is a chronic inflammatory condition which may affect any part of the GI tract from the mouth to the anus but has a particular tendency to affect the terminal ileum. The disease can involve one small area of the gut such as the terminal ileum, or multiple areas with relatively normal bowel in between ('skip lesions'). It may also be extensive, involving the whole of the colon and/or small bowel.

Ulcerative colitis can affect the rectum alone (proctitis), can extend proximally to involve the sigmoid and descending colon ('left-sided colitis'), or may involve the whole colon ('total colitis'). In some of these patients there is also inflammation of the distal terminal ileum ('backwash ileitis').

Macroscopic changes

In Crohn's disease the involved bowel is usually thickened and narrowed. There are deep ulcers and fissures in the mucosa, producing a cobblestone appearance. Fistulas and abscesses may be seen. An early sign is aphthoid ulceration which can be seen endoscopically.

In ulcerative colitis the mucosa looks reddened, inflamed and bleeds easily. In severe disease there is extensive ulceration, with the adjacent mucosa appearing as inflammatory polyps. In fulminant disease most of the mucosa is lost, leaving a few islands of oedematous mucosa (mucosal islands) and toxic dilatation occurs. On healing, the mucosa can return to normal, although there is usually some residual glandular distortion.

Microscopic changes

In Crohn's disease the inflammation extends through all layers of the bowel whereas in ulcerative colitis a superficial inflammation is seen. In Crohn's disease there is an increase in chronic inflammatory cells, lymphoid hyperplasia and in 50–60% of patients granulomas are present. These granulomas are non-caseating epithelioid cell aggregates with Langhans's giant cells.

In ulcerative colitis the mucosa shows a chronic inflammatory cell infiltrate in the lamina propria. Crypt abscesses and goblet cell depletion are also seen.

The differentiation between these two diseases is made not only on the basis of clinical and radiological data but also on the histological differences seen in the rectal and colonic mucosa obtained by biopsy (Table 4.12).

CLINICAL FEATURES

Crohn's disease

The major symptoms are of diarrhoea, abdominal pain and weight loss. Constitutional symptoms of malaise, lethargy, anorexia, nausea, vomiting and a low grade fever may be present. Despite the recurrent nature of this condition, many patients remain well and have an almost normal lifestyle. However, patients with extensive disease may have frequent recurrences necessitating multiple hospital admissions.

The clinical features are very variable and depend partly on the region of the bowel that is affected. The disease may present insidiously or acutely. The abdominal pain may be colicky, suggesting obstruction, but it usually has no special characteristics and sometimes in colonic disease only minimal discomfort is present. Diarrhoea is present in 80% of all cases and in colonic disease may contain blood, making it difficult to differentiate from ulcerative colitis. Steatorrhoea can be present in small bowel disease. Some patients (15%) present with only anorexia, weight loss and general ill health, with an absence of any other GI symptoms.

Crohn's disease may present as an emergency with acute right iliac fossa pain mimicking appendicitis. If laparotomy is undertaken, an oedematous, reddened terminal ileum is found. There are many other causes of an acute ileitis, e.g. infections such as *Yersinia*. Crohn's disease is the cause of approximately 10%.

Examination. Physical signs are few, apart from loss of weight and general ill-health. Aphthous ulceration of the mouth is often seen. Abdominal examination is often normal, although tenderness and a right iliac fossa mass are occasionally found. This mass is due either to inflamed loops of bowel that are matted together or to an abscess. A careful examination of the anus should always be made to look for oedematous anal tags, fissures or perianal abscesses. These abnormalities are particularly common (80%) in colonic involvement.

Other extra-gastrointestinal features of inflammatory bowel disease should be looked for, e.g. erythema nodosum, arthritis, iritis (see below).

Sigmoidoscopy should always be performed in a patient with Crohn's disease. With small bowel involvement the rectum may appear normal, but a biopsy must be taken as non-specific histological changes may sometimes be found in the mucosa. Even with extensive colonic Crohn's disease the rectum may be spared and be relatively normal, but patchy involvement with an oedematous haemorrhagic mucosa can be present and should be biopsied.

Ulcerative colitis

The major symptom in ulcerative colitis is diarrhoea with blood and mucus, sometimes accompanied by lower abdominal discomfort. General features include malaise, lethargy and anorexia. Aphthous ulceration is seen. The disease can be mild, moderate or severe, and runs a course of remissions and exacerbations. Ten per cent of patients have persistent chronic symptoms, although some patients may have only a single attack.

Table 4.12 Histological differences between Crohn's disease and ulcerative colitis.

	Crohn's disease	Ulcerative colitis
Inflammation	Deep (transmural) Patchy	Superficial Continuous
Granulomas	++	Rare
Goblet cells	Present	Depleted
Crypt abscesses	+	++

When the disease is confined to the rectum, blood mixed with the stool, urgency and tenesmus are common. There are normally very few constitutional symptoms but patients are nevertheless greatly inconvenienced by the frequency of defecation.

In an acute attack patients have bloody diarrhoea, passing 10–20 liquid stools per day. Diarrhoea also occurs at night, with urgency and incontinence which is severely disabling for the patient. Occasionally blood and mucus alone are passed.

The definition of a severe attack is given in Table 4.13. The patient may be very ill and needs careful monitoring in hospital with prompt treatment to avoid the development of complications such as septicaemia, toxic dilatation and perforation.

Examination. In general there are no specific signs in ulcerative colitis. The abdomen may be slightly distended or tender to palpate. The anus is usually normal. Rectal examination will show the presence of blood. Sigmoidoscopy is always abnormal and shows an inflamed, bleeding, friable mucosa. A biopsy should be taken for histological diagnosis.

Extra-gastrointestinal manifestations
These occur with both diseases and some are related to the intestinal disease activity (see Table 4.14).

INVESTIGATION

Blood tests
Anaemia is common and is usually the normocytic normochromic anaemia of chronic disease. Deficiency of iron and/or folate also occurs. Despite terminal ileal involvement in Crohn's disease, megaloblastic anaemia due to B_{12} deficiency is unusual, although the B_{12} level can be low. There is often a raised ESR and a raised white cell count. Hypoalbuminaemia is present in severe disease.

Table 4.13 Definition of a severe attack of ulcerative colitis.

Stool frequency	> 6 stools per day with blood
Fever	> 37.5°C
Tachycardia	> 90 per minute
ESR	> 30 mm per hour
Anaemia	Haemoglobin < 10 g·dl^{-1}
Albumin	< 30 g·l^{-1}

Table 4.14 Extra-gastrointestinal manifestations of inflammatory bowel disease.

	Per cent of cases	
	Crohn's disease	Ulcerative colitis
Eyes		
Uveitis		
Episcleritis	4	4
Conjunctivitis		
Joints		
Monoarticular arthritis	14	11
Ankylosing spondylitis*		
Skin		
Erythema nodosum	2	2
Pyoderma gangrenosum	1	3
Vasculitis		
Liver†*		
Fatty change	Common	Common
Pericholangitis	19	25
Sclerosing cholangitis	<1	12
Chronic active hepatitis	Uncommon	Uncommon
Cirrhosis	7	19
*Kidney**		
Stones	30	—
*Gallbladder**		
Stones	30	5 (normal)

* These manifestations are not related to disease activity.
† Biochemical abnormalities are common, but clinically overt disease is uncommon.

Liver function tests may be abnormal. Blood cultures are required if septicaemia is suspected.

Stool cultures
These should always be performed on presentation if diarrhoea is present.

Radiology
In Crohn's disease a small bowel follow-through shows an asymmetrical alteration in the mucosal pattern with deep ulceration and areas of narrowing (string sign) largely confined to the ileum (Fig. 4.20). Skip lesions with normal bowel in between are also seen. A barium enema is necessary to demonstrate large bowel involvement. Early changes consist of aphthous ulceration (Fig. 4.21a); this involvement is again usually patchy, with deep ulceration developing later.

In ulcerative colitis a barium enema will show the extent of the disease (Fig. 4.21b), but it is not always possible to distinguish between ulcerative colitis and Crohn's disease. In long-standing disease the colon is shortened and narrowed. A plain abdominal x-ray should be performed if toxic dilatation is suspected.

Colonoscopy
This is not always essential but is sometimes necessary to delineate the exact extent of the disease. It is also useful for obtaining biopsies from the whole colon and ileum to differentiate between Crohn's disease and ulcerative colitis. In ulcerative colitis it is used to detect premalignant mucosal dysplasia.

Small bowel function tests (see p. 176)
When Crohn's disease involves the small bowel, other tests may be necessary, e.g. a breath test for bacterial overgrowth or a test for vitamin B_{12} absorption.

DIFFERENTIAL DIAGNOSIS

Crohn's disease has to be considered in the differential diagnosis of all chronic diarrhoeas, malabsorption and malnutrition. It is also a differential diagnosis of small stature in children (see p. 710). A small bowel follow-through usually differentiates it from other forms of small bowel disease. Ileocaecal tuberculosis is common in Asia and Africa. Lymphomas cause a major diagnostic difficulty.

Colitis, both ulcerative and Crohn's, must be differentiated from amoebic and ischaemic colitis as well as infective causes of diarrhoea. The latter are becoming commoner in homosexuals (gay bowel disease) and should be suspected if multiple or unusual organisms are found. A rare cause of a colitis is Behçet's disease, which also gives orogenital ulceration.

TREATMENT

Medical management
Some patients require only symptomatic treatment. Diarrhoea can be controlled with agents such as codeine phosphate 30–60 mg three times daily, diphenoxylate with atropine 1–2 tablets four times

Fig. 4.20 Small bowel follow-through showing narrowing and ulceration of the terminal ileum (arrow) in Crohn's disease.

(a)

Fig. 4.21 (a) Double contrast barium enema showing early aphthous ulceration in Crohn's disease. Note the asymmetrical pattern. (b) (*facing page*) Double contrast barium enema showing the fine ulceration and tubular colon of ulcerative colitis.

daily or loperamide 4 mg three times daily. Patients with more severe disease require specific medical therapy and acute attacks often require admission to hospital. Medical therapy relies mainly on anti-inflammatory and immunosuppressive drugs. The mechanism of action of these drugs in inflammatory bowel disease is unknown and treatment is largely empirical.

Anaemia will improve as the patient gets better, but appropriate haematinics, e.g. ferrous sulphate 400 mg daily or folic acid 5 mg daily may be required.

Crohn's disease. Acute attacks require oral corti-costeroids 30–60 mg daily. On this regimen patients usually improve quickly and the steroid dosage can then be reduced. Sulphasalazine (see below) is used in patients with colonic involvement. Azathioprine (2 mg·kg^{-1} daily) is an immunosuppressive agent which has been shown to be helpful in maintaining the steroid-induced remission, although it has not gained universal acceptance. Patients with colonic involvement can also be given rectal steroids (see

below). Metronidazole (800 mg three times daily) and co-trimoxazole (two tablets twice daily) are useful in severe perianal disease due to their antibacterial action.

Elemental diets (see p. 143) or parenteral nutrition can induce remissions, usually in small gut disease. They improve nutrition, allow the bowel to 'rest', and reduce antigen load to the bowel. Their mode of action and efficacy is under clinical trial.

Some patients in remission may not require therapy, but others need small doses of steroids to suppress the disease activity.

Ulcerative colitis. Severe attacks require careful management in hospital as the mortality of this condition is still high.

All patients with ulcerative colitis are treated with sulphasalazine, initially in a dose of 3–4 g daily reducing to a maintenance dose of 2 g daily. In mild cases it may induce a remission. Its main role, however, is to reduce the number of relapses when taken long term. Sulphasalazine consists of a 5-

(b)

aminosalicylic acid (5ASA) attached to sulpha-pyridine as a carrier. This combination is broken down in the colon by bacteria to release the active agent, 5ASA. Sulphasalazine may induce nausea and has some reversible side-effects, including haemolytic anaemia, skin rashes and infertility in men. These are produced by the sulphapyridine and recently new forms of slow-release 5ASA without sulphapyridine have been developed. These are likely to supersede sulphasalazine.

Mild attacks and proctitis can be treated with local rectal steroids in the form of enemas (prednisolone-21-phosphate 20 mg) or a 10% hydrocortisone foam.

Moderate attacks are treated with oral pred-nisolone 30–40 mg daily. Patients with their first attack or who do not respond quickly should be admitted to hospital. In severe attacks, high dose corticosteroids in the form of prednisolone 60 mg, hydrocortisone 100 mg i.v. 6-hourly or cortico-trophin (synthetic ACTH) 1–2 mg i.m. are given. In addition, dehydration and electrolyte disturbances should be corrected by intravenous therapy.

Accompanying septicaemia, which is usually due to gram-negative bacteria, should be treated with anti-biotics. Surgical treatment may be necessary if there is no improvement.

The main complication of severe ulcerative colitis and Crohn's colitis is toxic megacolon (see below).

Surgical management
Crohn's disease. Approximately 80% of patients will require an operation at some time during the course of their disease. Nevertheless, surgery should be avoided if at all possible and only minimal resections undertaken, as recurrence (15% per year) is almost inevitable. The indications for surgery are:
● Failure of medical therapy, with acute or chronic symptoms producing ill-health
● Complications, e.g. toxic dilatation, obstruction, perforation, abscesses
● Failure to grow in children

In most patients with small bowel disease, surgical treatment consists of resection and end-to-end anastomosis. The surgery for colonic disease is similar to that for ulcerative colitis (see below).

Ulcerative colitis. This disease is confined to the colon and therefore colectomy is curative.

Indications for surgery are the same as those for Crohn's disease, although complications of the disease are less common. In addition, a prophylactic colectomy is sometimes performed in patients who have a high cancer risk.

Surgery for ulcerative colitis and colonic Crohn's disease consists of protocolectomy with ileostomy or colectomy with an ileorectal anastomosis. Ileo-anal anastomoses are currently under evaluation.

Protocolectomy with an ileostomy is the standard operation in which the colon and rectum are removed and the ileum is brought out through an opening in the right iliac fossa and attached to the skin. The patient wears an ileostomy bag which is stuck on to the skin over the ileostomy spout. This bag requires to be emptied once or twice daily. This is compatible with a near normal lifestyle. Stoma-care therapists are readily available with help and advice.

Problems associated with ileostomies include:
● Mechanical problems
● Dehydration, particularly in hot climates
● Psychosexual problems
● Infertility in men
● Recurrence in Crohn's disease

A *colectomy with an ileorectal or ileo-anal anastomosis* is used to avoid ileostomy. Ileorectal anastomosis leaves a diseased rectum in situ and frequent diar-rhoea still occurs. With an ileo-anal anastomosis a pouch of ileum is formed which acts as a reservoir and the patient is continent with only a few bowel motions per day. The recurrence rate in Crohn's disease may be higher than with an ileostomy and

therefore the ileo-anal operation is used for ulcer-ative colitis only and is still being evaluated.

COMPLICATIONS

These are similar in both conditions but vary in frequency. Crohn's disease, with its transmural inflammation, has a higher incidence of fistulas, fissures and abscess formation.

Perforation
This is a rare but serious complication that occurs in association with toxic megacolon. In Crohn's disease local perforations may occur, forming walled off abscesses, and occasionally small bowel perforation gives rise to peritonitis.

Haemorrhage
Massive haemorrhage is rare.

Toxic dilatation
Toxic dilatation may occur during an acute severe attack of colitis. The diagnosis should be suspected in a patient with a severe episode (see above) who develops abdominal distension. A plain abdominal x-ray (Fig. 4.22) will show a dilated thin-walled colon which is gas-filled and contains mucosal islands. Treatment is as for a severe attack of colitis plus daily abdominal x-rays and measurements of abdominal girth. If the patient does not settle in 48 h with high-dose corticosteroids, emergency surgery should be performed. When mucosal islands are present the risk of perforation is high, as is the mortality, and many favour immediate surgery without medical therapy.

Carcinoma
The incidence is increased in both conditions. In Crohn's disease the incidence of carcinoma is only marginally increased and does not influence management. In ulcerative colitis the risk of car-cinoma of the colon in a patient who has had total colitis for more than 10 years is much greater than it is for the general population. It is suggested that regular sigmoidoscopy and colonoscopy with biop-sies may detect early premalignant changes. The degree of surveillance necessary is currently under study.

COURSE AND PROGNOSIS

Crohn's disease
These patients have recurrent relapses and virtually all have a significant relapse over a 20-year period. The mortality rate is variable, but generally appears to be at least twice as high as that seen in the normal population. Most deaths are associated with surgery. Despite this, many patients lead a normal life. Crohn's disease in childhood causes growth retardation.

Fig. 4.22 Plain abdominal X-ray showing toxic dilatation in ulcerative colitis. The arrows indicate mucosal islands. Note the barium in the rectum. The enema was stopped as it is contraindicated in toxic dilatation.

Ulcerative colitis

The course and prognosis is variable. In proctitis it is very good; only 10% of these cases go on to develop more extensive disease. On the other hand, severe fulminant disease still carries a 15–25% mortality. The mortality is reduced if the acute attack is treated promptly and surgery performed if no improvement occurs in the first 2–3 days.

Overall, because many cases are mild, the mortality of this disease is not much greater than the mortality rates for the general population, in contrast to Crohn's disease.

There is no particular risk to mother or child during pregnancy in either form of inflammatory bowel disease.

The colon and rectum

Structure

The large intestine starts at the caecum, on the posterior medial wall of which is the appendix. The colon is made up of ascending, transverse, descending and sigmoid parts, which join the rectum at the rectosigmoid junction.

The muscle wall consists of an inner circular layer and an outer longitudinal layer. The outer layer is incomplete, coming together to form the taenia coli, which produce the haustral pattern seen in the normal colon.

The mucosa of the colon is lined by epithelial cells with crypts but no villi, so that the surface is flat. The mucosa is full of goblet cells. A variety of cells, mainly lymphocytes and macrophages, are found in the lamina propria.

The blood supply to the colon is from the superior and inferior mesenteric vessels. Generally there are good anastomotic channels, but the caecum and splenic flexure are areas where ischaemia can occur.

The rectum is about 12 cm long. Its interior is divided by three crescentic circular muscles producing shelf-like folds. These are the rectal valves and can be seen at sigmoidoscopy.

The anal canal is surrounded by an internal and an external sphincter.

Physiology

The main role of the colon is the absorption of water and electrolytes (see Table 4.15). Approximately 2 l of fluid passes the ileocaecal valve each day. The absorption of fluid and electrolytes takes place mainly in the right side of the colon, and only about 150 ml is passed in the faeces.

The role of the rectum and anus in defecation is complex. The rectum is usually empty and collapsed; the entry of faeces from the colon produces relaxation of the internal sphincter and the puborectalis muscle. This decreases the acute angle between the rectum and the anal canal. When the rectum contains approximately 100 ml of faeces the urge to defecate is experienced. The rectum is emptied by relaxation of the external anal sphincter (under voluntary control) and an increase in intra-abdominal pressure.

Diverticular disease

Diverticula are frequently found in the colon and occur in 50% of patients over the age of 50. They are most frequent in the sigmoid, but can be present over the whole colon.

The term *diverticulosis* indicates the presence of diverticula; *diverticulitis* implies that these diverticula are inflamed. It is perhaps better to use the more general term *diverticular disease*, as it is often difficult to be sure whether the diverticula are inflamed. The precise mechanism of diverticular formation is not known. There is thickening of the muscle layer and because of high intraluminal pressures pouches of mucosa extrude through the muscular wall through weakened areas near blood vessels to form diverticula. Diverticular disease seems to be related to the low-fibre diet eaten in the Western hemisphere.

Diverticulitis occurs when faeces obstruct the neck of the diverticulum, causing stagnation and allowing bacteria to multiply and produce inflammation. This can then lead to bowel perforation (peridiverticulitis), abscess formation, fistulas into adjacent organs, or even generalized peritonitis.

CLINICAL FEATURES AND MANAGEMENT

Diverticular disease is asymptomatic in 90% and is usually discovered incidentally; no treatment is required.

It may present with pain in the left iliac fossa, sometimes associated with either constipation or the passage of frequent loose stools. On examination there may be tenderness in the left iliac fossa. Rectal examination and sigmoidoscopy are normal. Diagnosis is made on barium enema examination (Fig. 4.23). Diverticula are often seen and can be an incidental finding, so care must be taken not to miss any other lesion such as a carcinoma. The symptoms are very similar to those of the irritable bowel syndrome and because both conditions are so common it is often difficult to distinguish between them. In practice, both conditions are treated symptomatically with a high-fibre diet, antispasmodic drugs (e.g. mebeverine 135 mg three times daily) and agents to regulate the bowel.

Acute diverticulitis almost always affects diverticula in the sigmoid colon. It presents with severe pain in the left iliac fossa, often accompanied by fever and constipation. These symptoms and signs are similar to appendicitis but on the left side. On examination there is tenderness, guarding and rigidity on the left side of the abdomen. Tachycardia and pyrexia are present and the white cell count shows a leucocytosis. An abdominal x-ray is performed to exclude free perforation.

COMPLICATIONS OF ACUTE DIVERTICULITIS

- *Abscess formation*, causing pain, pyrexia, and a palpable tender mass in the left iliac fossa
- *Perforation*, leading to generalized peritonitis (see p. 200)
- *Fistula formation* into the bladder, causing dysuria

Table 4.15 Input and output of water and electrolytes in the gastrointestinal tract.

	Water (ml)	Sodium (mmol)	Potassium (mmol)
Input			
Diet	1500	150	80
GI secretions	7500	1000	40
Total	9000	1150	120
Output			
Faeces	150	5	12
Ileostomy (adapted)	500–1500	60–120	4

Fig. 4.23 Double contrast barium enema showing diverticular disease (the diverticula are arrowed). Note the mucosal hypertrophy.

or pneumaturia, or into the vagina, causing discharge; the diverticular disease is often chronic, without evidence of acute inflammation

- *Intestinal obstruction* (see p.201). Acute attacks are treated with bowel rest, intravenous fluids and antibiotics, e.g. ampicillin and metronidazole. Most attacks settle on this regimen, but a few require emergency surgery, which usually consists of a defunctioning colostomy to be followed later by resection.

Acute episodes do not necessarily recur and elective surgery is mainly reserved for patients with intestinal obstruction or fistulae.

- *Rectal bleeding.* Diverticular disease can produce rectal bleeding, which is sometimes massive, particularly from right-sided diverticula. In most cases the bleeding stops and the cause of the bleeding can be established by x-ray, colonoscopy and sometimes angiography. In rare cases emergency colectomy is necessary.

Simple constipation

This is a major problem that is so common that it need not be considered as a disease. The long-standing constipation which is common in young women does not usually require investigation, but a change in bowel habit in the middle-aged or elderly does need investigation. A rectal examination should always be performed. The differential diagnosis is from other causes of constipation (see Table 4.16).

TREATMENT

Laxatives should be avoided if at all possible and the patient should be encouraged to take a high-fibre diet. Glycerol suppositories, which can be used by the patient, are often useful.

Megacolon

This term is used to describe a number of congenital and acquired conditions in which the colon is dilated. In many instances it is secondary to chronic constipation and in some parts of the world Chagas' disease is a common cause.

All young patients with megacolon should have Hirschsprung's disease excluded. In this disease, which presents in the first years of life, an aganglionic segment of the rectum gives rise to constipation and subacute obstruction. Occasionally Hirschsprung's disease affecting only a short segment of the rectum can be missed in childhood and a full-thickness rectal biopsy should be performed in adult patients with megacolon to exclude it. Pressure studies show failure of relaxation of the internal sphincter, which is diagnostic of Hirschsprung's disease. This disease can be successfully treated surgically.

Treatment of megacolon is similar to simple constipation, but saline washouts and manual removal of faeces are sometimes required.

Table 4.16 Causes of constipation.

Simple
Obstruction
Painful anal conditions
Drugs, e.g. opiates, aluminium antacids
Hypothyroidism, hypercalcaemia
Depression
Immobility
Hirschsprung's disease (occasionally in the adult)

Pneumatosis cystoides intestinalis

This is a rare condition in which multiple gas-filled cysts are found in the submucosa of the intestine, chiefly the colon. The cause is unknown but many cases are associated with chronic bronchitis and some with peptic ulceration. Patients are usually asymptomatic, but abdominal pain and diarrhoea does occur and occasionally the cysts rupture to produce a pneumoperitoneum. This condition is diagnosed on x-ray of the abdomen, barium enema or at sigmoidoscopy, when a globular mass is seen.

Treatment is often unnecessary, but continuous oxygen therapy will help to disperse the largely nitrogen-containing cysts.

Ischaemic disease of the colon (ischaemic colitis)

This commonly presents in the older age group (over 50 years) with sudden onset of abdominal pain and the passage of bright red blood with or without diarrhoea. There may be signs of shock and there is sometimes evidence of other cardiovascular disease. This condition has also been described in young women on the contraceptive pill.

On examination the abdomen is distended and tender. Sigmoidoscopy is normal apart from the presence of blood. Investigations include an abdominal x-ray to exclude perforation. 'Thumb-printing'—a characteristic sign for ischaemic disease—can be seen on a barium enema performed when the patient is well; strictures can also be seen.

The differential diagnosis is of other causes of acute colitis, but these can usually be excluded on the basis of the sigmoidoscopy findings.

TREATMENT

Most patients with this condition settle on symptomatic treatment. A few develop gangrene and perforation and require urgent surgery. Some develop strictures.

Anorectal conditions

These important conditions largely present to surgeons. The major conditions presenting initially to the physicians include:

Pruritus ani
Pruritus ani, or an itchy bottom, is common and often no cause is found. Treatment consists of good personal hygiene and keeping the area dry. Secondary causes include any local anal lesions such as haemorrhoids, infestation, e.g. threadworm (*Enterobius vermicularis*), or fungal infection, e.g. candidiasis. The latter condition often occurs secondary to the use of hydrocortisone creams, which should be avoided.

Haemorrhoids

Haemorrhoids usually produce rectal bleeding and pruritus ani. They are the commonest cause of rectal bleeding (Table 4.17) but if minor require no treatment. Diagnosis is made on proctoscopy.

Anal fissures

Anal fissures cause painful defecation and minor rectal bleeding and can often be seen in the anal margin on inspection. Treatment is by application of a local anaesthetic gel. Chronic fissures require dilatation.

Faecal incontinence

This can be a major problem in the elderly, infirm or demented patient. It is often secondary to impaction. Some of the major factors responsible are rectal prolapse, carcinoma of the rectum and diarrhoea from any cause. The patient should be carefully examined and investigation and treatment instituted as appropriate.

Faecal impaction

This occurs in the elderly with constipation. It can lead to overflow incontinence. It usually requires manual removal of faeces, and care to prevent recurrences (see constipation).

Solitary rectal ulcer

These ulcers occur in young adults and produce bowel irregularity and rectal bleeding with the passage of mucus. The cause is unclear, but many seem to be due to excess straining at stool with prolapse of the rectal mucosa (descending perineal syndrome).

Rectal examination is usually normal but sigmoidoscopy reveals redness or an ulcer approximately 10 cm from the anal margin on the anterior rectal wall. It often has an appearance not unlike a carcinoma.

Histology is diagnostic; there are non-specific inflammatory changes with bands of smooth muscle extending into the lamina propria.

Treatment is unsatisfactory and many cases run an indolent chronic course with continuation of symptoms. Local steroids may help and surgical

excision should be avoided. Patients should be advised to stop straining on defecation.

Rectal prolapse

In this common condition affecting children and the elderly the rectal mucosa prolapses through the anus due to excessive straining. Initially prolapse occurs only during defecation, but later ulceration, mucosal discharge and faecal incontinence can occur. Surgical treatment is required in complete prolapse.

Diarrhoea

With true diarrhoea there is an increase in stool weight of greater than 300 g per day. This is usually accompanied by increased stool frequency. Patients often interpret diarrhoea differently (see p. 150).

Mechanisms

Osmotic diarrhoea. The gut mucosa acts as a semipermeable membrane and fluid enters the bowel if there are large quantities of non-absorbed hypertonic substances in the lumen. This occurs because:

- The patient has ingested a non-absorbable substance, e.g. a purgative such as magnesium sulphate or lactulose
- The patient has generalized malabsorption
- The patient has a specific malabsorption, e.g. disaccharidase deficiency or glucose–galactose malabsorption

The volume of diarrhoea produced by these mechanisms is reduced by the absorption of fluid by the ileum and colon. The diarrhoea stops when the patient stops eating or the malabsorptive substance is discontinued.

Secretory diarrhoea. In this disorder there is both active intestinal secretion of fluid and electrolytes as well as decreased absorption. The mechanism of intestinal secretion is shown in Fig. 4.24a. Common causes of secretory diarrhoea are:

- Enterotoxins, e.g. cholera, *E. coli* (thermolabile or thermostable toxin) (p. 31)
- Hormones, e.g. vasoactive intestinal peptide in the Verner–Morrison syndrome
- Bile salts (in the colon) following ileal resection
- Fatty acids (in the colon) following ileal resection
- Some laxatives, e.g. dioctyl sodium sulphosuccinate

With secretory diarrhoea the stool volumes may be very high. Food does not affect the diarrhoea and it therefore continues during fasting.

Inflammatory diarrhoea (mucosal destruction). Diarrhoea occurs because of damage to the intestinal

Table 4.17 Causes of rectal bleeding.

Cause	Type of bleed
Common (75%) Haemorrhoids Anal fissures	Small but recurrent
Less common (25%) Diverticular disease	Large but infrequent
Ischaemic colitis Polyps Carcinoma	Small but persistent
Inflammatory bowel disease	Usually with diarrhoea

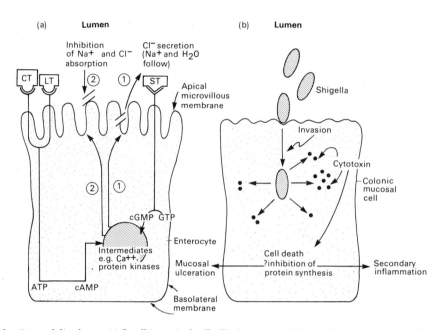

Fig. 4.24 Mechanisms of diarrhoea. (a) Small intestinal cell. Cholera toxin (CT) and the heat-labile *E. coli* enterotoxin (LT) share the same receptor and activate the adenylate cyclase pathway. This activates intermediates, e.g. Ca^{++} and protein kinases, which act on the apical microvillous membrane to cause Cl^- secretion (1) and inhibition of Na^+ and Cl^- absorption (2). The heat-stable *E. coli* enterotoxin (ST) has a different receptor and acts through cGMP to produce the same effect. In both mechanisms, stimulation occurs without invasion. (b) Colonic mucosal cell. This demonstrates the mechanisms by which an invasive pathogen, e.g. *Shigella*, acts. Following penetration the pathogens generate cytotoxins which lead to mucosal ulceration and cell death.

mucosal cell so that there is a loss of fluid, blood, etc. In addition, there is defective absorption of fluid and electrolytes. Common causes are infective conditions, e.g. dysentery due to *Shigella*, and inflammatory conditions, e.g. ulcerative colitis (see Fig. 4.24b).

Abnormal motility (usually not true diarrhoea). Diarrhoea in the irritable bowel syndrome is due to abnormal colonic motility. Diabetic, post-vagotomy and hyperthyroid diarrhoea are all due to abnormal motility of the upper gut. In many of these cases the volume and weight of the stool is not all that high, but frequency of defecation occurs; this therefore is not true diarrhoea.

Some causes of diarrhoea are shown in Table 4.18.

Acute diarrhoea (excluding cholera, which is discussed on p. 29)
Diarrhoea of sudden onset is very common, often short-lived and requires no investigation or treatment. This type of diarrhoea is seen after dietary indiscretions, but diarrhoea due to viral agents also lasts 24–48 h. The causes of infective diarrhoeas are shown on p. 31. Traveller's diarrhoea, which affects people travelling outside their own countries, particularly to Third World countries, usually lasts 2–5

Table 4.18 Causes of diarrhoea.

Acute
Dietary indiscretion
Infective
    Food poisoning—see p. 33
    Viral
    Other organisms
Traveller's diarrhoea—see p. 31
    E. coli
    Giardia lamblia
    Shigella
    Entamoeba histolytica

Chronic
Inflammatory bowel disease
Parasitic/fungal
Gay bowel disease
Malabsorption
Gut resection
Drugs
Diverticular disease
Colonic neoplasia
Endocrine
    Pancreatic tumours, e.g. gastrinoma
    Thyrotoxicosis
    Diabetic neuropathy
Faecal impaction—in the elderly
Irritable bowel disease (often not increased volume)

days; it is discussed on p. 31. Clinical features associated with the acute diarrhoeas include fever, abdominal pain and vomiting. If the diarrhoea is particularly severe, dehydration can be a problem; the very young and very old are at special risk from this. Investigations are necessary if the diarrhoea has lasted more than one week. Stools (up to three) should be sent immediately to the laboratory for culture and examination for ova, cysts and parasites. A sigmoidoscopy and rectal biopsy should be performed. If the diagnosis has still not been made, radiological studies should be performed.

Oral fluid replacement is of prime importance in the treatment. Special oral rehydration solutions, e.g. sodium chloride and glucose powder (see Table 1.16, p. 30), are available for use in severe episodes of diarrhoea in infants. These compounds were initially developed for use in cholera but are valuable in all severe diarrhoeas. Anti-diarrhoeal drugs are thought to impair the clearance of any pathogen from the bowel but may be necessary for short-term relief, e.g. codeine phosphate 30 mg four times daily or loperamide 2 mg three times daily.

Chronic diarrhoea
This always needs investigation (see Fig. 4.25). All patients should have a sigmoidoscopy and rectal biopsy. Whether the large or the small bowel is investigated first will depend on the clinical story of,

for example, bloody diarrhoea or steatorrhoea. The investigations and treatment are described under the individual diseases.

Some other causes of diarrhoea
Purgative abuse. This is usually seen in females who surreptitiously take high-dose purgatives and are often extensively investigated for chronic diarrhoea. The diarrhoea is usually of high volume (> 1 l/day). Sigmoidoscopy may show a pigmented mucosa, a condition known as *melanosis coli.* Histologically the rectal biopsy shows pigment-laden macrophages in patients taking an anthraquinone purgative (e.g. Senokot). Melanosis coli is also seen in people taking regular purgatives in normal doses. Phenolphthalein laxatives can be detected by pouring an alkali, e.g. sodium hydroxide, on the stools, which then turn pink; a magnesium-containing purgative will give a high faecal magnesium content. A barium enema shows loss of haustral patterns and there may be mild abnormalities of absorption tests and a low serum potassium. Management is difficult as the patient usually denies purgative ingestion. If the diagnosis is suspected, a locker or bed search, while the patient is out of the ward, may occasionally be necessary. The patient needs psychiatric help.

Pseudomembranous colitis (antibiotic-associated diarrhoea). This colitis develops following the use of

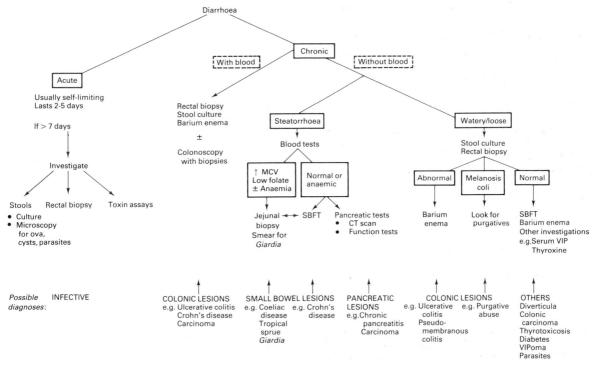

Fig. 4.25 Flow diagram for the investigation of diarrhoea. Rectal biopsies are obtained via a sigmoidoscope, and the macroscopic appearances of the mucosa should be noted. SBFT = small bowel follow-through; VIP = vasoactive intestinal polypeptide.

antibiotics such as lincomycin, ampicillin and cephalosporins. Diarrhoea occurs in the first few days after taking the antibiotic or even up to six weeks after stopping the antibiotic.

Sigmoidoscopy usually shows multiple yellow plaques and inflammation; histology shows inflammation, sometimes with a pseudomembrane. Treatment, if necessary, is with vancomycin 125–500 mg four times daily for 1–2 weeks or metronidazole 400 mg three times daily. *Clostridium difficile* (see p. 26) and its toxin are found in the stools.

Functional bowel disease

This is the general term used to embrace two syndromes:
● Non-ulcer dyspepsia
● The irritable bowel syndrome

These conditions are extremely common, making up 60–80% of patients seen in a gastroenterology clinic. The two conditions overlap, with some symptoms being common to both. In general, however, the term *non-ulcer dyspepsia* is given to patients complaining of indigestion, wind, nausea, heartburn, i.e. dyspepsia, when no ulcer is found. It can be difficult on the history to differentiate it from the symptoms of gastric or duodenal ulceration, but typically patients with ulcers have nocturnal pain and respond to antacids. Barium studies or endoscopy are usually performed to exclude ulceration, but are probably unnecessary in those under 35 years. Treatment is by reassurance. Antacids and H_2-receptor antagonists can be tried, but are probably of little benefit apart from the placebo effect. Metoclopramide 10 mg three times daily may be helpful.

The irritable bowel syndrome is the term now used for all other types of functional bowel disease.

The irritable bowel syndrome

CLINICAL FEATURES

In the classical irritable bowel syndrome, pain is situated in the left iliac fossa and is usually relieved by defecation or the passage of wind. The patient may complain of constipation or diarrhoea with the passage of frequent small-volume stools and a feeling of incomplete emptying of the rectum. Stools may be ribbon-like or rabbity in appearance. True watery diarrhoea suggests organic disease. The pain, however, can occur in any part of the abdomen and the bowel habit may be normal.

The length of history is usually long, with frequent recurrent episodes and long symptom-free intervals. The patient may give a history of recurrent episodes of abdominal pain as a child. Mild episodes of pain

occur frequently in the normal population and are usually disregarded and therefore undiagnosed. The patient with the irritable bowel syndrome looks well despite frequent episodes of pain, some of which can be very acute and require hospital admission to rule out an acute abdominal condition.

AETIOLOGY

The exact cause of the irritable bowel syndrome is not known, but the symptoms do seem to be produced by a combination of disordered gut motility and increased tenderness of the gut.

Psychological factors are important and most patients find the symptoms are exacerbated by stress. Some patients are depressed, which may be missed unless carefully looked for.

EXAMINATION

Examination reveals no abnormality. Rectal examination and sigmoidoscopy should be performed. Although sigmoidoscopy shows a normal mucosa, air insufflation may reproduce the pain. If diarrhoea is a feature, a rectal biopsy should be performed, even if the mucosa looks normal, to help rule out inflammatory bowel disease.

INVESTIGATION

The amount of investigation varies in individual patients. A young girl with pain in the left iliac fossa exacerbated by stress will require no investigation. Conversely, an elderly person who had developed pain or diarrhoea for the first time must be fully investigated, with a full radiological assessment, before the diagnosis of functional bowel disease is made.

Traps for the unwary
● *Beware of false correlations.* Diverticular disease is common in the elderly and because diverticular disease is seen on the barium enema it must not be assumed to be the cause of the pain. Hiatus hernias are also common findings and are also often asymptomatic.
● *Gynaecological problems* must be excluded; on the other hand, it must not be assumed that all lower abdominal pain in women is due to some gynaecological problem. Many unnecessary operations are carried out as a consequence.
● *Recurrent pain in the right iliac fossa* is not due to chronic appendicitis but to the irritable bowel syndrome.
● *Recurrent pain in the right hypochondrium* is usually not due to gallbladder disease but to the irritable bowel syndrome.
● *Abdominal bruits* are common and abdominal pain should not be ascribed to ischaemic bowel on this basis alone.

MANAGEMENT

- Explanation of the symptoms and their mechanism often helps and patients must be reassured of the benign nature of the condition. Cancer phobia must be dispelled. The patient has to learn to live with his symptoms as they tend to be recurrent.
- A high-fibre bran diet may help some patients.
- Antispasmodics, e.g. mebeverine, may be given.
- Underlying stress and depression should be treated.

The acute abdomen

This section deals with acute abdominal conditions which cause the patient to be hospitalized within a few hours of the onset of their pain. It is important to make the diagnosis as quickly as possible to reduce morbidity and mortality. Although a specific diagnosis should be attempted, the immediate problem in management is to decide whether an 'acute abdomen' exists or not.

History

Pain
The onset, site, type and subsequent cause of the pain should be determined as accurately as possible.

Usually the pain is fairly rapid in onset, but if there is a perforation of a hollow viscus, e.g. a perforated duodenal ulcer, the pain is particularly sudden in onset. Acute intestinal ischaemia also presents with acute pain, whereas inflammatory conditions, e.g. appendicitis, produce a more gradual onset of pain. In intestinal obstruction the pain is typically colicky in nature, whereas with peritonitis the pain is continuous and may be made worse by movement.

The site of the pain can help in determining the organ involved: generally upper abdominal pain is produced by lesions of the upper GI tract and lower abdominal pain by lesions of the lower GI tract. It must, however, be remembered that the GI tract is not fixed and, for example, the appendix may not always be in the right iliac fossa.

Vomiting
Vomiting accompanies any acute abdominal pain: it is persistent with a high obstructive lesion of the gut.

Physical examination

The general condition of the patient should be noted. Does he look ill? Is he shocked? Because fluid is lost from the vascular compartment into the peritoneal cavity or into the lumen of the bowel, hypovolaemia frequently occurs, causing pale, cold skin, especially the nose, a weak rapid pulse, and hypotension.

Abdomen
Signs of peritonitis. The abdomen should be examined gently. Sites of tenderness and the presence or absence of guarding should be noted. Guarding is involuntary spasm of the abdominal wall and it indicates peritonitis. This can be localized to one area or it may be generalized, involving the whole abdomen.

Rebound tenderness occurs when the palpating hand is removed from the abdomen suddenly. The pain is due to sudden movement of the inflamed peritoneum.

Signs of obstruction. The main findings are distension of the abdomen due to gas in the bowel and increased bowel sounds due to increased bowel movement. High-pitched (tinkling) bowel sounds indicate small bowel obstruction.

Absent bowel sounds suggest peritoneal involvement (peritonitis) in addition to obstruction and may be seen in intestinal ischaemia or strangulated bowel.

It is essential that the hernial orifices are examined if intestinal obstruction is suspected.

Pelvic and rectal examinations. These can be very helpful, particularly in diagnosing gynaecological causes of an acute abdomen, e.g. a ruptured ectopic pregnancy. Rectal examination may detect localized tenderness or blood in the stools, which is suggestive of a vascular lesion.

Other observations
- Tongue—furred in most acute abdominal disease
- Temperature—fever is more common in acute inflammatory processes
- Urine—examine for:
  (a) Glucose and ketones (ketoacidosis can present with acute pain)
  (b) White cells (to exclude acute pyelonephritis)
  (c) Porphyrins (porphyria is a rare cause of abdominal pain)
- Think of other conditions, e.g.
  (a) Diabetes mellitus (ketoacidosis)
  (b) Pneumonia (referred pain)
  (c) Myocardial infarction (referred pain)
  (d) Lead poisoning
  (e) The irritable bowel syndrome (this can produce acute severe pain)

Investigation

- *Blood count*—raised white cell count likely in inflammatory conditions.
- *Serum amylase*—high levels of greater than five times normal indicate acute pancreatitis. Raised levels below this can occur in any acute abdomen

and should not be considered diagnostic of pancreatitis.
- *Serum electrolytes*—not particularly helpful for diagnosis, but useful for general evaluation of the patient.
- *X-ray of the abdomen*—an erect and supine x-ray of the abdomen are useful to detect air under the diaphragm (perforation) or dilated loops of bowel or fluid levels suggestive of obstruction.

SPECIFIC CONDITIONS

Acute appendicitis

This is the commonest surgical emergency. It affects all age groups from the very young to the very old and appendicitis should always be considered in the differential diagnosis if the appendix has not been removed.

Acute appendicitis mostly occurs when the lumen of the appendix becomes obstructed with a faecolith; however, in some cases there is only generalized acute inflammation. If the appendix is not removed at this stage, gangrene occurs with perforation, leading to a localized abscess or to generalized peritonitis.

CLINICAL FEATURES

All patients have abdominal pain; in many it starts vaguely in the centre of the abdomen, becoming localized to the right iliac fossa in the first few hours. There is nausea, some vomiting and occasional diarrhoea. Because of the variable position of the appendix, symptoms and signs differ.

Examination of the abdomen reveals tenderness in the right iliac fossa, with guarding due to the localized peritonitis. Rectal examination shows tenderness to the right. There may be a tender mass in the right iliac fossa.

Laboratory tests are unhelpful, except that the white cell count may be raised. An ultrasound examination may be useful in localizing a mass.

In the differential diagnosis all abdominal conditions must be considered, and in children and young adults non-specific mesenteric lymphadenitis may mimic appendicitis. Acute terminal ileitis (see p. 185) also gives similar symptoms and signs. The exact diagnosis may be difficult to make, but if there is a reasonable possibility of it being acute appendicitis, laparotomy should be performed.

Generalized peritonitis still causes a significant mortality and morbidity and early surgery is a better option in suspected acute appendicitis than a 'wait and see' policy. Nevertheless, functional bowel disease can present acutely and must always be considered.

If an appendix mass is present, the patient is treated conservatively. The pain subsides over a few days and the mass usually disappears over a few weeks. Appendectomy is recommended at a later date to prevent further acute episodes.

Acute peritonitis

Localized peritonitis
There is virtually always some degree of localized peritonitis with all acute inflammatory conditions of the GI tract, e.g. acute appendicitis, acute cholecystitis. Pain and tenderness are largely features of this localized peritonitis. The treatment is for the underlying disease.

Generalized peritonitis
This is still a serious condition resulting from irritation of the peritoneum due to infection, e.g. perforated appendix, or from chemical irritation due to leakage of intestinal contents, e.g. perforated ulcer. In the latter case superadded infection gradually occurs; *E. coli* and *Bacteroides* are the commonest organisms.

The peritoneal cavity becomes acutely inflamed, with production of an inflammatory exudate which spreads throughout the peritoneum leading to intestinal dilatation and paralytic ileus.

Acute peritonitis should not be allowed to develop and will not do so if the underlying conditions are treated promptly.

CLINICAL FEATURES

In perforation the onset is sudden, with acute severe abdominal pain, followed by general collapse and shock. The patient may improve temporarily, only to become worse later as generalized toxaemia occurs.

When the peritonitis is secondary to inflammatory disease, the initial features are those of the underlying disease. Peritonitis is always treated surgically, with initial treatment of the patient's general condition, including insertion of a nasogastric tube, intravenous fluids and antibiotics. Surgery has a twofold objective:
- Drainage of the abdominal cavity
- Specific treatment of the underlying condition

COMPLICATIONS

Any delay in treatment of peritonitis produces more profound toxaemia and septicaemia. In addition, local abscess formation occurs and should be suspected if the patient continues to remain unwell with a swinging fever, high white cell count and continuing pain. Abscesses are commonly pelvic or subphrenic. Both are now localized chiefly by ultrasound examination; treatment is with antibiotics and drainage in the case of a subphrenic abscess.

Intestinal obstruction

Most intestinal obstruction is due to a mechanical block. Sometimes the bowel does not function, leading to paralytic ileus. This occurs temporarily after most abdominal operations and with peritonitis. Some causes of intestinal obstruction are shown in Table 4.19.

Obstruction of the bowel leads to bowel distension above the block, with increased secretion of fluid into the distended bowel. Bacterial contamination occurs in the distended stagnant bowel. In strangulation the blood supply is impeded, leading to gangrene, perforation and peritonitis unless urgent treatment of the condition is undertaken.

CLINICAL FEATURES

The patient complains of colicky abdominal pain, vomiting and constipation without passage of wind. In upper gut obstruction the vomiting is profuse, but in lower gut obstruction it may be absent.

Examination of the abdomen reveals distension, with increased bowel sounds. Examination of the hernial orifices must be performed.

X-ray of the abdomen reveals distended loops of bowel with fluid levels.

MANAGEMENT

Initial management is by nasogastric intubation to decompress the bowel and replacement of fluid loss by intravenous fluids (mainly isotonic saline).

Laparotomy with removal of the obstruction is necessary in most instances and if the bowel is gangrenous due to strangulation, gut resection will be required.

A few patients, e.g. those with Crohn's disease, may have recurrent episodes of subacute intestinal obstruction which can be managed conservatively.

Rarely the clinical features of obstruction are produced by a condition in which the nerve plexuses of the bowel are damaged—intestinal pseudo-obstruction. This condition is managed conservatively.

Volvulus of the sigmoid colon can be managed by the passage of a rectal tube to unkink the bowel, but recurrent volvulus may require sigmoid resection.

Acute intestinal ischaemia

Mesenteric artery occlusion, either from an embolus or from thrombosis in an arteriosclerotic artery, leads to gut ischaemia and, if not dealt with promptly, necrosis of the intestine.

The patient presents with severe abdominal pain and vomiting. Bloody diarrhoea is a helpful indicator of the diagnosis but does not occur for some time. The abdomen is usually tender and bowel sounds are absent. The diagnosis must be considered in any elderly patient with arteriosclerotic disease or in patients with atrial fibrillation. Early surgery may prevent gut necrosis, but sometimes massive resection of the dead gut is required to save the patient's life.

Mesenteric venous thrombosis occurs mainly in patients who have circulatory failure and can lead to gut necrosis. Often the patient is extremely ill from his underlying condition, but surgery may be necessary if the patient is fit enough.

The peritoneum

The peritoneal cavity is a closed sac lined by mesothelium. It normally contains a little fluid which allows the intra-abdominal organs to move freely. Some conditions that can affect the peritoneum are shown in Table 4.20.

Peritonitis can be acute or chronic, as seen in tuberculosis. Most cases of infective peritonitis are secondary to gastrointestinal diseases, but it occasionally occurs without intra-abdominal sepsis in ascites due to liver disease. Very rarely, fungal and parasitic infections can also cause primary peritonitis, e.g. amoebiasis, candidiasis. Peritonitis is discussed further on p. 200.

Table 4.19 Some causes of intestinal obstruction.

Constriction from the outside, e.g.
bowel entrapped in a hernia
adhesions
volvulus, particularly of sigmoid colon
Bowel disease obstructing the lumen, e.g.
carcinoma
Crohn's disease
diverticular disease
Luminal obstruction, e.g.
foreign body
gallstones

Table 4.20 Diseases of the peritoneum.

Infective (bacterial) peritonitis
Secondary to gut disease, e.g. appendicitis, perforation of any organ
Chronic peritoneal dialysis
Spontaneous, usually in ascites with liver disease
Tuberculosis
Neoplasia
Secondary deposits, e.g. from ovary, stomach
Primary mesothelioma
Vasculitis
Connective tissue disease

The peritoneum can be involved by *secondary malignant deposits* and the commonest cause of ascites in a young to middle aged woman is an ovarian carcinoma.

A *subphrenic abscess* is usually secondary to infection in the abdomen and is characterized by fever, malaise, pain in the right or left hypochondrium and shoulder-tip pain. A plain abdominal x-ray shows gas under the diaphragm, impaired movement of the diaphragm on screening and a pleural effusion. Ultrasound is usually diagnostic.

Ascites is associated with all diseases of the peritoneum. The fluid which collects is an exudate with a high protein content. It is also seen in liver disease. The mechanism, causes and investigation of ascites are discussed on p. 235.

Tuberculous peritonitis

This is usually due to reactivation of a tuberculous focus in the peritoneum with concurrent pulmonary, intestinal or genital TB. It is often seen in debilitated patients and alcoholics. Usually the onset is insidious, with fever, anorexia and weight loss. Abdominal pain is common, accompanied by ascites (75%) or an abdominal mass caused by an inflamed mesentery.

Diagnosis is made by examination of the peritoneal fluid, which shows an increase in lymphocyte count; occasionally tubercle bacilli are seen on staining. Culture of the fluid should be performed.

At laparoscopy the peritoneum is seen to be studded with tubercles which can be biopsied and sent for culture and histology. Treatment is with conventional chemotherapy (see p. 602) for 18 months to 2 years.

Retroperitoneal fibrosis

This is a rare condition in which there is a marked fibrosis over the posterior abdominal wall and retroperitoneum. The aetiology is usually unknown but it has been associated with the drug methysergide and occasionally with the carcinoid syndrome. The disease usually presents in middle age with malaise, fever, and loss of weight. There is often anaemia and a raised ESR. The major complication is urinary tract obstruction from ureteric involvement, which may require surgery.

Tumours of the gastrointestinal tract

THE OESOPHAGUS

Benign tumours

Leiomyomas are the commonest benign tumours. They are usually discovered accidentally and they do not often produce symptoms.

Carcinoma

The majority of malignant tumours occur in the middle (50%) and lower third (25%) of the oesophagus. The tumours are usually squamous but adenocarcinoma occurs in the lower third and at the cardia, arising from the fundus of the stomach or from localized areas of columnar epithelium in the lower oesophagus resulting from long-standing reflux (Barrett's oesophagus). The incidence of carcinoma varies throughout the world, being high in China, parts of Africa and in the Caspian regions of Iran (where the incidence is the highest observed for any type of cancer anywhere in the world). In the UK it is 5–10 per 100 000 or 2.5% of all malignant disease. The variation in incidence throughout the world is greater than for any other carcinoma and is unusual in that sharp differences occur in regions very close to one another. Dietary and other environmental causes have been looked for, but so far none has been unequivocally proved. Carcinoma of the oesophagus is commoner in men and there is an increased incidence in heavy drinkers of alcohol as well as heavy smokers. Predisposing factors include Plummer–Vinson syndrome, achalasia, Barrett's oesophagus and the familial condition of tylosis (hyperkeratosis of palms and soles).

CLINICAL FEATURES

Carcinoma of the oesophagus occurs mainly in those aged 60–70 years. Dysphagia is the commonest single symptom and is progressive. Initially there is difficulty in swallowing solids, but eventually dysphagia for liquids also occurs. Benign strictures, on the other hand, initially produce intermittent dysphagia. Impaction of food causes pain, but more persistent pain implies infiltration.

The lesion is usually ulcerative, extending around the wall of the oesophagus to produce a stricture. Direct invasion of the surrounding structures rather than widespread metastases occurs, and at presentation 50% have regional lymph node involvement. Weight loss, due to the dysphagia as well as to anorexia, frequently occurs. The oesophageal obstruction eventually causes difficulty in swallowing saliva, and coughing and aspiration into the lungs is common.

Signs are often absent. Weight loss, anorexia and lymphadenopathy are occasionally found.

INVESTIGATION

Barium swallow is the initial investigation (Fig. 4.26). Oesophagoscopy provides histological or cytological proof of the carcinoma; 90% of oesophageal carcinomas can be confirmed with this technique. Computed tomography is useful to outline the size of the tumour and to evaluate mediastinal spread.

TREATMENT

The overall results are poor (2% 5-year survival) and only symptomatic and palliative treatment is a realistic possibility. Dilatation of the stricture and the placing of a tube to keep the oesophagus open is the usual therapy and can be performed via an endo-scope. Surgery carries a high morbidity and mortality and little chance of anything but palliation. Radiotherapy can be used for squamous carcinoma with limited success. Recently oesophageal tumours have been photocoagulated using a laser beam directed through an endoscope. This may prove a useful palliative technique.

THE STOMACH

Benign tumours

The commonest benign tumour is a leiomyoma. This tumour is usually discovered by chance, but it can occasionally ulcerate and produce haematemesis. Treatment is surgical removal.

Gastric polyps are uncommon and are again found usually by chance. They produce no symptoms. The commonest are regenerative or hyperplastic polyps, which are often multiple and require no treatment. Rarely adenomatous polyps are found and endoscopic removal is recommended because of possible malignant potential. There is no good evidence that gastric cancers arise from pre-existing adenomas (in contrast to colonic polyps).

Carcinoma

Carcinoma of the stomach is the commonest malignant tumour of the GI tract and is the third most common fatal cancer in the UK. The frequency varies throughout the world, being high in Japan and Chile and relatively low in the USA.

In the UK 20 per 100 000 males are affected per year. The world-wide incidence of gastric carcinoma appears to be falling, even in Japan, for no obvious cause. The incidence increases with age and more men than women are affected. The reason for the difference in incidence is unclear but it may be due to genetic, dietary or environmental factors:
- Carcinoma is more common in people of blood group A.
- Japanese who emigrate to the USA still have a high incidence, but this decreases in succeeding generations.
- The incidence is higher in lower socioeconomic groups.
- Dietary factors that have been suggested include alcohol, spicy foods and more recently nitrate ingestion. Nitrates can be converted into nitrosamines by bacteria at neutral pH and nitrosamines are known to be carcinogenic in animals. Nitrosamines are present in the stomach of patients with achlorhydria, who have an increased cancer risk.

Possible precancerous conditions
Benign gastric ulcers do not develop into gastric cancer. It can, however, be difficult to differentiate a

Fig. 4.26 Barium swallow showing carcinoma of the oesophagus. There is an irregular narrowed area (arrow) at the lower end of the oesophagus.

benign ulcer from a malignant ulcer as even malignant ulcers can partially heal on medical treatment. For these reasons it was originally thought that gastric ulcers could become malignant.

Pernicious anaemia carries a small increased risk of developing gastric carcinoma. Gastric atrophy present in the body and fundus of the stomach of these patients may be a precancerous lesion.

Many gastric cancers develop in areas of *atrophic gastritis* and also areas of *intestinal metaplasia*. Intestinal metaplasia and chronic gastritis are also found in the resected stomach and there is an increased incidence of gastric cancer after partial gastrectomy (especially with a gastrojejunostomy). This increased incidence is the same whether the gastric resection was for a gastric or duodenal ulcer.

Screening
Gastric cancer has an appalling prognosis despite treatment, and in an attempt to improve this, earlier diagnosis has been advocated. Unfortunately earlier diagnosis does not necessarily mean longer survival. The patient is merely operated on at an earlier date and although the survival may appear longer, death will still occur at the same time from the point of genesis of the cancer (called lead time bias). In Japan, mass screening with mobile x-ray units has increased the proportion of early gastric cancers diagnosed. Early gastric cancer is defined as a carcinoma which is confined to the mucosa or submucosa. It is associated with 5-year survival rates of approximately 90%. In a large series of patients with gastric cancer from the UK, only 0.7% were identified as having early gastric cancer and therefore screening would not be warranted.

An effective screening procedure needs:
● To be cheap
● To be acceptable to all social groups so that they attend for examination
● To have a good discriminatory index from benign lesions
● To result in an improvement in prognosis

Unless all these criteria are fulfilled, screening is unwarranted except possibly in individuals with an increased risk for the disease. Nevertheless, even in this high-risk group, screening asymptomatic subjects would not be justified as the overall benefit is minimal.

An alternative approach to screening asymptomatic patients is to investigate symptomatic patients as quickly as possible. At the present time the mean interval between the onset of symptoms and attendance at hospital is approximately 6–9 months. However, dyspepsia is very common in the general population without any gastric lesions and it would obviously be impractical for every dyspeptic member of the general population to consult a physician. Even if they did, most primary physicians would think it unjustified to arrange a complicated series of investigations on the first visit.

Thus the detection of early gastric cancer in symptomatic patients is not a feasible proposition at the present time.

PATHOLOGY

Most gastric cancer occurs in the antrum and is almost invariably adenocarcinoma. The tumours are ulcerating lesions with heaped up, rolled edges. Sometimes they may be fungating polypoid lesions and if present in the fundus may infiltrate into the oesophagus and cause dysphagia. Lastly, the carcinoma may be diffuse with extensive submucosal spread, which may result in the picture of 'linitis plastica' (Fig. 4.27).

CLINICAL FEATURES

Symptoms
The commonest symptom is epigastric pain, which is indistinguishable from the pain of peptic ulcer disease, both being relieved by food and antacids. The pain can vary in intensity, but may be constant and severe. Most patients with carcinoma of the stomach have advanced disease at the time of presentation, and also have nausea, anorexia and weight loss. Vomiting is frequent and can be severe if

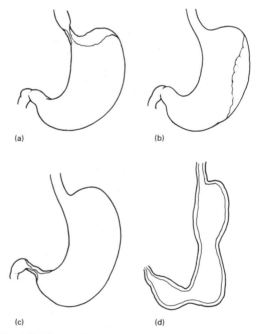

(a)   (b)

(c)   (d)

Fig. 4.27 Diagrammatic representation of various gastric carcinomas. (a) Fundal carcinoma extending into oesophagus. (b) Ulcerating carcinoma of the body. (c) Carcinoma of the antrum. (d) Diffuse infiltrating carcinoma (linitis plastica).

the tumour is near the pylorus. Dysphagia can occur with tumours involving the fundus (see Fig. 4.27). Gross haematemesis is unusual, but anaemia from occult blood loss is frequent.

Patients can present with metastases causing abdominal swelling due to ascites or jaundice due to liver involvement. Metastases also occur in bone, brain and lung, producing appropriate symptoms.

Signs

Nearly 50% of patients have a palpable epigastric mass with abdominal tenderness. Often weight loss is the only feature. A palpable lymph node is sometimes found in the supraclavicular fossa (Trousseau's sign) and signs of metastases are present in up to one-third of patients. Carcinoma of the stomach is the cancer most frequently associated with dermatomyositis and acanthosis nigricans.

INVESTIGATION

Barium meal
A good-quality, double-contrast barium meal has a diagnostic accuracy of up to 90%. The carcinoma is usually seen as a filling defect or an irregular ulcer with rolled edges. With the infiltrating type, the x-ray may show a rigid stomach.

Gastroscopy
Gastroscopy is sometimes performed as the primary procedure and has the advantage that biopsies can be performed for histological assessment and to exclude lymphoma. Positive biopsies can be obtained in almost all cases of obvious carcinoma, but a negative biopsy does not necessarily rule out the diagnosis. For this reason 8–10 biopsies should be taken from around the ulcer margin and its base. Superficial brushings for cytology will further improve the diagnostic rate.

Measurement of gastric secretion
This is seldom performed. Achlorhydria only occurs in 25% of patients with gastric cancer.

TREATMENT

Surgery for stomach cancer gives only a 10% 5-year survival rate; this figure has not changed over the past 25 years. Total gastrectomy is now seldom performed since the operative morbidity is high and the 5-year survival rate no better than subtotal or partial gastrectomy. Sixty-five per cent of cases are found to be inoperable at the time of surgery, but a palliative resection is usually performed to prevent obstruction and haemorrhage and to relieve the patient's immediate symptoms.

Treatment with chemotherapy has made little impact and is currently not justifiable apart from in clinical trials. Survival may be prolonged by a few months but the serious toxicity of the drugs limits their use.

THE SMALL INTESTINE

The small intestine is relatively resistant to the development of neoplasia and only 3–6% of all GI tumours and less than 1% of all malignant lesions occur in the small bowel. The reasons for the rarity of tumours is unknown. Explanations include the fluidity and relative sterility of small bowel contents and the rapid transit time, reducing the time of exposure to potential carcinogens. It is also possible that the high population of lymphoid tissue and secretion of IgA in the small intestine protects against malignancy.

Benign tumours

Adenomas, leiomyomas or lipomas are rarely found and are usually asymptomatic and picked up incidentally.

Peutz–Jeghers syndrome consists of mucocutaneous pigmentation (circumoral, hands and feet) and gastrointestinal polyps and has a Mendelian dominant inheritance. The brown buccal pigment is characteristic of this condition. The polyps which are hamartomas can occur anywhere in the GI tract, but are most frequent in the small bowel. They may bleed or cause intussusception. Rarely they become malignant. Treatment is by individual polypectomy. Multiple polypectomies may have to be performed, but bowel resection should be avoided.

Malignant tumours

Adenocarcinoma of the small intestine is found most frequently in the duodenum in the periampullary region and in the jejunum. Lymphomas are most frequently found in the ileum. These are of the non-Hodgkin's type and must be distinguished from generalized lymphoma involving the gut secondarily.

Predisposing factors
Coeliac disease. There is an increased incidence of lymphoma and adenocarcinoma of the small bowel in coeliac disease. There are no identifiable risk factors predisposing to malignancy, although the increased cell turnover found may be important. There is no evidence that treatment with a gluten-free diet protects against the development of malignancy.

Crohn's disease. There is a small increase in the incidence of adenocarcinoma of the small bowel in Crohn's disease.

Alpha-chain disease. This occurs mainly in areas surrounding the Mediterranean, in South America and in the Far East. It is related to poor hygiene and intestinal infestation. There is a proliferation of plasma cells in the lamina propria of the small bowel. These produce IgA heavy chains which can be detected in the gut mucosa by immunofluorescence as well as in the serum. The disease develops into lymphoma and therefore chemotherapy is given.

CLINICAL FEATURES

Patients present with abdominal pain, diarrhoea, anorexia, weight loss and symptoms of anaemia.

There may be a palpable mass and a small-bowel follow-through will detect most lesions. Laparotomy is required on many occasions to help with the diagnosis and to obtain tissue for histology and sometimes for resection. Treatment is often with resection, radiotherapy and chemotherapy.

Carcinoid tumours

These are discussed on p. 208.

THE LARGE INTESTINE

Colon polyps and polyposis syndromes (see Table 4.21)

A polyp is an elevation above the mucosal surface. The majority of colorectal polyps are adenomas with malignant potential. Polyps range in size from a few millimetres to 10 cm in diameter. They may be single or multiple and in the polyposis syndromes hundreds may be found.

Non-neoplastic polyps
Metaplastic (hyperplastic) polyps. These are commonly found in the rectum and produce no symptoms. They are usually small and need no treatment. The larger ones need to be removed for histological identification.

Inflammatory polyps. These are seen in the healing phase following an acute attack of colitis (e.g. ulcerative, Crohn's, schistosomal). They are often numerous and vary in size and shape. The larger ones can cause bleeding and need to be removed for histological identification.

Hamartomatous polyps. These are juvenile or Peutz–Jeghers in type. Hamartomatous polyps are commonly large and stalked. The Peutz–Jeghers polyps have characteristic fibromuscular fronds radiating between the disorganized mucosal crypts, whilst juvenile polyps show mucus retention cysts.

Juvenile polyps are a cause of bleeding and intussusception. They are confined to the colon. There is no evidence that these polyps have malignant potential.

Peutz–Jeghers polyps are usually multiple. They can occur in the large intestine where they bleed, producing chronic anaemia. Other non-neoplastic polyps are less common and are shown in Table 4.21.

In the Cronkhite–Canada syndrome polyps are

Table 4.21 Classification of colorectal polyps.

	Solitary	Multiple (polyposis syndromes)
Non-neoplastic		
Hamartomas	Peutz–Jeghers	Peutz–Jeghers syndrome
	Juvenile (mucus retention)	Juvenile polyposis
Inflammatory	Lymphoid	Benign lymphoid polyposis
	Inflammatory	Inflammatory polyps, e.g.
		ulcerative colitis
		Crohn's disease
		schistosomiasis
Miscellaneous	Metaplastic (hyperplastic)	Metaplastic polyposis
	Connective tissue polyps	Cronkhite–Canada syndrome
	Fibroma	
	Leiomyoma	
	Lipoma	
	Neurofibroma	
Neoplastic		
	Adenomas	Familial adenomatous
	Tubular	polyposis
	Tubulovillous	
	Villous	
	Carcinoid	
		Malignant lymphoid polyposis

associated with ectodermal abnormalities such as alopecia, nail dystrophy and skin hyper-pigmentation.

All of these polyps must be distinguished from adenomas, which have malignant potential.

Neoplastic polyps

Adenomas occur in about 10% of the population in the Western World but are rare elsewhere in the world. Genetic and environmental factors have been implicated, but no definite aetiological factors have been identified.

Polyps rarely produce symptoms and most are diagnosed on x-ray or on colonoscopy performed for other reasons. Large polyps may bleed intermittently and cause anaemia. Large sessile villous adenomas of the rectum can present with profuse diarrhoea and hypokalaemia.

The frequency with which invasive carcinoma occurs in adenomas increases with the size of the polyp and most if not all colonic carcinomas originate as adenomas. Once a polyp has been found on x-ray or endoscopy it is usually removed endoscopically. Further polyps may develop and continuous surveillance is necessary.

Familial adenomatous polyposis. For this high-risk group a prophylactic proctocolectomy with ileo-anal anastomosis is performed. Constant surveillance is still necessary. Screening of relatives is essential from the age of 12 years and if polyps are found proctocolectomy is performed at 20 years of age.

Gardner's syndrome is a variant of this condition. In addition to adenomatosis there are mesodermal tumours (e.g. dermoid tumours, osteomas of the skull).

Colorectal carcinoma

Adenocarcinoma of the colon is the second commonest tumour in the UK. The incidence increases with age, the average age at diagnosis being 60–65 years. The disease is rare in Africa and Asia and this is thought to be largely environmental rather than racial. There is a correlation between the consumption of meat and animal fat and colonic cancer. Western diets are low in fibre and the resulting intestinal stasis increases the time for which any potential carcinogen is in contact with the bowel wall. The bacterial flora in the colon is also affected by different diets, particularly in amount of fibre present, and recent speculation is that certain bacteria convert bile acids to potential carcinogens. Ulcerative colitis (see p. 190) and familial polyposis are predisposing factors.

PATHOLOGY

Two-thirds of carcinomas occur in the rectosigmoid area. The tumour, which is usually a polypoid mass with ulceration, spreads by direct infiltration through the bowel wall. It then invades the lymphatics and blood vessels with early spread to the liver. Widespread metastases, e.g. to the lung, can occur.

CLINICAL FEATURES

Alteration in bowel habit, with or without abdominal pain, is a common symptom of left-sided colonic lesions. Rectum and sigmoid carcinomas usually bleed, blood being mixed in with the stool. Carcinoma of the caecum may become large and still remain asymptomatic. It can present simply as an iron-deficiency anaemia.

Any change in bowel habit or bleeding per rectum must be investigated, particularly in the older age group.

Clinical examination is usually unhelpful, but a mass may be palpable. With liver metastases, hepatomegaly is found. Digital examination of the rectum is essential and sigmoidoscopy should be performed in all cases.

INVESTIGATION

Double-contrast barium enema is still the investigation of choice, but good preparation to ensure that the colon is free of faeces is essential. Colonoscopy is used for confirmation of doubtful lesions and to obtain specimens for histological examination.

Occult blood tests have been used for mass screening but are of no value in hospital practice (see p. 170).

TREATMENT

This is surgical, with resection and end-to-end anastomosis if possible. Anastomosis is now possible with all but the most distal rectal carcinomas, when colostomy is necessary. The 5-year survival rate is 50% overall, but in tumours confined to the mucosa (i.e. Dukes grade A classification) the survival is over 95%.

Chemotherapy is sometimes used when metastases are present, but results are poor.

ENDOCRINE TUMOURS

Most tumours arise in the pancreas from APUD (*a*mine *p*recursor *u*ptake and *d*ecarboxylation) cells and are sometimes called apudomas.

Pancreatic endocrine tumours can occur in association with other endocrine tumours, particularly parathyroid adenoma and pituitary adenoma, as part of multiple endocrine adenomatosis (see p. 742).

Endocrine tumours predominantly secrete one hormone which produces its clinical effect, but other hormones are often synthesized and can be detected either in the blood or in the resected tumour.

Gastrinoma (Zollinger–Ellison syndrome)

These tumours mainly arise from G cells in the pancreas and secrete large amounts of gastrin. This stimulates maximal gastric acid secretion, so that the main clinical problem is peptic ulceration. Peptic ulcers occur in the usual areas of the stomach and duodenum and also in the jejunum. The ulcers are often large and deep and sometimes multiple. Haemorrhage and perforation can occur, particularly immediately after surgery has been performed for an apparently straightforward duodenal ulcer.

Diarrhoea due to the low pH in the upper intestine is also a common feature. Jejunal mucosal abnormalities are also seen. A high serum gastrin confirms the diagnosis. Acid studies show high acid output.

Treatment has been revolutionized since the introduction of H_2-receptor antagonists. These are now given in high doses to reduce acid output. A new drug, omeprazole, which inhibits the H^+–K^+ proton pump necessary for acid secretion, has recently been introduced. Surgery is reserved for removal of the primary tumour only. This may be demonstrated by scans or local venous sampling for gastrin. These tumours are malignant but grow slowly.

Carcinoid tumours

These originate from the argentaffin cells of the intestine. They make up 10% of all small bowel neoplasms, the commonest sites being in the appendix, terminal ileum and the rectum. It is often difficult to be certain histologically whether a particular tumour is benign or malignant. Clinically most carcinoid tumours are asymptomatic until metastases are present. Ten per cent of carcinoid tumours in the appendix present as acute appendicitis, the inflammation being secondary to obstruction.

Carcinoid syndrome

This syndrome occurs in only 5% of patients with carcinoid tumours and only when there are liver metastases. Patients complain of spontaneous or induced bluish red flushing, predominantly on the face and neck. This can lead to permanent changes with telangiectasis. Gastrointestinal symptoms consist of abdominal pain and recurrent watery diarrhoea. Cardiac abnormalities are found in 50% of patients and consist of pulmonary stenosis or tricuspid incompetence.

Examination of the abdomen reveals hepatomegaly, and ultrasound examination confirms the presence of secondary deposits.

Biochemical abnormalities. Some of the features of the carcinoid syndrome are partly due to the tumour producing serotonin (5-hydroxytryptamine; 5HT). Its breakdown product 5-hydroxyindole-acetic acid is readily measured in the urine.

The diarrhoea and cardiac complications are probably caused by this agent, but the cutaneous flushing is thought to be produced by one of the kinins such as bradykinin which is known to cause vasodilatation, bronchospasm and increased intestinal motility. Phenoxybenzamine, an alpha receptor antagonist, reduces flushing.

Surgery is the best treatment for localized carcinoid tumours and can be used for liver involvement to reduce the bulk of tumour and symptoms. Selective embolization of hepatic metastases via the hepatic artery can be used, but may be accompanied by massive liver necrosis and release of 5HT. The serotonin antagonist cyproheptadine 4 mg four times daily helps with the diarrhoea. Parachlorophenylalanine, an inhibitor of tryptophan 5-hydroxylase, also helps the diarrhoea in some patients. Chemotherapy is also used for symptomatic treatment of the carcinoid syndrome. Most patients survive for 5–10 years after diagnosis.

Other endocrine tumours

Vipomas. These rare pancreatic tumours produce severe intestinal secretion and watery diarrhoea leading to dehydration. Vasoactive intestinal peptide (VIP) is a neurotransmitter which stimulates adenyl cyclase to produce intestinal secretion. Plasma concentrations of VIP are very high and are diagnostic. Levels of pancreatic polypeptide (PP) hormone are also raised. The role of peptide histidine isoleucine (PHI), levels of which are also raised in this condition, is uncertain but this hormone may be involved in secretion.

Corticosteroids help reduce the stool volume, but an attempt should be made to localize the tumour and, if possible, it should be resected.

Glucagonomas. These are alpha-cell tumours of the pancreas which produce pancreatic glucagon. The patients have diabetes mellitus and a unique characteristic necrolytic migratory erythematous rash. The diagnosis is made by measuring pancreatic glucagon in the serum.

Enteroglucagonoma. A tumour originating in the right kidney has been described which produces marked hypertrophy of the villi in the jejunum.

Somatostatinomas. These have also been described; they produce diabetes, steatorrhoea and weight loss.

Medullary carcinoma of the thyroid. This tumour secretes calcitonin (see p. 718) and is a rare cause of diarrhoea.

Islet cell tumours. These are described on p. 768.

Further reading

Booth CC & Neale GR (1985) *Disorders of the Small Intestine.* Oxford: Blackwell Scientific.

Bouchier IAD, Allan RN, Hodgson HJF & Keighley MRB (1984) *Textbook of Gastroenterology.* London: Baillière Tindall.

Clinics in Gastroenterology—a series published by WB Saunders, London.

Cotton PB & Williams CB (1980) *Practical Gastrointestinal Endoscopy.* Oxford: Blackwell Scientific.

Johnson LR (ed.) (1981) *Physiology of the Gastrointestinal Tract*, Vols 1 and 2. New York: Raven Press.

Kirshner JB & Shorter RG (eds) (1980) *Inflammatory Bowel Disease.* Philadelphia: Lea & Febiger.

Morson BC & Dawson IMP (1979) *Gastrointestinal Pathology.* Oxford: Blackwell Scientific.

Sleisenger MH & Fordtran JS (1983) *Gastrointestinal Disease: Pathophysiology, Diagnosis, Management*, 3rd edn. Philadelphia: WB Saunders.

5

Liver, Biliary Tract and Pancreatic Diseases

Introduction

In the Western World, alcohol is the major cause of liver disease, whilst elsewhere the hepatitis B virus is still the most significant factor. Vaccines against hepatitis B viruses have been developed and hold a promise for possible eradication of this disease. Health education and the improvement of social conditions should also help stop the spread of other viral infections.

New imaging techniques such as ultrasound, CT scanning and endoscopic retrograde cannulation of the biliary tree enable the liver and biliary tree to be visualized with precision, resulting in earlier diagnosis and the avoidance of exploratory laparotomy.

Results of liver transplantation continue to improve and may in the future be of value, albeit limited, in the treatment of liver problems.

The liver and biliary tract

Structure

Liver

The liver, the largest organ in the body, is situated in the right hypochondrium. Its upper border lies between the fifth and sixth ribs and its lower border can sometimes be palpated below the right costal margin on inspiration. The liver is divided into two main lobes—right and left. The right is larger and also contains the quadrate and caudate lobes. Riedel's lobe is an extension of the lateral portion of the right lobe and it can occasionally be felt in a normal abdomen.

The blood supply to the liver is via two main vessels:
- The hepatic artery, which is a branch of the coeliac axis and supplies 25% of the total blood flow

- The portal vein, which drains the gastrointestinal tract and the spleen

Both vessels enter the liver at the porta hepatis and the blood is distributed via the portal tracts into the sinusoids throughout the liver. Fifty per cent of the total oxygen supply is via the portal venous system.

Each liver lobe is divided into polyhedral lobules containing a central vein and peripheral portal tracts (see Fig. 5.1). The hepatic artery and portal vein, which lie in the portal tracts, pass blood to the central vein via the sinusoids. These sinusoids are lined by endothelial cells, Kupffer's cells (phagocytic cells) and fat storage cells and are separated by plates of liver cells (hepatocytes). The space that lies between the sinusoids and hepatocytes (space of Disse) contains fluid which drains to the lymphatics in the portal tracts.

Biliary system

Bile canaliculi form a network between the hepatocytes. These join at the periphery of the hepatic lobules to form thin intralobular bile ductules, which

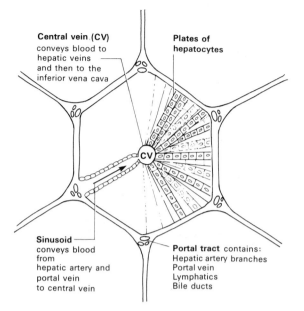

Central vein (CV) conveys blood to hepatic veins and then to the inferior vena cava

Plates of hepatocytes

Sinusoid conveys blood from hepatic artery and portal vein to central vein

Portal tract contains: Hepatic artery branches Portal vein Lymphatics Bile ducts

Fig. 5.1 Diagram of a liver lobule.

in turn enter the interlobular bile ductules in the portal tracts. These then combine to form the right and left hepatic ducts, which leave each liver lobe. The hepatic ducts join at the porta hepatis to form the common hepatic duct. The cystic duct connects the gallbladder to the lower end of the common hepatic duct. The gallbladder lies under the right lobe of the liver and stores and concentrates hepatic bile; it has a capacity of approximately 50 ml. The common bile duct is formed by the combination of the cystic and hepatic ducts and is approximately 8 mm wide, narrowing at its distal end to pass into the duodenum. The common bile duct and pancreatic duct open into the second part of the duodenum through a common channel at the ampulla of Vater. The lower end of the common bile duct contains the muscular sphincter of Oddi, which contracts rhythmically and prevents bile entering the duodenum in the fasting state.

Functions of the liver

Protein metabolism

Synthesis
The liver is the principal site of synthesis of all circulating proteins apart from gamma globulins, which are produced in the reticuloendothelial system. Plasma contains 60–80 g·l^{-1} of protein, mainly in the form of albumin, globulin and fibrinogen.

Albumin has a half-life of 16–24 days and 10–12 g are synthesized daily. Its main functions are first to maintain the intravascular oncotic (colloid osmotic) pressure, and second to transport water-insoluble substances, e.g. bilirubin, hormones, fatty acids and drugs. Reduced synthesis of albumin over prolonged periods produces hypoalbuminaemia and is seen in chronic liver disease and malnutrition. Hypoalbuminaemia is also found in hypercatabolic states, e.g. trauma with sepsis, and with excessive loss, e.g. nephrotic syndrome, protein-losing enteropathy.

Transport or carrier proteins such as transferrin and caeruloplasmin, and other proteins, e.g. alpha-1-antitrypsin and alpha-fetoprotein, are also produced in the liver.

The liver also synthesizes all coagulation factors (see Chapter 6) apart from factor VIII, i.e. fibrinogen, prothrombin, factors V, VII, IX, X, XIII, and components of the complement system. Most factor VIII is produced in the reticuloendothelial system.

Degradation (nitrogen excretion)
Amino acids, the products of protein absorption, are degraded by transamination and oxidative deamination to produce ammonia, which is then converted to urea in the Krebs cycle and excreted by the kidneys. This is a major pathway for the elimination of nitrogenous waste. Failure of this process occurs in severe liver disease.

Carbohydrate metabolism

Glucose homeostasis and the maintenance of the blood sugar is an important function of the liver. It stores approximately 80 g of glycogen. In the fasting state, blood glucose is maintained either by glucose released from the breakdown of glycogen (glycogenolysis) or by newly synthesized glucose (gluconeogenesis). Sources for gluconeogenesis are lactate, pyruvate, amino acids from muscles (mainly alanine and glutamine), and glycerol from lipolysis of fat stores. In prolonged starvation, ketone bodies and fatty acids are used as alternative sources of fuel and the body tissues adapt to a lower glucose requirement (see Chapter 3).

Lipid metabolism

Fats are insoluble in water and are transported in the plasma as protein/lipid complexes (lipoproteins). These are discussed in detail on p. 770.

The liver plays a major role in the metabolism of lipoproteins. It synthesizes very low density lipoproteins (VLDLs) and high density lipoproteins (HDLs). HDLs are the substrate for lecithin–cholesterol acyltransferase (LCAT), which catalyses the conversion of free cholesterol to cholesterol ester (see below). Hepatic lipase catabolizes chylomicrons and VLDLs and is also involved in the metabolism of

HDL phospholipid and triglycerides. The liver and kidney are the major sites of HDL catabolism. Low-density lipoproteins (LDLs) are degraded by the liver after uptake by specific cell surface receptors.

Triglycerides may be of dietary origin, but are also formed in the liver from circulating free fatty acids and glycerol and incorporated into VLDLs. Cholesterol may also be of dietary origin, but most is synthesized from acetyl-CoA mainly in the liver, intestine, adrenal cortex and skin. It occurs either as free cholesterol or esterified with fatty acids, this reaction being catalysed by LCAT. This enzyme is reduced in severe liver disease, increasing the free cholesterol to ester ratio, which alters membrane structures. One result of this is the red cell abnormalities, e.g. burr cells, seen in chronic liver disease. Phospholipids, e.g. lecithin, are also synthesized in the liver.

The complex interrelationships between protein, carbohydrate and fat metabolism are shown in Fig. 5.2.

Bile acid metabolism

Bile acids are synthesized in hepatocytes from cholesterol. The rate-limiting step in their production is that catalysed by cholesterol–7α–hydroxylase. They are excreted into the bile and then pass into the duodenum. The two primary bile acids—cholic acid and chenodeoxycholic acid (see Fig. 5.3)—are conju-gated with glycine or taurine (in a ratio of 3:1 in man) and this process increases their solubility. Intestinal bacteria convert these acids into secondary bile acids—deoxycholic acid and lithocholic acid. Approximately 95% of the bile acids are reabsorbed in the terminal ileum, pass back to the liver in the portal blood, and are re-excreted into the bile (the enterohepatic circulation) (Fig. 5.4). As the bile acid pool is relatively small (3–5 g) and up to 40 g are excreted daily into the bile, the entire bile pool recycles through the enterohepatic circulation six to eight times a day. Approximately 10–20% of the pool is lost daily and synthesis of new bile acids only compensates for this loss.

Bile acids act as detergents; their main function is lipid solubilization. Bile acid molecules contain both a hydrophilic and a hydrophobic end. In aqueous solutions they aggregate to form micelles, with their hydrophobic (lipid-soluble) ends in the centre. Lipid, chiefly cholesterol, is taken up within these micelles to form mixed micelles. Bile acids also solubilize dietary fat in the intestinal lumen in a similar manner.

Bilirubin metabolism

Bilirubin is produced mainly from the breakdown of mature red cells in the Kupffer's cells of the liver and in the reticuloendothelial system. Fifteen per cent of bilirubin comes from the catabolism of other haem-

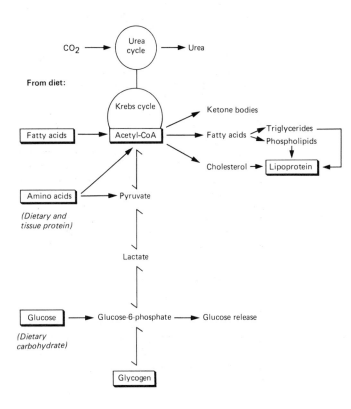

Fig. 5.2 Interrelationships of protein, carbohydrate and lipid metabolism in the liver.

Fig. 5.3 Primary and secondary bile acids. All bile acids are normally conjugated with glycine or taurine.

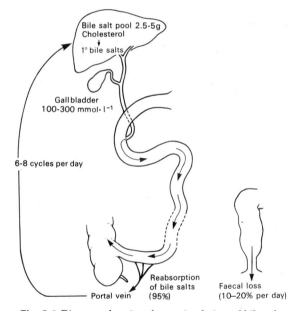

Fig. 5.4 Diagram showing the re-circulation of bile salts.

and Z proteins, carry the bilirubin to the endoplasmic reticulum of hepatocytes, where it is conjugated with glucuronic acid and excreted into bile. The microsomal enzyme uridine diphosphoglucuronyl transferase catalyses the formation of bilirubin mono- and then di-glucuronide. This conjugated bilirubin is water soluble and is actively secreted into the bile canaliculi and excreted into the intestine with the bile. It is not absorbed from the small intestine because of its large molecular size. In the terminal ileum, bacterial enzymes hydrolyse the molecule, releasing free bilirubin, which is then reduced to urobilinogen. Some of this is excreted in the stools as stercobilinogen. The remainder is absorbed by the terminal ileum, passes to the liver via the enterohepatic circulation, and is re-excreted into the bile. Urobilinogen bound to albumin enters the circulation and is excreted in the urine via the kidneys. When hepatic excretion of conjugated bilirubin is impaired, a small amount of conjugated bilirubin is found strongly bound to serum albumin. It is not excreted by the kidney and accounts for the continuing hyperbilirubinaemia for a short time after cholestasis has resolved.

Hormone and drug inactivation

The liver catabolizes hormones such as insulin, glucagon, oestrogens, growth hormone, glucocorticoids and parathormone. It is the most important site for the metabolism of drugs (see p. 246) and alcohol (see p. 241). Fat-soluble drugs are converted to water-soluble substances, which facilitates their excretion in the bile or urine.

containing proteins such as myoglobin, cytochromes and catalases.

Normally, 250–300 mg of bilirubin are produced daily. The iron and globin are removed from the haem and are re-utilized. Biliverdin is formed from the haem and this is reduced to form bilirubin. The bilirubin produced is unconjugated and water insoluble, and is transported to the liver attached to albumin. In the liver, transporter substances, the Y

Immunological function

The reticuloendothelial system of the liver contains many immunologically active cells such as the phagocytic Kupffer's cells and also a little lymphoid tissue in the portal tracts. The liver acts as a 'sieve' for the bacterial and other antigens carried to it via the portal tract from the gastrointestinal tract. These antigens appear to be phagocytosed and degraded without the production of antibody. This process does not allow the antigens to reach other antibody-producing sites in the body and thereby prevents adverse immunological reactions. The reticuloendothelial system is also thought to play a role in tissue repair, T and B cell interaction, and cytotoxic activity in disease processes.

Investigation

Investigative tests can be divided into:
- Tests to assess liver function
- Imaging techniques to define gross anatomy
- Liver biopsy for histology
- Other tests, e.g. haematological

Liver function tests

Most liver function tests are markers of liver disease and not actual tests of 'function' per se. These tests are usually abnormal in hepatobiliary disease, but normal values do not necessarily exclude severe disease. Recognized patterns of test abnormalities may occur in some diseases, but considerable overlap occurs.

Routine tests

A routine blood sample sent to the laboratory for liver function tests will be processed by an automated multichannel analyser to produce serum levels of bilirubin, aminotransferases, alkaline phosphatase, gamma glutamyl transferase and serum proteins. Subsequent investigations are often based on these tests.

Bilirubin. In the serum, bilirubin is normally almost all unconjugated. Increased serum bilirubin is usually accompanied by other abnormalities of liver function. Determination of whether the bilirubin is conjugated or unconjugated is only necessary in congenital disorders of bilirubin metabolism (see below) or to exclude haemolysis.

Aminotransferases. These enzymes (often referred to as transaminases) are present in hepatocytes and leak into the blood with liver cell damage. The two enzymes measured are:

- *Aspartate aminotransferase* (AST), which was previously known as serum glutamic oxaloacetic transaminase (SGOT). This is a mitochondrial enzyme and is also present in heart, muscle, kidney and brain. High levels are seen in hepatic necrosis, cardiac infarction, muscle injury and congestive cardiac failure.
- *Alanine aminotransferase* (ALT), which was previously known as serum glutamic pyruvic transaminase (SGPT). This is a cytosol enzyme and is more specific for the liver than AST.

Alkaline phosphatase (AP). This is present in the canalicular and sinusoidal membranes of the liver, but is also present in many other tissues, e.g. bone, intestine and placenta. If necessary, its origin can be determined by electrophoretic separation of isoenzymes or, alternatively, if there is also an abnormality of, for example, gamma glutamyl transferase, the alkaline phosphatase can be presumed to come from the liver.

Serum alkaline phosphatase is raised in cholestasis from any cause, whether intra- or extra-hepatic disease. Increased alkaline phosphatase is synthesized and leaks into the blood. In cholestatic jaundice, levels may be up to four to six times the normal limit. Raised levels may also occur in conditions with infiltration of the liver, e.g. metastases, and in cirrhosis, frequently in the absence of jaundice. The highest serum levels due to liver disease (>1000 iu) are seen with hepatic metastases and primary biliary cirrhosis.

Gamma glutamyl transferase (γ-GT). This is a microsomal enzyme. Its activity can be induced by drugs such as phenytoin and by alcohol. If the alkaline phosphatase is normal, a raised γ-GT is a good guide to alcohol intake and can be used as a screening test (see p. 892). Mild elevation of the γ-GT is common even with a small alcohol consumption and does not necessarily indicate liver disease. In cholestasis, the γ-GT rises in parallel with the alkaline phosphatase as it has a similar pathway of excretion.

Serum proteins. Serum albumin is a sensitive marker of synthetic function and is a valuable guide to the severity of chronic liver disease. A falling serum albumin is a bad prognostic sign.

Hyperglobulinaemia occurs in chronic liver disease. This is thought to be due to reduced phagocytosis by sinusoidal and Kupffer's cells of the antigens absorbed from the gut, which then stimulate antibody production in the spleen and lymph nodes. In chronic liver disease, immunoglobulins are formed by lymphoid and plasma cells which infiltrate the portal tracts. The routine plasma electrophoretic strips contain immunoglobulins in the beta and gamma regions. In cirrhosis there is beta–gamma fusion due to an increase in the faster-moving globulins; the diagnostic value of these strips is, however, limited. In primary biliary cirrhosis the predominant serum immunoglobulin raised is IgM, and in autoimmune chronic active hepatitis it is IgG. This latter finding is of help in the diagnosis.

Other liver function tests
5-Nucleotidase (5NT). This enzyme shares the same pathway of excretion as alkaline phosphatase and is therefore mainly of value in deciding whether a raised alkaline phosphatase is due to bone or liver disease, i.e. if the 5NT is also raised, the raised alkaline phosphatase is of liver origin.

Prothrombin time (PT). This is a marker of synthetic function. Because of its short half-life, it is a sensitive indicator of both acute and chronic liver disease. It is important to exclude vitamin K deficiency as the cause of a prolonged PT by giving an intravenous bolus (10 mg) of vitamin K. Vitamin K deficiency commonly occurs in biliary obstruction, as the low intestinal concentration of bile salts results in poor absorption of vitamin K.

Bromsulphalein (BSP) test. This is now very rarely performed. The liver normally clears BSP from the blood. The level of BSP in the blood after an intravenous injection of BSP is a guide to hepatocellular damage. A second recirculation peak occurs in the congenital hyperbilirubinaemia of the Dubin–Johnson syndrome. Anaphylactic reactions may occur.

Alpha-fetoprotein. This is normally produced by the fetal liver. With the more sensitive radioimmunoassay techniques, very low levels can be detected in normal individuals and moderately raised levels in patients with hepatitis or chronic liver disease. Its reappearance in increasing and high concentrations in the adult indicates hepatocellular carcinoma. Increased concentrations in pregnancy in the blood and amniotic fluid suggest neural-tube defects of the fetus. Blood levels are also raised in teratomas.

Immunological tests
There are no specific antibodies to the liver that are routinely measured. Three autoantibodies can, however, be of some help in diagnosing chronic active hepatitis (CAH) and primary biliary cirrhosis (PBC). These antibodies are antinuclear factor (ANF), antimitochondrial antibodies (AMA), and anti-smooth-muscle antibodies (SMA). ANF is present in 80% of patients with CAH not due to viral hepatitis. Ninety-five per cent of patients with PBC have AMA, as opposed to less than 1% of patients with large duct obstruction. ANF and AMA may also occur in other connective tissue and autoimmune disorders.

SMA is an IgM antibody and is present in 70% of patients with hepatitis B surface antigen negative

CAH and 50% with PBC. It is also present in low titre in many liver diseases, including viral hepatitis. Useful tests for certain liver diseases are shown in Table 5.1.

Imaging techniques

The main aim of these investigations is to delineate the anatomy of and to look for any abnormality in the liver or biliary tree.

Plain x-rays of the abdomen
These are used to detect:
- Gallstones (10% contain enough calcium to be seen)
- Air in the biliary tree, usually due to a fistula between the intestine and the gallbladder
- Pancreatic calcification
- Calcification of the gallbladder (porcelain gallbladder)—rare

Ultrasound examination
This non-invasive, safe and relatively cheap technique involves the analysis of the reflected ultrasound beam detected by a probe moved across the abdomen. The normal liver appears as a homogeneous transonic area. The gallbladder, common bile duct, portal vein and other structures in the abdomen can be visualized.

This technique is most valuable in the jaundiced patient. The size of the common bile duct and intrahepatic ducts can be accurately estimated, thereby

Table 5.1 Useful tests for certain liver diseases.

Test	Disease
Antinuclear factor	Chronic active hepatitis Primary biliary cirrhosis (occasionally)
Antimitochondrial antibody	Primary biliary cirrhosis Chronic active hepatitis (occasionally)
Antismooth muscle antibody	Chronic active hepatitis Primary biliary cirrhosis
Viral markers (IgG and IgM)	Hepatitis A and B
Alpha-fetoprotein	Primary hepatocellular carcinoma
Serum iron, saturated iron binding capacity, ferritin	Haemochromatosis
Serum and urinary copper, serum caeruloplasmin	Wilson's disease
Alpha-1-antitrypsin	Cirrhosis (±emphysema)

distinguishing extrahepatic biliary obstruction from other, intrahepatic causes of jaundice. Gallstones can be detected in the gallbladder with 95% accuracy (Fig. 5.5), but may be missed in the common bile duct. The size and patency of the portal and hepatic veins can be assessed. Changes in liver architecture, e.g. cirrhosis, can be detected, as well as space-occupying lesions of more than 1 cm in diameter. Other abdominal masses can be delineated, and biopsies can be obtained under ultrasonic control.

Computed tomography (CT)

This technique is extremely useful in detecting the site of abdominal masses. Pancreatic disease, enlargement of regional lymph nodes, and lesions in the porta hepatis can be visualized. Abnormalities of size and shape as well as focal lesions of the liver can be detected. CT can detect calcification not seen on plain x-rays. It is not as good as ultrasound for biliary tract disease, but has advantages in obese subjects and in detecting ascites. As with ultrasound, biopsies can be taken under CT control.

Cholecystogram

This is still the most frequent investigation used to outline the gallbladder in the uncomplicated case, although it is being replaced by ultrasound in many centres. Tablets of iopanoic acid are taken the night before the x-ray. This is absorbed from the gut, conjugated in the liver, secreted in bile, and concentrated in the gallbladder, which opacifies homogeneously. Radiolucent gallstones are shown in Fig. 5.6. A fatty meal is given, which makes the gallbladder contract. The bile ducts can be outlined on some occasions.

The gallbladder is frequently not visualized with this technique due to disease, a blocked cystic duct, or because the contrast medium has not been absorbed. The dye is excreted by the liver via the same mechanism as bilirubin, so that non-visualiza-

Liver

Hepatic duct

Portal vein

Acoustic shadowing

Gallbladder with wall of normal thickness

Collection of small gallstones

Fig. 5.5 An ultrasound showing a gallstone.

Fig. 5.6 Cholecystogram showing gallstones.

tion will also occur in the jaundiced patient and in the patient with liver disease. A cholecystogram should not be performed in these situations. If non-visualization occurs, this test can be repeated after some days using a double dose of iopanoic acid, but it is now more usual to do an ultrasound examination.

Intravenous cholangiography

This technique is being replaced by ultrasound and endoscopic retrograde cholangiopancreatography (ERCP). It was particularly useful in patients after cholecystectomy to visualize the biliary duct. The contrast medium meglumine ioglycamate given intravenously is secreted by the liver into the biliary tree. It will not be excreted in the presence of jaundice or liver disease.

Scintiscanning

Technetium-99m (^{99m}Tc) colloid scan. This colloid, when injected intravenously, is taken up by the reticuloendothelial cells of the liver and spleen. It can show space-occupying lesions, and a generalized

decrease in uptake is found in parenchymal disease of the liver.

Since the introduction of ultrasound this technique has been used less frequently. Currently its main uses are in:

- Advanced cirrhosis, in which there is poor uptake in the liver and most of the colloid is taken up in the spleen and bone marrow
- Alcoholic hepatitis, in which there is virtually no uptake in the liver owing to Kupffer's cell damage by alcohol

^{99m}Tc-HIDA scan. ^{99m}Tc-HIDA (an imino-diacetic acid derivative) is taken up by the hepatocytes and excreted rapidly into the biliary system. Its main uses are in the diagnosis of:

- Acute cholecystitis
- Hepatitis due to biliary atresia in the neonatal period

Gallium-67 (^{67}Ga) scan. This agent is concentrated in areas of inflammation and can be used in the detection of abscesses.

Endoscopic retrograde cholangiopancreatography (ERCP)

This technique is used to outline the biliary and pancreatic ducts, particularly in the presence of jaundice (see p. 223). It involves the passage of an endoscope into the second part of the duodenum and cannulation of the ampulla. Contrast is injected into both systems and the patient is screened radiologically. Contrast medium with a low iodine content of 1.5 mg·ml^{-1} is used for the common bile duct, so that gallstones are not obscured; a higher iodine content of 2.8 mg·ml^{-1} is used for the pancreatic duct. In addition, other diagnostic and therapeutic procedures can be carried out:

- Removal of common bile duct stones after a diathermy cut to the sphincter has been performed to facilitate their withdrawal
- Obtaining samples for cytology, in particular for pancreatic malignancy
- Draining the biliary system by passing a tube (stent) through an obstruction

Complications include cholangitis, and broad-spectrum prophylactic antibiotics should be given to all patients with suspected obstruction. Pancreatitis can occur and ERCP is usually not performed if a pseudocyst of the pancreas is suspected.

Percutaneous transhepatic cholangiography (PTC)

Under a local anaesthetic a fine, flexible needle is passed into the liver. Contrast is injected slowly until a biliary radicle is identified and then further contrast is injected to outline the whole of the biliary tree. The main use of PTC is in jaundiced patients who have been shown to have dilated intrahepatic ducts demonstrated on ultrasound. Here it is almost always successful and can delineate the cause of the obstruction. Antibiotic cover should be given to avoid cholangitis. This technique is often a prelude to surgery, but if the lesion is likely to be malignant, a tube can be passed through the lesion to bypass the obstruction. Contraindications are as for liver biopsy (see below). The main complications are bleeding and cholangitis with septicaemia.

Angiography

This can be performed by selective catheterization of the coeliac axis and hepatic artery, and is useful for detecting the abnormal vasculature of hepatic tumours. The portal vein can be demonstrated with increased definition using subtraction techniques and spleno-portography (by direct splenic puncture) is now rarely performed. In a recently developed technique called digital vascular imaging (DVI), contrast given intravenously or intra-arterially can be detected in the portal system using computerized subtraction analysis. Attempted visualization of the hepatic veins by venography is particularly important in the diagnosis of the Budd–Chiari syndrome. Hepatic venous cannulation also allows an indirect measurement of portal pressure to be made, although this has seldom been shown to be of any diagnostic or therapeutic value.

Magnetic resonance imaging

This technique is being used for the detection of liver masses. It involves the imaging of the magnetic spin of protons (H^+) of different tissues.

Liver biopsy

This is the only means by which a diagnosis of intrinsic liver disease can be confirmed. It is a simple, relatively safe procedure which can be performed either on a day-case or overnight-stay basis. The indications and contraindications are shown in Table 5.2. There are many contraindications, and a biopsy should not be undertaken lightly. The mortality rate is less than 0.02%.

Needle biopsy of the liver

This should only be performed by experienced doctors and with sterile precautions.

- The patient's coagulation status (prothrombin time, platelets) is checked.
- The patient's blood group is checked and serum saved for cross-matching.
- The patient lies on his back at the edge of the bed.
- The liver margins are delineated using percussion.
- Local anaesthetic is injected at the point of maximum dullness in the mid-axillary line through the intercostal space during expiration. Anaesthetic (1% lignocaine, approximately 5 ml) should be injected down to the liver capsule.
- A tiny cut is made in the skin with a scalpel blade.
- A special needle (Menghini, Trucut or Surecut) is used to obtain the liver biopsy whilst the patient holds his breath in expiration.
- The biopsy is laid on filter paper and placed in 10% formalin. If a culture of the biopsy is required it should be placed in a sterile pot.
- The patient should be observed, with pulse and blood pressure measurements taken regularly for 6 h.

Table 5.2 Indications and contraindications for liver biopsy.

Indications
Liver disease
Unexplained hepatomegaly
Some cases of jaundice (see p. 223)
Persistently abnormal liver function tests
Occasionally in acute hepatitis (see p. 225)
Cirrhosis
Drug-related liver disease
Infiltrations
Tumours—primary or secondary
Systemic disease
Screening relatives of patients with certain diseases,
e.g. haemochromatosis
Pyrexia of unknown origin
Usual contraindications to needle biopsy
Uncooperative patient
Prolonged prothrombin time (more than 3 s)
Platelets $<80 \times 10^9/l$
Ascites
Obstructive jaundice

Liver biopsy is sometimes performed during laparoscopy under local or general anaesthesia through a small incision in the abdominal wall. This procedure has the advantage that the whole peritoneum can be inspected after CO_2 insufflation (pneumoperitoneum). Biopsies can be taken from diseased peritoneal areas as well as from the liver.

Biopsies can also be performed via the inferior vena cava using the transjugular route in patients with a prolonged prothrombin time.

Complications

These are usually minor and include abdominal or shoulder pain which settles with analgesics. Minor intraperitoneal bleeding is common but this settles spontaneously. Rare complications include major intraperitoneal bleeding, pleurisy and perihepatitis, biliary peritonitis, haemobilia and transient septicaemia. Haemobilia produces biliary colic, jaundice and melaena within three days of the biopsy.

Haematological tests

Anaemia may be present. The red cells are often macrocytic and can have abnormal shapes—target cells and spur cells—due to membrane abnormalities. Vitamin B_{12} levels are normal or high, and folate levels are often low due to poor dietary intake.

- Bleeding produces a hypochromic, microcytic picture.
- Alcohol causes macrocytosis, sometimes with leucopenia and thrombocytopenia.
- Hypersplenism results in pancytopenia.
- Cholestasis can often produce abnormal-shaped cells and also deficiency of vitamin K.
- Haemolysis accompanies acute liver failure and jaundice.

Symptoms of liver disease

Acute liver disease

Acute liver disease may be asymptomatic and anicteric. For example, an abnormality such as raised aminotransferases may be found during a routine biochemical screen.

Symptomatic acute liver disease, which is often viral, produces generalized symptoms of malaise, anorexia and fever. Jaundice may appear as the illness progresses.

Chronic liver disease

Patients may be asymptomatic or complain of non-specific symptoms. Specific symptoms include:
- Abdominal distension due to ascites, ankle swelling and fluid retention
- Haematemesis and melaena from gastrointestinal haemorrhage
- Pruritus due to cholestasis; this is often an early symptom of primary biliary cirrhosis
- Breast swelling, loss of libido and amenorrhoea due to endocrine dysfunction
- Confusion and drowsiness due to neuro-psychiatric complications

Signs of liver disease

Acute liver disease

There may be few signs apart from jaundice and an enlarged liver. Jaundice is a yellow coloration of the skin and mucous membranes and is best seen in the conjunctivae. In the cholestatic phase of the illness, pale stools and dark urine are seen. Spider naevi and liver palms usually indicate chronic disease but they can occur in severe acute disease.

Chronic liver disease

The possible physical signs are shown in Fig. 5.7. However, it is possible for the physical examination to be normal in patients with chronic liver disease.

Common signs
The skin. The chest and upper body may show spider naevi. These are telangiectases which consist of a central arteriole with radiating small vessels. They are found in the distribution of the superior vena cava, i.e. above the nipple line. They are also found in pregnancy. In haemochromatosis the skin may have a slate-grey appearance.

The hands may show palmar erythema, which is a non-specific change indicative of a hyperdynamic circulation; it may also be seen in pregnancy, thyrotoxicosis or rheumatoid arthritis. Clubbing occasionally occurs, and a Dupuytren's contracture is often seen in alcoholic cirrhosis.

Xanthomas (cholesterol deposits) may be seen in the palmar creases or above the eyes in primary biliary cirrhosis.

The abdomen. Initial hepatomegaly will be followed by a small liver in well established cirrhosis.

Splenomegaly is usually taken as an indication of portal hypertension.

The endocrine system. Gynaecomastia (occasionally unilateral) and testicular atrophy may be found in males. The cause of gynaecomastia is complex, but it is probably related to altered oestrogen metabolism or to treatment with spironolactone.

In *decompensated cirrhosis*, additional signs that can be seen are:
- Jaundice
- Ascites with or without peripheral oedema
- Evidence of portosystemic encephalopathy (PSE) (see p. 236), including drowsiness, stupor, fetor hepaticus and a flapping tremor of the outstretched hands
- Collateral veins and veins around the umbilicus (caput medusae) (rare)

Jaundice

Jaundice (icterus) is detectable when the serum bilirubin is greater than 30–60 mmol·l^{-1} (>3 mg·100 ml^{-1}). The usual division of jaundice into pre-

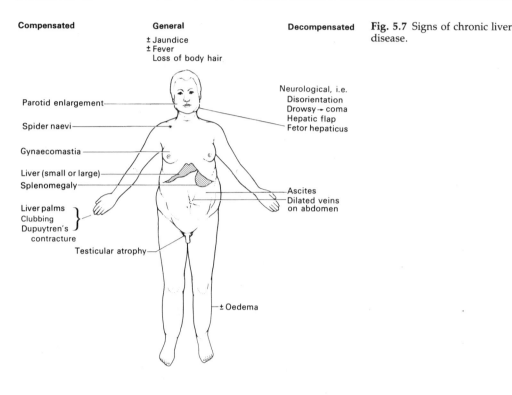

Compensated

General
±Jaundice
±Fever
Loss of body hair

Decompensated

Parotid enlargement

Spider naevi

Gynaecomastia

Liver (small or large)
Splenomegaly

Liver palms ⎫
Clubbing   ⎬
Dupuytren's ⎭
contracture

Testicular atrophy

Neurological, i.e.
Disorientation
Drowsy → coma
Hepatic flap
Fetor hepaticus

Ascites
Dilated veins
on abdomen

±Oedema

Fig. 5.7 Signs of chronic liver disease.

hepatic, hepatocellular and obstructive (cholestatic) is an oversimplification as mixed pictures are often seen; the latter two in particular often occur together. Jaundice will therefore be considered under the following headings:

- Haemolytic jaundice
- Congenital hyperbilirubinaemias
- Cholestatic jaundice, including parenchymal liver disease and large duct obstruction

Haemolytic jaundice

The increased breakdown of red cells (see p. 274) leads to an increase in production of bilirubin. The resulting jaundice is usually mild (serum bilirubin of 68–102 mmol·l^{-1}[4–6 mg·100 ml^{-1}]) as normal liver function can easily handle the increased bilirubin derived from excess haemolysis. Unconjugated bilirubin is not water soluble and therefore will not pass into the urine, hence the term 'acholuric jaundice'. Urinary urobilinogen is increased.

The causes of haemolytic jaundice are those of haemolytic anaemia (see p. 276). The clinical features depend on the cause; anaemia, jaundice, splenomegaly, gallstones and leg ulcers may be seen.

Investigations show features of haemolysis (see p. 276). The level of unconjugated bilirubin is raised, but the serum alkaline phosphatase, protein and albumin are normal. Serum haptoglobins are low.

The differential diagnosis is from other forms of jaundice (see p. 222).

Congenital hyperbilirubinaemias (non-haemolytic)

The commonest is Gilbert's syndrome. The others —Crigler–Najjar, Dubin–Johnson and Rotor syndromes—are rare (see Table 5.3).

Gilbert's syndrome
This is the commonest familial hyperbilirubinaemia and affects 2–5% of the population. It is asymptomatic and is usually detected as an incidental finding of a slightly raised bilirubin (3–5 mg·dl^{-1}; 51–85 mmol·l^{-1}) on a routine check. No signs of liver disease are seen. There is a family history of jaundice in 5–15% of patients. The aetiology of the syndrome is multifactorial, and many abnormalities of bilirubin handling have been demonstrated. It is possible that this condition merely represents one end of the normal distribution curve.

The major importance of establishing this diagnosis is to inform the patient that this is not a serious disease and to prevent unnecessary investigation in the future. Investigations show only a raised unconjugated bilirubin, which rises on fasting and during a mild illness. The reticulocyte count is normal. Rarely a liver biopsy needs to be performed to exclude intrinsic liver disease; this will be normal. No treatment is necessary.

Table 5.3 Congenital hyperbilirubinaemias.

	Inheritance	Age at presentation	Prognosis	Defect	Liver histology	Bile in urine	Other findings	Treatment
Unconjugated bilirubin								
Gilbert's syndrome	Autosomal dominant	Mainly young adult, but can be any	Excellent	↓ Bilirubin uptake ↓ Glucuronyl transferase ↓ Red cell survival	Normal	No	—	None
Crigler–Najjar syndrome								
Type I	Autosomal recessive	Neonate	Fatal (due to kernicterus)	No glucuronyl transferase	Normal	No	—	None
Type II	Autosomal dominant	Neonate	Survive to adult life	↓ Glucuronyl transferase	Normal	No	—	Phenobarbitone if necessary
Conjugated bilirubin								
Dubin–Johnson syndrome	Autosomal recessive	Any	Good	↓ Bilirubin excretion	Melanin deposition	Yes	Non-filling gallbladder. BSP test shows secondary rise at 2h	None
Rotor syndrome	? Autosomal dominant	Variable (usually childhood)	Good	↓ Bilirubin uptake ↓ Storage of bilirubin	Normal	Yes	Non-filling gallbladder. BSP test abnormal at 45 min; no secondary rise	None

Cholestatic jaundice

This can be divided into:
- *Intrahepatic cholestasis*, due to the swelling of hepatocytes and oedema in parenchymal liver damage (hepatocellular) or to an excretory dysfunction of the bile canaliculi at a cellular level
- *Extrahepatic cholestasis*, due to large duct obstruction of bile flow at any point in the biliary tract distal to the bile canaliculi

The causes are shown in Table 5.4.

Clinically there is jaundice with pale stools and dark urine. The bilirubin in the serum is conjugated.

Intrahepatic and extrahepatic cholestatic jaundice must be differentiated, as their clinical management is entirely different.

THE DIFFERENTIAL DIAGNOSIS OF JAUNDICE

HISTORY

A careful history may give a clue to the diagnosis. Patients should be asked a series of questions, keeping in mind that certain causes of jaundice are more likely in particular categories of people. A young person is more likely to have hepatitis and therefore questions about drug and alcohol abuse and homosexuality are important. An elderly person with gross weight loss is more likely to have a carcinoma.

All patients may complain of malaise, but abdominal pain only occurs in biliary obstruction with gallstones or sometimes with an enlarged liver, when the pain is due to distension of the capsule.

The following aspects of the history should be covered; questions should be appropriate to the particular situation:

- *Duration of illness*—a history of jaundice with prolonged weight loss in an older patient suggests

malignancy; a short history, particularly with a prodromal illness of malaise, suggests a hepatitis
- *Recent contact with jaundice*—suggests hepatitis A
- *Drug addiction, homosexuality, injections and transfusions*—all increase the chances of hepatitis B
- *Alcohol consumption*—a careful history of drinking habits is important, although many patients often lie about the actual amount they drink
- *Drugs taken*, particularly in the last 2–3 months —many drugs cause jaundice (see p. 248)
- *Travel abroad* to areas with increased hepatitis risks
- *Recent anaesthetics*—e.g. halothane may cause jaundice
- *Family history*—patients with, for example, Gilbert's disease may have family members who get recurrent jaundice
- *Recent surgery* on the biliary tract or for carcinoma
- *Occupation*—farm and sewage workers used to be at risk for leptospirosis, but this is now rare
- *Fevers or rigors*—suggestive of cholangitis or possibly a liver abscess

CLINICAL EXAMINATION

The signs of acute and chronic liver disease should be looked for (see p. 219). Certain additional signs may be useful:
- *Hepatomegaly*—a smooth tender liver is seen in hepatitis and with extrahepatic obstruction, but a knobbly irregular liver suggests metastases. Causes of hepatomegaly are shown in Table 5.5.

Table 5.5 Causes of hepatomegaly.

'Apparent'
Low-lying diaphragm
Reidel's lobe
Cirrhosis—early
Inflammation
Hepatitis
Schistosomiasis
Abscesses—pyogenic or amoebic
Cysts
Hydatid
Polycystic
Metabolic
Fatty liver
Amyloid
Glycogen storage disease
Haematological
Leukaemias
Lymphoma
Myeloproliferative disorders
Tumours—primary and secondary carcinoma
Venous congestion
Heart failure
Hepatic vein occlusion
Biliary obstruction—particularly extrahepatic

Table 5.4 Causes of cholestatic jaundice.

Extrahepatic
Common duct stones
Carcinoma
Head of pancreas
Ampulla
Bile duct
Biliary stricture
Pancreatitis ± pseudocyst
Sclerosing cholangitis
Intrahepatic
Viral hepatitis
Drugs
Alcoholic hepatitis
Cirrhosis—any type
Pregnancy
Recurrent idiopathic cholestasis
Some congenital disorders

- *Splenomegaly* indicates portal hypertension in patients when signs of chronic liver disease are present. It is also seen occasionally in viral hepatitis.
- *Ascites* is found in cirrhosis, but can also be due to carcinoma (particularly ovarian) and many other causes (see Table 5.12, p. 235).
- *A palpable gallbladder* can suggest a carcinoma of the pancreas obstructing the bile duct.
- *Generalized lymphadenopathy* suggests a lymphoma.

INVESTIGATION

Jaundice is not a diagnosis and the cause should always be sought.

A flow diagram for investigation of jaundice is shown in Fig. 5.8. An ultrasound should always be performed to exclude extrahepatic obstruction (Fig. 5.9) unless the patient is young and there is a clear history of hepatitis.

The blood tests referred to in Fig. 5.8 include:
- *Liver function tests*. In hepatitis the AST tends to be high early in the disease, with only a small rise in the alkaline phosphatase. Conversely, in extra-

Fig. 5.9 Ultrasound. A longitudinal oblique view across the porta hepatis showing a dilated common bile duct (arrow). The tubular structure behind this is the portal vein.

hepatic obstruction the alkaline phosphatase is high, with a smaller rise in AST. These findings cannot however be relied on alone to make a diagnosis in an individual case. The prothrombin time is often prolonged in long-standing liver disease, and the serum albumin is low.
- *Haematological tests*. These are helpful in a haemolytic jaundice. A raised white count may indicate infection, e.g. cholangitis. A leucopenia often occurs in viral hepatitis, while abnormal mononuclear cells suggest infectious mononucleosis or toxoplasmosis; a Monospot test should be performed for the former.
- *Other blood tests*. These include viral studies for hepatitis, e.g. hepatitis A and B, cytomegalovirus, autoimmune antibodies, e.g. ANF, AMA (for primary biliary cirrhosis) and alpha-fetoprotein for a hepatoma.

Acute liver disease

Acute parenchymal liver damage can be caused by many agents (Fig. 5.10). If there is widespread damage of hepatocytes, the normal liver architecture may collapse. The extent of hepatocellular damage may be extremely variable.

Pathology

Histological changes are essentially similar whatever the cause. The hepatocytes become swollen and have a granular appearance. Necrosis is mainly centrilobular. The lobules and portal tracts are infiltrated with mononuclear cells. Centrizonal cholestasis is found, but fatty change is usually

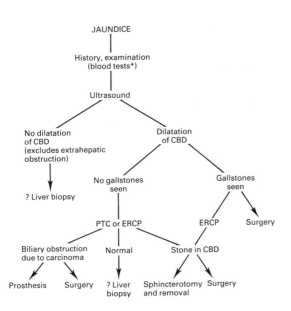

Fig. 5.8 Investigation of jaundice. PTC = percutaneous transhepatic cholangiography; ERCP = endoscopic retrograde cholangiopancreatography; CBD = common bile duct.

The choice between ERCP and PTC often depends on local expertise. ERCP is frequently the first choice as sphincterotomy and stone removal can be performed. In duct obstruction due to, for example, a carcinoma, a prosthesis or stent can be inserted.

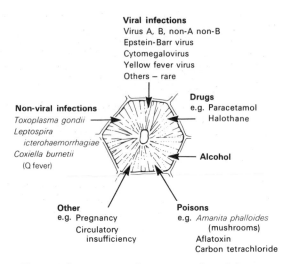

Viral infections
Virus A, B, non-A non-B
Epstein-Barr virus
Cytomegalovirus
Yellow fever virus
Others – rare

Drugs
e.g. Paracetamol
Halothane

Non-viral infections
Toxoplasma gondii
Leptospira
   icterohaemorrhagiae
Coxiella burnetii
   (Q fever)

Alcohol

Other
e.g. Pregnancy
Circulatory
   insufficiency

Poisons
e.g. *Amanita phalloides*
   (mushrooms)
Aflatoxin
Carbon tetrachloride

Fig. 5.10 Some causes of acute parenchymal damage.

absent. Dead hepatocytes become shrunken to form eosinophilic Councilman bodies. With more severe damage the reticulin framework collapses, causing the central veins and portal tracts to become linked ('bridging'). In massive necrosis, as is seen in fulminant hepatic failure, whole lobules are destroyed. In certain types of hepatitis due to toxins such as alcohol or that seen in pregnancy, fatty change may be a feature.

VIRAL HEPATITIS

The differing features of the common forms of viral hepatitis are summarized in Table 5.6.

In hepatitis A the damage is due to the virus itself, but in hepatitis B it is due to an immunological reaction to the virus.

Hepatitis A

EPIDEMIOLOGY

This is the commonest type of viral hepatitis and causes 20–40% of clinically apparent hepatitis. It occurs world-wide, often in epidemics. The disease is commonly seen in the autumn and affects children and young adults. Spread of infection is mainly by the faecal–oral route and arises from the ingestion of contaminated food (e.g. shellfish, clams) or water. Lower socioeconomic classes are affected more frequently, possibly due to overcrowding and poor sanitation. There is no carrier state.

HEPATITIS A VIRUS

Hepatitis A virus (HAV) (Fig. 5.11) is excreted in the faeces of infected persons for about 2 weeks before the onset of the illness and for up to 7 days after. The disease is maximally infectious just before the onset of jaundice. HAV particles can be demonstrated in the blood, but viraemia does not persist beyond the acute phase of the disease. The disease affects other parts of the body as well as the liver, e.g. the heart, pancreas, gastrointestinal tract and spleen.

Table 5.6 Summary of the features of hepatitis A, B and non-A non-B.

	A	B	Non-A non-B
Virus	RNA 27 nm	DNA 42 nm	DNA ? >2 viruses
Spread: Faecal Blood Vertical Saliva Sexual	Yes Rare No Yes Occasionally	No Yes Yes Yes Yes	No Yes Yes ? No ?
Incubation	Short (2–3 weeks)	Long (1–5 months)	Intermediate
Age	Young	Any	Any
Carrier state	No	Yes	Yes
Chronic liver disease	No	Yes	Yes
Liver cancer	No	Yes	? Yes
Mortality (acute)	<0.5%	1–5%	1–3%
Immunization: Passive	Normal immunoglobulin i.m. (0.04–0.06 ml·kg^{-1})	Hyperimmune serum	—
Active	—	Vaccine	—

Fig. 5.11 Schematic diagram of the hepatitis A virus.

CLINICAL FEATURES

The pre-icteric or prodromal phase lasts up to 2 weeks. The viraemia causes the patient to feel unwell, with nausea, vomiting, diarrhoea, anorexia, headaches, malaise and a distaste for cigarettes. Fever is usually mild and there may be upper abdominal discomfort. There are few physical signs at this stage; the liver is tender but not enlarged initially.

After one or two weeks the patient becomes icteric (although some may never do so) and symptoms often improve. The appetite returns and the patient feels better. As the jaundice deepens the urine becomes dark and the stools pale due to intra-hepatic cholestasis. The liver is moderately enlarged and the spleen is palpable in about 10% of patients. Occasionally tender lymphadenopathy is seen, with a transient rash in some cases. Thereafter the jaundice lessens and in the majority of cases the illness is over within 3–6 weeks. Relapses occasionally occur, with the return of jaundice. Rarely the disease may be very severe, with fulminant hepatitis, liver coma and death. The sequence of events after hepatitis A exposure is shown in Fig. 5.12.

INVESTIGATION

Liver function tests
In the prodromal stage the serum bilirubin is usually normal. However, there is bilirubinuria and increased urinary urobilinogen. A raised serum AST,

which can sometimes be very high, precedes the jaundice.

In the icteric stage the serum bilirubin reflects the level of jaundice. Serum AST reaches a maximum 1–2 days after the appearance of jaundice, and may rise above 500 iu·l^{-1}. Serum alkaline phosphatase is usually less than 300 iu·l^{-1}.

After the jaundice has subsided, the AST may remain elevated for some weeks and occasionally up to 6 months; a liver biopsy should be performed after this time interval.

Haematological tests
There is leucopenia with a relative lymphocytosis. Very rarely there is a Coombs'-positive haemolytic anaemia or an associated aplastic anaemia. The prothrombin time is prolonged in severe cases. The ESR is raised.

Other tests
- *Antibodies to HAV.* IgG antibodies are common in the general population over the age of 50 years, but an anti-HAV IgM implies an acute infection. Measurement of these antibodies is now becoming routine and they are now almost always looked for in cases of acute jaundice in the UK.
- *Ultrasound.* In an older patient, bile duct obstruction should be excluded.
- *Liver biopsy.* This is only indicated when there is doubt about the diagnosis.

DIFFERENTIAL DIAGNOSIS

This is from all other causes of jaundice but, in particular, from other types of viral and drug-induced hepatitis. Ultrasound has become extremely valuable in these patients to exclude biliary obstruction and hence avoid an unnecessary and potentially dangerous laparotomy.

COURSE AND PROGNOSIS

The prognosis is excellent, with most patients making a complete recovery. The mortality in young adults is 0.1% but it increases with age. Death is usually due to fulminant hepatic necrosis (see p. 228). During convalescence 5–15% of patients may have relapse of the hepatitis but this settles spontaneously. Occasionally a more severe jaundice with cholestasis will run a prolonged course of 7–20 weeks and is called cholestatic viral hepatitis.

There is no reason to stop alcohol consumption, other than for the few weeks when the patient is ill. Patients may complain of debility for several months following resolution of the symptoms and biochemical parameters. This is known as the post-hepatitis syndrome; it is a functional illness. Treatment is by reassurance. Hepatitis A never progresses to chronic liver disease.

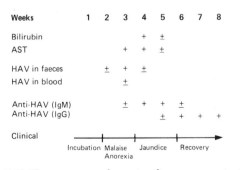

Fig. 5.12 The sequence of events after exposure to the hepatitis A virus (HAV).

TREATMENT

There is no specific treatment; rest and dietary measures are unhelpful. Corticosteroids have no benefit. Admission to hospital is not usually necessary. The condition is notifiable.

PREVENTION AND PROPHYLAXIS

Contacts and persons without antibodies travelling to endemic areas abroad may be protected for approximately three months by an injection of normal immunoglobulin (0.04–0.06 ml·kg^{-1} i.m.), which should be repeated on continued exposure. The most effective prophylactic measure is good hygiene and improved sanitation, as the virus is excreted in the faeces. The virus is resistant to chlorination but is killed by boiling water for 10 minutes.

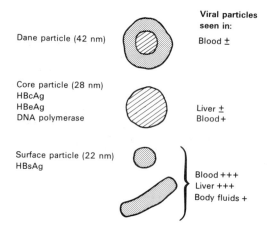

Fig. 5.13 The antigenic components of the hepatitis B virus.

Hepatitis B

The hepatitis B virus was identified by Blumberg in 1965 when he found an antibody in the serum of a patient (who had had multiple blood transfusions) which reacted with an antigen in the blood of an Australian aborigine. Subsequently this antigen was found in patients with viral hepatitis.

EPIDEMIOLOGY

The virus is present world-wide but the incidence of the carrier state varies from country to country. Britain and the USA have a carrier rate of 0.1%, but it rises to 10–15% in parts of Africa and the Far East. The virus can only be transmitted within the human population and there is no evidence that blood sucking vectors such as mosquitos spread the infection as the virus does not replicate in arthropods.

Spread of this virus is by the intravenous route, e.g. transfusion of infective blood or contaminated needles used by drug addicts, tattooists or acupuncturists, or by close personal contact, e.g. sexual intercourse, particularly in homosexuals. The virus can be found in semen and saliva. Vertical transmission from mother to child during parturition or soon after birth is the most important means of transmission world-wide.

HEPATITIS B VIRUS

Under electron microscopy, a number of particles are seen (Fig. 5.13). The whole virus is the Dane particle, which consists of an inner core formed by the liver cell nucleus and an outer surface coat (HBsAg) produced by multiplication in the cytoplasm. The inner core contains double-stranded DNA, DNA polymerase, the core antigen (HBcAg) and the e antigen (HBeAg) (Fig. 5.14). Small spheres and

Fig. 5.14 Schematic diagram of the hepatitis B virus.

tubules (100 nm long) of excess viral protein also contain the hepatitis surface antigen (HBsAg).

The virus only replicates in the liver and there is evidence to suggest that it becomes integrated with the host nuclear protein. This may be an important link in the development of hepatoma. HBsAg particles have further antigenic determinants on their surface known as a, d, y, w and r. Combinations of these subdeterminants, e.g. adw, adr, ayw and ayr, are useful in epidemiology for studying geographical differences. For example, in France the major subdeterminant is b, whilst in Greece it is y.

Delta virus
This is a defective virus which requires the hepatitis B virus for its propagation. It may be seen transiently in acute hepatitis B in drug addicts, but its major interest is that it can cause recurrent hepatitis in hepatitis B positive patients. It is usually spread parenterally and if chronic is usually associated with progressive disease. Antibodies to the delta virus are seen.

CLINICAL FEATURES

The sequence of events following infection are shown in Fig. 5.15. Clinical features are the same as those found in hepatitis A infection. In addition, a serum-sickness-like immunological syndrome may be seen with transient rashes, e.g. urticaria or a maculopapular rash, and polyarthritis affecting small joints occurs in up to 25% of cases in the prodromal period. Fever is usual. The illness may be more severe than hepatitis A. Extrahepatic immune complex mediated conditions such as an arteritis or glomerulonephritis are occasionally seen.

INVESTIGATION

This is generally the same as for hepatitis A.

Specific tests
The markers for hepatitis B are shown in Fig. 5.13. HBsAg is looked for routinely. If it is found, a full viral profile is then performed.

COURSE

The majority of patients recover completely, but some go on to develop chronic hepatitis (see p. 229) or become asymptomatic carriers (Fig. 5.16). The outcome depends upon several factors, including the virulence of the virus, and the immuno-competence and age of the patient.

Chronic asymptomatic carriers
Following an acute hepatitis B infection, approximately 5–10% of patients will not clear the virus and

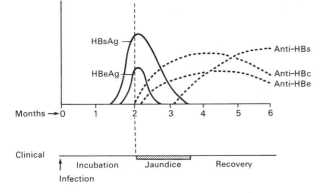

Fig. 5.15 Time course of the events and serological changes seen following infection with hepatitis B virus.

Antigens: HBsAg appears in the blood from about 6 weeks to 3 months after an acute infection. It may then disappear or persist. Its presence indicates a current or chronic infection as well as a carrier state. HBcAg is not usually seen in the blood. HBeAg rises early and usually declines rapidly. It correlates with increased severity and infectivity of the disease and its persistence correlates with the development of chronic liver disease or the carrier state.

Antibodies: Anti-HBs appears late and indicates immunity. Anti-HBc is the first antibody to appear and high titres of IgM anti-HBc suggest an acute and continuing viral replication. It persists for many months. Anti-HBe appears after anti-HBc and its appearance relates to a decreased infectivity, i.e. a low risk.

		Markers	Liver function tests	Liver histology
	Resolved	HBsAb	NAD	NAD
Acute hepatitis HBsAg HBcAg HBeAg	Chronic liver disease	HBsAg HBcAb HBeAg	Abnormal	Chronic active hepatitis Chronic persistent hepatitis Cirrhosis
	Carrier (5%)	HBsAg HBeAb HBcAb	NAD	NAD

Fig. 5.16 Clinical course of hepatitis B infection showing the blood markers, liver function and liver histology. NAD = no abnormality detected.

will become carriers. Alternatively asymptomatic patients with no history of an acute hepatitis and normal liver function tests may also be chronic carriers. There is a vast geographical variation in the incidence of carriers (see p. 226). In the UK, carriers are usually discovered incidentally on blood tests, e.g. when they are screened for donating blood for transfusion or when attending genital medicine clinics. Carriers with HBeAg or DNA polymerase in the serum (and thus having active viral replication) are highly infective.

Certain patients with immune deficiency, e.g. those with Hodgkin's disease, lymphomas or Down's syndrome, on immunosuppressive therapy, or on long-term dialysis, may become carriers. The carrier status is also increased among other patients in long-term mental institutions. Standard precautions to avoid accidental punctures should be taken by the staff if such patients require dental or medical treatment.

The prognosis of the carriers is uncertain, but most remain HBsAg positive. Some may seroconvert, i.e. develop HBe antibodies, and therefore are a low infective risk to others. Some patients may carry the virus for many years without developing chronic liver disease, whereas others, particularly those with the e antigen, may go on to develop chronic hepatitis and cirrhosis and there is an increased risk of hepatocellular carcinoma.

TREATMENT AND PREVENTION

There is no specific treatment. There is some evidence that corticosteroids may lead to a failure to clear the virus. Anti-viral agents e.g. interferon and vidarabine, are being assessed but their exact role is, as yet, unclear. This therapy should be considered for young heterosexual HBeAg-positive individuals who are likely to spread the infection beyond their immediate community.

Blood transfusion laboratories now have scrupulous procedures to exclude hepatitis B infected blood and most transfusion hepatitis is now due to non-A non-B hepatitis.

Prophylaxis is possible. If a person has been accidentally punctured by an infected needle, an intramuscular injection of hyperimmune serum globulin prepared from blood containing anti-HBs should be given. Unfortunately this is not available everywhere. The injection must be given soon after exposure, preferably within 24 h, but even then the protection from hepatitis is not certain.

A hepatitis B vaccine is now available which can provide active immunization in 95% of individuals. It should be considered for people at special risk, e.g. doctors, patients with haemophilia or on dialysis, spouses and sexual partners of chronic hepatitis B carriers, drug addicts and homosexuals. All babies of hepatitis B positive mothers must be given active and passive immunization at birth.

Non-A non-B hepatitis

No specific virus or viruses have as yet been identified as the cause of non-A non-B hepatitis. The existence of this condition became evident with the ability to test for hepatitis A and B viruses, cytomegalovirus and Epstein–Barr virus. Recently, transmission of non-A non-B hepatitis in primates has been achieved and viral particles have been identified.

Non-A non-B hepatitis accounts for 15–20% of cases of sporadic hepatitis and about 75% of cases of post-transfusion hepatitis in North America. Epidemiologically it is like hepatitis B, but with a slightly shorter incubation period. Clinical features are like those of hepatitis A and B. It is transmitted by blood and blood products and is therefore seen in drug addicts and patients who have received multiple transfusions. A chronic carrier state can follow infection in a high proportion and chronic liver disease may develop; hepatoma can occur.

Fulminant hepatic failure

This is a rare but often life-threatening syndrome due to acute hepatitis from any cause. Acute viral hepatitis and drugs, e.g. paracetamol overdose, monoamine oxidase inhibitors, isoniazid, halothane anaesthesia, are the two commonest aetiological factors. Rarely it occurs in pregnancy, Wilson's disease or Reye's syndrome in children, or following poisons, e.g. carbon tetrachloride. The reason why fulminant hepatic failure develops is unknown.

Histologically there is massive necrosis of the whole liver lobule. Severe fatty degeneration is seen in pregnancy, Reye's syndrome or lymphoma, or following tetracycline administration.

CLINICAL FEATURES

Examination shows a jaundiced patient with the physical signs of hepatic encephalopathy (see p. 236). The mental state varies from slight drowsiness, confusion and disorientation (grades I and II) to unresponsive coma (grade IV) with convulsions. Ascites and oedema may occur; splenomegaly is uncommon. A small liver is usually found, but hepatomegaly may occur with a fatty liver or lymphoma. Neurological examination shows spasticity and extensor plantar responses. Fever, sweating, hypotension and renal failure also occur.

INVESTIGATION

This is as for acute liver disease. The prothrombin time is the most useful index of severity and when very high indicates a poor prognosis. The AST is high initially, but is not a useful indicator of the course of the disease. The serum albumin falls and an

EEG is sometimes helpful in grading the encephalopathy.

TREATMENT

There is no specific treatment. Supportive therapy as for hepatic encephalopathy (see p. 237) is necessary. Cerebral oedema is the major cause of death, and when signs of raised intracranial pressure are present, 20% mannitol (1 g·kg^{-1} body weight) should be infused intravenously; this dose may need to be repeated. Dexamethasone is of no value. Hypoglycaemia, hypokalaemia and hypocalcaemia should be anticipated and corrected with 10% dextrose infusion (checked by 2-hourly Dextrostix testing), potassium and calcium. Haemorrhage may be a problem and patients are given H$_2$-receptor antagonists to prevent gastrointestinal bleeding. Infection should be treated with suitable antibiotics, and renal and respiratory failure treated as appropriate. Charcoal haemoperfusion has been used, but its value has not been proved and it may be hazardous.

Fulminant hepatic failure should be treated in an intensive care unit.

COURSE AND PROGNOSIS

In mild cases (grades I and II), two-thirds of the patients will survive. The outcome of severe cases (grades III and IV) is related to the aetiology. In special units 70% of patients with paracetamol overdosage and grade IV coma survive, as do 30–40% of patients with hepatitis A or B. The survival is almost nil in those with non-A non-B hepatitis.

ACUTE HEPATITIS DUE TO OTHER VIRUSES

Infectious mononucleosis (see p. 53)
Infectious mononucleosis is due to the Epstein–Barr virus. Mild jaundice associated with minor abnormalities of the liver function tests is extremely common, but 'clinical' hepatitis is rare. The patient complains of sore throat, fever and malaise. Lymphadenopathy and splenomegaly may be present. A Paul–Bunnell test or Monospot test is usually positive and atypical lymphocytes are present in the peripheral blood. Treatment is symptomatic. Splenic rupture is a rare complication.

Toxoplasmosis (see p. 74)
Toxoplasmosis produces a similar clinical picture to infectious mononucleosis, with abnormal liver function tests. Similarly clinical hepatitis can occur. The Paul–Bunnell test is negative.

Cytomegalovirus (see p. 53)
Cytomegalovirus can cause acute hepatitis, particularly in patients with poor immune responses. The

virus may be isolated from the urine. The liver biopsy shows intranuclear inclusions and giant cells.

Yellow fever (p. 58)
This viral infection is carried by the mosquito *Aedes aegypti* and causes acute hepatic necrosis. There is no specific treatment.

Herpes simplex (see p. 52)
Very occasionally the herpes simplex virus causes a generalized acute infection, particularly in the immunosuppressed patient. Liver biopsy shows extensive necrosis. Antiviral agents have been used for treatment.

Other infectious agents
Abnormal liver function tests are frequently found in a number of acute infections. The abnormalities are usually mild and have no clinical significance.

Chronic hepatitis

This is defined as any hepatitis lasting 6 months or longer and the classification is usually based on histological grounds. There are three forms:
● Chronic persistent hepatitis
● Chronic lobular hepatitis
● Chronic active hepatitis

CHRONIC PERSISTENT HEPATITIS

Chronic persistent hepatitis (CPH) is a benign condition with a good prognosis and must be distinguished from the more serious chronic active hepatitis (CAH). Patients are often male and are usually asymptomatic. Physical examination shows minimal hepatomegaly but no signs of chronic liver disease. Laboratory findings show a moderately raised AST, but the alkaline phosphatase, albumin and globulin are normal. HBsAg may be positive, but the HBeAg is usually negative. Diagnosis is made on a liver biopsy, which shows a marked chronic inflammatory cell infiltrate in enlarged portal tracts. Slender septa may extend into the parenchyma. The basic liver architecture is undisturbed and piecemeal necrosis does not occur (see below). Treatment is unnecessary. Months or years may pass before spontaneous resolution occurs. The majority of patients do not develop CAH or cirrhosis.

CHRONIC LOBULAR HEPATITIS

Chronic lobular hepatitis is an uncommon condition. Patients present with acute hepatitis, and the course is one of remissions and exacerbations. Patients are usually male. The condition can follow a type B or a non-A non-B hepatitis. Autoantibodies may be present. Histology of the liver biopsy resembles acute viral hepatitis and there is intralobular inflammation and necrosis. The condition responds to corticosteroids and patients do not go on to develop cirrhosis.

CHRONIC ACTIVE HEPATITIS

Chronic active hepatitis (CAH) was formerly called aggressive hepatitis. The causes are shown in Table 5.7. There are four distinct types:

CAH positive for HBsAg

Three per cent of patients with acute viral hepatitis B progress to CAH. The cause of continued liver damage is unknown, but defective immunological responses, mainly 'T' cell responses, are thought to be involved. There is no association with autoimmune disease or any particular genetic markers. It occurs mainly in older men and it is often not preceded by an acute attack. The condition may be asymptomatic or may present as a mild, slowly progressive hepatitis. Fifty per cent present with established chronic liver disease.

Investigations show a moderately raised bilirubin and AST, and a slightly raised alkaline phosphatase. Smooth muscle antibodies may be present in low titre; mitochondrial antibodies are absent. HBsAg is positive and e antigen is usually present.

Histology of the liver shows inflammatory cells spreading into the liver parenchyma from enlarged portal tracts. The limiting plate of parenchymal cells around the portal tracts is destroyed. In severe forms, small groups of hepatocytes are isolated into rosettes by fibrous septa. The destruction of these hepatocytes is called piecemeal necrosis. With the distortion of the liver architecture and the regeneration of nodules, cirrhosis may result. The hepatocytes have a ground glass appearance on a

Table 5.7 Causes of chronic active hepatitis.

Viral
Hepatitis B
Hepatitis non-A non-B
Autoimmune
Drugs, e.g. methyldopa, oxyphenisatin (withdrawn in UK)
Hereditary
Alpha-1-antitrypsin deficiency
Wilson's disease
Others
Inflammatory bowel disease—ulcerative colitis
Alcohol—rarely

haematoxylin and eosin stain and HBsAg can be confirmed on orsein or immunofluorescent stains.

TREATMENT

Corticosteroids are not used for this condition. Trials with antiviral agents, e.g. acyclovir, have shown some success in sero-converting patients with the e antigen to HBe antibody positivity. This may result in remission of the disease.

PROGNOSIS

The progression is slow and remission may occur. Established cirrhosis is associated with a poor prognosis. Primary liver cell carcinoma is a frequent association and is one of the commonest carcinomas in hepatitis B endemic areas such as the Far East.

CAH with ANF-positive and autoimmune features, but HBsAg negative

This was called 'lupoid' hepatitis because LE cells were found in the blood in 15% of cases. It occurs more frequently in young (10–20 years) and middle-aged women. There is an association with other autoimmune diseases, e.g. pernicious anaemia, thyroiditis and Coombs'-positive haemolytic anaemia, and 60% are associated with HLA-B8,DR3.

The cause is unknown, but many immunological abnormalities are seen. Humoral disturbances are associated with a hypergammaglobulinaemia (mainly IgG) and autoantibodies to nuclear factor and smooth muscle. The association with other diseases (see above) suggests immune complex formation and deposition. CAH produced by some drugs (see below) may also be associated with the production of autoantibodies. Suppressor T cell function is impaired and this may play a part in the pathogenesis.

The onset may be insidious, but 25% present as acute hepatitis. Alternatively, patients can be asymptomatic for years and the signs of chronic liver disease are discovered on a routine examination. Amenorrhoea is common. Examination shows the signs of chronic liver disease, hepatosplenomegaly, cutaneous striae, acne, hirsuties and bruises. Jaundice may be present. In advanced cases the complications of cirrhosis occur. An ill patient can also have features of an autoimmune disease, with a fever, migratory polyarthritis, glomerulonephritis, pleurisy, pulmonary infiltration or fibrosing alveolitis. The 'sicca' syndrome can occur (see p. 335).

INVESTIGATION

The hallmark of this condition is positive antibodies against nuclei, smooth muscle, and occasionally mitochondria. Serum bilirubin, globulins and aminotransferases are very high. Histology of the liver biopsy shows the changes found in hepatitis B positive CAH with piecemeal necrosis, but without the hepatitis B staining.

TREATMENT

Prednisolone 30 mg is given daily for 2 weeks, followed by a maintenance dose of 10–15 mg daily. Azathioprine 2 mg.kg^{-1} daily may be added and may allow the prednisolone dosage to be reduced.

COURSE AND PROGNOSIS

Remissions and exacerbations occur but most patients will go on to develop cirrhosis. Fifty per cent of patients will die of liver failure within 5 years if no treatment is given. The prognosis can be considerably improved with steroid therapy, underlining the importance of establishing this diagnosis by liver biopsy and immune markers.

CAH due to non-A non-B hepatitis

When CAH due to hepatitis B or autoimmune disease has been excluded and no other cause is found, the condition is usually assumed to be due to non-A non-B hepatitis. Corticosteroids are unhelpful.

CAH due to other causes

CAH can be caused by other agents, e.g. drugs (Table 5.14, p. 248).

Cirrhosis

Cirrhosis results from the necrosis of liver cells followed by fibrosis and nodule formation. The liver architecture is distorted and this interferes with the liver blood flow and function. This derangement produces the clinical features of portal hypertension and impaired liver cell function.

AETIOLOGY

The causes of cirrhosis are shown in Table 5.8. Alcohol is now the commonest cause in the Western World, but hepatitis B is the commonest cause world-wide. In the UK, no cause is found in approximately 30% of cases (cryptogenic cirrhosis). Young patients with cirrhosis must be carefully investigated as the cause may be treatable, e.g. Wilson's disease.

Table 5.8 Causes of cirrhosis.

Common
Alcohol
Idiopathic (cryptogenic)
Chronic active hepatitis due to
 hepatitis B
 hepatitis non-A non-B

Others
Biliary cirrhosis
 Primary
 Secondary
Chronic active hepatitis (autoimmune)
Haemochromatosis
Hepatic venous congestion
Budd–Chiari syndrome
Wilson's disease
Drugs, e.g. methotrexate
Alpha-1-antitrypsin deficiency
Fibrocystic disease
Intestinal bypass operations
Galactosaemia
Glycogen storage disease
Veno-occlusive disease

PATHOLOGY

Histologically two types have been identified (see Fig. 5.17):
● *Micronodular cirrhosis*, where the regenerating nodules are usually less than 3 mm in size and are

Micronodular cirrhosis

Macronodular cirrhosis

Fig. 5.17 Diagram showing the histology of different types of cirrhosis.

surrounded by fibrous septa, and the condition uniformly involves all lobes. This type is often caused by alcohol damage.

- *Macronodular cirrhosis*, where the nodules are of variable size and normal lobules may be seen within the larger nodules. This type is often seen following hepatitis B infection.

A mixed picture with small and large nodules is sometimes seen and an aetiological cause cannot necessarily be inferred from the pathological picture.

SYMPTOMS AND SIGNS

These are described on p. 219.

INVESTIGATION

Assessment
Liver function tests vary, depending on the aetiology and clinical severity of the disease, but can be normal. In most cases there is at least a slight elevation of the alkaline phosphatase and serum aminotransferases. In decompensated cirrhosis the bilirubin, AST and alkaline phosphatase are all raised. A low serum albumin indicates severe disease. The serum gamma globulin is usually raised as the damaged liver cannot clear the intestinal antigens. The gamma globulin level is particularly high in patients with autoimmune CAH.

Haematological tests are discussed on p. 219.

The serum sodium can be low in severe disease because of dilution secondary to failure of free water clearance.

Causes
Blood tests, e.g. HBsAg and autoantibodies, are necessary to establish the cause. Rarely tests include estimation of iron, copper and alpha-1-antitrypsin.

Liver biopsy is usually necessary to confirm the diagnosis and to give an indication of the severity. The core of liver obtained often fragments and sampling errors occur in macronodular cirrhosis. The cause of cirrhosis may be obvious, e.g. presence of fat indicative of alcohol, but occasionally special stains are necessary, e.g. iron for haemochromatosis, copper for Wilson's disease. Copper content should be estimated in a sample of the biopsy where indicated.

Complications
A barium swallow and meal is performed to look for oesophageal or gastric varices, although endoscopy is preferred in many centres, particularly if bleeding from varices is suspected.

Ultrasound or CT scan is occasionally necessary when a hepatoma is suspected because of clinical deterioration or the presence of a raised serum alpha-fetoprotein.

MANAGEMENT

Management is that of the complications seen in decompensated cirrhosis and patients should be followed-up in order to detect complications as early as possible.

There is no treatment that will arrest or reverse the cirrhotic changes, although progression may be halted by correcting the cause (see below). Patients with compensated cirrhosis should lead a normal life and no particular diet is helpful. Alcohol should be avoided, although if the cirrhosis is not due to alcohol small amounts are not harmful.

COURSE AND PROGNOSIS

This is extremely variable depending on many factors, including the aetiology and the presence of complications. Poor prognostic indicators are given in Table 5.9. Development of any complication usually worsens the prognosis. In general, the 5-year survival rate is approximately 50%, but this also varies depending on the aetiology and the stage at which the diagnosis is made.

COMPLICATIONS AND EFFECTS OF CIRRHOSIS

These are shown in Table 5.10.

Table 5.9 Poor prognostic indicators in cirrhosis.

Blood tests
Low albumin (<25 g·l^{-1})
Low serum sodium (<120 mmol·l^{-1})
Prolonged prothrombin time
Clinical
Persistent jaundice
Failure of response to therapy
Ascites
Haemorrhage from varices, particularly with poor liver function
Neuropsychiatric complications developing with progressive liver failure
Small liver
Persistent hypotension
Aetiology, e.g. cryptogenic cirrhosis is worse than alcoholic cirrhosis (in a patient who has stopped drinking)

Table 5.10 Complications and effects of cirrhosis.

Portal hypertension and gastrointestinal haemorrhage
Ascites
Portosystemic encephalopathy
Renal failure
Hepatoma (primary liver cell carcinoma)

Portal hypertension and gastrointestinal haemorrhage

The portal vein is formed by the union of the splenic and superior mesenteric veins. The pressure within it is normally 5–10 mmHg. Collaterals between the portal and systemic circulation develop when the pressure rises above 14 mmHg. The main sites for these portosystemic anastomoses are the oesophagus and stomach, the rectum, the left renal vein, the lumbar veins, the ovarian or testicular veins, and the veins of the anterior abdominal wall. The formation of these collaterals produce 'varices', commonly at the oesophagogastric junction.

The causes of portal hypertension can be classified according to the site of obstruction (see Table 5.11). Portal hypertension can result from:
- Blockage of the portal vein before the liver
- Distortion of the liver architecture, which can be pre-sinusoidal, e.g. in schistosomiasis, or post-sinusoidal, e.g. in cirrhosis
- Venous blockage outside the liver (rare), e.g. in Budd–Chiari syndrome, veno-occlusive disease or constrictive pericarditis

CLINICAL FEATURES

In a patient with chronic liver disease, portal hypertension is suspected if there is splenomegaly and/or ascites. Patients can present with ascites, encephalopathy, or gross haematemesis or melaena from rupture of oesophageal or gastric varices. Occasionally a coincidental peptic ulcer may be the cause of the bleeding. In alcoholics, particularly, the bleeding can be from the Mallory–Weiss syndrome (see p. 170). Portosystemic anastomoses in other sites only rarely bleed.

Table 5.11 Causes of portal hypertension.

Extrahepatic
Portal vein thrombosis

Intrahepatic
Cirrhosis
Hepatitis (alcoholic)
Idiopathic non-cirrhotic portal hypertension (subtle liver disease)
Schistosomiasis
Partial nodular transformation
Congenital hepatic fibrosis
Myelosclerosis (extramedullary haemopoiesis)

Posthepatic
Budd–Chiari syndrome
Veno-occlusive disease
Right heart failure—rare
Constrictive pericarditis

MANAGEMENT OF VARICEAL HAEMORRHAGE

After the diagnosis has been made:

1 Assess the general condition of patient—pulse and blood pressure.
2 Insert an intravenous line and obtain blood for grouping and cross-matching, haemoglobin, urea, prothrombin time, electrolytes and liver function tests.
3 Restore blood volume with plasma expanders or blood transfusion if possible. These measures are discussed in more detail in the treatment of shock (p. 636).
4 A useful emergency procedure is to reduce the portal vein pressure:
- *Vasopressin* 20 units in 50–100 ml of 5% dextrose given intravenously over 20 minutes followed by a continuous infusion of 0.4 units per minute will help control bleeding in 50–60% of cases, partly by constricting the splanchnic vessels and thus reducing portal pressure and flow. Care is needed in patients with ischaemic heart disease as vasoconstriction may cause angina or even myocardial infarction. If the vasopressin is active (it has a limited shelf-life), the patient will complain of abdominal colic, evacuate his bowels and have facial pallor due to the generalized constriction of arterioles.
- *Terlipressin* (triglycyl-lysine vasopressin) is a precursor of vasopressin and has a longer half-life and fewer side-effects. An intravenous bolus of 2 mg should be given every six hours.

For the 40–50% of patients who continue to bleed, the following measures are used:

5 *Direct pressure over varices.* Tamponade can be applied using a Sengstaken–Blakemore tube. The tube is passed into the stomach and the gastric balloon is inflated with water containing a radio-paque substance. The tube is pulled up tight against the oesophagogastric junction and the oesophageal balloon is then inflated. The tube is then fixed by the side of the mouth. As soon as the patient's condition is stable, emergency sclerotherapy should be performed. If this is not available, the balloons can be left inflated for 24 h, but the oesophageal balloon should then be deflated to avoid ischaemic damage. Following this, the gastric balloon is deflated within 24 h and the tube removed, but it may be reinserted at any time if further bleeding occurs. With both balloons inflated the patient is unable to swallow and care should be taken to prevent aspiration. One type of tube available has an aspiration tube above the oesophageal balloon to suck out secretions in the proximal oesophagus and pharynx. A plain radiograph should always be requested to check the site of the tube (Fig. 5.18).

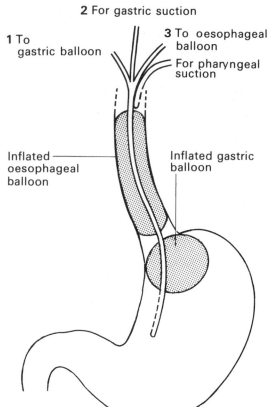

2 For gastric suction

1 To gastric balloon

3 To oesophageal balloon

For pharyngeal suction

Inflated oesophageal balloon

Inflated gastric balloon

Fig. 5.18 X-ray and diagram of a Sengstaken–Blakemore tube in-situ.

Vasoconstriction and balloon tamponade are only temporary measures and the rebleeding rate is high. More definitive procedures are required; these are described below.

6 *Sclerotherapy.* This is now the treatment of choice. It is used in the acute situation either alone or in conjunction with balloon tamponade.

The varices are injected via a flexible or rigid endoscope. A needle is passed down the endoscope and the varices are injected with a sclerosing agent. Repeat sclerotherapy is performed after 24 h if bleeding recurs (see below).

7 *Measures to prevent encephalopathy.* Portosystemic encephalopathy (PSE) can be precipitated by a large bleed (since blood contains protein). Preventative measures are described below. In addition blood should be aspirated from the stomach —see below.

8 *Emergency surgery.* This may be required if medical measures fail to stop the bleeding, but should be avoided if possible as the mortality rate is high. Oesophageal transection with anastomosis using a universal stapling gun, gastric transection, and undersewing of varices are accepted procedures.

Emergency portacaval shunts are seldom performed.

LONG-TERM MANAGEMENT OF GASTROINTESTINAL BLEEDING

Medical

Beta-blockade with propranolol in doses that achieve a 25% reduction in pulse rate has been shown to cause a reduction in the portal vein pressure. It is currently being assessed for use in the prevention of rebleeding.

Recurrent sclerotherapy performed weekly until varices have disappeared has been shown to reduce the recurrence of bleeding and to decrease mortality. In most cases this is now the accepted way of managing patients with variceal haemorrhage. Follow-up sclerotherapy should be performed at intervals to keep the varices ablated.

Surgical

Elective portacaval anastomosis in patients who have bled is performed less often than previously because of its long-term complication of PSE. A good prognostic guide is the Child's classification (A, B or C), which is based on the presence of jaundice, ascites and encephalopathy, and the level of the serum albumin. Young patients with good liver function (Child's grade A) have a low operative mortality (0–5%) but are still liable to encephalopathy. Other patients with poor liver functions (albumin < 30 g·l^{-1}, bilirubin > 50 mmol·l^{-1} and ascites—Child's grade C) have a very high operative risk. The most common 'shunts' performed today are an end-to-side portacaval anastomosis or a selective distal splenorenal shunt (Warren shunt), which maintains hepatic blood flow via the superior mesenteric vein.

PROGNOSIS OF A VARICEAL BLEED

This depends on the severity of the underlying liver disease. The mortality of the first bleed is 30%, with a similar mortality in the survivors when they rebleed. In general, patients with stable liver disease have an overall survival rate of 90% at 5 years, while patients with poor liver function, e.g. jaundice, ascites and encephalopathy, have a 50% 1-year survival rate.

OTHER CAUSES OF PORTAL HYPERTENSION (see Table 5.11)

Extrahepatic causes
Extrahepatic blockage is due to portal vein thrombosis. The cause is usually unidentifiable but there may be a history of neonatal sepsis of the umbilical vein. Patients usually present with bleeding, often at a young age. They have normal liver function and, because of this, their prognosis following bleeding is excellent. A splenectomy should never be performed as it may be possible to perform a splenorenal shunt in adult life. Treatment is usually with repeated sclerotherapy.

Intrahepatic causes
Although cirrhosis is the commonest intrahepatic cause of portal hypertension, other causes include:

- *Non-cirrhotic portal hypertension* or subtle change liver disease. Patients present with portal hypertension and variceal bleeding but without cirrhosis. Histologically, the liver shows broad fibrous bands. The aetiology is unknown, but arsenic, vinyl chloride and other toxic agents have been implicated in some cases. A similar disease has been described in India. The liver lesion does not progress and the prognosis is therefore good.
- *Partial nodular transformation*. This is a very rare condition of unknown aetiology. Portal hypertension may arise due to non-cirrhotic nodules in the hilar region. It is not progressive and the prognosis is better than in patients with cirrhosis.

Posthepatic causes
Prolonged severe heart failure with tricuspid incompetence and constrictive pericarditis can both lead to portal hypertension. The Budd–Chiari syndrome is described on p. 242.

Ascites

Ascites is the presence of free fluid in the peritoneal cavity. The causes are shown in Table 5.12. In cirrhosis the actual mechanism of the production of ascites is unclear, but it probably results from a combination of the effects of hepatocellular failure and portal hypertension.

Plasma aldosterone is increased and this initiates sodium and water retention. This results in an expanded extracellular fluid, which 'overflows' into the peritoneal cavity due to localizing factors, i.e. increased portal pressure, reduced plasma oncotic

Table 5.12 Causes of ascites divided according to the type of ascitic fluid.

Straw-coloured
Malignancy—commonest cause
Cirrhosis
Infective
Tuberculosis
Following intra-abdominal perforation—any bacteria may be found, e.g. *E. coli*
'Spontaneous' in cirrhotics
Hepatic vein obstruction (Budd–Chiari syndrome)—protein level high in fluid
Chronic pancreatitis
Constrictive pericarditis
Meigs' syndrome
Hypoproteinaemia, e.g. nephrotic syndrome
Chylous
Obstruction of main lymphatic duct, e.g. by carcinoma—chylomicrons are present
Haemorrhagic
Malignancy
Ruptured ectopic pregnancy
Abdominal trauma
Acute pancreatitis

pressure (low albumin) and impaired lymph drainage. The increase in plasma aldosterone is a result of increased plasma renin produced in the kidney, probably due to an alteration in blood distribution in the kidney. Later, a fall in the extracellular fluid volume produces decreased renal perfusion and this may also increase sodium retention via the renin–aldosterone system. Urinary sodium is less than 5 mmol·day^{-1} and serum sodium is often low, partly due to the diuretics used. However, the total body sodium stores are increased due to the increased extracellular sodium space. Free water excretion is also reduced due to the proximal tubular reabsorption of sodium.

CLINICAL FEATURES

Ascites can develop suddenly or insidiously over months. Shifting dullness can be demonstrated. Peripheral oedema is usually seen. A pleural effusion is found in 6% of patients with cirrhosis and is usually right-sided. Patients often require hospital admission for diagnosis of the cause of the ascites and its treatment.

INVESTIGATION

A diagnostic tap, taking 10–20 ml of ascitic fluid, should be performed. The fluid is usually straw-coloured and should be sent to the laboratory for:
- Cells—the total white count and differential are both raised in infection (> 250 cells per mm^3 indicates infection).
- Protein—rarely exceeds 30–40 g·l^{-1} (a transudate) in portal hypertension. An exudate (> 30–40 g·l^{-1}) suggests a malignant, infective or pancreatic cause. A high protein can also been seen in the Budd–Chiari syndrome and chronic constrictive pericarditis, i.e. hepatic venous hypertension.
- Gram stain and culture for bacteria and acid-fast bacilli
- Cytology for malignant cells

MANAGEMENT

Ascites is generally treated unless it is minimal. The aim is to treat the ascites slowly so as to avoid complications; a weight loss of 1 kg per day is safe. The rate of ascitic fluid reabsorption is only 700–900 ml per day and if the diuresis is more than 3 l per day, hypovolaemia will result. This leads to decreased renal perfusion and uraemia.

The management is as follows, together with daily weighing and measurement of the 24-h urine output:
- *Bed rest*. This increases renal perfusion and potentiates a diuresis.
- *Diet*. This should be low in sodium, the amount of restriction depending on the severity of the liver disease. A 'no added salt' diet contains 80 mmol per day, whilst a strict 'salt-free' diet contains 22–40 mmol. The diet should be adequate in calories and protein content. Fluid restriction to 1 l can be helpful, particularly when hyponatraemia is present.
- *Diuretics*. The use of these in cirrhosis is associated with many complications, e.g. electrolyte disturbances, encephalopathy and renal failure. It is probably best to start with a combination of an aldosterone-antagonist, e.g. spironolactone (200 mg daily), and either triamterene (100–500 mg daily) or amiloride (10–60 mg daily), which act on the distal nephron. Most patients will respond to this combination, but some will require a powerful loop diuretic such as frusemide 80–120 mg daily.

Therapeutic paracentesis and drainage is used occasionally when the abdominal discomfort is severe. In addition, an initial paracentesis is now often used to reduce the stay in hospital. However, care must be taken to avoid hypoalbuminaemia and volume depletion. Complications of this procedure include infection, haemorrhage, perforation and encephalopathy.

Portosystemic encephalopathy (PSE)

The term portosystemic encephalopathy (PSE) refers to a chronic neuropsychiatric syndrome secondary to chronic liver disease. This condition occurs with cirrhosis but a similar acute encephalopathy can occur in acute fulminant hepatic failure (see p. 228). PSE is seen in patients with portal hypertension due to spontaneous 'shunting' or in patients following a portacaval shunt operation. Encephalopathy is potentially reversible. The mechanism is unknown but several factors are thought to play a part. In cirrhosis, the blood bypasses the liver via the collaterals and the 'toxic' metabolites pass directly to the brain to produce the encephalopathy. Many 'toxic' substances have been suggested as the causative factor, including ammonia, free fatty acids, mercaptans and false neurotransmitters (octopamine). Increased blood levels of aromatic amino acids (tyrosine and phenylalanine) and reduced branch-chain amino acids (valine, leucine and isoleucine) also occur. Nevertheless, ammonia seems to play a major role. Ammonia is produced by the breakdown of protein by intestinal bacteria and a high blood ammonia is seen in most patients. It may alter the blood–brain barrier and allow 'toxins' to interfere with cerebral metabolism. The factors which can precipitate PSE are shown in Table 5.13.

CLINICAL FEATURES

An acute onset often has a precipitating factor (see Table 5.13). The patient becomes increasingly drowsy and comatose.

Table 5.13 Factors precipitating portosystemic encephalopathy.

High dietary protein
Gastrointestinal haemorrhage
Constipation
Infection
Diuretic therapy
Drugs, e.g. narcotics
Paracentesis (large amounts)
Hypokalaemia
Portacaval shunt operations

Chronically, there is a disorder of personality, mood and intellect, with a reversal of normal sleep rhythm. These changes may be fluctuating and a history from a relative must be obtained. The patient is irritable, confused, disorientated and has slow slurred speech. General features include nausea, vomiting and weakness. Convulsions and coma occur as the encephalopathy becomes more marked. Hyperventilation and pyrexia are seen.

Signs include fetor hepaticus (a sweet smell to the breath) and a coarse flapping tremor seen when the hands are outstretched and the wrists hyperextended (asterixis). There is a constructional apraxia and the patient cannot write or draw, for example, a five-pointed star. Mental function can be assessed by using the serial sevens test (see p. 870). A trail making test (the ability to join numbers and letters with a pen within a certain time—a standard psychological test for brain dysfunction) is prolonged and is a useful bedside test to assess encephalopathy.

INVESTIGATION

See p. 214. Additional investigations include:
- *Electroencephalogram (EEG).* This shows a decrease in the frequency of the normal alpha waves (8–13 Hz) to delta waves (1.5–3 Hz). These changes occur before coma supervenes.
- *Blood ammonia.* This is occasionally useful in the differential diagnosis of the cause of the coma and to follow the course of the PSE.

MANAGEMENT

Management consists of restricting protein intake and sterilizing the bowel.

Immediate
- Identify and remove the possible precipitating cause, e.g. drugs with cerebral depressant properties.
- Give purgation and enemas to empty the bowels of nitrogenous substances. Lactulose (10–30 ml three times daily) is an osmotic purgative which

reduces the colonic pH and limits ammonia absorption. Hypernatraemia can result from water loss.
- Institute a protein-free diet, with adequate calories, given if necessary via a fine bore nasogastric tube.
- Give the antibiotic neomycin orally in a dose of 1 g four times daily. Neomycin can also be used in retention enemas. It is mainly unabsorbed, but in the long-term it can produce deafness.
- Stop or reduce diuretic therapy.
- Correct any electrolyte imbalance.
- Give intravenous fluids.
- Treat any infection.

Long-term
- Increase protein in the diet to a limit of tolerance (20–50 g) as the encephalopathy improves.
- Avoid constipation.
- Give lactulose 10–30 ml three times daily and neomycin 2 g daily.
- Avoid precipitating factors, e.g. drugs, over-diuresis.

COURSE AND PROGNOSIS

Acute encephalopathy, often seen after fulminant hepatic failure, has a very poor prognosis as the disease itself has a high mortality. In cirrhosis, chronic PSE is very variable and the prognosis is that of the underlying liver disease.

Renal failure (hepatorenal syndrome)

Renal failure occurs in hepatocellular failure and is thought to result from changes in renal blood flow due to renal vasoconstriction. The kidneys are histologically normal. The syndrome often occurs in end-stage alcoholic cirrhosis. The serum urea and creatinine levels rise progressively and the serum sodium is less than 120 mmol·l^{-1}.

TREATMENT

Diuretics should be withdrawn and fluids restricted. Nephrotoxic drugs should be avoided. The prognosis is poor.

Primary hepatocellular carcinoma (hepatoma)

This is dealt with on p. 245.

TYPES OF CIRRHOSIS

Alcoholic

This is discussed in the section on alcoholic liver disease (see p. 241).

Primary biliary cirrhosis (PBC)

This is a chronic disorder in which there is a progressive destruction of bile ducts, eventually leading to cirrhosis. It predominantly affects women (female to male ratio = 8:1) who are middle-aged. It used to be considered rare but is now being diagnosed more frequently in its milder forms. PBC has been called 'chronic non-suppurative destructive cholangitis'; this term is more descriptive of the early lesion and emphasizes that true cirrhosis only occurs in the later stages of the disease.

AETIOLOGY

The aetiology is unknown but immunological mechanisms are thought to play a part. Antibodies to nuclear factor (ANF), mitochondria (AMA) and smooth muscle (SMA) are found in high frequency in PBC as well as other conditions with disturbed immunity such as chronic active hepatitis and cryptogenic cirrhosis. However, the presence of AMA in high titre is unrelated to the clinical or histological picture and may play no part in its pathogenesis. Although damage to bile ducts is a feature, antibodies to bile ductules are not specific to PBC. Cell-mediated immunity is impaired (demonstrated both in vitro and by skin testing) and this suggests that sensitized T lymphocytes might be involved in producing damage. There may be a defect in the immunoregulation, as a decrease in T suppressor cells may allow cytotoxic T cells and B cells to produce damage to the bile ducts.

CLINICAL FEATURES

Asymptomatic patients may be discovered on routine examination to have hepatomegaly, a raised serum alkaline phosphatase or autoantibodies.

The earliest symptom is pruritus, often preceding jaundice by a few years. When jaundice appears hepatomegaly is usually found.

In the later stages there is jaundice with severe pruritus. On examination the patient is jaundiced and pigmented, xanthelasma or other deposits of cholesterol may be seen, usually around the eyes and in the creases of the hands, and there is hepatosplenomegaly.

ASSOCIATIONS

Connective tissue diseases occur with increased frequency. Renal tubular acidosis and membranous glomerulonephritis may occur. The 'sicca complex' (dry eyes and mouth) is seen in 70% of cases.

INVESTIGATION

- A high serum alkaline phosphatase is often the only abnormality in the liver function tests.

- Mitochondrial antibodies are seen in over 95% of patients with PBC, but it should be remembered that they are also seen in 30% of patients with HBsAG-negative CAH. Other non-specific antibodies, e.g. antinuclear factor and smooth muscle, may also be present.
- The serum IgM may be very high.
- Liver biopsy shows characteristic histological features of portal tract inflammation, a paucity of bile ducts, bile ductular proliferation, centrilobular cholestasis and granuloma formation, usually with cirrhosis.

DIFFERENTIAL DIAGNOSIS

This is from other causes of cirrhosis but, in addition, extrahepatic biliary obstruction should be excluded. Primary sclerosing cholangitis (see p. 253) also produces a similar clinical picture and should be considered.

Hepatic granulomas are also seen in sarcoidosis, tuberculosis, schistosomiasis, drug reactions (e.g. phenylbutazone), brucellosis, parasitic infestation (e.g. strongyloidiasis), and other conditions.

TREATMENT

There is no specific therapy of proven benefit. Azathioprine, corticosteroids and penicillamine have all been tried without beneficial effect, and corticosteroids are contraindicated because of bone thinning.

Fat-soluble vitamins (A, D and K) may be required in the deeply jaundiced patient as malabsorption occurs.

Pruritus is difficult to control, but cholestyramine one 4 g sachet three times daily can be helpful, although it is unpalatable.

COMPLICATIONS

The complications are those of cirrhosis. Rarely bone pain due to osteomalacia and a peripheral neuropathy can also occur.

COURSE AND PROGNOSIS

This is very variable. Asymptomatic patients and those presenting with pruritus will survive for more than 10–15 years. Symptomatic patients with jaundice have a more rapidly progressive course and die of liver failure or bleeding varices in approximately 5 years. Transplantation is becoming an accepted form of treatment for these patients.

Secondary biliary cirrhosis

Cirrhosis can result from prolonged (for months) large duct biliary obstruction. Causes include bile duct strictures, gallstones (p. 249) and sclerosing cholangitis (p. 253). An ultrasound examination, followed by ERCP or PTC is performed to outline the ducts and any remedial cause dealt with surgically.

Haemochromatosis

Idiopathic haemochromatosis (IHC) is an inherited disease characterized by excess iron deposition in various organs leading to eventual fibrosis and functional organ failure.

AETIOLOGY

The underlying metabolic defect is unknown, but abnormal enterocyte function resulting in inappropriate levels of iron absorption has been suggested (see p. 264). IHC is inherited as an autosomal recessive with only homozygotes manifesting the clinical features of the disease. It is associated with HLA-A3 and B14. Dietary intakes of iron and chelating agents (ascorbic acid) are probably also important. Iron overload may be present in alcoholics, but alcohol excess per se does not cause IHC. There is a history of excess alcohol intake in 25% of patients. The iron accumulation is gradual and occurs throughout life.

PREVALENCE

Prevalence of homozygotes varies between 0.3 and 0.5%, with a heterozygote frequency of 9–14%.

PATHOLOGY

The iron content is particularly increased in the liver and pancreas (50–100 × normal), but is also increased in all other organs, e.g. the endocrine glands, heart and skin. Gonadal function is impaired despite a low testicular iron content.

Histologically the liver shows extensive pigmentation and fibrosis, with iron deposition in dense, fibrous septae forming a network surrounding groups of lobules. Early in the disease, iron is deposited in the periportal hepatocytes (in pericanalicular lysosomes). Later it is distributed widely throughout the lobules, biliary duct epithelium, Kupffer's cells and connective tissue. Cirrhosis with nodularity is a late feature.

CLINICAL FEATURES

The course of the disease depends on a number of features, including sex, dietary iron intake, presence of associated hepatotoxins (especially alcohol) and genotype. Overt clinical manifestations occur more frequently in men; the reduced incidence in women is probably explained by physiological blood loss and a smaller dietary intake of iron. Most affected individuals present in the fifth decade. The classic triad of bronze skin pigmentation (owing to melanin deposition), hepatomegaly and diabetes mellitus is only present in cases of gross iron overload. Other more common features include gonadal atrophy, lethargy and loss of libido.

Hypogonadism secondary to pituitary dysfunction is the commonest endocrine feature. Deficiency of other pituitary hormones is also found, but symptomatic endocrine deficiencies are exceedingly rare. Cardiac manifestations, particularly heart failure and arrhythmias, are common, especially in younger patients. Calcium pyrophosphate is deposited asymmetrically in both large and small joints (chondrocalcinosis), leading to an arthropathy. The exact relationship of chondrocalcinosis to iron deposition is uncertain.

COMPLICATIONS

Thirty per cent of patients with cirrhosis will develop primary hepatocellular carcinoma (HCC). HCC has not been described in non-cirrhotic patients in whom the excess iron stores have been removed. This has important implications for early diagnosis.

INVESTIGATION

Homozygotes
- The serum iron is elevated ($> 30\,\mu\mathrm{mol}\cdot\mathrm{l}^{-1}$), with a reduction in the total iron binding capacity and complete or almost complete transferrin saturation ($> 70\%$).
- The serum ferritin is elevated (usually > 500 $\mu\mathrm{g}\cdot\mathrm{l}^{-1}$), and there is evidence of excessive parenchymal deposition.
- There is excessive excretion of iron following administration of chelating agents.
- Liver function tests are often normal, even with established cirrhosis.

Heterozygotes
Heterozygotes may have normal biochemical tests or modest increases in serum iron transferrin saturation ($> 50\%$) or serum ferritin (usually $< 400\,\mu\mathrm{g}\cdot\mathrm{l}^{-1}$).

Liver biopsy
This is important in defining the extent of tissue damage, assessing tissue iron, and measuring the hepatic iron concentration ($> 180\,\mu\mathrm{mol}\cdot\mathrm{g}^{-1}$ dry weight of liver indicates haemochromatosis).

Mild degrees of parenchymal iron deposition in patients with alcoholic cirrhosis can often cause confusion with true homozygous IHC. It is highly likely that many of this former group are heterozygotes for the haemochromatosis gene.

Magnetic resonance imaging is still being investigated for use as a screening test and shows early promise.

Causes of secondary iron overload such as multiple transfusions must be excluded.

TREATMENT AND MANAGEMENT

Venesection

Venesection prolongs life and may reverse tissue damage; the risk of malignancy still remains. All patients should have excess iron removed as rapidly as possible. This is achieved using venesection of 500 ml performed twice weekly. During venesection, serum iron and ferritin and the MCV should be monitored. These fall only when available iron is depleted. Three or four venesections per year are required to prevent reaccumulation of iron. Serum ferritin should remain within the normal range. Liver biopsy is usually repeated to ensure removal of iron and to assess progress of hepatic disease.

Manifestations of the disease usually improve or disappear, except for diabetes, testicular atrophy and chondrocalcinosis. The requirements for insulin often diminish in diabetic patients. Testosterone replacement is often helpful.

Chelation therapy

In rare patients who cannot tolerate venesection (because of severe cardiac disease or anaemia), chelation therapy with desferrioxamine either intermittently or continuously by infusion has been successful in removing iron.

Screening of relatives

In all cases of IHC it is important to screen all first degree family members to detect early and asymptomatic disease. Serum ferritin is an excellent test with only occasional false-positives in hepatocellular necrosis and rare false-negatives in some family studies.

Wilson's disease (hepatolenticular degeneration)

This is a very rare inborn error of copper metabolism which results in copper deposition in various organs to produce cirrhosis and degeneration of the basal ganglia of the brain. It is potentially treatable and all young patients with cirrhosis should be screened for this condition.

Copper metabolism. Dietary copper is absorbed from the stomach and upper small intestine. It is transported to the liver loosely bound to albumin. Here it is incorporated into caeruloplasmin, a glycoprotein synthesized in the liver, and secreted into the blood. Copper is normally lost in the bile.

AETIOLOGY

It is inherited as an autosomal recessive gene and occurs world-wide, particularly in countries where consanguinity is common. The basic problem is a failure to excrete copper but, although there is a low serum caeruloplasmin, the precise defect remains unknown.

PATHOLOGY

The histology is not diagnostic and varies from that of chronic active hepatitis to macronodular cirrhosis. Stains for copper show a periportal distribution but this can be unreliable (see below). The basal ganglia are damaged and show cavitation, the kidneys show tubular degeneration, and erosions are seen in bones.

CLINICAL FEATURES

Children usually present with hepatic problems, whilst young adults have more neurological problems, such as tremor, dysarthria, involuntary movements and eventually dementia (see p. 830).

Signs are of chronic liver disease with neurological signs of basal ganglia involvement. A specific sign is the Kayser–Fleischer ring, which is due to copper deposition in Descemet's membrane in the cornea. It appears as a greenish brown pigment at the corneoscleral junction just within the cornea. Identification of this ring frequently requires slit-lamp examination. It may be absent in young children. Very rarely the Kayser–Fleischer ring may be seen in cryptogenic cirrhosis.

INVESTIGATION

The serum copper and caeruloplasmin are usually reduced, but can be normal. The 24-h urinary copper is usually increased. The diagnosis depends on the measurement of the amount of copper in the liver, although high levels of copper are also found in the liver in chronic cholestasis. Measurement of ^{64}Cu incorporation into the liver may be helpful. Haemolysis and anaemia may be present.

TREATMENT

Long-term penicillamine, approximately 1 g daily, is effective in chelating copper and leads to clinical and biochemical improvement. Toxic side-effects of the drug are unusual and include skin rashes, leucopenia and renal damage. Urine copper levels should be monitored. All siblings and children of patients should be screened. Homozygotes may have the above physical signs, Kayser–Fleischer rings and a low serum caeruloplasmin. Symptomless homozygous relatives should be treated.

PROGNOSIS

Early diagnosis and effective treatment have improved the outlook. Neurological damage is, however, permanent. Death is from liver failure, bleeding varices or intercurrent infection.

Alpha-1-antitrypsin deficiency (see also p. 579)

A deficiency of alpha-1-antitrypsin is sometimes associated with liver disease and pulmonary emphysema (particularly in smokers). Alpha-1-antitrypsin (a protease inhibitor) is synthesized in the liver and comprises 90% of serum alpha-1-globulin seen on electrophoresis.

Clinically, deficiency may present as a cholestatic jaundice in the neonate (neonatal hepatitis) or with signs of chronic liver disease in the young adult. It is inherited as an autosomal dominant gene.

INVESTIGATION

- The serum alpha-1-antitrypsin is low.
- *Liver biopsy.* Periodic acid–Schiff (PAS) positive, diastase-resistant globules are seen in the hepatocytes. These can be shown to be alpha-1-antitrypsin using immunodiagnostic techniques.
- *Phenotypes.* The glycoprotein is characterized on its electrophoretic mobility as medium (M), slow (S) or very slow (Z). The Pi (protease inhibitor) M is the normal type, and is associated with serum levels of alpha-1-antitrypsin of 2–4 g·l^{-1}. Homozygotes for the protease inhibitor Z (i.e. PiZZ) have low alpha-1-antitrypsin levels and are seriously affected with liver disease. Heterozygotes (PiSZ, PiMZ, etc.) exist and may develop signs of deficiency.

TREATMENT

There is no treatment apart from dealing with the complications of liver disease. Patients should be advised to stop smoking (see p. 579).

Alcoholic liver disease

In this section only a description of the pathology and clinical features of the liver disease will be given. The amounts needed to produce liver damage, alcohol metabolism, and other clinical effects of alcohol are described on p. 146.

PATHOLOGY

Alcohol can produce a wide spectrum of liver disease from fatty change to hepatitis and cirrhosis.

Fatty change
The metabolism of alcohol produces fat in the liver. This is minimal with small amounts of alcohol, but with larger amounts the cells become swollen with fat (steatosis) giving, eventually, a Swiss cheese effect on haematoxylin and eosin stain. Steatosis can also be seen in obesity, diabetes, starvation, and occasionally in chronic illness. There is no liver cell damage and therefore in general this is not precirrhotic. The fat disappears on stopping alcohol.

In some cases collagen is laid down around the central hepatic veins and this can sometimes progress to cirrhosis without a preceding hepatitis.

Alcoholic hepatitis
Here there is necrosis of liver cells and infiltration with polymorphonuclear leucocytes. A dense perinuclear eosinophilic material called Mallory's hyaline is sometimes seen in hepatocytes. Steatosis is also present. Mallory's hyaline is suggestive of but not specific for alcoholic damage as it can also be found in other liver diseases, such as Wilson's disease and PBC. Alcoholic hepatitis usually goes on to become cirrhosis if alcohol consumption continues.

Alcoholic cirrhosis
Destruction and fibrosis with regenerating nodules produces cirrhosis. There is bridging fibrosis between portal tracts and terminal hepatic veins. Fat may be present, with the additional features of alcoholic hepatitis.

CLINICAL FEATURES

Fatty liver
There are often no symptoms or signs. Vague abdominal symptoms of nausea, vomiting and diarrhoea are due to the more general effects of alcohol on the GI tract. Hepatomegaly, sometimes huge, can occur together with other features of chronic liver disease.

Alcoholic hepatitis
The clinical features vary in degree:
- The patient may be well, with few symptoms, the hepatitis only being apparent on the liver biopsy in addition to fatty change.
- Mild to moderate symptoms of ill health, occasionally with mild jaundice, may occur. Signs include all the features of chronic liver disease. Liver function tests are deranged and the diagnosis is made on a liver biopsy.
- In the severe case, usually superimposed on patients with alcoholic cirrhosis, the patient is ill, with jaundice and ascites. Abdominal pain is frequently present, with a high fever associated with the liver necrosis. On examination there is deep jaundice, hepatomegaly, sometimes splenomegaly, and ascites with ankle oedema. The signs of chronic liver disease are also present.

Alcoholic cirrhosis

This represents the final stage of liver disease from alcohol abuse. Nevertheless, patients can be very well with few symptoms. On examination, there are usually signs of chronic liver disease. The diagnosis is confirmed by liver biopsy.

Usually the patient presents with one of the complications of cirrhosis. In many cases there are features of alcohol dependence (see p. 892) as well as evidence of involvement of other systems, e.g. peripheral neuropathy.

INVESTIGATION

Fatty liver

An elevated MCV often indicates heavy drinking. Liver function tests show mild abnormalities, with elevation of both aminotransferase enzymes. The γ-GT level is a sensitive test for determining whether the patient is taking alcohol. With severe fatty infiltration, marked changes in all liver function tests can occur.

Liver biopsy is the only way to assess the degree of liver damage.

Alcoholic hepatitis

Investigations show a leucocytosis with markedly deranged liver function tests, with elevated:
- Bilirubin
- Aspartate and alanine aminotransferases
- Alkaline phosphatase
- Prothrombin time

A low serum albumin may also be found. Rarely, hyperlipidaemia with haemolysis (Zieve's syndrome) may occur.

The prolonged prothrombin time makes liver biopsy impossible in the severe form. In these severe cases the mortality is at least 50%, and with a prothrombin time twice the normal, progressive encephalopathy and renal failure the mortality approaches 90%.

Alcoholic cirrhosis

Investigations are as for cirrhosis in general.

MANAGEMENT AND PROGNOSIS

Fatty liver

In all but the mild cases the patient is advised to stop drinking; the fat will disappear and the liver function tests usually return to normal. Small amounts of alcohol can be drunk subsequently as long as the patient is aware of the problems and can control his consumption.

Alcoholic hepatitis

In severe cases the patient is confined to bed. Treatment for encephalopathy and ascites is commenced. Patients should be fed either by a fine bore nasogastric tube or intravenously. Nitrogen solutions enriched with branched chain amino acids, e.g. leucine, isoleucine and valine, may be helpful. Vitamins B and C should be given by injection. Corticosteroids are often given, but controlled trials have shown them to be of little benefit.

Patients are advised to stop drinking for life as this is undoubtedly a precirrhotic condition. The prognosis is variable and, despite abstinence, the liver disease is progressive in many patients. Conversely, a few patients continue to drink heavily without developing cirrhosis.

Alcoholic cirrhosis

The acute management is described on p. 232.

Again all patients are advised to stop drinking for life. Abstinence from alcohol results in an improvement in prognosis, with a 90% 5-year survival, but with continued drinking this falls to 60%. With advanced disease (i.e. jaundice, ascites and haematemesis) the 5-year survival rate falls to 35%, with most of the deaths occurring in the first year.

Hepatoma is a complication in men in approximately 10–15% of cases.

Budd–Chiari syndrome

In this condition there is obstruction to the venous outflow of the liver due to occlusion of the hepatic vein. In one-third of patients the cause is unknown, but specific causes include hypercoagulability states such as polycythaemia vera, taking the contraceptive pill, or leukaemia. Other causes include occlusion of the hepatic vein due to posterior abdominal wall sarcomas, renal or adrenal tumours, hepatomas, hepatic infections (e.g. hydatid cyst), congenital venous webs, radiotherapy, or trauma to the liver.

The acute form presents with abdominal pain, nausea, vomiting, tender hepatomegaly and ascites. The liver biopsy shows centrilobular congestion. In the chronic form there is an enlarged liver, mild jaundice, ascites, a negative hepatojugular reflex, and splenomegaly with portal hypertension.

INVESTIGATION

Investigations show a high protein content in the ascitic fluid and characteristic histology on liver biopsy. With isotopic scanning of the liver there is uptake only in the caudate lobe, which has a different venous drainage. Venography may demonstrate the thrombosed vein.

TREATMENT

Ascites should be treated as well as any underlying cause, e.g. polycythaemia. Congenital webs should be resected surgically. A side-to-side portacaval or spenorenal anastomosis may decompress the congested liver, with considerable improvement in the clinical state of the patient. A peritoneal–jugular LeVeen shunt is occasionally useful.

DIFFERENTIAL DIAGNOSIS

A similar picture can be produced by inferior vena caval obstruction, right-sided cardiac failure or constrictive pericarditis, and appropriate investigations should be performed.

PROGNOSIS

The prognosis depends on the aetiology but some patients can survive for several years.

Veno-occlusive disease

This is due to injury of the hepatic veins and presents clinically like the Budd–Chiari syndrome. It was originally described in Jamaica, where the ingestion of the toxic alkaloids in bush tea (made from plants of the genera *Senecio*, *Heliotropium* and *Crotolaria*) caused toxic damage to the hepatic veins. It can be seen in other parts of the world and nowadays is also associated with the use of antimitotic drugs and hepatic irradiation.

Fibropolycystic diseases

These diseases are usually inherited and lead to the presence of cysts or fibrosis in the liver, kidney, and occasionally the pancreas and other organs.

Polycystic disease of the liver

Adult

This usually presents in middle age with abdominal swelling or right hypochondrial discomfort. It can also be detected by ultrasound scanning or may only be discovered at autopsy. There may or may not be hepatomegaly and bilateral irregular palpable kidneys. It is inherited as an autosomal dominant. The cysts are of variable size and consist of thin-walled cavities containing clear fluid or altered blood. Liver function is normal and complications such as oesophageal varices are very rare. The prognosis is excellent and is often dependent on whether the kidneys are involved.

Child

Childhood polycystic disease is inherited in a different way from the adult type. It is an autosomal recessive condition presenting in the first few months of life. Renal involvement is common, with cystic changes in the renal tubules.

Congenital hepatic fibrosis

In this rare condition the liver architecture is normal but there are broad collagenous fibrous bands extending from the portal tracts. It is often inherited as an autosomal recessive condition, but can also occur sporadically. It usually presents in childhood with hepatosplenomegaly and portal hypertension is common. It may present later in life and can be misdiagnosed as cirrhosis. A wedge biopsy of the liver may be required to confirm the diagnosis. The outlook is good and the condition should be distinguished from cirrhosis. Patients who bleed do well after variceal sclerotherapy or a portacaval anastomosis because of their good liver function.

Congenital intrahepatic biliary dilatation (Caroli's disease)

In this rare, non-familial disease there are saccular dilatations of the intra- or extrahepatic ducts. It can present at any age, although usually in childhood, with fever, abdominal pain and recurrent attacks of cholangitis with gram-negative septicaemia. Jaundice and portal hypertension are absent. Diagnosis is by ultrasound, PTC or ERCP.

Solitary non-parasitic cysts

These are rare and probably a variant of polycystic disease.

Liver abscess

Pyogenic abscess

These abscesses are uncommon, but may be single or multiple. The commonest cause used to be a portal pyaemia from intra-abdominal sepsis, e.g. appendicitis or perforations, but now in many cases the aetiology is not known. Biliary sepsis, particularly in the elderly, is a common cause. Other causes include trauma, bacteraemia and direct extension from, for example, a perinephric abscess.

The commonest organism found is *Escherichia coli*. Other organisms include *Streptococcus faecalis*, *Proteus vulgaris* and *Staphylococcus aureus*. *Streptococcus milleri* and anaerobic organisms such as *Bacteroides* are now more frequently seen. Often the infection is mixed. Failure to culture an organism may be due to previous antibiotic therapy or inadequate anaerobic culture.

CLINICAL FEATURES

Some patients are not acutely ill and present with malaise lasting several days or even months. Others can present with fever, rigors, anorexia, vomiting, weight loss and abdominal pain. In these patients a gram-negative septicaemia with shock can occur. On examination there may be little to find. Alternatively, the patient may be toxic, febrile and jaundiced. In such patients, the liver is tender and enlarged and there may be signs of a pleural effusion, or a pleural rub, in the right lower chest.

INVESTIGATION

Patients are often investigated as a 'pyrexia of unknown origin' (PUO) and in the mild chronic case most investigations will be normal. Often the only clue to the diagnosis is a raised serum alkaline phosphatase.

The serum bilirubin is usually raised. There is a normochromic normocytic anaemia, usually accompanied by a polymorphonuclear leucocytosis. The ESR is often raised. The serum B_{12} is very high as vitamin B_{12} is stored in and subsequently released from the liver.

Blood cultures are positive in only 30% of cases.

Imaging
Ultrasound has superceded radionuclide scans for detecting filling defects. A chest x-ray will show elevation of the right hemidiaphragm, with a pleural effusion in the severe cases.

MANAGEMENT

Aspiration of the abscess should be attempted under ultrasound control. Antibiotics should initially cover gram-positive, gram-negative and anaerobic organisms until the causative organism is identified.

Further drainage via a large bore needle under ultrasound control or surgically should almost always be performed if a localized abscess is found. The underlying cause must also be treated.

PROGNOSIS

The overall mortality depends on the nature of the underlying pathology and is approximately 50% in the ill elderly patient. A unilocular abscess in the right lobe has a better prognosis. Scattered multiple abscesses have a very high mortality with only one in five patients surviving.

Amoebic abscess (see p. 80)

This condition occurs world-wide and must be considered in patients travelling from endemic areas. *Entamoeba histolytica* (see p. 79) can be carried from the bowel to the liver in the portal venous system. Portal inflammation results, with the development of multiple microabscesses and eventually single or multiple abscesses. Clinically the onset is usually gradual but may be sudden. There is fever, anorexia, weight loss and malaise. There is often no history of dysentery. On examination the patient looks ill and has tender hepatomegaly and signs of an effusion or consolidation in the base of the right side of the chest. Jaundice is unusual.

INVESTIGATION

This is as for pyogenic abscess, plus:
- Serological tests for amoeba, e.g. haemagglutination inhibition, amoebic complement fixation test, ELISA. These are always positive, particularly if there are bowel symptoms, and remain positive after a clinical cure and therefore do not indicate current disease. A negative test, however, is good evidence against an amoebic abscess.
- Diagnostic aspiration of a fluid looking like anchovy sauce

TREATMENT

Metronidazole 800 mg three times daily is given for 10 days. Some physicians recommend repeated aspirations in addition.

COMPLICATIONS

Complications include rupture, secondary infection and septicaemia.

Non-viral infections of the liver

Schistosomiasis (see p. 89)

Schistosoma mansoni and *S. japonicum* affect the liver but *S. haematobium* rarely does so. During their life cycle the ova reach the liver via the portal system and obstruct the portal branches, producing granulomas, fibrosis and inflammation but not cirrhosis. Clinically there is hepatosplenomegaly and presinusoidal portal hypertension, which is particularly severe with *S. mansoni*.

Investigations show a raised alkaline phosphatase, and ova can be found in the stools (centrifuged deposits) and in rectal and liver biopsies. Skin tests and other immunological tests often have false results and may also be positive because of past infection.

Treatment is with praziquantel or oxamniquine.

Hydatid disease (see p. 95)

Cysts caused by *Echinococcus granulosus* are single or multiple. They usually occur in the lower part of the right lower lobe. The cyst has three layers: an outside layer derived from the host, an intermediate laminated layer, and an inner germinal layer which buds off brood capsules to form daughter cysts.

Clinically there may be no symptoms or a dull ache and swelling in the right hypochondrium. Investigations show a peripheral eosinophilia and a positive hydatid complement fixation test or haemagglutination. The Casoni skin test is no longer used because of its lack of specificity. Plain abdominal x-ray may show calcification of the outer coat of the cyst. Ultrasound and CT scan demonstrate a space-occupying lesion and may show diagnostic daughter cysts.

Needle aspiration should *not* be performed because of the risk of dissemination or fatal anaphylaxis.

Treatment is usually surgical, with removal of the cyst intact if possible after first sterilizing the cyst with formalin or alcohol. Medical treatment, e.g. with merbendazole, is unhelpful because penetration into large cysts is variable. Chronic calcified cysts can be left.

Complications include rupture, secondary infection and involvement of other organs.

The prognosis without any complications is good, although there is always the risk of rupture. Preventative measures are important, including deworming of pet dogs and prevention of pets from eating infected carcasses where possible.

Jaundice in pregnancy

Liver function is not impaired in pregnancy. Any liver disease from whatever cause can occur incidentally and coincide with pregnancy. For example, viral hepatitis accounts for 40% of all cases of jaundice during pregnancy. Pregnancy does not necessarily exacerbate established liver disease, but it is uncommon for women with advanced liver disease to conceive. There are, however, certain types of jaundice which are particularly associated with pregnancy. Three main types are seen:

Acute fatty liver of pregnancy

This is a rare, serious condition of unknown aetiology. It presents in the last trimester with symptoms of fulminant hepatitis, i.e. jaundice, vomiting, abdominal pain, possibly haematemesis and coma. Liver histology shows fine droplets of fat (microvesicules) in the liver cells with little necrosis. Immediate delivery of the child may save both baby and mother, but the maternal and fetal mortality is about 75%. The prognosis is good for those who survive. Treatment is as for liver failure.

Recurrent intrahepatic cholestasis

Patients present with pruritus and a mild jaundice, usually during the last trimester of pregnancy. There is a cholestatic jaundice with dark urine and pale stools. It does not affect the health of the mother or fetus and disappears within two weeks of delivery. Jaundice will recur during subsequent pregnancies and may also occur if the patient takes the contraceptive pill. The aetiology is unknown, but it may be a cholestatic response to a steroid produced in pregnancy. A particularly high incidence is seen in South America and Scandinavia.

Toxaemias of pregnancy

Raised serum alkaline phosphatase and aminotransferases are common, but jaundice is rare; if it occurs it is mainly haemolytic. Occasionally fulminant hepatic failure can occur.

Liver tumours

The commonest liver tumour is a secondary (metastatic) tumour, particularly from the gastrointestinal tract, breast or bronchus.

Primary liver tumours may be benign or malignant. The commonest are malignant.

MALIGNANT TUMOURS

Hepatocellular carcinoma (hepatoma)

This is one of the commonest cancers world-wide, although it is rare in the West.

AETIOLOGY

Carriers of hepatitis B have an extremely high risk of developing hepatoma. In areas where the hepatitis B virus is prevalent, 90% of patients with this cancer are hepatitis B positive. Cirrhosis is present in over

80% of these patients. Primary liver cancer is also associated with other forms of cirrhosis, e.g. alcoholic cirrhosis and haemochromatosis. Males are affected more than females; this may account for the high incidence seen in haemochromatosis and low incidence in PBC. Other suggested aetiological factors are aflatoxin (a metabolite of a fungus found in groundnuts) and androgenic steroids, and there is an association with the contraceptive pill.

PATHOLOGY

The tumour is either single or occurs as multiple nodules throughout the liver. Histologically it consists of cells resembling hepatocytes. It can metastasize via the hepatic or portal veins to the lymph nodes, bones and lungs.

CLINICAL FEATURES

Hepatoma usually presents below the age of 50 years. The clinical features include weight loss, anorexia, fever, an ache in the right hypochondrium and ascites. The rapid development of these features in a cirrhotic patient is suggestive of hepatoma. On examination, an enlarged irregular tender liver may be felt.

INVESTIGATION

Alpha-fetoprotein is usually raised. Radioisotope or ultrasound scans show large filling defects in 90% of cases. A liver biopsy, particularly under ultrasonic control, is performed for diagnosis.

TREATMENT

Surgical resection is occasionally possible. Chemotherapy and radiotherapy are unhelpful.

PROGNOSIS

Survival is seldom more than 6 months.

Cholangiocarcinoma

Cholangiocarcinomas can be extrahepatic (see p. 253) or intrahepatic. Intrahepatic adenocarcinomas arising from the bile ducts account for approximately 10% of primary tumours. They are not associated with cirrhosis or hepatitis B. In the Far East they may be associated with infestation with *Clonorchis sinensis*. The clinical features are similar to primary hepatocellular carcinoma except that jaundice is frequent with hilar tumours. Treatment is unsuccessful and patients usually die within 6 months.

BENIGN TUMOURS

The commonest benign tumour is a haemangioma. This is usually found incidentally.

Hepatic adenomas are associated with oral contraceptives. They can present with abdominal pain or intraperitoneal bleeding.

Miscellaneous conditions of the liver

Reye's syndrome

This syndrome is of unknown aetiology, but recently it has been associated with aspirin consumption in childhood. It consists of an acute encephalopathy with cerebral oedema and diffuse microvesicular fatty infiltration of the liver. It occurs mainly in children and the mortality rate is 50%.

Benign recurrent intrahepatic cholestasis

This condition often presents in children and consists of bouts of cholestatic jaundice with pruritus. Jaundice may last for weeks or months. There is no treatment; cholestyramine 12 g daily may help relieve the itching.

Indian childhood cirrhosis

This condition of children is seen in the Indian subcontinent. The cause is unknown. Eventually there is development of a micronodular cirrhosis with excess copper in the liver.

Hepatic porphyrias

These are dealt with on p. 777.

Drugs and the liver

Drug metabolism

The liver is the major site of drug metabolism. Drugs are converted from fat-soluble to water-soluble substances which can be excreted in the urine or bile. This metabolism of drugs is mediated by a group of mixed-function enzymes, including cytochrome P450, located on the smooth endoplasmic reticulum of the liver cell. It takes place in two stages:
- Phase I metabolism involves oxidation, reduction or demethylation of the drug.
- Phase II involves the conjugation of the deriva-

tives produced in Phase I with glucuronide, sulphate and glutathione. These conjugates are excreted in the urine and bile as they cannot be reabsorbed by renal tubular or bile ductular cells.

Factors affecting drug metabolism

The microsomal enzyme system. The *speed* of metabolism of drugs is dependent on the microsomal enzyme system. Certain drugs, e.g. phenytoin, barbiturates and alcohol, can themselves increase the activity of these enzymes such as cytochrome P450, i.e. cause 'enzyme induction', and are known as 'inducing agents'. Therapy with any of these drugs will produce increased metabolism of the drug and consequently a reduction in its effectiveness. Equally, if two drugs are metabolized by the same microsomal enzymes, metabolism of both drugs will be reduced, prolonging their actions.

Route of administration. Many drugs are partially inactivated on passage through the liver (first-pass effect). If this is pronounced drugs taken orally are inactive.

Liver blood flow. The rate of removal of the drug from the liver is influenced by the liver blood flow.

Competitive inhibition. Some drugs compete with bilirubin at various stages:
● Uptake by the liver, e.g. rifampicin
● Conjugation, e.g. novobiocin
● Excretion into the bile canaliculus, e.g. oral contraceptives

Drug hepatotoxicity

Many drugs impair liver function and drugs should always be considered as a cause when mildly abnormal liver function tests are found. Damage to the liver by drugs is usually classified as being either predictable (or dose-related) or non-predictable (not dose-related) (see p. 651). This classification should not be used rigidly as there is considerable overlap and many mechanisms may be involved in the production of damage.

Biochemical pathways
When a small amount of a hepatotoxic drug whose effect is dose-dependent, e.g. paracetamol, is ingested, a large proportion of it undergoes conjugation with glucuronide and sulphate, whilst the remainder is metabolized by microsomal enzymes to produce toxic derivatives which are immediately detoxified by conjugation with glutathione. If larger doses are ingested, the former pathway becomes saturated and the toxic derivative is produced at a faster rate. Once the hepatic glutathione is depleted, large amounts of the toxic metabolites accumulate and produce damage.

The 'predictability' of drugs to produce damage can, however, be affected by metabolic events preceding their ingestion. For example, chronic alcoholics may become more susceptible to liver damage because of the enzyme-inducing effects of alcohol, or ill or starving patients may become susceptible because of the depletion of hepatic glutathione produced by starvation. Many other factors such as environmental or genetic effects may be involved in determining the 'susceptibility' of certain patients to certain drugs.

Immunological mechanisms
These can be involved in the production of hepatic cell damage by certain drugs. The toxic metabolite produced by the microsomal enzymes may bind to the liver cell protein, thereby altering its antigenicity. The production of antibody against this will lead to immunologically mediated damage. An example of this mechanism is halothane-induced hepatic necrosis, which requires prior sensitization of the patient to halothane, although direct toxicity may also play a part.

Other pointers for the involvement of immunological mechanisms are the development of skin rashes, fever and arthralgia (serum sickness syndrome) following ingestion of certain drugs. Eosinophilia and circulating immune complexes and antibodies may occasionally be detected.

Hepatic damage

The type of damage produced by various drugs is shown in Table 5.14. The diagnosis of these conditions is usually by exclusion of other causes. Most reactions occur within three months of starting the drug. Monitoring liver function tests in patients on long-term treatment, e.g. antituberculosis therapy, is advisable. If a drug is suspected to be causing hepatic damage, it should be stopped immediately. Liver biopsy is of limited help in confirming the diagnosis, but occasionally hepatic eosinophilia may be seen. Sometimes diagnostic challenge with subtherapeutic doses of the drug is required after the liver function tests have returned to normal to prove the diagnosis.

Individual drugs

Paracetamol
In high doses paracetamol produces liver cell necrosis (see above). The toxic metabolite binds irreversibly to liver cell membranes. Overdosage is discussed on p. 665.

Halothane
This commonly used anaesthetic agent rarely produces a hepatitis in patients having repeated exposures. The mechanism is thought to be a hypersensitivity reaction. An unexplained fever occurs

Table 5.14 Some drugs producing hepatic damage. Percentages indicate the proportion of patients who develop abnormal liver function tests.

Type of reaction	Drug
Hepatocellular damage:	
Dose-dependent	Paracetamol Salicylates Tetracycline

Dose-independent	Antidepressants:
	   Monoamine-oxidase inhibitors (1%) (particularly iproniazid)
	   Tricyclic antidepressants (<1%)
	Antituberculous drugs
	   Isoniazid (10–20%)
	   Para-aminosalicylic (PAS) (5%)
	   Pyrazinamide or ethambutol (10%)
	   Rifampicin
	Anticonvulsants and antispasmodics
	   Phenytoin
	   Dantrolene (1–2%)
	   Carbamazepine
	   Phenobarbitone
	   Sodium valproate
	Anti-inflammatory drugs
	   Indomethacin
	   Non-steroidals
	Antibiotics (uncommon)
	   Penicillins
	   Sulphonamides
	Anaesthetics
	   Halothane (20% with repeated exposures)
	Cardiovascular drugs
	   Amiodarone
	   Methyldopa (5%)
	   Perhexiline maleate
	Antifungal drugs
	   Ketoconazole

Cholestasis	
Pure cholestasis	Oral contraceptives Synthetic anabolic steroids
Cholestatic hepatitis	Chlorpromazine (1%) Erythromycin estolate (38%) Antirheumatic drugs, e.g. sodium aurothiomalate Antithyroid drugs, e.g. carbimazole Hypoglycaemic drugs, e.g. chlorpropamide (25%)
Fatty change	Tetracycline
Hepatic fibrosis	Methotrexate
Chronic active hepatitis	Methyldopa Nitrofurantoin Sulphonamides Oxyphenisatin (withdrawn)
Granulomatous reaction	Sulphonamides (long-acting) Methotrexate Hydralazine Allopurinol Chlorpropamide
Liver tumours and peliosis hepatis	17α-Alkylated synthetic androgens (hepatocellular carcinomas) Oral contraceptives (benign adenomas)

approximately 10 days after the second or subsequent halothane anaesthetic and is followed by jaundice, typically with a hepatitic picture. Most patients recover spontaneously but there is a high mortality in severe cases. There are no chronic sequelae.

Steroids

Cholestasis is caused by natural and synthetic oestrogens as well as methyltestosterone. These agents interfere with canalicular biliary flow and cause a pure cholestasis. Cholestasis is rare with the contraceptive pill because of the low dosage used. However, the contraceptive pill is associated with an increased incidence of gallstones, hepatic adenomas (rarely hepatic carcinomas), the Budd–Chiari syndrome and peliosis hepatis. The latter condition, which also occurs with anabolic steroids, consists of dilatation of the hepatic sinusoids to form blood-filled lakes.

Phenothiazines

Phenothiazines, e.g. chlorpromazine, can produce a cholestatic picture due to a hypersensitivity reaction. It occurs in 1% of patients, usually within 4 weeks of starting the drug. Typically it is associated with a fever and eosinophilia. Recovery occurs on stopping the drug.

Anti-tuberculous chemotherapy

Isoniazid produces elevated aminotransferases in 10–20% of patients. Hepatic necrosis with jaundice occurs in a smaller percentage. The hepatotoxicity of isoniazid appears to be related to acetylator status as the damage is due to the metabolites.

Rifampicin produces a hepatitis, usually within 3 weeks of starting the drug, particularly in patients on high doses.

Pyrazinamide produces abnormal liver function tests and, rarely, liver cell necrosis.

Drug prescribing in patients with liver disease

The metabolism of drugs is impaired in severe liver disease (with jaundice and ascites) as the removal of many drugs depends on liver blood flow and the integrity of the hepatocyte. In general, therefore, the effect of drugs is prolonged by liver disease and also by cholestasis. This is further accentuated by portosystemic shunting, which diminishes the first-pass extraction of drugs. With hypoproteinaemia there is decreased protein-binding of some drugs and bilirubin competes with many drugs for the binding sites on serum albumin. In patients with portosystemic encephalopathy, care must be taken in prescribing drugs with a central depressant action.

Gallstones

Bile secretion

Bile consists of water, electrolytes, bile acids, cholesterol and phospholipids. Two processes are involved in bile secretion:
- In the *bile salt-dependent process* there is active secretion of bile salts; water and electrolytes follow down an osmotic and electrical gradient.
- In the *bile salt-independent process*, bile flow is linked to sodium transport, which is dependent on Na^+-K^+ ATPase activity.

Bile ductules reabsorb and secrete bicarbonate, the secretion being stimulated by secretin. The average total bile flow is approximately 1 l per day. The mucosa of the gallbladder absorbs 80–90% of the water and electrolytes, but is impermeable to bile acids and cholesterol. The bile thus concentrated is stored in the gallbladder in the fasting state. Following a meal, cholecystokinin is secreted by the duodenal mucosa and stimulates contraction of the gallbladder and relaxation of the sphincter of Oddi, so that bile enters the duodenum. An adequate bile flow is dependent on bile salts being returned to the liver by the enterohepatic circulation.

Incidence of gallstones

Gallstones are present in 10–20% of the population in the Western Hemisphere, but the exact prevalence is unknown. Gallstones are rare in the Far East and Africa. They occur twice as frequently in young women than in men but the difference decreases with increasing age.

Types of gallstones

Gallstones can be divided into those composed of cholesterol and those composed of bile pigment. Cholesterol stones, which account for 80% of all gallstones in the Western Hemisphere, contain more than 70% cholesterol, often with some bile pigment and calcium (mixed stones). Pure cholesterol stones are often solitary.

Cholesterol gallstones. Cholesterol is partly derived from dietary sources. In addition, it is synthesized, chiefly in the liver, but also in the small intestine, skin and adrenals. The rate-limiting step in cholesterol synthesis is β-hydroxy-β-methylglutaryl-CoA (HMGCoA) reductase, which catalyses the first step, i.e. the conversion of acetate to mevalonate. The cholesterol formed is secreted into bile. Unesterified cholesterol is insoluble in water and is held in solution in bile by the formation of mixed micelles composed of cholesterol, bile salts and phospholipid.

Cholesterol stones develop in bile which has an excess of cholesterol relative to bile salts and phospholipids (supersaturated bile). This could occur because of excess of cholesterol or because of a decrease in bile salts. There is a reduced bile salt pool in patients with cholesterol gallstones and the pool circulates more frequently. This may account for the reduction in the rate-limiting cholesterol-7α-hydroxylase found in some patients (feedback inhibition) (see p. 213).

Diminished bile salt synthesis is not the only cause of supersaturated bile; there appears to be an increase in HMGCoA reductase with an increase in cholesterol secretion into bile.

It is likely that factors other than cholesterol saturation are required to form gallstones, as saturated bile is found in normal subjects during an overnight fast. Other factors involved in gallstone formation include the rate of cholesterol crystallization and the state of the gallbladder. Mucus may possibly contribute to the formation of a nidus around which stones can develop. The role of infection is unknown. Definite risk factors for gallstones are shown in Table 5.15.

Bile pigment stones. These stones contain calcium salts of bilirubin, phosphate and carbonate, and the biliary lipids are normal. Little is known about their formation, except in haemolysis, where there is increased bilirubin production. In the Far East bile pigment stones are associated with infection of the biliary tract.

Clinical presentation of gallstones (Fig. 5.19)

The majority of gallstones remain in the gallbladder and are asymptomatic.

A gallstone may impact in the neck of the gallbladder or in the cystic duct, leading to biliary colic or acute cholecystitis.

Finally, gallstones may pass into the common bile duct, giving rise to biliary obstruction, which produces biliary colic and sometimes cholestatic jaundice. Bacterial infection can occur and produce cholangitis.

Table 5.15 Risk factors for cholesterol gallstones.

Age
Sex (F > M)
Obesity
Diet, e.g. high in animal fat
Drugs, e.g. contraceptive pill
Ileal disease or resection

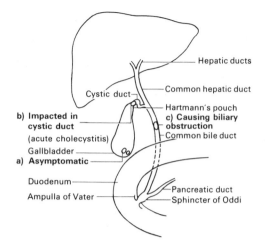

Fig. 5.19 Diagram of the gallbladder and biliary tree showing sites at which gallstones can cause clinical problems.

Rarely a gallstone may perforate through the wall of an inflamed gallbladder into the intestine, producing a fistula.

Gallstones do not give rise to any other symptom complex, and the idea that they produce indigestion, chronic right hypochondrial pain or intolerance to fatty food is based on a false correlation. Gallstones and upper abdominal symptoms are both common, so great care must be taken to establish that the two are truly related. Fair, fat, fertile females of 40 have the same chance of having gallstones as the rest of the general population (10–20%). Thus if they are investigated regardless of symptoms, gallstones will obviously be seen frequently by chance alone.

Asymptomatic (silent) gallstones

Gallstones may be discovered accidentally when a patient is being investigated for some other reason. They require no treatment, as the natural history is for them to remain asymptomatic, with only 18% having symptoms over a 15-year period.

Acute cholecystitis

PATHOPHYSIOLOGY

In over 90% of cases, the gallbladder contains gallstones. Initially there is obstruction to the neck of the gallbladder or the cystic duct by an impacted stone, leading to distension and inflammation. The inflammation is usually sterile, but within 24 h gut organisms can be cultured from the gallbladder. Occasionally the inflammation may be mild and quickly subsides, leaving a gallbladder distended by mucus (mucocele). In this situation the patient may only have slight abdominal pain with a palpable gallbladder.

More commonly, however, the inflammation is more severe, involving the whole wall and giving rise to localized peritonitis and acute pain. The gall-bladder may be distended by pus (an empyema). Very occasionally acute gangrenous cholecystitis occurs, with perforation and a more generalized peritonitis.

CLINICAL FEATURES

The disease is classically seen in females aged 20 to 40 years, but it can occur at any age. The main symptoms are severe pain in the epigastrium and right hypochondrium. The pain is constant and lasts anything up to 24 h and can radiate to the back and shoulder. It may be accompanied by nausea and vomiting.

EXAMINATION

The patient is usually ill, with a fever and shallow respirations. Right hypochondrial tenderness is present, being worse on inspiration (Murphy's sign). There is guarding and rebound tenderness. Jaundice is occasionally present, but usually this implies a stone in the common duct.

INVESTIGATION

- *Blood count.* A moderate leucocytosis is found.
- *Biochemistry.* The serum bilirubin, alkaline phosphatase and aspartate aminotransferase may be slightly raised.
- *X-ray.* A plain abdominal x-ray shows gallstones in 10% of cases.
- *Ultrasound examination.* This will often reveal gallstones.
- *HIDA scintiscan.* This is extremely valuable and shows blockage of the cystic duct.

Further investigation of the biliary tract is usually left until the patient recovers from the acute episode.

DIFFERENTIAL DIAGNOSIS

The differential diagnosis includes other abdominal emergencies, such as a perforated peptic ulcer, retrocaecal appendicitis and acute pancreatitis. Right basal pneumonia and myocardial infarction must also be considered.

MANAGEMENT

The majority of patients improve with conservative management consisting of bedrest, nil by mouth and intravenous fluids, with the addition of an antibiotic, usually ampicillin or co-trimoxazole. In all but the mild cases pain relief with an opiate is required.

In the absence of vomiting, the patient can soon tolerate oral fluids and nasogastric aspiration

is not often required. Signs of complications such as generalized peritonitis or gangrene of the gall-bladder (which causes increasing pain and fever) are an indication for surgery, particularly in the elderly.

Cholecystectomy within days of the acute attack has been advocated for all patients who are not an anaesthetic risk. A firm diagnosis can usually be made using a HIDA scan. Alternatively, cholecystectomy can be performed 2–3 months later. There is little to choose between the two approaches, although early surgery means only one hospital visit and no possibility of a recurrent attack while awaiting surgery to be performed, and does not increase operative morbidity or mortality.

Chronic cholecystitis

There is no doubt that gallbladders studied histologically can show signs of chronic inflammation and occasionally a small, shrunken gallbladder is found either radiologically or on ultrasound examination. There are, however, no symptoms and signs that can conclusively be shown to be due to chronic cholecystitis and this clinical diagnosis should therefore not be made. Most patients with chronic right hypochondrial pain suffer from functional bowel disease.

Common bile duct stones

These may be asymptomatic or they may present with any one or all of the triad of abdominal pain, jaundice and fever. The pain is usually severe and situated in the epigastrium and right hypochondrium (see p. 151).

The pain may be accompanied by vomiting. It usually lasts for a few hours and then clears up, only to return days, weeks or even months later. In between attacks the patient is well.

The jaundice is variable in degree, depending on the amount of obstruction. The urine is dark and the stools pale. High fevers and rigors indicate cholangitis.

The liver is moderately enlarged if the obstruction lasts for more than a few hours. Prolonged biliary obstruction or repeated attacks lead to secondary biliary cirrhosis, but this is now rare.

INVESTIGATION

- *Blood count.* A leucocytosis is present.
- *Blood cultures.* These may grow an intestinal organism (*E. coli*, *S. faecalis*).
- *Liver function tests.* These indicate a cholestatic picture (see p. 222), with a raised conjugated bilirubin and alkaline phosphatase in the serum and relatively normal serum aminotransferases.
- *Prothrombin time.* This may become elevated over a few weeks due to poor vitamin K absorption.

- *X-ray.* A plain abdominal x-ray may reveal gallstones.
- *Ultrasound examination.* This may reveal a dilated common bile duct and sometimes gallstones (see p. 216).
- *ERCP.* This may be needed to confirm the diagnosis (Fig. 5.20).

DIFFERENTIAL DIAGNOSIS

The differential diagnosis includes all causes of jaundice.

MANAGEMENT

The acute episode is allowed to settle and the serum bilirubin usually falls to normal levels. During this stage the patient only requires pain relief, but occasionally antibiotics are necessary.

The serum alkaline phosphatase falls slower than the serum bilirubin, and if the patient is seen some time after an acute attack, elevation of this enzyme may be the only evidence of biliary tract disease.

Following ultrasonic examination, surgery or endoscopic removal of the stones should then be considered (see below).

Occasionally in the very ill patient with jaundice, immediate surgery may be necessary to relieve the pressure in the bile duct. Acute renal failure is a recognized complication of surgery and all such severely ill patients should be treated prophylactically with intravenous mannitol infusion during the operative period.

TREATMENT OF GALLSTONES

Cholecystectomy

This is a safe procedure with a mortality of less than 0.1% in experienced hands. An increased mortality occurs in obese and elderly patients.

Post-cholecystectomy syndrome
Some patients continue to complain of right hypochondrial pain, flatulence, indigestion and intolerance to fatty foods after cholecystectomy, despite a normal radiological appearance of the biliary tree. In the vast majority of these patients the wrong diagnosis was originally made and the patient was suffering from functional bowel disease, the gallstones being an incidental finding. The occurrence of severe pain with jaundice suggests a retained stone in the common duct.

Exploration of the common duct

The duct should be explored at operation in all patients with a history of jaundice or in whom the history suggests biliary colic. The duct is opened and examined with a choledochoscope, if available, and cholangiography performed. This procedure increases the mortality of the operation over that of simple cholecystectomy. All stones must be removed.

A T-tube is placed in the common bile duct at operation and bile is allowed to drain through it. Prior to removal of the T-tube, further cholangiography is performed to see whether any stones remain.

Retained stones

These can be removed via the T-tube if still in position, using an endoscope, or can be dissolved chemically by the infusion of mono-octanoin down the T-tube.

Removal via the T-tube. Removal of stones is possible through a large T-tube (14 French gauge) using a steerable catheter under fluoroscopic control.

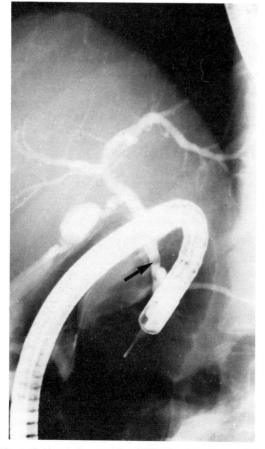

Fig. 5.20 X-ray showing an ERCP. The bile duct and the pancreatic duct are outlined by dye. There is a gallstone at the lower end of the common bile duct (arrow).

Endoscopic removal. Stones can be removed from the common bile duct following a sphincterotomy in two ways:
- They can be allowed to pass naturally through the enlarged opening.
- They can be removed endoscopically using a Dormia basket.

The latter technique is used chiefly for patients who are found to have common duct stones after a cholecystectomy. It is also used in the frail, elderly patient with an intact gallbladder and symptoms of a common duct stone.

Gallstone dissolution

Cholesterol gallstones can be dissolved by the bile acids chenodeoxycholic acid and ursodeoxycholic acid, which increase cholesterol solubility in bile. They only dissolve radiolucent stones in a functioning gallbladder and not calcified stones.

Gallstone dissolution takes anything from 6 months to 2 years and when the treatment is stopped the gallstones recur. Chenodeoxycholate also produces diarrhoea. For these reasons, as well as the cost, medical therapy is not recommended for the majority of patients with symptoms of gallstone disease and dissolution is rarely advocated.

COMPLICATIONS OF GALLSTONES

- Cholangitis and obstructive jaundice (see above)
- Carcinoma of the gallbladder
- Pancreatitis (p. 255)
- Gallstone ileus and biliary enteric fistula. Gallstones can occasionally erode through the wall of the gallbladder into the intestine. They can cause obstruction, mainly in the terminal ileum, but occasionally in the duodenum.

Tumours of the biliary tract

Primary carcinoma of the gallbladder

This adenocarcinoma represents < 1% of all cancers. It occurs chiefly in those over 70 years of age and is commoner in females. Gallstones are usually present but a definite relationship is uncertain. The presenting features are of jaundice and occasionally right hypochondrial pain. A mass may be palpable in the right hypochondrium. The diagnosis is often made at operation and cholecystectomy is performed if possible. Few patients survive 1 year.

Cholangiocarcinoma (see p. 246)

This sometimes affects the extrahepatic biliary tree, giving rise to jaundice. Surgery, if possible, is the only effective treatment. Alternatively, a stent or tube can be passed through the obstruction during PTC or ERCP. The prognosis is poor.

Periampullary tumours

These tumours arise from the common bile duct, the ampulla of Vater or the head of the pancreas. All give rise to obstructive jaundice. Carcinoma of the ampulla can sometimes be resected, with a 40% 5-year survival rate (compare with pancreatic carcinoma, p. 258).

Miscellaneous conditions of the biliary tract

Primary sclerosing cholangitis

Primary sclerosing cholangitis results from inflammation and fibrosis of the bile ducts leading to multiple areas of narrowing throughout the biliary system. The cause is unknown.

Fifty per cent of patients have inflammatory bowel disease. In such cases there may not be any symptoms and the diagnosis is suggested by a raised serum alkaline phosphatase. Symptoms are pruritus, jaundice and occasionally abdominal pain. Portal hypertension can develop.

An ERCP will show the multiple strictures. Treatment is unsatisfactory. In half of the patients the disease runs a benign course. Steroids and azathioprine are of unproven value and should be avoided because of their side-effects.

Acute cholangitis

This is due to bacterial infection of the bile ducts and is always secondary to bile duct abnormalities. The common causes are common duct stones, biliary strictures, neoplasms, or following ERCP in the presence of large duct obstruction.

The symptoms are fever, often with a rigor, upper abdominal pain and jaundice. All three symptoms are present in 70% of cases. Older patients can present with collapse and gram-negative septicaemia.

Specific signs may be minimal but tenderness over the liver occurs.

When all three symptoms are present the diagnosis is not difficult, but the patient can present with only a fever and an accompanying leucocytosis.

Blood cultures are often positive (usually for *E. coli*) and a severe gram-negative septicaemia can occur.

Treatment is with intravenous amoxycillin 1 g 6-hourly with intravenous gentamicin 2–5 mg·kg^{-1} daily in divided doses for severe cases.

Suppurative cholangitis can occur as a complication. The fever continues and shock develops despite adequate antibiotics. Urgent decompression of the duct should be performed endoscopically or surgically.

Non-calculous cholecystitis

Occasionally cholecystitis occurs in diabetes mellitus, polyarteritis nodosa and systemic infections.

Cholesterolosis of the gallbladder

In this condition deposits of cholesterol are seen in the mucosal wall, producing a fine yellow pattern on a red background (strawberry gallbladder). Cholesterol stones may or may not be present. The relationship to symptoms is unclear.

Adenomyomatosis of the gallbladder

This may be found as an incidental finding on a cholecystogram and consists of thickening of the mucosal and muscle layers with the presence of Rokitansky–Aschoff sinuses, often associated with small gallstones. It does not usually produce symptoms.

Choledochal cyst

This is a congenital cystic dilatation of the extra-hepatic bile ducts producing jaundice and abdominal pain. Fifty per cent of the patients do not present until early adult life. Treatment is surgical.

Haemobilia

Haemobilia can occur due to hepatic trauma, sometimes due to a tumour, and rarely after liver biopsy. Blood enters the biliary tree and either produces obstructive jaundice or gastrointestinal bleeding.

The pancreas

Structure and function

The pancreas extends retroperitoneally across the posterior abdominal wall from the second part of the duodenum to the spleen. The head is encircled by the duodenum; the body, which forms the main bulk of the organ, ends in a tail which lies in contact with the spleen. The main pancreatic duct usually joins the common bile duct to enter the duodenum as a single duct at the ampulla of Vater. The main pancreatic duct has many tributary ductules and gradually tapers towards the tail of the pancreas.

Exocrine cells form 98% of the human pancreas. The pancreatic acinar cells synthesize the pancreatic enzymes and form a ductal system that eventually joins into the main pancreatic duct.

The main regulators of pancreatic exocrine secretion are the hormones secretin and cholecystokinin (CCK). Enzymes produced are amylase, lipase, colipase, phospholipase and proteases (trypsinogen and chymotrypsinogen). The proteases are secreted in the inactive form but are then activated in the duodenum by enterokinase. The secretions also contain water and electrolytes, chiefly sodium bicarbonate.

The endocrine pancreas consists of hormone-producing cells arranged in nests or islets—the islets of Langerhans. They do not connect directly to the duct system. There are four main types of islet cell and these have different secretory granules in their cytoplasm:
- The beta cell, which is the commonest cell, produces insulin
- Alpha cells produce glucagon
- D cells produce somatostatin
- PP cells produce pancreatic polypeptide (PP)

Investigation (see Table 5.16)

Endocrine function

Assessment of endocrine function is only useful if a hormone-secreting tumour is suspected and the serum measurements are often diagnostic. Plasma PP is raised with all endocrine tumours. The glucose tolerance test is seldom performed as it is affected by so many parameters.

Exocrine function

- *Serum amylase measurement* is useful in acute disease but is of no value in chronic disease.
- *Measurement of duodenal enzymes*, either after hormone stimulation or after food, is only sometimes helpful in the diagnosis of chronic pancreatitis because of the large reserve in enzyme capacity. A tube is passed into the duodenum and pancreatic secretions are collected after stimulation. Stimulation with secretin or CCK causes a rise in bicarbonate and enzyme, e.g. trypsin levels, which are low with chronic disease. The differential

Table 5.16 Investigations available for the assessment of pancreatic disease.

Exocrine
Serum amylase
Duodenal enzymes after:
   Hormone stimulation with CCK and secretin
   Food stimulation (Lundh meal)
Fat excretion
   Faecal fat (see p. 176)
   Breath tests

Endocrine
Serum levels of:
   Insulin
   Glucagon
   Pancreatic polypeptide
Glucose tolerance test measuring glucose and insulin

Visualization of the pancreas
Abdominal x-ray—to detect calcification
Barium meal—to show an abnormal duodenal loop
Ultrasound ⎫ To demonstrate size and presence of calcification, tumours,
CT scan   ⎬ pseudocyst (NB. Percutaneous biopsies can be taken.)
ERCP—to examine the ductular system
Angiography—to detect tumours

diagnosis between pancreatic tumour and pancreatitis is difficult. These tests have been largely superseded by imaging techniques. The Lundh test is performed in a similar fashion, the stimulation being produced by a meal. Measurement of trypsin and lipase is undertaken. These are low in chronic pancreatitis. The Lundh meal test is particularly useful in the investigation of steatorrhoea.

- *Faecal fat estimation* is performed to demonstrate steatorrhoea. A breath test can also be used; here the amount of $^{14}CO_2$ in expired air is measured following oral ingestion of a labelled fatty acid compared with a labelled triglyceride (e.g. ^{14}C-oleic acid compared with ^{14}C-triolein). Impaired triglyceride absorption with normal fatty acid absorption indicates that pancreatic disease is the cause of the steatorrhoea.

Visualization of the pancreas

This now largely depends on ultrasound examination and CT scan to detect pancreatic size and shape, and the presence of cysts or tumours. An ERCP can be used to outline the pancreatic ducts. Selective catheterization of the splenic artery shows irregularity and encasement in carcinoma.

A combination of two or three tests is often necessary and none of the investigations is diagnostic. Fine needle aspiration of any abnormality discovered can be performed under ultrasound or CT scan control. The presence of malignant cells in the aspirate indicates tumour but,

of course, a negative sample does not exclude malignancy.

Pancreatitis

Classification
The Marseilles classification divides pancreatitis into:

- Acute pancreatitis ⎫ Full recovery of
- Acute recurrent   ⎬ the gland to
  pancreatitis   ⎭ normal
- Chronic pancreatitis ⎫
- Chronic relapsing   ⎬ Permanent damage
  pancreatitis   ⎭

Aetiology
Acute pancreatitis is associated with gallstone disease, possibly alcohol, and a number of less common causes, as shown in Table 5.17.

Alcohol undoubtedly damages the pancreas and can cause an acute 'episode' of pancreatitis. However, the gland has almost invariably been previously damaged by alcohol, so that it is more correct to use the term 'chronic relapsing pancreatitis' for acute episodes seen in heavy alcohol consumers. In contrast, gallstones cause acute pancreatitis which may be recurrent, but they are rarely

Table 5.17 Causes of pancreatitis.

Acute
Gallstones
? Alcohol
Viral infections, e.g. coxsackie B, mumps
Ischaemia
Pancreatic tumours
Hyperparathyroidism
Hyperlipidaemia
Drugs, e.g. corticosteroids, azathioprine
Iatrogenic, e.g. post-surgical, post-ERCP
Idiopathic

Chronic
Alcohol (> 85%)
Protein–energy malnutrition
Hyperlipidaemia
Idiopathic

associated with chronic pancreatitis with permanent damage to the gland.

Acute pancreatitis

PATHOGENESIS

The exact mechanism by which pancreatic necrosis occurs is unclear. Associated gallstones are mainly found in the gallbladder and only occasionally in the common bile duct. Reflux of bile up the pancreatic duct associated with occlusion of the ampulla may play a role in the pathogenesis. Autodigestion of the pancreas by proteolytic enzymes (particularly trypsin and phospholipase A) released in the pancreas rather than in the intestinal lumen may also be involved in the pathogenesis. Active enzymes could digest cell membranes, leading to proteolysis, oedema, vascular damage and necrosis. The mildest form of pancreatitis is characterized by intestinal oedema with an inflammatory exudate (oedematous pancreatitis), while in the severe form there is pancreatic necrosis and haemorrhage (haemorrhagic pancreatitis).

CLINICAL FEATURES

These vary depending on the severity of the attack. In all patients the principal symptom is abdominal pain which is usually localized to the epigastrium or upper abdomen. It may radiate to the back between the scapulae. The pain will vary from mild discomfort to excruciating pain in severe cases. Rarely, acute pancreatitis can occur in the absence of pain.

Nausea and vomiting accompany the pain in most cases.

Physical examination may reveal tenderness, guarding and rigidity of the abdomen, with varying degrees of shock depending on the severity of the attack. Rarely, body wall ecchymoses, e.g. umbilical

(Cullen's sign) or in the flanks (Turner's sign), occur. The remaining clinical features depend on the local and systemic complications that occur (Table 5.18).

Local pancreatic complications can occur with mild attacks of pancreatitis, but systemic complications only occur with severe attacks.

INVESTIGATION AND DIAGNOSIS

The clinical manifestations are so varied that pancreatitis must be considered in the differential diagnosis of all causes of upper abdominal pain. Most present as an acute abdomen and differentiation from an acute perforated ulcer is the most difficult, as both may give rise to abdominal rigidity.

The diagnosis of acute pancreatitis depends on the serum amylase. A raised serum amylase level can be seen in other acute abdominal emergencies such as acute cholecystitis and perforated peptic ulcer, but if the serum amylase level is five times greater than normal, acute pancreatitis is very likely. However, the serum amylase cannot be entirely relied upon and must be evaluated in conjunction with the history and physical signs; if there is doubt about the diagnosis exploratory laparotomy must be performed to exclude a potentially fatal but treatable non-pancreatic lesion.

Peritoneal aspiration and lavage, with estimation of amylase in the peritoneal fluid obtained, is particularly useful in difficult cases. Ultrasound or CT

Table 5.18 Complications of acute pancreatitis.

Pancreatic
  Pseudocyst
  Abscess
  Ascites

Intestinal
  Paralytic ileus
  GI haemorrhage

Hepatobiliary
  Jaundice

Systemic
  Metabolic
    Malnutrition
    Hypocalcaemia
    Hypoglycaemia
  Haematological
    Disseminated intravascular coagulation
    Portal vein thrombosis
  Renal
    Acute renal failure
  Cardiovascular
    Circulatory failure (shock)
  Respiratory
    Hypoxic acute respiratory failure

Fat necrosis

scan may reveal a swollen pancreas, and an x-ray may show gallstones, all of which help with the diagnosis.

The differential diagnosis includes all acute abdominal conditions.

Factors indicating the severity, which is assessed chiefly on blood investigations, are given in Table 5.19.

TREATMENT

Nasogastric suction is necessary to reduce vomiting and abdominal distension even in mild cases. All feeding is stopped and in severe cases nothing is given by mouth for weeks and intravenous nutrition is required (see p. 143). Water and electrolyte replacement and analgesia with an opiate (other than morphine) are necessary. No form of drug therapy has been shown to help and the efficacy of peritoneal lavage which is sometimes used for severe cases is in doubt.

Management of shock plus respiratory failure (see p. 635) is required.

LOCAL COMPLICATIONS

Pseudocysts (see also p. 258)
These are uncommon in the acute attacks and do not usually require treatment per se. Large collections persisting for weeks can be aspirated or removed surgically.

Pancreatic abscesses
Secondary infection of a peripancreatic collection of fluid may occur, usually after about 2 weeks. The clinical features are persistent fever, leucocytosis and abdominal distension, with a possible palpable mass. Patients are usually very ill with the accompanying respiratory, cardiac and renal problems.

Surgical drainage with vigorous antibiotic therapy and general support of the patient is required as the disease has a long clinical course of several months.

Pancreatic ascites
This is usually associated with chronic pancreatitis.

Table 5.19 Factors indicating severe pancreatitis and a poor prognosis.

Age	>55 years
WBC	$>16 \times 10^9/l$
Blood urea	>16 mmol$\cdot$l^{-1}
Serum albumin	<30 g$\cdot$l^{-1}
Serum calcium	<2 mmol$\cdot$l^{-1}
P_aO_2	<60 mmHg (8.0 kPa)

PROGNOSIS

The mortality rate varies from 1% in mild cases to 50% in severe cases. With multiple complications and the presence of all the bad prognostic signs, the mortality is nearer 100%. The patients who recover may have recurrent attacks, depending on the aetiology and whether accompanying gallstones are dealt with.

Chronic pancreatitis

PATHOGENESIS

The majority of cases occur as a result of high alcohol consumption and it is in these cases that the pathology has been most studied. The earliest change appears to be deposition of protein plugs within pancreatic ducts. These then lead to ductular dilatation followed by acinar atrophy. There is some accompanying infiltration but this is variable. Extensive fibrous tissue is deposited near the pancreatic ducts. Eventually only a few acinar and islet cells remain, with widely dilated pancreatic ducts. Intraluminal calcification of the protein plugs occurs, leading to stone formation.

Chronic pancreatitis is not reversible but it is possible that the disease will arrest if the patient stops drinking. However, because patients often continue to take small amounts of alcohol, the disease is most often progressive.

CLINICAL FEATURES

The major symptom is abdominal pain situated mainly in the epigastrium and upper abdomen and radiating to the back. The pain can be severe; in some cases it is comparable to that occurring in acute pancreatitis.

Continuing episodes of pain may occur; sometimes these are mild and of brief duration. In other cases there may be chronic pain interspersed by acute episodes (relapsing pancreatitis). The relationship to alcohol is variable; nevertheless, some acute episodes seem to be precipitated by heavy alcohol consumption.

The abdominal pain is accompanied by severe weight loss due to anorexia.

Steatorrhoea occurs when the secretion of pancreatic lipase is reduced by 90%. It occurs in about half the patients. The development of diabetes is more common. The steatorrhoea is often severe, and the patient may notice drops of oil in the lavatory pan. Both diabetes and steatorrhoea occur more commonly with calcified pancreatitis.

Less common presentations include biliary obstruction with jaundice and occasionally cholangitis. Obstruction of the splenic vein can lead to portal hypertension.

INVESTIGATION

This includes assessment of some of the endocrine and exocrine functions as outlined earlier, as well as visualization of the pancreas. The serum amylase is of little value in chronic pancreatitis but may be raised during an acute episode of pain.

Patients with pain are investigated using ultrasound or CT scan, which show abnormalities in size and the presence of calcification not seen on a plain x-ray. An ERCP is also useful in these patients to confirm the diagnosis. Dilatation of the pancreatic duct, sometimes with stones or stenotic areas, can be identified. Early cases are difficult to diagnose and a combination of all tests with a strong clinical suspicion is necessary.

Patients presenting with steatorrhoea require a Lundh test to estimate exocrine function (see p. 255).

DIFFERENTIAL DIAGNOSIS

Carcinoma of the pancreas must be suspected, particularly when the history is short; occasionally laparotomy may be necessary to distinguish between these two conditions.

TREATMENT

In alcoholic pancreatitis the patient should stop drinking alcohol.

The pain needs to be controlled, often with narcotics, with the problem of addiction. Surgery is used for the treatment of intractable pain, pancreatic resection combined with drainage of an obstructed pancreatic duct into the small bowel being required. The use of surgery is controversial; good results are only obtained in a small number of cases, usually those who stop drinking.

Steatorrhoea is treated with a low-fat diet, pancreatic supplements, e.g. pancreatin 2–4 g with each meal, and cimetidine 400 mg twice daily. Diabetes mellitus is treated with diet, oral hypoglycaemic agents and/or insulin as appropriate. The insulin requirement is greater than in idiopathic diabetes, and patients may experience frequent or severe hypoglycaemia. This may be because pancreatic glucagon is lacking.

COMPLICATIONS

The commonest complication is a pancreatic pseudocyst. These are found very frequently if careful ultrasound examinations are performed. Small cysts require no treatment. Large cysts can give rise to increased pain, nausea and vomiting 3–4 weeks after the onset of the most recent attack of pain. A smooth, tender mass may be palpable and the cyst can be easily identified using ultrasound. Surgical treatment has been used for most large pseudocysts, but a more conservative approach, with aspiration and close follow-up using ultrasound examination, can now be advocated.

Pancreatic ascites occurs, usually in alcoholic pancreatitis, when there is a communication between the pancreatic duct and the peritoneal cavity. The amylase content of the ascitic fluid is high.

A good prognosis depends on complete alcohol abstention.

Carcinoma of the pancreas

The incidence of pancreatic carcinoma is steadily increasing in Western countries. This tumour is now the fourth commonest cause of cancer death in the USA. The incidence increases with age and most patients are over 60 years of age. Males are affected more than females.

There are no known aetiological factors, but the increasing incidence has been attributed to an increase in both smoking and the consumption of alcohol. Excess coffee ingestion has also been implicated.

Most carcinomas of the pancreas are adenocarcinomas arising from duct epithelium. In 60% of cases the tumour is in the head of the pancreas. The tumour spreads locally to involve lymph nodes and the liver.

CLINICAL FEATURES

Carcinoma of the head of the pancreas or the ampulla of Vater presents with painless jaundice due to obstruction of the common duct. However, most patients will have pain at some time in the course of their disease. Weight loss also occurs.

Carcinoma of the body or tail of the pancreas presents with abdominal pain, anorexia and weight loss. The pain is often a dull, boring pain which radiates through to the back. It may be relieved by sitting forward. Jaundice is rare. Diabetes may occur and there is an increased incidence of thrombophlebitis.

In carcinoma of the head of the pancreas examination will reveal jaundice with the dilated gallbladder sometimes being palpable (Courvoisier's sign). A dilated gallbladder is not found with gallstone disease because of the accompanying chronic inflammation of the gallbladder.

A palpable mass can be felt in 20% of patients, with hepatomegaly being present in most cases eventually.

INVESTIGATION

The glucose tolerance test may indicate diabetes; other haematological or biochemical tests are not helpful.

Diagnosis is now usually made using ultrasound or CT scan, but in almost all cases by the time the tumour is visualized resection is impossible. Duodenoscopy with ERCP may detect tumour of the head of the pancreas or of the ampulla.

DIFFERENTIAL DIAGNOSIS

The differential diagnosis includes all causes of painless jaundice and persistent upper abdominal pain in the elderly.

TREATMENT

Resection of the tumour with total pancreatectomy is not usually possible and as this operation carries a very high mortality and morbidity it is seldom attempted. Jaundice from carcinoma of the head of the pancreas is usually relieved by a bypass procedure. This is either achieved surgically where the common duct or the gallbladder is anastomosed to the jejunum or endoscopically with the placement of a stent. If an ampullary carcinoma is found at operation it may be possible to resect it. Ampullary tumours have a better prognosis than pancreatic carcinomas.

Most patients with pancreatic carcinoma are dead within 9 months. Chemotherapy and radiotherapy are not helpful.

Cystic fibrosis (see p. 585)

(see p. 585)

This is the commonest cause of pancreatic disease in childhood. It is inherited as an autosomal recessive condition. The basic defect is a dysfunction of all exocrine glands, which produce thick viscoid secretions causing cystic dilatation of the ducts. Increased numbers of patients are now surviving into adult life because of improved therapy. Treatment is required for their pancreatic insufficiency and respiratory problems. Steatorrhoea is treated with a low-fat diet, pancreatic supplements and cimetidine.

Further reading

Howat HT & Sarles H (1979) *The Exocrine Pancreas*. London: WB Saunders.

Thomas HC & Jewell DP (1979) *Clinical Gastrointestinal Immunology*. Oxford: Blackwell Scientific.

Scheuer PJ (1980) *Liver Biopsy Interpretation*, 3rd edn. London: Baillière Tindall.

Schiff L (1975) *Diseases of the Liver*, 4th edn. Philadelphia: Lippincott.

Sherlock S (1985) *Disease of the Liver and Biliary System*, 7th edn. Oxford: Blackwell Scientific.

Wright R, Millward-Sadler GH, Alberti KGMM & Karran S (1985) *Liver and Biliary Disease*, 2nd edn. London: Baillière Tindall.

6

Diseases of the Blood

Introduction

Blood disorders are widely prevalent throughout the world.

Prevalence of anaemia

In the United Kingdom anaemia is seen mainly in:
- Children under 5 years of age
- Pregnant women
- Social classes 4 and 5
- The elderly

Anaemia is frequent in tropical and Third World countries, and the cause is often multiple; iron-deficiency anaemia is widely distributed, particularly in association with malnutrition and hookworm infestation. Hereditary anaemias are also very common. Thalassaemias affect populations in a wide band eastwards from the shores of the Mediterranean Sea through the Middle East to the Indian sub-continent and south-east Asia (see Fig. 6.13, p. 277). Sickle cell anaemia is found frequently in the black African population, in the Caribbean and in the USA.

Blood

Blood consists of:
- Red cells
- White cells
- Platelets
- Plasma, in which the above elements are suspended

Plasma is the liquid component of blood, which contains soluble fibrinogen. Serum is what remains after the formation of the fibrin clot.

The formation of blood

Around the third week of development of the embryo, blood islands are formed in the yolk sac. These produce primitive blood cells, which become the first haemoglobin synthesizing cells or erythroblasts. In the third month, these cells migrate to the liver and spleen, which become the chief sites of erythropoiesis until after birth. Erythropoiesis starts in the bone marrow from about the fifth month in utero; this is known as *medullary erythropoiesis*. Red cells made elsewhere are produced by *extramedullary erythropoiesis*.

At birth erythropoiesis occurs in the marrow of nearly every bone. As the child grows, the marrow cavity starts to be replaced by fat, so that, in the adult, red cell production is confined to the ends of the long bones, the axial skeleton, the ribs and the skull. Only if the demand for red cells increases and persists do the areas of red marrow extend once again. Pathological processes which obliterate the bone marrow cause extramedullary erythropoiesis to recommence in the liver or spleen.

All peripheral blood cells are derived from a single stem cell. Experiments on these pluripotent stem cells suggest that they divide and eventually produce cells which are 'committed' to producing a single cell line. Fig. 6.1 shows some of these stages which produce:
- Red cells
- Platelets
- Monocytes, neutrophils and eosinophils
- Possibly the lymphoid series

Studies on bone marrow cultures have shown that there are colony-forming units (spleen) (CFU-S), which form other recognizable red cell precursors of the marrow, i.e. burst-forming units (BFU) and colony-forming units (CFU), under the influence of erythropoietin. Similar white cell precursors, known as colony-forming units (granulocyte) (CFU-GM), also exist.

The names of a number of haemopoietic progenitor cells, the stimuli to which these respond and their role are given in Table 6.1.

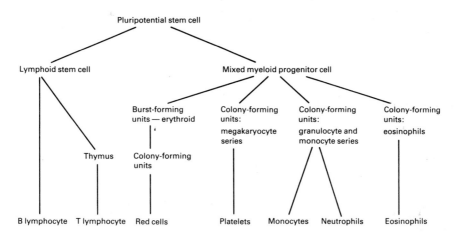

Fig. 6.1 The pluripotential stem cell. From Hoffbrand AV & Pettit JE (1984) *Essential Haematology*, 2nd edn. Oxford: Blackwell Scientific. With permission.

Table 6.1 Haemopoietic progenitor cells.

Cell	Stimulus	Role
Colony forming unit, spleen (CFU-S)	Environmental factors	Pluripotent stem cell
Colony forming unit, culture (CFU-C) or colony forming unit, granulocyte (CFU–GM)	Factors from other cells	Committed progenitor of granulopoiesis
Burst-forming units, erythropoiesis (BFU-E)	Erythropoietin	Committed progenitor cells of early erythropoiesis
Colony forming units, erythropoiesis (CFU-E)	Erythropoietin	Committed progenitor cells of late erythropoiesis

Proliferation of bone marrow cells results in the formation of cells with different functions. Some produce haemoglobin, others immunoglobulin, and some have special biological functions, for example, phagocytosis.

The normal adult values for the cells in peripheral blood are given in Table 6.2.

Table 6.2 Normal ranges for an automated cell count (parameters are based on the 95% values of 180 healthy adults aged 18–30 years).

	Male	Female
Hb (g·dl^{-1})	14.0–17.7	12.2–15.2
PCV (haematocrit) (l·l^{-1})	0.42–0.53	0.36–0.45
RCC ($\times 10^{12}$/l)	4.5–6.0	3.9–5.1
MCV (fl)	80–96	
MCH (pg)	27–33	
MCHC (g·dl^{-1})	32–35	
WCC ($\times 10^9$/l)	4.0–11.0	
Platelets ($\times 10^9$/l)	150–400	

The red cell

Erythropoiesis

Red cells pass through several stages to maturity. They begin as pronormoblasts, develop into basophilic normoblasts, and then, as haemoglobin synthesis starts within them, they start to become polychromatic and finally orthochromatic normoblasts, containing progressively more haemoglobin. As the cells develop they become smaller, and the nucleus is lost. Cells containing residual ribosomal RNA are called reticulocytes. These cells remain in the marrow for about 24 h and then are released into the circulation, where they lose their RNA and become mature erythrocytes, which are non-nucleated biconcave discs. Usually not more than 2% of the red cells in the peripheral blood are reticulocytes. Throughout the maturation of red cells, some 10% of the cells are lost; these lost cells are said to be produced by 'ineffective erythropoiesis'.

Factors affecting erythropoiesis

Erythropoiesis is stimulated by erythropoietin, which is produced mainly in the kidney. Its production is stimulated by a decreased oxygen tension in the blood. Thus people living at high altitudes have a higher number of red cells (polycythaemia) than those living at sea level. Even in a normal subject, anoxia, whatever the cause, will produce an increase in marrow activity to about eight times the normal value.

Other requirements for normal erythropoiesis
- Iron for haemoglobin synthesis
- Vitamin B_{12} and folate for normal DNA synthesis
- Other vitamins—B_6, ascorbic acid and riboflavin
- Trace metals (zinc, copper and cobalt)
- Hormones—androgens and thyroxine

Haemoglobin synthesis

Each red cell contains haemoglobin, which is a special protein able to carry oxygen to the tissues and return carbon dioxide from the tissues to the lungs. The binding of oxygen to haemoglobin is regulated by 2,3-diphosphoglycerate (2,3-DPG), which is an intermediate in red cell glycolysis. The concentration of 2,3-DPG affects the haemoglobin oxygen dissociation curve (see Fig. 6.17, p. 626); an increased concentration shifts the curve to the right.

Haemoglobin synthesis occurs in the mitochondria of the developing red cell. The complex biochemical reactions which occur are shown in Fig. 6.2. The major rate-limiting step is the formation of δ-aminolaevulinic acid (ALA) by ALA synthetase, which converts glycine and succinic acid to ALA. This reaction is inhibited by haem and stimulated by erythropoietin. Pyrrole rings are formed and then grouped in fours to produce protoporphyrins. Finally iron is inserted to form haem. Haem is then inserted into the globin chains to form haemoglobin.

Each normal adult haemoglobin molecule, Hb A, has a molecular weight of 68 000 and consists of two alpha and two beta polypeptide chains. Two other haemoglobins, Hb F and Hb A_2 are found in small amounts in the blood of adults. Details of the structure of these and other haemoglobins are discussed on p. 278.

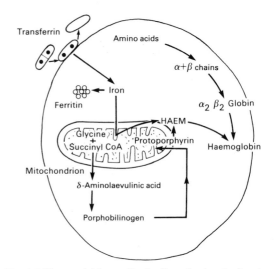

Fig. 6.2 Haemoglobin synthesis. Transferrin attaches to a surface receptor. Iron is released and transported to the mitochondrion, where it combines with protoporphyrin to form haem. Haem combines with α and β chains (formed on ribosomes) to make haemoglobin. From Hoffbrand AV & Pettit JE (1984) *Essential Haematology*, 2nd edn. Oxford: Blackwell Scientific. With permission.

A summary of normal red cell production, function and destruction is given in Fig. 6.3.

Anaemia

Anaemia is present when there is a decrease in the number of circulating red cells, a decrease in the amount of haemoglobin in the blood, or a haematocrit below the normal range. Alterations in the haemoglobin and haematocrit may occur as a result of changes in the plasma volume, as shown in

Definitions in haematology			Normal
Mean corpuscular volume (MCV)	=	$\dfrac{\text{haematocrit}}{\text{red cell count}}$	80–96 fl
Mean corpuscular haemoglobin (MCH)	=	$\dfrac{\text{haemoglobin} \times 10}{\text{red cell count}}$	27–33 pg
Mean corpuscular haemoglobin concentration (MCHC)	=	$\dfrac{\text{haemoglobin} \times 100}{\text{haematocrit}}$	32–35 g·dl^{-1}

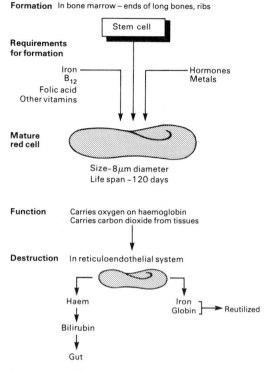

Formation   In bone marrow – ends of long bones, ribs

Stem cell

**Requirements
for formation**

Iron ——————————— Hormones
B₁₂   Metals
Folic acid
Other vitamins

**Mature
red cell**

Size – 8 μm diameter
Life span – 120 days

Function   Carries oxygen on haemoglobin
Carries carbon dioxide from tissues

Destruction   In reticuloendothelial system

Haem   Iron ⎤
                              Globin ⎦ ——→ Reutilized

Bilirubin

Gut

Fig. 6.3 Red cell production, function and breakdown.

Fig. 6.4. A reduction in the plasma volume will lead to a spuriously high haematocrit; this is seen in the clinical condition of stress polycythaemia. A high plasma volume, such as in pregnancy, may produce a spurious anaemia.

After a major bleed anaemia may not be apparent for several days until the plasma volume returns to normal.

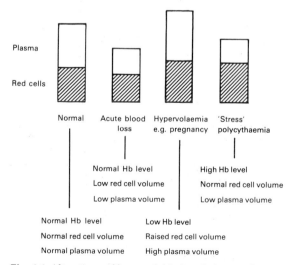

Plasma

Red cells

| Normal | Acute blood loss | Hypervolaemia e.g. pregnancy | 'Stress' polycythaemia |

Normal Hb level   High Hb level
Low red cell volume   Normal red cell volume
Low plasma volume   Low plasma volume

Normal Hb level   Low Hb level
Normal red cell volume   Raised red cell volume
Normal plasma volume   High plasma volume

Fig. 6.4 Alterations of haemoglobin in relation to plasma.

CLINICAL FEATURES

Patients with anaemia may be asymptomatic. A very slowly falling haemoglobin allows for haemodynamic compensation and enhancement of the oxygen-carrying capacity of the blood. A rise in 2,3-DPG causes a shift of the oxygen dissociation curve to the right, so that oxygen is more readily given up to the tissues. Where blood loss is more rapid or severe, particularly in elderly people, symptoms may occur.

Symptoms (all non-specific)
- Fatigue ⎤   NB Very common in the
- Headaches ⎦   normal population.

- Faintness
- Breathlessness
- Angina of effort
- Intermittent claudication
- Palpitations

Signs
Non-specific signs include:
- Pallor
- Tachycardia
- A full pulse
- Systolic flow murmur
- Cardiac failure
- Ankle oedema
- Rarely papilloedema and retinal haemorrhage in an acute bleed (can be accompanied by blindness)

Specific signs of the different types of anaemia will be discussed in the appropriate section. Examples include:
- Koilonychia—spoon-shaped nails seen in iron deficiency anaemia
- Jaundice—found in haemolytic anaemia
- Bone deformities—found in thalassaemia major
- Leg ulcers—occur in association with sickle cell disease

It must be emphasized that anaemia is not a diagnosis, and a cause must be found.

CLASSIFICATION

The various types of anaemia, classified in terms of the appearance of the red cells, are shown in Fig. 6.5. There are three major types of anaemia:
- Hypochromic microcytic with a low mean corpuscular volume (MCV)
- Normochromic normocytic with a normal MCV
- Macrocytic with a high MCV

Where there are both large and small red cells, a dimorphic anaemia is said to be present. This may, for example, be seen in coeliac disease, where both iron and folic acid are not being absorbed.

Fig. 6.5 Classification of red cell appearances; (a)–(i) refer to Fig. 6.6

INVESTIGATIONS

Blood investigations
A low haemoglobin should always be considered in relation to:

- The white cell count
- The platelet count
- The reticulocyte count (as this indicates marrow activity)

Special investigations
A bone marrow aspiration from the sternum or posterior iliac crest is performed to:

- Confirm a diagnosis made from a peripheral blood count
- Determine the cellularity of the marrow
- Determine the type of erythropoiesis, for example normoblastic or megaloblastic
- Determine the proportion of the various cell lines
- See whether the marrow is infiltrated
- Determine the size of the iron stores

A marrow trephine, a biopsy of the bone marrow, may be performed to allow the structure of the bone trabeculae to be examined. It enables the degree of myelofibrosis or the presence of tumour to be confirmed.

TECHNIQUES FOR OBTAINING BONE MARROW

Aspiration

- Site—usually sternum.
- Give local anaesthetic injection.
- Use special bone marrow needle (e.g. Salah).
- Aspirate marrow.
- Make smear on a glass slide.
- Stain with:
  (a) Romanovsky technique
  (b) Perl's reaction for iron
- *Indications* include any blood disorder, PUO, malignant diseases

Trephine

Performed if 'dry tap' obtained with aspiration.
- Site–usually posterior iliac crest.
- Give local anaesthetic injection.
- Use special needle (e.g. Jamshidi—longer and wider than for aspiration)
- Obtain core of bone.
- Fix in formalin; decalcify—this takes a few days.
- Stain with:
  (a) Haematoxylin and eosin
  (b) Reticulin stain

Microcytic anaemia

Iron deficiency is the commonest cause of this type of anaemia in the world. Thalassaemia also causes a microcytic hypochromic anaemia and is described on p. 277.

Iron

Dietary intake
The average daily diet in the United Kingdom con-

tains 15–20 mg of iron, but normally only 10% of this is absorbed. Absorption is increased, however, in iron deficiency. Iron is contained in many foods, e.g. liver, green vegetables, flour, eggs, meat and milk. Inorganic iron is usually present in the diet in the ferric form, whilst most organic iron is contained in haem.

Absorption
This takes place in the duodenum and jejunum. The absorption of iron is a complex process; some of the factors influencing it are shown in Table 6.3.

Table 6.3 Factors influencing iron absorption.

Ferrous iron is absorbed better than ferric.

Gastric acidity helps to keep iron in the ferrous state and soluble in the upper gut.

Reducing agents, e.g. ascorbic acid, increase iron absorption.

Inorganic iron is absorbed better than organic iron.

Iron absorption is increased with low iron stores and decreased in iron overload.

Increased erythropoietic activity, e.g. bleeding, haemolysis, high altitude, increases absorption.

Alcohol increases absorption.

Formation of insoluble complexes with phytate or phosphate decreases iron absorption.

There is increased absorption in primary haemochromatosis.

The iron content of the body is kept within narrow limits and its loss and intake are finely balanced. The precise mechanisms by which iron is absorbed and transported across the epithelial cell are uncertain but its absorption appears to be closely related to the total iron stores of the body.

Iron is taken up into the intestinal epithelial cell both from the serosal and the mucosal surfaces and enters a labile pool where it is available for transfer to plasma. Excess iron in the intestinal cell is joined to apoferritin to form ferritin. Ferritin is lost into the gut lumen when the intestinal cell is shed. In iron deficiency, the amount of iron in the labile pool is low and more iron enters the cell and is transported to the portal vein. In iron overload, the amount of iron in the labile pool is high and therefore less iron is absorbed and more ferritin is formed and shed into the lumen. Iron enters the plasma in the ferric form and becomes bound to transferrin.

Transport in the blood
Normal serum iron is about 11–30 $\mu mol \cdot l^{-1}$; there is a diurnal rhythm with high levels in the morning. Iron is transported in the plasma bound to transferrin, a beta globulin which is synthesized in the liver. Each molecule binds two atoms of ferric iron, and normally transferrin is one-third saturated. Most of the iron bound to transferrin comes from macrophages in the reticuloendothelial system and not from iron absorbed by the intestine. Transferrin-bound iron becomes attached by specific receptors to erythroblasts and reticulocytes in the marrow and the iron is removed (Fig. 6.2).

Ferritin is only present in the plasma in small amounts.

Iron stores
Iron is stored in the tissues as ferritin and haemosiderin; stores normally amount to 1000–1500 mg. In an average man, 20 mg of iron, chiefly obtained from red cell breakdown, is incorporated into haemoglobin every day. About two-thirds of the total body iron is in the circulation as haemoglobin (2.5–3 g in normal adult man); small amounts are found free in the plasma, with some in myoglobin and enzymes.

Requirements
Each day 0.5–1 mg of iron are lost in the faeces, urine and sweat. Menstruating women lose 40 ml of blood per menstrual period, an average of about 0.7 mg of iron per day of menstruation. Blood loss through menstruation in excess of 100 ml will usually result in iron deficiency as it cannot be compensated for by increased iron absorption from the gut. The demand for iron also increases during growth and pregnancy.

In the normal adult the iron content of the body remains relatively fixed. Increases in the body iron content (haemochromatosis) are classified into primary and secondary forms. Primary (idiopathic) haemochromatosis is discussed on p. 239, and secondary haemochromatosis (transfusion siderosis) on p. 279.

Iron deficiency

Iron-deficiency anaemia develops when there is an inadequate amount of iron for haemoglobin synthesis. Haemoglobin formation is maintained as long as possible until all the iron stores are depleted; during this time *latent iron deficiency* is said to be present.

CAUSES OF IRON DEFICIENCY

- Poor intake
- Decreased absorption
- Increased demands
- Blood loss

Most iron deficiency occurs from blood loss. Premenopausal women are always in a state of precarious iron balance due to menstruation. The commonest cause of iron deficiency world-wide is blood loss from the gastrointestinal tract due to hookworm infestation.

CLINICAL FEATURES

The symptoms of anaemia are described on p. 263. Other clinical features occur as a result of tissue iron deficiency. These are mainly epithelial changes induced by the effect of inadequate iron in the cells:
- Brittle nails
- Spoon-shaped nails (koilonychia)
- Atrophy of the papillae of the tongue
- Angular stomatitis

- Brittle hair
- A syndrome of dysphagia and glossitis (Plummer–Vinson or Paterson Brown Kelly syndrome)
- Rarely, in severe iron deficiency, parotid gland enlargement, splenomegaly and failure to grow

The diagnosis of iron-deficiency anaemia relies on a good clinical history with questions about dietary intake, regular self-medication with aspirin (which may give rise to gastrointestinal bleeding) and the presence of blood in the faeces (which may be a sign of haemorrhoids or carcinoma of the lower bowel). No examination of an iron-deficient patient is complete without a rectal examination and proctoscopy. In women a careful inquiry about the duration of periods, the occurrence of clots and the number of sanitary towels or tampons used should be made.

INVESTIGATION

Blood count and film
A characteristic blood film is shown in Fig. 6.6. The red cells are microcytic (MCV<80 fl) and hypochromic (MCH<27 pg). There may be poikilocytosis (variation in shape) and anisocytosis (variation in size). Target cells and hypersegmentation of polymorphs have been reported.

Serum iron and iron-binding capacity
The values for serum iron and iron-binding capacity in iron deficiency are included in Fig. 6.7; the serum iron falls and the total iron-binding capacity rises compared with normal. Iron deficiency is regularly present when the percentage saturation (i.e. serum iron divided by total iron binding capacity) falls below 19%.

Serum ferritin
The level of serum ferritin reflects the amount of stored iron, probably more accurately than the saturation of the serum iron-binding capacity does. The normal value for serum ferritin is $5.8–120 \text{ nmol·l}^{-1}$ ($15–250 \text{ μg·l}^{-1}$); it is usually lower in females than in males.

Bone marrow
Erythroid hyperplasia with ragged normoblasts are seen in the marrow in iron deficiency. Staining with potassium ferrocyanide does not show the characteristic blue granules of stainable iron in the cells in the interstitium of the marrow.

Other investigations
These will be indicated by the clinical history and examination; investigations of the gastrointestinal tract are often required.

DIFFERENTIAL DIAGNOSIS

The presence of anaemia with microcytosis and hypochromasia does not necessarily infer iron deficiency. The differential diagnosis is outlined in Table 6.4.

TREATMENT

The correct management of iron deficiency is to find and treat the underlying cause.

Enough iron must be given not only to restore the haemoglobin level to normal but also to replace the body's iron stores. Oral iron is all that is required in most cases. Preparations such as ferrous sulphate 600 mg daily and ferrous gluconate 600 mg daily are

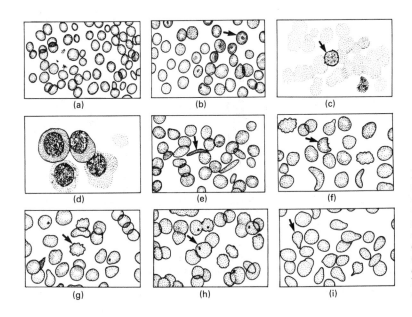

Fig. 6.6 Shapes of red cells.
(a) Hypochromic microcytic cells.
(b) Microcytes and target cells (arrowed) in thalassaemia. (c) Ring sideroblast (arrowed).
(d) Megaloblasts (in marrow).
(e) Sickle cell (arrowed).
(f) Schistocyte (arrowed). (g) Burr cell (arrowed). (h) Howell–Jolly body (arrowed). (i) Tear drop cell (arrowed) of myelofibrosis.

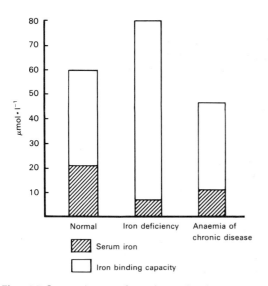

Fig. 6.7 Serum iron and total iron-binding capacity. Chronic diseases causing anaemia include renal failure, carcinoma and connective tissue disorders.

Table 6.4 Causes of hypochromasia and microcytosis.

Iron-deficiency anaemia

Thalassaemia

Defects of haem synthesis as a result of poisoning due to:
  Lead
  Pyrizinamide
  Isoniazid

Pyridoxine-responsive anaemia

Sex-linked hypochromic anaemia

Sideroblastic anaemia

Anaemias of chronic disease

both absorbed well. Various additions such as ascorbic acid and succinic acid bring no clinical benefit. If the patient has side-effects from iron medication, reducing the dose is all that is required. Prescribing expensive iron compounds, particularly the slow release ones, is a waste of money.

Patients who have general intolerance of oral preparations, even at low doses, and who have chronic diseases may require parenteral iron. Iron dextran can be given in doses of 50–250 mg daily by deep intramuscular injections. There is no justification for large intravenous infusions of iron, which are dangerous and unnecessary.

The correction of iron deficiency can be monitored using the reticulocyte count in the blood.

Sideroblastic anaemia

Sideroblastic anaemias are genetic or acquired disorders characterized by dyserythropoiesis and iron overload. They can be classified as shown in Table 6.5. In sideroblastic anaemia there is a disordered accumulation of iron in the erythroblasts. A ring of iron is formed round the nucleus which can be seen with Prussian blue stain (Fig. 6.6c).

In sideroblastic anaemia, a dimorphic peripheral blood film with both normal and microcytic cells is seen. The small cells result from the ineffective synthesis of haemoglobin as a result of failure in the formation of haem. Failure to produce protoporphyrin results in iron not being taken up to form haem, and iron accumulates in the cell.

TREATMENT

Some patients respond when drugs or alcohol are withdrawn if these are the causative agents. In some cases folic acid or pyridoxine may improve iron utilization.

Lead poisoning

Lead poisoning may produce a hypochromic or haemolytic anaemia, and the bone marrow may show ring sideroblasts (Fig. 6.6). Haem and globin synthesis are inhibited by lead. Lead inhibits several enzymes, including δ-aminolaevulinic acid (ALA) synthetase and pyrimidine 5'-nucleotidase. A deficiency of the latter enzyme interferes with the normal depolarization of ribosomal RNA. These factors lead to the characteristic appearance of punctate basophilia on ordinary staining. Treatment consists of removing the patient (very often a child) from the source of lead, and the use of chelating agents. Lead poisoning is discussed in more detail on p. 669.

Table 6.5 Classification of sideroblastic anaemia.

Congenital
X-linked disease—transmitted by females

Acquired
Primary or idiopathic
Secondary:
  Drugs, e.g. isoniazid, phenacetin
  Alcohol
  Lead
  Myeloproliferative disorders
  Leukaemias
  Secondary carcinoma
  Other systemic disorders, e.g. connective tissue
    diseases

Normocytic anaemia

This is seen as the 'anaemia of chronic disease'. Many chronic inflammatory conditions, such as rheumatoid arthritis, Crohn's disease and systemic lupus erythematosus, and neoplastic diseases are associated with a mild anaemia which is normocytic and normochromic in type. Both the serum iron and the total iron-binding capacity are low, in contrast to the raised total iron-binding capacity in iron-deficiency anaemia. Iron stores are usually normal, and consequently the anaemia does not respond to iron therapy, but only improves with treatment of the underlying disorder.

Macrocytic anaemia

Megaloblastic anaemia

Megaloblastic anaemia is characterized by the presence in the bone marrow of erythroblasts with delayed nuclear maturation because of defective DNA synthesis (megaloblasts). These megaloblasts are large and have a large immature nucleus; the cytoplasm stains dark blue with a Romanowsky stain. The nuclear chromatin pattern has an open stippled appearance. Associated with this abnormality of the red cell series are characteristic abnormalities of white cells; for example, giant metamyelocytes are seen. These megaloblastic changes occur in:

● Vitamin B_{12} deficiency
● Folic acid deficiency
● A small group of megaloblastic anaemias which do not appear to have deficiency of either vitamin B_{12} or folate

Haematological values
Anaemia may be present. Characteristically there is an MCV of >96 fl. The peripheral blood film shows macrocytes with hypersegmented polymorphs. If severe, there may be neutropenia and thrombocytopenia.

VITAMIN B_{12}

Vitamin B_{12} is synthesized by certain microorganisms, and animals and humans are ultimately dependent on this source. It is found in meat, fish, eggs and milk, but not in plants. Vitamin B_{12} is not usually destroyed by cooking. The average daily diet contains 5–30 μg of vitamin B_{12}, of which 1–5 μg are absorbed. The average adult stores some 1000 μg in the liver, and, as the daily loss is small, it may take up to 5 years after absorptive failure before B_{12} deficiency develops.

Structure
The planar group, which has a central cobalt atom, is called a corrin; derivatives are called corrinoids, of which cyanocobalamin (vitamin B_{12}) and hydroxy-cobalamin are two examples (Fig. 6.8). Vitamin B_{12} is a coenzyme for the biochemical reactions shown in Fig. 6.9. In the absence of vitamin B_{12}, N^5-methyltetrahydrofolate is not converted to N^5,N^{10}methylenetetrahydrofolate, which is necessary for the action of thymidylate synthetase. In this way DNA production is impaired.

Absorption and transport
In the gut lumen, vitamin B_{12} initially combines with an R binder to form the R binder complex. This is broken down by pancreatic juice to liberate B_{12}, which then binds with intrinsic factor. Intrinsic factor is a glycoprotein with a molecular weight of over 44 000 which is found in gastric juice. It combines with vitamin B_{12} and carries it to specific receptors on the surface of the mucosa of the ileum. B_{12} is then liberated and binds to these receptors, but intrinsic factor remains in the lumen. B_{12} is then transported from the enterocytes by the glycoprotein transcobalamin II (TC II) to the marrow. In serum, B_{12} is mainly bound to TC I (70–90%) and some to TC III (<10%), but neither protein plays a role in delivering B_{12} to the marrow. TC I and TC III are derived from granulocytes and thus a rise in serum B_{12} is seen in myeloproliferative disorders.

Fig. 6.8 The chemical structure of vitamin B_{12} (cyanocobalamin). (a) The molecular structure. (b) A three-dimensional representation. From Beck WS (1962) *New England Journal of Medicine* 266: 708. With permission.

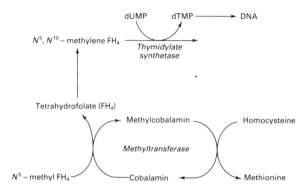

Fig. 6.9 Important biochemical reactions of vitamin B_{12}.

Pernicious anaemia

There are a number of causes of vitamin B_{12} deficiency (Table 6.6). One of the commonest in adults is pernicious anaemia (PA).

Pernicious anaemia is a disease of unknown aetiology, although it is known to have an autoimmune basis. Atrophy of the gastric mucous membrane occurs, with failure of intrinsic factor production and consequently vitamin B_{12} malabsorption.

PATHOGENESIS

This is a disease of the elderly with 1 in 800 of the population over 60 years being affected in the United Kingdom. It can be seen in all races, but is particularly common in Nordic, fair-haired and blue-eyed people. There is an association with other autoimmune diseases, particularly thyroid disease, Addison's disease and vitiligo. Approximately one-half of

Table 6.6 Causes of vitamin B_{12} deficiency.

Low dietary intake Vegans

Impaired absorption
Stomach
    Pernicious anaemia
    Gastrectomy

Small bowel
    Coeliac disease
    Tropical sprue
    Bacterial overgrowth
    Ileal disease or resection

Pancreas
    Chronic pancreatic disease
    Zollinger–Ellison syndrome

Miscellaneous and rare
Fish tapeworm (*Diphyllobothrium latum*)
Congenital deficiency
    Intrinsic factor
    Transcobalamin III
Nitrous oxide (inactivates B_{12})

all patients with PA will have thyroid antibodies. There is possibly a higher incidence of gastric carcinoma in patients with PA than in the general population.

Parietal cell antibodies are present in virtually all patients with PA; 50% of patients also have antibodies to intrinsic factor. Two types of intrinsic factor antibodies are found, but their role is uncertain:
- Type 1 or blocking antibody, which inhibits binding of intrinsic factor to B_{12}
- Type 2 or precipitating antibody, which inhibits the binding of the B_{12}–intrinsic factor complex to its receptor site in the ileum

B_{12} deficiency may rarely occur in children due to abnormal or absent intrinsic factor.

PATHOLOGY

Gastric atrophy (see p. 161) is present, with plasma cell and lymphoid infiltration. The histological abnormality can be improved by corticosteroid therapy, which supports an autoimmune basis for the disease.

CLINICAL FEATURES

The clinical features are those of anaemia, weight loss and neurological syndromes. The onset of PA is usually insidious and patients frequently have a very low haemoglobin before symptoms of anaemia develop.

The neurological changes are of greatest importance; if left untreated, the changes can be irreversible. The neurological abnormalities only occur with very low levels of serum B_{12} (less than 60 $ng \cdot l^{-1}$) and can occasionally occur in patients who are not clinically anaemic.

The classical neurological features are those of a peripheral neuropathy progressively involving the posterior and lateral columns of the spinal cord. Patients present with symmetrical paraesthesia in the fingers and toes, early loss of vibration sense and proprioception, and progressive weakness and ataxia. Paraplegia may result.

Mental changes can be present, with somnolence, irritability and psychosis occasionally being seen. Dementia also occurs. Smokers may suddenly become blind because of the cyanide in tobacco destroying the last reserves of cyanocobalamin.

Examination reveals an anaemic patient. Occasionally the skin has a lemon-yellow tint due to hyperbilirubinaemia. There may be signs of bleeding and heart failure, and hepatosplenomegaly is occasionally found. The patient usually has a low-grade fever; the reason for this is unknown.

A red sore tongue (glossitis) and angular stomatitis are sometimes present. Purpura due to thrombocytopenia is also seen.

Neurological examination may reveal the signs of peripheral neuropathy and, less often, the signs of subacute combined degeneration of the cord (see p. 859).

INVESTIGATION

The peripheral blood film shows the features of a megaloblastic anaemia as described on p. 268. The serum vitamin B_{12} is below the normal level of 160 ng·l^{-1}. The serum bilirubin is often raised as a result of increased haemolysis.

The bone marrow shows the typical features of megaloblastic erythropoiesis (Fig. 6.6d).

Serum vitamin B_{12} can be assayed using microbiological or radioisotope dilution techniques. Concurrent estimation of the serum folate and serum iron will show normal or high levels. A rapid fall in either of these following the administration of vitamin B_{12} is an early indication of successful B_{12} therapy. Treatment can also be monitored using the reticulocyte count.

In an elderly patient with clinical features of pernicious anaemia, a macrocytic blood film and a low vitamin B_{12} level are sufficient evidence to make the diagnosis. In the younger patient, full investigations are required.

Absorption tests
The absorption of B_{12} can be measured using the Schilling test. This test is satisfactory if patients can be trusted to collect urine specimens correctly, but this may not be the case, particularly in the elderly. It may also give an inaccurate result when renal function is poor. Whole body counting apparatus gives a much more reliable measurement of the absorption of B_{12} and should be used whenever possible. A radioactive dose of B_{12} is given orally and the total body activity is measured. The level of radioactivity is also counted not less than 7 days later to measure how much vitamin B_{12} has been retained.

Gastrointestinal investigations
In PA there is marked gastric atrophy with achlorhydria and intubation studies can be per-

---

Schilling test

Part I

- Give 1 μg ^{58}Co–B_{12} orally to fasting patient.
- Give 1000 μg B_{12} (non-radioactive) by intramuscular injection to saturate B_{12}-binding proteins and to flush out ^{58}Co–B_{12}.
- Collect urine for 24 h.
- Normal subjects excrete more than 10% of the radioactive dose.

If abnormal:

Part II

- Repeat part I after giving oral intrinsic factor capsules.

Result

- If excretion still abnormal, lesion is in the terminal ileum or there is bacterial overgrowth.
- If excretion now normal, diagnosis is pernicious anaemia.

---

formed to confirm this. Endoscopy or barium meal examination of the stomach are occasionally necessary to exclude a gastric neoplasm.

DIFFERENTIAL DIAGNOSIS

Vitamin B_{12} deficiency must be differentiated from other causes of megaloblastic anaemia, principally folate deficiency, but usually this is quite clear from the blood level of these two vitamins. The more common differential diagnosis is between PA and other causes of vitamin B_{12} deficiency; these are briefly indicated below:
- *Vegans.* These are patients who are strict vegetarians and eat no meat or animal products. A careful dietary history should be obtained.
- *Gastrointestinal disease.* Any disease involving the terminal ileum or bacterial overgrowth in the small bowel produce vitamin B_{12} deficiency.

FOLIC ACID

Folic acid was first found in spinach leaves and is widely distributed in plants. It is formed from three building blocks: a pteridine (similar to xanthopterin), para-aminobenzoic acid and glutamic acid (Fig. 6.10). Folates with additional glutamate radicals (polyglutamates) are the form of folate present in most foods. Polyglutamates are broken down to monoglutamates in the upper gastrointestinal tract and during the absorptive process these are then converted to methyltetrahydrofolate.

Pteroylglutamic acid (folic acid)

Tetrahydrofolate (FH$_4$)

Fig. 6.10 The structure of folic acid and tetrahydrofolate.

The biochemistry of tetrahydrofolate is very important, as it serves as an intermediate carrier of hydroxymethyl ($-CH_2OH$), formyl ($-CHO$) and methyl ($-CH_3$) groups, which take part in a large number of enzyme reactions. The mechanisms of action of antimetabolite and immunosuppressive drugs depend on the inhibition of these reactions.

Dietary intake
The body obtains its folate from green vegetables such as spinach or broccoli, and offal, such as liver or kidney. Folate is destroyed by cooking. The daily requirement is about 100 μg.

Folate deficiency

The causes of folate deficiency are shown in Table 6.7. The main cause is poor intake. Folate stores are not usually reduced by excessive utilization or malabsorption, but both these mechanisms can precipitate folate deficiency in a patient with an inadequate diet. Unlike Vitamin B$_{12}$, body reserves of folate are low; on a deficient diet folate deficiency rapidly develops over the course of about 4 months.

Approximately one-fifth of the cases of megaloblastic anaemia occurring in Great Britain are due to folic acid deficiency associated with factors such as old age, poverty, alcoholism or regular medication with antiepileptic drugs such as phenytoin (Table 6.7). The use of parenteral feeding without folic acid supplementation may lead to the development of severe folate deficiency.

CLINICAL FEATURES

Patients with folate deficiency may be asymptomatic. Symptoms, if present, are those of anaemia. Polyneuropathy is seen rarely.

Table 6.7 Causes of folate deficiency.

Nutritional (major cause)
Poor intake:
    Old age
    Poor social conditions
    Starvation
    Alcohol excess (also causes impaired utilization)

Poor intake due to anorexia:
    Gastrointestinal disease, e.g.
        partial gastrectomy
        coeliac disease
        Crohn's disease
    Cancer

Excess utilization
Physiological:
    Pregnancy
    Lactation
    Prematurity

Pathological:
    Haematological disease with excess red cell
        production, e.g. haemolysis
    Malignant disease with increased cell turnover
    Inflammatory disease
    Metabolic disease, e.g. homocystinuria
    Haemodialysis or peritoneal dialysis

Malabsorption
Occurs in small bowel disease, but the effect is minor compared with that of anorexia

Antifolate drugs
Anticonvulsants
    Phenytoin
    Primidone
Methotrexate

INVESTIGATION

A routine blood count shows a raised MCV with or without accompanying anaemia.

The bone marrow shows a characteristic megaloblastic erythropoiesis.

Blood measurements
Serum folate can be assayed microbiologically using the *Lactobacillus casei* method. Contamination of specimens with other bacteria or with antibiotics leads to false results. Normal levels of serum folate are 3–15 μg·l^{-1}. The amount of folate in the red cells is a better measure of tissue folate; the normal range is 165–600 μg·ml^{-1}.

Deoxyuridine suppression test
Folate and vitamin B$_{12}$ are needed in order to be able to use deoxyuridine to produce DNA. A single carbon unit is added to deoxyuridine to form thymidine, which is then used to build DNA. If necessary, preformed thymidine can be used to form DNA via the so-called salvage pathway.

The uptake of tritiated thymidine added to marrow in vitro can give an indication of the severity and type of deficiency. In a normoblastic marrow, the thymidine requirement is supplied by methylating deoxyuridine, and there is little requirement for preformed tritiated thymidine. In a megaloblastic marrow, however, much more tritiated thymidine is used. If B$_{12}$ is added to the incubated marrow, and this suppresses the uptake of tritiated thymidine, it suggests that B$_{12}$ is the cause of the deficiency. Alternatively, if folate is added and corrects the deficiency, then folate deficiency is the cause of the megaloblastosis. This is a rapid and useful method of determining the nature of the vitamin deficiency which is causing megaloblastosis.

Further investigations
In many cases of folate deficiency the cause is not obvious from the clinical picture or dietary history. Occult gastrointestinal disease should then be suspected (see Chapter 4) and appropriate investigations performed.

TREATMENT AND PREVENTION OF MEGALOBLASTIC ANAEMIA

Treatment depends on the type of deficiency. Blood transfusion is not indicated in chronic anaemia; indeed, it is dangerous to transfuse elderly patients, as heart failure may be precipitated.

Vitamin B$_{12}$ deficiency
This is treated with hydroxycobalamin 1000 µg intramuscularly to a total of 5000–6000 µg over the course of 3 weeks; 1000 µg is then necessary every 3 months for the rest of the patient's life. Clinical improvement should occur within 48 h and a reticulocytosis can be seen some 5 to 7 days after starting therapy. Neurological improvement may take 6–12 months, but long-standing lesions may be irreversible.

In patients who have had a total gastectomy or an ileal resection, vitamin B$_{12}$ should be monitored, and if low levels occur prophylactic vitamin B$_{12}$ injections should be given.

Folate deficiency
This is corrected by giving 5 mg of folic acid daily; the same haematological response as seen after treatment of vitamin B$_{12}$ deficiency occurs.

Prophylactic folate is justifiable in pregnancy, and is usually given in combination with iron.

OTHER CAUSES OF MEGALOBLASTIC ANAEMIA

Rare congenital deficiencies of enzymes can produce megaloblastic anaemia, but there is no response to the administration of either vitamin B$_{12}$ or folate.

Orotic aciduria, in which there is a defect in pyrimidine synthesis, is one example.

Macrocytosis without megaloblastic anaemia

A raised MCV with macrocytosis on the peripheral blood film can occur with a normoblastic rather than a megaloblastic bone marrow. Common causes of macrocytosis include:
- Alcohol
- Liver disease
- Reticulocytosis
- Hypothyroidism
- Aplastic anaemia

Macrocytosis occurs in chronic liver disease and with alcohol due to interference with red cell membrane formation. Alcohol is a frequent cause of a raised MCV in an otherwise normal individual. An increased number of reticulocytes leads to a raised MCV because they are large cells.

In all these conditions, normal levels of vitamin B$_{12}$ and red cell folate will be found.

Anaemia due to marrow failure (aplastic anaemia)

Aplastic anaemia is defined as aplasia of the bone marrow with peripheral blood pancytopenia. It is an uncommon but serious condition which may be inherited but more commonly is acquired.

MECHANISMS

Aplastic anaemia is due to a reduction in the primitive progenitor or stem cells (see Fig. 6.1) together with a fault in differentiation. Failure of red cell production or cell renewal at a later stage may also occur, resulting in such isolated deficiencies as the absence of red cells (pure red cell aplasia). Suppression of stem cells by subsets of the lymphocyte series, in particular the suppressor T cells, has been implicated in aplastic anaemia.

CAUSES

A list of causes of aplasia is given in Table 6.8. There is good circumstantial evidence to incriminate a number of drugs in the development of aplastic anaemia; these probably account for the gradual

Table 6.8 Causes of aplastic anaemia.

Congenital Fanconi's anaemia
Acquired Chemicals, e.g. benzene Drugs—see Table 6.9 Insecticides Ionizing radiation Infections, e.g. viral hepatitis, measles Miscellaneous infections, e.g. tuberculosis Thymoma Pregnancy Unknown

increase in the incidence of this condition in recent times (Table 6.9).

In pregnancy and hepatitis, the prognosis is grave, with a mortality rate of 90% in the former and 60% in the latter. In patients with tuberculosis in whom pancytopenia and hypoplasia of the marrow

Table 6.9 Drugs associated with marrow aplasia.

Anticancer drugs (always cause aplasia if dose high   enough) Mercaptopurine Busulphan Cyclophosphamide Doxorubicin Methotrexate Cyclophosphamide
Anti-inflammatory and anti-rheumatic drugs Phenylbutazone ⎱ Oxyphenbutazone ⎰ Withdrawn in the UK Gold compounds Indomethacin
Anti-epileptic drugs Phenytoin Troxidone Primidone
Antidiabetic drugs Tolbutamide Chlorpropamide
Antithyroid drugs Carbimazole Methylthiouracil Propylthiouracil Potassium perchlorate
Tranquillizers Chlorpromazine Prochlorperazine Promazine
Antihistamines Chlorpheniramine
Antibiotics Chloramphenicol Sulphonamides

is recognized, successful treatment of the infection leads to haematological recovery. In thymoma, removal of the tumour may be effective in restoring the blood count to normal. The rare congenital aplastic anaemia (also known as Fanconi's anaemia) is inherited as a recessive trait. It is associated with skeletal, renal and central nervous system abnormalities.

CLINICAL FEATURES

The clinical manifestations of marrow failure are anaemia, bleeding and infection. Physical findings include ecchymoses, bleeding gums and epistaxis. Mouth infections are common, particularly fungal infections. Lymphadenopathy, splenomegaly and hepatomegaly are rare in aplastic anaemia.

INVESTIGATION

The laboratory diagnosis is made on the basis of:
- A low haemoglobin, a white cell count below 0.5 $\times 10^9$/l and a platelet count of less than 20×10^9/l (i.e. pancytopenia)
- The virtual absence of reticulocytes
- A hypocellular or aplastic bone marrow with clusters of lymphocytes and large fat spaces
- An elevated serum iron, and a failure to utilize radioactive iron

DIFFERENTIAL DIAGNOSIS

This is from other causes of pancytopenia (Table 6.10).

TREATMENT AND PROGNOSIS

The course of aplastic anaemia can be variable, ranging from a rapid spontaneous remission to a persistent increasingly severe deficiency of all formed elements in the blood, which may lead to death through haemorrhage or infection. The most reliable

Table 6.10 Causes of pancytopenia.

Aplastic anaemia
Megaloblastic anaemias

Bone marrow infiltration or replacement
  Hodgkin's and non-Hodgkin's lymphoma
  Acute leukaemia
  Myeloma
  Secondary carcinoma
  Myelofibrosis

Hypersplenism
Systemic lupus erythematosus
Disseminated tuberculosis
Paroxysmal nocturnal haemoglobinuria

determinants for the prognosis are the number of neutrophils, reticulocytes, platelets, and non-myeloid cells present.

Bad prognostic features
- A neutrophil count of $<0.4 \times 10^9/l$
- A platelet count of $<20 \times 10^9/l$
- A reticulocyte count of $<10 \times 10^9/l$ (0.1%)
- Non-myeloid cells comprising >80% of the cells in the bone marrow

Patients who show any three of these four features for 3–4 weeks have less than a 50% chance of survival beyond 6 months. These patients should be considered for bone marrow transplantation.

Patients with aplastic anaemia should be treated at specialist centres. Supportive care together with transfusion of red cells and platelets should be given. Adult patients are treated with high dose methylprednisolone, antilymphocyte serum and bone marrow transplantation. There is little evidence that androgens have any value except in the Blackfan–Diamond type of aplastic anaemia in children.

Bone marrow transplantation
The bone marrow donor must be closely matched with the recipient. The donor is usually a sibling or identical twin who is HLA-identical and mixed lymphocyte culture (MLC) unreactive. The recipient's bone marrow is treated with intensive chemo- and/or radiotherapy, the latter given as total body irradiation (TBI). The donor marrow cells are then infused intravenously and repopulate the marrow cavity. Rejection is prevented by immunosuppression with various cytotoxic agents or cyclosporin. A successful engraftment occurs in about 70% of patients given transplants for aplastic anaemia.

Graft-versus-host disease (GVHD), both acute and chronic, is still a problem. It affects the skin, liver and gut in particular and is due to an imbalance of T lymphocyte subsets. Its impact has been greatly reduced with cyclosporin therapy.

Haemolytic anaemia

The normal red cell is a remarkably plastic, biconcave disc which is capable of changing shape as it circulates in the bloodstream. The red cell normally survives about 120 days, but in haemolysis the cell survival times are considerably shortened (Fig. 6.11).

Consequences of haemolysis

The shortening of red cell survival can lead to anaemia. However, compensatory mechanisms

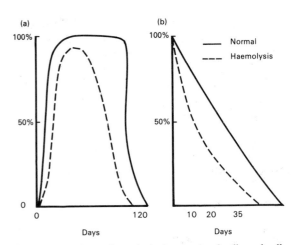

Fig. 6.11 Patterns of survival of normal red cells and cells affected by haemolysis. (a) Cohort of red cells labelled with ^{14}C-glycine. (b) Red cells of mixed ages labelled with ^{51}Cr.

result in an increase in red cell production. If the red cell loss can be contained within the marrow's capacity for increased output (which is usually eight times normal or more), then a haemolytic state can exist without the presence of anaemia. In chronic conditions the area and volume of bone marrow can gradually be increased, but the cells are released prematurely and therefore contain remnants of RNA (reticulocytes).

Red cell breakdown leads to a rise in serum bilirubin, a fall in the serum haptoglobin, and a rise in urine urobilinogen (resulting from bilirubin breakdown in the intestine). The peripheral blood film shows changes of macrocytosis, spherocytosis and abnormal red cell fragments in addition to the reticulocytosis.

Sites of haemolysis

Intravascular haemolysis
When red cells are rapidly destroyed within the circulation, haemoglobin is liberated. This is removed mainly by circulating haptoglobin and also haemopexin until these are used up. Any remaining haemoglobin circulates partly as free haemoglobin, but more commonly as methaemoglobin attached to albumin, forming methaemalbumin. On spectrophotometry of the plasma, methaemalbumin forms a characteristic band; this is the basis of Schumm's test.

Some haemoglobin is lost in the urine, although small amounts are reabsorbed by the renal tubules. In the renal tubular cell haemoglobin is broken down and the iron combines with a storage protein to form haemosiderin. This is of low molecular weight and can be excreted in the urine, where it can be detected in the spun sediment using the Prussian blue reaction.

Extravascular haemolysis

In extravascular haemolysis, the red cells are removed from the circulation by macrophages in the reticuloendothelial system, particularly the liver and spleen. The haemolysis is usually not so severe, but when it occurs chronically it leads to hypertrophy of the organ involved; consequently in long-term extravascular haemolysis the spleen may become palpable.

Mechanisms of haemolysis

Abnormalities of the red cell membrane

The red cell membrane is constantly being renewed and changed in its lipid composition. In addition, red cells can alter their shape by gaining surface or volume, or by losing surface or volume. The conditions and types of cells produced by such changes are shown diagrammatically in Fig. 6.12. For example, in

Fig. 6.12 Abnormalities of red cell surface area, volume and shape. HE = hereditary elliptocytosis; HS = hereditary spherocytosis; HPP = hereditary pyropoikilocytosis; LCAT = lecithin cholesterol acyltransferase. From Beck WS (ed) (1984) *Hematology*, 3rd edn. Massachusetts: MIT Press. With permission.

liver disease there is reduction in the surface area relative to the volume, and therefore the cell becomes less deformable and spherocytic in shape. In hereditary spherocytosis the red cell also loses membrane, so that the ratio of surface area to volume decreases and the cells become spherocytes. Such cells cannot pass through the reticuloendothelial system of the spleen with ease, and are therefore sequestrated there. If the cells become covered with antibody, they will also be susceptible to sequestration within the spleen due to interaction with macrophages and are thus taken out of the circulation.

Abnormal haemoglobin

Red cells with abnormal haemoglobins, for example in sickle cell disease or thalassaemia, are all much less deformable than normal cells, and are consequently sequestrated in the spleen. In glucose-6-phosphate dehydrogenase deficiency, the red cells are unable to prevent the oxidation and denaturing of haemoglobin by certain drugs; again the red cell is less deformable.

Abnormalities of the vessel wall

In certain conditions in which the capillaries and vessel walls are abnormal, the fragile red cells can be damaged and bizarre circulating fragments can be seen. This may occur in disseminated intravascular coagulation (see Fig. 6.6).

Evidence for haemolysis

Increased red cell breakdown leads to:
- Elevated serum bilirubin
- Excess urinary urobilinogen
- Reduced plasma haptoglobin
- Abnormal red cell fragments in peripheral blood

Increased red cell production leads to:
- Reticulocytosis
- Erythroid hyperplasia of the bone marrow

Having established that haemolysis is occurring, it is then necessary to assess the severity and site of the red cell destruction and also the cause. The frequency of blood transfusion is a practical way of assessing severity. Survival times measured using chromium-51 will also give an indication of the severity of the haemolysis, and, if external body counting is used, areas of red cell destruction such as the spleen can be localized.

Raised levels of plasma haemoglobin, low or absent haptoglobin and the presence of methaemalbumin will suggest an intravascular site for the haemolysis. Various laboratory studies will be carried out to determine the type of haemolytic anaemia. The causes of haemolytic anaemias are shown in Table 6.11.

Table 6.11 Causes of haemolytic anaemias.

INHERITED

Red cell membrane defect
Hereditary spherocytosis
Hereditary elliptocytosis

Haemoglobin abnormalities
Thalassaemia
Sickle cell disease

Metabolic defects
Glucose-6-phosphate dehydrogenase deficiency
Pyruvate kinase deficiency

ACQUIRED

Immune
Autoimmune
Isoimmune (Rh or ABO incompatibility)
Drugs, e.g. penicillin

Non-immune
Membrane defects:
    Paroxysmal nocturnal haemoglobinuria
    Liver disease
    Renal disease
Mechanical:
    Damaged vessels
    Valve prosthesis
    March haemoglobinuria

Miscellaneous
Infections
Drugs and chemicals
Hypersplenism

Inherited haemolytic anaemias

RED CELL MEMBRANE DEFECTS

Hereditary spherocytosis (HS)

Hereditary spherocytosis is a disease in which the red cell surface is reduced. The cell membrane has a defect in the structural protein spectrin which results in the cell losing membrane as it passes through the spleen. The surface to volume ratio is decreased, and the cells become spherocytes. The red cell membrane is also more permeable to sodium ions.

HS is a relatively common haemolytic anaemia, affecting 1 in 5000 caucasians. It is inherited in an autosomal dominant manner, but in 25% of patients neither parent is affected. This is explained by incomplete penetrance, spontaneous mutation, or possibly some form of additional recessive inheritance.

CLINICAL FEATURES

The condition may present with jaundice at birth. However, the onset of jaundice can sometimes be delayed for many years. The patient may eventually develop anaemia, splenomegaly and ulcers on the leg. The latter occur only rarely in children, but are common in adults. Hypertrophy of the bone in the skull and of the maxillary sinuses occurs, and in moderately severe cases growth is impaired. As in many haemolytic anaemias, the course of the disease may be interrupted by aplastic and megaloblastic crises. Aplastic anaemia commonly occurs after infections, whereas megaloblastic anaemia is the result of folate depletion due to hyperactivity of the bone marrow. Chronic haemolysis leads to the formation of pigment gallstones (see p. 250).

INVESTIGATION

- Anaemia is usually mild, but occasionally can be severe.
- The blood film shows macrocytes, reticulocytes and spherocytes.
- There is evidence of haemolysis, e.g. the serum bilirubin and urinary urobilinogen will be raised.

Osmotic fragility

When red cells are placed in solutions of increasing hypotonicity, they take in water, swell, and eventually lyse. A normal biconcave disc is able to tolerate imbibition of water more readily than the spherocyte. This increased osmotic fragility can be demonstrated when the cells are incubated in their own plasma for 48 h. Such fragility is also seen in other haemolytic disorders, but the direct Coombs' test is negative in spherocytosis.

TREATMENT

The spleen, which is the site of cell destruction, is removed in all but the mildest cases. In childhood it is best to avoid splenectomy, as sudden overwhelming fatal infections, usually due to encapsulated organisms such as pneumococci, may occur. If it is necessary to carry out splenectomy, the child should be given long-term prophylactic penicillin until his early 20s, and should also receive polyvalent anti-pneumococcal vaccine every 3–4 years.

Following splenectomy the spherocytosis remains but the haemoglobin usually returns to normal as the red cells are no longer destroyed.

Hereditary elliptocytosis

This disorder of the red cell membrane is inherited in an autosomal dominant manner. It is similar to HS, although the red cells are elliptical. Only a minority of patients have anaemia, and the haemolysis is usually mild.

HAEMOGLOBIN ABNORMALITIES

Thalassaemia

The thalassaemias (Greek *thalassa* = sea) are anaemias found in people living on the shores of the Mediterranean. Affected people live in a broad tract of land from the Mediterranean through the Middle East, the Indian subcontinent and into south-east Asia (Fig. 6.13).

Thalassaemia is a condition in which there is a deficiency in the synthesis of the globin chains of haemoglobin. In addition, the accumulation of abnormal chains within the red cell leads to its early destruction.

The structure of haemoglobin

Normal adult haemoglobin is made up of two polypeptide chains, the alpha and beta chains, which have 141 and 146 amino acids, respectively. These are folded so that haem molecules can be held within the folds, and yet are able to reversibly combine with oxygen. Adult haemoglobin has two alpha chains and two beta chains. In early embryonic life, haemoglobins Gower 1, Gower 2 and Portland are produced. Later, fetal haemoglobin (haemoglobin F), which has two alpha and two gamma chains, is produced (Table 6.12). Four globin genes are required to control alpha chain production (see Fig. 6.14); two are present on each haploid genome (genes derived from one parent). These are situated close together on chromosome 16. The genes for controlling the non-alpha chains are close together on chromosome 11.

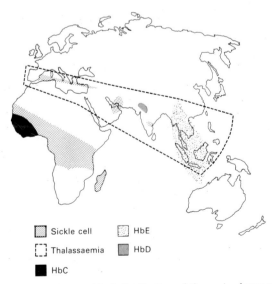

▨ Sickle cell	▦ HbE
⬚ Thalassaemia	▨ HbD
■ HbC	

Fig. 6.13 Geographical distribution of the major haemoglobin abnormalities.

Table 6.12 Fetal and adult haemoglobins.

Haemoglobin	Structure	Comment
A	α_2, β_2	Comprises 92% of adult haemoglobin.
A_{1c}	α_2 (β–NH glucose)	Comprises 5% of adult haemoglobin. This glycosylated haemoglobin is increased in patients with uncontrolled diabetes.
A_2	α_2, δ_2	Comprises about 2% of adult haemoglobin. Elevated in β-thalassaemia.
F	α_2, γ_2	Normal haemoglobin in fetus from 3rd to 9th month. Increased in β-thalassaemia.
H	β_4	Found in α-thalassaemia. Biologically useless.
Barts	γ_4	Comprises 100% of haemoglobin in homozygous α-thalassaemia. Biologically useless.

In normal development, suppression of genes occurs so that genes for gamma chains are suppressed at the end of fetal life, and beta chains rather than gamma chains are then produced. Furthermore, the rate of alpha and beta chain production is normally arranged so that the right numbers of each are produced. If an excess of alpha chains occurs, these precipitate in the red cell, forming inclusions which may lead to the early destruction of the cell.

Abnormal haemoglobin production
The production of haemoglobin is deranged if:
- The genes for production of the constituent chains are deleted or suppressed
- The messenger RNA activity is inhibited
- The chain is unstable and cannot be utilized

In addition to abnormalities of globin chain production, structural abnormalities of haemoglobin can occur, as in, for example, haemoglobin S. The two inherited defects of thalassaemia and abnormal haemoglobin often occur together.

In *β-thalassaemia* either no beta chains are produced (β^0) or beta chain production is impaired (β^+). Since alpha chain production is normal, alpha chains will combine with any beta chains available, leaving the excess alpha chains to combine with whatever delta or gamma chains are being produced. Thus, with a decrease in beta chain production, increased quantities of haemoglobin A_2 and haemoglobin F will be found (see Table 6.12). Table 6.13 shows the molecular defects and findings in the homozygote and heterozygote for the common types of β-thalassaemia.

The severity of the thalassaemia will depend on the amount of haemoglobin A_2 and F present. Clinically β-thalassaemia can be divided into:
- Thalassaemia major, with severe anaemia
- Thalassaemia intermedia, with moderate anaemia rarely requiring transfusion
- Thalassaemia minor, the symptomless heterozygous carrier state

The abnormalities in *α-thalassaemia* are complex but again there are two main forms. In one there is a deletion of only one alpha chain gene (due to a molecular defect) and therefore some alpha chains are produced (α^+). In the other there is deletion of both alpha chain genes (α^0), and no alpha chains are produced (Table 6.13). In the heterozygous state some alpha chains are produced, but in the homozygous state only haemoglobin Barts (γ_4) is present. Haemoglobin Barts cannot carry oxygen and is therefore incompatible with life (see Tables 6.12 and 6.13).

Less commonly an abnormal alpha chain with

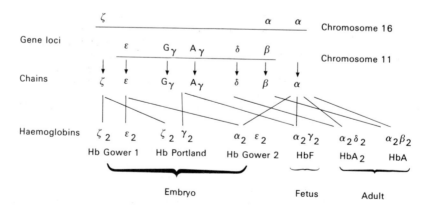

Fig. 6.14 Genetic control of human haemoglobin. From Weatherall DJ (1983) Other anaemias resulting from defective red cell maturation. In Weatherall DJ, Ledingham JGG & Warrell DA (eds) *Oxford Textbook of Medicine*, pp. 19.40–19.53. Oxford: Oxford University Press. With permission.

Table 6.13 Findings and molecular defects in some types of β- and α-thalassaemia.

Type of thalassaemia	Findings in homozygote	Findings in heterozygote	Molecular defect
β^+	Thalassaemia major A + F + A$_2$	Thalassaemia minor Hb A$_2$ raised	Reduced β-chain mRNA Abnormal mRNA processing
β^0	Thalassaemia major F + A$_2$	Thalassaemia minor Hb A$_2$ raised	Unknown, possibly gene deletions
α^+	Thalassaemia minor 5–10% Hb Barts at birth	Thalassaemia minor 1–2% Hb Barts	Deletion of one α-chain gene
α^0	Hydrops 80% Hb Barts at birth Fatal	Thalassaemia minor 5–10% Hb Barts at birth	Deletion of both α-chain genes

From Weatherall DJ (1983) Other anaemias resulting from defective cell maturation. In Weatherall DJ, Ledingham JGG and Warrell DA (eds) *Oxford Textbook of Medicine*, pp. 19.40–19.53. Oxford: Oxford University Press. With permission.

many extra amino acids may be produced, resulting in the formation of haemoglobin Constant Spring. This should be included in the differential diagnosis of α^+-thalassaemia.

In some patients with a marked reduction in alpha chains (α^+) more beta chains are produced. There is therefore some physiologically normal haemoglobin A, but also some haemoglobin H (β$_4$), which is physiologically useless.

Other chain deletions, apart from alpha and beta, may occur, producing syndromes with various clinical expressions.

β-Thalassaemia
Children affected by severe β-thalassaemia (thalassaemia major) present during the first few years of life with:
- Failure to thrive
- Intermittent infection
- Severe anaemia
- Extramedullary haemopoiesis which soon leads to hepatosplenomegaly and bone expansion, giving rise to the classical thalassaemic facies (Fig. 6.15)

Bone x-rays in these children show the 'hair on end' arrangement of bony trabeculation (Fig. 6.15).

There is wide variation in the severity of these clinical features. In thalassaemia intermedia the symptoms may vary from virtually none to a severe anaemia with splenomegaly and bone deformities. Recurrent leg ulcers, gallstones and infections are also seen in this group of thalassaemias.

Investigation. The following are found:
- *The blood count* shows a moderate to severe anaemia with reduced MCV and MCH. The reticulocyte count is raised. The white cell count and number of platelets are normal unless hypersplenism is present.
- *The blood film* shows a hypochromic and predominantly microcytic picture. Additional

features of autosplenectomy (Howell–Jolly bodies; see Fig. 6.6) can be present.
- *The iron binding capacity* is saturated, with high ferritin levels (after multiple transfusions).
- *Haemoglobin electrophoresis* shows an increase in Hb F. Hb A is absent in β^0. Hb A$_2$ is normal or slightly increased (Fig. 6.16).

Treatment. Children should be regularly transfused to keep the haemoglobin above 10 g·dl^{-1}. Blood transfusion may be required every 6–8 weeks. If the requirement for transfusion becomes more frequent, and there is evidence of red cell destruction, then splenectomy should be considered. If splenectomy is performed, prophylaxis against infection with encapsulated organisms is required as outlined on p. 277.

Iron must be removed from the tissues by the use of an effective chelating agent. The best available is desferrioxamine, and this is given as a 12-h infusion, the total dose being dependent on the age and size of the child. It is important to monitor the condition of the lens as reversible cataract may occur with desferrioxamine treatment.

Folic acid is given to counteract the deficiency produced by the overactive bone marrow. Ascorbic acid is also given as it helps to increase iron chelation.

Repeated transfusions will allow normal development, but the iron overload caused by this may lead to damage of the endocrine glands, pancreas and the myocardium by the time patients reach adolescence. Iron overload should be periodically assessed by measuring the serum ferritin.

This is the commonest cause of iron overload (transfusion siderosis), but it can also be seen in aplastic anaemia and refractory anaemias of various types.

β-Thalassaemia trait (heterozygous thalassaemia minor). This common carrier state is asymptomatic. There is no anaemia, but the red cells are hypochromic and microcytic. It may therefore be confused

(a)

(b)

(c)

Fig. 6.15 (a) A child with thalassaemia, showing the typical features. (b) Skull x-ray of a child with β-thalassaemia showing the 'hair on end' appearance. (c) X-ray of hand showing expansion of the marrow and a thinned cortex.

with iron deficiency. However, it can be easily distinguished by the fact that the serum iron, the serum ferritin and the iron stores are normal. Iron must not be given to these patients.

α-Thalassaemia

This gives rise to two chief clinical syndromes:
- *Homozygous α⁰ thalassaemia.* This is incompatible with life—all the haemoglobin is Hb Barts. Infants are either still-born at 28–40 weeks or die very

shortly after birth. They are pale, oedematous and have enormous livers and spleens—a condition called hydrops fetalis. It is associated with toxaemia of pregnancy and with obstetric problems.
- *Haemoglobin H disease.* HbH precipitates in red cells and is therefore removed by the spleen. The resulting haemolysis produces splenomegaly. The anaemia is variable but most patients survive to adult life.

Origin HbA$_2$ HbS   HbF   HbA

Normal

Sickle cell trait

Sickle cell anaemia

β-Thalassaemia trait

β-Thalassaemia major

Fig. 6.16 Patterns of haemoglobin electrophoresis.

GENERAL MANAGEMENT OF THALASSAEMIA

Recognition of the heterozygous states and family counselling should provide a basis for reducing the incidence of thalassaemia major. For example, 25% of the offspring of two parents with thalassaemia trait will have severe thalassaemia. Screening programmes using samples of fetal blood for the investigation of the rate of alpha, beta and gamma chain synthesis can pick up homozygous fetuses, and abortion can be offered.

Sickle syndromes

The most important haemoglobin variant is haemoglobin S, in which there is a substitution of glutamine for valine in the sixth position on the beta chain. This results from a single base change in the DNA coding for the amino acid. The variant is inherited in an autosomal dominant manner. Homozygous sickle cell disease and heterozygous sickle cell trait are inherited on Mendelian lines. The disease occurs mainly in Africans, but is also found in India, the Middle East, the Caribbean and the southern United States (Fig. 6.13). Sickle cell trait protects against *Plasmodium falciparum* malaria.

CLINICAL FEATURES

Sickle cell trait

Patients with less than 40% of haemoglobin S have no symptoms unless they are subjected to anoxia, e.g. during anaesthesia.

Sickle cell anaemia

In this condition, which represents the homozygous state, more than 75% of the haemoglobin is Hb S. The red cells spontaneously change to a sickle shape

due to the crystallization of haemoglobin in long crystals or tactoids which distort the cell (see Fig. 6.6). The cells are unable to pass freely through the normal capillary circulation and obstruction of small vessels occurs, followed by infarction in the bone, abdominal organs, lungs and brain. The condition can mimic a number of medical and surgical emergencies, such as acute intestinal obstruction or pleurisy.

Many patients do not suffer severe symptoms most of the time, but are nevertheless subject to acute painful episodes due to infarction, haemolytic or aplastic crises (following infections, particularly those due to parvoviruses), or acute sequestration, when the liver or spleen become engorged with sickle cells. Acute splenic sequestration is a very important feature and may be fatal in young children; early recognition allows prompt treatment. The hand and foot syndrome, in which there is painful swelling of the digits of the hands and feet, is quite common in children. Complications at an older age include:

● Septic necrosis of the bone, with osteomyelitis often being due to *Salmonella*
● Papillary necrosis affecting the kidney and producing haematuria
● Sequential infarction of the spleen leading to autosplenectomy
● A susceptibility to encapsulated organism infections such as pneumococcal septicaemia or meningitis
● A large heart, often symptomless and only discovered on chest x-ray
● Cerebral damage, resulting in focal epileptic fits
● Painful priapism

INVESTIGATION

There is usually an anaemia together with an elevated reticulocyte count. Sickling of red cells may be seen in the blood film, or may be induced in the presence of sodium metabisulphite.

The diagnosis may be confirmed on haemoglobin electrophoresis (Fig. 6.16). In Hb SS, no Hb A is found but Hb F is present. If unusually large amounts of Hb F are found, the patient may have sickle cell thalassaemia.

The parents of the affected child will show the features of sickle cell trait.

MANAGEMENT

No specific medication has been found to prevent sickling. Painful crises of sickle cell anaemia are produced by infections, dehydration or low oxygen tension, or by a variety of other factors including cold; these situations should be avoided or treated quickly. The repeated attacks of pain associated with crises must be adequately controlled with effective analgesics.

In elective operations, or before obstetric delivery, repeated transfusions may reduce the proportion of circulating haemoglobin S.

The sudden increase in spleen and liver size due to sequestration can be watched for in babies known to be suffering from sickle cell anaemia. Transfusion and splenectomy may be life-saving.

PROGNOSIS

Patients with Hb SS frequently die in the first few years of life from either infection or episodes of sequestration. There may, however, be marked individual variation in the severity of the disease. Genetic counselling is important.

Other haemoglobinopathies

There are many haemoglobin variants (e.g. Hb C, D, E), many of which are not associated with clinical manifestations. Some patients may have associated haemoglobinopathies, for example, sickle cell thalassaemia. Haemoglobin C disease may also be associated with haemoglobin S and this haemoglobin SC disease is associated with an increased likelihood of thrombosis. This may lead to life-threatening episodes of thrombosis during or following delivery. The condition should be treated by exchange transfusion.

METABOLIC DISORDERS OF THE RED CELL

It has already been noted how important it is for the red cell to 'keep its figure' if it is to perform satisfactorily. If the sodium or potassium content of the cell varies, then the water content, and consequently the shape, will also alter. There are therefore cation 'pumps' in the cell wall which maintain the correct balance by the outward transport of sodium at a rate of approximately 3 $mmol \cdot l^{-1} \cdot h^{-1}$ and the inward transport of potassium at about 2 $mmol \cdot l^{-1} \cdot h^{-1}$. These cation pumps require ATP. The concentration of calcium is also regulated by a pump requiring ATP. The intracellular calcium is almost undetectable normally, but if the pump fails calcium accumulates, and a spiculated cell is formed, which then dies.

The red cell does not have a nucleus, mitochondria or any of the intracellular apparatus needed for the production of protein, in particular enzymes. At its birth it receives a package of enzymes, and when these are used up the cell dies. Inherited defects in the amount of some of the enzymes render the cell vulnerable to oxidants of various types. This will result in shortened red cell survival.

Energy for the cell is produced from glucose metabolism along two pathways (Fig. 6.17):

- The Embden–Meyerhof glycolytic pathway
- The hexose monophosphate shunt pathway

About 90% of glucose is metabolized by the former, and 10% by the latter. The importance of the hexose monophosphate shunt is that it maintains glutathione (GSH) in a reduced state. Once the reduced form of GSH becomes unavailable, haem can be oxidized to methaemoglobin.

Glucose-6-phosphate dehydrogenase deficiency

The enzyme glucose-6-phosphate dehydrogenase (G-6-PD) holds a vital position in the hexose monophosphate shunt. Deficiency of this enzyme is a common condition which presents with a haemolytic anaemia and affects millions of people throughout the world, particularly in Africa, around the Mediterranean, the Middle East and south-east Asia. The gene for G-6-PD is sex-linked, being carried on the X chromosome. The deficiency therefore mainly affects males. It may also be carried by females, who show half the normal red cell values for the enzyme.

G-6-PD has a number of variants. About 10% of African and North American black people carry the variant known as G-6-PD Gd^{A-}. G-6-PD Gd^{A-} is a labile enzyme which is found in small quantities. Young cells have normal enzyme activity, whilst older cells are grossly deficient. Haemolysis is self-limiting as the bone marrow compensates by increasing its output. On the other hand, in the variety seen in Mediterranean peoples, G-6-PD Gd^{Med}, both the young and old red cells have very poor catalytic activity, and following an oxidant shock the haemoglobin level may fall precipitately; death may follow unless the condition is recognized and the patient transfused urgently.

The haemolytic anaemia associated with G-6-PD deficiency became generally recognized in World War II when black American troops fighting in malarial areas were given prophylactic antimalarials such as primaquine. These powerfully oxidant drugs resulted in oxidation of haem to methaemoglobin. Many drugs have been found to do this; a list of these and other causes is given in Table 6.14. Infections, acute illnesses such as diabetic acidosis, and ingestion of fava beans will also precipitate haemolysis in patients who have the deficiency (favism).

CLINICAL FEATURES

The differential diagnosis of jaundice and mild haemolysis in babies should include G-6-PD deficiency. In those with G-6-PD Gd^{A-} or Gd^{Med}, jaundice, dark urine and pallor develop within a day or so of exposure to one of the causes listed in Table 6.14. In blacks with G-6-PD Gd^{A-} a chronic haemolysis persists for some time after such exposure.

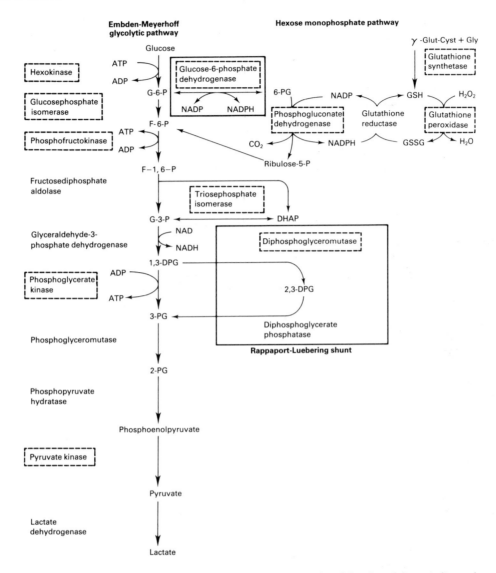

Fig. 6.17 Metabolic pathways (simplified) in the red cell. Enzymes enclosed by dotted lines indicate documented hereditary deficiency diseases. G = glucose; F = fructose; P = phosphate; DPG = diphosphoglycerate; PG = phosphoglycerate; DHAP = dihydroxyacetone phosphate; GSH = reduced glutathione; GSSG = oxidized glutathione.

INVESTIGATION

- The blood count is normal between attacks.
- During an attack, the blood film shows small fragmented cells, Heinz bodies (see Fig. 6.6) and a reticulocytosis.
- There is evidence of haemolysis (see p. 276).
- G-6-PD deficiency can be detected using several screening tests, such as demonstration of the ability of G-6-PD deficient cells to reduce dyes, producing a change in colour. The level of the enzyme may also be directly assayed.

TREATMENT

- Any offending drugs should be stopped.
- Blood transfusion may be life-saving. In the usual forms of G-6-PD deficiency splenectomy is not helpful.

Pyruvate kinase deficiency

This deficiency is the next most common after G-6-PD deficiency, but affects thousands rather than millions of people. The site of the defect is shown in

Table 6.14 Causes of haemolysis in glucose-6-phosphate dehydrogenase deficiency.

Infections
Acute illnesses, e.g. diabetic acidosis
Fava beans (not seen with G-6-PD Gd^{A-})

Drugs
  Analgesics, e.g.
    acetylsalicylic acid
    phenacetin (withdrawn in the UK)
    acetanilide
  Antimalarials, e.g.
    primaquine
    pyrimethamine
    quinine
    chloroquine
    pamaquin
  Antibacterials, e.g.
    most sulphonamides
    dapsone
    nitrofurantoin
    nitrofurazone
    furazolidone
  Miscellaneous drugs, e.g.
    vitamin K
    probenecid
    nalidixic acid
    chloramphenicol
    quinidine
    dimercaprol
    phenylhydrazine
    aminosalicylic acid

Fig. 6.17. It is inherited in an autosomal recessive manner. Homozygotes have haemolytic anaemia, splenomegaly and a low pyruvate kinase activity; this may be present at birth and continues throughout life.

INVESTIGATION

- The patients are anaemic, with a Hb of 5–10 g·dl^{-1}. Because the anaemia is long standing, the oxygen dissociation curve is shifted as a result of the rise in intracellular 2,3-diphosphoglycerate (Fig. 6.17).
- The blood film shows distorted cells and a reticulocytosis.
- Autohaemolysis is increased; this is not prevented by the addition of glucose to the red cells, in contrast to hereditary spherocytosis.
- Pyruvate kinase, if assayed, is low.

TREATMENT

Where anaemia is causing severe symptoms, a splenectomy may be helpful.

In addition to G-6-PD and pyruvate kinase deficiencies, there are a number of rare enzymic deficiencies which need specialist study. In practice, the only treatment available in these conditions is judicious blood transfusion.

Acquired haemolytic anaemia

These anaemias may be divided into those due to immune, non-immune, or other causes (see Table 6.11).

Mechanisms of haemolysis
- Antibody may be produced against red cells. This renders them liable to splenic sequestration and destruction.
- Drugs may lead to haemolysis by:
  (a) The formation of a drug–red cell complex which is antigenic and produces an antibody (i.e. which acts as a hapten). Penicillin or cephalosporins can produce haemolytic anaemia in this way.
  (b) The formation of a drug–plasma protein complex. This is adsorbed onto the red cell and then antibody and complement become attached. A good example of this is the drug quinine.
  (c) Directly inducing an autoimmune haemolytic anaemia. An example of this is the anaemia produced by methyldopa.
- Cells may be destroyed by valve prostheses or by changes in the capillary wall induced by various disease processes.
- Red cells may be destroyed by organisms such as *Plasmodium* or *Clostridium welchii*.

IMMUNE HAEMOLYTIC ANAEMIA

Immune haemolytic anaemia may be autoimmune or isoimmune.

Autoimmune haemolytic anaemias are acquired disorders in which the body produces antibodies against its own cells. Antibody or components of complement bind to the patient's red cells, which are then phagocytosed and removed from the circulation by macrophages of the reticuloendothelial system. These anaemias are characterized by the presence of a positive Coombs' test, which detects the protein on the cell surface (Fig. 6.18).

Autoimmune haemolytic anaemias are divided into 'warm' or 'cold' types, depending on whether the antibody attaches to the red cells at body temperature (37°C) or at 4°C. The major features and the causes of these two forms of autoimmune haemolytic anaemia are shown in Table 6.15.

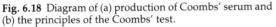

Fig. 6.18 Diagram of (a) production of Coombs' serum and (b) the principles of the Coombs' test.

'Warm' autoimmune haemolytic anaemias

CLINICAL FEATURES

These anaemias may occur at all ages and in both sexes. They can present as a short episode of anaemia or jaundice, or may progress to an intermittent chronic pattern. Usually, the spleen becomes palpable. Infections or folate deficiency may provoke a profound fall in the haemoglobin level. In more than 50% of cases, the cause remains unknown. They may be associated with lymphoid malignancies or diseases such as rheumatoid arthritis and systemic lupus erythematosus.

INVESTIGATION

- There is evidence of haemolytic anaemia.
- Spherocytosis is present as a result of red cell damage. A reduction in the surface membrane leads to microspherocytosis.
- The direct Coombs' test is positive, with IgG or IgA being found on the surface of the red cells. Antibodies are best detected at 37°C.
- The condition may be associated with thrombocytopenia (Evans' syndrome).
- Neutropenia may occur.

TREATMENT AND PROGNOSIS

Corticosteroids (e.g. prednisolone in doses of 60–80 mg daily) are usually effective. Blood transfusions may be required until spontaneous remission, with the disappearance of the antibody, occurs. Rarely splenectomy may be necessary if there is no response to the steroids. Treatment of the underlying condition, for example, the treatment of chronic lymphatic leukaemia by cytotoxic drugs, may be an important factor in controlling the condition.

'Cold' autoimmune haemolytic anaemia

CLINICAL FEATURES

The patient presents with a haemolytic anaemia which may be acute. In addition, there may be peripheral circulatory symptoms such as Raynaud's phenomenon due to the associated vascular haemolysis. Often the cause is unknown, but this condition may be associated with an acute *Mycoplasma pneumoniae* infection. The antibodies are IgM in type and attach to the red cells in the

Table 6.15 Causes and major features of autoimmune haemolytic anaemias.

	Warm	Cold
Temperature at which antibody attaches to red cells:	37°C	4°C
Type of antibodies:	IgG (IgA)	IgM
Direct Coombs' test:	Strongly positive	Positive
Causes of primary condition:	Idiopathic Evans syndrome	Idiopathic
Causes of secondary condition:	Autoimmune disorders, e.g. systemic lupus erythematosus Lymphomas Chronic lymphatic leukaemias Hodgkin's disease Carcinomas Drugs, e.g. methyldopa	Infections, e.g. infectious mononucleosis, *Mycoplasma pneumoniae* Other viral infections (rare) Lymphomas Paroxysmal cold haemoglobinuria

peripheral circulation when the blood temperature falls. Thus, the anaemia may be precipitated by exposure to cold.

Paroxysmal cold haemoglobinuria (PCH) is a rare condition associated with common childhood infections such as measles, mumps or chickenpox. In these patients intravascular haemolysis is associated with a complement-fixing antibody, the Donath–Landsteiner antibody.

INVESTIGATION

Investigations similar to those used in 'warm' auto-immune haemolytic anaemia can be carried out. In addition:
- Red cells agglutinate in the cold or at room temperature.
- Serum antibodies are usually IgM in type and show specificity to the I antigen which is present on the red cell surface.
- The direct Coombs' test shows only C3 complement on red cells.
- Spherocytosis is less well marked.

TREATMENT

Patients should avoid cold, and should be advised to wear gloves and keep their feet warm. Sometimes specific treatment with chlorambucil may be helpful.

Haemolytic disease of the newborn (HDN)

This is an *isoimmune* haemolytic anaemia which is due to the passage of IgG antibodies from the maternal circulation via the placenta into the fetus, where they destroy the fetal red cells. This condition was commonly due to incompatibilities in the rhesus blood group system. However, since the mechanism of HDN has been understood, rhesus incompatibility has become less common due to the attempts made to prevent immunization of the mother by giving IgG anti-D globulin to rhesus-negative mothers shortly after delivery or abortion. Therefore, when HDN does occur, it is now much more likely to be due to ABO blood group antibodies than to rhesus antibodies.

CLINICAL FEATURES

These may vary from mild to severe.

Mild
The infant has a mild anaemia; jaundice may or may not be present.

Moderate
There is usually severe anaemia with jaundice. The infant has hepatosplenomegaly, oedema and cardiac failure. There is a high unconjugated bilirubin of more than 250 mmol·l^{-1}. At this level, bile pigment deposition occurs in the basal ganglia and gives rise to kernicterus. This results in mental deficiency, deafness, epilepsy and spasticity.

Severe
In the most extreme form of the disease, the condition is incompatible with life. The child is delivered with the characteristic appearance of hydrops fetalis.

INVESTIGATION

Prenatally
Sensitization of the rhesus-negative mother occurs at delivery by fetal rhesus-positive cells entering the maternal circulation. Mothers who are rhesus-negative should therefore have their serum tested for anti-D antibodies at 3 months and then monthly during the third trimester. A rising titre is an indication for amniocentesis to assess the level of jaundice in the fetus. A fetus severely affected before 33 weeks will need an intrauterine blood transfusion carried out in a special care unit.

At birth
A sample of cord blood is obtained. This shows:
- Anaemia with a high reticulocyte count
- A rhesus-D positive blood group
- A positive direct Coombs' test
- A raised bilirubin

TREATMENT

Management of the baby
After 33 weeks, induction of labour with exchange transfusion is necessary in severe cases. This will raise the Hb level, and reduce the level of antibody and bilirubin. The blood used should be freshly donated rhesus-negative blood.

In mild cases phototherapy has been used to convert bilirubin to harmless biliverdin. Biliverdin can be excreted by the kidneys and this therefore reduces the chance of kernicterus.

Prevention of rhesus immunization in the mother
IgG anti-D globulin 250–300 μg intramuscularly should be given to rhesus-D negative mothers within 72 h of delivery or abortion. A useful simple check to assess whether immunization has occurred is whether fetal cells can be found in the maternal blood using the Kleihauer test. The test relies on the acid elution of all except fetal Hb from red cells. Consequently, in a blood film prepared from the mother, the only cells that will remain stained are those containing fetal Hb derived from the fetus.

NON-IMMUNE HAEMOLYTIC ANAEMIA

Paroxysmal nocturnal haemoglobinuria (PNH)

This is a rare acquired red cell defect in which a proportion of the red cells are sensitive to destruction by activated complement. These cells are continually haemolysed intravascularly. It may complicate aplastic anaemia, and it is associated with a tendency to thrombosis.

CLINICAL FEATURES

Patients present with haemolysis and abdominal pain, which may be precipitated by infection, iron therapy or surgery. Because intravascular haemolysis is more common at night, the urine voided first thing in the morning may be dark in colour. The condition may be complicated by thrombotic episodes, giving acute abdominal pain, myocardial infarction or stroke. The pathophysiology of PNH is shown in Fig. 6.19.

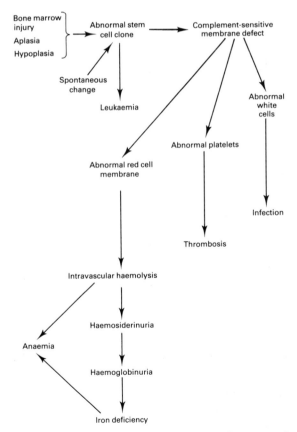

Fig. 6.19 Pathophysiology of paroxysmal nocturnal haemoglobinuria. From Beck WS (ed) (1984) *Hematology*, 3rd edn. Massachusetts: MIT Press. With permission.

INVESTIGATION

- There is evidence of haemolysis. A raised reticulocyte count will accompany a severe anaemia.
- Haemosiderinuria is present. The iron can be detected using potassium ferrocyanide in spun-down urinary sediment.
- Cells from a patient with PNH lyse more readily in acidified serum than do normal cells (Ham's test). PNH cells also lyse in solutions of sucrose.
- The peripheral blood film may show leucopenia and thrombocytopenia in addition to anaemia. PNH should be suspected if the bone marrow, instead of showing hypoplastic features, is active.

TREATMENT

There is no specific treatment for PNH. Very occasionally, if the abnormal cell clone disappears, complete spontaneous recovery may occur.

In severe anaemia, blood transfusion may be necessary. Filtered (leucocyte-depleted) blood is used in order to prevent transfusion reactions and acceleration of the haemolysis. The possibility of using bone marrow transplantation is being explored.

Anticoagulants are used in thrombotic episodes.

MISCELLANEOUS CAUSES OF ACQUIRED HAEMOLYTIC ANAEMIA

Drug-induced haemolysis

Many drugs and chemicals can induce haemolysis by direct action. Examples of such drugs are sulphonamides, phenacetin, aminosalicylic acid and sulphasalazine.

Infections

Plasmodium falciparum rarely produces an acute intravascular haemolysis (blackwater fever, see p. 77). Bacterial infections with *Clostridium welchii* may also cause intravascular haemolysis.

Other

Direct damage to the red cell, either by heat (as in extensive burns) or as the result of mechanical trauma, for example when the red cell is battered against a mitral valve prosthesis, may result in haemolytic anaemia. All the features of haemolysis are present, and, in addition, the loss of haemosiderin in the urine gives rise to iron deficiency. Sometimes red cell destruction may occur when capillaries are damaged by disease, so that the red cells are broken and fragmented. This condition is known as microangiopathic haemolytic anaemia. It is associated with a number of other diseases, including arteritis, disseminated carcinoma, malignant hypertension and the haemolytic uraemic syndrome. It can be accompanied by disseminated intravascular coagulation.

Non-leukaemic myeloproliferative disorders

The 'myeloproliferative syndrome' originally referred to an increase in each of the marrow elements: white cells, red cells, megakaryocytes and fibroblasts. The term was an attempt to explain the interrelationships that could be seen, for example, between such diseases as polycythaemia vera and myelofibrosis. Erythroid hyperplasia can eventually be overtaken and superseded by fibroblastic proliferation, so that almost one-third of patients with polycythaemia vera become myelofibrotic. Originally abnormalities of granulocytes were included in this group of disorders, but erythroid leukaemia and granulocytic leukaemia are now known to be distinct pathological entities. The relationship between the marrow stem cells and the various pathological entities is shown in Fig. 6.20.

Polycythaemia

Polycythaemia is defined as a haemoglobin level greater than 18 g·dl^{-1}, a red cell count above 6×10^{12}/l, and a PCV >0.55 l·l^{-1}. The red cell volume is greater than 36 ml·kg^{-1} in males and 32 ml·kg^{-1} in females.

A diminished plasma volume may result from a number of causes, such as dehydration, and leads to haemoconcentration and an apparent raised haemoglobin and PCV. True polycythaemia must be distinguished from this; this can only be done by measurement of the red cell volume. The causes of polycythaemia are given in Table 6.16.

Secondary polycythaemia is due to an increased level of erythropoietin. This may be due to an appropriate increase in secretion in response to anoxia, or may be due to inappropriate production of erythropoietin by, for example, a tumour such as a renal carcinoma.

PRIMARY POLYCYTHAEMIA

Polycythaemia vera (PV)

This condition is caused by a chronic sustained proliferation of the erythroid population of the bone marrow. It is due to a fundamental alteration in the progenitor cells, as the level of erythropoietin is normal. The increased red cell volume increases blood viscosity, but this is compensated for by an increased plasma volume and cardiac output. When the haematocrit is very high (>0.65 l·l^{-1}) these compensating mechanisms break down and there is an increase in the frequency of myocardial infarction and stroke. In PV there is also an abnormality of the platelets which results in the formation of minor thrombi, aggravating the tendency to thrombosis and infarction.

CLINICAL FEATURES

The onset is insidious. It usually presents in patients over 60 with tiredness, depression, vertigo, tinnitus and visual disturbance. It should be noted that these symptoms are also common in the normal popula-

Table 6.16 Causes of polycythaemia.

PRIMARY
Polycythaemia vera
SECONDARY
Due to an appropriate increase in erythropoietin
High altitude
Lung disease
Cardiovascular disease (right-to-left shunt)
Heavy smoking
Increased affinity of haemoglobin, e.g. familial polycythaemia
Due to an inappropriate increase in erythropoietin
Renal disease, renal cell carcinoma, Wilms' tumour
Hepatocellular carcinoma
Adrenal tumours
Cerebellar haemangioblastoma
Massive uterine fibroma
RELATIVE
Stress or spurious polycythaemia
Dehydration
Burns

Fig. 6.20 The non-leukaemic myeloproliferative disorders.

tion over the age of 60, and consequently PV is easily missed. These features, together with hypertension, angina, intermittent claudication and a tendency to bleed are suggestive evidence for PV. Severe itching after a hot bath or when the patient is warm is common. Gout due to increased cell turnover may be a feature, and peptic ulceration occurs in a minority of patients.

Physical signs
The patient usually is plethoric, and has a deep dusky cyanosis of the tongue. Injection of the conjunctivae is commonly seen. The spleen is often palpable, and the liver is usually enlarged.

INVESTIGATION

- The haemoglobin is above 18 g·dl^{-1} and the PCV in excess of 0.55 l·l^{-1}. There is an elevated white cell and platelet count in many patients.
- The bone marrow shows erythroid hyperplasia and abnormal megakaryocytes.
- The red cell volume measured by chromium-51 is increased. Measurement of plasma volume shows normal or increased values.
- Serum uric acid levels may be raised.
- The leucocyte alkaline phosphatase (LAP) is high.
- Vitamin B_{12} binding protein is also high.

DIFFERENTIAL DIAGNOSIS

The existence of an increased red cell volume should be established, and the causes of secondary polycythaemia excluded. Intravenous pyelograms should be carried out in patients with polycythaemia to exclude a renal cause for the disease.

COURSE AND MANAGEMENT

The unmodified course of PV is not seen nowadays, but death from thrombosis, infarction and haemorrhage occur early in the untreated patient. Treatment is now aimed at keeping the PCV below 0.5 l·l^{-1}. These are three types of treatment:

- *Venesection.* This will successfully relieve many of the symptoms of PV. Iron deficiency is a common complication.
- *Radioactive phosphorus-32.* In addition to reducing the haematocrit, phosphorus-32 will lower a high platelet count, and therefore reduce the tendency to haemorrhage and thrombosis. One dose may give control for up to 18 months, but the administration of phosphorus-32 makes the patient liable to radiation-induced acute leukaemia.
- *Chemotherapy.* Drugs such as busulphan and hydroxyurea are effective. They also bring the possibility of secondary malignancy, but because of ease of control and general safety, hydroxyurea is now being used quite frequently.

There is no generally agreed scheme for the use of these treatment modalities in PV. Patients treated with venesection alone were found to die earlier than those treated with phosphorus-32, and leukaemia occurred in patients treated with venesection alone, phosphorus-32 or chlorambucil. However, the incidence of leukaemia was greater with chlorambucil and this agent should probably not be used. One current policy is therefore to manage polycythaemia with venesection alone if possible. However, if there is a high platelet count, this can be treated initially with a chemotherapeutic agent (preferably hydroxyurea); if this fails to control the condition, phosphorus-32 may be given in doses of 5–7 mCi $(1.8 \times 10^8$–2.6×10^8 Bq). The total cumulative dose of phosphorus-32 to which a patient is exposed should not be in excess of 15 mCi (5.5. $\times 10^8$ Bq).

Allopurinol is given to block uric acid production. The pruritus is lessened by avoiding very hot baths. Sometimes cimetidine is very effective in relieving distressing pruritus. Antihistamines have largely proved unsuccessful.

It should be noted that patients with PV have a high operative risk; 75% of patients have severe haemorrhage following surgery, and 30% of these patients die. If the surgery is elective, the polycythaemia should· be controlled first. In an emergency, reduction of the haematocrit by venesection and fluid replacement must be carried out.

PROGNOSIS

Polycythaemia frequently develops into myelosclerosis or acute myeloid leukaemia as part of the natural history of the disease.

'Stress' polycythaemia (Gaisböck's syndrome)

This condition was originally thought to be stress-induced. The red cell volume is normal but, as the result of a decreased plasma volume, there is a 'relative' polycythaemia. 'Stress' polycythaemia is commoner than PV, and occurs in middle-aged men, particularly those who are obese and hypertensive and who smoke. The higher the PCV, the greater the risk of arterial thrombotic episodes; the condition often presents as cardiovascular problems such as myocardial or cerebral ischaemia. For this reason, it may be justifiable to venesect the patient until the PCV is normal. Sometimes the PCV then remains stabilized. Smoking must be stopped.

SECONDARY POLYCYTHAEMIAS

The causes of these are shown in Table 6.16. The treatment is that of the precipitating factor; for example, renal or posterior fossa tumours need to be resected. Complications are similar to those seen in PV, including thrombosis, haemorrhage and cardiac failure, but myeloproliferative disease does not develop.

Myelosclerosis (myelofibrosis)

In this condition there is fibrosis in the bone marrow and extramedullary haemopoeisis in the liver and spleen. It develops in about 30% of patients with PV or may arise de novo. The terms myelosclerosis and myelofibrosis are interchangeable.

CLINICAL FEATURES

The disease presents insidiously with lethargy, weakness and weight loss. Patients often complain of a 'fullness' in the upper abdomen due to the large spleen. Severe pain related to respiration may indicate perisplenitis secondary to splenic infarction, and pain in the bones and attacks of gout can complicate the illness. Bruising and bleeding occurs in the thrombocytopenic patient.

Signs
- Anaemia
- Fever
- Massive splenomegaly

Other conditions which must be considered when massive splenomegaly is seen are chronic myeloid leukaemia, chronic malaria, kala-azar or, rarely, Gaucher's disease.

INVESTIGATION

- There is anaemia with leucoerythroblastic features. Poikilocytes and red cells with characteristic tear drop forms (see Fig. 6.6i) are seen. The white cell count may be over $100 \times 10^9/l$, and the differential white cell count may be very similar to that seen in chronic granulocytic leukaemia; later leucopenia may develop.
- The platelet count may be very high, but in later stages thrombocytopenia occurs.
- Bone marrow aspiration is usually unsuccessful and this gives a clue to the presence of the condition. A bone marrow trephine is necessary to show the markedly increased fibrosis and islands of hypercellularity.
- The Philadelphia chromosome is absent; this helps to distinguish myelosclerosis from most cases of chronic granulocytic leukaemia.
- The leucocyte alkaline phosphatase is normal or high.
- A high serum urate is present.
- Low serum folate levels occur due to the increased activity of marrow tissue.

DIFFERENTIAL DIAGNOSIS

Fibrosis of the marrow, often with a leucoerythroblastic anaemia, can occur secondary to malignant infiltration with metastatic carcinoma, chronic granulocytic leukaemia or lymphoma. It can also occur post-irradiation. These secondary causes of myelosclerosis should be excluded.

Myelosclerosis should also be differentiated from chronic granulocytic leukaemia.

TREATMENT

This consists of general supportive measures such as blood transfusion, folic acid by mouth, analgesics and allopurinol. Cytotoxics and radiotherapy have been used to reduce splenic size, but these have little value; hydroxyurea is the commonest drug used. If the spleen becomes very large and painful, and transfusion requirements are high, it may be advisable to perform splenectomy.

PROGNOSIS

Patients may survive for 5 to 20 years. Death may occur from leukaemic change.

Essential thrombocythaemia

This is a very rare condition which is closely related to PV. The patient has $>1000 \times 10^9/l$ platelets in the peripheral blood. It presents with bruising, bleeding and cerebrovascular symptoms. Initially splenic hypertrophy may be seen, but as the condition progresses, recurrent thromboses due to the increased number of platelets reduce the size of the spleen and it may atrophy.

Essential thrombocythaemia has to be distinguished from secondary thrombocythaemia which is seen in haemorrhage, in infiltration of the bone marrow with malignancy, post-splenectomy and in other forms of the myeloproliferative syndrome.

Treatment is with phosphorus-32 or busulphan.

Hypersplenism

This can result from splenomegaly due to any cause. It is commonly seen with splenomegaly due to portal hypertension, rheumatoid arthritis (Felty's syndrome) and lymphoma. Hypersplenism produces:
- Pancytopenia

- Haemolysis due to sequestration and destruction of red cells in the spleen
- Increased plasma volume due to pooling of red cells in the enlarged spleen

Treatment is often dependent on the underlying cause, but splenectomy is sometimes required for severe anaemia or thrombocytopenia.

Blood groups

The blood groups are determined by antigenic structures on the surface of red cells. The presence of these antigens is under genetic control and they are therefore of value in paternity testing. More than 400 antigenic determinants are known to exist. The ABO and rhesus (Rh) systems are the groups of major clinical importance, although other groups may also be responsible for haemolytic transfusion reactions and haemolytic disease of the newborn. Table 6.17 shows some of the main blood group systems.

ABO system

The ABO blood group system was discovered in 1900 by Landsteiner, who took blood from six colleagues and noted whether agglutination took place when washed cells and serum were mixed together on a tile. In the ABO system, three genes are involved—A, B and O—but only two, A and B, produce red cells which are antigenic. This is because the A and B genes control enzymes that alter the basic antigenic glycoprotein present on the red cell, which is known as the H substance. Presence of the A gene results in conversion of the H substance to the A marker by the addition of N-acetyl galactosamine, and the B gene is responsible for the

conversion of the H substance to the B marker by the addition of D-galactose. The O gene leaves the H substance unchanged and therefore not antigenic. Antibodies can thus only be formed against A or B markers (see Table 6.18). The ABO markers are found on most body cells and are also secreted in fluids such as saliva, gastric juice, plasma and semen, under the control of secretor genes.

A or B antigens on the red cells will invoke IgG antibodies if transfused into an incompatible recipient, or if the cells cross the placenta during pregnancy.

The rhesus system

Antisera prepared in rabbits against the red cells of the rhesus monkey react with the blood of about 85% of Caucasian people. The system is complex, with C, D and E antigens; the reaction with the D antigen determines whether a patient is Rh(D) positive or Rh(D) negative. Immune antibodies directed against the D antigen can result from transfusion or may cross the placenta during pregnancy. They are of major importance in haemolytic disease of the newborn.

Blood transfusion

Transfusion of blood is a relatively safe procedure. Voluntary blood donations from donors who have been screened for syphilis, hepatitis and HIV are a safe and effective method of providing whole blood, packed red cells, albumin, fresh frozen plasma, cryoprecipitate, platelets and granulocyte concentrates, and immunoglobulins. Red cells of rare groups can be stored for a long time by keeping them at $-80°C$ with the addition of glycerol, but usually blood is stored at 4°C.

Selection and cross-matching of blood for transfusion
- The ABO and Rh(D) group of the patient is determined.
- The patient's serum is screened for atypical antibodies using saline techniques at room temperature (this excludes the presence of 'cold' antibodies, mainly IgM). Screening should also be carried out up to 37°C as IgG antibodies may cause agglutination at this temperature.

Table 6.17 The most important blood groups.

System	Frequency of antibodies
ABO	Very common
Rhesus	Common
Kell	Occasional
Duffy	Occasional
Kidd	Occasional
Lutheran	⎫
Lewis	⎪
P	⎬ Rare
MNS	⎪
Ii	⎭

Table 6.18 Definition of blood groups A, B and O using two antigens, anti-A and anti-B.

Blood group	Antigens in red cells	Antibodies in serum
O	None	Anti-A and anti-B
A	A	Anti-B
B	B	Anti-A
AB	A and B	None

- A blood donor of the same ABO and Rh(D) type is selected.
- The patient's serum is cross-matched with the donor red cells using saline techniques at room temperature and up to 37°C.

The hazards of blood transfusion (Table 6.19)
The hazards of blood transfusion are mainly haematological, and consist of:
- *Alloimmunization.* Antibodies may be produced against red cell antigens (ABO, Rh(D) and others), leucocytes, platelets and plasma proteins.
- *Incompatibility:*
  (a) ABO incompatibility may lead to intra-vascular haemolysis. Extravascular haemo-lysis may also occur.
  (b) Leucocyte and platelet incompatibility gives rise to febrile reactions, pulmonary symp-toms such as cough and dyspnoea, or post-transfusion purpura.

Other immediate complications are circulatory over-load, air embolism, thrombophlebitis, citrate tox-icity, hyperkalaemia and, when very large quantities of blood have been given, clotting abnormalities (see p. 636).

As a late consequence of blood transfusions, infections such as hepatitis, malaria, cytome-galovirus, acquired immunodeficiency syndrome (AIDS), and, rarely these days, syphilis, have been reported. Iron overload due to transfusion is dis-cussed on p. 279.

Severe intravascular haemolysis. The most serious com-plication of blood transfusion is incompatibility lead-ing to severe intravascular haemolysis. This pro-duces rigors, lumbar pain, substernal tightness, dyspnoea, a fall in blood pressure, haemoglobinuria and renal failure. Bleeding due to disseminated

Table 6.19 Hazards of blood transfusion.

Haemolytic transfusion reactions due to:
   Clerical error
   Mismatched blood
   Antibodies

Bacterial or pyrogen contamination

Circulatory failure due to overload

Thrombosis or air embolism due to faulty technique

Transmission of infection:
   Non-A non-B hepatitis
   Acquired immunodeficiency syndrome
   Malaria   ⎫ rare
   Hepatitis B ⎭

Transfusion haemosiderosis with multiple transfusions

Bleeding and electrolyte changes with massive trans-fusion of stored blood

intravascular coagulation (DIC) is a bad prognostic sign. The only effective treatment of this emergency is to stop the infusion and support the patient by maintaining the blood pressure and renal function.

The white cell

The five types of leucocytes found in peripheral blood are polymorphonuclear leucocytes (neutrophil granulocytes), eosinophil granulocytes, basophil granulocytes, lymphocytes and monocytes. Polymorphonuclear leucocytes originate in the bone marrow and are carried to tissues via the blood, where they are involved in phagocytosis. In contrast, lymphocytes are involved in immune defence, and may continue to circulate between the lymphatic tissue and the bloodstream.

NEUTROPHILS

The neutrophil granulocyte originates in the bone marrow as a myeloblast. This large undifferentiated cell gives rise to the promyelocyte and myelocyte, which contain characteristic granules. The nuclei then become lobulated, the number of lobes increas-ing with age. The neutrophils thus formed are then stored for up to 10 days, but are available for immed-iate release into the bloodstream in response to stimuli. Immature white cells are released when a rapid response (i.e. within hours) occurs in acute infection (described as a 'shift to the left' on a blood film).

Function
The prime function of the neutrophil granulocyte is to ingest and kill bacteria. Neutrophils are particu-larly effective if the bacteria are first coated with protein or opsonized. Bacteria are ingested into vacuoles, where they are subjected to enzymic destruction which requires the generation of hydro-gen peroxide. An accumulation of degenerate neutrophils gives rise to pus.

Neutrophil leucocytosis

A rise in the number of neutrophils to $>10 \times 10^9/l$ occurs in bacterial infections or as a result of tissue damage. It may also be seen in pregnancy, during exercise and after corticosteroid administration, due to early release of neutrophils from marrow stores (Table 6.20). In any tissue necrosis, a leucocytosis is produced and this may be accompanied by a pyrexia due to the production of a leucocyte pyrogen. The pyrexia and leucocytosis accompanying a myo-cardial infarction are a good example of this and may

Table 6.20 Causes of neutrophil leucocytosis.

Bacterial infection
Tissue necrosis, e.g. myocardial infarction
Corticosteroid therapy
Leukaemia
Myeloproliferative disease
Leukaemoid reaction
Leucoerythroblastic anaemia

be wrongly attributed to infection. A leukaemoid reaction (the overproduction of white cells, many of them primitive) may occur in severe infections, tuberculosis, or malignant infiltration of the bone marrow. In leucoerythroblastic anaemia, e.g. due to marrow infiltration with neoplasia, erythroblasts and primitive white cells are found in the peripheral blood.

Neutropenia and agranulocytosis

Neutropenia is defined as a circulatory neutrophil count below $1.5 \times 10^9/l$. A virtual absence of neutrophils is called agranulocytosis. The causes are given in Table 6.21. It may be a feature of severe infections with typhoid fever, virus infections or hypersplenism. It may also occur as a result of the administration of various drugs, including sulphonamides, phenothiazine, carbimazole and phenytoin. Neutropenia commonly complicates vitamin B_{12} or folate deficiency. In Felty's syndrome, rheumatoid arthritis is complicated by splenomegaly and profound neutropenia. This makes these patients very liable to infection.

In chronic granulomatous disease, neutrophils can ingest bacteria but, because of an enzyme defect which stops the production of hydrogen peroxide, certain organisms such as staphylococci, *Candida* and *Aspergillus* cannot be killed. The patient suffers from recurrent infections which are eventually fatal.

Table 6.21 Causes of neutropenia.

Racial (neutropenia is common in black races)
Viral infection
Severe bacterial infection, e.g. typhoid
Felty's syndrome
Megaloblastic anaemia
Drugs (for drugs causing marrow aplasia, see Table 6.9)
Pancytopenia from any cause (see Table 6.10)

CLINICAL FEATURES

Infections are frequent. A characteristic glazed mucositis occurs in the mouth and ulceration is common. Septicaemia complicates the condition.

INVESTIGATION

The blood film shows marked neutropenia, and the bone marrow confirms the absence of cells from the neutrophil granulocyte series.

TREATMENT

All current drug therapy should be stopped. Infection may require antibiotic therapy.

EOSINOPHILS

These are characterized by large cytoplasmic granules which stain brightly with eosin. The role of the eosinophil is uncertain. Eosinophilia is said to occur when the number of eosinophils is $>0.4 \times 10^9/l$ in the peripheral blood. It is associated with a wide variety of disorders. The eosinophil seems to play some part in the response to infections with helminths and protozoa. The causes of eosinophilia are listed in Table 6.22.

Table 6.22 Causes of eosinophilia.

Parasitic infestations, e.g.
Ascaris
Strongyloides
Allergic disorders, e.g.
Hayfever (allergic rhinitis)
Other hypersensitivity reactions, including drug reactions
Skin disorders, e.g.
Urticaria
Pemphigus
Eczema
Pulmonary disorders, e.g.
Bronchial asthma
Tropical pulmonary eosinophilia
Allergic bronchopulmonary aspergillosis
Polyarteritis nodosa (Churg-Strauss syndrome)
Malignant disorders
Lymphoma
Carcinoma
Melanoma
Eosinophilic leukaemia
Miscellaneous, e.g.
Hypereosinophilic syndrome
Sarcoidosis
Hypoadrenalism
Eosinophilic gastroenteritis

BASOPHILS

The physiological role of the basophil is not known. It is, however, associated with acute hypersensitivity reactions and life-threatening urticaria, asthma, and anaphylactic shock. Basophils are usually few in number, but are significantly increased in chronic granulocytic leukaemia and myelosclerosis.

MONOCYTES

These are precursors of tissue macrophages and are often involved in immune responses. Monocytes spend only a few hours in the blood, but can continue to proliferate in the tissues for many years. Macrophages are widely distributed through the reticuloendothelial system.

LYMPHOCYTES

Lymphocytes form nearly half the circulating white cells. They originate in the lymph glands, spleen, Peyer's patches, bone marrow and thymus. Circulating lymphocytes are small cells, a little larger than red cells, with a dark-staining central nucleus. There are two main types: the thymus-dependent or T lymphocytes, which are concerned with cellular immunity and form about 70% of the circulating lymphocytes, and the 'bursa dependent' or B lymphocytes, which are concerned with humoral immunity (see p. 113).

Lymphocytosis occurs in response to virus infections, particularly Epstein–Barr virus, which causes the illness known as infectious mononucleosis or glandular fever. It may also be seen in cytomegalovirus infection. It may occur following immunization against various childhood illnesses, and is seen in chronic infections such as tuberculosis and syphilis. Acute viral infections, pertussis and brucellosis also produce a lymphocytosis.

Bleeding disorders

In bleeding disorders there is abnormal bleeding due to impairment of haemostasis. Blood is normally separated by the endothelial cell from the activators of haemostasis.

Haemostasis

Haemostasis is achieved by the following processes (Fig. 6.21):

Vascular damage
When a vessel is injured and the endothelial cell lining damaged, the vessel constricts and platelets adhere at once to the exposed collagen.

Platelet aggregation
Platelets aggregate at the site of injury, resulting in release of substances such as nucleotides and

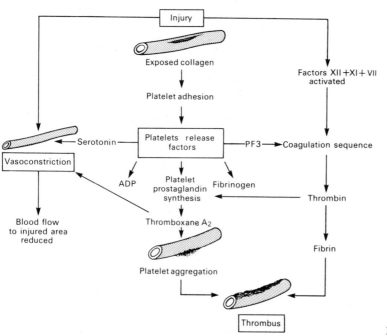

Fig. 6.21 Haemostasis.

serotonin, all of which contribute to haemostasis. Platelets also expose a surface membrane phospholipid (PF-3), which is necessary to activate both the intrinsic and common pathways of coagulation (Fig. 6.22). Platelet aggregation is enhanced by thrombin generated during coagulation. Platelets are also essential for the formation of a firm fibrin clot.

Central to these actions is the activation of platelet prostaglandin synthesis and the formation of thromboxane A_2 (Fig. 6.23), which increases aggregation. Prostacyclin (PGI_2) is synthesized by the vascular endothelial cell and prevents platelet aggregation on the normal vascular endothelial cell. PGI_2 formation is also stimulated by thrombin and may play a role in limiting coagulation to the site of damage.

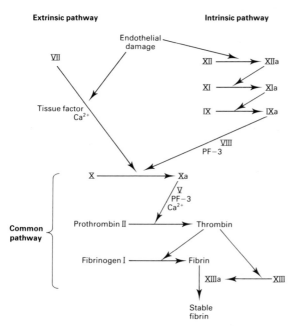

Fig. 6.22 Coagulation sequence.

Coagulation and fibrinolysis
Coagulation involves a series of enzymatic reactions leading to the conversion of soluble fibrinogen to fibrin clot. All of the enzymes except factor XIII are serine proteases and hydrolyse peptide bonds.

In the extrinsic pathway, tissue factors (lipoproteins released from damaged cells) together with factor VII and calcium ions activate factor X. In the intrinsic pathway, factor XII is activated by contact with the injured surface, and this activates factors XI and IX. Activated factor IX together with factors VIII and PF-3 are able to activate factor X. Factor X is therefore the start of a common pathway (Fig. 6.22). Its active form, Xa, together with factor V, PF-3 and calcium ions, forms a 'thromboplastin' which converts prothrombin to thrombin.

Thrombin hydrolyses the peptide bonds of fibrinogen to form fibrin. At the same time with calcium it activates factor XIII, which then stabilises the fibrin.

Clotting factors and platelets are both necessary for formation of a firm clot.

Coagulation is localized to the site of damage by circulating inhibitors of thrombin such as antithrombin III (AT III). This inactivates the serine proteases by forming stable complexes with them. Thrombin also complexes with the endothelial cell via a receptor protein, thrombomodulin. This increases the rate of generation of the active protein C, which destroys the coagulant properties of factors V and VIII.

Fibrinolysis, which helps to restore vessel patency, also occurs in response to vascular damage. Activated factor XII interacts with a kallikrein–kinin system, plasminogen and factor XI. The stable precursor plasminogen (Fig. 6.24) is then activated to form the serine protease plasmin, which hydrolyses fibrin, fibrinogen and other proteins.

Fibrin degradation products (FDPs) are readily measured in blood. Inhibitors of activation and of plasmin are present in blood and limit fibrinolysis.

Extravascular factors
These are important for haemostasis in situations

Fig. 6.23 Prostaglandin synthesis (simplified). TXA_2 = thromboxane A_2.

Fig. 6.24 Fibrinolytic system. Inhibitors of activation and of plasmin limit the process.

such as tonsillectomy, dental extraction and after parturition.

Investigation of bleeding disorders

Although the final diagnosis of a bleeding disorder may depend on laboratory tests, it is often indicated by the history and physical examination. The simple question 'Do you stop bleeding normally after tooth extraction?' gives valuable information.

Laboratory investigation
A blood count and film show the number of platelets, any morphological abnormality and may identify a blood disease such as leukaemia.

Bleeding time (BT) is a useful test in vascular disorders and disorders of platelet function. It depends mainly on capillary function, as well as platelet numbers and function. The bleeding time is determined by applying a sphygmomanometer cuff to the arm and inflating it to 40 mmHg. Three small lancet cuts are made in the skin of the forearm. Bleeding normally stops within 10 minutes.

The Hess or capillary resistance test parallels the BT but is less useful. In this test the sphygmomanometer cuff is inflated to 100 mmHg for 5 minutes. Development of purpura is abnormal.

Coagulation tests are performed on blood collected into citrate solution, which exactly neutralizes calcium ions and prevents clotting. The two most widely used tests are the prothrombin time (PT) and the partial thromboplastin time with kaolin (PTTK). The PT is measured using plasma recalcified with a tissue factor. This test is sensitive to depletion of factors in the extrinsic and common pathways (Fig. 6.22). A normal prothrombin time is 10–14 s. It is used to monitor oral anticoagulant treatment, and as a coagulation and liver function test. In the PTTK test plasma is recalcified with cephalin (a platelet substitute), and kaolin is added for maximal activation of clotting factors. The normal PTTK is 30–40 s. It is sensitive to factors in the intrinsic and common pathways (Fig. 6.22) and is valuable for screening for possible coagulation defects as well as control of heparin treatment.

Several other tests may be needed, such as estimation of fibrinogen and fibrin degradation products (FDPs), coagulation factor assays, especially for factor VIII, platelet function tests, and occasionally tests of the fibrinolytic system.

The purpuras

The purpuras are a group of disorders associated with superficial capillary bleeding, mainly in skin and mucous membranes, due to thrombocytopenia, platelet functional disorders or increased capillary permeability. A purpuric rash consists of small purplish red spots which do not fade on pressure. When they are confluent they are called ecchymoses.

THROMBOCYTOPENIC PURPURA

This is caused by either reduced platelet production in the marrow or excessive peripheral destruction of platelets (Table 6.23). Bleeding is uncommon with a count above 50×10^9/l.

Idiopathic thrombocytopenic purpura (ITP)

This is an autoimmune disorder which is commoner in women. An autoantibody (IgG) to platelets is found in 70% of patients. The sensitized platelets are removed by the reticuloendothelial system. The antibodies can cross the placenta, causing neonatal

Table 6.23 Causes of thrombocytopenia.

Impaired production
Marrow infiltration
Leukaemia
Tumours
Myelosclerosis
Myeloma
Marrow damage
Chemotherapy
Chemicals
Alcohol
Drugs
Aplastic anaemia
B_{12}/folate deficiency
Excessive destruction
Immune
Idiopathic thrombocytopenic purpura
Autoimmune haemolytic anaemia
Systemic lupus erythematosus
Drugs
Coagulation
Disseminated intravascular coagulation
Thrombotic thrombocytopenic purpura
Haemolytic uraemic syndrome
Massive transfusion
Sequestration
Hypersplenism
Haemangioma

thrombocytopenia. Subjects transfused with plasma from patients with ITP also develop thrombocytopenia.

CLINICAL FEATURES

The acute form is commonly seen in children following a viral infection and usually remits spontaneously. In adults it presents insidiously with a purpuric rash and superficial bruising. Epistaxis and menorrhagia are common.

Physical examination is normal except for evidence of bleeding. Splenomegaly is rare.

INVESTIGATION

Anaemia is uncommon and the only blood abnormality is thrombocytopenia, the platelet count usually being less than $20 \times 10^9/l$ in acute cases. The bone marrow is normal except for increased numbers of megakaryocytes with few associated platelets. Secondary causes of thrombocytopenia must be looked for. Platelet antibodies can be demonstrated in 70% of cases.

TREATMENT

The main aim of treatment is to reduce the level of autoantibody and reduce the removal of antibody-sensitized platelets. Initial treatment is with large doses of prednisolone, about 60 mg daily in an adult, with cautious reduction of the dose as remission occurs. This is successful in 75% of patients, but relapses occur. Splenectomy is used if steroids fail and is successful in over 50%. However, splenectomy should not be performed in young children because of the risk of subsequent infection.

Intravenous infusion of high-dose IgG sometimes produces a rapid increase in platelet count, as IgG blocks Fc receptors on macrophages. This increase in the number of platelets may be sustained.

Some refractory patients respond to azathioprine or vincristine. Platelet transfusions are used in ill, bleeding patients. However, because of the presence of antibody, these transfused platelets survive no longer than the patient's own platelets.

Secondary thrombocytopenic purpura

Secondary thrombocytopenic purpura may be due to a wide variety of causes (Table 6.23). Onset may be gradual or acute with bruising and excessive bleeding after injury, sometimes without a purpuric rash.

Drugs may cause thrombocytopenia as part of a general marrow depression. Isolated thrombocytopenia is sometimes due to an autoantibody produced against a drug–plasma protein antigen. Antigen–antibody complexes attach to platelets which are then removed by the reticuloendothelial system.

Platelet functional disorders

These are usually associated with excessive bruising and bleeding and, in some of the acquired forms, with thrombosis. The platelet count is normal or increased (thrombocythaemia), but the bleeding time is prolonged. Congenital forms are rare. Acquired forms of platelet dysfunction are seen in association with:
- Myeloproliferative disorders with morphologically abnormal platelets
- Uraemia and liver disease
- Paraproteinaemias which alter platelet aggregation and adherence
- Drugs, e.g. aspirin, dipyridamole and sulphinpyrazone. Aspirin inhibits prostaglandin synthetase and thereby interferes with platelet aggregation; because of this, aspirin is used in small dosages in thromboembolic disease.
- Von Willebrand's disease, in which there is platelet functional impairment caused by inherited abnormality of factor VIII

NON-THROMBOCYTOPENIC PURPURA

The causes of non-thrombocytopenic purpura are shown in Table 6.24. There is increased capillary permeability resulting in purpura and sometimes a prolonged bleeding time. Conditions include:
- *Hereditary haemorrhagic telangiectasia.* This is a rare disorder with autosomal dominant inheritance. Dilatation of capillaries and small arterioles produces characteristic small red spots on the skin and

Table 6.24 Causes of non-thrombocytopenic purpura.

Congenital
Congenital hereditary haemorrhagic telangiectasia (Osler–Weber–Rendu disease)
Ehlers–Danlos syndrome
Acquired
Severe infections
Septicaemia
Meningococcal infections
Measles
Typhoid
Allergic
Henoch–Schönlein purpura
Connective tissue disorders (SLE, rheumatoid arthritis)
Drugs
Steroids
Sulphonamides
Others
Senile purpura
Easy bruising syndrome
Autoerythrocytic sensitization
Paraproteinaemias

in the nose, mouth and gastrointestinal tract. Treatment by cautery may be needed for epistaxis. Chronic gastrointestinal bleeding is the major problem and the site of bleeding may be hard to localize.

- *Purpura due to infections*. This is usually due to damage to the vascular epithelium.
- *Easy bruising syndrome*. This occurs in young women. The purpura may be extensive. The cause is unknown and all investigations are normal. Recovery is spontaneous.
- *Senile purpura* and *purpura due to steroids*. These are both due to atrophy of the vascular supportive tissue.
- *Henoch–Schönlein purpura*. This usually occurs in children. It is a Type III hypersensitivity reaction which is often preceded by an acute infection. In addition to widespread purpura, abdominal pain, arthritis, haematuria and nephritis are present. Recovery is usually spontaneous.

Coagulation disorders

These may be hereditary or acquired. Hereditary disorders are uncommon and usually involve the deficiency of one factor only. Acquired disorders are commoner and almost always involve several coagulation factors.

HEREDITARY COAGULATION DISORDERS

Isolated deficiencies of all factors have been described, but 90% of cases are due to factor VIII deficiency.

Structure of factor VIII
Factor VIII is a complex protein made up of a small protein molecule (VIII:C) with coagulant activity and a larger protein molecule (VIIIR:Ag) which is associated with platelet function, particularly their adhesion to exposed collagen. Von Willebrand's factor (VIII:WF) is part of the VIIIR:Ag molecule. All these various components are necessary for coagulation.

Haemophilia A

In haemophilia, VIII:C is depleted; the other components of factor VIII are normal. It is inherited as an X-linked trait. The locus for this gene has been assigned to the long arm of the X chromosome. Therefore only males are affected. The incidence varies from 1 in 5000 to 1 in 10 000 of the population.

CLINICAL FEATURES

The most severely affected have factor VIII levels of less than 2% of normal. Haemarthroses which are often spontaneous and lead to arthritic changes are the most characteristic feature of haemophilia. Severe bleeding follows injury and isolated bleeding may occur into muscles, kidney, the mouth or neck. In patients with higher levels of factor VIII, spontaneous bleeding is rare.

INVESTIGATION

The main laboratory findings are shown in Table 6.25. Female carriers are identified by the family history and a low VIII:C compared with normal. Recently, DNA analysis of the VIII:C gene has provided an accurate method for carrier detection, and prenatal diagnosis with genetic counselling is now possible.

TREATMENT

Bleeding is treated by administration of factor VIII by intravenous infusion. In haemarthroses it may suffice to raise the level to 30% of normal, but for severe injuries, surgery and dental extractions the levels must be at least 60%. Factor VIII has a short half-life, so it must be administered twice daily. It is given as cryoprecipitate of normal plasma or as factor VIII concentrate.

Fibrinolytic inhibitors like tranexamic acid aid haemostasis, but these should not be given with renal bleeds as they may lead to the production of unlysable clots. Desmopressin (DDAVP) produces a rise in coagulant factor VIII and may be adequate for any mild bleed.

COMPLICATIONS

Boys with haemophilia are referred to special centres for advice on education, occupation and other social problems. Home treatment with factor VIII con-

Table 6.25 Blood changes in haemophilia, von Willebrand's disease and vitamin K deficiency.

	Haemophilia	von Willebrand's disease	Vitamin K deficiency
Bleeding time	Normal	↑	Normal
PT	Normal	Normal	↑
PTTK	↑ +	↑ ±	↑
FVIII:C	↓ ++	↓	Normal
FVIII:WF	Normal	↓	Normal
FVIIIR:Ag	Normal	↓	Normal

centrate is now possible and has reduced the incidence of haemarthrosis.

About 10% of severe haemophiliacs develop antibodies to factor VIII, making them refractory to treatment.

Following numerous transfusions there is a high incidence of hepatitis B infection and a risk of acquired immunodeficiency syndrome (AIDS). These risks are being reduced by heat treatment of plasma; it may eventually be possible to produce factor VIII by bioengineering methods.

Von Willebrand's disease

In this disease there is a reduced level of all the factor VIII components. It is inherited as an autosomal dominant disorder and therefore affects both sexes. It is usually less severe than haemophilia and haemarthroses are rare. Bleeding follows minor injury or surgery and menorrhagia and epistaxis are often seen.

INVESTIGATION

The observation that ristocetin aggregates platelets only in the presence of factor VIII:WF forms the basis for assay of factor VIII:WF (see Table 6.25).

TREATMENT

Fresh plasma or cryoprecipitate is administered intravenously when bleeding occurs or prophylactically before surgery.

Christmas disease (haemophilia B)

This is caused by a deficiency of factor IX. The inheritance and clinical presentation are identical to those for haemophilia A, but the incidence is only about 10% of that of haemophilia A. Christmas disease is treated with factor IX concentrates.

ACQUIRED COAGULATION DISORDERS

Vitamin K deficiency

Vitamin K is necessary for the carboxylation of factors II, VII, IX and X and without it these factors are unable to bind calcium and exert their coagulant function. Deficiency of vitamin K may be due to:
- Inadequate stores, as in haemorrhagic disease of the newborn or protein–energy malnutrition (see p. 132)
- Malabsorption of vitamin K, which particularly occurs in cholestatic jaundice as it is a fat-soluble vitamin and therefore bile salts are required for its absorption
- Oral anticoagulant drugs, which are vitamin K antagonists

The PT and PTTK are prolonged (Table 6.25) and there may be bruising, haematuria, and gastrointestinal or cerebral bleeding. Bleeding is treated with phytomenadione (a vitamin K) 10 mg intramuscularly or intravenously, which will restore coagulation factors to normal within 24 h. Severe bleeding is treated with fresh plasma. Vitamin K is administered prophylactically to all premature neonates.

Liver disease

Liver disease can result in coagulation defects for a number of reasons:
- With hepatocellular damage many coagulation factors are depleted because of poor liver function. The prothrombin time is prolonged. Vitamin K is not helpful, but is generally given because of accompanying malabsorption.
- Cholestasis, either intra- or extrahepatic, leads to malabsorption of vitamin K, with a decrease in the vitamin K dependent factors, i.e. II, VII, IX and X. The prothrombin time is prolonged and intramuscular vitamin K is required.
- Portal hypertension leads to splenomegaly, hypersplenism and a decreased platelet count.
- Acute liver failure is associated with disseminated intravascular coagulation (DIC) (see p. 301) and platelet abnormalities. Fresh frozen plasma is given if bleeding occurs.

Multiple transfusion syndrome

Stored blood contains few platelets and labile coagulation factors are depleted. After large rapid transfusions the PT, PTTK and platelet count should be checked, and fresh plasma, and possibly platelets, given if indicated.

Thrombosis

A thrombus is formed within the circulation by an aggregation of various components of blood. Thrombi are soluble; bits broken off are known as emboli. Thromboembolic disease is much more common than abnormal bleeding and may affect arteries, veins or the heart.

Arterial thrombosis

This usually occurs in atheromatous vessels but is also seen in normal arteries at sites of turbulent blood flow. Platelets adhere to diseased surfaces and the thrombus formed consists mainly of platelets with a small amount of fibrin, a *white thrombus*.

Anticoagulants will not prevent the formation of

thrombi composed mainly of platelets. Drugs inhibiting platelet function such as aspirin and dipyridamole may prevent further thrombosis.

Arterial emboli may derive from mural thrombi in the left ventricle, from the left atrium in mitral valve disease, or from the surface of prosthetic heart valves. They also arise from the aorta and large vessels, particularly the carotid arteries. Anticoagulants may prevent further embolization when the embolus comes from the heart.

Venous thrombosis

This often occurs in normal veins. Important causes are stasis and hypercoagulability. Stasis accompanies immobilization from any cause, e.g. after surgery or childbirth. Stasis permits accumulation of activated coagulation factors and limits their dispersal, preventing contact with inhibitors. A *red thrombus* is formed, consisting mainly of red cells and fibrin. Emboli are thrown off from newly formed areas of thrombus. A common clinical problem is pulmonary embolism from a thrombosis in the deep veins of the thighs or pelvis following childbirth or surgery.

Predisposing factors include local damage by cannulation and injections, varicose veins, surrounding inflammation, a previous history of thrombosis and advanced age. Increased blood viscosity is associated with both venous and arterial thrombosis and may be produced by changes in blood cells, as in polycythaemia, thrombocythaemia or sickle cell anaemia, or by high levels of plasma protein, as in myeloma or macroglobulinaemia. Depletion of inhibitors of coagulation has also been linked with venous thrombosis; examples include ATIII deficiency and reduced activity of vein wall plasminogen activator in malignant disease, obesity and women on the contraceptive pill. The roles of platelets, the protein C system and prostacyclin release are at present uncertain.

The clinical features and diagnosis are discussed on p. 549.

PREVENTION AND TREATMENT

Many blood changes have been described in venous thrombosis, but it is not possible to predict by laboratory tests whether an individual will suffer a thrombosis in the same way that bleeding can be predicted. Risk situations are well recognized. Preventive treatment consists mainly of promoting mobility in all cases and administration of anticoagulants when there is a special risk.

Anticoagulant treatment
Thrombi in veins usually resolve naturally. Anticoagulant treatment aims to prevent further thrombosis and prevent embolization while resolution takes place.

Heparin. This mucopolysaccharide has a direct and immediate action on coagulation in vivo and in vitro. It potentiates the irreversible complex formation between ATIII and the activated clotting factors, e.g. thrombin, factors Xa, XIIa and XIa.

Heparin is given by intravenous or subcutaneous injection and has a half-life of about 90 min. Dosage depends on whether it is being used for prophylaxis or treatment of established thrombosis. In the latter case 20 000–50 000 units daily are administered intravenously to prolong the PTTK or whole-blood clotting time to twice the normal value. Subcutaneous heparin is used prophylactically when venous thrombosis is likely to occur, e.g. after a myocardial infarction. The dose is then 5000–10 000 units 12-hourly.

The main complication is bleeding. This is treated by stopping the heparin. Only very occasionally is it necessary to give the heparin antidote protamine. Prolonged heparin treatment may cause osteoporosis.

Oral anticoagulants. The drugs used are coumarins or indanediones. These inhibit hepatic synthesis of vitamin K dependent factors II, VII, IX and X. They take at least 48 h to produce a therapeutic effect.

The most widely used drug is warfarin. Dosage is controlled by PT tests, which should be kept at two to four times normal if British Standard Thromboplastin (Manchester) is used. The initial dose is 10 mg, and maintenance doses are usually 1–10 mg daily. The PT is measured daily for the first few days until stability is achieved.

Many drugs interact with warfarin (see Chapter 14). Warfarin is largely bound to serum albumin, the free unbound warfarin being the active component. Any drug which interferes with this binding will potentiate the anticoagulant effect; examples include aspirin and indomethacin.

Warfarin is metabolized by the mixed function oxidases in the liver and induction of these enzymes by, for example, alcohol increases warfarin breakdown. Finally, drugs like aspirin which inhibit platelet function affect warfarin anticoagulation.

Side-effects other than bleeding are rare. Overdosage is common, but does not always cause bleeding and usually responds to reduction or stoppage of the tablets. With anything other than minor bleeding, vitamin K or fresh plasma is given.

Thrombolytic therapy
Heparin followed by warfarin is effective treatment in preventing further cases of venous thrombosis and pulmonary embolism, but does not affect established thrombi. The fibrinolytic system can be activated, inducing thrombolysis, by the administration of streptokinase or urokinase. These drugs are very expensive and there is a risk of bleeding when they are given systemically. Streptokinase is now becoming standard therapy during the first 6 h fol-

lowing a myocardial infarct. The introduction of streptokinase directly into the thrombosed vessel is being used for arterial thrombosis.

Disseminated intravascular coagulation (DIC)

DIC occurs in a number of conditions when coagulation factors from both pathways are activated. This activation generates thrombin which aggregates platelets, leading to platelet consumption and thrombocytopenia. Intravascular thrombin generates fibrin, thus depleting fibrinogen, prothrombin and other coagulation factors. In addition, fibrinolysis is stimulated, producing fibrin degradation products (FDPs), which further inhibit platelet function and fibrin polymerization (Fig. 6.25).

If the vascular endothelium is extensively damaged, surface contact stimulates platelet and tissue factors which then activate both coagulation and fibrinolysis. In DIC there is failure of inhibition of coagulation and secondary fibrinolysis follows.

CLINICAL FEATURES

The clinical presentation varies from no bleeding to complete haemostatic failure with widespread haemorrhage. This can occur from the mouth, nose or venepuncture sites, and the skin shows widespread ecchymosis. The patient is often acutely ill and shocked, but the clinical severity will vary according to the initiating factors.

CAUSES

These are varied and include abruptio placentae, amniotic fluid embolism, retained dead fetus, septic abortion, disseminated malignant disease, septicaemia, acute leukaemia, incompatible transfusion and anoxia.

INVESTIGATION

The diagnosis is initially suggested by the underlying condition. The PT is prolonged and the platelet count is reduced. The fibrinogen level is also reduced and FDPs are usually raised. A blood film may show fragmented red cells.

TREATMENT

Treatment may not be necessary. Bleeding requires infusion of fresh plasma and perhaps platelets. Heparin in low dosage to prevent intravascular coagulation is sometimes given in malignant disease and leukaemia, but its use is controversial. Fibrinolytic inhibitors like tranexamic acid should not be used in DIC as dangerous fibrin deposition may result.

Further reading

Beck WS (1985) *Hematology*, 4th edn. Cambridge, Massachusetts: MIT Press.

Biggs R & Rizza CR (1984) *Human Blood Coagulation, Haemostasis and Thrombosis.* Oxford: Blackwell Scientific.

Bothwell TH, Charlton RW, Cook JD & Finch EA (1980) *Iron Metabolism in Man.* Oxford: Blackwell Scientific.

Chanarin I (1979) *The Megaloblastic Anaemias.* Oxford: Blackwell Scientific.

Dacie JV (1985) *The Haemolytic Anaemias,* 3rd edn. London: Churchill Livingstone.

Ingram GIC, Brozovic M & Slater NGP (1982) *Bleeding Disorders.* Oxford: Blackwell Scientific.

Pennington D, Rush B & Castaldi P (eds) (1978) *de Gruchy's Clinical Haematology in Medical Practice,* 4th edn. Oxford: Blackwell Scientific.

Weatherall DJ & Clegg JB (1981) *The Thalassaemia Syndromes,* 3rd edn. Oxford: Blackwell Scientific.

Wintrobe MM (1981) *Clinical Hematology.* Philadelphia: Lea and Febiger.

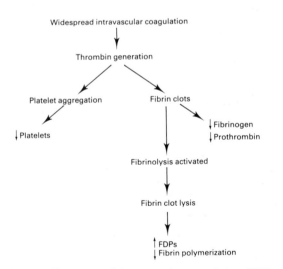

Fig. 6.25 Disseminated intravascular coagulation (DIC). FDP = fibrin degradation products.

7

Medical Oncology

Introduction

Cancer is a widely prevalent disease and is only second to cardiovascular disease as a cause of death in Western countries. It is not confined to the elderly; for example, it is the commonest disease causing of death in children over the age of 1 year in Britain.

The commonest cancers are malignant neoplasms of epithelial linings of organs such as the gut and the bronchi; these are called *carcinomas*. Malignancies arising from the mesenchyme, the *sarcomas*, are much less common, except in children. *Leukaemia* and *lymphoma* form a third important group. The management of cancer frequently involves more than one specialist, including the surgeon, radiotherapist and medical oncologist.

Haematological malignant disease is dealt with in this chapter; tumours of specific organs are covered in the appropriate chapters.

Aetiology and epidemiology of cancer

A wide variety of factors have been identified as being responsible for cancer, but in the vast majority of commonly occurring neoplasms, a single cause has not been discovered. Table 7.1 shows a list of possible factors. The role of these in producing cancers is discussed in the appropriate chapters. It is very likely that more than one factor is involved in tumour induction; for example it has been shown that asbestos and cigarette-smoking are synergistic in producing lung cancer.

Table 7.1 Possible factors in the causation of cancer.

Inheritance
Abnormal gene (e.g. dominant inheritance in retinoblastoma)

Environmental
Smoking
Ionizing radiation
Drugs – alkylating agents
Diet – aflatoxins
Alcohol
Occupation and chemicals (see Table 7.3)
Viruses

The changing incidences of three major cancers are shown in Fig. 7.1. The increase in lung cancer is directly related to the number of cigarettes smoked. The reason for the decline in stomach cancer is unknown.

Geographical factors
Geographical factors may play a part in determining the incidence of cancer. Scotland, England and Wales have the highest death rate from cancer in the world, largely as a result of the contribution made by carcinoma of the bronchus. Table 7.2 shows the variation in incidence of different tumours related to their geographical site. An example is the very high incidence of liver cancer, hepatoma, seen in parts of Mozambique; this has been traced to the ingestion of a toxic material called aflatoxin, which is formed by a mould on the groundnuts that form part of the diet.

Clustering of certain malignancies may give vital clues as to the aetiology of the condition. For example, the T cell leukaemias described in the southern

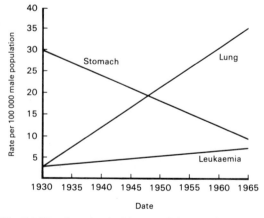

Fig. 7.1 The changing incidences of three major cancers.

Table 7.2 Variations in cancer incidence.

Types of primary cancer	Ratio of incidences (high : low)	High incidence area	Low incidence area
Liver	1000 : 1	Lourenço Marques Mozambique	Birmingham, UK
Oesophagus	200 : 1	Ghurjen in Kazakhstan	Netherlands
Nasopharynx	100 : 1	Chinese in Singapore	Chile
Bronchus	40 : 1	Liverpool, UK Birmingham, UK	Uganda
Stomach	30 : 1	Japan	Mozambique
Melanoma	10 : 1	New Zealand	Iceland

part of Japan and in the West Indies proved to be due to a virus.

Occupational factors
The first description of occupation playing a role in the development of cancer was by Percival Pott in 1775, who described scrotal epitheliomas in young chimney sweeps. These were subsequently shown to be due to carcinogenic hydrocarbons in soot and poor personal hygiene. A list of some of the most important industrially related cancers is given in Table 7.3.

Pathology of malignancy

Diagnosis of malignancy must be based on a biopsy of the tumour. The differences between the malignant cell and its normal counterpart are given in Table 7.4. Virtually all tumours begin as one abnormal cell. A single cell which transforms into a malignant cell may grow slowly in the epithelium over a number of years, giving rise to a carcinoma in situ (e.g. as occurs in carcinoma of the cervix). The growth then may become more aggressive and invade blood vessels. The next stage involves tumour-induced angiogenesis. This allows the tumour to grow rapidly, and it becomes clinically detectable. Tumours initially invade their local surroundings. As they do so, they infiltrate blood vessel walls and liberate cells into the circulation. These

Table 7.3 Industrially related cancers.

Agent	Occupation	Cancer
Ultraviolet light	Farmer, sailor	Skin
Soot, tar, oil	Chimney sweep	Skin
β-Naphthylamine	Chemical worker	Bladder
Asbestos	Insulation worker	Mesothelioma
Benzene	Varnisher, glueworker	Leukaemia
Vinyl chloride	PVC manufacturer	Liver

Table 7.4 Differences between benign and malignant cells.

Benign	Malignant
Non-invasive	Invasive
Highly differentiated	Poorly differentiated
Mitoses rare	Mitoses common
Slow growth	Rapid growth
No anaplasia	Anaplasia
No metastases	Metastases

cells are deposited into other tissues such as the liver and lungs to form micrometastatic disease. The continuing growth of a tumour and the burden of metastatic deposits eventually kill the patient. Fig. 7.2 shows how a relatively short interval may exist between clinically demonstrable disease and death, and how difficult it is, theoretically, to detect cancer early.

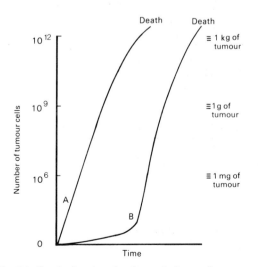

Fig. 7.2 Graph showing the theoretical growth curves of two tumours. A = rapid growth; B = dormant phase.

Staging malignant diseases

Prognosis is equally important to the patient as diagnosis. One of the major determinants for prognosis in most tumours is the stage that has been reached by the tumour. Staging is essentially a shorthand notation, generally understood, which describes whether the tumour is confined to the tissue of origin, has spread locally, or has metastasized. One of the most widely adopted is the TNM (tumour, node, metastasis) classification, which is applied to tumours such as breast cancer, carcinoma of the stomach and a wide variety of other cancers. Specific staging classifications have been developed for some tumours; for example, Hodgkin's disease is classified according to the Ann Arbor staging scheme, which incorporates not only the stage of the disease, but also the symptoms that have accompanied it (see Table 7.14, p. 322).

The TNM and allied methods of staging have been of great value in an era when surgery has dominated the diagnosis and treatment of patients. It is likely that as surgery becomes less important as the initial treatment these staging classifications will be modified. Although anatomical staging is important, the effect of the tumour on the patient has also to be taken into account, as this proves to be a powerful determinant for the patient's survival. David Karnowsky introduced the idea of a performance scale. The scale that he used is shown in Table 7.5. The Karnowsky performance scale is a powerful indicator of prognosis, it may allow the patient's performance as a result of treatment to be monitored, and it gives a measure of the treatment's toxicity.

Table 7.5 Karnowsky performance status.

100	Normal; no complaints
90	Able to carry on normal activity. Minor symptoms of disease
80	Normal activity with effort. Some symptoms of disease
70	Cares for self. Unable to carry on normal activity or to work
60	Requires occasional assistance but is able to care for most of own needs
50	Requires considerable assistance and frequent medical care
40	Disabled. Requires special care and assistance
30	Severely disabled. Hospitalization indicated, although death not imminent
20	Very sick. Hospitalization necessary, active supportive treatment necessary
10	Moribund. Fatal processes progressing rapidly

Measuring response to treatment

Response to treatment can be objective or subjective. A subjective response is one perceived by the sufferer. This term may therefore be applied to relief of pain, malaise and depression. An objective response is one that the observer makes, and is usually associated with some form of measurement, such as the size of a lump, the size of the spleen, or the width of a mediastinal shadow on a chest x-ray. Terms used to evaluate the response of tumours are given in Table 7.6.

The aim of all tumour treatment is to produce a complete response in a solid tumour, or complete remission in a haematological malignancy for without these patients will never be cured. A complete response in a solid tumour is the clinical disappearance of all evidence of malignancy with no evidence of tumour presence using the appropriate investigations. Complete remission is a term more commonly used in haematological malignancies, e.g. leukaemia, where, in addition to the absence of symptoms and signs of leukaemia (a normal peripheral blood count), a bone marrow aspiration with histological proof of the absence of any disease is required to confirm complete remission.

Assessing cure rates

Survival of a patient for 5 years used to be equated with cure, particularly when tumours were amenable to surgery, e.g. carcinoma of the colon. Recently, the terms 'median survival' and 'median duration of remission' have come into use; examples of these are shown in Fig. 7.3. The curve in Fig. 7.3b shows a plateau in the remission duration curve, which would infer that a proportion of the patients treated by that particular therapy are being cured. Statistical methods using life table curves are now of great importance in the assessment of therapeutic programmes.

Table 7.6 Definitions of response.

Complete response	Complete disappearance of all detectable disease
Partial response	More than 50% reduction in the size of the tumour
No response	No change or less than 50% reduction
Progressive disease	Increase in size of tumour at any site

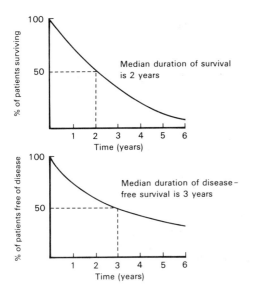

Fig. 7.3 Graphs showing examples of 'median survival' and 'median duration of remission'.

PRINCIPLES OF CHEMOTHERAPY

The use of drugs to attempt to cure cancer is relatively recent.

Alkylating agents
The discovery that nitrogen mustard, a derivative of the sulphur mustard war gases used in World War I, could cause regression in the size of lymphoid tissue opened the era of the treatment of disseminated cancer. Various congeners of nitrogen mustard were then produced, all with the ethylenimine group which is able to alkylate a wide variety of intracellular substances, including DNA. Most of the available alkylating agents are listed in Table 7.7. These drugs are 'radiomimetic', i.e. they produce damage of DNA by breaking up the molecule and by causing cross-linkages, so preventing cell division.

Antimetabolites
Another group of agents are the so-called 'anti-metabolic' drugs. Methotrexate, a compound very similar to folic acid, combines so tightly with the enzyme dihydrofolate reductase that it completely inhibits this enzyme, which is concerned with initiating DNA production. Methotrexate was the first of a large number of synthetic antimetabolic agents, and has been shown to produce temporary remission in childhood lymphoblastic leukaemia. More recently the administration of very high doses of methotrexate in order to achieve high cell kill has been made possible by the discovery that folinic acid can rescue normal cells. A number of antimetabolites are listed in Table 7.7. These agents act by interrupt-

Table 7.7 Antitumour agents.

Alkylating agents
Mustine hydrochloride (HN$_2$)
Chlorambucil
Cyclophosphamide
Melphalan
Dacarbazine (DTIC)
Nitrosoureas
Busulphan

Antimetabolites
Methotrexate
Mercaptopurine
Fluorouracil
Thioguanine
Cytarabine

Antitumour agents derived from plants
Vinblastine ⎫
Vincristine ⎬ Vinca alkaloids
Etoposide ⎭

Antitumour antibiotics

Actinomycin D
Daunorubicin
Doxorubicin
Bleomycin
Mitomycin C

Miscellaneous drugs of importance

Cisplatin derivatives
Hexamethylmelamine
Procarbazine
Hydroxyurea
Asparaginase

Hormones and antihormones

Oestrogens
Progestagens
Steroids
Tamoxifen
Aminoglutethimide
Buserelin

ing metabolic pathways or by substitution of various key sites in the DNA molecule.

Agents derived from plants
The periwinkle plant produces the two vinca alkaloids vinblastine and vincristine (Table 7.7). These are poisons which damage the protein tubules of the spindle of the cell during the process of cell division. Other powerful anticancer agents derived from plants include the epipodophyllotoxins such as etoposide.

Agents derived from bacteria
In the search for antibacterial agents, some species of *Streptomyces* were found to produce antitumour substances. The most important of these antitumour antibiotics are listed in Table 7.7. These may affect

cell division by damaging DNA. Actinomycin D, for example, forms complexes in the DNA helix, preventing separation and replication.

Miscellaneous drugs
Some miscellaneous but important drugs are also listed in Table 7.7.

Combination of anticancer drugs

In many tumours it has been shown that the proportion of tumour cells killed is related directly to the dose of the anticancer drug. Reduction of the number of cancer cells is usually measured in 'logs' (e.g. a decrease from 10^{12} to 10^{11} tumour cells is a decrease of one log) or in millions of cells killed. It is usual for the proportion of cells killed to remain constant with each dose of anticancer agent. Thus a number of doses of drug are needed in order to achieve the elimination of the cancer. Cancer drugs also have a powerful effect on normal tissues. It is therefore beneficial to combine two drugs which are additive or synergistic in their antitumour effect but which have different toxicities. A good example of this is the combination of vincristine, which is neurotoxic, and prednisolone, which has no neurotoxicity; the resulting summation of their antitumour properties is shown in Fig. 7.4. Multidrug regimens have become widely used in leukaemia, lymphoma and solid tumours such as testicular teratoma and the common childhood malignancies. Since the dose-limiting factor is often damage to the haemopoietic system, recent techniques in which the bone marrow is removed, stored and then administered after the cessation of chemotherapy have enabled even larger doses of cytotoxic drugs to be given.

Fig. 7.4 Remission rates in children with acute lymphoblastic leukaemia showing the summation of antitumour properties when two drugs are combined. P = prednisolone; V = vincristine.

Intermittent drug administration

The administration of chemotherapeutic drugs in 'pulses' allows the restoration of normal tissues between doses, as normal tissues repair more rapidly than tumour tissue. With pulses of drugs, recovery and growth of the tumour will lag behind normal tissue repair, and each course can have additive effect despite the relatively narrow therapeutic index for anticancer drugs (Fig. 7.5).

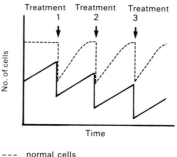

Fig. 7.5 Effects of multiple courses of cytotoxic chemotherapy (see text). From Priestman TJ (1977) *Cancer Chemotherapy—An Introduction.* Barnet: Montedison Pharmaceuticals. With permission.

Exploitation of the action of drugs on cell kinetics

On first principles it would appear an advantage for drugs, when used in combination, to affect different parts of the cell cycle. The cell, after dividing, rests for a while (Fig. 7.6); the interval, or gap, between mitosis and the onset of synthesis of the double quantity of DNA required for cell division is called G_1. Combining drugs that affect G_1, synthesis and mitosis might be more effective in killing the tumour. However, early attempts to exploit cell kinetics in this way have not been very successful.

Fig. 7.6 Diagram showing cell kinetics. M = mitosis; G_1 = gap 1; G_2 = gap 2; G_0 = phase out of cycle; S = synthesis.

Adjuvant therapy

When a patient first presents with a tumour, it is very likely that small amounts of tumour tissue have already spread to rest in the lungs, liver, bone marrow and other sites. This micrometastatic disease consists of relatively few cells with a good blood supply, and might be particularly amenable to the action of anticancer drugs. If, therefore, the primary tumour is removed, and chemotherapy is given to destroy the micrometastatic disease, the long-term survival and cure is improved. This was dramatically demonstrated in the childhood renal sarcoma, Wilms' tumour, when actinomycin D given after nephrectomy doubled the number of children with this condition who survived. Chemotherapy used in this way is known as adjuvant therapy, and has been employed in a number of other childhood tumours.

Treatment of malignancy in sanctuary sites

A 'sanctuary site' is the term used to indicate that micrometastatic disease has involved a site which is not accessible to conventional drug therapy. An example of this is the leukaemic infiltration of the meninges in children with acute lymphoblastic leukaemia (Fig. 7.7). Because of the blood/brain barrier agents such as vincristine and prednisolone do not enter the subarachnoid space in sufficient quantity to eliminate all the leukaemic cells, and are therefore ineffective in preventing the development of leukaemic meningeal infiltration. In order to treat these cells, intrathecal methotrexate or cranial irradiation is required.

Drug toxicity

Chemotherapeutic agents cause a wide variety of toxic side-effects, sometimes of considerable severity. It is therefore very important to be aware of the effects that can be produced by these drugs. A useful classification of such reactions is whether they are early, intermediate or late, and whether they are general or specific. Most chemotherapeutic drugs affect rapidly dividing tissues, and consequently are toxic to the bone marrow, the lining of the gut and the hair follicles (Table 7.8).

Drug resistance

Drug resistance is said to occur when a tumour is no longer sensitive to a drug and starts to regrow. Tumour growth may occur either because a group or 'clone' of cells that has never responded to the drugs is selected and becomes dominant, or because the tumour cells which were originally responsive are now able to circumvent the activity of the cytotoxic drug. For example, a tumour cell can, with repeated exposure, acquire the ability to reduce the amount of antitumour agent it takes up. Most antimetabolites work by inhibiting enzymes, and with repeated exposure these enzymes may decrease their affinity for the agent. In some cases the gene responsible for the production of the enzyme affected by the drug is

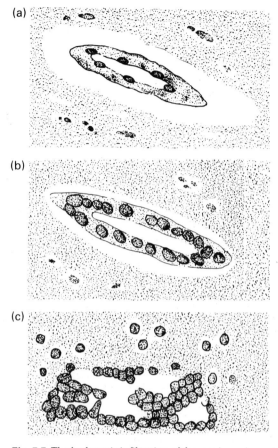

(a)

(b)

(c)

Fig. 7.7 The leukaemic infiltration of the meninges in acute lymphoblastic leukaemia. (a) A post-capillary venule, showing the pial–glial membrane. (b) Blast cells are seen in the vessel wall. (c) The pial–glial membrane is destroyed and blast cells are seen in the grey matter.

reduplicated, more enzyme is produced, and the effect of the drug, e.g. methotrexate, is thus diminished.

PRINCIPLES OF ENDOCRINE THERAPY

Many organs, particularly those associated with reproduction, are under hormonal control. Consequently, when tumours develop in such organs, manipulation of the hormonal environment may result in regression of the tumours. 'Hormone therapy' may be either the attempted removal of the source of a normal hormone, the administration of antihormone, or even the administration of other hormone substances. In general, hormonal therapy is not curative. It does, however, have the advantage of achieving long-term control with either little or no unpleasant side-effects in some patients. One exam-

Table 7.8 Classification of therapeutic toxicity.

Problems seen with most drugs	Specific problems (causative drugs in parentheses)
Immediate (hours)	
Nausea and vomiting	Haemorrhagic cystitis (cyclophosphamide)
Local tissue necrosis	Hypocalcaemia (mithramycin)
Phlebitis	Facial flushing (mithramycin)
Hyperuricaemia	Radiation reaction (actinomycin D, doxorubicin)
Anaphylaxis	Fever and chills (bleomycin)
Early (days to week)	
Leucopenia	Paralysis (vinca alkaloids)
Thrombocytopenia	Hypercalcaemia (oestrogen, tamoxifen)
Alopecia	Psychosis (steroids)
Stomatitis	Disseminated intravascular coagulation (asparaginase)
Diarrhoea	Pancreatitis (asparaginase)
	Fluid retention (steroids)
	Influenza syndrome (dacarbazine [DTIC])
	Pulmonary fibrosis (methotrexate, bleomycin)
	Cerebellar ataxia (fluorouracil, cytarabine in high doses)
	Ototoxicity (platinum compounds)
	Renal toxicity (platinum compounds)
Delayed (weeks to months)	
Anaemia	Peripheral neuropathy (vinca alkaloids)
Aspermia	Cardiac necrosis (anthracyclines)
Hepatocellular damage	Constipation (vinca alkaloids)
Hyperpigmentation	Cushing's syndrome (steroids)
Pulmonary fibrosis	Inappropriate ADH secretion (cyclophosphamide, vinca alkaloids)
	Masculinization (androgens)
	Feminization (oestrogens)
	Jaundice (6-mercaptopurine)
	Addisonian symptoms (busulphan)
Late	
Sterility	Hepatic fibrosis (methotrexate)
Hypogonadism	Encephalopathy (methotrexate)
Acute leukaemia	Carcinoma of bladder (cyclophosphamide)
Lymphoma	Osteoporosis (steroids)
Other second primary malignant tumours	

ple is in breast tumours, where hormone therapy may be the treatment of choice.

Tumours of the breast, prostate, endometrium and thyroid respond to specific hormones. Carcinoma of the prostate responds to orchidectomy, which removes the source of testosterone, but this tumour will also respond to oestrogens, and more recently has been shown to be responsive to buserelin (see below). Endometrial carcinomas can be treated with medroxyprogesterone, and some thyroid cancers respond to thyroid hormone, which causes suppression of the thyroid stimulating hormone. Leukaemia and lymphoma may respond to steroid hormones because of the general, and poorly understood, lympholytic effect of these agents.

The importance of cell-surface receptors for hormones, and the determination of their presence in the malignant cell, has been demonstrated. The binding of a hormone to a receptor and the translocation of the hormone–receptor complex into the nucleus, where it reacts with the DNA, is shown diagrammatically in Fig. 7.8. This mechanism can be seen in the 80% of patients with breast cancer who

Fig. 7.8 Mechanism of the cell receptor system. A hormone H combines with a receptor and the complex is transported to the nucleus where it reacts with DNA.

have receptors for oestrogens or progesterone. Hormone manipulation of breast cancer includes the administration of oestrogen, the use of the anti-oestrogen tamoxifen, the eradication of endogenous oestrogen production by oophorectomy, and by the use of aminoglutethimide which produces a 'medical' adrenalectomy. More recently, the use of buserelin, a long-acting analogue of gonadotrophin releasing hormone, which down-regulates pituitary gonadotrophin production and consequently depresses the level of gonadal hormone, appears to have an effect in premenopausal women with breast cancer.

Haematological malignant disease

THE LEUKAEMIAS

These diseases are characterized by the proliferation of a single malignantly transformed progenitor cell in the haemopoietic system. Acute leukaemia is a condition which, if untreated, has a rapidly fatal course. Chronic leukaemia has a more prolonged natural history, but the disease usually ends in death. These definitions are now less secure, for with modern effective treatments many patients with acute leukaemia survive for long periods of time, and some are cured.

CLASSIFICATION

There are two major types of acute leukaemia:
- Acute lymphoblastic leukaemia (ALL)
- Acute non-lymphocytic leukaemia (ANLL) —sometimes also called acute myelogenous leukaemia (AML)

The more chronic forms of these conditions are:
- Chronic granulocytic leukaemia (CGL)
- Chronic lymphatic leukaemia (CLL)

INCIDENCE

The commonest childhood leukaemia is acute lymphoblastic in type—some 80% of children with leukaemia suffer from this form. In adults the commonest acute leukaemia is ANLL, while ALL is less common. With increasing age, CLL becomes very much more frequent. The relative frequencies of acute and chronic leukaemias at different ages are shown in Table 7.9.

Table 7.9 Percentage of leukaemia at different ages.

| Type | Percentage of patients in age group | | |
	0–14 years	15–49 years	50+ years
All leukaemias	20	20	60
Acute	35	23	42
Chronic	4	15	81

From Gunz FW & Henderson ES (eds) (1983) *Leukemia*, 4th edn. New York: Grune and Stratton. With permission.

AETIOLOGY

The aetiology of the majority of leukaemias in humans remains unknown.

Genetic factors
Genetic factors are known to be important, as there is a low frequency of ALL in black children, a high incidence of leukaemia in the identical twin who has a sibling affected with acute leukaemia, and an increased risk of developing acute leukaemia in children with Down's syndrome (who have chromosomal abnormalities).

Environmental factors
These include:
- Radiation (there is an increased incidence of leukaemia in survivors of the atomic bomb in Hiroshima)
- Chemicals, e.g. benzene
- Drugs (phenylbutazone) and chemotherapeutic agents, e.g. alkylating drugs
- Viruses, e.g. human leukaemia virus type I (HTLV-I), which was first discovered in Japanese with T cell leukaemia and hypercalcaemia

Acute leukaemia

Cellular types
Acute lymphoblastic leukaemia (ALL). The blast cells involved may vary. They have been classified histologically into L1, L2 and L3 types as shown in Fig. 7.9. Some differences have been noted between the clinical presentation and prognosis of ALL L3 compared with the other two forms, but morphological distinction is not always easy, and this differentiation has not been of great clinical use. Far more useful has been the recognition of the different markers on the surface of the lymphocyte; the different types present in various leukaemias are shown in Table 7.10. These phenotypic markers have proved to be of considerable importance in assessing the likelihood of response and the long-term outlook.

Acute non-lymphocytic leukaemia (ANLL). In this condition the morphology and cell cytochemistry of the leukaemic blasts have been more helpful than cell

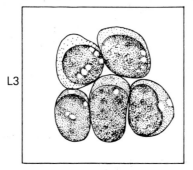

Fig. 7.9 The FAB classification of lymphoblastic leukaemia. In L1 the cells are small with scanty cytoplasm. In L2 the cells are larger with more abundant cytoplasm. In L3 the cells are large with characteristic vacuolation.

surface phenotypes in differentiating the clinical forms of the disease. The French–American–British (FAB) classification of ANLL is given in Table 7.11.

CLINICAL FEATURES

Symptoms
The history is usually short, and consists of:
- Symptoms of anaemia and malaise
- Acute infections such as mouth ulceration, sore throat, pneumonia, perianal and skin infections
- Painful and enlarging lymphadenopathy

- Bruising and bleeding
- Bone pain—this is particularly common in children with ALL
- Symptoms due to infiltration of tissues with leukaemic blast cells, e.g. marked gum hypertrophy in ANLL
- Headache, nausea, vomiting and blurred vision, as a result of raised intracranial pressure

Signs
These may be relatively few, but commonly they are:
- Pallor
- Bruising, petechial haemorrhages, bleeding gums and gum hypertrophy
- Lymphadenopathy
- Splenomegaly and hepatomegaly
- Haemorrhages in the optic fundi, occasionally with a characteristic central white deposit in the middle of the fundal haemorrhage, a classic feature of leukaemic retinopathy

Rarely, the patient may present with signs of meningeal leukaemia. In boys, hard enlarged testicles indicate that the testes have become infiltrated with leukaemic tissue.

INVESTIGATION

Examination of a peripheral blood film and of the bone marrow are essential. Because the disease may spread to the meninges, the CSF should also be examined, either at diagnosis or early in the course of treatment. Tests of renal function, serum uric acid, serum calcium and serum electrolytes, particularly potassium, should be performed. Blood cultures are necessary, and a chest x-ray is required to determine the presence of a mediastinal mass. Preparation for therapy will include blood grouping, coagulation studies and blood grouping of parents and siblings.

Diagnostic features
- There is a normochromic and normocytic anaemia.
- The white cell count may be normal or raised; very occasionally only a few blast cells may be seen in the peripheral blood, or none at all.
- The platelet count is usually reduced.
- Bone marrow examination shows a hypercellular marrow with characteristic blasts in the trail of the fragments on the microscope slide.
- The CSF should be examined on a cytospin. The prepared sediment will contain blast cells if meningeal leukaemia is present.

TREATMENT

The specific treatment programmes for the various forms of leukaemia will be considered, but it is important to note that they are steadily evolving and rapidly becoming obsolete. The supportive care and

Table 7.10 Phenotypes of childhood and adult leukaemia.

	Type of leukaemia			
	Common ALL (non-T non-B ALL)	T cell ALL	B cell CLL	ANLL
Anti-CALL	+	–	–	–
Anti-HLA-DR	+	–	+	+
Anti-TdT	+	+	–	–
Rosette formation	–	+	–	–
Anti-T	–	+	–	–
Surface immunoglobulin	–	–	+	–

CALL = common ALL antigen; TdT = terminal deoxynucleotidyl transferase; anti-T = anti-thymic antigen. Rosettes are formed with sheep red cells. From Hoffbrand AV & Pettit JE (1984) *Essential Haematology*, 2nd edn. Oxford: Blackwell Scientific. With permission.

preparation of the patient before specific therapy is probably as important to the patient's survival as the combination of drugs that is used.

Where there is rapid destruction of leukaemic cells, liberation of phosphates and other intracellular components results in hyperphosphataemia, hypercalcaemia, hyperkalaemia and hyperuricaemia—the so-called *tumour lysis syndrome*. It may be rapidly fatal. It is avoided by hyperhydration before administering chemotherapy and careful biochemical monitoring at frequent intervals.

Therapeutic strategy for ALL
This includes:
● Correction of dehydration
● The treatment of hyperuricaemia with intravenous fluids and allopurinol, a xanthine oxidase inhibitor
● The treatment of anaemia and thrombocytopenia by red cell and platelet transfusions
● Leukapheresis. This may be necessary in the presence of a high blast count (> 50 × 10⁹/l).
● Control of infection with the appropriate antibiotics
● Specific therapy. This should only be given in units with experience of managing acute leukaemia and where a particular programme is being followed.

There are three phases of therapy for ALL:
1 *Induction of remission.* This is carried out with a combination of four drugs, usually vincristine, prednisolone, an antitumour antibiotic such as doxorubicin or daunorubicin, and asparaginase. When remission is achieved, the further eradication of residual lymphoblasts is attempted by consolidation therapy. This uses drugs which are active against leukaemia but have not been given during induction.
2 *Cranial prophylaxis.* This usually consists of giving intrathecal methotrexate and cranial irradiation,

except in the very young; this is the standard regimen by which all others are judged. More recently, chemotherapy alone using methotrexate, cytarabine and corticosteroids has been used. In very young children, in whom there is evidence that cranial irradiation may cause brain damage, radiation is only given after completion of treatment.
3 *Continuation or maintenance therapy.* Once the bulk of tumour is reduced to a minimum, and disease abolished in sanctuary sites, continuation or maintenance therapy is given for a period of about 2 years. This comprises methotrexate and mercaptopurine given orally on an outpatient basis. During this time children are encouraged to lead a normal life, returning to school and all normal activities.

Management of relapse. Relapse of acute leukaemia can occur in three sites:
● *Bone marrow relapse.* This is the major cause of failure of therapy, and if it occurs while the child is on continuation therapy, the outlook is grave. The reinduction of remission and the use of total body irradiation supported by allogeneic bone marrow transplantation (see p. 274) is the only therapy known to produce long-term survival and possible cure. Bone marrow transplantation trials are currently under evaluation; only limited success has been achieved in this situation because of leukaemia recurrence in the marrow.
● *Relapse in the central nervous system.* This is much less frequent. It must be treated with intrathecal drugs and with craniospinal irradiation. If the blasts can be cleared from the CSF and bone marrow remission maintained, then about one-third of patients may become long-term survivors.
● *Testicular relapse.* This is sometimes seen as an isolated phenomenon, particularly during the

Table 7.11 FAB Classification of acute non-lymphocytic leukaemia.

FAB class	Common name	Morphology	Stains*	Electron microscopic features	Auer rods
M1	Acute myelocytic leukaemia without differentiation	Myeloblasts predominant; distinct nucleoli; few granules	MP+ SBB+ NSE−	Few granules	Rare
M2	Acute myelocytic leukaemia with differentiation	Myeloblasts and promyelocytes predominant; further maturation abnormal	MP+ SBB+ NSE−	Few to several granules	Few to several
M3	Acute promyelocytic leukaemia	Promyelocytes predominate; hypergranular	MP+ SBB+ NSE−	Many granules	Many, may be in clusters
M4	Acute myelomonocytic leukaemia	Myelocytic and monocytic maturation evident; may be peripheral	MP+ SBB+ NSE+	Granules in myelocytic cells; ribosomal lamella complexes in monocytic cells	Rare
M5	Acute monocytic leukaemia with differentiation	Promonocytes predominant; large cerebriform nuclei	MP− SBB− NSE+	Ribosomal lamella complexes	Not seen
M5A	Acute monoblastic leukaemia with differentiation	Completely undifferentiated blast cells	MP− SBB− NSE+	Ribosomal lamella complexes	Not seen
M6	Erythroleukaemia	Bizarre, multinucleated, megaloblastic erythroblasts predominate; myeloblasts also present	MP+† SBB+ NSE− PAS+‡	Ferritin granules‡	May be found in myeloblasts

* MP = myeloperoxidase; SBB = Sudan black B; NSE = Non-specific esterase; PAS = periodic acid–Schiff.
† In myeloblasts.
‡ In malignant erythroblasts.
From Wiernik PH (ed.) (1985) *Contemporary Issues in Clinical Oncology. Leukemias and Lymphomas.* New York: Churchill Livingstone. With permission.

first year off therapy, but it is usually a warning of general systemic relapse and has to be treated promptly. The outlook is good if the testes are treated with irradiation and the patient given reinduction therapy and a further period of maintenance treatment.

Prognostic factors. In childhood ALL the following are poor prognostic factors:
● The height of the initial leucocyte count. The greater the number of cells present, the worse the prognosis.
● The presence of central nervous system involvement at diagnosis
● Massive enlargement of nodes, liver or spleen
● Age below 2 years, or above 10 years
● Thymic enlargement
● The presence of T or B cell markers on the blast cells. These are probably not independent of the features recorded above.

All these factors must be taken into account in assessing the outlook in a particular child, but of greatest importance is the use of appropriate specific treatment and good supportive care.

Therapeutic strategy for ANLL
ANLL has to be carefully distinguished from other haematological conditions in which the bone marrow is infiltrated with blast cells, e.g. 'refractory anaemia with an excess of blasts' (RAEB). This latter condition, which is an example of a myelodysplastic syndrome, may be managed more satisfactorily by supportive care with blood transfusion and antibiotics than by specific chemotherapy, particularly in the elderly patient.

Principles of therapy. The aim is to secure complete remission by means of specific therapy. In ANLL this means ablating the bone marrow, and therefore a period of intensive support, including the administration of blood products and antibiotics, is required. Induction therapy usually includes an antitumour antibiotic, such as doxorubicin or daunorubicin, in conjunction with cytarabine. Other effective agents are steroids and vincristine; some other antimetabolites are less effective. The continuation treatments used for ALL are considered to be less effective in ANLL. The survival curves in a series of patients treated for ANLL in one unit are shown in Fig. 7.10. The best survival is seen with short-term intensive chemotherapy.

Types of acute leukaemia which require special management
Hypergranular promyelocytic leukaemia. Patients with hypergranular promyelocytic leukaemia (M3 on the FAB classification, see Table 7.11) present with severe bleeding problems. Severe bruising around the site of a venepuncture may be the first presenting

Fig. 7.10 Graph showing the survival of patients with ANLL treated with different types of therapy.

sign. This haemorrhagic state is due to disseminated intravascular coagulation (DIC) (see p. 301). It may be present at diagnosis, but can also be precipitated by therapy, when breakdown of the promyelocytes within the circulation results in an explosive production of fibrin, depletion of fibrinogen, and platelet aggregation.
　Initially treatment consists of:
● Platelet transfusion
● Maintaining the fibrinogen level with fresh frozen plasma
● Heparin

It is important to control the condition before specific cytotoxic therapy is started.

Hairy cell leukaemia. A rare form of leukaemia which is characterized by blast cells with cytoplasmic processes on the surface ('hairy' cells) is now recognized. It is associated with giant splenomegaly. It has proved to be resistant to usual forms of specific therapy for leukaemia, but recently has been shown to respond to interferon and to deoxycorformycin.

SURVIVAL

Children
Remission is achieved in more than 90% of children with ALL, and remission alone is now no longer the criterion by which success is measured. Disease-free remission after 5–6 years is a much better indication of the success of any treatment programme. The overall survival of children with all types of lymphoblastic leukaemia varies between 40 and 60%. Children with blast cells showing the common ALL antigen, so-called CALLA-positive acute leukaemia, may achieve higher survival rates, in the region of 70%, whilst children with T cell leukaemia do very much worse than the average.

Adults
The remission rate in adults with ALL is of the order of 70%. Long-term survival is, however, much less

satisfactory than in children, with only 15–20% surviving more than 5 years.

In ANLL, patients between the ages of 15 and 60 years may now have remission rates of between 75 and 80%, and in major centres using intensive chemotherapy, survival at 4 years is of the order of 30%. Since relapses are rare after that time, many of these patients may well be cured.

Chronic granulocytic leukaemia (CGL)

This is a relatively uncommon form of leukaemia which occurs in middle-aged and elderly people. It occurs in the myeloproliferative syndromes, which include polycythaemia vera, myelofibrosis, essential thrombocytosis and erythroleukaemia. It is characterized by the presence of the Philadelphia chromosome (see below).

CLINICAL FEATURES

- Often of insidious onset (may only be discovered on a routine blood count)
- Anaemia
- Bruising and bleeding manifestations
- Pain or discomfort due to a very large spleen, which may cause gastrointestinal disturbance
- Sweating, fever and loss of weight as the result of a high metabolic rate

Physical signs
- Anaemia
- Lymphadenopathy (uncommon)
- A large spleen (common)
- Haemorrhage and thrombosis; bruising, bleeding and priapism may occur
- Gout

INVESTIGATION

- The blood count initially may show a normal haemoglobin level, but eventually a normocytic, normochromic anaemia develops with an Hb of 9–10 g·dl^{-1}.
- The white cell count is greater than 50×10^9/l.
- The blood film shows an abundance of neutrophils, but myelocytes and even a few blast cells are present.
- The platelet count is normal or sometimes elevated.
- The bone marrow shows a hypercellular marrow with the granulocyte precursors markedly increased.
- A chromosome preparation shows the Philadelphia chromosome (Fig. 7.11).
- The leucocyte alkaline phosphatase (LAP) is very low.
- Levels of serum vitamin B$_{12}$ and B$_{12}$ binding proteins are elevated.

PROGNOSIS

Philadelphia-positive chronic granulocytic leukaemia is a distinct entity with a relatively slow progression. Median survival is about 35 months. The disease terminates with a blast phase (when acute transformation into blast cells occurs), or occasionally myelofibrosis becomes the dominant picture.

TREATMENT

The drugs of choice are busulphan and hydroxyurea. These are given to relieve symptoms, control the blood count and reduce the spleen size. Although

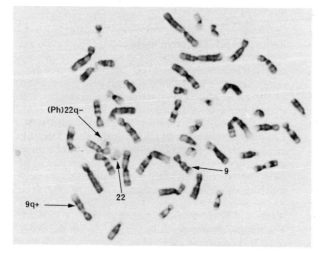

Fig. 7.11 Philadelphia chromosome. This is formed by a reciprocal translocation of part of the long arm (q) of chromosome 22 to chromosome 9. It is seen in 90–95% of patients with chronic granulocytic leukaemia. The karyotype is expressed as 46XX, t(9; 22)(q34; q11).

these drugs are effective, the median survival of CGL has not altered in the last 30 years. The management of the blast crisis is also very unsatisfactory. Treatment programmes used in ANLL may achieve remission but this is of short duration. Splenectomy does not alter the course of the disease, but can relieve discomfort. Bone marrow transplantation has been successful in a few young patients with CGL, but this treatment is only currently considered in patients under 40 years of age.

Chronic lymphatic leukaemia (CLL)

This is a disease of late middle-aged and elderly people, and is responsible for the rise in acute leukaemia that is being seen in the increasingly aged population in the Western World. It is a rare disease in the Far East, even in Japan where the proportion of elderly people resembles that seen in the West. It is a disorder of B cells, with accumulation of mature lymphocytes in the tissues and peripheral blood.

In a few cases the lymphocytes are T cells and skin involvement can occur.

CLINICAL FEATURES

The onset is insidious with:
- Lethargy
- Fever and sweating
- Loss of weight

Signs
- Moderate enlargement of lymph nodes in the neck, axilla and groin
- Splenic and hepatic enlargement, but not usually massive

INVESTIGATION

- There is usually a mild anaemia of the normochromic, normocytic type.
- The white cell count is $> 15 \times 10^9/l$, of which more than 40% are lymphocytes.
- The platelet count is usually normal.

As the disease progresses, the anaemia may become more severe, and the number of lymphocytes in the peripheral blood gradually increases until counts as high as $1000 \times 10^9/l$ may occur. Anaemia may suddenly become more severe as a result of Coombs' positive haemolysis.

STAGING

The Rai staging system is helpful, and gives an indication of prognosis (Table 7.12). Patients with Stage 0 have a median survival of 150 months, with the other stages having a poorer prognosis.

Table 7.12 The Rai staging system in chronic lymphatic leukaemia.

Stage	Definition
0	Lymphocytes $15 \times 10^9/l$ Lymphocytes 40% or more No enlarged lymph nodes, splenomegaly or hepatomegaly Normal Hb and platelets
I	Stage 0 + enlarged lymph nodes
II	Stage 0 + enlarged lymph nodes, splenomegaly or hepatomegaly
III	As Stage 0, I or II, but Hb <11 g·dl^{-1}
IV	As Stage 0, I, II or III + platelets <100 $\times 10^9/l$

TREATMENT

Patients in the early stage of the disease may not need any therapy. When symptoms develop, single drug therapy with oral chlorambucil is effective. Other useful drugs are cyclophosphamide and prednisolone. Intensive chemotherapy does not benefit these patients.

Radiotherapy should be avoided in the early stages of the disease, unless there is a specific indication, e.g. mediastinal obstruction, as it may result in loss of bone marrow reserve.

Infections due to reduced humoral immunity may occur as the B cell malignancy suppresses the normal immunoglobulin production. Potent intravenous preparations of gamma globulin are now available and are being assessed as prophylactic therapy.

VARIANT FORMS OF LEUKAEMIA AND LYMPHOMA OF T CELL ORIGIN

Very rare forms of malignancy in which the cell is of T cell origin are:
- Mycosis fungoides (see also p. 942)
- The Sézary syndrome (see p. 942)
- Peripheral T cell lymphoma
- Adult T cell leukaemia

The first three conditions may manifest themselves as a skin condition with progressive infiltration. The skin is usually erythematous, indurated and there may be intensive pruritus. These conditions show bone marrow and peripheral blood infiltration by characteristic T cells at some stage during their development. Adult T cell leukaemia is unique in that a specific virus, HTLV I, has been identified as its cause in humans.

THE LYMPHOMAS

These are malignant tumours of the lymphoreticular system. There are two main types histologically: Hodgkin's disease and non-Hodgkin's lymphoma.

Hodgkin's disease

This was first described by Thomas Hodgkin in 1832. It is characterized by aggressive enlargement of the lymph nodes, with hyperplasia, infiltration with histiocytes and lymphocytes, and the presence of characteristic cells described by Sternberg and Reed (Fig. 7.12).

EPIDEMIOLOGY

It is a rare disease in children, where it affects boys twice as often as girls, but with increasing age both sexes become equally affected. It appears to have an early peak of incidence in the twenties and a later peak in middle-age.

CLINICAL FEATURES

Hodgkin's disease commonly presents with enlargement of the cervical lymph nodes. However, cervical lymphadenopathy is a common finding in children and adults; the differential diagnosis is shown in Table 7.13. Glands elsewhere may also be enlarged, e.g. in the axilla or inguinal region, and are classically painless and 'rubbery'. Patients may also present with constitutional symptoms of weakness, fatigue and anorexia. Other clinical features of Hodgkin's disease are:
- Fever and sweating
- Pruritus
- Loss of weight
- Alcohol-induced pain at the site of the enlarged node

These clinical symptoms are usually seen in more advanced stages of the disease, particularly intermittent fever with drenching sweats. The so-called classical Pel–Ebstein fever, which consists of a few days of high pyrexia followed by apyrexia for a few days, is very rarely seen. Symptoms due to involvement of other organs, e.g. bone, lung and skin, may also be seen.

Examination reveals lymphadenopathy, hepatomegaly, and sometimes splenomegaly.

INVESTIGATION

Haematological findings may be unhelpful in the early stages. Later, a normochromic, normocytic anaemia with a raised ESR is characteristic. With marrow infiltration a leucoerythroblastic anaemia may occur. White cell levels can be raised, with occasional eosinophilia.

Biochemical findings show hypercalcaemia, hyperuricaemia, and slightly abnormal liver function tests due to liver involvement.

A chest x-ray may show mediastinal lymphadenopathy or pulmonary infiltration. Lymphangiography is commonly employed to show infiltration of the iliac, para-aortic and coeliac nodes,

Table 7.13 Differential diagnosis of cervical lymph node enlargement.

Infections
Acute:
  Pyogenic infections
  Infective mononucleosis
  Toxoplasmosis
  Cytomegalovirus infection
  Infected eczema
  Cat scratch fever
  Acute childhood exanthema

Chronic:
  Tuberculosis
  Syphilis
  Sarcoidosis
  HIV infection

Connective tissue disorders
Rheumatoid arthritis

Drug reactions
Phenytoin

Primary lymph node malignancies
Hodgkin's disease
Non-Hodgkin's lymphoma
Chronic lymphocytic leukaemia
Acute lymphoblastic leukaemia

Secondary malignancies
Nasopharyngeal
Thyroid
Laryngeal
Lung
Breast
Stomach

Miscellaneous
Sinus histiocytosis

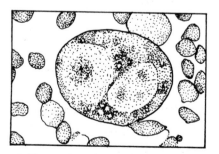

Fig. 7.12 The Sternberg–Reed cell.

but this is now less frequently used in non-Hodgkin's lymphoma where it has been replaced by CT scanning as this is rapid and non-invasive. However, in Hodgkin's disease when it is intended to proceed to laparotomy, lymphangiography should still be carried out. CT scanning of the chest is also helpful, particularly for identifying a tumour placed behind the heart in the mediastinum.

The diagnosis of Hodgkin's disease rests on the biopsy of a suitable node. If possible, a whole node should be removed, handled as little as possible, and placed immediately into fixative after incising the capsule.

Histological classification

There are four histological types of Hodgkin's disease:
- Lymphocyte-predominant, where there is heavy lymphocytic infiltration of the node
- Nodular sclerosing, where the gland is infiltrated with fibrous tissue
- Mixed cellularity, in which both lymphocytes and histiocytes are present
- Lymphocyte-depleted, in which there may be few or no lymphocytes present

STAGING

The current staging classification for Hodgkin's disease is shown in Table 7.14. Staging has been of great value in determining the prognosis and appropriate treatment.

TREATMENT

There are two effective treatments for Hodgkin's disease:
- Radiotherapy
- Chemotherapy using combinations of four or more active drugs

Radiotherapy

Radiotherapy is curative in Hodgkin's disease if all the disease sites are within the radiation field and an adequate dosage is given. In preparing a patient for radiotherapy alone, therefore, it is still necessary, in addition to the investigations noted above, to carry out a staging laparotomy with sampling of the para-aortic, iliac and coeliac nodes, removal of the spleen and a liver biopsy. Lymphangiography or CT scanning alone do not obviate the necessity for a laparotomy to obtain pathological staging of the disease. Treatment of stage IA or IIA with radiotherapy has an excellent prognosis, with more than 80% of patients showing long-term survival and probable cure.

Chemotherapy

Patients who have evidence of disseminated disease in stage IIIB or IV do not require a laparotomy, but should be treated with chemotherapy. It is the policy of some units to treat all patients with B symptoms (see Table 7.14) and those with stage III or IV disease with chemotherapy. Complete responses are seen in 90% of patients. Of those patients who achieve a complete response, 80% of those with stage IIIB disease and 60% of those with stage IV are alive after 10 years. A number of multidrug regimens for the treatment of Hodgkin's disease are now available; these are listed in Table 7.15.

Failure to achieve a complete response, or a relapse soon after a complete response has been achieved, is a very bad prognostic factor, and there are few long-term survivors in this group.

In children, the danger of splenectomy producing a susceptibility to overwhelming and fatal infection and the gross disturbance produced by extended field high-dose radiotherapy have resulted in the use of combined modality therapy: chemotherapy and lower-dose in-field radiotherapy

Table 7.14 Ann Arbor staging classification for Hodgkin's disease. The absence or presence of fever, night sweats, and/or unexplained loss of 10% or more of body weight in the 6 months preceding admission are indicated in all stages by the suffix letters A or B, respectively.

Stage	Definition
I	Involvement of a single lymph node region (I) or a single extralymphatic organ or site (I_E)
II	Involvement of two or more lymph node regions on the same side of the diaphragm (II) or localized involvement of an extralymphatic organ or site and of one or more lymph node regions on the same side of the diaphragm (II_E)
III	Involvement of lymph node regions on both sides of the diaphragm (III), which may also be accompanied by involvement of the spleen (III_S) or by localized involvement of an extralymphatic organ or site (III_E) or both (III_{SE})
IV	Diffuse or disseminated involvement of one or more extralymphatic organs or tissues, with or without associated lymph node involvement

Table 7.15 Combination chemotherapy for Hodgkin's disease.

Combination therapy regimen	Dosage	Route	Days when administered
MOPP			
Mustine (HN$_2$)	6 mg·m^{-2}	i.v.	1 and 8
Vincristine (Oncovin)	1.0–1.4 mg·m^{-2}	i.v.	1 and 8
Procarbazine	100 mg·m^{-2} daily	oral	1–14
Prednisolone	40 mg·m^{-2} daily	oral	1–14

14-day cycles separated by 14-day rest periods.
Usually 6 cycles.
Prednisolone in 1st and 4th cycles only.

MVPP			
Mustine (HN$_2$)	6 mg·m^{-2}	i.v.	1 and 8
Vinblastine	6 mg·m^{-2}	i.v.	1 and 8
Procarbazine	100 mg·m^{-2} daily	oral	1–14
Prednisolone	40 mg·m^{-2} daily	oral	1–14

14-day cycles separated by 28-day rest periods.
Usually 6 or more cycles.
Prednisolone given in all cycles.

ABVD			
Doxorubicin (Adriamycin)	25 mg·m^{-2}	i.v.	1 and 14
Bleomycin	10 mg·m^{-2}	i.v.	1 and 14
Vinblastine	6 mg·m^{-2}	i.v.	1 and 14
Dacarbazine (DTIC)	150 mg·m^{-2} daily	i.v.	1–5

14-day cycles separated by 14-day rest periods.

Chl.VPP			
Chlorambucil	6 mg·m^{-2} daily	oral	1–14
Vinblastine	6 mg·m^{-2}	i.v.	1 and 8
Procarbazine	100 mg·m^{-2} daily	oral	1–14
Prednisolone	40 mg daily	oral	1–14*

14-day cycles separated by a 14-day rest period.

* Reduced appropriately in children.

are given and laparotomy is avoided. Centres using this therapy report a greater than 95% overall survival after 5 years.

Non-Hodgkin's lymphoma

This is a tumour of lymphoreticular tissue derived from malignant clones of B or T cells. Presentation at extra-nodal sites such as Waldeyer's ring (tonsils, adenoids and nasopharyngeal glands), the gut or skin, is common.

CLINICAL FEATURES

Lymphadenopathy is again the outstanding feature, but the involved sites may be non-contiguous. Mediastinal lymph node involvement is less common, except in the T cell type of lymphoma. Abdominal lymph node involvement is common, and splenomegaly and hepatomegaly may occur early in the disease.

Wasting, fever and sweating may occur. Pruritus is uncommon, but nodular infiltration of the skin may be seen.

INVESTIGATION

- A normochromic, normocytic anaemia is seen with a raised ESR. Advanced cases show a leucoerythroblastic picture.
- Liver function tests may be abnormal if there is liver involvement.
- A chest x-ray, CT scan of the abdomen and, if necessary, a CT scan of the chest will show lymph node involvement.
- A bone marrow biopsy may show infiltration by lymphoid tissue

As in Hodgkin's disease, the most important investigation is the biopsy of a lymph node from an accessible site, with careful preservation of its architecture. In addition to formalin fixation, imprints of the gland may be prepared. Cell suspensions from the lymph node may be helpful in phenotyping.

Histological classification

There are two main systems of pathological classification:

- *Rappaport classification.* This was an early classification in which the essential prognostic difference between lymphomas showing a nodular or follicular pattern and a diffuse pattern of infiltration of the node was recognized. Patients who had nodes with a nodular pattern of infiltration did better than those with a diffuse pattern of infiltration. A better understanding of the biology of the cells contributing to the lymphoma has enabled a second classification to be developed.
- *Kiel classification.* This was described by Lennert in 1978 and is now finding wide acceptance. The major features of this classification are shown in Table 7.16.

The Kiel classification divides lymphomas into low grade and high grade malignancy. Centroblastic/centrocytic lymphomas with small cells have a good prognosis. Centroblastic lymphomas have a poor prognosis. Nearly all follicular and diffuse lymphomas derive from B lymphocytes. The blastic lymphomas are either lymphoplasmacytoid (some of which may produce monoclonal paraproteins) or centroblastic in type. In some patients who are young and present with mediastinal masses, the lymphoma has been shown to be derived from T cells; these have an especially poor prognosis.

TREATMENT

There is as yet no agreement as to the best way to treat these diseases. Patients with low grade non-Hodgkin's lymphomas who have been carefully staged and found to be stage I may be cured by local radiotherapy to the involved areas and adjacent nodes. Patients with favourable histology and stage II disease may also do well if local radiotherapy is given together with adjuvant chlorambucil.

Treatment of generalized disease

Favourable histology. Patients who have disseminated disease with a favourable histological type are currently not curable, although their prognosis may be good, with a median survival of 50% at 8 years. The aim of treatment is to control symptoms. This is done by the periodic use of short pulses of a single chemotherapeutic agent. Although multiple drug regimens, such as cyclophosphamide, vincristine and prednisolone (Table 7.17), may produce a slightly improved response rate, in randomized studies the overall survival has been no better than with single agents. On occasions, when local disease is producing severe symptoms, radiotherapy may be an effective method of treatment.

High grade non-Hodgkin's lymphoma. Paradoxically this may be curable and consequently should be treated with high-dose multidrug regimens such as cyclophosphamide, doxorubicin, vincristine and prednisolone (Table 7.18). Cranial prophylaxis with cranial irradiation and intrathecal methotrexate is

Table 7.16 Histological classification of non-Hodgkin's lymphoma.

Kiel classification	Rappaport equivalent
Low grade malignancy	
ML lymphocytic (CLL and others)	ML well differentiated lymphocytic, diffuse
ML lymphoplasmacytoid (immunocytic)	ML lymphocytic type with dysproteinaemia Lymphoproliferative diseases with dysproteinaemia
ML centrocytic	ML lymphocytic, well or poorly differentiated, nodular or diffuse
ML centroblastic/centrocytic (follicular, follicular and diffuse, or diffuse)	ML lymphocytic, histiocytic/lymphocytic or histiocytic, well or poorly differentiated, nodular or diffuse
High grade malignancy	
ML centroblastic	ML histiocytic, nodular or diffuse ML undifferentiated, nodular or diffuse
ML lymphoblastic (Burkitt type, convoluted cell type, or others)	ML undifferentiated ML poorly differentiated lymphocytic, diffuse
ML immunoblastic	ML histiocytic, diffuse

ML = malignant lymphoma; CLL = chronic lymphatic leukaemia.

From Lennert K (1978) *Malignant Lymphomas other than Hodgkin's Disease.* Berlin: Springer.

Table 7.17 Therapy for low-grade non-Hodgkin's lymphoma.

Drug	Dose	Administered
Chlorambucil	10 mg daily	Day 1 to day 42
		Day 56 to day 60
		Day 74 to day 88
		Day 102 to day 116
OR		
'CVP' combination chemotherapy		
Cyclophosphamide	400 mg·m^{-2} daily	Day 1 to day 5
Vincristine	1.4 mg·m^{-2}	Day 1
Prednisolone	100 mg·m^{-2} daily	Day 1 to day 5
Courses are given every 21 days.		

necessary. In T cell lymphomas or any high grade lymphoma with a large bulk of tumour, care must be taken to mitigate the effects of tumour lysis syndrome in the manner already described for acute leukaemia (see p. 311). With intensive multidrug therapy, the 5-year survival rate of adults with disseminated non-Hodgkin's lymphoma is of the order of 30%. In children it is higher, 5-year survival rates of 60–75% being reported in many series.

Burkitt's lymphoma

Burkitt's lymphoma was first described in African children presenting with massive jaw lesions, extranodal abdominal involvement, and ovarian tumours. It is endemic in areas of central Africa where there is a high incidence of the Epstein–Barr virus and in those areas where insect vectors and malaria are rife. There is an abnormality in chromosome 14. A child with African Burkitt's lymphoma is shown in Fig. 7.13.

The tumour is very sensitive to radiation and chemotherapy, but has a tendency to relapse.

Fig. 7.13 A child with Burkitt's lymphoma.

Table 7.18 Therapy for high-grade non-Hodgkin's lymphoma.

Drug	Dose	Route	Administered
CHOP Chemotherapy			
Cyclophosphamide	600 mg·m^{-2}	i.v	Day 1
Doxorubicin (hydroxydaunorubicin)	40 mg·m^{-2}	i.v.	Day 1
Vincristine (Oncovin)	1.4 mg·m^{-2}	i.v.	Day 1
Prednisolone	40 mg·m^{-2} daily	Oral	Day 1 to day 5
Courses are given every 21 days.			
MACOP Chemotherapy			
Cyclophosphamide	1 g·m^{-2}	i.v.	Day 1
Doxorubicin (Adriamycin)	50 mg·m^{-2}	i.v.	Day 1
Vincristine (Oncovin)	1.6 mg·m^{-2}	i.v.	Day 1
Prednisolone	100 mg·m^{-2} daily	Oral	Day 1 to day 5
Methotrexate	12.5 mg·m^{-2}	i.t.*	Day 7
Methotrexate†	300 mg·m^{-2}	i.v.	Day 10

* i.t. = intrathecal
† With folinic acid rescue: 15 mg folinic acid 6-hourly after 24 h for eight doses

Paraproteinaemias

Common clinical conditions associated with paraproteinaemia are:
● Multiple myeloma
● Waldenström's macroglobulinaemia
● Monoclonal gammopathy of undetermined significance (MGUS)
● Plasma cell leukaemia (very rare)

Paraproteinaemias are usually but not always associated with the presence of circulating paraprotein which is homogeneous and biologically inactive. Paraproteins are demonstrated by a single dark staining band on serum electrophoresis, which is referred to as an 'M' or monoclonal band. The relative frequencies of these so-called monoclonal gammopathies are given in Table 7.19.

The paraprotein is produced by abnormal cells which arise from a single clone and therefore produce monoclonal immunoglobulin. When there is an accumulation in the serum of either IgG, IgA or rarely IgD producing cells, the disease is known as multiple myeloma and the abnormal cells producing these immunoglobulins are plasma cells. The frequency with which the different immunoglobulins are produced in myeloma is given in Table

Table 7.19 Relative frequencies of monoclonal gammopathies.

	Percentage of total
Plasma cell myeloma:	
Multiple myeloma—symptomatic	60
Multiple myeloma—indolent	3
Localized plasmacytoma	2
Waldenström's macroglobulinaemia	10
Heavy chain disease	<1
Monoclonal gammopathy of undetermined significance (MGUS)	20
Primary amyloidosis	<5

Table 7.20 Relative frequencies of paraproteins in myeloma.

Paraprotein	Percentage of cases of myeloma
IgG	55
IgA	25
Light chain	18
IgD	1
Biclonal	1

7.20. An excess of light chains, which are either kappa or lambda in type, are excreted in the urine as Bence Jones protein.

In Waldenström's macroglobulinaemia there is an accumulation of IgM, which is produced by plasmacytoid lymphocytes. Excess monoclonal immunoglobulins are also seen in leukaemia (IgG or IgM) and in MGUS, where there is a monoclonal spike on electrophoresis but no evidence of multiple myeloma or Waldenström's macroglobulinaemia.

Multiple myeloma

CLINICAL FEATURES

Multiple myeloma is a disease of the elderly, the median age of presentation being 60 years. Men are affected slightly more often than women, and it occurs three times as often in blacks as in caucasians.

Symptoms
● Backache is very common, occurring in more than 80% of patients with myeloma. Vertebral collapse may lead to loss of height and paraplegia.
● There may be symptoms of anaemia.
● Recurrent infections occur. A history of sinus infections or pneumonia is common.
● Patients may present with renal failure, which may sometimes be secondary to hypercalcaemia and dehydration.
● There may be a bleeding diathesis, due either to thrombocytopenia or to the interference of the circulating paraprotein with clotting.
● There may be associated amyloid disease.
● There may be the symptoms of hyperviscosity, with pre-coma or coma, visual failure or heart failure. Hyperviscosity is particularly common in IgM myeloma, but may also occur in IgA or IgD myeloma.

INVESTIGATION

Three criteria required for the diagnosis of myeloma are:
● The presence of a paraprotein in the serum
● The presence of Bence Jones protein in the urine
● The presence of lytic lesions in the bone

The presence of any two of these features makes the diagnosis of myeloma very likely. Infiltration of the bone marrow with plasma cells may occur in myeloma, but is not diagnostic. Fig. 7.14 shows myeloma cells.

Other investigations
A normochromic, normocytic anaemia is common with rouleaux formation. There may be neutropenia and thrombocytopenia in advanced disease. The ESR is elevated, usually above 100 mm·h^{-1}.

A raised serum calcium is seen in one-third of

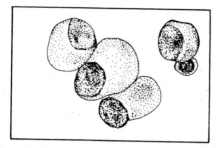

Fig. 7.14 Myeloma cells—large cells with an eccentric nucleus and a perinuclear halo.

Fig. 7.15 Myeloma affecting the skull. Note the rounded lytic translucencies produced by infiltration of the skull with myeloma cells.

patients on presentation. The alkaline phosphatase is normal in more than 85% of patients; a raised alkaline phosphatase is a bad prognostic feature, as also is a low serum albumin. About one-fifth of patients have evidence of renal failure on presentation. This is usually associated with heavy excretion of light chains in the urine, though other factors such as hypercalcaemia, hyperuricaemia, amyloidosis and infiltration of the kidney with myeloma tissue, may contribute to the renal failure.

Radiology
Radiology in myeloma may show characteristic features, e.g. the appearance of the skull shown in Fig. 7.15. Lytic lesions in the bone may also be caused by the common carcinomas of breast and bronchus, and the rarer carcinomas of thyroid and kidney.

PATHOLOGY

The complex pathology of myeloma is summarized in Fig. 7.16.

PROGNOSIS

The prognosis will depend on the amount of tumour present. Myeloma is difficult to stage, but schemes

dependent on radiology and quantitation of 'M' protein, the presence of anaemia, renal failure and hypercalcaemia have been devised and give a good indication of the outlook. The presence of severe anaemia or renal failure at presentation is a poor prognostic factor; in the presence of severe renal failure or a severe anaemia, half the patients are dead after 9 months. In good prognosis myeloma, where these features are not present, the median survival is of the order of 5 years.

TREATMENT

General management

Pain may be severe and require urgent treatment. If it is due to a local lesion, radiotherapy will give prompt relief.

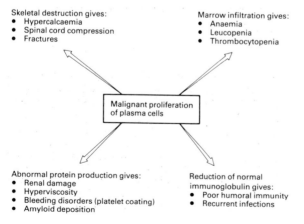

Skeletal destruction gives:
• Hypercalcaemia
• Spinal cord compression
• Fractures

Marrow infiltration gives:
• Anaemia
• Leucopenia
• Thrombocytopenia

Malignant proliferation of plasma cells

Abnormal protein production gives:
• Renal damage
• Hyperviscosity
• Bleeding disorders (platelet coating)
• Amyloid deposition

Reduction of normal immunoglobulin gives:
• Poor humoral immunity
• Recurrent infections

Fig. 7.16 The pathological consequences of plasma cell proliferation in myeloma.

Lytic lesions in the bone may predispose to pathological fractures; these may be prevented by the insertion of metal pins.

Patients presenting with severe renal failure require correction of the hypercalcaemia (see p. 737) and dehydration by intravenous fluids (more than 3 l daily), and steroids; with such treatment restoration of the renal function is usually prompt and successful. Other agents used to treat hypercalcaemia, such as calcitonin, mithramycin and diphosphonates, should be considered if the serum calcium fails to be controlled.

Anaemia and thrombocytopenia should be treated by transfusions of blood and platelets, but are more likely in the long term to respond to specific measures.

If the patient presents with paraplegia with bone destruction and the diagnosis is unknown, it is usual for surgery to be carried out in order to make a histological diagnosis. If the diagnosis is already known, the immediate use of dexamethasone in high dosage (12 mg in 24 h) is the treatment of choice. A myelogram is then performed to delineate the extent of the block and is followed by radiotherapy.

Hyperviscosity syndromes are treated using plasmapheresis.

Specific therapy
Specific chemotherapy with melphalan or cyclophosphamide has been shown to increase the median duration of survival from 7 to 30 months for large numbers of patients. Melphalan is given in courses at 3-weekly intervals, starting with 10 mg daily together with prednisolone 40 mg daily for 5 days. The courses can be gradually extended until further increase is prevented by the falling white cell count. Intensive multidrug regimens which have included doxorubicin, nitrosoureas and vincristine have been shown to produce slightly better response rates, but currently the evidence that they increase survival is dubious. More recently, in special centres with supportive care, the intensive use of high doses of melphalan has produced durable remissions in patients with bad prognosis myeloma.

Waldenström's macroglobulinaemia

This is a condition commonly seen in elderly men. It is more benign than myeloma, and is characterized by the production of monoclonal IgM paraprotein.

CLINICAL FEATURES

These are:
- Fatigue and weight loss of insidious onset
- Hyperviscosity (see p. 288)
- Bleeding tendency
- Anaemia
- Hepatomegaly and splenomegaly

INVESTIGATION

- There is usually a normochromic, normocytic anaemia with rouleaux formation.
- IgM paraprotein is found in the serum.
- The bone marrow shows infiltration with lymphoplasmacytoid cells.
- The ESR is often very raised to over 140 $mm \cdot h^{-1}$.
- Radiology shows an absence of lytic lesions.

TREATMENT

The progress of this disease can be very slow and specific treatment may not be required immediately. Supportive care with blood transfusion and antibiotics for infections will be needed. Specific treatment with alkylating agents such as cyclophosphamide or chlorambucil is usually given. Plasmapheresis is required for the symptoms of hyperviscosity.

Monoclonal gammopathy of undetermined significance (MGUS)

This used to be referred to as 'benign monoclonal gammopathy', but since a proportion of these patients go on to develop lymphoma or myeloma, this term is no longer appropriate.

Patients are usually elderly. A paraprotein is present in the blood, but the level is $< 2 \ g \cdot l^{-1}$. Patients are usually well, with no anaemia, renal impairment, skeletal lesions or Bence Jones protein in their urine. Serial estimations of the paraprotein should show no further increase. Specific therapy is not necessary and, as these patients are often elderly, it is important to recognize this condition and not put them at risk by giving them chemotherapy. The condition has to be distinguished from the rare form of indolent myeloma, which also may not need immediate specific therapy.

Amyloidosis

This is a complex condition and the mechanisms underlying the production of proteins are heterogeneous. Amyloid in tissues appears as an amorphous homogeneous hyalin-like substance which stains pink with haematoxylin and eosin and red with Congo red. With the latter stain it also shows a green fluorescence in polarized light. Amyloid consists of a network of fibrils. Amyloidosis can be classified according to the nature of the protein involved.

Immunocyte-related amyloidosis

In this variety the amyloid deposits (AL) consist of immunoglobulin fragments of light chains (the L in AL stands for light chain). The amyloidosis may be primary, when no cause is found, or may be associated with the lymphoproliferative diseases described above, e.g. myeloma, Waldenström's macroglobulinaemia or non-Hodgkin's lymphoma.

CLINICAL FEATURES

The clinical features are related to the organs involved, patients presenting with heart failure, nephrotic syndrome, purpura or bleeding, peripheral neuropathy or weight loss. Weakness and paraesthesia of the hand may occur due to the carpal tunnel syndrome. On examination a characteristic feature is macroglossia. Hepatomegaly and occasionally splenomegaly are seen.

INVESTIGATION

The diagnosis is made on the presence of the characteristic histological features mentioned above in a biopsy of the rectum or gums. The bone marrow may show plasma cells in primary amyloidosis or a lymphoproliferative disorder. A paraproteinaemia and light chains in the urine may be seen as a result of associated conditions.

TREATMENT

Treatment is symptomatic or is of the associated cause.

Reactive systemic amyloidosis

In reactive systemic amyloidosis, the amyloid (AA) is composed of protein A, which is a precursor of normal active-phase serum protein. This type of amyloidosis, which used to be known as secondary amyloidosis, involves the spleen, liver, kidney and adrenal glands. It is associated with long-standing chronic infections (e.g. tuberculosis), inflammation (e.g. rheumatoid arthritis), malignancy (e.g. Hodgkin's disease), and also occurs in familial Mediterranean fever (FMF).

Clinically there is hepatosplenomegaly. Hepatic failure and renal failure with renal vein thrombosis or the nephrotic syndrome may develop.

Other types of amyloidosis

Other types of amyloid can be identified on the basis of their biochemical structure. Proteins other than AL and AA have been identified. Amyloid may be limited to one organ, e.g. the heart, skin, lungs or brain. Localized deposits can also occur, for example in medullary carcinoma of the thyroid, insulinoma,

gastrinoma and myeloma kidney. Such deposits are also seen in the elderly. Various hereditary familial systemic amyloidoses apart from FMF also occur, e.g. Portuguese type I neuropathic amyloidosis.

Treatment of 'solid tumours'

Some non-haematological tumours can now be cured by chemotherapy. These include choriocarcinoma, testicular cancer and a number of childhood tumours such as Wilms' tumour, rhabdomyosarcoma, Ewing's sarcoma and osteosarcoma. Other tumours respond to chemotherapy, with resultant relief of symptoms and prolongation of life, e.g. small cell carcinoma of the bronchus, carcinoma of the breast and carcinoma of the ovary. It is beyond the scope of this chapter to give a detailed description of the presentation and investigation of these tumours, but a brief comment on current status of treatment programmes is included.

Testicular cancer

This is the commonest malignancy in young men between the age of 20 and 35 years. Disseminated teratoma of the testis was previously uniformly fatal. Currently, the use of vinblastine, bleomycin and more recently cisplatin has increased the survival rate to 66–80%.

Carcinoma of the breast

It is now accepted that breast cancer is probably a disseminated disease from its clinical onset, and that medical treatment is appropriate for the management of manifestations of the disease and its symptoms. There is little evidence that either chemotherapy or endocrine manipulation prolongs survival, but considerable relief of symptoms can be achieved.

Since neither chemotherapy nor endocrine therapy is curative in breast cancer, the principle should be to give the least toxic modality of treatment first; this should usually be endocrine manipulation. Tamoxifen has proved an effective and very tolerable form of treatment both in pre- and post-menopausal breast cancer. For patients who respond to hormonal manipulation, other agents such as aminoglutethimide which produces a medical adrenalectomy, may be helpful in relapse.

If endocrine therapy is not effective, or if the liver or bones are involved, chemotherapy should be considered. Doxorubicin and cyclophosphamide have been very effective when used in combination. The alopecia, stomatitis and cardiotoxicity, however, has limited acceptability of such treatment. A combination of cyclophosphamide, methotrexate and fluorouracil (CMF) also produces a high response rate.

The ability to affect overt breast cancer has stimulated the use of chemotherapy in an adjuvant setting over the past decade. Long-term experience, however, has shown very little evidence that multidrug adjuvant chemotherapy can produce more than a 10% increase in survival, and that this increase has often been achieved at the cost of considerable side-effects. More recently, a randomized trial of tamoxifen, with which there were no serious side-effects, has indicated that there is improved survival in the group treated postoperatively with this drug.

Terminal care and pain control

In many types of cancer the time comes when specific treatment is no longer effective. Therapy intended to cure has to be abandoned, and the patient enters the phase of terminal or long-term care. It is important not to look on this phase as the end of treatment. Indeed, surgery, chemotherapy or radiotherapy may still be required for palliation. The focus of treatment is now on symptom control, and the constant monitoring of pain, nausea, diarrhoea, constipation, insomnia, breathlessness, cough, anxiety and depression is essential if the patient is to be managed optimally.

Pain relief is a matter of skill. Local lesions in bone may respond dramatically to radiotherapy. Generalized bone pain may be relieved by steroids. Pain related to compression of nerves may be helped by local nerve blocks or cordotomy; newly developed techniques of epidural infusions or injections of steroid are also promising.

Analgesia must be given regularly and in sufficient dosage. Addiction is not a problem in the terminally ill and medical and nursing staff should not be inhibited in giving diamorphine or morphine in adequate amounts to control pain. The patient should not have to ask for analgesia, as the principle of administration is that analgesia should be given to prevent the onset of pain. It therefore needs to be given regularly, and the dose and time interval adjusted so that the patient remains pain-free. Drugs ascending in potency can be used. Paracetamol and dihydrocodeine may be used initially. When these become ineffective, dipipanone with cyclizine may be substituted, moving on to morphine or heroin for severe pain. Long-acting oral morphines are now available and are useful in patients to whom it is difficult to give parenteral therapy. It should be remembered that pain relief is not only a matter of giving analgesic drugs—sometimes a frank talk with an explanation to the patient of the reason for the pain and of the various measures which can now be used to suppress it may give considerable benefit.

Anorexia, nausea and vomiting are often troublesome symptoms in the terminally ill. Obstructive vomiting should be relieved by a nasogastric tube. Metoclopramide, cyclizine or chlorpromazine may be helpful in preventing nausea. Small doses of steroid may be of value, and the appetite-inducing effects of drugs like medroxyprogesterone are currently being studied. Constipation is a symptom which causes considerable misery, particularly in the elderly, and this may be made worse by analgesia. Regular mild aperients may help, but enemas may be necessary at the beginning of treatment with analgesics. Cough is relieved by methadone or diamorphine. Dyspnoea is a very difficult symptom to control and it is often related to anxiety. Diazepam and reassurance may be helpful. Anxiety and depression also often respond to sympathetic and patient discussion, but if this is not effective tricyclic antidepressants should be used.

The aim of terminal care is constantly to assist the patient. The first question should be 'What is the cause of the symptom and is it related to the cancer?' If it is not then it may well be alleviated. Heart failure, asthma and other common medical conditions can occur in a cancer patient as in any other, and these conditions should be treated. If the symptoms are due to the cancer, then it is important to identify the most distressing and to relieve them rapidly. Terminal care is exacting for the doctor and nursing staff but can be rewarding if carried out effectively.

Further reading

Goldman JM & Preisler HD (eds) (1984) *Leukaemias*. London: Butterworth.

Gunz FW & Henderson ES (eds) (1983) *Leukemia*, 4th edn. New York: Grune and Stratton.

Hoffbrand AV & Lewis SM (eds) (1981) *Postgraduate Haematology*, 2nd edn. London: Heinemann.

Kaplan HS (1980) *Hodgkin's Disease*. Cambridge, Massachusetts: Harvard University Press.

Lennert K (1978) *Malignant Lymphomas other than Hodgkin's Disease*. Berlin: Springer.

Saunders C & Baines M (1983) *Living with Dying. The Management of Terminal Disease*. Oxford: Oxford University Press.

Wiernik PH (ed.) (1985) *Contemporary Issues in Clinical Oncology. Leukemias and Lymphomas*. New York: Churchill Livingstone.

Yarbro JW (ed.) *Seminars in Oncology*. Orlando, Florida: Grune and Stratton.

Rheumatology and Bone Disease

Introduction

Rheumatology is concerned with medical disorders of the locomotor system; these can be divided into three categories: arthritis, back pain and soft tissue rheumatism. Most of these diseases are seen worldwide, although the prevalence of individual conditions varies. Rheumatological diseases constitute a major part (approximately 20%) of the workload of a primary care physician. The major complaints are pain and disability, arising not only from the joints, but also from the surrounding soft tissues.

The normal joint
The structure of a typical synovial joint is shown in Fig. 8.1. The joint itself is made up of two articulating bone surfaces, each covered with articular cartilage, and a fibrous capsule lined by synovium. The space within the joint is filled with synovial fluid which acts as a lubricant. Inflammation of the above structures is described as arthritis. The term arthropathy is sometimes used to describe joint disease of any type. The joint is surrounded by so-called 'soft tissues', including tendons, ligaments and bursae. The specialized junction of tendon and bone is called an enthesis; this can also become inflamed.

Rheumatological terminology
The main terms used in rheumatology are outlined in Table 8.1.

Table 8.1 Rheumatological terms.

Term	Meaning
Monarticular	One joint involved
Polyarticular	Many joints involved
Oligoarticular or pauciarticular	Two, three or four joints involved
Migratory	Arthritis moving from joint to joint
Arthralgea	Joint pain without swelling
Small joints	Joints of hands and feet
Large joints	Any other joint
Sero-positive arthritis	Rheumatoid factor present in serum
Sero-negative arthritis	Rheumatoid factor absent in serum
Sero-negative spondyloarthropathies	HLA-B27 associated diseases, e.g. ankylosing spondylitis, Reiter's disease, psoriatic arthritis

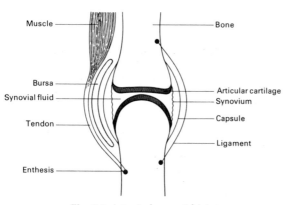

Muscle — Bone
Bursa
Synovial fluid — Articular cartilage
— Synovium
Tendon — Capsule
— Ligament
Enthesis

Fig. 8.1 A typical synovial joint.

CLINICAL FEATURES

History

The main features are listed in Table 8.2, and some of these points are discussed below.

Background information. This may be helpful in assessing the type of arthritis. For example:

- *Age.* Osteoarthritis commonly presents over 50 years of age.
- *Sex.* Rheumatoid arthritis is commoner in women, whilst Reiter's syndrome is commoner in men.
- *Race.* Some arthropathies are particularly associated with diseases occurring in particular races, e.g. in sickle cell disease.
- *Occupation.* This can be an important factor in soft tissue rheumatism or osteoarthritis.

Joint pain. The type of pain is of little help, as all joint pains feel much the same to the patient. The following points are of some value:

- *Duration.* For example, a long history is suggestive of rheumatoid arthritis, whilst a short history may suggest gout.
- *Onset.* Some conditions start suddenly.
- *Precipitating factors.* For example, injury may lead to arthritis, diuretic therapy can produce gout, and a sore throat precedes rheumatic fever.
- *Characteristics:*
  (a) Site of the pain—this usually indicates the site of the pathology (although hip disease may present with knee pain).
  (b) Radiation—e.g. pain from a lesion of the cervical and lumbar spine will give pain in the distribution of the affected roots.
  (c) Severity—e.g. excruciating pain is characteristic of acute gout.
  (d) Activity—joint pains are often made worse by activity and relieved by rest.
  (e) Diurnal variation—pain due to inflammation is characteristically worse in the mornings and improves during the day.
  (f) Episodic nature—the frequency, regularity and duration of attacks should be noted.

Other joint symptoms. The following should be inquired about:

- *Morning stiffness.* This is seen in inflammatory arthropathies. The duration of stiffness gives some guide to the activity of the inflammatory process.
- *Joint swelling.* This always indicates disease.
- *Pattern of joint involvement.* For example, recurrent attacks in the big toe are suggestive of gout.
- *Joint swelling.* This always indicates disease.
- *Clicking and creaking of the joint.* These are not important and can be felt in normal joints.
- *Disability.* This is a very individual problem. One patient may continue all activities, whilst another with the same degree of pain may be confined to bed or chair.

Associated non-articular symptoms. These are seen in many types of arthritis; for example, nodules or pleural effusions are seen in rheumatoid arthritis. Alternatively, systemic diseases such as ulcerative colitis may have an associated arthritis.

Past medical history. This may be helpful in the diagnosis, e.g. trauma or psoriasis.

Family history. Some conditions run in families, e.g. diseases associated with HLA-B27. Patients with ankylosing spondylitis may have relatives with ulcerative colitis. Patients with psoriatic arthritis do not necessarily have psoriatic skin lesions, but may give a family history of psoriasis.

Social history. The occupation of the patient may have a bearing on his arthritis. In addition, the development of a chronic arthritis has a major influence on the lifestyle of the patient and his family.

Treatment record. A record of the previous treatments tried and their success is important for the future management.

Examination of joints

There are three stages in the examination of an individual joint: *look at it*, *feel it* and *move it*.

Inspection will reveal swelling, deformities, changes in the overlying skin, e.g. erythema, and abnormalities of the surrounding structures, e.g. wasting of muscle or swelling of bursae.

Palpation will reveal the nature of any observed swelling as well as the presence or absence of warmth and tenderness, which are cardinal signs of inflammation. There are three types of joint swelling:

- A hard or bony swelling
- An effusion
- Synovial thickening

Table 8.2 Main features in the history of a patient with arthritis.

Background information
Main complaint
Pain, e.g. situation, radiation
Other symptoms, e.g. stiffness
Resultant problems
Pattern of joint involvement
Associated symptoms
Past medical history
Family history
Social history
Previous treatment

The presence of an effusion can be demonstrated by fluctuation or by a patella tap in the knee joint. A firm non-fluctuant swelling is characteristic of synovial thickening.

Movement of a joint may produce pain or crepitus—a sensation of grating which is characteristic of osteoarthritis. The range of movement should be noted. Excessive abnormal movement is called instability. Posture and gait should also be assessed.

Movement of joints is described in terms of flexion, extension, abduction, adduction and rotation. Deformities are described as valgus (pointing inwards) or varus (pointing outwards).

A system of examination should be followed so that no joint is missed.

INVESTIGATION (see Table 8.3)

Investigations are often unnecessary in patients with rheumatic complaints. In patients with tennis elbow, osteoarthritis and many other conditions, the diagnosis can be made on the basis of history and examination findings. There are no diagnostic tests in osteoarthritis and tests are only requested to exclude some other condition.

Erythrocyte sedimentation rate (ESR)
This is a simple but non-specific test which provides a guide to the activity of inflammation in a patient with arthritis. It is characteristically raised in inflammatory conditions such as rheumatoid arthritis. It is normal in osteoarthritis.

Tests for rheumatoid factor
Rheumatoid factors are autoantibodies found in the serum, usually of the IgM class, which are directed against human IgG. They are detected by agglutination of either latex particles (the latex test) or sheep

red cells (Fig. 8.2). The major value of rheumatoid factor tests is in the diagnosis of rheumatoid arthritis (Table 8.4). The latex test is quicker and easier to perform; it is more sensitive, and therefore more often positive, but is less specific than the sheep red cell test.

Fig. 8.2 Rheumatoid factor tests. The carrier particles used are latex in the latex test (which is positive in a titre of > 1:20) and sheep red cell coated with rabbit immunoglobulin in the Rose–Waaler test (differential agglutination test; DAT) and the sheep red cell agglutination test (SCAT) (which is positive in a titre of > 1:16).

Table 8.4 Conditions in which rheumatoid factor is found in the serum.

Diseases involving joints
Rheumatoid arthritis (80%)
Sjögren's syndrome (100%)
Systemic lupus erythematosus (50%)
Systemic sclerosis (30%)
Mixed connective tissue disease
Chronic infections (low titres), e.g.
Tuberculosis
Malaria
Infective endocarditis
Infectious mononucleosis
'Normal' population
Elderly
Relatives of patients with rheumatoid arthritis
Miscellaneous
Chronic active hepatitis (HBsAg-negative)
Fibrosing alveolitis

Table 8.3 Investigations in rheumatic diseases. (Most diagnoses are made on the history and examination.)

Useful tests
ESR
Rheumatoid factor
Antinuclear antibodies
Serum uric acid
Synovial fluid examination
X-rays
Occasionally useful tests
White blood count
Alkaline phosphatase
ASO titre—in rheumatic fever
Protein electrophoresis, immunoglobulin, urinalysis for Bence Jones protein, bone marrow—for myeloma
Complement
Arthroscopy
Synovial biopsy
Bone scan
HLA-B27

Antinuclear antibodies (see Fig. 8.3)
Antinuclear antibodies in the serum are detected using immunofluorescent staining of the nuclei of a tissue such as rat liver or human cells in tissue culture. The test is positive in most patients with systemic lupus erythematosus.

An increasing number of more specific antinuclear antibodies are being discovered.

Tissue containing   Serum from patient   Anti-human globulin
nuclei, e.g liver   containing anti-   labelled with
              nuclear antibodies   fluorescent label

Fig. 8.3 Immunofluorescent antinuclear antibody test. Control serum with no antinuclear antibodies does not fluoresce. Different patterns of nuclear fluorescent staining are seen (see text) which correlate with the presence of antibodies to a number of nuclear antigens.

A low titre of 1:10 is weakly positive and of little significance. A high titre is seen in systemic lupus erythematosus (SLE) (>95%), mixed connective tissue disease (9%), systemic sclerosis (50+%), rheumatoid arthritis (30%), Sjögren's syndrome (<80%), juvenile chronic arthritis (30%), and other diseases including polyarteritis nodosa (occasionally) and drugs producing an SLE-like syndrome, e.g. hydralazine.

Antibodies against double-stranded DNA. These can be detected using the FARR test, a radioimmunoassay measuring the percentage antibody binding of added labelled double-stranded DNA. Antibodies are found in about 50% of cases of systemic lupus erythematosus, but seldom in any other condition. They are therefore a much more specific test than antinuclear antibodies. They are also associated with more severe disease and renal involvement.

Antibodies against extractable nuclear antigen. IgG class antibodies against soluble nuclear antigens are frequently measured. A large number of these antibodies have been described, e.g. anti-Sm in systemic lupus erythematosus, and anti-Ro and anti-La in Sjögren's syndrome.

Other antibodies
Nucleolar staining suggests antibody to nucleolar RNA and is seen in scleroderma. Centromere staining is seen in the CRST syndrome (p. 344)

Serum uric acid
A raised serum uric acid is a good confirmatory test for gout, but is not diagnostic. A low level of uric acid excludes gout. In known cases of gout, the uric acid level is helpful in deciding treatment (see p. 353).

Synovial fluid examination
The characteristics of synovial fluid in normal and diseased joints are shown in Table 8.5. When synovial fluid is obtained from a joint, it should first be inspected and its volume, colour and viscosity noted. It should be divided into three portions for:
- White cell count and differential
- Polarized light microscopy
- Bacteriological examination

Polarized light microscopy reveals the presence of negatively birefringent crystals in gout. In pyrophosphate arthropathy, crystals of calcium pyrophosphate, which are weakly positively birefringent, are seen. Crystals of hydroxyapatite are too small to be seen on polarized light microscopy and need to be identified using electron microscopy. Gram stain may identify organisms in septic arthritis, but the fluid should also be cultured.

X-rays
X-rays show characteristic abnormalities in many rheumatic conditions; these are described in the appropriate sections. Degenerative changes are present in almost everyone by the age of 65 years and their presence on an x-ray therefore does not necessarily have clinical significance.

X-rays are of little value in acute conditions such as septic arthritis.

Table 8.5 Typical synovial fluid changes in some rheumatic diseases.

	Normal	Osteoarthritis	Rheumatoid arthritis	Septic arthritis	Gout	Pyrophosphate arthropathy
Appearance:	Clear viscous fluid	Increased volume; viscosity retained	Sometimes turbid, yellow or green in colour; viscosity lost	Turbid; low viscosity	Clear; low viscosity	Clear; low viscosity
White blood cells ($\times 10^6$/l):	<200 Mononuclear	3000 Mononuclear	30 000 Neutrophils	100 000 Neutrophils	10 000 Neutrophils	10 000 Neutrophils
Crystals:	None	5% have pyrophosphate	None	None	Needle-shaped, negatively birefringent	Brick-shaped, positively birefringent
Culture:	Sterile	Sterile	Sterile	Positive	Sterile	Sterile

Occasionally useful tests (see Table 8.3)
- The white blood cell count is useful in cases of infections and leukaemia presenting with arthritis.
- A raised serum alkaline phosphatase is characteristic of Paget's disease (p. 367), but is also sometimes seen in active rheumatoid arthritis and polymyalgia rheumatica.
- A monoclonal protein band on electrophoresis is found in myeloma, a condition which characteristically presents with back pain and a high ESR. The diagnosis may be confirmed by finding Bence Jones protein in the urine and abnormal plasma cells on bone marrow examination.
- A raised antistreptolysin-O (ASO) titre indicates recent streptococcal infection. Very high levels are characteristic of rheumatic fever.
- A high serum iron or ferritin level occurs in haemochromatosis, which may present with arthritis.
- A low serum complement may be found in the active phase of systemic lupus erythematosus.
- Arthroscopy is useful for the demonstration of mechanical lesions in the knee joint such as a torn meniscus and if necessary a synovial biopsy can be obtained during the procedure. This investigation is particularly useful in persistent monoarticular arthritis, e.g. in tuberculosis.
- A bone scan is useful in demonstrating malignant deposits. Increased uptake also occurs around osteoarthritic joints and also in inflammatory arthropathies, but these abnormalities can usually be distinguished from malignant disease.
- The histocompatibility antigen HLA-B27 is found in 96% of patients with ankylosing spondylitis and only 5% of normal people in the UK. There are marked differences between the incidence of the antigen in different populations which roughly parallel the frequency of ankylosing spondylitis. In addition, about 60% of patients with Reiter's disease are B27 positive.

Arthritis

The causes of arthritis are given in Table 8.6.

OSTEOARTHRITIS

Osteoarthritis (OA) is the commonest type of arthritis, occurring in about 10% of the population as a whole and in 50% of those over 60. It is a disease of cartilage, which becomes eroded and progressively thinned as the disease proceeds.

The pattern of development of joint disease in osteoarthritis is additive. The disease moves slowly

Table 8.6 Main causes of arthritis.

Osteoarthritis
Rheumatoid arthritis
Connective tissue disorders 　Systemic lupus erythematosus 　Polymyositis/dermatomyositis 　Systemic sclerosis
Polymyalgia rheumatica
Crystal deposition diseases 　Gout 　Pyrophosphate arthropathy 　Acute calcific periarthritis
Infective arthritis
Reactive arthritis
Ankylosing spondylitis
Juvenile arthritis, e.g. Still's disease
Arthritis associated with other diseases, e.g. psoriasis
Rare rheumatic diseases

from joint to joint and also progresses very slowly (in most cases) within individual joints. Its greatest impact is on weight-bearing joints such as the hips and knees and involvement of these joints is the commonest cause of disability in an elderly population.

AETIOLOGY AND PATHOGENESIS

Most OA is primary but in a small proportion of patients there is an obvious cause. The causes of secondary OA are listed in Table 8.7. Certain factors should be considered in primary OA:
- *Age*. OA was thought to be a gradual wearing down of joints as part of the ageing process. However, it does not affect all elderly persons and can also occur in the young. It has been shown that the cartilage in older people is biochemically different in those with OA.
- *Mechanical factors*. Damage to the joints, for example due to trauma and fractures through the articular surfaces, exercise or surgical meniscectomy, predisposes to OA.
- *Genetic factors*. The incidence of OA varies in different races and a familial tendency is often seen.
- *Obesity*. OA is more common in the obese.
- *Biochemical abnormalities*. OA is increased in patients with, for example, acromegaly, suggesting a metabolic or hormonal basis.
- *Diet*. There is no definite evidence for this being a factor in the genesis of OA, apart from over-eating leading to obesity.

Table 8.7 Causes of secondary osteoarthritis.

Congenital abnormalities of joints
Hypermobility
Congenital dysplasias

Structural disorders in children
Slipped femoral epiphysis
Perthes' disease

Trauma and mechanical problems
Intra-articular fractures
Meniscectomy
Obesity
Recurrent dislocation
Occupational hazards (e.g. repetitive actions)

Crystal deposition disease and metabolic abnormalities of cartilage
Pyrophosphate arthropathy
Ochronosis
Haemochromatosis

Avascular necrosis, e.g.
Sickle cell disease
Corticosteroid therapy
Caisson disease

Other conditions in which cartilage is destroyed, e.g.
Septic arthritis
Recurrent haemarthrosis
Inflammatory arthropathy such as rheumatoid arthritis

Neuropathic causes
Diabetes mellitus
Peripheral nerve lesions
Tabes dorsalis
Syringomyelia

PATHOLOGY

Changes in the articular cartilage occur first. There is loss of proteoglycans which form the ground substance, and an increase in hydration and cellular proliferation. This leads to the development of cracks and fissures; this process is known as fibrillation. Collagen fibrils, which are normally parallel to the surface, become disarranged.

Cartilage is lost from the articular surfaces and as a result the synovial tissues become thickened. There is increased activity and remodelling of subchondral bone; osteophytes (outgrowths of bone and cartilage) are formed and the surface of the joint becomes mineralized and hard (eburnation). Bone cysts, which are areas of relative porosis, show up as lucent areas on x-ray and occur adjacent to the joints.

EPIDEMIOLOGY

OA occurs throughout the world and has occurred throughout the history of mankind.

It often begins at about 50 years. It is twice as common in women as in men. It is particularly common in British populations, but this has nothing to do with climate, latitude or longitude and is therefore presumably genetic. OA is uncommon in black populations; when it does occur, it usually affects the knees and hand involvement is rare.

CLINICAL FEATURES

Symptoms
Pain, typically in the knees, hips or hands, is the major symptom. It is worse in the evenings and on movement, and is helped by rest. Initially the pain may be intermittent, but later it becomes constant and severe. There is morning stiffness (usually lasting less than 30 minutes) and stiffness after sitting. Eventually there is limitation of movement of the involved joint. Acute exacerbations, particularly in the knee, produce inflammation and swelling of the joint.

Signs
Early in the disease there may be no signs, but in most cases crepitus and swelling are present. Swelling is either due to an effusion or can be hard and bony. Acute exacerbations produce a warm, tender joint with an effusion.

There is limitation of both active and passive movement. Muscles surrounding the joint are wasted.

Joint deformities due to bony remodelling and cartilage damage are seen in the hands, knees and feet.

Hands. Bony swellings occur at the distal interphalangeal joints of the fingers (Heberden's nodes) and also at the proximal interphalangeal joints (Bouchard's nodes). When the small joints are affected they are hot, swollen and tender; when distal interphalangeal joints are affected in this way they are sometimes called 'hot Heberden's nodes'. In the later stages of the disease, inflammation disappears, leaving knobbly swellings.

The pattern of joint involvement in the hand is shown in Fig. 8.4. The first carpometacarpal joints are also sometimes involved. Bony swelling of the first carpometacarpal joint makes the hand appear square.

Knees. A fixed flexion deformity with joint instability is common. Bony outgrowths occur from the femoral condyles and upper end of tibia.

Feet. Deformity of the first metatarsophalangeal joint produces restriction of movement (hallux rigidus) and a valgus deformity (hallux valgus).

Hips. The hip joints are commonly affected, causing limitation of movement.

Arthritis of other joints, e.g. elbows and shoulders,

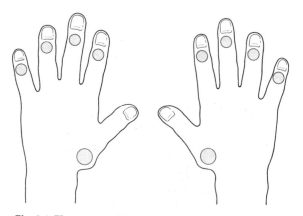

Fig. 8.4 The pattern of hand involvement in osteoarthritis. Bony swelling of the first carpometacarpal joints gives rise to the appearance of 'square hands'.

rarely occurs. Osteoarthritis is characterized by inflammation of joints but, unlike rheumatoid arthritis, there is no systemic involvement. Thus there are no non-articular features and no systemic illness.

DIFFERENTIAL DIAGNOSIS

The pattern of hand involvement should be contrasted with that of rheumatoid arthritis (see below), in which metacarpophalangeal and proximal interphalangeal joint involvement is usual and the distal interphalangeal joints are characteristically spared. The pattern of involvement of other joints in OA is contrasted with that in rheumatoid arthritis in Fig. 8.5. The number of joints affected in OA is much less than in rheumatoid arthritis and is usually only one to four sites.

Apophyseal joints in the cervical and lumbar spine are not uncommonly involved but it is difficult to distinguish OA in this site from chronic disc disease (see p. 362).

INVESTIGATION

X-ray changes
The x-ray changes in osteoarthritis are shown in Fig. 8.6. Narrowing of the joint space is due to loss of cartilage and is the most important change. It is accompanied by the formation of osteophytes at the margin of the joints, sclerosis of the underlying bone and cyst formation. In addition there is often calcification, which takes one of two forms:
- Linear calcification, which is characteristic of pyrophosphate deposition (see p. 354)
- Spotty calcification, which is characteristic of hydroxyapatite deposition

The formation of these crystals may contribute to the inflammation of osteoarthritis.

Osteoarthritis   Rheumatoid arthritis

Fig. 8.5 The pattern of joint involvement in osteoarthritis compared with rheumatoid arthritis. Both conditions are usually bilateral and symmetrical in distribution.

Blood tests
There are no diagnostic markers for OA. The ESR is normal and there are no biochemical abnormalities. Rheumatoid factor and antinuclear antibodies are negative; remember, positive tests can occur non-specifically in the elderly.

Synovial fluid (see Table 8.5)
Although not routinely performed, hydroxyapatite crystals can be demonstrated in the fluid by electron microscopy in a small proportion of cases. Pyrophosphate crystals can be demonstrated in 5% of cases.

MANAGEMENT

The nature of the condition, treatment and prognosis should be discussed with the patients.

There are three main types of treatment: drugs, physical measures and surgery.

Drug treatment
There is no specific therapy to control the disease process. Simple analgesics and non-steroidal anti-inflammatory drugs (NSAIDs) are used to control symptoms. The latter are more effective because of the part played by inflammation in OA. Systemic corticosteroid therapy is not used. Drugs such as gold and penicillamine which are used for rheumatoid arthritis are not effective in OA.

Intra-articular corticosteroids can be used for very painful and inflamed joints. Injection should be preceded by aspiration of any fluid in the joint.

Fig. 8.6 X-ray changes in osteoarthritis of the knee.

Labels on figure: Narrowing of joint space; Periarticular bone sclerosis; Osteophyte; Cyst

Physical therapy
The application of heat to an osteoarthritic joint may provide pain relief. Exercises are useful to maintain muscle power and are especially required for the quadriceps muscle in patients with knee involvement. Hydrotherapy is particularly useful for the hip joint, sometimes enabling a stiff joint to be mobilized and providing symptomatic relief. A walking stick may be useful for a patient with involvement of one hip or knee and should be held in the opposite hand.

Surgery
The greatest advance in the management of osteoarthritis has been joint replacement. Patients with severe disease of the hip can now have a total hip replacement which increases mobility and relieves pain. Knees can also be successfully replaced. For disease of the first carpometacarpal joint, the trapezium can be removed or replaced with a plastic prosthesis. The first metatarsophalangeal joint can also be removed (excision arthroplasty) or replaced.

RHEUMATOID ARTHRITIS

Rheumatoid arthritis (RA) is a common, chronic, systemic disease producing:

- A symmetrical inflammatory polyarthritis
- Extra-articular involvement, e.g. in the lungs and many other organs
- Severe disability in young adults in the prime of life
- Progressive joint damage
- A high morbidity which requires considerable resources in terms of doctors, drugs and surgery

PATHOLOGY

RA is a disease of the synovium. There are two main pathological characteristics—inflammation and proliferation. The synovium shows signs of a chronic inflammatory reaction with infiltration of lymphocytes, plasma cells and macrophages. It then proliferates and grows out over the surface of the cartilage, producing a tumour-like mass called 'pannus'.

The subcutaneous nodules seen in RA have a central area of necrosis surrounded by a palisade of macrophages and fibrous tissue. Similar lesions occur in the pleura, pericardium and lung. The lymph nodes are often hyperplastic.

PATHOGENESIS

The cause of RA is unknown. Toxic substances produced by the inflammatory reaction in the synovium are thought to lead to the destruction of cartilage, the characteristic feature of progressing RA.

Many immunological disturbances are seen, and RA is considered to be an autoimmune disease for the following reasons:

- Autoantibodies are seen:
  - (a) Rheumatoid factor—this is an antibody of any class, but predominantly IgM, directed against the patient's IgG (see Fig. 8.2). It is also found in other diseases and therefore may play little part in the pathogenesis of RA.
  - (b) Antinuclear antibodies (see Fig. 8.3)
  - (c) Antibodies against cytoplasmic antigens in the cytoskeletal structure, e.g. vimentin and keratin
- Immune complexes are common in the synovial fluid and the circulation.
- Synovial fluid also contains locally synthesized immunoglobulins and lymphokines.
- There is a defect in cell-mediated immunity.

In view of these abnormalities, a series of events can be postulated for the production of damage. Any unknown foreign antigen, perhaps even a virus, in the joint will be processed by antigen-presenting cells (see p. 109) and cause the local production of antibodies. Antigen–antibody complexes are formed and these attract neutrophil polymorphs into the synovial fluid and activate the complement system. The neutrophils and macrophages phagocytose the immune complexes and release chemical mediators of acute inflammation such as lymphokines, lysosomal enzymes, prostaglandins and leukotrienes. Continued inflammation stimulates the synovium to proliferate and spread over the joint as 'pannus', whilst the enzymes destroy the cartilage and bone.

Although it is tempting to ascribe the pathogenesis to a primary immunological event, the above abnormalities may, nevertheless, merely be secondary to the process of inflammation and proliferation.

EPIDEMIOLOGY

RA affects about 2% of the population world-wide and is just as common in tropical countries as in cold, damp Britain. It is about three times as common in women than in men. It can begin at any age from 10 to 70 years, but it most often starts between the ages of 30 and 40. There is an increased incidence in those with a family history of RA (5–10%), and an association between HLA-DR4 and seropositive RA has been described.

CLINICAL FEATURES

RA usually presents with the insidious onset of pain and stiffness in the small joints of the hands and feet, which eventually leads to the characteristic bilateral symmetrical peripheral polyarthritis. Less often it can present as arthritis of a single joint such as the knee.

Approximately 15% of patients have an acute onset. This can occur in the elderly and is sometimes called explosive RA.

General symptoms
Patients often feel tired and unwell. The pain is worse in the mornings on waking, improves as the day goes on and gets worse again in the evenings. Pain at night with disturbed sleep is common. With active RA, patients may remain stiff for several hours after waking.

Joints
Affected joints are swollen, often warm, but are seldom red. The swelling is soft and made up of effusion and synovial proliferation. Actively inflamed joints are stiff, painful and tender. There may be muscle wasting. The pattern of joint involvement is shown in Fig. 8.5. Sites which may be involved include the hands and feet, wrists and ankles, knees and elbows, the shoulders and the cervical spine. The dorsal and lumbar spines are not involved.

The hips. The hip joint is involved in about 50% of patients. This seldom occurs at the onset of the disease but usually develops within the first few years.

The hands and wrists. The pattern of joint involvement is shown in Fig. 8.7. In contrast to OA, the distal interphalangeal joints are only involved in 30% of cases. Early in the disease there is spindling of the

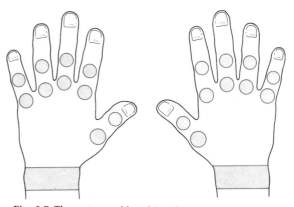

Fig. 8.7 The pattern of hand involvement in rheumatoid arthritis.

fingers, with swellings in the metacarpophalangeal and wrist joints. Tenosynovitis at the wrists can produce the carpal tunnel syndrome due to entrapment of the median nerve. Later, with progressive disease activity, there is weakening of joint capsules, muscle wasting and rupture of the tendons. These changes may produce the characteristic deformities shown in Fig. 8.8.

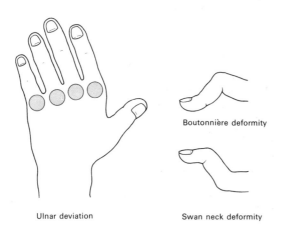

Fig. 8.8 Characteristic hand deformities in rheumatoid arthritis.

The feet and ankles. Deformities similar to those seen in the hands and wrists occur. There is lateral deviation of the toes and subluxation of the metatarsophalangeal joints so that the heads of the metatarsals become palpable in the soles of the feet. Patients often describe a sensation of walking on marbles.

The knees. Synovial effusions, weakening of the capsule and quadriceps wasting produce an unstable knee joint. Valgus or varus deformities may be seen. The synovial space may expand to form a Baker's cyst in the popliteal fossa. If the joint ruptures posteriorly, the synovial fluid passes into the calf and, being an irritant, produces pain and swelling in the muscle. This may be mistaken for a deep vein thrombosis, but the diagnosis can be confirmed with an arthrogram.

The cervical spine. Changes in the cervical spine occur in the majority of patients and, although many are asymptomatic, a few patients may have gross neurological signs. Atlanto-axial subluxation occurs in a quarter of hospital patients.

Progression and prognosis of joint involvement
The activity and rate of progression of joint changes in RA are very variable. New joints appear to get involved in an additive pattern in most cases. The pattern of joint involvement is established within months of its onset. Partial remissions and relapses follow. In some, the disease is mild with little or no progression. In others, the characteristic deformities and complications occur. About 10% of patients become seriously disabled and 40% develop significant disability.

Palindromic rheumatism. This consists of short episodes of joint pain and stiffness lasting up to seven days. Wrists, knees, ankles and elbows are usually involved, with good recovery between attacks. Some cases progress to typical RA.

Non-articular features (Fig. 8.9)
Soft tissues surrounding joints. Rheumatoid nodules are found in about 20% of cases. They are most often felt on the surface of the ulnar just below the elbow, but they can appear almost anywhere.

The olecranon and other bursae may be swollen, and a tendon sheath swelling over the dorsal surface of the wrist is not uncommon. Tenosynovitis, particularly affecting the flexor tendons in the palm of the hand, can cause trigger finger and may contribute to flexion deformities.

There is wasting of muscles around affected joints, particularly in the hands.

The eyes. Sjögren's syndrome is the commonest eye problem in RA, occurring in about 15% of cases. It comprises dry eyes (keratoconjunctivitis sicca), a dry mouth (xerostomia) and rheumatoid arthritis. This syndrome is occasionally seen in other connective tissue disorders, e.g. systemic lupus erythematosus. The lacrimal and salivary glands are infiltrated with lymphocytes and plasma cells, suggesting that this syndrome is probably part of the immunological process of rheumatoid disease. The development of dry eyes is particularly important because tear production protects the cornea. Artificial tears such as hypromellose 0.3% eye drops should be prescribed.

Scleritis may occur, causing a painful red eye. Scleromalacia presents as a bluish discoloration of the sclera around the iris; perforation rarely occurs.

The nervous system. The commonest neurological abnormality associated with RA is carpal tunnel syndrome. This condition is described on p. 856

The most serious neurological abnormality results from atlanto-axial subluxation. In this condition, rheumatoid involvement of an adjacent bursa lead to weakening of the transverse ligament of the atlas. This in turn allows the odontoid process to separate from the anterior arch of the atlas and to move posteriorly when the patient flexes his neck, with potential infringement on the cervical cord. Atlanto-axial subluxation is a common x-ray finding, but cervical cord compression is fortunately rare.

A polyneuropathy can also occur, causing glove and stocking sensory loss and sometimes motor weakness. It is usually symmetrical and often involves the legs.

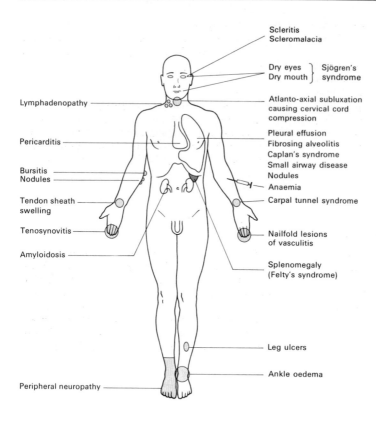

Sceritis
Scleromalacia

Dry eyes ⎫ Sjögren's
Dry mouth ⎭ syndrome

Atlanto-axial subluxation
causing cervical cord
compression

Pleural effusion
Fibrosing alveolitis
Caplan's syndrome
Small airway disease
Nodules

Anaemia

Carpal tunnel syndrome

Nailfold lesions
of vasculitis

Splenomegaly
(Felty's syndrome)

Leg ulcers

Ankle oedema

Lymphadenopathy

Pericarditis

Bursitis
Nodules

Tendon sheath
swelling

Tenosynovitis

Amyloidosis

Peripheral neuropathy

Fig. 8.9 The non-articular manifestations of rheumatoid arthritis.

Multiple mononeuropathy (mononeuritis multiplex) can also occur as a result of vasculitis.

The spleen, lymph nodes and blood. Palpable lymph nodes are common in RA, usually in the distribution of affected joints. The spleen may be enlarged. RA and splenomegaly with neutropenia which leads to repeated infections and weight loss is known as Felty's syndrome; skin pigmentation also occurs.

Anaemia is almost universal in RA and is proportional to the activity of the inflammatory process. The anaemia may be:
- Normochromic normocytic—the anaemia of chronic disease
- Iron deficient—due to gastrointestinal blood loss from analgesic ingestion
- Haemolytic (positive Coombs' test)
- Part of a pancytopenia due to hypersplenism in Felty's syndrome

A thrombocytosis rarely occurs and can correlate with articular disease activity.

The lungs. The lung is commonly affected; the abnormalities are described in detail on p. 606. They include:
- Pleural effusion—this is the commonest lung problem and occurs in approximately 10% of men

but is less common in women. It may occur before the onset of RA.
- Diffuse fibrosing alveolitis—rare
- Rheumatoid nodules in the lungs—can be up to 3 cm in diameter
- Caplan's syndrome—the occurrence of nodular pulmonary fibrosis in patients with RA exposed to various industrial dusts
- Obliterative bronchiolitis—irrespective of smoking history

The heart. A pericardial rub is often heard in patients with RA (up to 30%). Pericarditis is seldom a clinical problem, but occasionally a large pericardial effusion causes tamponade. Constrictive pericarditis is rare.

An endocarditis and myocarditis causing conduction defects may occur, but are rare.

The kidneys. RA is a common cause of amyloidosis affecting the kidneys. It usually presents as proteinuria and may go on to renal failure or to the nephrotic syndrome. Analgesic nephropathy is also seen (see p. 396).

The liver. There may be mild non-specific abnormalities of liver structure and function. In the presence of Felty's syndrome the liver may show nodular regenerative hyperplasia, which can lead to portal hypertension.

The skin. The skin is not directly involved in RA, but leg ulcers may occur, particularly in patients with Felty's syndrome and in those with a vasculitis. Vasculitis most often appears as nail fold lesions in the hands and, very occasionally it produces gangrene of the fingers or toes. Ankle oedema is often seen in active RA and is due to increased vascular permeability.

INVESTIGATION

X-ray changes
The x-ray changes in RA are shown in Fig. 8.10. The characteristic lesion is an erosion, which has the appearance of a mouse-bite on the surface of the affected bone. Erosions are best seen in x-rays of the hands and feet. Other changes include loss of joint space, which indicates thinning of the cartilage. There is porosis of the periarticular bone and cysts are sometimes seen. In advanced disease, destruction of bone ends and occasionally ankylosis occurs.

Full blood count
A full blood count in RA shows anaemia (see above) and an ESR raised in proportion to the activity of the inflammatory process.

Other tests
Tests for rheumatoid factor are positive in about 80% of cases, and antinuclear antibodies in about 30%.

Aspirated synovial fluid will show the changes outlined in Table 8.5. Fluid from a suddenly painful rheumatoid joint should always be aspirated and cultured, as septic arthritis is a complication of RA (see p. 348).

MANAGEMENT (see Table 8.8)

Stage 1
The first stage involves making the diagnosis and telling the patient about the condition. Many patients have already heard tales of horrific disabilities and should therefore be reassured that only a few patients suffer from severe problems and that the prospects of treatment are good. All the aspects of a patient's lifestyle should be reviewed, including his home, work and leisure activities. In general, a

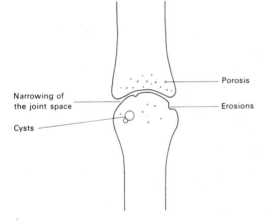

Fig. 8.10 X-ray changes in rheumatoid arthritis. Erosions are best seen in the small joints of the hands and feet.

Table 8.8 Stages in the management of rheumatoid arthritis.

Stage 1
Making the diagnosis, telling the patient
Joint protection and maintenance
Management planning

Stage 2
Symptomatic treatment with NSAIDs and other
  measures

Stage 3
The control of the disease with long-term suppressive
  drugs

Stage 4
Regular supervision and the management of
  complications

Stage 5
Rehabilitation of the disabled patient

patient's lifestyle should not be disrupted and he should be encouraged to continue a full, normal and busy life.

Physical activity does not increase the rate of deterioration of joints in RA, and since patients are particularly at risk of developing progressive joint stiffness and deformity, they should undertake simple exercises to maintain joint mobility and muscle power. Restriction of movement is particularly likely to occur in the shoulders, while flexion deformities are more likely to occur in the knees. Both of these problems are easier to prevent than correct.

Plans must be made for the continuing care of a patient with RA. Most will require some supervision for many years, even if the disease is mild.

Stage 2
The second stage of treatment is devoted to the relief of symptoms. NSAIDs are the mainstay of such treatment and are more effective than simple analgesics. Corticosteroids are effective, but are seldom used because of their side-effects.

In explosive RA in the elderly, small doses of prednisolone (less than 10 mg daily) are effective; the dose can be reduced over the years. In the younger patient, however, much larger doses of prednisolone, often for long periods, are necessary to control symptoms and therefore side-effects are commonly seen.

There is large variation in an individual's response to NSAIDs. It is often necessary to try a number of different drugs for a particular patient before finding one which provides adequate relief of symptoms. Each compound should be given for about 1 week to assess its affects. Drugs with a low incidence of side-effects, a good safety record and a convenient dosage schedule should be tried first. Aspirin no longer fulfils these requirements and has

been replaced as a first line of treatment by newer NSAIDs, e.g. naproxen 500 mg twice daily.

The relief of night pain and morning stiffness is particularly important in RA. A single capsule of slow-release indomethacin (75 mg) or a suppository taken on retiring usually produces dramatic relief of symptoms on the following day. This can be given in addition to regular daytime therapy or may be sufficient alone. If patients require additional relief, a simple analgesic can be taken as required. Aspirin or paracetamol are ideal for this purpose, but many patients prefer to use a combination such as dextro-propoxyphene and paracetamol.

A period of rest in hospital is often useful either to produce a remission of the disease or to encourage a dispirited disabled patient. Localized rest for individual joints can be provided with splints, which are particularly useful for the wrist. Intra-articular corticosteroid injections are of value for particularly troublesome joints.

Stage 3
The third stage consists of giving long-term suppressive drug therapy with drugs such as penicillamine. This is required with:
● Progressive disease
● Troublesome extra-articular problems
● Failure of NSAIDs to control symptoms
● Excessive corticosteroid therapy being used to control the disease

Suppressive compounds take several months to relieve symptoms and NSAIDs should initially be prescribed as well. Their action on joints is accompanied by improvement in extra-articular features, e.g. the disappearance of nodules and a reduction in the ESR and the rheumatoid factor titre. In some cases they produce either a complete remission or very effective suppression of the disease activity. This type of treatment should therefore be considered early in the course of the disease before joint deformities have developed. Drugs available for long-term suppressive therapy in RA are shown in Table 8.9. Unfortunately it is difficult to predict which patients will benefit from this treatment. The mechanism of action of these drugs is unknown.

Penicillamine and gold are usually used as the first line of treatment, although recent trials have shown sulphasalazine to be of value. Sulphasalazine should be given in the enteric-coated form because patients with RA are particularly liable to experience nausea with this drug.

Immunosuppressive drugs such as azathioprine are also equally effective but, because of their potential side-effects, are usually only used in patients over the age of 45 and in those who have failed to respond to gold or penicillamine. Chloroquine and hydroxychloroquine are milder and safer and can be used for the less severe case. All of these drugs have side-effects and patients require regular supervision,

Table 8.9 Drugs used in long-term suppressive therapy for rheumatoid arthritis.

Drug	Usual dose	Side-effects
Penicillamine	250 mg daily	Rash Loss of taste Thrombocytopenia Proteinuria
Gold (sodium aurothiomalate)	50 mg weekly i.m.	Stomatitis Dermatitis Thrombocytopenia
Azathioprine	50 mg twice daily	Neutropenia Nausea and vomiting Infections, e.g. herpes zoster
Hydroxychloroquine	400 mg daily	Retinopathy
Sulphasalazine	1 g twice daily	Nausea Depression Male infertility

including blood and sometimes urine checks. Patients should be informed of the side-effects, and told to report symptoms such as sore throat, rash or deterioration in vision immediately. The antimalarial drugs chloroquine and hydroxychloroquine may affect the eyes and vision must be checked regularly.

Stage 4
Regular supervision is required to assess the course of the disease and to watch for complications.

Non-articular complications. These may require treatment. For example, the patient who develops carpal tunnel syndrome (see p. 856) will require an injection of corticosteroid into the tendon sheath or surgical decompression of the median nerve.

Social and domestic complications. These require discussion and the patient may require considerable help, particularly with finding a suitable occupation and coping with domestic responsibilities.

Articular complications. Joints may become stiff and painful and require intra-articular injections of corticosteroids and exercises to mobilize the joint and improve muscle power. Deformities can also sometimes be corrected by steroid injections and exercises.

Rupture of the knee joint is treated with aspiration, injection of corticosteroid and rest. A Baker's cyst behind the knee does not itself require treatment since it merely reflects inflammatory changes in the knee joint. Steps should be taken to control the activity of the disease in the affected knee.

Painful feet may be treated with insoles; metatarsal bar insoles are particularly useful for subluxed metatarsal heads. More complex foot deformities may require special shoes such as space shoes.

At this stage in the disease replacement surgery plays an increasingly important role in the management of a patient with a wrecked joint. Not only can hips be replaced, but also knees, shoulders, elbows and the small joints of the hands.

Excision arthroplasty is of value in two situations. First, the painful subluxed metatarsal heads in the feet can be excised (Fowler's operation) and the lateral deviation of the toes corrected at the same time. Second, the head of the ulnar can be excised at the wrist, often relieving pain and allowing better movement. Osteotomy is occasionally used at the knee joint to relieve pain and correct deformity.

Stage 5
Despite all treatments, the disease can continue to progress and become disabling. Priorities in treatment then need to change. Attention should be focussed on the patients' symptoms and on trying to make their lives as comfortable as possible. All aspects of the patient's treatment and way of life should be reviewed. It may be useful to visit their homes and institute modifications and appliances in the house or provide a wheelchair. In general, steps should be taken to preserve as much as possible of all aspects of the patient's life. Successful management can make an enormous difference to the overall lifestyle of rheumatoid patients.

CONNECTIVE TISSUE DISEASES

The relationships between systemic lupus erythematosus, systemic sclerosis, and polymyositis and dermatomyositis are shown in Fig. 8.11. The collective term 'connective tissue disease' means little but, since the aetiology of these conditions is unknown, it is difficult to suggest a better alternative. The diseases have a number of features in common, including the occurrence of arthritis or

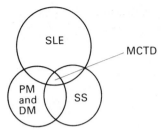

Fig. 8.11 The family of connective tissue diseases: systemic lupus erythematosus (SLE), polymyositis (PM), dermatomyositis (DM), systemic sclerosis (SS) and mixed connective tissue disease (MCTD).

arthralgia, multisystem involvement, vasculitis and immunological abnormalities such as circulating autoantibodies and immune complex deposition. Features of all three diseases appear in mixed connective tissue disease.

Systemic lupus erythematosus

Systemic lupus erythematosus (SLE) is the commonest of the connective tissue disorders and is characterized by the presence in the serum of antibodies against nuclear components (ANA). It is a multi-system disease, with arthralgia and rashes as the commonest clinical features, and cerebral and renal disease as the most serious problems.

EPIDEMIOLOGY

The disease probably affects about 0.1% of the population and is thus about 20 times less common than RA. It is much commoner in coloured races, with a prevalence of up to 1 in 250 amongst black women. It is about nine times as common in women than men, with a peak incidence between 20 and 40 years.

PATHOGENESIS

The cause of SLE is unknown, but many factors are thought to play a part:

- *Immunological abnormalities* (see Table 8.10). Humoral antibodies against nuclei (see p. 329), cytoplasmic components and double-stranded DNA have been demonstrated, as have other organ-specific (e.g. antithyroid) antibodies. These antibodies suggest a defect of suppressor T cell function, which normally prevent production of autoantibodies. Circulating immune complexes, made up of nuclear antigens and antinuclear antibodies, have been demonstrated and their deposition in tissues may cause renal disease and vasculitis. A number of these immunological changes may well be secondary to the disease process.

Table 8.10 Immunological abnormalities in systemic lupus erythematosus.

Humoral—antibodies to:
Human IgG—rheumatoid factor
Nuclear protein—anti-DNA (double- and single-stranded), anti-RNA, anti-RNP
Smooth muscle—anti-Sm
Cytoplasm
Organ, e.g. specific antibodies to thyroid
Leucocytes, platelets
Red cells
Clotting factor
Cryoglobulins
Anticoagulants (lupus anticoagulant)
Cardiolipin—false-positive tests for syphilis
Circulating immune complexes

Cell-mediated immune defects, e.g.
Reduced suppressor T cell activity

- *Viral aetiology.* No virus has been isolated, but approximately two-thirds of household contacts of SLE patients have lymphocytotoxic antibodies. These antibodies are also found following some viral infections. In animal models a virus has been identified, and it is known that viruses can alter nuclear proteins and make them antigenic. This alteration of nuclear protein has also been shown to occur with ultraviolet light.
- *Genetic factors.* There is an increased incidence of SLE, other connective tissue diseases and immunological disorders in relatives of patients with SLE. Patients with complement deficiencies, which are associated with changes near the HLA region, have an increased risk of developing SLE. There are other weak HLA associations, but their importance is subject to debate.
- *Sex.* There is a female preponderance.
- *Drugs.* Certain drugs can produce an SLE-like picture, e.g. hydralazine and procainamide. They may act by altering double-stranded DNA.

PATHOLOGY

SLE is characterized by a widespread vasculitis affecting capillaries, arterioles and venules. Fibrinoid (an eosinophilic amorphous material) is deposited along blood vessels and tissue fibres. The synovium of joints may be oedematous and may contain fibrinoid deposits. Haematoxylin bodies (rounded haematoxylin-stained areas) are seen in inflammatory infiltrates.

Lesions of other organs are described in the appropriate chapters.

CLINICAL FEATURES (Fig. 8.12)

SLE is extremely variable in its manifestation and most of the clinical features are due to the consequences of vasculitis. Mild cases may present only

General
Fever (80%)
Depression

Skin
Photosensitivity ⎫
Butterfly rash ⎬
Vasculitis ⎫
Purpura ⎬
Urticaria ⎭

Chest (50%)
Pleurisy/effusion
Restrictive lung defect

Raynaud's phenomenon

Joints (90%)
Aseptic necrosis of hip
Arthritis in small joints

Nervous system (60%)
Fits
Hemiplegia
Ataxia
Peripheral neuropathy
Cranial nerve lesions

Heart (40%)
Pericarditis
Endocarditis
Aortic valve lesions

Abdominal pain

Renal disease (50%)
Glomerulonephritis (all types)

Myopathy

Blood (75%)
Anaemia (normochromic normocytic
   or haemolytic Coombs positive)
Leucopenia
Thrombocytopenia

Fig. 8.12 Clinical features of systemic lupus erythematosus.

with arthralgia, whilst in severe cases there may be multi-system involvement.

General features. Fever is common in exacerbations, occurring in up to 80% of cases. Patients complain of malaise and tiredness.

The joints. Joint involvement is the commonest clinical feature (>90%). Patients often present with symptoms which sound like rheumatoid arthritis. Pain is often severe, but the joints may appear clinically normal, although sometimes there is slight soft tissue swelling surrounding the joint. Aseptic bone necrosis, possibly related to corticosteroid therapy, may be seen. Myalgia is common, but true myositis also occurs.

The skin. This is affected in 80% of cases (see p. 931). Erythema in a butterfly distribution on the cheeks of the face and across the bridge of the nose is characteristic. Vasculitic lesions on the finger tips and around the nail folds, purpura and urticaria occur. In one-third of cases there is photosensitivity and prolonged exposure to sunlight can lead to exacerbations of the disease. Livedo reticularis, palmar and plantar rashes, pigmentation and alopecia may be seen. Raynaud's phenomenon is common and may precede the development of arthralgia and other clinical problems by years.

Discoid lupus is a benign variant of the disease in which skin involvement is often the only feature, although systemic abnormalities may occur with time. The rash is characteristic and appears on the face as well-defined erythematous plaques which progress to scarring and pigmentation (see p. 931).

The lungs. Up to two-thirds of patients will have lung involvement sometime during the course of the disease (see p. 606). Recurrent pleurisy and pleural effusions (exudates) are the commonest manifestations. Pneumonitis and atelectasis may be seen; eventually a restrictive lung defect develops. Rarely pulmonary fibrosis occurs.

The heart. This is involved in over 40% of cases. Pericarditis, with small pericardial effusions detected by echocardiography, is common. A mild myocarditis also occurs. Aortic valve lesions and a cardiomyopathy can rarely be present. Endocarditis involving the mitral valve (Libman–Sacks syndrome) is very rare.

The kidneys. These are affected in 30–50% of cases. Proteinuria (>1g per 24 h) is common. The renal histological lesions consist of minimal change, proliferative changes (either focal, diffuse or crescentic) or a membranous glomerulonephritis (see p. 386). Most patients with or without renal disease have immune complex deposits in their kidneys.

Hypertension may occur due to progression to either the nephrotic syndrome or renal failure.

The nervous system. Involvement of the nervous system occurs in 60% of cases. There may be a mild depression, but occasionally more severe psychiatric disturbances occur. Epilepsy, cerebellar ataxia, aseptic meningitis, cranial nerve lesions, cerebrovascular accidents or peripheral neuropathy may be seen. These lesions may be due to vasculitis or immune complex deposition.

The eyes. Retinal lesions include cytoid bodies, which appear as hard exudates, and haemorrhages. Blindness is uncommon. Sjögren's syndrome may be seen.

The gastrointestinal system. SLE often causes gastrointestinal symptoms, although these are usually not a major presenting feature. Symptoms include nausea, vomiting, anorexia and diarrhoea.

Drug-induced SLE
This is usually characterized by arthralgia and mild systemic features, rashes and pericarditis, but seldom renal or cerebral disease. It usually disappears when the drug causing it is stopped.

INVESTIGATION

- A full blood count shows anaemia (usually normochromic normocytic), neutropenia and thrombocytopenia. An autoimmune haemolytic anaemia may occur. There may be a history of idiopathic thrombocytopenia. The ESR is raised in proportion to the disease activity.
- Antinuclear antibodies are positive in almost all cases. Double-stranded DNA binding is specific for SLE, although it is only present in 50% of cases, particularly those with severe systemic involvement, e.g. renal disease.
- Rheumatoid factor is positive in half of the patients.
- Serum complement levels are reduced during active disease. C-reactive protein is normal. Immunoglobulins are raised (usually IgG and IgM).
- Characteristic histological abnormalities are seen in biopsies from, for example, the kidney.

Immunofluorescence of skin biopsies will show immunoglobulin and complement deposition at the dermoepidermal junction; this is known as the positive band test.

MANAGEMENT

Drug therapy
Systemic corticosteroid therapy is the mainstay of treatment in SLE, although patients with mild disease and arthralgia can be managed with NSAIDs. In cases where steroids are required, they should be used in small doses for short periods just sufficient to suppress the disease in order to minimize complications. Active SLE, with fever and pleurisy, should be treated with prednisolone 30 mg daily, the dose being reduced over the course of a few weeks to a maintenance level of around 5–10 mg daily. It may be possible to stop treatment in such a patient within a few months.

Two other types of drug are used in the management of SLE:
- The antimalarial drug chloroquine (150 mg daily) is useful for suppressing the disease activity in patients with minor manifestations such as arthralgia which cannot be controlled with NSAIDs or troublesome skin lesions. Ocular toxicity may occur (Table 8.9).
- Immunosuppressive drugs are used for patients with more serious disease manifestations such as renal disease, usually in combination with steroids. Azathioprine ($2\,mg\cdot kg^{-1}$ daily) is most often used; chlorambucil is an alternative and cyclophosphamide is reserved for patients with life-threatening disease. Immunosuppressive drugs also have a useful steroid-sparing effect.

General management
Patients should be told about their disease and its management. Patients with photosensitivity problems should avoid excessive exposure to sunlight.

There is no major contraindication to pregnancy. However, there is an increased rate of fetal loss and complications may arise during the pregnancy; specialist care should therefore be available.

COURSE AND PROGNOSIS

An episodic course is characteristic, with exacerbations and complete remissions which may last for long periods of time. These remissions may occur even in patients with renal disease. A chronic course is occasionally seen. Earlier estimates of the mortality in SLE were exaggerated; 5-year survival rate is about 95%. In most cases the pattern of the disease becomes established in the first few years; if serious problems have not developed in this time, they are unlikely to do so. The arthritis is usually intermittent. Chronic progressive destruction of joints as seen in RA and OA does not occur, but a few patients develop deformities such as ulnar deviation.

Systemic sclerosis

This is a multi-system disease which predominantly affects the skin and presents with Raynaud's phenomenon in over three-quarters of cases. It is less common than SLE. The major features distinguishing systemic sclerosis from polymyositis and SLE are shown in Fig. 8.13. It is commoner in women than men (3:1) and can appear at any age under 50 years.

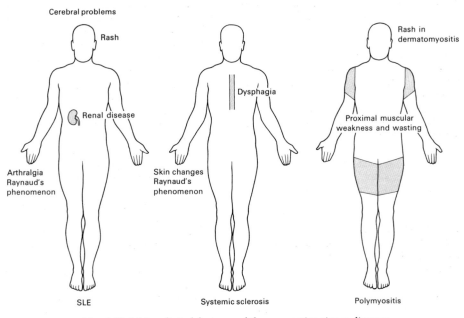

Fig. 8.13 Major clinical features of the connective tissue diseases.

PATHOLOGY

In the early phase the skin is oedematous, with perivascular lymphocytic infiltration and degeneration of collagen fibres. Later there is an increase in collagen. Small blood vessels show intimal proliferation and obliteration. Progressive fibrosis is the major feature of visceral involvement.

AETIOLOGY

The aetiology of systemic sclerosis is unknown. Abnormalities in both humoral and cellular immunity have been documented. A positive speckled or nucleolar antinuclear antibody is found in up to 60% of patients. Familial cases have been documented, and HLA–B8,DR3 has been reported to occur with greater frequency in systemic sclerosis. Occupational factors may be involved; for example, workers with polyvinyl chloride can develop a similar disease.

CLINICAL FEATURES

The involvement of various organs is shown in Table 8.11.

The skin. The cutaneous changes which occur are described on p. 932. Sclerosis of the skin can lead to beaking of the nose and difficulty in opening the mouth. Other changes seen in the skin include telangiectasis, pigmentation or depigmentation,

Table 8.11 Involvement of various organs in systemic sclerosis.

Organ	Involved in:
Skin	90%
Vascular system— Raynaud's phenomenon	80%
Oesophagus	80%
Lungs	45%
Heart	40%
Kidneys	35%
Joints	25%
Muscle	20%

ulceration and calcinosis. Raynaud's phenomenon often occurs; it is described on p. 548.

The gastrointestinal system. Oesophageal involvement is almost invariable, although only half of these patients will have symptoms of heartburn or dysphagia. A barium swallow may show delayed peristalsis, dilatation or stricture formation, but oesophageal manometry is the most sensitive test. This shows lack of distal oesophageal peristalsis and a reduced oesophageal sphincter pressure.

The small bowel can be involved, producing malabsorption from bacterial overgrowth due to dilatation and atony. Dilatation and atony may also affect the colon.

The joints and muscles. The fibrotic process can affect tendons, causing flexion deformities of the fingers. The small joints of the hands are affected in 25% of patients, particularly in the early stages of the disease. Soft tissue swelling of the fingers produces 'sausage fingers'. Progressive changes in joints are not seen.

Myopathy and myositis occur and EMG abnormalities are common.

The lungs (see also p. 607). Lower lobe fibrosis leads to cyst formation and honeycombing in advanced cases. Gas transfer and restrictive ventilatory defects are seen. Aspiration pneumonia and pulmonary hypertension may occur.

The heart. Diffuse myocardial fibrosis with arrhythmias (in 25%) and conduction defects may occur. Effusions accompany pericardial disease.

The kidneys. This is the most serious manifestation of the disease and is caused by an obliterative endarteritis of renal vessels. It can cause renal failure and malignant hypertension.

The eyes. Sjögren's sydrome with keratoconjunctivitis sicca may be seen.

Variants of systemic sclerosis
- Morphoea—see p. 932
- CR(E)ST syndrome—consists of calcinosis (C), Raynaud's phenomenon (R), oesophageal involvement (E), sclerodactaly (S) and telangiectasia (T). Antinuclear antibodies to the centromere are found in the blood
- Mixed connective tissue disease—see p. 345

INVESTIGATION

- Antinuclear antibodies are often positive. Antinucleolar and anti-centromere antibodies are specifically elevated. A positive rheumatoid factor is found in 30% of cases.
- A normochromic normocytic anaemia can be seen. An acquired haemolytic anaemia with 'cold' agglutinins may occur. The ESR may be raised.
- X-rays of the hands may show deposits of calcium around the fingers. In severe cases there is erosion and resorption of the tufts of the distal phalanges.
- A barium swallow to detect oesophageal involvement is often a useful confirmatory test.

TREATMENT

No treatment has been shown to influence the progress of this condition. Management is therefore symptomatic.

PROGNOSIS

In some patients the disease is mild, whilst in others it is severe and complicated by systemic features such as renal disease. The mean 5-year survival rate is 50%.

Polymyositis and dermatomyositis

Polymyositis is a disorder of muscle in which the pathological features are necrosis of muscle fibres together with evidence of regeneration and inflammation, particularly around blood vessels. It presents with proximal muscular weakness and wasting. When this is accompanied by a rash, it is called dermatomyositis. Its incidence is comparable with that of systemic sclerosis, i.e. it is less common than SLE. It occurs at any age, even in children, but with a peak incidence in adults aged between 30 and 60 years. It is twice as common in women than in men.

AETIOLOGY

This is unknown, but immunological and viral factors have been suggested. Dermatomyositis is associated with an increased incidence of carcinoma of the bronchus in men or of the ovary in women, mainly in patients presenting after 50 years.

CLINICAL FEATURES

The major feature of polymyositis is muscle weakness and wasting affecting the proximal muscles of the shoulder and pelvic girdles. It may be very acute in onset, particularly in children, and is sometimes accompanied by myoglobinuria. In the chronic form there is gradually progressive muscular weakness. Muscle pain and tenderness are found in about one-half of the cases, but weakness is the chief complaint. The rash of dermatomyositis is characteristic (see p. 933). As in other connective tissue tissue diseases, systemic features are often found:
- Arthralgia or arthritis occur in about half of all patients and may be the presenting feature, occurring before the onset of the muscular symptoms. The small joints of the hands are particularly affected, but the arthritis may extend in a distribution resembling that of rheumatoid arthritis. Joints are often swollen, but the arthritis is intermittent and not progressive.
- Dysphagia is found in 50% of cases and is due to oesophageal muscle involvement.
- Raynaud's phenomenon is common.

- Sjögren's syndrome and respiratory problems may occur.

INVESTIGATION

The diagnosis of polymyositis is made on the basis of three tests, two of which at least should be positive.
- *Muscle enzymes.* Serum creatine phosphokinase and aldolase are raised and can be used to follow the disease progress during treatment.
- *Electromyography (EMG).* Short polyphasic motor potentials, sometimes spontaneous fibrillation and high frequency repetitive discharges (see p. 863) are almost pathognomonic of polymyositis.
- *Muscle biopsy.* This shows necrosis of muscle fibres with swelling and disruption of muscle cells. Vacuolation, fragmentation and fibrosis of the fibres are seen, with thickening of the blood vessels. There are also inflammatory changes.

Other tests
- The ESR is usually raised. A normochromic normocytic anaemia and a polymorphonuclear leucocytosis are seen in acute cases.
- Serum antinuclear antibodies and tests for rheumatoid factor may be positive.

MANAGEMENT

Systemic corticosteroids, starting with 60 mg of prednisolone daily and reducing to a maintenance dose of about 15 mg daily, are used. In most cases this produces a gradual remission of the disease. Physiotherapy may be required to restore muscle power. Treatment is required for a variable period, usually months but sometimes years. Some patients fail to respond to steroids, and immunosuppressive drugs such as methotrexate or occasionally azathioprine may be required.

PROGNOSIS

Fifty per cent of affected children die within 2 years. In adults the prognosis is obviously better in those without a malignancy.

Mixed connective tissue disease

This is rare. The existence of such a disorder emphasizes the overlap between the connective tissue diseases and it may not itself be a distinct entity. It is a useful term for cases with features of more than one of the connective tissue diseases together with high titres of antibody to extractable nuclear antigens such as RNA. Like the other conditions, it affects women more often than men and presents in young adults.

Clinical features include arthralgia, Raynaud's phenomenon, proximal muscle weakness and wasting, and a puffy swelling of the skin of the hands which somewhat resembles the changes occurring in scleroderma. Other features of systemic lupus erythematosus, polymyositis or scleroderma may appear, but serious problems such as renal disease are unusual.

The condition tends to be benign and often responds well to small doses of prednisolone.

VASCULITIS

The 'vasculitides' encompass a wide range of diseases with considerable overlap between them. Many classifications have been suggested; one of these is based on the size of the vessels. Large vessel disease includes giant cell arteritis (see below) and Takayasu's disease (p. 548). Polyarteritis nodosa is a systemic arteritis involving medium-sized vessels. Small vessel vasculitis occurs in the connective tissue diseases such as systemic lupus erythematosus and rheumatoid arthritis as well as in infections such as subacute bacterial endocarditis. This vasculitis may be responsible for some of the clinical features of these conditions. Skin lesions are usually associated with small vessel vasculitis.

Polyarteritis nodosa

Polyarteritis nodosa (PAN) is a rare condition and, unlike other connective tissue diseases, it usually presents in middle-aged men. Pathologically there is a fibrinoid necrosis of blood vessel walls and microaneurysm formation. These changes give rise to the clinical manifestations of multi-system disease with progressive organ failure, infarction and haemorrhage.

CLINICAL FEATURES

Initial features are non-specific, being fever, malaise, weight loss, myalgia and arthralgia. Later the most characteristic features are renal impairment, hypertension, peripheral neuropathy, lung disease and cardiac problems, including arrhythmia, heart failure and myocardial infarction. The peripheral neuropathy in vasculitic disorders characteristically takes the form of a mononeuritis multiplex (p. 857). A migratory arthralgia or arthritis and fever are seen, and abdominal pain, with evidence of vasculitis in the liver and gastrointestinal tract, is common. Death is usually from renal disease.

INVESTIGATION

The ESR is raised, but the diagnosis depends upon either histological examination of biopsy material from an affected organ or angiographic demonstration of microaneurysms in hepatic, intestinal or renal vessels.

TREATMENT

Treatment is with corticosteroids, usually in combination with immunosuppressive drugs such as azathioprine.

Essential mixed cryoglobulinaemia

In this disorder a cutaneous vasculitis is associated with cryoglobulinaemia. It is exacerbated by exercise and the cold, and there is an association with hepatitis B infection. Multi-system involvement occurs as in other connective tissue disorders.

Vasculitis associated with granulomas

Two forms of vasculitis associated with granulomas also occur. *Wegener's granulomatosis* classically consists of the triad of upper respiratory tract granuloma, fleeting pulmonary shadows, and glomerulonephritis; it is discussed on p. 386. The *Churg–Strauss syndrome*, in which there is eosinophilic infiltration, mainly of the lungs, is described on p. 609.

Polymyalgia rheumatica and giant cell arteritis

Polymyalgia rheumatica and giant cell arteritis (also known as temporal or cranial arteritis) can be regarded as two conditions at the ends of a spectrum, with giant cell arteritis as the basic pathological lesion (see Fig. 8.14). The cause is unknown. Occasionally the syndrome is due to some underlying condition, e.g. a severe infection or a malignancy.

CLINICAL FEATURES

Polymyalgia rheumatica is characterized by pains and morning stiffness in the proximal muscles of the shoulder and pelvic girdle, and a high ESR.

The onset is sudden. It is rare before the age of 50 years and usually occurs in those aged 60 to 70 years. Women are three times more commonly affected than men. Severe pains and weakness occur in the girdle muscles and also in the muscles of the cervical and lumbar spines. The hands and feet are never

affected. Early morning stiffness often causes difficulty in getting out of bed. Systemic symptoms include malaise, anorexia, weight loss and a low-grade fever. Restriction of movement of the shoulders and hips is characteristic. The distribution of the muscle involvement is bilateral and symmetrical. Occasionally it may involve the limb muscles. There may be no physical signs if the patient is examined in the afternoon when the stiffness has worn off.

Headache, particularly if localized and accompanied by temporal tenderness and loss of pulsation, suggests a temporal arteritis (see p. 847), which can occur with polymyalgia.

INVESTIGATION

- The ESR is usually raised to a very high level (around 100 mm·h^{-1}), but returns to normal with treatment.
- There is a mild normochromic normocytic anaemia.
- Tests for rheumatoid factor are negative, though false-positive results are found particularly in older people.
- Alkaline phosphatase levels are sometimes raised, but return to normal with treatment.

There is no specific test. It is not usual to carry out a temporal artery biopsy in polymyalgia, although a giant cell arteritis can be demonstrated in 40% of cases. Temporal artery biopsy is often performed in temporal arteritis, but is not necessary in classic cases.

MANAGEMENT

Corticosteroids are the treatment of choice in polymyalgia rheumatica, starting with 15 mg of prednisolone daily. NSAIDs are less effective and, as they do not control the arteritis, should not be used. Treatment should be started immediately the diagnosis is made and before waiting for the results of tests in order to prevent irreversible blindness, although this is rare in the absence of temporal arteritis. With steroid therapy, patients feel better within days, though mobilization of stiff shoulders may take a month or two. The dose of prednisolone is slowly reduced over the course of the next 2 years in increments not exceeding 1 mg and at intervals not exceeding 1 month. Relapses are common. In most patients it is possible to stop treatment after 2–4 years.

DIFFERENTIAL DIAGNOSIS OF ARTHRITIS IN THE ELDERLY

Common conditions are summarized in Fig. 8.15. Osteoarthritis is common from the age of 50 onwards

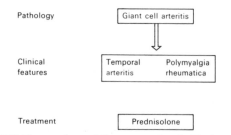

Fig. 8.14 The spectrum of disease associated with giant cell arteritis.

OSTEOARTHRITIS

POLYMYALGIA
RHEUMATICA

Pyrophosphate
arthropathy

Gout

Rheumatoid
arthritis

Septic arthritis

Fig. 8.15 The differential diagnosis of arthritis in the elderly.

but is easily distinguished from polymyalgia rheumatica by its less dramatic onset, peripheral distribution and normal ESR; if there is any doubt, a 1-week trial of prednisolone should be given.

Rheumatoid arthritis can begin in elderly patients. It is often sudden in onset, with very dramatic joint inflammation ('explosive' rheumatoid arthritis). Unlike the disease in young patients, it often responds very well to small doses of steroids (prednisolone 10–15 mg daily) and has a good prognosis.

Pyrophosphate deposition is common in elderly patients, typically presenting as a painful swollen knee.

Gout and septic arthritis are other causes of acute problems in the elderly.

ARTHRITIS IN CHILDREN (see Fig. 8.16)

Joint pain is a common problem in childhood, but arthritis is fortunately rare. Benign limb pain in childhood is sometimes called 'growing pain' and, though meaningless, this is probably a convenient term which parents readily accept.

Juvenile chronic arthritis is a general term used to cover a group of diseases in which an exact diagnosis is not always possible. There are three main types: Still's disease, juvenile rheumatoid arthritis and juvenile ankylosing spondylitis.

Still's disease

This is the commonest type of juvenile chronic arthritis, accounting for about 70% of cases. It is entirely distinct from rheumatoid arthritis, being distinguished by a number of clinical features and negative tests for rheumatoid factor. There are two peaks in the age of onset: the first and largest is between the ages of 2 and 5 years and the second between the ages of 10 and 15. Still's disease occasionally begins after the age of 16, and rarely in the 20s. The disease is often episodic, with bouts of fever and arthritis. It can be divided into three subtypes:

- *The systemic type* is usually seen in children under the age of 5. They present with a high fever, a characteristic rash and various other features, including lymphadenopathy, splenomegaly and pericarditis. Arthritis or arthralgia are minor features of the illness and may be absent. Arthritis may, however, develop later in the course of the disease.
- *The pauciarticular or oligoarticular type* of Still's disease affects up to four of the large joints such as the hips, knees or ankles. These patients are particularly liable to chronic iritis, which may lead to blindness without any preceding symptoms. Antinuclear antibodies are often positive and provide a useful warning that iritis may develop. Slit lamp examination should be performed at regular intervals in these patients.
- *Polyarticular Still's disease* presents with a bilateral symmetrical polyarthritis not unlike that of rheumatoid arthritis, but with less prominent and less frequent involvement of the small joints of the hands and feet.

JUVENILE CHRONIC ARTHRITIS:
Still's disease (systemic,
   oligoarticular or
   polyarticular)
Juvenile rheumatoid arthritis
Juvenile ankylosing spondylitis

OTHER TYPES:
Infections, e.g. tuberculosis, rubella
Rheumatic fever
Henoch-Schönlein purpura
Traumatic arthritis
Hypermobility syndrome
Leukaemia
Sickle cell disease
Psoriatic arthritis
SLE and connective tissue disorders
Transient synovitis of the hip

Fig. 8.16 The differential diagnosis of arthritis in children.

DIAGNOSIS

The non-articular features of Still's disease mentioned above are often helpful in making a diagnosis. A high swinging fever is also characteristic. This can be misleading to the unwary as it suggests the possibility of infection.

The joints themselves are swollen, but pain and tenderness are much less prominent than in adult rheumatoid arthritis. The ESR is usually raised and there is frequently an anaemia.

TREATMENT

Treatment is with NSAIDs as in rheumatoid arthritis. Gold and penicillamine are effective, but probably in a smaller proportion of cases than in rheumatoid arthritis. Corticosteroids should be avoided because of their effect on growth. It is important to protect the joints and prevent deformity during relapses, particularly as spontaneous remissions occur in 85% of patients before the age of 20 years. Long periods of rest and splinting of joints may be necessary. The patient's education and normal lifestyle should be continued if possible.

Juvenile rheumatoid arthritis

Rheumatoid arthritis may begin before the sixteenth birthday. The clinical features are identical to those of adults and tests for rheumatoid factor are usually positive. However, the prognosis is much worse than in adults. Juvenile rheumatoid arthritis accounts for about 15% of cases of juvenile chronic arthritis.

Juvenile ankylosing spondylitis

This accounts for 15% of cases of juvenile chronic arthritis. It is the most benign of the subtypes, and usually presents between the ages of 10 and 15. A peripheral arthritis occurs, with the lower limb joints being particularly affected. Joints are swollen and painful in the acute stage, but often respond well to anti-inflammatory drugs and usually settle within a few years. These patients may develop iritis and there may be other features of HLA-B27 associated diseases. Back pain is not a prominent feature at this age. A family history of ankylosing spondylitis or related diseases is sometimes helpful in the diagnosis. Tests for rheumatoid factor are negative. Although the arthritis usually resolves, 50% of these patients go on to develop ankylosing spondylitis in adult life.

Other conditions

Other types of arthritis which are seen in childhood are summarized in Fig. 8.16.

Some soft tissue syndromes particularly affect children; one of these is Osgood–Schlatter's disease, which is characterized by localized pain over the tibial tubercle and is often seen in athletic teenagers.

A mysterious condition called transient synovitis of the hip which causes hip pain may give rise to concern because of the possibility of tuberculosis or other serious conditions. It presents as painful limitation of movement of one hip, and usually resolves within a few weeks or months.

INFECTIVE ARTHRITIS

Infection of joints is fortunately uncommon but is important because of the damage it produces. The possibility of infection as a cause of arthritis must always be kept in mind. If its presence is suspected, synovial fluid must be obtained for culture. Infection with pyogenic organisms (septic arthritis) can be caused by a number of bacteria, including mycobacteria (see below). Arthritis also occurs with viral infections and less commonly from infection with spirochaetes or fungi.

Apart from direct infection, arthritis can also occur as a result of an immunological reaction to infection elsewhere. This is called reactive arthritis (see p. 350).

Septic arthritis

Septic arthritis results from infection of joints with pyogenic organisms, of which *Staphylococcus aureus* is the commonest. It can also occur with other types of staphylococci, pneumococci, gonococci or gram-negative bacilli.

Organisms reach the joint in septic arthritis via the bloodstream, sometimes from an identifiable site of infection such as otitis media or a boil. Less commonly, infection spreads from osteomyelitis adjacent to the joint or the organism is introduced directly as a result of trauma, surgery or intra-articular injection.

Septic arthritis particularly occurs at the extremes of life and in immunologically compromised individuals, e.g. patients receiving immunosuppressive drugs or with rheumatoid arthritis.

CLINICAL FEATURES

The clinical features of septic arthritis are similar for all the different causative organisms. The presentation is usually dramatic. The patient typically presents with a single painful joint, usually the knee. The joint is red, warm and swollen with a demonstrable effusion. Fever is usual and there may be evidence of infection elsewhere.

In rheumatoid arthritis, the presentation may be misleading; patients are often afebrile and do not necessarily have a systemic reaction or a leucocytosis. Any suddenly painful joint in a patient with rheumatoid arthritis should be aspirated to exclude infection.

Systemic and local reactions can also be absent in patients receiving corticosteroids.

INVESTIGATION

- Aspiration of the joint is the only important diagnostic manoeuvre (Table 8.5). The synovial fluid is often purulent and typically contains about 100×10^9/l white blood cells, predominantly neutrophils. A Gram stain may show the presence of organisms. Culture of the fluid, including special techniques for detecting anaerobes and gonococci, usually gives a definitive answer.
- There may be a leucocytosis.
- Blood culture may be positive.
- X-rays are of no value in the diagnosis of septic arthritis; they become abnormal only when joint destruction is advanced.

TREATMENT

This should be started immediately the diagnosis is made, as cartilage destruction can occur within a few days of the onset of the joint infection and the situation can be life-threatening. The joint should be immobilized.

Antibiotic therapy
The choice of antibiotic will depend upon the organism concerned. If the identification of this is delayed, 'blind' therapy should be started immediately with a slow i.v. infusion of flucloxacilin 500 mg 6-hourly together with clindamycin 300 mg i.v. 6-hourly or fusidic acid 500 mg 8-hourly by mouth. Antibiotics given by the intramuscular or intravenous route will pass into joints, especially when they are inflamed; antibiotics should not be injected intra-articularly. Antibiotic levels in the synovial fluid should be checked during the acute illness. Antibiotics should be continued for 6 weeks.

Drainage
Drainage of infected joints is best achieved by needle aspiration, which should be performed daily until no further fluid is obtainable. For inaccessible joints such as the hip, surgical drainage may be required. If infection is allowed to continue, debris collects within the joint which cannot be removed with a needle and this delays recovery. In these circumstances, the effusion will fail to resolve and surgical debridement will be required.

PROGNOSIS

The resolution of septic arthritis with complete recovery usually occurs within a few days or weeks.

Specific types of bacterial arthritides

Tuberculous arthritis
One per cent of patients with tuberculosis have skeletal involvement. Tuberculous arthritis affecting children is usually due to the primary stage of the disease. In adults, it is invariably secondary to pulmonary or renal disease and is due to haematogenous spread to the subchondral bone or the spinal intervertebral discs. Predisposing factors for tuberculous arthritis are those for developing TB anywhere in the body, e.g. alcoholism, diabetes mellitus or any other chronic debilitating disease.

Pathology. The synovial membrane and periarticular tissues become inflamed and oedematous; histologically caseating granulomas are seen. Later there is destruction of cartilage and this may lead to fibrous ankylosis. When the spine is involved, the infection may track along the fascial planes to produce a psoas abscess.

Clinical features. There is usually a monoarticular arthritis affecting the hip or knee (30%) or the sacroiliac or other joints (20%); in 50% of patients there is spinal involvement. There is an insidious onset of pain and dysfunction of the joint, with swelling and restriction of movement, associated with general symptoms of malaise, anorexia and night sweats. Occasionally an allergic (i.e. not infective) polyarthritis is seen in tuberculosis.

Diagnosis. The mycobacterium may be cultured from the synovial fluid; however, negative results do not exclude the diagnosis. X-rays may initially only show slight abnormality, but later there is a narrowing of the joint space and bony erosions.

Treatment. Drug treatment is as for tuberculosis elsewhere (see p. 602). The joint should be immobilized in the acute phase. If infection is allowed to continue, the effusion cannot be aspirated via a needle because of debris and surgical debridement is necessary.

Meningococcal arthritis
Meningococcal arthritis usually occurs as part of a generalized septicaemia. It is a migratory polyarthritis and organisms cannot usually be recovered from the synovial fluid. Joint destruction does not occur. This type of arthritis is due to circulating immune complexes containing meningococcal antigens. Occasionally the effusion is purulent and contains meningococcal organisms. Treatment is with penicillin.

Gonococcal arthritis
Gonococcal arthritis is similar to meningococcal arthritis. It particularly affects young adult females and also homosexual men. It presents with a mildly

inflammatory polyarthritis. It is usually asymmetrical and occasionally migratory. A useful clue to the diagnosis is the presence of small pustular skin lesions, often near the affected joints. The organism can be recovered from the bloodstream and in 25% of cases from the joints. In the remainder the arthritis is a reaction to the infection, and is probably immunologically mediated.

If neglected, gonococcal septicaemia may go on to produce a typical septic arthritis. Treatment is with penicillin 1g daily for 2 weeks.

Salmonella arthritis

Salmonella infection differs from septic arthritis in being polyarticular. It is also less dramatic than septic arthritis and is therefore easily missed. It particularly occurs with types of *Salmonella* that invade the bloodstream rather than staying within the gastrointestinal tract. Gastrointestinal features may therefore be minor or absent, deflecting attention away from the correct diagnosis.

Treatment with systemic antibiotics, e.g. amoxycillin 500 mg 6-hourly, is curative.

Lyme disease (see p. 48)

Arthritis is seen in patients with Lyme disease in the USA.

Viral arthritis

A number of different viral infections cause arthritis which is immunologically mediated. The commonest and most important is *rubella*, where the virus can occasionally be isolated from the joint. Arthritis is particularly a complication of the disease in young adult females, occurring in 15% of cases. Arthritis may follow either rubella or the rubella vaccine. It begins a few days after development of the rash, or 2 weeks after vaccination. It may be associated with other complications such as lymphadenopathy. It presents as a bilateral, symmetrical polyarthritis, closely resembling rheumatoid arthritis, for which it is often mistaken. However, it resolves within a few weeks in most cases. Occasionally there is persistent or recurrent arthralgia which may continue for years. Treatment is symptomatic.

Arthritis may also complicate *mumps*. A few large joints are typically affected and, as in rubella, the condition is self-limiting.

Arthralgia and sometimes arthritis may be features of the prodromal stage of *hepatitis B infection*, but resolve when the jaundice appears. As in meningococcal arthritis, this prodromal syndrome is associated with circulating immune complexes.

Transient polyarthritis is also seen in *infectious mononucleosis*, *chickenpox* and other viral infections.

Fungal infections

Fungal infections of joints occur rarely. Actinomycosis can affect the mandible or vertebrae. Bone abscesses may be seen. Destructive joint lesions can also occur with blastomycosis. A benign polyarthritis accompanied by erythema nodosum occasionally occurs in coccidioidomycosis and histoplasmosis. Culture of purulent synovial fluid and skin tests for fungi may help the diagnosis.

ARTHRITIS FOLLOWING INFECTION

Much more common than direct infection of joints is a condition in which arthritis is associated with an immunological reaction to infection. This is sometimes called reactive arthritis. There are two different types; these are summarized in Table 8.12. Rheumatic fever and Henoch–Schönlein purpura follow streptococcal infections and predisposition to these disorders is not related to the presence of the antigen HLA-B27. By contrast, HLA-B27-positive individuals are particularly likely to develop reactive arthritis following enteric or venereal infection; these are sometimes known as seronegative spondyloarthropathies.

Reiter's syndrome

This syndrome consists of the triad of a seronegative reactive arthritis, non-specific urethritis and conjunctivitis. Two types are recognized:
- Following a gastrointestinal infection with *Shigella*, *Salmonella*, *Yersinia* or *Campylobacter*
- Post-venereal infection. About 2% of patients attending clinics for genital medicine with venereal disease have Reiter's syndrome.

The male to female ratio is 20:1 and most cases occur in young adults. HLA-B27 is present in up to 80% of

Table 8.12 Classification of arthropathies following infections.

HLA-B27 association:	HLA-B27 associated	Not associated with HLA-B27
Type of infection:	Enteric or venereal	Streptococcal
Resulting arthropathies:	Reactive arthritis Reiter's syndrome	Rheumatic fever Henoch–Schönlein purpura

cases. An HLA-B27-positive male has a 20% risk of developing the disease following a dysenteric infection.

CLINICAL FEATURES (Fig. 8.17)

The arthritis begins within 2 weeks of the enteric or venereal infection, which may have been mild and asymptomatic. The joints of the lower limb are particularly affected in an asymmetrical pattern; the knees, ankles and feet are the commonest sites. The wrists and other joints of the upper limbs are occasionally involved, and there may be localized pain and tenderness in the spine due to sacroiliitis. The arthritis is often very acute at presentation, but resolves over the course of a few months.

Achilles tendonitis and plantar fasciitis are common. Nail dystrophy with subungal keratosis may lead to shedding of the nails.

The urethritis is associated with a sterile urethral discharge and mild dysuria. Prostatism can occur. Circinate balanitis, a superficial penile lesion characterized by a circle of erythema with a pale centre, may occur.

The conjunctivitis is usually mild and bilateral, resolving spontaneously. It occurs in only one-third of patients. Acute anterior uveitis develops later in the disease, in approximately 10% of patients.

Keratoderma blennorrhagica is seen in 10% of patients with post-venereal Reiter's syndrome. It is characterized by intense scaling of the skin of the soles of the feet, resembling pustular psoriasis.

Patients with Reiter's syndrome have a low-grade fever. Very rarely cardiac (e.g. pericarditis, aortitis), respiratory (mainly pleurisy) or neurological (peripheral neuropathy) complications occur.

DIAGNOSIS

The diagnosis in these conditions is entirely clinical; there are no diagnostic blood tests. The ESR is raised in the acute stage. Tests for rheumatoid factor and other autoantibodies are negative. X-rays are of no value in the acute stage of the disease, though signs of sacroiliitis may appear with the development of ankylosing spondylitis. Aspirated synovial fluid is inflammatory in nature, with a high polymorphonuclear leucocyte count; it is sterile.

TREATMENT

Treatment is with NSAIDs such as indomethacin. It is often useful to aspirate acutely inflamed joints and to inject them with a corticosteroid preparation.

PROGNOSIS

Though the acute arthritis resolves within a few months, there is a very high incidence of long term problems. About 50% of patients with Reiter's syndrome will go on to develop recurrences of arthritis, iritis or ankylosing spondylitis. Recurrent synovitis is the commonest problem and typically presents with effusions in the knee. Recurrences are not necessarily associated with further enteric or venereal infection and are not associated with progressive deterioration of joints.

Rheumatic fever (see p. 511)

This post-streptococcal condition is associated with a migratory polyarthritis. A joint such as the wrist or elbow becomes acutely painful and swollen for about 2 days. As resolution occurs, another joint becomes involved. The arthritis lasts for a few weeks or months, but eventually resolves completely without any long-term problems.

Henoch–Schönlein purpura (see p. 298)

This also follows a streptococcal infection. It presents as a generalized purpuric rash associated with abdominal pain and a symmetrical polyarthritis, and lasts for a few weeks.

CRYSTAL DEPOSITION DISEASES

Three types of crystal are deposited in joints; each is associated with a characteristic clinical syndrome (Fig. 8.18):

- *Monosodium urate deposition* is associated with acute gout, typically affecting the big toe.
- *Calcium pyrophosphate deposition* causes many dif-

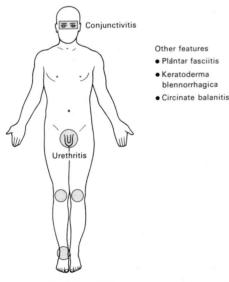

Conjunctivitis

Other features
- Plantar fasciitis
- Keratoderma blennorrhagica
- Circinate balanitis

Urethritis

Asymmetrical oligoarthritis

Fig. 8.17 The clinical features of Reiter's syndrome.

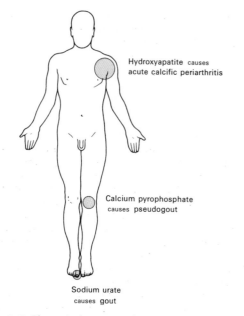

Hydroxyapatite causes
acute calcific periarthritis

Calcium pyrophosphate
causes pseudogout

Sodium urate
causes gout

Fig. 8.18 The typical patterns of joint involvement seen in crystal deposition disease.

ferent syndromes including pseudogout, which most often affects the knee.
- *Hydroxyapatite deposition* causes acute calcific periarthritis and most often affects the shoulder.

In addition, calcium pyrophosphate and hydroxyapatite crystals are found in the joints of patients with osteoarthritis and may contribute to the inflammation.

Gout

Gout is an abnormality of uric acid metabolism which results in the deposition of sodium urate crystals in:
- Joints—causing acute gouty arthritis
- Soft tissue—causing tophi and tenosynovitis
- Urinary tract—causing urate stones

The biochemical abnormality is hyperuricaemia resulting from over-production or under-excretion of uric acid. A high dietary intake of purines can be an additional factor, but does not in itself produce hyperuricaemia.

Uric acid production
Uric acid is the last step in the breakdown pathway of nucleoprotein and purines. The last two steps—the conversion of hypoxanthine to xanthine and xanthine to uric acid—are catalysed by the enzyme xanthine oxidase.

Uric acid excretion
Uric acid is completely filtered by the glomerulus, 100% is then reabsorbed in the proximal tubule and 75% is secreted by the distal tubule. Some post-secretory reabsorption also takes place.

Pathogenesis of hyperuricaemia
In 75–90% of patients with gout the cause of hyperuricaemia is impaired excretion. In idiopathic (primary) gout, increased synthesis also occurs. Conditions in which hyperuricaemia occurs are shown in Table 8.13.

CLINICAL FEATURES

Gout is predominantly a disease of men. Hippocrates was the first to note that it does not occur in men before puberty or in women until after the menopause. It is a disease which mostly begins in middle life. About one-third of patients give a family history of the disease and at least 50% are regular alcohol drinkers. Gout is common in the upper social classes and in certain races, e.g. Polynesians. Asymptomatic hyperuricaemia is 10 times more common than gout.

There are two stages in the natural history of the disease. First, recurrent acute attacks of arthritis occur. Secondly, the attacks fail to resolve com-

Table 8.13 Causes of hyperuricaemia.

Impaired excretion of uric acid
Idiopathic (primary) gout
Chronic renal disease (clinical gout unusual)
Drug therapy, e.g. thiazide diuretics, low-dose aspirin
Hypertension
Lead toxicity
Primary hyperparathyroidism
Hypothyroidism
Increased lactic acid production from alcohol, exercise, starvation,
Glucose-6-phosphatase deficiency (interferes with renal excretion)

Increased production of uric acid
Idiopathic (primary) gout
Increased purine synthesis de novo due to:
  hypoxanthine-guanine-phosphoribosyl transferase (HGPRT) reduction (an X-linked inborn error causing the Lesch–Nyhan syndrome)
  Phosphoribosyl-pyrophosphate synthetase overactivity
Glucose-6-phosphatase deficiency with glycogen storage disease type I (patients who survive develop hyperuricaemia due to increased production as well as decreased excretion)

Increased turnover of purines
Myeloproliferative disorders, e.g. polycythaemia vera
Lymphoproliferative disorders, e.g. leukaemia
Others, e.g. carcinoma, severe psoriasis

pletely and there are persistent symptoms associated with the permanent deposition of urate in and around joints; this stage is known as chronic tophaceous gout.

The typical acute attack begins suddenly in the early hours of the morning with excruciating pain in the big toe. Attacks may be precipitated by a traumatic event such as:

- A surgical operation (hence postoperative arthritis is usually gout)
- Dietary or alcoholic excess
- Starvation
- Drugs, e.g. thiazide diuretics

In 25% of attacks, a joint other than the big toe is the site of the disease. Joints of the lower limb are most often affected, including the toes, ankles and knees. Occasionally attacks occur in the upper limb, particularly in the distal interphalangeal joints of the fingers. One joint only is affected in 90% of attacks.

Signs
The typical gouty joint is red, warm, swollen and exquisitely tender. The presence of tophi in the ear lobes or around joints may provide a clue to the correct diagnosis, but they usually occur in the later stages of the disease by which time the nature of the problem is obvious.

Associated features
Patients with gout have a higher than expected incidence of vascular disease, hypertension and renal disease. Renal disease may be due to uric acid stones or very rarely to deposition of uric acid in the kidney itself, a condition known as chronic hyperuricaemic nephropathy (see p. 397). However, most often the renal disease is due to hypertension and vascular disease, which are genetic associations of gout rather than complications of hyperuricaemia.

INVESTIGATION

- The affected joint is aspirated and the synovial fluid examined under polarized-light microscopy. In acute gout, the presence of long needle-shaped negatively birefringent crystals is diagnostic. The test takes just a few minutes and is the best way to make the diagnosis.
- The serum uric acid has a number of limitations as a diagnostic test. It takes time, and a high incidence of false-positive and false-negative results may make interpretation difficult. Acute gout never occurs with a serum uric acid in the lower half of the normal range. However, in the first few attacks, which are the most difficult to diagnose, the serum uric acid is often only towards the upper limit of normal. The level may also fall after an acute attack. Thus a normal serum uric acid does not exclude the diagnosis of gout. Similarly, a high level alone is not diagnostic. However, the serum uric acid is useful in monitoring treatment.
- Causes for the hyperuricaemia should be investigated.

MANAGEMENT

Acute attacks
Acute gout is treated with anti-inflammatory drugs:

- Indomethacin 50 mg three to four times daily should produce substantial relief within 24–48 h, when the dose should be reduced to 25 mg three to four times daily. The attack should resolve completely within a few weeks. Azapropazone or naproxen are alternatives which may be used.
- Colchicine works slowly and produces diarrhoea; it is now rarely used.
- Intramuscular ACTH (corticotrophin) is very effective in difficult cases.
- Effusions in large joints should be aspirated and a corticosteroid injected to reduce inflammation.

Long-term therapy
Long-term therapy should be considered only after the acute attack has settled. Simple measures include:

- Weight reduction
- Reduction in alcohol intake
- Avoidance of foods containing high levels of purine, e.g. game
- Good fluid intake
- Withdrawal of drugs such as salicylates and thiazides

Drugs. Allopurinol (a xanthine oxidase inhibitor) is the drug of choice and should be used, usually for life, for:

- Recurrent acute attacks
- Tophi or chronic gouty arthritis
- Renal stones
- Very high serum uric acid levels (>9 mg·100ml^{-1} or 0.55 mmol·l^{-1})
- Prophylaxis when treating malignant disease

Allopurinol should not be started for 4 weeks after the last acute attack. It may precipitate acute gout and should initially be given with an anti-inflammatory drug (e.g. indomethacin) for the first few months to prevent flare-ups. Colchicine 0·5 mg twice daily is an alternative.

The dosage of allopurinol is 300 mg daily, which should be sufficient to bring the serum urate down to normal levels. In renal disease 100 mg daily is given. Side-effects are uncommon and include skin rashes. The tophi disappear with the reduction in serum urate.

Probenecid, a uricosuric drug, is occasionally used.

Pyrophosphate arthropathy

This condition is associated with the deposition of calcium pyrophosphate dihydrate in joints. The acute attacks of crystal synovitis which occur in about 25% of patients with the disease are known as pseudogout.

Pyrophosphate arthropathy is a disease of older people, with the typical age of onset being 60 years. It is equally common in men and women.

CLINICAL FEATURES

The commonest manifestation of pyrophosphate arthropathy is osteoarthritis; this occurs in about 50% of cases. It is not dissimilar to primary osteoarthritis, but tends to be polyarticular, sometimes with involvement of unusual joints such as the wrist. The course of osteoarthritis associated with pyrophosphate deposition may be punctuated by attacks of pseudogout. The aetiology of pyrophosphate arthropathy is unknown but there is an association with primary hyperparathyroidism, haemochromatosis, hypophosphatasia and true gout.

Acute attacks most commonly affect the knee, but they can affect various other joints, usually large ones and mainly one at a time. The attacks begin suddenly with pain and swelling. The affected joint is warm and swollen with a large effusion. The attack resolves within weeks or months, but recurs at irregular intervals. Patients may have other changes associated with osteoarthritis such as Heberden's nodes.

Occasionally pyrophosphate deposition is entirely asymptomatic. Rarely it causes a polyarthritis resembling rheumatoid arthritis, a severe destructive arthritis of weight-bearing joints, an acute spinal syndrome or polymyalgia rheumatica.

INVESTIGATION

- The serum calcium is normal.
- The ESR may be raised during an attack.
- Aspiration of synovial fluid and identification of crystals by polarized-light microscopy is diagnostic. Calcium pyrophosphate crystals are smaller than urate crystals. They are brick-shaped and positively birefringent, and are therefore easily distinguished from urate crystals.
- X-rays of the knee and occasionally the wrist may show linear calcification lying between and parallel to the articular surface (chondrocalcinosis articularis). X-rays may also show changes of osteoarthritis, with joint space narrowing and osteophyte formation.

MANAGEMENT

Pyrophosphate arthropathy is not as easy to treat and control as gout. Rest and aspiration of as much fluid as possible from an affected joint and an injection of corticosteroid are helpful. NSAIDs are less effective than in gout, but may be required in patients with osteoarthritis.

Acute calcific periarthritis

This syndrome is associated with deposition of hydroxyapatite in the soft tissues around joints. It is the least common of the crystal deposition diseases, but is by no means rare. It typically occurs in adults aged about 40 years and is equally common in men and women.

The shoulder joint is the commonest site, but it can affect the small joints of the hands and feet, the wrists, the knees and other joints. When the big toe is affected the condition is often confused with gout. There is a sudden onset of pain which is often very severe. The affected joint is red, warm and swollen, and there is sometimes a small effusion. The attack resolves within days or weeks, but attacks recur at irregular intervals.

X-rays are diagnostic: there is a rounded well-defined radiopaque deposit in the soft tissue adjacent to the joint. Hydroxyapatite crystals are too small for identification by polarized-light microscopy. Electron microscopy is required to demonstrate the crystals, but is not a routinely available investigation.

Treatment is with NSAIDs such as indomethacin. Potent analgesics such as opiates are sometimes required in the acute stage. It is often useful to inject the affected joint or soft tissues with a combination of local anaesthetic and corticosteroid. It is seldom, if ever, necessary to remove the calcific deposit.

ARTHRITIS ASSOCIATED WITH OTHER DISEASES

Gastrointestinal disease

Enteropathic synovitis occurs in 11% of patients with ulcerative colitis and 14% of patients with Crohn's disease. This type of arthritis is always related to the activity of the underlying disease, although in a small proportion of cases it is the first manifestation of underlying bowel problems. The aetiology is unknown, but deposition of immune complexes in the joint may play a part. Enteropathic synovitis usually affects the knees and ankles as a mono- or asymmetrical pauciarthritis. It presents with painful swollen joints and large effusions. Attacks last for a few months only and resolve without joint damage. Enteropathic synovitis should be distinguished from ankylosing spondylitis. The latter occurs in about 5% of patients with inflammatory bowel disease, but is an associated lesion rather than a complication of the bowel disease and therefore is not related to disease activity. Other non-articular features of inflammatory bowel disease, e.g. iritis, may be present.

X-rays of affected joints are normal and investigations are otherwise unhelpful. The first priority for treatment is to control the underlying inflammatory bowel disease. Aspiration and injection of affected joints and oral anti-inflammatory drugs may help the symptoms while the underlying disease is being brought under control.

Chronic active hepatitis may be accompanied by an arthralgia which is like that seen in systemic lupus erythematosus. Joint pain occurs in a bilateral, symmetrical distribution, with the small joints of the hands being prominently affected. Joints usually look normal but sometimes there is a slight soft tissue swelling. These patients often have positive tests for antinuclear antibodies and sometimes other features of connective tissue disorders such as Sjögren's syndrome.

Whipple's disease (see p. 182) is accompanied by a fever and an arthralgia.

Malignant disease

Hypertrophic pulmonary osteoarthropathy
Hypertrophic osteoarthropathy is most often associated with carcinoma of the bronchus. It is a non-metastatic complication and may be the presenting feature of the disease. It occurs only rarely with other conditions which cause clubbing. It is seen most often in middle-aged men, who present with pain and swelling of the wrists and ankles. Other joints are occasionally involved.

The diagnosis is made on the presence of clubbing of the fingers, which is usually gross, and periosteal new bone formation along the shafts of the distal ends of the radius, ulnar, tibia and fibula seen on x-ray. A chest x-ray usually shows the malignancy.

Treatment should be directed at the underlying carcinoma; if this can be removed, the arthritis disappears. NSAIDs may help to relieve the symptoms.

Other disorders
Secondary gout occurs in conditions such as chronic granulocytic leukaemia. Pain in the shoulder or back may be referred from malignant disease of the chest or abdomen. Secondaries around the joints may present with pain, but primary joint tumours are very rare. A synovioma presents as a painless soft tissue swelling adjacent to joints. It is highly malignant but extremely rare.

Skin disease

Psoriatic arthritis
This is a seronegative arthritis occurring in 10% of patients with psoriasis. The aetiology is unknown, but there is an increased incidence of HLA-B27 and of a history of psoriasis in the family.

The skin lesion, which is described on p. 908, may be minimal. The nail changes of psoriasis are usually present (85%). Differing patterns of arthritis are seen:

- The commonest pattern of psoriatic arthropathy is a polyarthritis affecting the small joints of the hands, including the distal interphalangeal joints, in an asymmetrical pattern. This is a mild but chronic condition, and in most cases is benign. It can usually be controlled with analgesics, but NSAIDs are sometimes necessary.
- Less often the pattern of the arthritis is similar to that in rheumatoid arthritis, i.e. a bilateral, symmetrical polyarthritis.
- Rarely the disease is rapidly progressive, producing destruction of the ends of the small bones of the hands and feet (arthritis mutilans), a condition which can also occur in rheumatoid arthritis. Because of the shortening of the bones of the fingers, there is an excess of soft tissue and the fingers can be pulled in and out like an opera glass, after which the condition is sometimes named.
- Finally, patients with psoriasis have an increased incidence of ankylosing spondylitis.

Blood tests are unhelpful in the diagnosis. The ESR is often normal and tests for rheumatoid factor are negative. X-rays may show characteristic changes in the terminal interphalangeal joints, with erosions and periarticular osteoporosis.

Treatment is with analgesic and anti-inflammatory drugs. In progressive cases, immunosuppressive drugs such as azathioprine are particularly effective. Gold is sometimes effective in psoriatic arthropathy, but penicillamine is not.

Erythema nodosum
Erythema nodosum (p. 916) is accompanied by arthritis in over 50% of cases. The knees and ankles are particularly affected and are swollen, red and tender. The arthritis subsides, along with the skin lesions, within a few months. Treatment is with NSAIDs or occasionally steroids.

Neurological disease

Neuropathic joints (Charcot's joints) are joints damaged by trauma as a result of the loss of the protective pain sensation. They were first described by Charcot in relation to tabes dorsalis. They are also seen in syringomyelia, diabetes mellitus and leprosy. The site of the neuropathic joint depends upon the localization of the pain loss:

- In tabes dorsalis, the knees and ankles are most often affected.
- In diabetes mellitus, the joints of the tarsus are involved.
- In syringomyelia, the shoulder is involved.

Neuropathic joints are not painful, although there may be painful episodes associated with crystal deposition. Presentation is usually with swelling and instability and eventually grotesque deformities appear.

The characteristic finding is a swollen joint with abnormal but painless movement. This is associated with neurological findings which depend upon the underlying disease, e.g. dissociated sensory loss in syringomyelia or peripheral neuropathy in diabetes. X-ray changes are characteristic with gross joint disorganization and bony distortion.

Treatment is symptomatic; surgery may be required in advanced cases.

Blood disease

Arthritis due to haemarthrosis is a common presenting feature of haemophilia. Attacks begin in early childhood in most cases and are recurrent. The knee is the commonest affected joint, but the elbows and ankles are sometimes involved. The arthritis can lead to bone destruction and disorganization of joints. Apart from replacement of factor VIII, affected joints require initial immobilization followed by physiotherapy to restore movement and measures to prevent and correct deformities.

Sickle cell crises are often accompanied by joint pain which particularly affects the hands and feet in a bilateral, symmetrical distribution. Affected joints usually look normal but are occasionally swollen. This condition may also be complicated by avascular necrosis (see below) and by *Salmonella* osteomyelitis.

Arthritis can also occur in acute leukaemia; it may be the presenting feature in childhood. The knee is particularly affected and is very painful, warm and swollen. Treatment is directed at the underlying leukaemia. Arthritis may also occur in chronic leukaemia, with leukaemic deposits in and around the joints.

Endocrine disorders

Hypothyroid patients may complain of pain and stiffness of proximal muscles, resembling polymyalgia rheumatica. They may also have carpal tunnel syndrome. Less often, there is an arthritis accompanied by joint effusions, particularly in the knees, wrists and small joints of the hands and feet. These problems respond rapidly to thyroxine.

In acromegaly an arthritis occurs in about 50% of patients. It resembles osteoarthritis and particularly affects the small joints of the hands and knees. It may be associated with the carpal tunnel syndrome.

In Cushing's disease back pain is common.

LESS COMMON ARTHROPATHIES

Amyloidosis (see p. 323)
Primary amyloidosis causes a polyarthritis resembling rheumatoid arthritis in distribution and which is also often associated with carpal tunnel syndrome and subcutaneous nodules.

Ankylosing vertebral hyperostosis (Forrestier's disease)
This is a condition of elderly people in which exuberant osteophytes are found in the spine, particularly the dorsal region. It is often asymptomatic, but it may be confused with ankylosing spondylitis. Sometimes there is stiffness and occasionally some discomfort. It may be associated with peripheral soft tissue problems associated with calcification, ossification and spur formation, when it is called diffuse idiopathic skeletal hyperostosis (DISH).

Avascular necrosis
In this condition bone infarction disrupts the surface of the joint and often leads to changes resembling osteoarthritis. The hip is particularly affected, for example, following fractures of the neck of the femur, perhaps because of its precarious blood supply. It also occurs in various systemic conditions, including sickle cell disease, prolonged steroid therapy, systemic lupus erythematosus, alcohol excess and Gaucher's disease. In deep-sea divers it may occur for no obvious reason (caisson disease), particularly in middle-aged men.

Avascular necrosis presents with a single painful joint. X-rays are usually diagnostic in the latter phases, showing rarefaction and dense bone in the subcortical areas with distortion of the epiphysis.

Behçet's syndrome
This is a rare condition characterized by oral and genital ulceration, iritis, and a polyarthritis of variable distribution which may be either chronic or episodic. There are many less common features of the disease, including erythema nodosum, pustular skin lesions, and neurological and gastrointestinal manifestations.

Drugs
Drugs may cause arthritis. Systemic lupus erythematosus may be induced by procainamide, hydralazine and other drugs. Certain drugs may also precipitate or aggravate gout.

Other minor syndromes may be caused by drugs; these are worth considering in a patient with unusual joint problems.

Familial Mediterranean fever
This condition occurs in certain ethnic groups, particularly Jews and Arabs. The aetiology is unknown. It is characterized by recurrent attacks of fever, arthritis and abdominal or chest pain due to pleurisy. The arthritis is usually monoarticular and attacks last

up to 1 week. The condition may be mistaken for palindromic rheumatism, but such attacks are not usually accompanied by fever. In familial Mediterranean fever, attacks can usually be prevented by regular treatment with colchicine 1.0–1.5 g daily. In general the disorder is benign but in some cases amyloidosis develops.

Hypermobility syndrome

Hypermobility syndrome occurs in children or young adults with lax joints. The musculoskeletal manifestations of this syndrome include recurrent attacks of joint pain and effusion, dislocation, ligamentous injuries, low back pain and premature osteoarthritis. Hypermobility is also associated with some rare congenital disorders such as the Ehlers–Danlos syndrome. Joints become stiffer with increasing age. Treatment should be directed at improving muscle power.

Osteochondritis dessecans

This is a rare condition of adolescent sportsmen in which there is separation of an avascular osteochondral fragment in the knee joint. It results in disruption of the joint surface and the formation of loose bodies within the joint. Osteoarthritis may develop.

Osteochondromatosis

In this condition foci of cartilage form within the synovial membrane. These foci become calcified and then ossified (osteochondromas). They may give rise to loose bodies within the joint. The condition occurs in a single joint of a young adult and x-rays are usually diagnostic. Treatment involves removal of loose bodies and synovectomy.

Pigmented villonodular synovitis

This is characterized by exuberant synovial proliferation which occurs either in joints or in tendon sheaths. The main manifestation in joints is recurrent haemarthrosis. Treatment is synovectomy. In tendons, the condition gives rise to a nodular mass which requires excision.

Relapsing polychondritis

Relapsing polychondritis is a rare condition of cartilage. It gives rise to a polyarthritis accompanied by chest disease due to tracheal or bronchial involvement. The diagnosis is often made on the basis of recurrent attacks of pain and swelling of the nose or external ear.

Subacute infective endocarditis

Subacute infective endocarditis (p. 524) may present with arthritis, which can occur in the early stages of the disease. Like other clinical features, the arthritis may be due to circulating immune complexes; direct infection of the joints is much less common. Asymmetrical arthritis of a few large joints is characteristic,

but other patterns may occur. Localized back pain associated with fever is another manifestation.

Temporomandibular pain dysfunction syndrome

This is a functional disorder of the temporomandibular joint associated with abnormalities of bite. It particularly occurs in anxious people who grind their teeth at night. It gives rise to pain and clicking in one or both temporomandibular joints. Treatment is dental correction of the bite.

Sarcoidosis (see p. 603)

A pauciarthritis frequently affecting the knees and ankles (often with erythema nodosum) is a common manifestation of this disease. Recovery occurs, usually with no joint deformity or destruction.

Hyperlipoproteinaemia type II (see p. 772)

This is associated with xanthomas in the tendons and a migratory polyarthritis.

Back pain

Back pain is extremely common. It can be mild and transient, or chronic and disabling. In many cases, the exact cause is not established. In Britain 375000 people lose some time from work each year because of back pain, an annual loss of 11.5 million working days, and back pain accounts for 6% of general practice consultations. Back pain is not usually serious and mostly resolves; in one survey 44% of cases resolved within a week and 12% within 2 months.

Most back pain can be readily diagnosed from a simple clinical history and physical examination. A diagnostic approach to back pain is shown in Table 8.14.

In many patients (30%) no cause will be found. It is foolish to label such patients as having 'spondylosis' or arthritis of the spine, terms which merely cause anxiety. It is better to use a term such as non-specific low back pain and explain to the patient what this means.

The back is a common site of psychogenic pain. If possible a positive diagnosis of psychogenic back pain, rather than a diagnosis by exclusion, should be made. Supportive treatment can then be given.

HISTORY

The following factors should be considered.

Site
- *Lumbar pain*. This is usually due to degenerative disease, disc prolapse and OA; these are not commonly seen in the thoracic spine.

Table 8.14 A diagnostic approach to back pain.

	Possible causes

1 Is it serious?	Infection
	    Septic discitis
	    Tuberculosis
	Malignancy
	    Metastases
	    Myeloma
	    Spinal tumour
	Referred pain

2 Is it inflammatory?	Ankylosing spondylitis

3 Is it disc disease?
    or osteoarthritis?
	Acute disc prolapse
	Chronic disc disease/osteo-
	    arthritis (spondylosis)

4 Is it bone disease?	Osteoporosis Osteomalacia Paget's disease Hyperparathyroidism Renal osteodystrophy

5 Is it a mechanical
    problem—perhaps
    amenable to surgery?
	Spondylolisthesis
	Spinal stenosis
	Posture
	Pregnancy
	Obesity
	Congenital abnormalities

6 Is it a soft tissue
    problem?
	Fibrositis, sprains and
	    strains

7 Is it psychogenic?	

If not, it is non-specific back pain.

- *Thoracic pain.* This is a characteristic site of osteoporotic crush fractures.

Radiation
Sciatic radiation of pain suggests root compression; however, sacroiliac pain can also radiate down the back of the thigh to the knee.

Onset
- Sudden, e.g. disc prolapse or mechanical injury
- Gradual, e.g. ankylosing spondylitis
- Over years—probably not serious

Aggravating factors
Pain in the back and leg on walking and relieved by stopping, suggestive of intermittent claudication, can be due to spinal stenosis.

Time pattern
- Disc disease is recurrent.
- Ankylosing spondylosis is chronic.

Associated symptoms
There may be evidence of disease elsewhere.

The past medical history and a family history should also be obtained.

The differences in the history given in inflammatory and in mechanical back pain are shown in Table 8.15.

EXAMINATION

Examination of the patient is summarized in Table 8.16.

INVESTIGATION (see Table 8.17)

In back pain investigations are less important than the history and examination. They can also be mis-

Table 8.15 Points of distinction between inflammatory and mechanical back pain.

	Inflammatory	Mechanical
Onset	Gradual	Sudden
Worst pain	In the morning	In the evening
Morning stiffness	Present	Absent
Effect of exercise	Relieves pain	Aggravates pain

Table 8.16 Examination of patients with back pain.

The back
Appearance—deformity
Movement
Palpation for tenderness

The nerve roots
Straight leg raising; femoral stretch test
Sensation; weakness
Reflexes; plantar responses

Complete physical examination ESSENTIAL
Look for abdominal masses, lymph nodes, iritis, etc.

Table 8.17 Investigations to consider in a patient with back pain.

X-rays

Blood count and ESR

Serum calcium, phosphate, alkaline phosphatase

Serum acid phosphatase

Protein electrophoresis; immunoglobulins

HLA-B27

Bone scan

Radiculogram

EMG

CT scan/magnetic resonance imaging

Discogram

leading; for example, degenerative changes are virtually always present in older people and may not be the cause of the pain.

X-rays are particularly useful for excluding bone disease. Normal x-rays usually exclude metastases but not invariably. They are of little value in acute disc disease, although a narrowed disc space is suggestive of disc involvement.

A radiculogram can be performed to demonstrate the spinal cord and nerve roots. It will detect large disc prolapses and spinal stenosis. However, it does not show the lateral recess which is the region of the intervertebral foramen in which osteophytes may compress the nerve root, giving rise to sciatica.

A CT scan or magnetic resonance imaging are being used more often for the detection of disc lesions.

Bone scans are useful to detect metastases; 'hot spots' will also appear at sites of degenerative disease, but these can usually be distinguished by the clinical features and accompanying x-ray appearances.

Blood tests
- ESR is a particularly useful investigation. A normal ESR makes a serious disease unlikely. A very high ESR suggests myeloma.
- Calcium, phosphate and alkaline phosphatase serum levels are measured to look for bone disease.
- Acid phosphatase is measured to look for secondary prostatic disease.
- Protein electrophoresis, immunoglobulins and bone marrow are performed to look for myeloma.

BACK PAIN DUE TO SERIOUS DISEASE

Back pain is seldom serious but nevertheless important because conditions such as infection are readily treatable. Some features that suggest serious back pain are shown in Table 8.18.

Spinal infections

Spinal infections include osteomyelitis, discitis and epidural abscess. Infections tend to affect the disc, while malignant processes affect the vertebra itself.

Table 8.18 Features which suggest that back pain is serious.

Recent onset
Weight loss
Symptoms elsewhere, e.g. cough
Localized pain in the dorsal spine
Fever
Raised ESR

Discitis can be due to pyogenic organisms such as *Staphylococcus aureus*, *Mycobacterium tuberculosis*, or rare organisms such as *Brucella*.

INVESTIGATION
- Blood count—leucocytosis, high ESR
- Blood culture
- Needle aspiration of joint for culture

TREATMENT

Immobilization and antibiotics are required, often for a long time.

Malignant disease

Bone metastases are classically from primaries in the bronchus, breast, kidney, thyroid or prostate. These are discussed on p. 369. Multiple myeloma produces osteolytic lesions of the spine (see p. 321). Primary tumours of the spinal cord are rarely causes of back pain (see p. 848).

Referred pain

Sources of referred pain are shown in Table 8.19.

INFLAMMATORY BACK PAIN

Ankylosing spondylitis

Ankylosing spondylitis is the most important cause of inflammatory back pain. It affects young adults, with men more commonly affected and more severely afflicted than women. It presents with back pain and morning stiffness, and is typically associated with sacroiliitis on x-ray. Other important associations include peripheral arthritis and non-articular features such as iritis.

It is a genetically-determined disease, susceptibility to which is related to the presence of HLA-B27. This antigen is found in about 5% of European people and 95% of patients with ankylosing spondylitis. Studies of large populations of B27-positive subjects such as blood donors suggest that about 20% of B27-positive individuals have ankylosing spondylitis or a related disease. The prevalence of ankylosing spondylitis in the population can thus be calculated as 1%. Since B27 is found equally in men and women, the incidence of the disease should also be equal. Population surveys using radiological sacroiliitis as the main criterion for diagnosis have shown both a much lower incidence than 1% and a male preponderance. It is now clear that there are many mild cases, especially in women, which present as pain and stiffness but with no other features. The presence of x-ray changes may not be essential for the diagnosis, although this remains controversial.

Table 8.19 Sources of referred pain in the back.

Kidney
Stones
Tumours
Infection
Hydronephrosis

Uterus
Dysmenorrhoea
Pelvic infection
Tumours

Ovary
Tumours
Cysts

Oesophagus
Oesophagitis
Carcinoma
Hiatus hernia

Stomach and duodenum
Peptic ulcer
Carcinoma

Pancreas
Pancreatitis
Carcinoma

Aorta
Aneurysm

Bowel
Diverticulitis
Abscess
Tumour

Gallbladder
Cholecystitis

The frequency of ankylosing spondylitis in different populations is roughly paralleled by the incidence of HLA-B27. Africans and Japanese have a low incidence of both B27 and ankylosing spondylitis. Some Indian tribes in America have a correspondingly higher incidence of both. HLA-B27 is the genetic marker of a family of diseases which includes Reiter's disease, iritis, inflammatory bowel disease, one type of juvenile chronic arthritis, and psoriasis. These associations are often helpful in the diagnosis of ankylosing spondylitis, since patients may give a family history of B27-related disorders.

CLINICAL FEATURES

The typical case presents with an insidious onset of low back pain in the late teens or early twenties. The pain is typically inflammatory in type (see Table 8.15). The first symptoms may arise from sacroiliitis, with pain in the buttocks and radiating down the back of both legs. Peripheral polyarthritis may also

occur; all the joints of the lower limbs are particularly affected. Plantar fasciitis may cause heel pain. Iritis occurs at some time in 30% of cases.

Inspection of the spine in a patient with ankylosing spondylitis reveals two characteristic abnormalities:
● Loss of lumbar lordosis and increased kyphosis
● Variable limitation of spinal flexion and a reduction in chest expansion

In addition, tenderness is commonly found around the pelvis and chest wall.

INVESTIGATION

The ESR is often raised. X-rays of the lumbar spine and pelvis are almost always abnormal. In the early stages, the sacroiliac joints are eroded, with irregular margins, and there is sclerosis of adjacent bone. As the disease advances, the sacroiliac joints may fuse. In the spinal column, the characteristic abnormality is a syndesmophyte which grows up or down from the margin of the vertebrae. There is calcification and ossification of the interspinous ligaments so that if syndesmophytes join together, the PA x-ray shows three continuous lines, the so-called tramline appearance. Vertebrae appear square as a result of the erosion of their corners. These changes are particularly seen at the dorsolumbar junction, but may occur throughout the spine.

HLA-B27 is only diagnostically helpful in the difficult case.

COURSE

In all but the mild cases there is progressive limitation of spinal movement over the course of a few years. In severe cases the spine becomes completely fused. There is a tendency for patients to develop a kyphosis, but this can usually be prevented. Despite the limitation of spinal movement, most patients are able to lead a normal active life and remain at work. In women, the disease is usually mild, with little restriction and no deformity.

MANAGEMENT

NSAIDs are very effective; indomethacin is often the best choice (75–100 mg at night). It is particularly useful in relieving night pain and morning stiffness. Useful alternatives include naproxen or flurbiprofen.

An exercise programme is essential to maintain movement, relieve symptoms and prevent deformity, particularly kyphosis. Exercises should be carried out at least twice daily. In addition, patients should be encouraged to take part in whatever sports they wish.

There is no evidence that penicillamine, gold or immunosuppressive drugs are effective in the management of ankylosing spondylitis. Radiotherapy has been used, but should seldom be necessary and carries a small risk of leukaemia.

A period of inpatient treatment may occasionally be required in difficult cases for diagnosis and physiotherapy. Surgery plays little part, but hip replacement is occasionally required.

DISC DISEASE

The term 'disc disease' is used to describe an acute syndrome in which disc prolapse causes conditions which are known to the layman as either lumbago or sciatica, depending upon the presence or absence of radiation of the pain to the areas supplied by the sciatic nerve. It is also used to describe a chronic syndrome in which back pain is associated with 'degenerative changes' on x-ray. This chronic syndrome is sometimes called spondylosis. Chronic disc disease is often associated with osteoarthritis of the apophyseal joints of the spine and it is difficult or impossible to separate the role of these two pathologies in the pathogenesis of symptoms. There is a very poor correlation between the presence of radiological changes and symptoms. Severe x-ray changes can be seen in patients without any appropriate symptoms and chronic back pain may also occur in patients with little radiological change.

Acute disc disease

Acute disc disease causes acute back pain (lumbago) with or without sciatic radiation (sciatica). The severity of this syndrome is enormously variable, from a brief and trivial episode to a long and difficult illness which occasionally requires surgical intervention. It is predominantly a disease of younger people, with a peak incidence between the ages of 20 and 40, since the disc degenerates with age and is no longer capable of prolapse in the elderly. In older patients, sciatica is more likely to be due to compression of the nerve root by osteophytes in the lateral recess of the spinal canal.

CLINICAL FEATURES

The back pain is sudden, often severe and often constant at first. Its onset may be associated with a feeling that something has 'gone' in the back. This may occur after some strenuous activity, typically with the back in forward flexion. The pain is often clearly related to position and at first the back may be fixed in forward flexion. The pain is aggravated by movement and by certain activities. The radiation of the pain and various examination findings are dependent upon the disc affected; these features are summarized in Table 8.20. The three lowest discs account for most cases of disc disease; in order of frequency, they are the L5/S1, L4/L5 and L3/L4 discs.

Examination
In a mild case, there may be no signs at all, but characteristic findings include loss of lumbar lordosis, sometimes a compensatory scoliosis (Fig. 8.19), and limitation of movement in all directions.

Fig. 8.19 Acute lumbar disc prolapse and sciatica, showing the area of the pain and the compensatory scoliosis.

Table 8.20 Symptoms and signs of common root compression syndromes produced by lumbar disc prolapse.

Root lesion	Pain	Sensory loss	Motor weakness	Reflex lost	Other signs
S1	From buttock down back of thigh and leg to ankle and foot	Sole of foot and posterior calf	Plantar flexion of ankle and toes	Ankle jerk	Diminished straight-leg raising
L5	From buttock to lateral aspect of leg and dorsum of foot	Dorsum of foot and anterolateral aspect of lower leg	Dorsiflexion of foot and toes	None	Diminished straight-leg raising
L4	Lateral aspect of thigh to medial side of calf	Medial aspect of calf and shin	Dorsiflexion and inversion of ankle; extension of knee	Knee jerk	Femoral stretch test

Nerve root compression leads to limitation of straight-leg raising on the side of the lesion. With involvement of the L3/4 disc, a positive femoral stretch test (raising the leg up backwards when the patient lies in a prone position) can also be elicited. Loss of an ankle or knee jerk may occur, depending upon the level of disc involved. Severe neurological problems such as foot drop or bladder or bowel dysfunction are fortunately rare.

INVESTIGATIONS

Investigations are of very limited value in disc disease. X-rays do not visualize the disc itself, although there may be narrowing at the level of the lesion. Radiculography and CT examination are usually reserved for patients in whom surgery is being considered.

MANAGEMENT

Treatment probably has little effect on the duration of the disease and is therefore aimed at the relief of symptoms and the maintenance of a reasonable way of life for the duration of the illness. Management therefore includes rest, and drugs and physical measures such as heat to relieve the pain. A few days of rest on a firm bed will be helpful in most cases in the acute stage. Long periods of rest are sometimes necessary, depending on the patient's progress.

Epidural corticosteroid injection may be considered in the acute early stage of the lumbar disc prolapse as it reduces pain. It requires admission to hospital and should be reserved for cases who fail to respond to simple conservative measures.

Physiotherapy is best avoided in the acute stage but is often required later. Very few patients require surgery for an acute disc unless there are severe or progressive neurological complications such as bladder or bowel dysfunction. Corsets are seldom required in patients with lumbar disc prolapse and are grossly over-prescribed. Fortunately many patients have the good sense not to wear them. A corset is sometimes helpful to provide immediate relief of symptoms in the acute stage of lumbar disc prolapse.

Once the acute stage has passed, the aim of treatment is the gradual mobilization of the patient and his back. Persistent stiffness can delay recovery and physiotherapy is often required. A particularly useful physiotherapy technique for mobilizing the lumbar spine is Maitland mobilization, which comprises gentle finger compression over the joints, with the oscillation amplitude being carefully graded to the response of the joint. It helps pain and stiffness, and may be combined with traction. At this stage it may also be useful to start a gentle exercise routine designed to restore lumbar spinal movement and muscle power. One physiotherapy regimen that is especially useful in patients with nerve root compression is the MacKenzie extension exercise regimen. This is a self-treatment method taught to the patient. It uses posture correction and particular repeated spinal movement exercises to relieve pain, restore joint function and prevent recurrence.

A corset is definitely not required at this stage in the treatment and if it has been prescribed earlier, it should now be withdrawn. Drugs are less necessary and should also be slowly reduced.

COURSE AND PROGNOSIS

Most cases of acute lumbar disc prolapse recover completely, though the process may take as long as a year. A small proportion of patients fail to recover and may require surgery. Further investigations, including a radiculogram and perhaps EMG, are required to pinpoint the lesion as closely as possible, thus improving the prospects of surgery. The simplest operation is removal of the prolapsed disc. Decompression may be achieved by laminectomy, and spinal fusion may be considered for recurrent cases.

Chronic disc disease and osteoarthritis

This very common syndrome is characterized by the presence of chronic low back pain associated with 'degenerative' changes in the lower lumbar discs and apophyseal joints. Pain in these cases is of the mechanical type and is typically aggravated by exercise, although there may be an inflammatory component, reflected in a brief period of morning stiffness. Sciatic radiation of the pain may occur and there may be a past history of acute disc prolapse. In many cases, the pain is long-standing and the prospects for cure are very limited. Nevertheless there are measures which will alleviate a difficult situation.

Analgesics and NSAIDs are widely used, as in acute disc disease. Diflunisal, 500 mg twice daily, which has good analgesic properties, is often preferred. Physiotherapy is helpful in mobilizing the stiff back, and an exercise regimen may be of value. Corsets should be avoided. These patients require advice about their way of life, methods of lifting, firm beds and other matters connected with the back.

There are many other ways of relieving pain, including acupuncture and transcutaneous nerve stimulation, which may occasionally help. Surgery may be considered, but the success rate in chronic disease is not high.

MECHANICAL PROBLEMS

There are two mechanical problems in the spine which are of particular importance because they are amenable to surgical treatment: spondylolisthesis and spinal stenosis.

Spondylolisthesis

This condition arises because of a defect in the pars interarticularis (the ligament joining two adjacent vertebrae) which may be either congenital or acquired. It gives rise to a slipping forward of one vertebra on another, most commonly at L4/L5. The acquired variety is usually the result of a fairly major traumatic episode which the patient will remember. A small spondylolisthesis is sometimes found in patients with degenerative disease of the lumbar spine and may contribute to the symptoms. The patients have mechanical pain which is not present on waking in the morning but develops as the day goes on and is aggravated by activities such as standing or walking. The pain may radiate to one or other leg and there may be signs of root irritation. More often there are no physical signs, though there may be some limitation of back movement. The diagnosis is confirmed by x-ray.

Small spondylolistheses are common, especially in patients with degenerative disease of the lumbar spine, and may be managed conservatively. It is appropriate to use simple analgesics to relieve the pain and there is no particular need for anti-inflammatory agents. A corset may provide support; this is one of the few indications for its use. A large spondylolisthesis causing severe pain, especially in a younger patient without associated degenerative changes, requires spinal fusion. This is usually a very successful procedure.

Spinal stenosis

This is sometimes called spinal claudication because of the resemblance of the symptoms to those of intermittent claudication due to vascular occlusion. The anatomical change in spinal stenosis is narrowing of the central canal, compressing the cauda equina. This can result from a variety of causes:
- Disc prolapse
- Degenerative osteophyte formation
- Tumour—rare
- Congenital narrowing of the spinal canal

The patient typically presents with pain in one or sometimes both legs. The absence of back pain makes the diagnosis difficult. The pain in the legs and buttocks develops after walking. The symptoms are relieved by rest and occasionally by leaning forward. There may be signs of root compression such as limitation of straight leg raising or absent reflexes; these may be transient after an episode of ischaemia.

If spinal stenosis is suspected, a radiculogram is required to confirm the diagnosis. Treatment is by surgical decompression.

Other mechanical problems

Bad posture is sometimes the cause of back pain. An exercise programme designed to improve posture will also therefore improve the pain. Such postural problems may be precipitated by congenital abnormalities of the spine such as a minor kyphoscoliosis. Obesity and presumably lack of activity sometimes appear to be relevant and weight-loss combined with an exercise programme may help.

SOFT TISSUE PROBLEMS

Back pain can arise from soft tissues, including the muscles, tendons and ligaments.

Sprains and strains

The relationship of symptoms to some unusual physical activity will usually make the diagnosis obvious. Spontaneous resolution is usual and may be aided by the use of a NSAID and soothing measures such as heat, ice packs or massage. Local injection of tender areas with steroidal local anaesthetic combinations may also be of value.

Sacroiliac strain. This usually results from some physical activity and is particularly common in people whose occupation requires lifting, such as nurses. The pain radiates from the sacroiliac joint to the buttock and sometimes down the back of the thigh. It is a sudden acute problem which usually resolves within a few weeks with rest, avoidance of lifting and NSAIDs. Unfortunately it has a great tendency to recur.

Coccyodynia

This is a soft tissue problem in which pain arises from the region of the coccyx, often in anxious women. Reassurance and protection with a soft ring cushion are usually sufficient treatment since the condition is self-limiting.

Fibrositis

This is described on p. 366.

PSYCHOGENIC BACK PAIN

Patients with psychogenic pain tend to be young adults; females are more often affected than males. In most cases there is no obvious psychiatric disorder. There is commonly a predisposing cause and a history of previous pain. Psychogenic back pain is accompanied by headaches and pains elsewhere. The patient has often been investigated in the past for various complaints, but no abnormalities have been found.

The pain is continuous and unvarying. There are few organic conditions of the back which are not relieved by rest and which continue unremittingly throughout the day. A history of treatment failures is also part of the characteristic description, and analgesics often fail to help.

The management of psychogenic pain is difficult. While reassurance about the absence of serious pathology is required, it is seldom sufficient. It is important to try to explain the situation and to explore possible mechanisms for it, but it is wise to try to avoid confrontation, which would simply drive the patient from one doctor to another. It is foolish to give an inappropriate physical diagnosis and even more foolish to predict a cure from treatment. Where there is depression, antidepressant drugs will probably help, but in most cases this is not a useful approach. In general, drugs have little part to play in this condition.

NON-SPECIFIC LOW BACK PAIN

This is an appropriate term for those cases which defy diagnosis with current knowledge and techniques. Patients will vary from those with acute pain which will quickly resolve to those with long-standing symptoms and little prospect of recovery. Without the possibility of definitive treatment, one must rely on simple symptomatic measures such as analgesic drugs.

NECK PAIN

Pain in the neck may be caused by rheumatoid arthritis, ankylosing spondylitis, soft tissue rheumatism or fibrositis. In addition, disc disease, both acute and chronic, the latter in association with osteoarthritis, may occur in the neck as well as in the lumbar spine. The three lowest cervical discs are most often affected and there is pain and stiffness of the neck with or without root pain radiating to the arm (see p. 860). Chronic cervical disc disease is known as cervical spondylosis.

Painful stiff necks are common clinical problems, often attributed, without much evidence, to disc disease. The essence of treatment is to mobilize the neck with physiotherapy techniques such as traction or Maitland mobilization. Pain may be relieved with simple analgesics. While cervical collars may be required in the acute stage of cervical disc prolapse and occasionally in patients with cervical spondylosis, they can also perpetuate the problem of a painful stiff neck when the right treatment is mobilization.

Soft tissue rheumatism

Soft tissue rheumatism is a convenient term for a number of conditions with similar features (Table 8.21). They cause musculoskeletal or joint pain which arises, not from the joint itself, but from surrounding structures such as the tendon sheaths and bursae. These conditions are benign and in most cases self-limiting. They are often regarded as trivial except by those who have them. Many are best treated by local corticosteroid injection rather than by anti-inflammatory drugs. It is also important to remove aetiological factors whenever possible; mechanical factors such as over-use and repetitive strain are probably particularly important.

Common soft tissue rheumatic syndromes are shown in Fig. 8.20.

Bursitis

There are numerous bursae around the body and any of these can become inflamed; olecranon bursitis (student's elbow) and prepatellar bursitis (housemaid's knee) are two examples. Bursitis may appear for no obvious reason or it can be secondary to trauma, repetitive injury or an arthritis such as rheumatoid arthritis or gout. Occasionally bursitis is due to infection, when aspiration may be necessary. In many cases no treatment is required other than protection of the inflamed site. Injection of corticosteroid may be useful, and, very occasionally, large and troublesome bursae may require excision. Ischial bursitis causes pain over the ischial tuberosity and makes sitting difficult. A ring cushion is usually helpful.

Tenosynovitis

Tenosynovitis can occur in any tendon sheath. The flexor tendons of the fingers are often affected and cause the condition known as trigger finger. Patients characteristically wake with one finger fixed in flexion. Some force is needed to extend the finger and this produces pain. There is a palpable nodule in the flexor tendon. Injection of this nodule with a corti-

Table 8.21 Types of soft-tissue rheumatism.

Bursitis
Tenosynovitis or peritendinitis
Enthesitis
Nerve compression
Periarthritis or capsulitis
Muscle tension and dysfunction

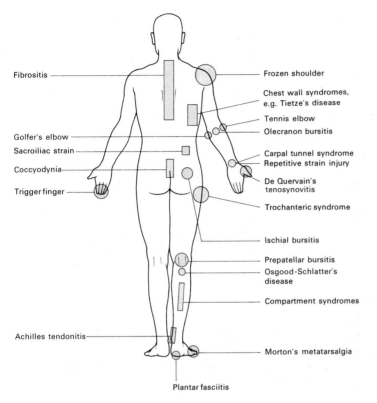

Fig. 8.20 Common soft tissue rheumatic syndromes.

Labels on figure:

Fibrositis

Golfer's elbow

Sacroiliac strain

Coccyodynia

Trigger finger

Achilles tendonitis

Plantar fasciitis

Frozen shoulder

Chest wall syndromes, e.g. Tietze's disease

Tennis elbow

Olecranon bursitis

Carpal tunnel syndrome
Repetitive strain injury

De Quervain's tenosynovitis

Trochanteric syndrome

Ischial bursitis

Prepatellar bursitis

Osgood-Schlatter's disease

Compartment syndromes

Morton's metatarsalgia

---

costeroid preparation usually provides relief.

De Quervain's tenosynovitis gives rise to pain in the anatomical snuff box and may be mistaken for osteoarthritis of the first carpometacarpal joint. The point of maximum tenderness should be injected with a combination of corticosteroid and local anaesthetic.

Enthesitis

The enthesis is the specialized area at the junction of tendons or ligaments and bone.

Inflammation of the junction of the common extensor origin of the muscles of the forearm and the lateral humeral epicondyle results in 'tennis elbow'. This condition is seldom due to tennis, more often it is caused by housework or some repetitive manual occupation. Often there is no obvious cause. There is pain in the elbow, but it is not clearly localized. However, on examination, the joint is normal and there is an area of exquisite tenderness over the lateral epicondyle. It is usually treated by injecting this tender area with a combination of corticosteroid and local anaesthetic. Since the condition resolves within a year or two whatever is done, in mild cases it may be best ignored.

Golfer's elbow is a similar problem at the junction of the origin of the flexor muscles of the forearm and the medial humeral epicondyle. Another common

site is the greater trochanter of the femur (trochanteric syndrome).

In plantar fasciitis, the inflammation arises on the undersurface of the heel at the origin of the plantar fascia. This common condition is best treated with a protective heel pad and normally resolves within a year or two.

Nerve compression syndromes

Carpal tunnel syndrome is described on p. 856. A similar condition in the foot, tarsal tunnel syndrome, gives rise to burning pain with pins and needles in the sole of the foot and toes. As in carpal tunnel syndrome, the pain is often worse at night and may wake the patient from sleep. In cases of diagnostic difficulty, nerve conduction studies will show a block at the appropriate level.

In Morton's metatarsalgia, pain arises from a digital nerve in the foot, usually between the third and fourth metatarsal heads. It is either due to a neuroma or to compression by a bursa. There is pain in the forefoot which radiates into the toes. It is usually aggravated by wearing shoes and relieved by removing them. Manual compression of the forefoot reproduces the symptoms. The condition sometimes responds to local injection and to the use of a metatarsal pad. If not, surgical exploration and excision of the bursa or digital nerve is required.

Frozen shoulder

This is a convenient term for a group of soft tissue syndromes which produce the same clinical picture—a painful stiff shoulder. Some people reserve the term for the later stage of the disease when the glenohumeral joint is completely immobile. Many other terms such as capsulitis are used to describe this condition, but without much pathological justification. In some cases, local tenderness points to a lesion such as supraspinatus tendonitis, bicipital tendonitis or subacromial bursitis. In most cases, however, it is not possible to identify a specific cause and differentiation makes little difference to the outcome or treatment.

Frozen shoulder is a common condition, with a peak incidence in older patients. It is usually but not always unilateral. There is pain in the shoulder which may radiate to the arm and is usually most troublesome at night. In most cases the condition appears without obvious cause but it may occasionally be related to over-use or injury. A similar clinical picture is produced by acute calcific periarthritis (see p. 354).

Examination shows restriction of glenohumeral movement. Analgesics, injection of the joint with a corticosteroid preparation and exercises to restore mobility are required.

Fibrositis

This is the term used to describe pain arising from muscles and muscle insertions. It may have a large psychogenic component. It begins in early adult life, with females being particularly affected. Widespread aches and pains are characteristic, moving from place to place, varying in severity, and often aggravated by cold and stress. The characteristic physical sign in patients with fibrositis is multiple areas of localized soft tissue tenderness known as trigger points. They are particularly found around the dorsal spine in the interscapular region, around the base of the neck, over both sacroiliac joints, over the lateral epicondyles of the elbows (resembling tennis elbow), and over the medial sides of both knees. Patients have a characteristic sleep disturbance, lacking the deepest type of sleep. Interruption of sleep in normal volunteers will reproduce the syndrome.

Blood tests and x-rays are normal. There is no consistent pathological abnormality. In some patients, crops of nodules appear in the muscles, but these have no definite pathological basis and are believed to be part of the functional abnormality.

The condition is chronic or recurrent and very difficult to treat. Reassurance is important but seldom sufficient. Physical therapy including heat and massage directed at trigger points is often the most effective symptomatic remedy. Local injection of trigger points with a combination of local anaesthetic and corticosteroid may also be useful.

Analgesic and anti-inflammatory drugs are often disappointing.

It is important to try to correct the sleep disturbance and antidepressant drugs may be of value. An exercise programme to improve physical fitness and an exploration of possible psychological factors may be additional helpful measures.

Chest pain

Musculoskeletal conditions are sometimes important in the differential diagnosis of chest pain. An important example is Tietze's disease. In this condition, pain arises from the costosternal junctions. It is usually unilateral and affects one, two or three joints. There is local tenderness, which helps to make the diagnosis. The condition is benign and self-limiting. It often responds well to anti-inflammatory drugs, or may be treated with local injections of corticosteroid and local anaesthetic.

Compartment syndromes

The muscles of the lower leg are enclosed in a compartment of fascia, with little room for expansion to occur. Compartment syndromes may be acute (anterior tibial syndrome), e.g. following exercise, or chronic, the former requiring immediate surgical decompression to prevent muscle necrosis. Chronic compartment syndromes produce pain in the lower leg which is aggravated by exercise and may therefore be mistaken for a vascular or neurological disorder.

Repetitive strain syndrome

Musculoskeletal pain is also a feature of an important group of occupational disorders known as repetitive strain or over-use syndromes. They particularly occur in occupations requiring repetitive manual work such as assembly work or keyboard operation. While this problem can occur at any site, it is particularly likely in the wrist. A wide range of clinical syndromes including conditions similar to frozen shoulder or tennis elbow can occur. It is important to recognize the nature of the problem as early as possible so that measures can be taken to prevent it by varying the nature of the patient's work, providing adequate breaks and correcting faulty equipment.

Bone disease

The structure, physiology and function of bone is described on p. 732. Table 8.22 shows the diseases of bone. Osteomalacia and osteoporosis are two

Table 8.22 Diseases of bone.

Osteomalacia and rickets (see p. 734)
Osteoporosis (see p. 735)
Paget's disease
Hyperparathyroidism (see p. 737)
Other hypercalcaemias
Disorders of collagen, e.g. Marfan's syndrome
(see p. 947)
Renal bone disease (see p. 419)
Infections
Neoplastic disease
Disorders of mucopolysaccharides, e.g. Hurler's
syndrome (see p. 776)
Skeletal dysplasias (achondroplasia)
Other hereditary diseases
Osteogenesis imperfecta
Osteopetrosis
Hypophosphatasia

important diseases which are described in Chapter 16.

Paget's disease

PATHOPHYSIOLOGY

There is greatly increased bone turnover with excessive osteoclastic resorption. These are partially compensated for by disorganized new bone formation. The cause of these changes is unknown, but a slow virus is a possible cause.

INCIDENCE

The disease is common in the UK, affecting 2–4% of the population in middle age and over 10% in the elderly. It is rare in Africa, the Middle and Far East and in Scandinavia. It is more common in men than in women.

CLINICAL FEATURES

The majority of patients with Paget's disease have no symptoms and the diagnosis, if made at all, is established coincidentally by x-ray or estimation of the serum alkaline phosphatase level.

When present, the major symptom is localized bone pain, which is often severe, continuous and unrelated to any exacerbating factors. While any part of the skeleton may be involved, common sites are the pelvis and lumbar spine, the skull and the long bones. Other effects, symptoms and signs are shown in Fig. 8.21a.

Bone deformity, especially in the weight-bearing long bones (Fig. 8.21b), and local warmth due to the increased blood flow through affected bones are often seen. Malignant transformation to osteogenic sarcoma occurs rarely.

INVESTIGATION

- X-ray appearances consist of a mixture of osteolytic and osteosclerotic areas (Fig. 8.21c), almost always with disruption of the normal trabecular pattern of bone. There is coarse trabeculation and expansion of the bone size. Small cortical fractures are found, and bowing may be seen in the tibia and femur.
- Isotope bone scanning identifies affected bones, though does not differentiate Paget's disease from other disorders (e.g. metastatic disease).
- Alkaline phosphatase of bone origin is increased (often to very high levels >1000 iu·l^{-1}) due to the excessive bone turnover. This increase may be minimal if bone involvement is very localized. Urinary hydroxyproline excretion, another marker of bone turnover, is also increased.

Calcium and phosphate levels are normal, except occasionally during immobilization; the parathormone level and vitamin D metabolism are also normal (Table 8.23).

TREATMENT

The incidental finding of asymptomatic Paget's disease does not require treatment. When pain is present, several lines of therapy are possible. Simple analgesics may be quite sufficient. If not, more specific therapy is available for pain and neurological complications.

The diphosphonate disodium etidronate (5–10 mg·kg^{-1} daily) is thought to be adsorbed onto hydroxyapatite crystals, preventing osteoclastic activity. Higher doses must only be used for very short periods (3 months or less), as excessive doses frequently lead to osteomalacia. Its long-term value is in doubt, but new intravenous diphosphonates may be more effective and safer.

Calcitonin (100 units s.c., two or three times weekly) inhibits bone resorption and turnover. It is extremely expensive, and clinical resistance because of antibody formation to the salmon and porcine preparations may limit its use. Side-effects following injection are flushing and mild nausea, sometimes accompanied by diarrhoea and vomiting, and can be disabling.

Infections of bone

Osteomyelitis

Staphylococcus is the organism responsible for 90% of cases of acute osteomyelitis (see p. 20). Other organisms include *Haemophilus influenzae* and *Salmonella*; infection with the latter may occur as a complication of sickle cell anaemia.

Osteomyelitis can be due either to metastatic haematogenous spread, e.g. from a boil, or to local infection. Malnutrition, debilitating disease and

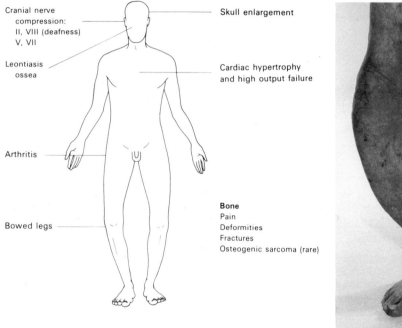

Cranial nerve
compression:
II, VIII (deafness)
V, VII

Leontiasis
ossea

Arthritis

Bowed legs

Skull enlargement

Cardiac hypertrophy
and high output failure

Bone
Pain
Deformities
Fractures
Osteogenic sarcoma (rare)

(a)

(b)

(c)

Fig. 8.21 Paget's disease. (a)
Clinical features. (b) Paget's disease
of the tibia showing bowing due to
increased bone growth. (c) X-ray
appearance of Paget's disease of
the pelvis.

Table 8.23 Serum biochemical findings in some bone diseases.

	Calcium	Phosphate	Alkaline phosphatase
Osteoporosis	N	N	N
Osteomalacia (and rickets)	N or ↓	N or ↓	↑
Paget's disease	N	N	↑ ↑
Hyperparathyroidism (and bone disease)	↑	↓	↑
Multiple myeloma	N or ↑	↓, N or ↑	N

N = normal; ↓ = low; ↑ = high.

decreased immunity may play a part in the pathogenesis.

Chronic osteomyelitis may follow an acute infection. Another variety of chronic osteomyelitis is due to infection being localized to form a chronic absc⸱ss within the bone (Brodie's abscess). Patients may be asymptomatic for months or years or may have intermittent local pain.

Treatment of osteomyelitis is with immobilization, antibiotics and surgical drainage.

Tuberculous osteomyelitis. This is usually due to haematogenous spread from a primary focus in the lungs or gastrointestinal tract. The disease starts in intra-articular bone. The spine is commonly involved (Pott's disease), with damage to the bodies of two neighbouring vertebrae leading to vertebral collapse and later abscess formation ('cold abscess'). Pus can track along tissue planes and discharge at a point far from the affected vertebrae. Symptoms consist of local pain and later swelling if pus has collected. Systemic symptoms of malaise, fever and night sweats occur. Treatment is as for pulmonary tuberculosis (see p. 602) together with immobilization.

Neoplastic disease

Malignant tumours of bone are shown in Table 8.24. The most common tumours are *metastases* from the bronchus, breast and prostate. Metastases from kidney and thyroid are less common. Symptoms are usually related to the anatomical position of the tumour, with local bone pain over the area. Systemic symptoms including malaise, pyrexia, and aches and pains occur and are sometimes related to the hypercalcaemia (see p. 737). The diagnosis of metastases can often be made from the history and examination, particularly if the primary has already been diagnosed. Symptoms from bony metastases may, however, be the first presenting feature.

INVESTIGATION

- Skeletal isotope scans can pick up bony metastases as 'hot' areas before radiological changes occur.
- X-rays may show metastases as osteolytic (or osteosclerotic) areas with bony destruction.
- Serum alkaline phosphatase (from the bone) is usually raised.
- Hypercalcaemia is seen in 10–20% of patients with malignancies. It is chiefly associated with metastases, but can also result from ectopic parathormone secretion.
- Serum acid phosphatase is raised in prostatic metastases.

TREATMENT

Treatment is usually symptomatic with analgesics. Local radiotherapy over bony metastases may help relieve the pain. Depending on the tumour, cytotoxic chemotherapy is occasionally helpful. Some tumours are hormone-dependent and a remission can be obtained by hypophysectomy or hormonal therapy. Occasionally pathological fractures require internal fixation.

Primary bone tumours are rare and usually seen in children and young adults.

Skeletal dysplasia

This is a heterogeneous group of disorders which affect the normal development of bone and cartilage and sometimes lead to shortness of stature.

Table 8.24 Malignant neoplasms of bone.

Metastases (osteolytic):
    Bronchus
    Breast
    Prostate (often osteosclerotic as well)
    Thyroid
    Kidney

Multiple myeloma

Primary bone tumours (rare; seen in the young), e.g.
    Osteosarcomas
    Fibrosarcomas
    Chondromas
    Ewing's tumour

Achondroplasia

Achondroplasia (dwarfism) is diagnosed in the first years of life. The disease is inherited in an autosomal dominant manner. The trunk is of normal length but the limbs are very short and broad. The vault of the skull is enlarged, the face is small and the nose bridge is flat. Intelligence is normal.

Other hereditary diseases

Osteogenesis imperfecta (fragilitas ossium, brittle bone syndrome)

This rare group of inherited disorders is due to an abnormality of connective tissue. The major feature is very fragile and brittle bones; other collagen-containing tissues are also involved, such as tendons, the skin and the eyes. Osteogenesis imperfecta tarda is a mild, dominantly inherited condition with milder bony derformities, blue sclerae, defective dentine, early-onset deafness, hypermobility of joints, and heart valve disorders. Severer forms present with multiple fractures and gross deformities. Prognosis is variable depending on the severity of the disease.

Osteopetrosis (marble bone disease)

This condition may be inherited in either an autosomal dominant or an autosomal recessive manner; the recessive type is severe and the dominant type is mild. In the severe form, bone density is increased throughout the skeleton but bones tend to fracture easily. Involvement of the bone marrow leads to a leucoerythroblastic anaemia. There is mental retardation and early death.

In the mild form there may only be x-ray changes, but fractures and infection can occur. The acid phosphatase level is raised.

Hypophosphatasia

This rare autosomal recessive condition is due to a deficiency of alkaline phosphatase and pyrophosphatase. It is not known where the primary defect lies, but it may be in the osteoblasts. It varies in severity from unmineralized bones in utero resulting in death, to rickets in infancy or recurrent fractures in adults.

Further reading

Currey HLF (1985) *Mason and Currey's Clinical Rheumatology*, 4th edn. London: Pitman Medical.

Huskisson EC & Hart FD (1987) *Joint Disease: All the Arthropathies*, 4th edn. Bristol: John Wright.

Kelly WN, Harris ED Jr, Ruddy S & Sledge CD (1985) *Textbook of Rheumatology*, 2nd edn. Philadelphia: WB Saunders.

Scott JT (ed.) (1986) *Copeman's Textbook of the Rheumatic Diseases*, 6th edn. Edinburgh: Churchill Livingstone.

Renal Disease

Renal function and structure

Despite the complexities of human metabolism and variations in diet and fluid intake, the milieu interieur of the body is remarkably constant. This principally results from the excretory and regulatory function of the kidneys. While not solely concerned with this (Table 9.1), the kidneys' paramount role is the elimination of waste material and the regulation of the volume and composition of body fluid. To effect this the kidneys have a unique system involving the free ultrafiltration of water and non-protein-bound low molecular weight compounds from the plasma and the selective reabsorption and/or excretion of these as the ultrafiltrate passes along the tubule.

The functioning unit is the nephron, of which there are approximately one million in each kidney.

Table 9.1 Functions of the kidney.

Excretory—excretion of waste products, drugs

Regulatory—control of body fluid volume and composition

Endocrine—production of erythropoietin, renin, prostaglandins

Metabolic—metabolism of vitamin D, small molecular weight proteins

A conventional diagrammatic representation is shown in Fig. 9.1a, and a physiological version in Fig. 9.1b.

An essential feature of renal function is that a large volume of blood—25% of cardiac output or approximately 1300 ml of blood per minute—passes through the two million glomeruli.

A hydrostatic pressure gradient of approximately 10 mmHg (a capillary pressure of 45 mmHg minus 10 mmHg of pressure within Bowman's space and 25 mmHg of plasma oncotic pressure) provides the driving force for ultrafiltration of virtually protein- and fat-free fluid across the glomerular capillary wall into Bowman's space and so into the renal tubule (Fig. 9.2).

The ultrafiltration rate (glomerular filtration rate; GFR) varies with age and sex but is approximately 120–130 ml per minute per 1.73 m^2 surface area in adults. This means that each day ultrafiltration of between 170 and 180 l of water and unbound small molecular weight constituents of blood occurs. The 'need' for this high filtration rate relates to the elimination of compounds present in relatively low concentration in plasma (e.g. urea).

The urinary excretion of such large volumes of water and electrolytes, with a consequential need to ingest huge amounts to stay in balance, is avoided by selective reabsorption of water, essential electrolytes and other blood constituents, such as glucose and amino acids, from the filtrate in transit along the nephron. Thus 60–80% of filtered water and sodium are reabsorbed in the proximal tubule along with virtually all the potassium, bicarbonate, glucose and amino acids (Fig. 9.1b). Further water and sodium chloride are reabsorbed more distally, and fine tuning of salt and water balance is achieved in the distal and collecting tubules under the influence of aldosterone and ADH. The final urine volume is thus 1–2 $l \cdot day^{-1}$. Calcium, phosphate, and magnesium are also selectively reabsorbed in proportion to need to maintain a normal electrolyte composition of body fluids. The urinary excretion of some compounds is more complicated. For example, potassium is freely filtered at the glomerulus, almost completely absorbed in the proximal tubule, and excreted in the distal tubule and collecting ducts. An important clinical consequence of this is that the ability to eliminate unwanted potassium is less dependent on GFR than is the elimination of urea or creatinine. Other compounds filtered and reabsorbed or

Fig. 9.1 (a) The principal parts of the nephron. (b) Sites of removal or addition of electrolytes from or into tubular fluid.

Fig. 9.2 Pressures controlling glomerular filtration. 1 = capillary hydrostatic pressure (45 mmHg). 2 = hydrostatic pressure in Bowman's space (10 mmHg). 3 = plasma protein oncotic pressure (25 mmHg). Arrows indicate direction of pressure gradient.

excreted to a variable extent include urate and many organic acids, including many drugs or their metabolic breakdown products. The more tubular secretion of a compound occurs, the less dependent elimination is on the GFR; penicillin and cephradine are examples of compounds secreted by the tubules.

Tubular function is also critical to the control of acid–base balance, bicarbonate being almost com-

pletely reabsorbed in the proximal tubule while hydrogen ions are eliminated more distally as ammonia (NH_3) or titratable acid (see p. 444).

Glomerular filtration rate (GFR)

In health the GFR remains remarkably constant due to intrarenal regulatory mechanisms. In disease, with a reduction in intrarenal blood flow, damage to or loss of glomeruli, or obstruction to the free flow of ultrafiltrate along the tubule, the GFR will fall and the ability to eliminate waste material and to regulate the volume and composition of body fluid will decline. This will be manifest as a rise in the blood level of urea or the plasma level of creatinine and in a reduction in *measured* GFR.

Uraemia

The concentration of urea or creatinine in blood or plasma respectively represents the dynamic equilibrium between production and elimination. In healthy subjects there is an enormous reserve of renal excretory function and blood urea and serum creatinine do not rise above the normal range until there is a reduction of 50–60% in the GFR. Thereafter, the level of urea depends both on the GFR and the production rate (Table 9.2). The latter is heavily influenced by protein intake and tissue catabolism. The level of creatinine is much less dependent on diet but is more related to age, sex and muscle mass. Once elevated, measurement of serum creatinine is a better guide to GFR than urea and, in general,

Table 9.2 Factors influencing blood urea levels.

PRODUCTION

Increased by:
High protein diet
Increased catabolism
   Surgery
   Infection
   Trauma
Steroid therapy
Tetracyclines

Decreased by:
Low protein diet
Reduced catabolism, e.g. old age

ELIMINATION

Increased by:
Elevated GFR, e.g. pregnancy

Decreased by:
Glomerular disease
Reduced renal blood flow
   Hypotension
   Dehydration
Urinary obstruction
Tubulo-interstitial nephritis

Fig. 9.3 Creatinine clearance versus serum creatinine. Note the serum creatinine does not rise above the normal range until there is a reduction of 50–60% in the glomerular filtration rate (creatinine clearance).

measurement of serum creatinine is a good way to monitor further deterioration in the GFR.

It must be re-emphasized that a normal blood urea or serum creatinine is *not* synonymous with a normal GFR.

Measurement of GFR
Measurement of the GFR is necessary to define the exact level of renal function. It is essential when the blood urea or serum creatinine are within the normal range.

Inulin clearance—the gold standard of physiologists—is not practical or necessary in clinical practice. The most widely used measurement is creatinine clearance, which closely approximates to inulin clearance (Fig. 9.3).

Measurement of creatinine clearance

- Urine is collected over 24 h for measurement of urinary creatinine; a 24-h collection diminishes collection errors.
- A plasma level of creatinine is measured sometime during the 24-h period.
- Given the rate of urine flow (V), the urine (U) and plasma (P) concentrations of creatinine, clearance is obtained from the formula:

$$\frac{U \times V}{P} \times 100$$

Where urine collections are difficult, e.g. with ileal conduits, or deemed inaccurate, the GFR may be measured by the single injection of compounds such as [^{51}Cr]-EDTA (ethylene diamine tetra-acetic acid) or [^{99}Tc^{m}]-DTPA (diethylene triamine penta-acetic acid), their excretion being primarily by glomerular filtration. Following intravenous injection of the compound, three blood samples are obtained at 2, 3 and 4 h (or rather longer intervals if the patient is oedematous or if renal failure is suspected). The GFR may then be calculated from the slope of the exponential fall in blood level of the compound.

TUBULAR FUNCTION

The major function of the tubule is the selective reabsorption or excretion of water and various cations and anions to keep the volume and electrolyte composition of body fluid normal.

The active reabsorption from the glomerular filtrate of compounds such as glucose and amino acids also takes place. Within the normal range of blood concentrations these substances are completely reabsorbed by the proximal tubule. However, if blood levels are elevated above the normal range, the amount filtered (filtered load = GFR × plasma concentration) may exceed the maximal absorptive capacity of the tubule and the compound 'spills over' into the urine. Examples of this occur with hyperglycaemia in diabetes mellitus or elevated plasma phenylalanine in phenylketonuria. Conversely, inherited or acquired defects in tubular function may lead to incomplete absorption of a *normal* filtered load, with loss of the compound in the urine (a lowered 'renal threshold'). This is seen in renal glycosuria, in which there is a genetically determined defect in tubular reabsorption of glucose. It is diagnosed by demonstrating glycosuria in the presence of normal blood sugar levels. Inherited or acquired defects in the tubular reabsorption of amino acids, phosphate, sodium, potassium and calcium also occur, either singly or in combination. Examples include cystinuria and the Fanconi syndrome (see p. 774). Tubular defects in the reabsorption of water (nephrogenic diabetes insipidus) or bicarbonate (proximal renal tubular acidosis; proximal RTA) and defective acidification of the urine (distal RTA) are dealt with on pp. 444 and 445.

ENDOCRINE FUNCTION

Renin–angiotensin system
The juxtaglomerular apparatus is made up of specialized arteriolar smooth muscle cells which are sited on the afferent glomerular arteriole as it enters the glomerulus (Fig. 9.1b). These cells secrete renin, which converts angiotensinogen in blood to angiotensin I. Renin release is controlled by:
- Pressure changes in the afferent arteriole
- Sympathetic tone
- Chloride and osmotic concentration in the distal tubule via the macula densa (Fig. 9.1b)
- Possibly local prostaglandin release

Angiotensin II, generated from angiotensin I, is both a vasoconstrictor and the most important stimulus for the release of aldosterone by the adrenal cortex. It may also modify intrarenal blood flow.

Erythropoietin
Erythropoietin is a glycoprotein produced principally by the kidney and is the major stimulus for erythropoiesis. Loss of renal substance with decreased erythropoietin production results in a normochromic, normocytic anaemia. Conversely, erythropoietin secretion may be increased, with resultant polycythaemia, in patients with polycystic renal disease, benign renal cysts or renal cell carcinoma.

Prostaglandins
Prostaglandin E_2 is the primary prostaglandin produced by the kidney and is known to be a powerful vasodilator agent. Its precise role in regulating intrarenal blood flow and its interaction with renin release remains unclear. It may also have some direct or indirect role in the renal handling of sodium and water.

Kallikrein–kinin system
The role of this system is not fully understood, but it probably also plays a part in the control of the distribution of renal blood flow and in salt and water excretion.

Natriuretic hormone
For many years there has been controversy as to the existence of a circulating natriuretic hormone. There is now considerable evidence that atrial tissue contains a group of peptides, at least one of which is a regulator of sodium balance—atrial natriuretic peptide (ANP). Intravenous infusion of ANP is followed by a marked natriuresis with a rise in GFR and a fall in blood pressure. The peptides appear to have four anti-renin/angiotensin system actions—reduced renin secretion, reduced aldosterone secretion, and opposition to the action of angiotensin II and to the sodium-retaining action of aldosterone on the renal tubule. Their role in the long-term regulation of sodium balance and blood pressure in man remains to be clarified.

METABOLIC FUNCTION

Vitamin D metabolism
Naturally occurring vitamin D_3 requires hydroxylation in the liver and again by the kidney to produce the metabolically active 1,25- or 24,25-dihydroxycholecalciferol. Loss of this metabolic activity in diseased kidneys results in renal osteodystrophy (see p. 419).

Protein and polypeptide metabolism
It is now clear that the kidney is a major site for the catabolism of many small molecular weight proteins and polypeptides, including many hormones such as insulin, parathormone and calcitonin. In renal failure the metabolic clearance of these substances is reduced and their half-life prolonged.

Tests for renal disease or malfunction

Renal disease is suspected if there are:
- Symptoms referable to the urinary tract
- Hypertension
- An elevated blood urea
- Abnormalities on urinalysis

THE URINE

Appearance

This is of little value in the differential diagnosis of renal disease except in the diagnosis of haematuria. Overt 'bloody' urine is usually unmistakable but should be checked using dip sticks (Stix testing). Very concentrated urine or urine containing pigments ingested in food or medicines may also appear dark or smoky urine. Urine which becomes dark on standing suggests the relatively rare condition of porphyria.

Smell

This is rarely important except in patients with infection, when a typical fishy odour may be noted.

Volume

In health, the volume of urine passed is primarily determined by diet and fluid intake. In temperate climates it lies within the range of 800–2500 ml per 24 h. The minimum amount passed to stay in fluid balance is determined by the amount of solute—mainly urea and electrolytes—being excreted and the maximum concentrating power of the kidneys. Thus on a normal diet some 800 mosmol of solute are passed daily. Since the maximum urine concentration is approximately 1200 mosmol·l^{-1}, the minimum volume of urine obligated by excretion of 800 mosmol of solute would thus be approximately 650 ml (Table 9.3). Fluid intake is generally greater than this, so that larger volumes of more dilute urine are passed. A diet rich in carbohydrate and fat and low in protein and salt results in a lower solute excretion and as little as 300 ml of urine per day may be required. Conversely, a high-salt, high-protein intake obligates a larger urine flow and, via the thirst mechanism, a higher fluid intake. The appropriateness of a given daily urine output must therefore be related to factors such as diet, body size and fluid intake.

In disease, impairment of concentrating ability requires increased volumes of urine to be passed, given the same daily solute output (Table 9.3). An increased solute output, e.g. in glycosuria or increased protein catabolism following surgery or associated with sepsis, also demands increased urine volumes.

The maximum urine output depends on the ability to produce a dilute urine. Intakes of 10 or even 20 l daily can be tolerated by normal man, but, given a daily solute output of 800 mosmol, require the ability to dilute to 80 and 40 mosmol·l^{-1} respectively. Where diluting ability is impaired, the ability to excrete large volumes of ingested water is also impaired.

Oliguria

Oliguria, usually defined as the excretion of less than 300 ml of urine per day, may be 'physiological', e.g. in patients with hypotension and hypovolaemia, where urine is maximally concentrated in an attempt to conserve water. More often, it is due to intrinsic renal disease or obstructive nephropathy (see p. 411).

Anuria (no urine) suggests urinary tract obstruction until proved otherwise; bladder outflow obstruction must always be considered first.

Polyuria

Polyuria is a persistent large increase in urine output, usually associated with nocturia. It must be distinguished from frequency of micturition with the passage of small volumes of urine. Documentation of fluid intake and output may be necessary. Polyuria is the result of an excessive (hysterical) intake of water, an increased excretion of solute, as in hyperglycaemia and glycosuria, or a defective renal concentrating ability.

Specific gravity and osmolality

The time-honoured measurement of specific gravity is of little value in clinical practice. Measurement of urine concentration is best done by osmometry and is only required under limited circumstances such as the differential diagnosis of oliguric renal failure or the investigation of polyuria or inappropriate ADH secretion.

pH

Measurement of urinary pH is rarely necessary except in the investigation and treatment of renal tubular acidosis (see p. 445).

Chemical (Stix) testing

Routine Stix testing of urine for blood, protein and sugar is obligatory in all patients suspected of having renal disease.

Table 9.3 Relationship between diet, kidney function and urine volume.

| | | Minimum urine volume required to excrete solute load (ml·24 hr^{-1}) | |
Diet	Approximate solute output (mosmol·$24h^{-1}$)	With normal urine concentration (maximum 1200 mosmol·kg^{-1})	In disease (impaired urine concentration—maximum 300 mosmol·kg^{-1})
Normal	800	667	2667
High protein/salt	1200	1000	4000
Low protein/salt	360	300	1200

Blood

Haematuria may be overt, with bloody urine, or microscopic and found only on chemical testing. A positive Stix test must always be followed by urine microscopy to confirm the presence of red cells and so exclude the relatively rare condition of haemoglobinuria (or the even more rare myoglobinuria). Bleeding may come from any site within the urinary tract (Fig. 9.4):

- Overt bleeding from the urethra is suggested when blood is seen at the start of voiding and then the urine becomes clear.
- Blood diffusely present throughout the urine comes from the bladder or above.
- Blood only at the end of micturition suggests bleeding from the prostate or bladder base.

Careful urine microscopy is mandatory as the presence of red cell casts is diagnostic of bleeding from the kidney, most often due to glomerulonephritis. In the absence of red cell casts, further investigations such as urine cytology, intravenous urography and cystoscopy are required to define the site of bleeding. Rarely, renal biopsy may be required (see p. 379).

Protein

Proteinuria is one of the most common signs of renal disease. Detection is now primarily by Stix testing. Most reagent strips can detect a concentration of $20 \text{ mg} \cdot \text{dl}^{-1}$ or more in urine. They react primarily with albumin and are relatively insensitive to globulin and Bence Jones proteins.

If proteinuria is confirmed on repeated Stix testing it should be quantitated by measurement of daily protein excretion in 24-h urine collections. Healthy adults excrete approximately 60–100 mg of protein per day, but up to 150–200 mg per day is within the acceptable range. Slightly higher values—up to 300 mg daily—may be excreted by adolescents. Proteinuria, while occasionally benign, always requires further investigation.

Glucose

Renal glycosuria is uncommon, so that a positive test for glucose always requires exclusion of diabetes mellitus.

Microscopy

This is an enormously valuable diagnostic tool which is commonly underused. Urine microscopy should be carried out in all patients suspected of having renal disease. Care must be taken to obtain a 'clean' sample of midstream urine. The presence of numerous skin squames suggests a contaminated, poorly collected sample which cannot be properly interpreted.

If a clean sample of urine cannot be obtained, suprapubic aspiration may be required in suspected urinary tract infections (see p. 393).

Collection of mid-stream specimens of urine (MSSU)

Female
- The patient's bladder should be full ('desperate to go').
- The patient removes underpants and *stands* over the toilet pan.
- The labia are separated using the left hand.
- The vulva is cleansed front to back with sterile swabs (optional).
- The patient voids downward into the toilet and continues until 'half-done'.
- *Without stopping the urine flow*, the sterile container is plunged into the stream of urine with the right hand. Only a small volume is required.
- The patient then completes voiding into the toilet.

Male
- The patient's bladder should be full.
- The foreskin, if present, is retracted.
- The glans penis is cleansed with a sterile swab (optional).
- The patient voids into the toilet until 'half-done'.
- *Without stopping the urine flow*, the sterile container is plunged into the stream of urine.
- The patient then completes voiding into the toilet.

White cells

The presence of 10 or more white blood cells (WBC) per millilitre in fresh unspun midstream urine samples is abnormal and indicates an inflammatory reaction within the urinary tract. Most commonly it is due to urinary tract infection (UTI), but it may also be found in sterile urine in patients during antibiotic

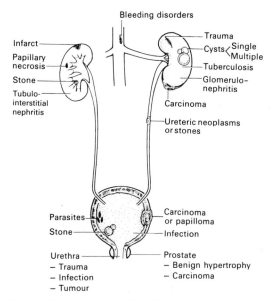

Fig. 9.4 Sites and causes of bleeding from the urinary tract.

treatment of urinary infection or within 14 days of treatment. Sterile pyuria also occurs in patients with stones, interstitial nephritis, papillary necrosis, tuberculosis, and interstitial cystitis (Hunner's ulcer), whether spontaneous or drug induced.

Red cells

The presence of one or more red cells in unspun urine samples results in a positive Stix test for blood and is abnormal. It is claimed that red cells of glomerular origin can be identified by their dysmorphic appearance, especially on phase-contrast microscopy, but this is not yet generally available or accepted.

Casts

These cylindrical bodies, which are moulded ('cast') in the shape of the distal tubular lumen, may be hyaline, granular or cellular. Hyaline casts and fine granular casts represent precipitated protein and may be seen in normal urine, particularly after exercise. More coarsely granular casts occur with pathological proteinuria in glomerular and tubular disease. Red cell casts—even one—always indicate renal disease. If red cells degenerate, a rusty coloured 'haemoglobin' granular cast is seen. White cell casts may be seen in acute pyelonephritis. They may be confused with the tubular cell casts which occur in patients with acute tubular necrosis.

Bacteria

The demonstration of bacteria on gram-staining of the centrifuge deposit of a clean-catch midstream urine sample is highly suggestive of urinary infection and can be of value in the *immediate* differential diagnosis of UTI. If accompanied by pyuria it may be accepted as evidence of UTI in the ill and febrile patient and treatment should be initiated. It must always be followed by quantitative urine culture (see p. 393) in order to confirm the diagnosis and to allow definition of bacterial antibiotic sensitivities.

Stix testing is of no value in the diagnosis of UTI as both blood and protein are absent in the urine of many patients with bacteriuria.

QUANTITATIVE TESTS OF RENAL FUNCTION

The use of blood urea, serum creatinine and GFR as measures of renal function is discussed on p. 372. Quantitation of proteinuria, including the investigation of selective proteinuria, is discussed on p. 389. Other quantitative tests of disturbed renal function such as measurements of urine output of calcium, sodium or potassium or urine acidification are described under the relevant disorders.

IMAGING TECHNIQUES

Plain x-ray

A plain radiograph of the abdomen is always taken prior to urography. Its main value is to identify renal calcification or radio-dense calculi in the kidney pelvis, line of the ureters or bladder (Fig. 9.5). Care must be taken in viewing the x-ray in order not to miss calculi obscured by bowel shadows or bone. Renal size and outline are best assessed during excretion urography or by ultrasound.

Excretion urography

This is also known as intravenous urography (IVU) or intravenous pyelography (IVP). If carefully executed and properly interpreted, the urogram is one of the most valuable diagnostic tools for the

Fig. 9.5 Calcification in the renal tract. Calculi can occur at any site.

investigation of renal disease. Carefully timed serial x-rays are taken of the kidneys and the full length of abdomen following the intravenous injection of an organic iodine-containing contrast medium. Films taken at the end of the injection show opacification of the parenchyma, allowing definition of size and renal outline. The kidneys are normally smooth in outline. In adults they measure 11–14 cm in length, differing by less than 2 cm. An irregular outline, whether due to local bumps or to cortical scarring, is abnormal. Reduction in size indicates chronic parenchymal disease.

The application of a compression band to the abdomen, designed to partially obstruct ureteral emptying, helps distension of the upper tracts. Special attention is paid to the size, shape and disposition of the calyces and pelvis for evidence of anatomical abnormality such as calyceal clubbing, abnormal dilatation, cavitation or filling defects. The significance of these are described under the particular diseases.

After 10–20 min, the compression bands are removed and full-length films are obtained before and after voiding to study emptying of the upper tract, ureters and bladder.

Retrograde urography

Following cystoscopy, preferably under screening control, a catheter is either impacted in the ureteral orifice or passed shortly up the ureter, and contrast medium is injected; this is followed by x-ray filming.

This technique is now primarily used to investigate lesions of the ureter and to define the site of obstruction shown on excretion urography or ultrasound.

Antegrade urography

Antegrade urography involves percutaneous puncture of a renal calyx, with the insertion of a fine catheter and the injection of contrast medium in an antegrade fashion. It is now the procedure of choice in patients with upper urinary tract obstruction demonstrated by ultrasound. It not only allows definition of the site of obstruction but also the catheter may be left in situ to allow urine drainage in oliguric patients.

Micturating cystourography (MCU)

This involves catheterization and the installation of contrast medium into the bladder. The patient is then screened and filmed during voiding to demonstrate or exclude vesico-ureteric reflux and to study bladder emptying. It is primarily used in children with recurrent infection (see p. 394) and in adults with disturbed bladder function, when it may be combined with urodynamic studies of bladder pressure and urethral flow.

Aortography or renal arteriography

These may be required to investigate extra- or intrarenal arterial disease and to investigate the presence and extent of renal tumours.

Renal venography

Renal venography may be required to diagnose renal vein thrombosis and, possibly as part of arteriography, to define extension of a tumour into the renal veins and vena cava.

Ultrasonography

Ultrasonography of the kidneys is playing an increasing role in the diagnosis of renal disease. It is of great value in the investigation of renal mass lesions and in screening for polycystic disease. Combined with plain x-rays it is supplanting the use of high-dose urography in the assessment of patients with unexplained renal failure (see p. 415). To be reliable it needs to be performed by an experienced and careful operator.

Computed tomography (CT)

Computed tomography has a valuable role in the diagnosis of renal tumours when this is not possible by ultrasound or excretion urography, and in the diagnosis of retroperitoneal masses. It is also valuable in defining the presence and spread of bladder or prostatic tumours.

RADIONUCLIDE INVESTIGATIONS

Gamma-emitting radioisotopes may be used to measure many aspects of renal function, e.g. GFR, renal blood flow, relative renal function, and transit times of filtrate across the parenchyma. Though these techniques are intellectually attractive as a possible means of accurately quantitating these various parameters of function, only a few have proved really valuable in routine clinical practice.

The radionuclides in common use are iodine-131 and -123, chromium-51 and technetium-99m. The radiopharmaceuticals to which the isotopes are attached may be excreted primarily by glomerular filtration ($[^{51}Cr]$-EDTA or $[^{99}Tc^m]$-DTPA) or by both filtration and tubular excretion (iodine-labelled hippuran or $[^{99}Tc^m]$-gluconate). $[^{99}Tc^m]$-dimercaptosuccinic acid (DMSA) fixes to proximal tubular cells but very little is excreted into the urine. This is of value in 'visualizing' the renal parenchyma.

Glomerular filtration rate (GFR)

Measurement of GFR is discussed on p. 373.

Relative kidney function

In patients with unilateral renal disease, whether due to obstruction or other causes, measurement of the contribution of each kidney to the total function may be of great value in planning treatment. This may be done using scintillation detector probes placed over each kidney or with a gamma camera. The uptake of intravenously administered isotope can be recorded and the relative uptake by each kidney calculated.

Renal blood flow

Renography has been used extensively to study renal blood flow. Its main role in clinical practice is in the investigation of patients in whom renal artery stenosis is suspected as a cause of hypertension, and in patients with severe oliguria (post-traumatic, post-aortic surgery, or after a kidney transplant) to establish whether and to what extent there is renal perfusion. Following the intravenous injection of $[^{131}I]$-hippuran, patients with unilateral renal artery stenosis have a delay in achieving a peak uptake in the affected kidney and the kidney contributes less than 42% to the total function. In patients with total renal artery occlusion, no kidney uptake of isotope is observed.

During studies patients must be well hydrated and must not have had diuretic treatment for 7 days prior to the examination.

Investigation of obstruction

Renography has been extensively used to study obstruction to the kidneys. The results obtained from overall uptake and outflow curves must, however, be treated with caution because of the large 'dead space' commonly contributed by dilated calyces and pelves. In recent years more sophisticated gamma-camera studies involving the use of $[^{99}Tc^m]$-DTPA, the selection of regions of interest over the renal parenchyma (whole kidney minus pelvis) and deconvolution analysis of results has allowed calculation of transit times of radionuclides through the kidney tissue—a more accurate measure of functional obstruction. Taken in conjunction with excretion urography, this is a most valuable investigation for planning and following up the surgical management of patients with upper tract obstruction.

Kidney visualization

Static imaging of the kidneys by the gamma camera following the intravenous injection of $[^{99}Tc^m]$-DMSA can be of great value in the differential diagnosis of a space-occupying lesion when its nature cannot be defined by excretion urography or ultrasonography.

TRANSCUTANEOUS RENAL BIOPSY

Transcutaneous renal biopsy has revolutionized our understanding of glomerular and tubulo-interstitial disorders (see p. 381), allowing definition of the nature of the parenchymal disease. Indications and contraindications for renal biopsy are shown in Table 9.4. Biopsy is best carried out under ultrasonographic control. Tissue must be examined by conventional histochemical staining, by electron microscopy and by immunofluorescence.

The complications of transcutaneous renal biopsy are shown in Table 9.5.

Table 9.4 Renal biopsy.

Indications
Nephrotic syndrome (with some exceptions)

Unexplained renal failure with normal-sized kidneys

Failure to recover from assumed reversible acute renal failure

Diagnosis of systemic disease with renal involvement such as sarcoidosis, amyloidosis (occasional indication only)

Asymptomatic proteinuria or haematuria (very occasional indication—justified only if knowledge of prognosis is essential)

Contraindications
Uncooperative patient

Single kidney (with the exception of transplant kidney, when biopsy is acceptable)

Small kidneys (technically difficult, histology hard to interpret, prognosis cannot be altered)

Haemorrhagic disorders (unless correctable temporarily or permanently, e.g. by Factor VIII administration in haemophilia)

Gross obesity or oedema (technical difficulties)

Uncontrolled hypertension

Table 9.5 Complications of transcutaneous renal biopsy.

Macroscopic haematuria—about 20%

Pain in the flank, sometimes referred to shoulder tip

Arteriovenous aneurysm formation—about 20%, almost always of no clinical significance

Profuse haematuria demanding blood transfusion—1–3%

Profuse haematuria demanding occlusion of bleeding vessel at angiography or nephrectomy—approximately 1 in 400

Introduction of infection

The mortality rate is about 0.1%

Transcutaneous renal biopsy

Before biopsy
- A coagulation screen is performed.
- The serum is grouped and saved for cross-matching.
- The patient is given a full explanation of what is involved.

During biopsy
- The patient lies prone with a hard pillow under his abdomen.
- The kidney is localized by ultrasound.
- Local anaesthetic is injected along the biopsy track.
- The patient holds his breath when the biopsy is performed.

After biopsy
- A pressure dressing is applied to the biopsy site and the patient rests in bed for 24 h.
- The fluid intake is maximized to prevent clot colic.
- The pulse and blood pressure are checked regularly.
- The patient is advised to avoid heavy lifting or gardening for 2 weeks.

Glomerulonephritis

Glomerulonephritis is a general term for a group of disorders in which:
- There is immunologically mediated injury to glomeruli
- The kidneys are involved symmetrically
- Secondary mechanisms of glomerular injury come into play following an initial immune insult (see below)
- The renal lesion may be part of a generalized disease, e.g. systemic lupus erythematosus

PATHOGENESIS

Two chief pathogenetic mechanisms are recognized:
- Deposition or in-situ formation of immune complexes
- Deposition of anti-glomerular basement membrane antibody

Both these pathogenetic mechanisms activate secondary mechanisms which produce glomerular damage.

Immune complex nephritis. Circulating antigen–antibody complexes (see p. 119) are deposited in the kidney or complexes are formed locally when circulating free antigen has become trapped in the glomerulus. The nature of the antigen involved in the complex formation is important in many instances.

The antigen may be:
- *Exogenous* (e.g. bacterial). For example, a nephritogenic Lancefield group A beta-haemolytic streptococcus can cause glomerulonephritis in previously healthy individuals.
- *Endogenous.* For example, patients with systemic lupus erythematosus may form antibodies to host DNA, leading to a glomerulonephritis.

Harmful immune complexes can also occur when there is impaired host ability to produce appropriate antibody. Certain strains of black mice regularly develop glomerulonephritis as a result of an impaired ability to produce antibody of appropriate quality or quantity, and it is possible that there may be human counterparts of this phenomenon.

Impaired ability on the part of the host to clear immune complexes from the circulation and deficiencies in the complement system are each associated with an increased incidence of glomerulonephritis.

Genetic factors may also be important and associations between certain immune complex nephritides and HLA markers are being recognized.

Anti-glomerular basement membrane (anti-GBM) antibody. Anti-GBM antibody reacts with an antigen in the glomerular basement membrane, producing glomerular damage. It is of the IgG type. The antibody can also react with alveolar capillary basement membrane (due to shared antigens) and can cause both lung haemorrhage and glomerulonephritis (Goodpasture's syndrome).

Secondary mechanisms of glomerular injury
Several events can be triggered by the above immunological insults. These are:
- Complement activation
- Fibrin deposition
- Platelet aggregation
- Inflammation with neutrophil-dependent mechanisms
- Activation of kinin systems

Immune complex or anti-GBM antibody deposition trigger these mechanisms to varying degrees, resulting in an increase in capillary permeability and glomerular damage.

In experimentally induced glomerulonephritis in animals, prior anticoagulation, prevention of complement activation, and depletion of polymorphonuclear leucocytes have all been shown to reduce the severity of the induced glomerular injury. However, in humans presenting with most forms of glomerulonephritis these measures do not help.

Cell-mediated mechanisms. T cell dysfunction may play a part in the production of lesions when immune complexes are not seen, e.g. focal glomerulo-sclerosis and minimal change disease. There is as yet no direct evidence for this mechanism in man.

CAUSES

In the majority of patients with immune complex mediated glomerulonephritis the cause is unknown, i.e. the nature of the antigen involved is not determined. Antigen derived from viruses, bacteria, parasites, drugs and from the host may be involved (Table 9.6). The reasons for the development of anti-GBM antibody are not known; viral damage to alveolar capillary basement membrane, rendering it antigenic, has been suggested as a possible cause.

PATHOLOGY

Macroscopic appearances
In acute glomerulonephritis, the kidneys are normal in size or enlarged and oedematous, and the surface of the kidney may show punctate haemorrhages.

In long-standing progressive chronic glomerulo-nephritis the kidneys may be normal in size or small with finely granular cortical scarring.

Microscopic appearances
Different immunological insults may induce similar or identical histological changes. For example, the immune complex mediated glomerulonephritis in mumps is not distinguishable from that following beta-haemolytic streptococcal infection. Conversely,

Table 9.6 Some causes of immune complex mediated glomerulonephritis.

Viruses:
  Mumps
  Measles
  Hepatitis B
  Epstein–Barr virus
  Coxsackievirus

Bacteria:
  Lancefield group A beta-haemolytic streptococci
  Streptococcus viridans (infective endocarditis)
  Staphylococci
  Treponema pallidum

Parasites:
  Plasmodium malariae
  Schistosoma

Host antigens:
  DNA (systemic lupus erythematosus)
  Cryoglobulin
  Malignant tumours

Drugs:
  Penicillamine

different histological responses may occur in the same disease process in different individuals, e.g. in systemic lupus erythematosus (see below).

The histological response to immune complex deposition probably depends on the size of the complexes, their rate of deposition and the efficiency of host clearance mechanisms.

Renal tissue, obtained at transcutaneous renal biopsy, is examined by:
- *Light microscopy* to assess the extent and histological type of disease. Immunoperoxidase methods may also be applied.
- *Electron microscopy* to define the type of disease and to correlate with immunofluorescence, e.g. to see the exact sites of deposits
- *Immunofluorescence* to assess the type of immunological injury

Immune complex deposition results in a diffuse granular pattern of staining, with IgG, IgM, IgA components of the complement system and, in addition, fibrin and fibrinogen all present (Fig. 9.6).

The presence of anti-GBM antibody produces a smooth linear pattern of staining for IgG (Fig. 9.7).

Fig. 9.6 Immunofluorescence showing immune complex deposition in a diffuse granular pattern.

Fig. 9.7 Immunofluorescence showing anti-glomerular basement membrane antibody deposition in a linear pattern typical of Goodpasture's syndrome.

All three methods of examination are necessary for proper histopathological assessment.

Histopathological types
There is not a complete correlation between the histopathological types and the clinical features of the disease; Table 9.7 shows the commonest associations.

Proliferative glomerulonephritis. Proliferative changes occur in many immune complex mediated nephritides and also in anti-GBM nephritis. It has the following subtypes:

- *Diffuse proliferative glomerulonephritis.* All the glomeruli are similarly affected; Fig. 9.8 shows the typical histological appearances. There is proliferation of endothelial and mesangial cells and several polymorphonuclear leucocytes are present. The glomerulus is swollen, packed with cells and bulges into the opening of the proximal tubule. A normal glomerulus is shown in Fig. 9.9 for comparison. Electron microscopy of the

lesions shows subepithelial humps present on the glomerular basement membrane (Fig. 9.10) and immunofluorescence shows granular deposits of immunoglobulin and C_3.

Fig. 9.9 A normal glomerulus.

Fig. 9.10 An electron micrograph showing immune complex mediated glomerulonephritis. EN = endothelial cell; FP = foot process; BM = basement membrane; EP = epithelial podocyte; D = electron-dense deposits (antigen–antibody complexes).

Fig. 9.8 A glomerulus showing proliferative glomerulonephritis.

Table 9.7 Correlation between the histological type of glomerulonephritis and the clinical picture.

Histological type	Most common clinical presentation
Proliferative glomerulonephritis:	
Diffuse	Acute nephritis
Focal segmental	Haematuria, proteinuria
With crescent formation (rapidly progressive glomerulonephritis)	Progressive renal failure
Mesangiocapillary (membranoproliferative)	Haematuria, proteinuria, nephritis or nephrotic syndrome
Membranous glomerulonephritis	Nephrotic syndrome in adults
Minimal change nephropathy	Nephrotic syndrome in children
Idiopathic focal glomerulonephritis with mesangial deposits of IgA	Asymptomatic haematuria
Focal glomerulosclerosis	Proteinuria or nephrotic syndrome

This type of glomerulonephritis, presenting as an acute nephritis, is commonly seen after a streptococcal infection (see below).

- *Focal segmental glomerulonephritis.* Only some of the glomeruli here show proliferative changes whilst others are normal, hence the term focal. The affected glomeruli show segmental involvement of the tufts, i.e. changes are present in one or more parts of the glomerulus.

  This condition may occur as a primary renal disease, but it is also seen in systemic lupus erythematosus, subacute infective endocarditis, with infected atrioventricular shunts (shunt nephritis), and in disorders with IgA deposits, e.g. Henoch–Schönlein purpura and IgA disease. A severe focal necrotizing form is seen in polyarteritis nodosa and Wegener's granulomatosis. Special subtypes (IgA disease and focal glomerulosclerosis) are discussed below.

- *Proliferative glomerulonephritis with crescent formation (rapidly progressive glomerulonephritis; RPGN)* (Fig. 9.11). The term 'crescent' is applied to an aggregate of macrophages and epithelial cells in Bowman's space. Crescents are associated with severe damage to the glomerular tuft and are seen in occasional glomeruli in several types of glomerulonephritis. However, if most glomeruli show crescents the glomerulonephritis is usually placed in this subtype, as clinical progression to renal failure is rapid.

  This condition is seen in both immune complex and anti-GBM antibody mediated nephritis. It particularly occurs in polyarteritis, Wegener's granulomatosis and Goodpasture's syndrome.

- *Mesangiocapillary (membranoproliferative) glomerulonephritis (MCGN).* In *type 1* there is mesangial cell proliferation, with mainly subendothelial immune complex deposition and apparent splitting of the capillary basement membrane, giving a 'tram-line' effect. It may be idiopathic or may occur with shunt nephritis. It can be associated with persistently reduced levels of C_3 and normal levels of C4.

In *type 2* there is mesangial cell proliferation with electron-dense, linear intramembranous deposits which usually stain for C_3 only. This type may be idiopathic or may occur after measles. Partial lipodystrophy (loss of subcutaneous fat in various parts of the body) may be seen.

MCGN affects young adults. Patients present with haematuria, proteinuria, the nephrotic syndrome or renal failure. Most patients eventually go on to develop renal failure over several years.

Membranous glomerulonephritis (Fig. 9.12). Thickening of the capillary basement membrane due to immune complex deposition is the main feature of this disease. In the majority of patients the antigenic component of the complex is unknown. Associations include systemic lupus erythematosus (where the antigen is host DNA), malignancy of the bowel and bronchus (tumour-derived antigen) and penicillamine therapy. *Plasmodium malariae* is a common cause in the tropics. Recently a strong association with HLA-DR3 has been found.

This condition occurs mainly in adults, predominantly in males. Patients present with proteinuria or frank nephrotic syndrome. Thirty per cent of patients undergo spontaneous remission, but the remainder eventually go on to develop chronic renal failure.

Minimal change glomerular lesion (minimal change nephropathy). This is not a true glomerulonephritis and is included here for convenience. In this condition the glomeruli appear normal on light microscopy. The only abnormality seen on electron microscopy is fusion of the foot processes of epithelial cells (podocytes). This is a non-specific finding and is seen in many conditions associated with proteinuria.

Neither immune complexes nor anti-GBM anti-

Fig. 9.11 Crescentic glomerulonephritis. Note 'epithelial' crescent at the periphery of the glomerulus (arrow).

Fig. 9.12 Membranous glomerulonephritis showing thickened basement membrane.

body can be demonstrated by immunofluorescence. However, the immunological pathogenesis of this condition is suggested by:

- Its response to steroids and immunosuppressive drugs
- Its occurrence in Hodgkin's disease, with remission following successful treatment
- Patients with the condition and family members having a higher incidence of asthma and eczema. Remission following desensitization or antigen avoidance has been described.

A suggested explanation for the proteinuria is the production by lymphocytes of a factor which increases glomerular permeability to protein.

Minimal change nephropathy occurs chiefly in children aged 2–4 years but it can occur in adults. Patients present with the nephrotic syndrome (see below). It does not lead to chronic renal failure.

Idiopathic focal glomerulonephritis with mesangial deposits of IgA (IgA disease, Berger's disease). This disease consists of focal proliferative glomerulonephritis and mesangial deposits of IgA. In some cases IgG, C_3 and properdin may also be seen in the glomerular mesangium.

Glomerulonephritis in Henoch–Schönlein purpura has a similar pathological picture.

This type of glomerulonephritis tends to occur in children and young adults. They present with recurrent haematuria, which is sometimes related to infection. The prognosis is usually good but up to 10% of patients eventually develop renal failure.

Focal glomerulosclerosis (FGS). This is a disease of unknown pathogenesis. It recurs in kidneys transplanted into affected individuals, often within hours of transplantation. A circulating factor may be involved. It presents as proteinuria or nephrotic syndrome and is usually resistant to steroid therapy. All age groups are affected.

On light microscopy, segmental glomerulosclerosis is seen, which later progresses to global sclerosis. The deep glomeruli at the corticomedullary junction are affected first. These may be missed on transcutaneous biopsy, leading to a mistaken diagnosis of minimal change glomerular lesion. Immunofluorescence may show deposits of C_3 and IgM in affected portions of the glomerulus, but non-specific fixation to damaged tissue, rather than immune complex deposition, may well be the explanation for this.

About 50% of patients progress to end stage renal failure within 10 years of diagnosis.

CLINICAL FEATURES

Glomerulonephritis presents in one of four ways:
- Asymptomatic proteinuria and/or microscopic haematuria

- Acute nephritic syndrome (see below)
- Nephrotic syndrome (see p. 387)
- Chronic renal failure (see p. 418)

Asymptomatic proteinuria and/or microscopic haematuria is discovered incidentally, e.g. at a routine medical examination. Some causes of haematuria are shown in Fig. 9.4. Overt haematuria may occur after exercise.

INVESTIGATION

Since false-positives are often obtained using the very sensitive Stix methods, the presence of significant proteinuria must be demonstrated by measuring the 24-h urinary output of protein on two consecutive occasions (see p. 376).

Urinary protein loss increases when in the erect position and 'postural' proteinuria can occur. Stix testing gives a negative result on urines passed early in the morning after rising, but positive results are seen during the day when the patient is mainly erect. Insurance companies do not tend to discriminate against those with postural proteinuria as the prognosis is usually good. Nevertheless, the majority of individuals with this condition have glomerulonephritis of some sort on renal biopsy.

Urine microscopy is performed to look for haematuria. A positive Stix test for blood may result from haematuria or haemoglobinuria. These can be differentiated on microscopy as red cells are only seen in patients with haematuria.

Further investigations will include:
- Urine microscopy for red cell casts
- Assessment of renal function by estimation of blood urea, serum creatinine and endogenous creatinine clearance
- Renal imaging, usually by excretion urography

Acute nephritic syndrome

This comprises:
- Haematuria (macroscopic or microscopic). Red cell casts are typically seen on urine microscopy.
- Proteinuria ⎫
- Hypertension ⎬ owing to salt retention and expansion of intravascular volume
- Oedema (periorbital, leg or sacral) ⎭
- Oliguria
- Uraemia

CLINICAL FEATURES

In classical post-streptococcal glomerulonephritis the patient, usually a child, will have suffered a streptococcal infection 1–3 weeks before the onset of the acute nephritic syndrome. Streptococcal tonsillitis or pharyngitis, otitis media or cellulitis may be responsible.

The infecting organism is a Lancefield group A beta-haemolytic streptococcus of a nephritogenic type. The latent interval between the infection and development of symptoms and signs of renal involvement reflects the time taken for immune complex formation and deposition and glomerular injury to occur.

INVESTIGATION

A list of investigations is given in Table 9.8.

If the clinical diagnosis of a nephritic illness is clear-cut, e.g. in post-streptococcal glomerulonephritis, renal imaging and renal biopsy are usually unnecessary. A biopsy is required if the diagnosis is uncertain, if the clinical features are unusual, or if renal failure is rapidly progressive, suggesting the presence of crescentic glomerulonephritis (RPGN).

MANAGEMENT

As spontaneous remissions usually occur, the aim of the management is to prevent patients dying from pulmonary oedema, uraemia or hypertensive encephalopathy whilst awaiting improvement in renal function.

Hospital admission is advisable for all adults and for children with oliguria and marked hypertension; levels of blood pressure that are of no risk to adults may be associated with hypertensive fits in the young.

Otherwise, hospital admission is not mandatory, providing the general practitioner is able to visit daily to examine the patient and check his blood pressure. Blood for measurement of urea or serum creatinine concentrations should be taken every few days.

Management in hospital

Most patients with renal disease who are admitted to hospital require:

- Daily recording of fluid intake and output
- Daily weighing (as a check on change in body fluid status)
- Regular measurement of blood pressure

Strict bedrest is unnecessary unless the patient feels ill, is severely hypertensive or has pulmonary oedema.

Dietary protein restriction is required if severe uraemia occurs, but salt restriction is always necessary. In oliguric patients, fluid restriction is necessary to maintain body weight at a level at which severe hypertension, pulmonary congestion and gross oedema are prevented.

Mild to moderate hypertension and oedema may respond to salt restriction and diuretic therapy, e.g. frusemide given orally or parenterally. Other hypotensive agents may be required. Beta-adrenergic receptor blocking therapy should be used with caution for hypertension as it may precipitate pulmonary oedema in those on the brink of heart failure due to the salt and water overload.

The prognosis in immune complex mediated glomerulonephritis is improved if the antigen responsible can be eradicated. In patients with post-streptococcal glomerulonephritis, a course of penicillin should be given.

Management of life-threatening complications
Hypertensive encephalopathy. In this condition the priorities are to maintain the airway and to reduce the blood pressure using a parenteral agent such as hydralazine 5–20 mg by slow intravenous infusion

Table 9.8 Investigation of acute nephritic syndrome.

Investigations	Positive findings
Urine microscopy	Red cells, red cell casts
Blood urea	May be elevated
Serum creatinine	May be elevated
Culture (throat swab, discharge from ear, swab from inflamed skin)	Nephritogenic organism—not always
Antistreptolysin-O titre	Elevated in post-streptococcal nephritis
C_3 level	May be reduced
Antinuclear antibody	Present in significant titre in systemic lupus erythematous
Creatinine clearance	Reduced
Urinary protein output	Increased
Chest x-ray	Cardiomegaly ⎤ not always Pulmonary oedema ⎦
Renal imaging	Usually normal
Renal biopsy	Glomerulonephritis

over 20 min. Fits should be controlled with parenteral diazepam (10 mg i.v.), but this may induce respiratory depression and facilities for resuscitation must be available.

Pulmonary oedema. This should be treated in the usual way (see p. 497). Because of the renal failure, high doses of potent diuretics such as frusemide given parenterally may be required. If this fails to produce a diuresis, salt and water may be removed osmotically by peritoneal dialysis, by ultrafiltration of blood alone, or by ultrafiltration combined with haemodialysis (see p. 418).

Severe uraemia. Peritoneal or haemodialysis will be required pending recovery of the renal function.

Outbreak of post-streptococcal glomerulonephritis in a closed community
Prophylactic penicillin (phenoxymethylpenicillin 500 mg daily) should be given to all individuals at risk, providing that they are not allergic to penicillin. If one member of a family living in overcrowded conditions develops the disorder, other members should be treated prophylactically. Evidence in support of long-term penicillin prophylaxis after the development of glomerulonephritis is lacking.

PROGNOSIS

Post-streptococcal glomerulonephritis
The prognosis in children is excellent. A small number of adults develop hypertension and/or renal impairment later in life. Therefore in older patients, an annual blood pressure check, and less frequently an estimation of serum creatinine, is a reasonable precaution, even after apparent complete recovery.

Acute glomerulonephritis of unknown cause
Here the prognosis is less good and the need for follow-up is correspondingly greater.

Rapidly progressive crescentic glomerulonephritis
Severe renal failure with oliguria and hypertension occurs within a few weeks or months of the onset of the illness. Corticosteroid treatment (to reduce glomerular inflammatory reaction), treatment with agents which prevent platelet aggregation, immunosuppression (e.g. with azathioprine or cyclophosphamide) and anticoagulants are used in combination. Such 'quadruple therapy' carries substantial risks but does appear to be of benefit in some patients. Repeated plasma exchange to remove circulating immune complexes or antibody may also be helpful. The prognosis is poor.

Goodpasture's syndrome (see p. 380)

This rare condition is mediated by anti-GBM antibodies. It presents with recurrent haemoptysis (see p. 610) and a severe progressive glomerulonephritis. Lung haemorrhage responds to repeated plasma exchange (which removes the anti-GBM antibodies) combined with immunosuppressive therapy. The effect of this treatment upon the glomerulonephritis is less clear-cut; when oliguria occurs or serum creatinine rises above $0.6-0.7$ mmol$\cdot$l^{-1}, renal failure is almost always irreversible.

The kidney in systemic disease

GLOMERULONEPHRITIS AS A PART OF SYSTEMIC VASCULITIS

Systemic lupus erythematosus (see p. 341)

Renal disease in systemic lupus erythematosus (SLE) is 10 times as common in women as in men. All varieties of histological abnormality are seen, ranging from a minimal change lesion to crescentic glomerulonephritis. The prognosis is better in patients with focal proliferative and membranous nephritis than in those with a diffuse proliferative lesion.

In acute SLE with severe renal involvement, high-dose steroid and immunosuppressive therapy is necessary. Long-term azathioprine and cyclophosphamide have a place in the prevention of kidney damage, but there is currently no certainty as to which categories of patient should be treated with these drugs.

Polyarteritis nodosa (see p. 345)

In this multi-system disorder aneurysmal dilatation of medium-sized arteries may be seen on renal arteriography. A focal proliferative glomerulonephritis with or without crescents can be present. The condition is commoner in men and in the elderly.

Corticosteroid therapy and immunosuppression with azathioprine or cyclophosphamide are of benefit.

Wegener's granulomatosis (see p. 606)

In this condition microscopic polyarteritis occurs together with necrotizing granulomatous lesions affecting the nasopharynx, lungs and kidneys. The necrotizing glomerular lesions do not appear to be due to immune complex deposition.

Corticosteroid treatment and cyclophosphamide are of benefit.

Systemic sclerosis (see p. 342)

Interlobular renal arteries are affected with intimal thickening and fibrinoid changes occur in afferent glomerular arterioles. Glomerular changes are non-specific. The pathogenesis is unknown and neither steroid nor immunosuppressive therapy is of value.

RENAL INVOLVEMENT IN OTHER DISEASES

Diabetes mellitus

Renal disease is a major complication of diabetes; it is discussed on p. 762.

Amyloidosis

The kidney is often affected in primary and secondary amyloidosis (see p. 324). Presentation is with asymptomatic proteinuria, nephrotic syndrome or renal failure.

PATHOLOGY

On light microscopy eosinophilic deposits are seen in the mesangium, capillary loops and arteriolar walls. Staining with Congo red renders these deposits pink and they show green birefringence under polarized light. Immunofluorescence is unhelpful but on electron microscopy the characteristic fibrils of amyloid can be seen. Primary and secondary renal amyloid are indistinguishable.

DIAGNOSIS

The diagnosis can often be made clinically when features of amyloidosis are present elsewhere. On excretion urography or ultrasound the kidneys are usually large. Renal biopsy is necessary in doubtful cases.

TREATMENT

Treatment of the underlying cause should be undertaken. Steroids and immunosuppression are of no proven value. The prognosis for renal function is poor in primary amyloid as well as in amyloid secondary to myelomatosis. The success of dialysis and kidney transplantation is dependent upon the extent of amyloid deposition in extrarenal sites, especially the heart.

Haemolytic uraemic syndrome (HUS)

This is a disorder of infancy and childhood which is characterized by intravascular haemolysis with red cell fragmentation (microangiopathic haemolysis, see p. 287), thrombocytopenia and acute renal failure. The syndrome often follows a febrile illness and it has been suggested that this triggers derangements of the coagulation system in susceptible individuals. Fibrin deposition is seen in the vascular endothelium, particularly in the renal arterioles and glomerular capillaries. Most children recover spontaneously.

Treatment with heparin, inhibitors of platelet aggregation, synthetic prostacyclins and plasma infusion and exchange has been employed, but so far there is no proof that these treatments are beneficial.

Thrombotic thrombocytopenic purpura (TTP)

This condition is characterized by the presence of widespread hyaline thrombi in small vessels. Young adults are most commonly affected. Microangiopathic haemolysis, renal failure and evidence of neurological disturbance are characteristically found. The pathogenesis is unknown. Some patients with TTP have underlying systemic lupus erythematosis or polyarteritis nodosa and there is clearly considerable overlap between HUS, TTP and the connective tissue disorders.

Nephrotic syndrome

The nephrotic syndrome consists of heavy urinary protein loss, hypoalbuminaemia and oedema. Hypercholesterolaemia is frequently, but not invariably, present.

PATHOPHYSIOLOGY

Urinary protein loss of the order of 3–5 g per day or more in an adult is required to cause hypoalbuminaemia. In children, proportionately less proteinuria results in hypoalbuminaemia.

The normal dietary protein intake in the UK is of the order of 70 g daily and the normal liver can synthesize albumin at a rate of 10–12 g daily. How then does a urinary protein loss of the order of 3–5 g daily result in hypoalbuminaemia? The explanation appears to be that in normal individuals there is some catabolism within the kidney of albumin filtered at the glomeruli. In nephrotic patients with heavy proteinuria catabolism is substantially increased, limiting the amount of protein appearing in the urine.

The mechanism of the proteinuria is complex. It occurs partly because structural damage to the glomerular basement membrane leads to an increase in the size and numbers of pores, allowing passage of more and larger molecules. Electrical charge is also involved in glomerular permeability. Fixed negatively charged components are present in the glomerular capillary wall, which repel negatively charged protein molecules. Reduction of this fixed charge occurs in glomerular disease and appears to be an important factor in the genesis of heavy proteinuria.

Pathogenesis of oedema in hypoalbuminaemia

The pathogenesis of the oedema is incompletely understood. A reduction in the concentration of osmotically active albumin molecules in the blood results in a reduction in the osmotic force which retains fluid within blood vessels, and salt and water escape into the extravascular compartment, i.e. oedema occurs. Such loss of salt and water results in a fall in blood volume and a reduction in pressure within afferent glomerular arterioles. This activates the renin–angiotensin–aldosterone system (see p. 739) and the consequent hyperaldosteronism promotes sodium and water reabsorption in the distal nephron, increasing the tendency to oedema. However, measurements of these various parameters do not always support this concept. The plasma renin activity in nephrotic patients is often normal and measured blood volume may be normal or high in nephrotic patients, even those without renal failure.

CAUSES (Table 9.9)

All types of glomerulonephritis can produce the nephrotic syndrome.

Minimal change glomerular disease accounts for more than 50% of cases of the nephrotic syndrome in childhood compared with approximately 20% of adult cases. In tropical areas minimal change is present in less than 10% of nephrotic children owing to the high incidence of nephrotic syndrome due to infections such as malaria. Minimal change disease does not progress to chronic renal failure (see p. 383).

Membranous glomerulonephritis occurs in systemic lupus erythematosus, as a complication of *Plasmodium malariae* infection, as a result of drugs (e.g. penicillamine) and in malignancy. The majority of cases are of unknown aetiology. Idiopathic membranous glomerulonephritis is commoner in men, in whom it also carries a worse prognosis than in women.

Table 9.9 Causes of the nephrotic syndrome.

All glomerulonephritides and minimal change glomerular lesions
Systemic vasculitides, mainly systemic lupus erythematosus
Diabetic glomerulosclerosis
Amyloidosis
Drugs
Allergies

Although proliferative glomerulonephritis is commoner than membranous disease, the latter is the commonest cause of nephrotic syndrome in adults in the UK.

Diabetic glomerular disease can also cause the nephrotic syndrome. The histological lesion seen on light microscopy in diabetes may comprise amorphous nodular deposits, which are not immune complexes, in the glomeruli or a diffuse glomerulosclerosis. There is associated glomerular basement membrane thickening.

Diabetes is also a cause of renal papillary necrosis, but patients with this lesion alone do not have sufficiently heavy proteinuria to become nephrotic.

Drugs

Many drugs can cause sufficiently heavy proteinuria to result in the nephrotic syndrome. Penicillamine, which in all probability combines with a plasma protein to form an antigen hapten, induces an immune complex mediated membranous glomerulonephritis. Troxidone, used in the treatment of absence seizures, may also cause heavy proteinuria. Various metals, whether used therapeutically (e.g. gold) or in industry (e.g. mercury and cadmium), can induce proteinuria severe enough to cause the nephrotic syndrome.

Allergic reactions

Reactions to many allergens such as poison ivy, pollens, bee stings and cow's milk may be associated with the nephrotic syndrome, but evidence of a causal relationship is lacking in most cases.

Most lists of causes of the nephrotic syndrome include renal vein thrombosis, but this is probably a complication rather than a cause of the syndrome. It is particularly likely to complicate membranous glomerulonephritis. In nephrotic patients the blood is more coagulable than normal and the circulation may be sluggish owing to hypovolaemia, both of which are likely to induce thrombosis. Estimates of the incidence of this complication range from 5% to approximately 50%.

Renal disorders not associated with the nephrotic syndrome

Proteinuria severe enough to cause the nephrotic syndrome is not a feature of reflux nephropathy (chronic atrophic pyelonephritis), chronic tubulo-interstitial nephritis, renal tuberculosis, polycystic disease or many other renal disorders.

HISTORY

The history may provide clues to the aetiology, e.g. exposure to a drug or allergen. Patients with minimal change lesions may give a history of atopy. There may be a family history of renal disease.

Patients with heavy proteinuria may have noted

that their urine has been frothy; the onset of the renal lesion can be timed from this observation.

EXAMINATION

Examination will reveal oedema; ascites may also be present, particularly in children. Genital oedema is sometimes seen. The oedema may involve the face (periorbital oedema) and arms.

Features of the underlying disorder may be evident, such as the butterfly facial rash of systemic lupus erythematosus or the neuropathy and retinopathy associated with diabetes mellitus.

Cardiac failure must be excluded; in cardiac failure the venous pressure is high, oedema is not usually present in the face, and the proteinuria is less severe.

Liver disease, and other causes of hypo-albuminaemia (Table 9.10), can also cause oedema and ascites and so careful examination to exclude these diseases should be performed.

INVESTIGATION

The presence of the nephrotic syndrome is established by measuring:
- The 24-h urinary protein
- The serum albumin concentration

Increased hepatic albumin synthesis is accompanied by increased cholesterol synthesis and there is an approximate reciprocal relationship between the serum albumin and the serum cholesterol concentration.

Renal function is assessed by measuring:
- The blood urea and serum creatinine
- The creatinine clearance, to determine the GFR

Further investigations are required to elucidate the cause:
- Microscopy of the urine may show red cells and red cell casts; the latter are virtually diagnostic of glomerulonephritis. Minimal change lesions do not usually result in red cells or red cell casts in the urine.
- Serum C_3 complement concentrations may be decreased in immune complex mediated glomerulonephritis.
- A throat swab and serum ASO titre may show evidence of streptococcal infection.

Table 9.10 Causes of hypoalbuminaemia.

Inadequate protein intake—protein-energy malnutrition
Failure of protein production—liver disease
Excessive protein loss—nephrotic syndrome, protein-losing enteropathy, extensive burns

- The presence of antinuclear factor and other antibodies may suggest systemic lupus erythematosus.
- In the nephrotic syndrome there is always a reduced serum albumin, commonly with an increase in the alpha- and beta-globulin fractions (Fig. 9.13) on serum and urinary electrophoresis. In myeloma abnormal protein bands may be found, including Bence Jones protein in the urine. Ten per cent of patients with myeloma have amyloid and can develop the nephrotic syndrome.
- The blood glucose level may suggest diabetes mellitus.
- The results of differential protein clearance measurement may indicate the cause. Blood and urine samples should be taken at the same time; a timed urine collection is not required. The clearance of a large molecular weight protein such as IgG is compared with that of a smaller molecule such as albumin or transferrin. A low ratio (selective protein leak) is found in minimal change glomerulopathy, early diabetes and renal amyloidosis. Severe glomerulonephritides, e.g. diffuse proliferative glomerulonephritis with crescent formation, are more typically associated with an unselective protein leak. Overlap between the groups exists.

Renal biopsy (see p. 379)
Transcutaneous biopsy is performed to make a histological diagnosis when management will be affected, particularly when the major question is whether a steroid-sensitive minimal change lesion is present or not. It is *not* indicated:
- In young children (particularly males) who have a highly selective protein leak, no hypertension and no red cells or red cell casts in the urine. The

Fig. 9.13 Serum electrophoresis in a normal person and a patient with nephrotic syndrome. Note the reduced albumin and increased alpha- and beta-globulin in the nephrotic patient.

diagnosis is almost certain to be a minimal change lesion so that a trial of steroids should be instituted first.

- In long-standing, insulin-dependent diabetes with associated retinopathy or neuropathy, since the diagnosis is not in doubt
- In patients on drugs such as penicillamine, which should be stopped first

MANAGEMENT

General measures

Initial treatment should be with dietary sodium restriction and a thiazide diuretic, e.g. bendroflu-azide 5 mg daily. Unresponsive patients require frusemide 40–120 mg daily with the addition of amiloride (5 mg daily), but the serum potassium concentration should be monitored carefully.

Patients are often hypovolaemic, and moderate oedema may have to be accepted in order to avoid postural hypotension.

A high-protein diet is usually given, but the efficacy of a high, as opposed to a normal, protein intake is unproven.

Infusion of albumin produces only a transient effect and is not normally required. Occasionally infusion is combined with diuretic therapy to initiate diuresis, which then often continues with diuretics alone.

Specific measures

The aim is to reverse the abnormal urinary protein leak.

Minimal change glomerular lesion. High-dose corti-costeroid therapy (prednisolone 60 mg per 1.73 m^2 daily for 8 weeks) corrects the urinary protein leak in more than 95% of children. Response rates in adults are significantly lower. Spontaneous remission also occurs and steroid therapy should, in general, be withheld if urinary protein loss is insufficient to cause hypoalbuminaemia or oedema.

In children, approximately one-third do not subsequently relapse. In both children and adults, if remission lasts for 4 years after steroid therapy, further relapse is very rare. About one-third of children have occasional relapses which respond to further corticosteroid therapy. The remainder relapse regularly when steroid therapy is withdrawn. In these patients, remission is induced with steroid therapy once more and a course of cyclophosphamide 3 mg·kg^{-1} daily is given for 6–8 weeks. This increases the likelihood of long-term remission. Steroid-unresponsive patients may also respond to cyclophosphamide. No more than two courses of cyclophosphamide should be prescribed in children because of the risk of side-effects, which include azoospermia.

Membranous glomerulonephritis. Spontaneous remis-sion does occur in this condition, particularly in women. Nevertheless, more than 50% of nephrotic patients with idiopathic membranous glomerulo-nephritis develop end stage renal failure within 10 years of diagnosis. Recent evidence suggests that high-dose corticosteroid therapy given on alternate days for 8 weeks may protect against deterioration in renal function to some extent. It may be best to reserve steroid treatment for those patients in whom the GFR is known to have declined rapidly.

Other causes. Remission occurs if the underlying disease can be treated. In patients with systemic lupus erythematosus, treatment with steroids and azathioprine usually induces long-term remission. Amyloidosis does not usually respond to therapy.

When the glomerular lesion causing the nephrotic syndrome progresses and the GFR declines, the degree of proteinuria often diminishes so that the hypoalbuminaemia and oedema improve.

Prevention and management of complications

Venous thrombosis. Hypovolaemia and a hypercoa-gulable state predispose to venous thrombosis. Prolonged bed rest should therefore be avoided.

Established venous thrombosis requires antico-agulant therapy. Once renal vein thrombosis has occurred prolonged anticoagulation is required.

Sepsis. Sepsis is an important cause of death in nephrotic patients. The increased susceptibility to infection is partly due to loss of immunoglobulin in the urine. Pneumococcal infections are particularly common.

Early detection and aggressive treatment of infec-tions rather than long-term antibiotic prophylaxis is the best approach.

Oliguric renal failure. A low blood volume and hypotension may lead to underperfused kidneys. Acute tubular necrosis may therefore readily develop when renal ischaemia occurs from other complications such as blood loss or septicaemia. In some patients uraemia appears to result from derangements in renal perfusion in the absence of hypotension.

Albumin infusion combined with mannitol or another diuretic may initiate a diuresis in oliguric renal failure.

Urinary tract infection

Urinary tract infection (UTI) is common in women, uncommon in men, and of special importance in children. If recurrent, it may be a cause of considerable morbidity; if complicated, it can cause severe renal disease including 'end-stage renal failure'. It is also a common source of life-threatening gram-negative septicaemia.

PATHOGENESIS

Infection is most often due to bacteria from the patient's own bowel flora (Table 9.11), but in 20–30% of young women it is due to *Staphylococcus saprophyticus* or *S. epidermidis*. Transfer to the urinary tract may be via the bloodstream, the lymphatics or by direct extension (e.g. from a vesico-colic fistula), but is most often via the ascending transurethral route (Fig. 9.14). For the latter route, three important steps are involved:

1 The periurethral area is heavily colonized with bacteria. This may be facilitated by the adhesion of bacteria to uro-epithelial surfaces by pili or fimbriae present on their surface. Previous UTIs may also predispose to further colonization, initiating a vicious circle. Other factors involved are unclear, although gross lack of personal hygiene, the wearing of nappies or sanitary towels, local infection (e.g. vaginitis) and the use of bubble baths or chemicals in bath water have all been incriminated.

2 Bacteria are transferred along the urethra to the bladder. This step is facilitated by catheterization or sexual intercourse. Spontaneous transfer along the short female urethra is easy, while the longer male urethra protects against transfer of bacteria to the bladder; in addition prostatic fluid has defensive bactericidal properties.

3 The most important step is the *establishment* and *multiplication* of bacteria within the bladder. Bladder urine is normally sterile, owing to bladder defence mechanisms which are the main protection against UTI. These include hydrokinetic and bladder mucosal factors. A high rate of urine flow and frequent and complete bladder emptying facilitate elimination of bacteria. Conversely, a low flow rate, infrequent and poor bladder emptying predispose to infection. Mucosal defence mechanisms are poorly understood. The establishment of infection may be facilitated by fimbriated bacteria adhering to the bladder uro-epithelium. This may be enhanced by previous damage to the uro-epithelium and opposed by mucosal factors which are as yet unknown. Neither humoral nor cell-mediated immune mechanisms have been shown to play any part in maintaining the sterility of bladder urine.

The first critical phase in the development of UTI is thus the entry and establishment of bacteria within the bladder. Extension of infection up the ureters to the kidneys is relatively easy and is facilitated by vesico-ureteric reflux and dilated hypotonic ureters. In terms of infection, and with the possible exception of renal carbuncles (see below), the urinary tract can be thought of as a continuous functional unit from the bladder to the kidney. Once infection is established it can pass up or down the system quite readily.

NATURAL HISTORY

UTI is commonly an isolated, never (or rarely) repeated event (Fig. 9.15). At least 50% of women will experience an episode of 'cystitis' at some time in their lives. Although often unpleasant, such single episodes of UTI rarely result in significant kidney damage. Recurrent or persistent infections are much more important.

Table 9.11 Organisms causing urinary tract infection in domiciliary practice.

Organism	Approximate frequency
Escherichia coli and other 'coliforms'	68% +
Proteus mirabilis	12%
*Klebsiella aerogenes**	4%
*Streptococcus faecalis**	6%
Staphylococcus saprophyticus or epidermidis†	10%

* More common in hospital practice.
† More common in young women (20–30%).

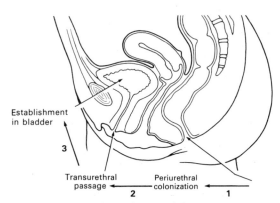

Fig. 9.14 Ascending infection of the urinary tract.

Fig. 9.15 The natural history of urinary tract infection.

Complicated versus uncomplicated infection

It is important to distinguish between UTI occurring in patients with functionally normal urinary tracts (with normal excretion urography) and UTI in patients with associated disease and/or abnormal tracts (Fig. 9.16). Persistent or recurrent infection in those with normal urinary tracts rarely, if ever, results in serious kidney damage and is known as 'uncomplicated UTI'.

Diabetes, analgesic abuse and sickle cell disease or trait can themselves cause kidney damage, but the potential for this increases when they are associated with infection.

Most important are those patients with stones, obstruction or vesico-ureteric reflux. These latter two groups are described as having 'complicated UTI'. UTI, especially infection with *Proteus*, may predispose to stone formation. Stones may cause kidney damage but more often result in obstruction to all or part of the collecting system. The combination of infection and obstruction results in severe, sometimes rapid, kidney damage (obstructive pyonephrosis) and is an important cause of gram-negative septicaemia, which may be immediately life-threatening.

Chronic pyelonephritis

Chronic pyelonephritis (also called atrophic pyelonephritis or reflux nephropathy) is now known to result from a combination of vesico-ureteric reflux and infection acquired in infancy or early childhood. Normally the vesico-ureteric junction acts as a one-way valve (Fig. 9.17), urine entering the bladder from above; the ureter is shut off during bladder contraction, thus preventing reflux of urine. In some infants and children—possibly even in utero—this valve mechanism is incompetent, bladder voiding being associated with variable reflux of a jet of urine up the ureter. A secondary consequence is incomplete bladder emptying, as refluxed urine returns to the bladder after voiding. This latter event predisposes to infection, and the reflux of infected urine leads to kidney damage. Typically there is papillary damage, interstitial nephritis and cortical scarring in areas adjacent to 'clubbed calyces' (Fig. 9.17). Diagnosis is based on excretion urography, which shows irregular renal outlines, clubbed calyces and a variable reduction in renal size. Reflux is confirmed by micturating cystourography (see p. 378). The condition may be unilateral or bilateral and affect all or part of the kidney.

Reflux usually ceases around puberty with growth of the bladder base. Damage already done persists and progressive renal fibrosis and further loss of function occurs in severe cases even though there is no further infection. This condition does not develop in the absence of reflux and does not begin in adult life. Chronic pyelonephritis acquired in infancy predisposes to hypertension in later life and, if severe, is a relatively common cause of end-stage renal failure in childhood or adult life. Early detection and treatment of infection, with or without ureteral re-implantation to create a competent valve, can prevent further scarring and allow normal growth of the kidneys.

Re-infection versus relapsing infection

When UTI is recurrent it is important to distinguish between relapse and re-infection.

Relapse is diagnosed by recurrence of bacteriuria with the *same* organism within 7 days of treatment and implies failure to eradicate infection (Fig. 9.18). It usually occurs in conditions in which it is difficult to eradicate the bacteria, e.g. stones, scarred kidneys, polycystic disease or bacterial prostatitis.

By contrast, in re-infection bacteriuria is absent after treatment for at least 14 days, usually longer, followed by recurrence of infection with the same or

Fig. 9.16 Complicated versus uncomplicated urinary tract infection.

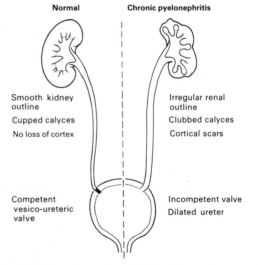

Fig. 9.17 Chronic pyelonephritis with vesico-ureteric reflux compared with the normal state.

Fig. 9.18 A comparison of re-infection, relapse and treatment failure in urinary tract infection.

different organisms. This is not due to failure to eradicate infection, but is the result of re-invasion of a susceptible tract with new organisms. Approximately 80% of recurrent infections are due to re-infection.

SYMPTOMS AND SIGNS

The most typical symptoms of UTI are:
- Frequency of micturition by day and night
- Painful voiding (dysuria)
- Suprapubic pain and tenderness
- Haematuria
- Smelly urine

These symptoms relate to bladder and urethral inflammation, commonly called 'cystitis', and suggest lower urinary tract infection. Loin pain and tenderness, with fever and systemic upset, suggest extension of the infection to the pelvis and kidney, known as pyelitis or pyelonephritis. However, localization of the site of infection on the basis of symptoms alone is unreliable.

UTI may also be present with minimal or no symptoms or may be associated with atypical symptoms such as abdominal pain, fever, or haematuria in the absence of frequency or dysuria.

In small children who cannot complain of dysuria, symptoms are often 'atypical'. The possibility of UTI must always be considered in the fretful, febrile sick child who fails to thrive.

Abacteriuric frequency or dysuria ('the urethral syndrome')
Symptoms of frequency and/or dysuria are *not* synonymous with UTI and 50% of symptomatic young women may have no demonstrable bac-

teriuria. Alternative causes include post-coital bladder trauma, vaginitis, atrophic vaginitis or urethritis in the elderly, and interstitial cystitis (Hunner's ulcer).

Careful history taking will identify a group with predominant frequency and passing small volumes of urine who have 'irritable bladders', possibly consequent on previous UTI or conditioned by psychosexual factors. Such patients must be distinguished from those with frequency due to polyuria. Repeated courses of antibiotics in patients with abacteriuric frequency or dysuria are quite inappropriate and detract from identifying the true nature of the problem.

DIAGNOSIS

The diagnosis must be based on *quantitative* culture of a clean catch midstream specimen of urine; more than 100 000 of the same organism per millilitre of urine indicates bladder infection ('significant bacteriuria'). Lower counts may be accepted as evidence of infection in patients passing large volumes of urine. If in doubt, urine must be obtained by suprapubic bladder aspiration, when any growth of a uropathogenic organism is evidence of infection. Pyuria is not a constant feature of UTI and its absence does not exclude the diagnosis (see p. 376).

SPECIAL INVESTIGATIONS

Excretion urography
Excretion urography is not indicated in women with one or two isolated episodes of UTI if post-treatment urinalysis, including microscopy and urine culture, are normal. If there are further attacks or if post-treatment urinalysis is abnormal, excretion urogra-

phy should be performed to identify or exclude anatomical or functional abnormalities predisposing to or complicating infection, e.g. impaired bladder emptying.

Excretion urography should be carried out in all males and children following a first proven episode of bacteriuria to identify complicating factors.

Micturating cystourography

Micturating cystourography is indicated in children with abnormal excretion urograms and may be required to evaluate abnormal bladder emptying at any age. Otherwise it is of no value in the management of UTI.

Cystoscopy

Cystoscopy in patients with known UTI has a very limited role, being indicated only to investigate abnormal bladder or ureteral emptying, or haematuria in bacteriuric women over the age of 40 years, bladder cancer becoming more common with age. It is more commonly performed in abacteriuric frequency or dysuria to exclude bladder lesions such as carcinoma or interstitial cystitis (Hunner's ulcer).

TREATMENT

Single isolated attack

Pre-treatment urine cultures are desirable. If symptoms are mild, symptomatic treatment with potassium citrate mixture (10 ml three times daily) can be given pending the result of urine culture. If symptoms are severe, treatment with 3–5 days of sulphafurazole (1 g three times daily), amoxycillin (250 mg three times daily), nitrofurantoin (50 mg three times daily) or trimethoprim (200 mg twice daily) should be started immediately without waiting for the result of urine culture. A high (2 l daily) fluid intake should be encouraged during treatment and for some weeks following.

Urinalysis, microscopy and culture should be repeated 5 days after treatment. 'Single shot' treatment with 3 g of amoxycillin, 1.92 g of co-trimoxazole or 2 g of sulphafurazole can be used for patients with bladder symptoms of less than 36 h duration who have no previous history of UTI.

If the patient is acutely ill with high fever, loin pain and tenderness (acute pyelonephritis) intravenous ampicillin or amoxycillin (1 g 6-hourly) or intravenous gentamicin (2–5 mg·kg^{-1} daily in divided doses) should be given, switching to a further 7 days' treatment with oral therapy as symptoms improve. Intravenous fluids may be required to achieve a good urine output.

Recurrent infection

Pre- and post-treatment urine cultures are mandatory to confirm the diagnosis and identify whether recurrent infection is due to relapse or re-infection.

In *relapse*, a search should be made for a cause, e.g. stones or scarred kidneys, and this should be eradicated if possible, for example by the removal of stones. Intense or prolonged treatment—intravenous or intramuscular aminoglycoside for 7 days or oral antibiotics for 4–6 weeks—is required. If this fails, long-term antibiotics are required.

Re-infection implies that the patient has poor defence systems; such patients must undertake prophylactic measures:
- A 2 l daily fluid intake
- Voiding at 2–3 h intervals with double micturition if reflux is present
- Voiding before bedtime and after intercourse
- Avoidance of bubble baths and other chemicals in bath water
- Avoidance of constipation, which may impair bladder emptying

Evidence of impaired bladder emptying on excretion urography requires urological assessment. If UTI continues to recur, treatment for 6–12 months with low dose prophylaxis (trimethoprim 100 mg, co-trimoxazole 480 mg, or nitrofurantoin 50 mg) is required; it should be taken last thing at night when urine flow is low.

Bacteriuria in pregnancy

The urine of pregnant women must always be cultured as 2–6% have asymptomatic bacteriuria. Failure to treat this may result in severe symptomatic pyelonephritis later in pregnancy, with the possibility of premature labour. Asymptomatic bacteriuria, particularly in the presence of previous renal disease, may predispose to pre-eclamptic toxaemia, anaemia of pregnancy, and small or premature babies. Therefore bacteriuria must always be treated and be shown to be eradicated. Re-infection may require prophylactic therapy. Tetracycline drugs must be avoided in pregnancy, as should trimethoprim in the first trimester and sulphonamides in the third.

Bacterial prostatitis

Bacterial prostatitis may cause relapsing infection and is difficult to treat. It presents as perineal pain, recurrent epididymo-orchitis and prostatic tenderness, with pus in expressed prostatic secretion. Treatment is with drugs that penetrate the prostate—trimethoprim, tetracyclines or erythromycins—for 4–6 weeks. Long-term low-dose treatment may be required.

Renal carbuncle

Renal carbuncle is an abscess in the renal cortex caused by a blood-borne staphylococcus, usually from a boil or carbuncle of the skin. It presents with high swinging fevers, loin pain and tenderness, and fullness in the loin. The urine shows no abnormality as the abscess does not communicate with the renal pelvis, more often extending into the perirenal tissue. Staphylococcal septicaemia is common. Diagnosis is by ultrasound. Treatment involves anti-bacterial therapy with flucloxacillin and surgical drainage.

Tuberculosis of the urinary tract

Tuberculosis of the urinary tract should still be kept in mind in patients presenting with frequency, dysuria or haematuria, particularly in the Asian immigrant population of the UK. Cortical lesions result from haematogenous spread in the primary phase of infection. Most heal, but in some infection persists and spreads to the papillae, with the forma-tion of cavitating lesions and the discharge of mycobacteria into the urine. Infection of the ureters and bladder commonly follows, with the potential for the development of ureteral stricture and a con-tracted bladder. Rarely, cold abscesses may form in the loin. In males the disease may present with testicular or epididymal discomfort and thickening.

Diagnosis depends on constant awareness, espe-cially in patients with sterile pyuria. Excretion urography may show cavitating lesions in the renal papillary areas, commonly with calcification. There may also be evidence of ureteral obstruction with hydronephrosis. Diagnosis of active infection depends on culture of mycobacteria from early morning urine samples.

The treatment is as for pulmonary tuberculosis (see p. 602); follow-up with excretion urography must be carried out as ureteral strictures may first develop in the healing phase.

Xanthogranulomatous pyelonephritis

This is an uncommon chronic interstitial infection of the kidney, most often due to *Proteus* spp., in which there is fever, weight loss, loin pain and a palpable enlarged kidney. It is usually unilateral and associ-ated with staghorn calculi. CT scanning shows up intrarenal abscesses as lucent areas within the kid-ney. Nephrectomy is the treatment of choice; anti-bacterial treatment rarely, if ever, eradicates the infection.

Tubulo-interstitial nephritis

Interstitial inflammation with tubular damage is a regular feature of bacterial pyelonephritis but, con-trary to former belief, it rarely, if ever, leads to chronic renal damage in the absence of reflux,

obstruction or other complicating factors. However, there is growing concern that tubulo-interstitial disease due to other causes is more common than was previously diagnosed. The major stimulus for this interest came from recognition that it could be due to analgesic abuse. Subsequently, tubulo-inter-stitial disease due to a variety of drugs has been recognized and this condition should be considered in all patients presenting with otherwise unex-plained renal failure. Presentation may be with acute, often oliguric renal failure or more commonly as chronic slowly progressive renal disease.

ACUTE TUBULO-INTERSTITIAL NEPHRITIS

Acute tubulo-interstitial nephritis is most often due to a hypersensitivity reaction to drugs (Table 9.12), most commonly drugs of the penicillin family and non-steroidal anti-inflammatory drugs (NSAIDs). Patients present with fever, arthralgia, skin rashes and acute oliguric or non-oliguric renal failure. There is a history of drug taking. Many have eosinophilia and eosinophiluria. Renal biopsy shows an intense interstitial cellular infiltrate, often including eosinophils, with variable tubular necrosis.

Treatment involves withdrawal of offending drugs. High-dose steroid therapy (prednisolone 60 mg daily) is commonly given but its efficacy has not been proved. Patients may require dialysis for management of the acute renal failure. Most patients have good recovery of kidney function, but some may be left with significant interstitial fibrosis.

Table 9.12 Common causes of acute tubulo-interstitial nephritis.

Penicillins
Sulphonamides
Non-steroidal anti-inflammatory drugs
Phenindione
Allopurinol

CHRONIC TUBULO-INTERSTITIAL NEPHRITIS

The major causes of chronic tubulo-interstitial nephritis are set out in Table 9.13. The patient usu-ally either presents with polyuria and nocturia, or is found to have proteinuria or uraemia. Proteinuria is usually slight (less than 1 g per day). Papillary necrosis with ischaemic damage to the papillae occurs in a number of interstitial nephritides, e.g. in analgesic abuse, diabetes mellitus, sickle cell disease or trait. The papillae can separate and be passed in the urine. Chronic tubulo-interstitial nephritis may be associated with microscopic or overt haematuria or sterile pyuria, and occasionally a sloughed papilla

Table 9.13 Causes of chronic tubulo-interstitial nephritis.

Common
Chronic pyelonephritis
Non-steroidal anti-inflammatory drugs
Diabetes
Sickle cell disease/trait
Cadmium or lead intoxication
Uncommon
Alport's syndrome
Balkan nephropathy
Irradiation
Sjögrens syndrome
Hyperuricaemic nephropathy

may cause ureteral colic or produce acute ureteral obstruction. The radiological appearances must be distinguished from those of chronic pyelonephritis (Fig.9.19).

Tubular damage to the medullary area of the kidney leads to defects in urine concentration and sodium conservation with polyuria and salt wasting. Fibrosis progressing into the cortex leads to loss of excretory function and uraemia.

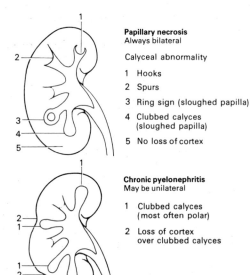

Papillary necrosis
Always bilateral

Calyceal abnormality

1 Hooks
2 Spurs
3 Ring sign (sloughed papilla)
4 Clubbed calyces (sloughed papilla)
5 No loss of cortex

Chronic pyelonephritis
May be unilateral

1 Clubbed calyces (most often polar)
2 Loss of cortex over clubbed calyces

Fig. 9.19 A comparison of the radiological appearances of chronic pyelonephritis and papillary necrosis.

Analgesic nephropathy

The chronic consumption of *large* amounts of analgesics (especially those containing phenacetin) leads to chronic tubulo-interstitial nephritis and papillary necrosis. This also seems to be true of NSAIDs.

In Australia, 20% of patients with end-stage renal failure have analgesic nephropathy.

CLINICAL FEATURES

Analgesic nephropathy is twice as common in women as in men and presents typically in middle-age. Patients are often depressed or neurotic. Presentation may be with anaemia, chronic renal failure, symptoms of urinary infection (which may be difficult to eradicate), haematuria, or urinary tract obstruction (due to sloughing of a renal papilla). Salt-and water-wasting renal disease may occur.

Chronic analgesic abuse also predisposes to the development of uro-epithelial tumours.

MANAGEMENT

The consumption of analgesics should be discouraged. If necessary, dihydrocodeine, paracetamol and aspirin alone are reasonable alternative choices. This may result in the arrest of the disease and even in improvement in function.

Urinary tract infection, hypertension (if present) and saline depletion will require appropriate management.

The development of flank pain or an unexpectedly rapid deterioration in renal function should prompt ultrasonography or urography to screen for urinary tract obstruction due to a sloughed papilla.

Balkan nephropathy

This is a chronic tubulo-interstitial nephritis endemic in the central Danube basin in Yugoslavia, Bulgaria and Rumania. Primarily restricted to rural areas, the cause is unknown. The disease is insidious in onset, with mild proteinuria progressing to renal failure in 3 months to 10 years. Patients exhibit a high incidence of uro-epithelial tumours. There is no treatment.

Other forms of chronic tubulo-interstitial nephritis are rare (see Table 9.13). Diagnosis of all forms depends on a careful history being taken, with special attention to drug taking and industrial exposure to nephrotoxins. In patients with unexplained renal impairment with normal-sized kidneys, renal biopsy must always be undertaken to exclude a treatable interstitial nephritis.

Hyperuricaemic nephropathy (gouty nephropathy)

Three patterns of renal disease have been described in patients with hyperuricaemia or hyperuricosuria:
● Gouty or chronic hyperuricaemic nephropathy

- Acute hyperuricaemic nephropathy
- Uric acid stone formation (see p. 400)

Uric acid nephrolithiasis is described on p. 400.

Chronic hyperuricaemic nephropathy

Considerable controversy surrounds the possible role of chronic hyperuricaemia as a cause of tubulo-interstitial disease and progressive renal damage. While uric acid 'tophi' may be found in the kidneys of patients with gout there is no convincing evidence that chronic hyperuricaemia per se causes progressive renal failure, nor that allopurinol treatment improves renal function. There is one important exception: a rare form of familial hyperuricaemia and gout occurring in adolescence is associated with renal impairment and allopurinol therapy both improves and protects kidney function.

Acute hyperuricaemic nephropathy

This is a well-recognized cause of acute renal failure in patients with marked hyperuricaemia due to lympho- or myeloproliferative disorders. This may occur prior to treatment but most often occurs on commencement of treatment, when there is rapid lysis of malignant cells, release of large amounts of nucleoprotein and increased uric acid production. Renal failure is due to intra- and extrarenal obstruction caused by deposition of uric acid crystals in the collecting ducts, pelvis and ureters. The condition is manifest in oliguria or anuria with increasing uraemia. There may be flank pain or colic. Plasma urate levels are above $0.75 \ \text{mmol} \cdot \text{l}^{-1}$ and may be as high as $4.5 \ \text{mmol} \cdot \text{l}^{-1}$. Diagnosis is based on the hyperuricaemia and the clinical setting. Ultrasound demonstrates extrarenal obstruction due to stones, but a negative scan does not exclude this where there is coexistent intrarenal obstruction.

PREVENTION

It is now regular practice to prescribe allopurinol 100–200 mg three times daily for 5 days prior to and continuing throughout treatment with radiotherapy or cytotoxic drugs. A high rate of urine flow must be maintained by oral or parenteral fluid and the urine kept alkaline by the administration of sodium bicarbonate 600 mg four times daily and acetazolomide 250 mg three times daily.

TREATMENT

Allopurinol treatment should be commenced immediately and a forced alkaline diuresis attempted with intravenous 1.4% sodium bicarbonate plus acetazolomide (500 mg dose, then 250 mg twice daily). In severely oliguric or anuric patients, dialysis is required to lower the plasma urate, which allows

urate to diffuse out of the obstructed collecting ducts into the peritubular capillaries. Percutaneous nephrostomy (see p. 406) may be required to relieve extrarenal obstruction due to stones in the pelvis or ureters. Such stones may subsequently be passed spontaneously or may require surgical removal (see p. 403).

Hypertension and the kidney

ESSENTIAL HYPERTENSION

PATHOPHYSIOLOGY

In *benign essential hypertension*, arteriosclerosis of major renal arteries and changes in the intrarenal vasculature (nephrosclerosis) occur:
- In small vessels and arterioles, intimal thickening with reduplication of the internal elastic lamina occurs and the vessel wall becomes hyalinized.
- In large vessels, concentric reduplication of the internal elastic lamina and endothelial proliferation produce an 'onion skin' appearance.
- Reduction in size of both kidneys may occur; this may be asymmetrical if one major renal artery is more affected by atheromatous change than the other.
- The proportion of sclerotic glomeruli is increased compared with age-matched controls.

Deterioration in excretory function accompanies these changes, but severe renal failure requiring protein restriction is unusual.

In *accelerated or malignant phase hypertension*:
- Arteriolar fibrinoid necrosis occurs, probably as a result of plasma entering the media of the vessel through splits in the intima.
- Fibrinoid necrosis in afferent glomerular arterioles is a prominent feature.
- Fibrin deposition within small vessels is often associated with thrombocytopenia and red cell fragmentation seen in the peripheral blood film (microangiopathic haemolytic anaemia).

Microscopic haematuria, proteinuria, usually of modest degree (1–3 g daily), and progressive uraemia occur. If untreated, less than 10% of patients survive 2 years.

MANAGEMENT

Management of benign essential and malignant hypertension is described on p. 543.

If treatment is begun before renal impairment has occurred, the prognosis for renal function is good. Stabilization or improvement in renal function with healing of intrarenal arteriolar lesions and resolution of microangiopathic haemolysis occur with effective treatment of malignant phase hypertension. Life-long follow-up of the patient is mandatory.

RENAL HYPERTENSION

Bilateral renal disease

Hypertension commonly complicates bilateral renal disease such as chronic glomerulonephritis, bilateral reflux nephropathy (chronic atrophic pyelonephritis of childhood), polycystic disease and analgesic nephropathy.

Two main mechanisms are responsible:
● Activation of the renin–angiotensin–aldosterone system
● Retention of salt and water with impairment in excretory function leading to an increase in blood volume and hence blood pressure

The second of these assumes greater importance as renal function deteriorates.

Hypertension occurs earlier, is more common and tends to be more severe in patients with renal cortical disorders such as glomerulonephritis than in those with disorders affecting primarily the renal interstitium, such as reflux or analgesic nephropathy.

Management is as for essential hypertension (see p. 543). Good control of the blood pressure is necessary to prevent further deterioration of renal function secondary to vascular changes produced by the hypertension itself.

Unilateral renal disease

A small proportion of cases of hypertension are due to unilateral renal disease. The main causes are:
● Unilateral renal artery stenosis due to fibromuscular hyperplasia or atheroma
● Unilateral reflux nephropathy (atrophic pyelonephritis)

Mechanism of hypertension
Unilateral renal ischaemia results in a reduction in the pressure in afferent glomerular arterioles. This leads to an increase in the production and release of renin from the juxtaglomerular apparatus (see p. 739).

INVESTIGATION

It is impractical to screen all patients with hypertension for unilateral renal disease. Those patients who do require investigation are described on p. 739.

In renal artery stenosis excretion urography shows a small kidney and a delayed and denser pyelogram on the side of the stenosis. This is a consequence of reduced renal perfusion pressure and prolonged nephron transit time on the side of the stenosis; salt and water reabsorption in the proximal tubule is increased. As a result the contrast medium is more concentrated on the side of the stenosis.

Significant stenoses may be present in the absence of urographic abnormality and can only be excluded by either selective renal arteriography or digital vascular imaging techniques.

Prediction of results of surgery
Divided renal function studies employing ureteric catheterization are now seldom used. Nevertheless, urine from the ischaemic kidney is more concentrated but has a lower sodium concentration than urine from the contralateral kidney. Inulin, creatinine and para-aminohippuric acid (PAH) clearances are decreased on the ischaemic side. The finding of significant ischaemia in one kidney with normal function in the contralateral kidney indicates a good prognosis after surgery.

The concentration of renin can be measured in each renal vein. If the ratio of renal vein renin concentration between the ischaemic and the contralateral kidney exceeds 1.6, correction of the stenosis is likely to be beneficial.

No single test or combination of tests predicts with complete accuracy the results of surgery in renal artery stenosis.

In patients with unilateral atrophic pyelonephritis, prediction of the outcome of nephrectomy is currently not possible. The case for nephrectomy is strengthened if isotope renography demonstrates the abnormal kidney to be making an insignificant contribution to overall excretory function, particularly if the patient is young and medical treatment has proved unsatisfactory.

TREATMENT

Treatment options in renal artery stenosis include transluminal angioplasty to dilate the stenotic lesion, reconstructive vascular surgery and nephrectomy. With good selection of patients more than 50% are cured or improved by intervention.

About one-third of patients with unilateral atrophic pyelonephritis benefit from nephrectomy.

Calculi and nephrocalcinosis

RENAL AND VESICAL CALCULI

Approximately 2% of the population in the UK have a urinary tract stone at any given time. A much higher prevalence of stone disease has been recorded elsewhere, notably in the Middle East. In the Western World, most stones occur in the upper urinary tract.

The incidence of bladder stones has declined in the UK since the eighteenth and nineteenth centuries, whereas in some Third World countries they are still common.

Most stones are composed of calcium oxalate and phosphate; these are commoner in men. Mixed infective stones, which account for about 20% of all calculi, are twice as common in women as in men. The overall male/female ratio of stone disease is 2:1.

Stone disease is frequently a recurrent problem. More than 50% of patients with a calculus will have formed a further stone or stones within 10 years. The risk of recurrence increases if a metabolic or other abnormality predisposing to stone formation is present and is not modified by treatment.

AETIOLOGY

It is in a sense surprising that stones are not universal since some constituents of urine are at times present in concentrations that exceed their maximum solubility in water. The presence of inhibitors of crystal formation in normal urine appears to be of importance in preventing stones.

Most stone-formers have no detectable metabolic defect, although microscopy of warm, freshly passed urine reveals both more and larger calcium oxalate crystals than are found in normal subjects. Factors predisposing to stone formation in these so-called 'idiopathic stone formers' are:
- A chemical composition of urine which favours stone crystallization
- The production of a concentrated urine as a consequence of dehydration associated with life in a hot climate or work in a hot environment
- Impairment of inhibitors which prevent crystallization in normal urine

Recognized causes of stone formation are listed in Table 9.14.

Table 9.14 Causes of urinary tract stone formation.

Dehydration
Hypercalcaemia
Hypercalciuria
Hyperoxaluria
Hyperuricaemia and hyperuricosuria
Infection
Cystinuria
Renal tubular acidosis
Primary renal disease (polycystic kidneys, medullary sponge kidneys)

Hypercalcaemia
If the GFR is normal, hypercalcaemia inevitably leads to hypercalciuria. The common causes of hypercalcaemia leading to stone formation are:
- Primary hyperparathyroidism
- Vitamin D ingestion
- Sarcoidosis

Of these, primary hyperparathyroidism (see p. 737) is the commonest cause of stones.

Hypercalciuria
This is by far the commonest metabolic abnormality detected in calcium stone-formers.

Approximately 8% of men excrete in excess of 7.5 mmol calcium per 24 h. Calcium stone formation is commoner in this group, but as most patients do not form stones the definition of 'pathological' hypercalciuria is arbitrary. A reasonable definition of pathological hypercalciuria is excretion of more than 7.5 mmol calcium per 24 h in males and more than 6.25 mmol calcium per 24 h in women.

Causes of hypercalciuria are:
- Hypercalcaemia
- An excessive dietary intake of calcium
- Excessive resorption of calcium from the skeleton, such as occurs with prolonged immobilization or weightlessness
- Idiopathic hypercalciuria

The majority of patients with idiopathic hypercalciuria can be shown to have increased absorption of calcium from the gut. Dietary calcium restriction in this group markedly reduces urinary calcium excretion. However, a proportion of these patients appear to have a renal tubular calcium leak with secondary compensatory hyperabsorption of calcium from the gut. Calcium restriction has less effect on urinary calcium excretion in this group.

Hyperoxaluria
Two inborn errors of glyoxalate metabolism that cause increased endogenous oxalate biosynthesis are known. Both are inherited in an autosomal recessive manner. In type I (primary hyperoxaluria) there is increased glycocholate excretion as well as hyperoxaluria. In type II L-glycerate excretion is increased. In both types, calcium oxalate stone formation occurs.

The prognosis is poor owing to widespread calcium oxalate crystal deposition in the kidneys. Renal failure typically develops in the late teens or early twenties.

Much commoner causes of mild hyperoxaluria are:
- Excess ingestion of high oxalate-containing food, such as spinach, rhubarb and tea
- Dietary calcium restriction, with compensatory increased absorption of oxalate
- Gastrointestinal disease, such as Crohn's disease, usually with an intestinal resection and/or an

ileostomy with associated increased absorption of oxalate from the gut. Dehydration secondary to fluid loss from the gut also plays a part in stone formation.

Hyperuricaemia and hyperuricosuria

Uric acid stones account for 3–5% of all stones in the UK, but in Israel the proportion is as high as 40%.

Uric acid is the end-point of purine metabolism. Hyperuricaemia (see p. 352) can occur as a primary defect, in idiopathic gout, and as a secondary consequence of increased cell turnover, e.g. in myeloproliferative disorders. Increased uric acid excretion occurs in these conditions, and stones will develop in some patients. Some uric acid stone formers have hyperuricosuria without hyperuricaemia.

Dehydration alone may also cause uric acid stones to form. Patients with ileostomies are at particular risk both from dehydration and from the fact that loss of bicarbonate from gastrointestinal secretions results in the production of an acid urine (uric acid is more soluble in an alkaline than an acid medium).

Some patients with calcium stones also have hyperuricaemia and/or hyperuricaciduria; it is believed the calcium salts precipitate upon an initial nidus of uric acid in such patients.

Urinary tract infection

Mixed infective stones are composed of magnesium ammonium phosphate together with variable amounts of calcium. Such stones are often large, forming a cast of the collecting system (staghorn calculus). They are believed to form as a result of infection of the urinary tract with organisms such as *Proteus mirabilis* which hydrolyse urea, with formation of the strong base ammonium hydroxide.

$$NH_2 \diagdown C{=}O + HOH \rightleftharpoons 2NH_3 + CO_2$$
$$NH_2 \diagup$$

$$NH_3 + HOH \rightleftharpoons NH_4OH \rightleftharpoons NH_4^+ + OH^-$$

The availability of ammonium ions and the alkalinity of the urine favour stone formation. An increased amount of mucoprotein resulting from infection also creates an organic matrix on which stone formation can occur.

Cystinuria

Cystinuria results in the formation of cystine stones. About 1% of all stones are composed of cystine.

Primary renal diseases

There is a moderate increase in prevalence of stone disease in patients with polycystic renal disease (see p. 424).

Medullary sponge kidney is another primary renal disorder associated with stones. In this congenital (though not inherited) condition there is dilatation of the collecting ducts with associated stasis and calcification (Fig. 9.20). Approximately 20% of these patients have hypercalciuria and a similar proportion have a renal tubular acidification defect.

Aetiology of bladder stones

Bladder stones are endemic in some Third World countries. The cause of this is unknown but dietary factors are probably important.

Stones forming in the bladder do so as a result of:
- Bladder outflow obstruction, e.g. urethral stricture, neuropathic bladder, prostatic obstruction
- The presence of a foreign body, e.g. catheters, non-absorbable sutures

(a)

(b)

Fig. 9.20 Medullary sponge kidney. (a) Plain film showing 'spotty' calcification in the renal areas. (b) After injection of contrast, the calcification is shown to be small calculi in the papillary zones.

Significant bacteriuria is usually found in patients with bladder stones.

Some stones found in the bladder have been passed down from the upper urinary tract.

PATHOLOGY

Stones may be single or multiple and vary enormously in size from sand-like minute particles to staghorn calculi or large stone concretions in the bladder. They may be located within the renal parenchyma or within the collecting system. Pressure necrosis from a large calculus may cause direct damage to the renal parenchyma and stones regularly cause obstruction, leading to hydronephrosis. They may ulcerate through the wall of the collecting system, including the ureter. A combination of obstruction and infection accelerates damage to the kidney.

CLINICAL FEATURES

Most people with urinary tract calculi are asymptomatic. Pain is the commonest symptom and may be sharp or dull, constant, intermittent or colicky.

When urinary tract obstruction is present measures which increase urine volume, such as copious fluid intake or diuretics, including alcohol, make the pain worse. Physical exertion may cause mobile calculi to move, precipitating pain and, occasionally, haematuria. Calyceal colic, i.e. pain resulting from movement of stones within the calyces, is a real entity, but whether small calyceal calculi are the cause of backache or not is often difficult to decide.

Ureteric colic occurs when a stone enters the ureter and either obstructs it or causes spasm during its passage down the ureter (Fig.9.21). This is one of the most severe pains known. Radiation from the flank to the iliac fossa and testis or labia in the distribution of the first lumbar nerve root is common.

Pallor, sweating and vomiting often occur and the patient is restless, tending to assume a variety of positions in an unsuccessful attempt to obtain relief from the pain. Haematuria often occurs. Untreated, the pain of ureteric colic typically subsides after a few hours.

When urinary tract obstruction and infection are present the features of acute pyelonephritis or of a gram-negative septicaemia may dominate the clinical picture.

Vesical calculi associated with bladder bacteriuria may present with frequency, dysuria and haematuria; severe introital or perineal pain may occur if trigonitis is present. A calculus at the bladder neck or an obstruction in the urethra may cause bladder outflow obstruction, resulting in anuria and painful bladder distension.

Physical examination should include a search for corneal or conjunctival calcification, gouty tophi and arthritis and features of sarcoidosis.

DIAGNOSIS AND INVESTIGATION

A history of possible aetiological factors should be obtained, including:
- Occupation and residence in hot countries likely to be associated with dehydration
- A history of vitamin D consumption
- Gouty arthritis

Calcified papillae may mimic ordinary calculi so that causes of papillary necrosis such as analgesic abuse should be considered.

Investigations should include a mid-stream specimen of urine for culture and measurement of the blood urea and electrolytes and serum creatinine and calcium levels.

Plain abdominal x-ray, renal tomography and excretion urography are the mainstay of diagnosis.

Pure uric acid stones are radiolucent. Mixed infective stones in which organic matrix predomin-

Fig. 9.21 X-ray showing acute left ureteric obstruction. Note the increased density of the nephrogram and the absence of a pyelogram on the left side 15 min after contrast injection. From Weatherall DJ, Ledingham JGG & Warrell DA (eds) (1987) *Oxford Textbook of Medicine*, 2nd edn. Oxford: Oxford University Press. With permission.

(a)   (b)

Fig. 9.22 X-rays showing a calculus. (a) The calculus is overlying bone on the left (easily missed). (b) The same patient 1 week later. The calculus has descended and is easily seen in the pelvis of the left side (arrowed).

ates are barely radiopaque. Calcium-containing and cystine stones are radiopaque. Calculi overlying bone are easily missed (Fig. 9.22). Staghorn calculi may be missed on excretion urography (Fig.9.23). Uric acid stones may present as a filling defect after injection of contrast medium (Fig.9.24). Such stones are readily seen on CT scanning (Fig. 9.25).

Excretion urography is carried out during the episode of pain; a normal urogram excludes the diagnosis of pain due to calculous disease. The uro-

Fig. 9.24 An excretion urogram showing a lucent filling defect (uric acid stone) in the left renal pelvis. The differential diagnosis includes a sloughed papilla and a transitional cell tumour.

PLAIN FILM   AFTER CONTRAST

Fig. 9.23 Staghorn calculus. X-ray appearances before and after contrast on the right side are identical owing to a staghorn calculus in a non-functioning right kidney. A plain film may be confused with those taken after contrast injection.

graphic appearances in a patient with acute left ureteric obstruction are shown in Fig. 9.21.

The urine of the patient should be sieved through muslin to trap any calculi passed for chemical analysis.

Fig. 9.25 CT scan showing a uric acid stone, which appears as a bright white lesion in the left kidney.

MANAGEMENT

Adequate analgesia should be given, e.g. morphine 15–30 mg i.m. repeated as necessary. A high fluid intake, if this can be tolerated, may help the stone to pass down the urinary tract.

Stones less than 0.5 cm in diameter usually pass spontaneously and can be left. Stones greater than 1 cm in diameter usually require surgery.

Persistent pain, frequent bouts of severe pain, or anuria are indications for operation. Surgery is also required if a stone has not moved for several weeks and is causing obstruction. Immediate action is required if complete or partial obstruction plus infection is present.

Stones may be removed by a cutting operation:
- Nephrolithotomy for renal calculi
- Pyelolithotomy for stones in the renal pelvis
- Ureterolithotomy for ureteric stones

Cutting operations can now be avoided by using either percutaneous nephrolithotomy or extra-corporeal shock-wave lithotripsy. In the former, stones in the calyces and renal pelvis are removed by creating a percutaneous track down to the collecting system followed by endoscopic removal along this track. In the latter, shock waves generated under water are focused upon the renal calculi, causing them to fragment. Most of the fragments then pass spontaneously via the urethra. Fragments which do not pass can be removed percutaneously.

Ureteric stones may be removed endoscopically or may be pushed up into the upper urinary tract to allow percutaneous nephrolithotomy or extra-corporeal shock-wave lithotripsy.

Large renal stones need to be reduced in bulk by percutaneous means before lithotripsy can be expected to be successful. Some staghorn calculi are best dealt with by open operation.

Bladder stones can be removed endoscopically. They may be dealt with by direct electrohydraulic disintegration at cystoscopy or may be gripped in a lithotrite and crushed, the stone fragments then being washed out. Open cystotomy is required for very large bladder stones.

INVESTIGATING THE CAUSE OF STONE FORMATION

In an elderly patient who has had a single episode with one stone, further investigation is not required. Younger patients and those with recurrent stone formation require detailed investigation.
- An excretion urogram is necessary to define the presence of a primary renal disease predisposing to stone formation.
- Significant bacteriuria may indicate mixed infective stone formation but relapsing bacteriuria may be a consequence of stone formation rather than the original cause.
- Chemical analysis of any stone passed may be of great value and may be all that is required to make a diagnosis of cystinuria or uric acid stone formation.
- Serum calcium concentration should be estimated and corrected for serum albumin concentration (see p. 734). Hypercalcaemia, if present, should be investigated further (see p. 737).
- Serum urate concentration is often, but not invariably, elevated in uric acid stone formers.
- A screening test for cystinuria should be carried out by adding sodium nitroprusside to a random unacidified urine sample; a purple colour indicates that cystinuria may be present. Urine chromatography is required to define the diagnosis precisely.
- Urinary calcium, oxalate and uric acid output should be measured in two consecutive carefully collected 24-h urine samples. After withdrawing aliquots for estimation of uric acid, it is necessary to add acid to the urine in order to prevent crystallization of calcium salts upon the walls of the collection vessel, which would give falsely low results for urinary calcium and oxalate.
- Plasma bicarbonate is low in renal tubular acidosis. The finding of a urine pH in excess of 5.3 in the face of metabolic acidosis is diagnostic of this condition (see p. 445).

PROPHYLAXIS

The age of the patient and the severity of the problem affect both the need for and the type of prophylaxis.

Idiopathic stone formers
Where no metabolic abnormality is present, the mainstay of prevention is maintenance of a high intake of fluid throughout the day and night. The aim should be to ensure a daily urine volume of 2–2.5 l, which requires a fluid intake in excess of this, substantially so in the case of those who live in hot countries or work in a hot environment. A large glass of water should be drunk before retiring for the night and on waking during the night if this occurs. Special dietary measures are not warranted, although avoidance of excessive consumption of calcium-rich dairy products seems sensible.

Idiopathic hypercalciuria

Dietary calcium restriction is the first measure to be taken; particular emphasis is placed on the restriction of milk, cheese, and white bread if this is fortified (as it is in the UK) with calcium and vitamin D. Vitamin D supplements should be avoided. Dietary calcium restriction results in hyperabsorption of oxalate and foods containing large amounts of oxalate should also be limited. The advice of a dietitian is invaluable.

A high fluid intake should be advised as for idiopathic stone formers. Patients who live in a hard water area may benefit from drinking softened water.

If hypercalciuria persists and stone formation continues, a thiazide, e.g. bendrofluazide 5 or 10 mg each morning, or sodium cellulose phosphate is used. The former reduces urinary calcium excretion by a direct effect upon the renal tubule and the latter binds calcium in the gut, thereby reducing calcium absorption. Bendrofluazide occasionally causes side-effects but is convenient to take and is inexpensive. Cellulose phosphate is not absorbed. Side-effects are mild diarrhoea and the consequences of absorption of sodium in patients with, for example, heart failure. For most patients, thiazide prophylaxis taken once daily proves more practicable than ingestion of sodium cellulose phosphate two or three times daily.

Mixed infective stones

Recurrent stones should be prevented by maintenance of a high fluid intake and meticulous control of bacteriuria. This will require long-term follow-up and may demand the use of long-term low-dose prophylactic antibacterial agents.

Uric acid stones

Dietary measures are probably of little value and are difficult to implement. Effective prevention can be achieved by the long-term use of the xanthine oxidase inhibitor allopurinol to maintain the serum urate and urinary uric acid excretion in the normal range. A high fluid intake should also be maintained. Uric acid is more soluble at alkaline pH and long-term sodium bicarbonate supplementation to maintain an alkaline urine is an alternative approach in those few patients unable to take allopurinol. However, alkalinization of the urine facilitates precipitation of calcium oxalate and phosphate.

Cystine stones

These can be prevented and indeed will dissolve slowly if there is obsessional attention to maintenance of a high fluid intake—5 l of water must be drunk each 24 h, and the patient must wake twice during the night to ingest 500 ml or more of water. Many patients cannot tolerate this regimen. An alternative, though potentially more troublesome, option is the long-term use of the chelating agent penicillamine; this causes cystine to be converted to the more soluble penicillamine–cysteine complex. Side-effects include drug rashes, blood dyscrasias and immune complex mediated glomerulonephritis and are by no means uncommon. In addition, the drug is expensive. It is, however, especially effective in promoting dissolution of cystine stones already present.

NEPHROCALCINOSIS

The term nephrocalcinosis means diffuse renal parenchymal calcification detectable radiologically (Fig. 9.26). The condition is typically painless. Hypertension and renal impairment commonly occur.

The main causes of nephrocalcinosis are listed in Table 9.15.

Dystrophic calcification occurs following renal cortical necrosis. In hypercalcaemia and hyper-

Fig. 9.26 An x-ray of nephrocalcinosis.

Table 9.15 Common causes of nephrocalcinosis.

Mainly cortical (rare)
Renal cortical necrosis (tram-line calcification)

Mainly medullary
Hypercalcaemia (primary hyperparathyroidism, hypervitaminosis D, sarcoidosis)
Renal tubular acidosis (inherited and acquired)
Primary hyperoxaluria
Medullary sponge kidney

oxaluria, deposition of calcium oxalate results from the high concentration of calcium and oxalate within the kidney.

In renal tubular acidosis (see p. 445) failure of urinary acidification and a reduction in urinary citrate excretion both favour calcium phosphate and oxalate precipitation, since precipitation occurs more readily in an alkaline medium and the calcium-chelating action of urinary citrate is reduced.

Treatment and prevention of nephrocalcinosis consists of treatment of the cause.

Urinary tract obstruction

The urinary tract may be obstructed at any point between the kidney and the urethral meatus. This results in dilatation of the tract above the obstruction. Dilatation of the renal pelvis is known as hydronephrosis.

AETIOLOGY

Obstructing lesions may lie within the lumen, in the wall of the urinary tract, or outside the wall, causing obstruction by external pressure. The major causes of obstruction are shown in Table 9.16. Overall the frequency is the same in men and women. However, in the elderly, urinary tract obstruction is more common in men owing to the frequency of bladder outflow obstruction.

PATHOPHYSIOLOGY

Obstruction with continuing urine formation results in:
- Progressive rise in intraluminal pressure
- Dilatation proximal to the site of obstruction
- Compression and thinning of the renal parenchyma, eventually reducing it to a thin rim and resulting in a decrease in the size of the kidney

CLINICAL FEATURES

Symptoms
Upper tract obstruction. Loin pain occurs and can be dull or sharp, constant or intermittent. It may be provoked by measures which increase urine volume and hence distension of the collecting system, such as a high fluid intake or diuretics, including alcohol.

Complete anuria is strongly suggestive of complete bilateral obstruction or complete obstruction of a single kidney.

Conversely, polyuria may occur in partial obstruction owing to impairment of renal tubular concentrating capacity. Intermittent anuria and

Table 9.16 Causes of urinary tract obstruction.

Within the lumen
Calculus
Blood clot
Sloughed papilla (diabetes; analgesic abuse; sickle cell disease or trait)
Tumour of renal pelvis or ureter
Bladder tumour
Within the wall
Pelvi-ureteric neuromuscular dysfunction (congenital, 10% bilateral)
Ureteric stricture (tuberculosis, especially after treatment; calculus; after surgery)
Uretero-vesical stricture (congenital; ureterocele; calculus; schistosomiasis)
Congenital megaureter
Congenital bladder neck obstruction
Neuropathic bladder
Urethral stricture (calculus; gonococcal; after instrumentation)
Congenital urethral valve
Pin-hole meatus
Pressure from outside
Pelvi-ureteric compression (bands; aberrant vessels)
Tumours (e.g. retroperitoneal tumour or glands, carcinoma of colon, diverticulitis, aortic aneurysm)
Retroperitoneal fibrosis
Accidental ligation of ureter
Retrocaval ureter (right-sided obstruction)
Prostatic obstruction
Tumours in pelvis (e.g. carcinoma of cervix)
Phimosis

polyuria indicates intermittent complete obstruction.

Infection complicating the obstruction may give rise to malaise, fever and septicaemia.

Bladder outflow obstruction. Symptoms may be minimal. Hesitancy, narrowing and diminished force of the urinary stream, terminal dribbling and a sense of incomplete bladder emptying are typical features. The frequent passage of small volumes of urine occurs if a large volume of residual urine remains in the bladder after urination. Incontinence of such small volumes of urine is known as 'overflow incontinence' or 'retention with overflow'.

Infection commonly occurs, causing increased frequency, urgency, urge incontinence, dysuria and the passage of cloudy smelly urine. It may precipitate acute retention.

Signs
Loin tenderness may be present. An enlarged hydronephrotic kidney may be palpable.

In acute or chronic retention the enlarged bladder may be felt or percussed.

Examination of the genitalia, rectum and vagina are essential since prostatic obstruction and pelvic malignancy are common causes of urinary tract obstruction. However, the apparent size of the prostate on digital examination is a poor guide to the presence of prostatic obstruction.

INVESTIGATION

Routine blood and biochemical investigations may be abnormal, e.g. there may be a raised blood urea or serum creatinine, hyperkalaemia, anaemia of chronic disease or blood in the urine, but the diagnosis of obstruction cannot be made on these tests alone and further investigations must be performed.

Ultrasonography

Diagnostic ultrasound is a reliable means of ruling out upper urinary tract dilatation. Ultrasound cannot distinguish a baggy, low-pressure unobstructed system from a tense, high-pressure obstructed one, so that false-positive scans are seen. However, a normal scan does rule out urinary tract obstruction.

Isotopic scans

Radioactive iodine-labelled hippuran is injected intravenously. The uptake, concentration and excretion of the radioactive compound by the kidney is assessed by scintillation detectors placed over the kidneys. In obstruction, as well as with a baggy, dilated but unobstructed collecting system, the excretory phase of the renogram is delayed.

Dynamic renal scintigraphy allows a distinction to be made between retention of isotope within the renal pelvis and prolongation of glomerular filtrate flow down the nephron; the latter is known as obstructive nephropathy.

With computer-assisted subtraction of blood background radioactivity, the absence of uptake of hippuran can be detected and indicates renal damage sufficiently severe to render correction of the obstruction unprofitable. Relative renal blood flow rates may similarly be deduced by background subtraction renography and this information may be helpful in deciding whether or not to operate upon a kidney damaged by long-standing obstruction.

Excretion urography

Excretion urography remains the most widely used investigation in the diagnosis of urinary tract obstruction. Properly carried out, urography can usually exclude obstruction even in the presence of severe renal failure, provided that a high dose of contrast medium, renal tomography and, if necessary, delayed films are employed.

A plain film is necessary to detect calcification. However, calculi overlying bone are easily missed.

In recent unilateral obstruction, the affected kidney is enlarged and smooth in outline. The nephrogram is delayed due to a reduction in the GFR. The calyces and pelvis fill with contrast medium later than on the normal side.

In time the nephrogram on the affected side becomes denser than normal, owing to the prolonged nephron transit time which allows greater than normal concentration of contrast medium within the tubules (this also occurs in unilateral renal artery stenosis). Later, the site of obstruction may be seen, with dilatation of the system proximal to the level of the block (Fig. 9.27).

A full-length film should be taken after an attempt at bladder emptying by the patient. Complete emptying indicates either that no obstruction to bladder outflow exists or that intravesical pressure can be raised sufficiently to overcome it. Apparent bladder outflow impairment may be the result of nervousness or embarrassment on the part of the patient or failure to carry out the x-ray before the bladder has refilled with contrast medium from above, or may be due to an atonic but non-obstructed bladder. Vesico-ureteric reflux can result in contrast medium returning to the bladder from above, giving the appearance of a partially full bladder.

Antegrade pyelography and ureterography

Percutaneous introduction of contrast medium directly into the renal pelvis or a calyx shows the pelvicalyceal system and ureter. This is being increasingly used to define the site and cause of obstruction. It can be combined with drainage of the collecting system by percutaneous needle nephrostomy.

Retrograde ureterography

Cystoscopy and catheterization of one or both ureters from below, followed by retrograde injection of contrast medium, is indicated if antegrade examination cannot be carried out or if there is the possibility of dealing with ureteric obstruction from below at the time of examination. The technique carries the risk of introducing infection into an obstructed urinary tract.

In obstruction due to neuromuscular dysfunction at the pelviureteric junction or retroperitoneal fibrosis, the collecting system may fill normally from below.

Cystoscopy, urethroscopy and urethrography

Obstructing lesions within the bladder and urethra can be seen directly by endoscopic examination.

Urethrography involves introducing contrast medium into the bladder by catheterization or suprapubic bladder puncture, and taking x-ray films during voiding to show obstructing lesions in the urethra. It is of particular value in the diagnosis of urethral valves and strictures.

Pressure-flow studies

Pressure changes within the bladder during filling and emptying can be recorded. Demonstration that a

Fig. 9.27 An x-ray taken 24 h after injection of contrast, showing a delayed nephrogram and pyelogram on the left side and dilatation of the system to the level of the block. By this time contrast medium has disappeared from the normal right side. From Weatherall DJ, Ledingham JGG & Warrell DA (eds) (1987) *Oxford Textbook of Medicine*, 2nd edn. Oxford: Oxford University Press. With permission.

high voiding pressure is required to maintain urine flow is indicative of bladder outflow obstruction. This may be combined with video cystography and urethrography to define the site of obstruction.

Normally, while the bladder is being filled there is only a small pressure rise before the voluntary initiation of urination. Uninhibited contractions of the detrusor muscle during filling may be seen in upper motor neurone bladder neuropathy, such as occurs in multiple sclerosis. Less commonly, a neuropathic bladder may be 'hypotonic', readily accepting large volumes of fluid before the initiation of weak contractions at a low intravesical pressure. A common cause of such lower motor neurone bladder neuropathy is diabetes mellitus.

Pressure-flow and video studies may enable a logical decision to be taken as to whether surgery to relieve bladder outflow impairment should be carried out.

TREATMENT

Aims
Treatment involves:
● Relieving the obstruction
● Treating the underlying cause
● Preventing and treating infection

The ultimate aim of treatment is to relieve symptoms and to preserve renal function.

Temporary external drainage of urine by nephrostomy may be valuable, as this allows time for further investigation when the site and nature of the obstructing lesion is uncertain and doubt exists as to the viability of the obstructed kidney, or when immediate definitive surgery would be hazardous.

Recent, complete upper urinary tract obstruction demands urgent relief to preserve kidney function, particularly if infection is present.

In contrast, with partial urinary tract obstruction, particularly if spontaneous relief is expected, e.g. by passage of a calculus, there is no immediate urgency.

Surgical management
This depends on the cause of the obstruction (see below). Dialysis may be required in the ill patient prior to surgery.

Nephrectomy or nephroureterectomy is justified when obstruction is due to malignant disease or when it is judged that no worthwhile amount of renal excretory function will be conserved by, or will return after, relief of obstruction.

Permanent urinary diversion is required when the obstruction cannot be relieved; in such cases malignant disease is usually present. Ureteric anastomosis to an ileal conduit opening on to the abdominal wall is often a satisfactory method of diversion. In some patients, obstruction is best relieved by the insertion of indwelling catheters or stents into the ureter. An obstruction high in the urinary tract may require a permanent nephrostomy.

In obstruction due to untreatable malignant disease it is wise to consider carefully whether urinary diversion is justified since this may exchange a pain-free death from renal failure for a painful one with malignant invasion of bones or nerves.

Diuresis usually follows relief of obstruction at any site in the urinary tract. Massive diuresis may occur due to previous sodium and water overload and the osmotic effect of retained solutes combined with a defective renal tubular reabsorptive capacity (as in the diuretic phase of recovering acute tubular necrosis). This diuresis is usually self-limiting, but a minority of patients will develop severe sodium,

water and potassium depletion requiring appropriate intravenous replacement. In milder cases oral salt and potassium supplements together with a high water intake are sufficient.

Specific causes of obstruction

Calculi
These are discussed on p. 398.

Pelvi-ureteric junction obstruction (Fig. 9.28)
This appears to result from a functional disturbance in peristalsis of the collecting system in the absence of mechanical obstruction. Typically a circular inelastic ring of collagen tissue is present at the pelvi-ureteric junction. Surgical attempts at correction of the obstruction by open or percutaneous pyeloplasty should be limited to patients with recurrent loin pain and those in whom serial excretion urography, back-

Fig. 9.28 An x-ray showing right pelvi-ureteric junction obstruction. From Weatherall DJ, Ledingham JGG & Warrell DA (eds) (1987) *Oxford Textbook of Medicine*, 2nd edn. Oxford: Oxford University Press. With permission.

ground-subtraction isotope renography or measurements of GFR indicate progressive kidney damage. Nephrectomy to remove the risk of developing pyonephrosis and septicaemia is indicated if long-standing obstruction has destroyed kidney function.

Obstructive megaureter
This childhood condition may only become evident in adult life. It results from the presence of a region of defective peristalsis at the lower end of the ureter adjacent to the ureterovesical junction. The condition is commoner in males. It presents with urinary tract infection, flank pain or haematuria. The diagnosis is made on excretion urography or, if necessary, ascending ureterography. Excision of the abnormal portion of ureter with reimplantation into the bladder is always indicated in children, and is indicated in adults when the condition is associated with evidence of progressive deterioration in renal function, bacteriuria which cannot be controlled by medical means or recurrent stone formation.

Retroperitoneal fibrosis
In this condition the ureters become embedded in dense retroperitoneal fibrous tissue with resultant unilateral or bilateral obstruction. The condition may extend from the level of the second lumbar vertebra to the pelvic brim. The incidence of the condition in men is three times that in women. The majority of cases are of unknown aetiology; it has been suggested that the fundamental problem is immunologically mediated peri-aortitis. Recognized associations are with retroperitoneal lymphoma, carcinoma of the bladder or colon, abdominal aortic aneurysm and prolonged exposure to the drug methysergide.

Malaise, back pain, normochromic anaemia, uraemia and a raised ESR are typical features. Excretion urography shows bilateral but usually asymmetrical obstruction to the ureter commencing at the level of the pelvic brim. A peri-aortic mass may be seen on a CT scan.

Obstruction is relieved surgically by ureterolysis. Biopsy should be performed at operation to determine whether or not there is an underlying lymphoma or carcinoma. Corticosteroids are of benefit, and in bilateral obstruction in frail patients it may be best to free only one ureter and to rely upon steroid therapy to induce regression of fibrous tissue on the contralateral side, since bilateral ureterolysis is a major operation. In some patients, surgery alone or steroid therapy alone may suffice, but in the majority both surgery and subsequent corticosteroid therapy appear to be necessary.

Response to treatment and disease activity are assessed by serial measurements of ESR and GFR supplemented by isotopic and imaging techniques including CT scanning. The latter method enables the size of the retroperitoneal mass to be assessed. Relapse after withdrawal of steroid therapy may

occur and treatment may need to be continued for years. Long-term follow-up is mandatory.

Benign prostatic hypertrophy
Benign prostatic hypertrophy is a common cause of urinary tract obstruction. It is described on p. 429.

Prognosis of urinary tract obstruction

The prognosis depends upon the cause and the stage at which obstruction is relieved. In obstruction, four factors influence the rate at which kidney damage occurs, its extent and the degree and rapidity of recovery of renal function after relief of obstruction. These are:
● Whether obstruction is partial or complete
● The duration of obstruction
● Whether or not infection occurs
● The site of obstruction

Complete obstruction for several weeks will lead to irreversible or only partially reversible kidney damage. If the duration of complete obstruction is several months, total irreversible destruction of the affected kidney will result.

Partial obstruction carries a better prognosis, depending upon its severity.

Bacterial infection coincident with obstruction rapidly increases kidney damage.

Obstruction at or below the bladder neck may induce hypertrophy and trabeculation of the bladder without a rise in pressure within the upper urinary tract, in which case the kidneys are protected from the effects of back-pressure.

Drugs and the kidney

Drug-induced impairment of renal function

Drug-induced impairment of excretory function may be pre-renal (resulting from impaired renal perfusion), renal (a consequence of renal parenchymal damage) or post-renal (resulting from urinary tract obstruction).

Pre-renal
Impaired perfusion of the kidneys can result from drugs which cause hypovolaemia and/or a decrease in cardiac output or from those which have a direct effect on renal blood flow, such as angiotensin-converting enzyme inhibitors.

Hypovolaemia can be caused by:
● Potent loop diuretics such as frusemide, especially in elderly patients
● Renal salt and water loss, e.g. from hypercalcaemia induced by vitamin D therapy

Cardiac decompensation due to beta-blockers is sometimes accompanied by impaired renal perfusion.

Renal
Several mechanisms of drug-induced renal damage exist and may coexist. These include:
- Acute tubular necrosis produced by direct nephrotoxicity. Examples include prolonged or excessive treatment with aminoglycosides (kanamycin, gentamicin, streptomycin), amphotericin B and cephaloridine, heavy metals or carbon tetrachloride. The combination of aminoglycosides or cephaloridine with frusemide is particularly nephrotoxic.
- Acute tubulo-interstitial nephritis with interstitial oedema and inflammatory cell infiltration. This cell-mediated hypersensitivity nephritis occurs with many drugs, including penicillins, particularly methicillin, sulphonamides and some NSAIDs. Papillary necrosis (Fig. 9.19) is seen.
- Chronic tubulo-interstitial nephritis due to drugs (see p. 395)
- Immune complex mediated glomerulonephritis. Examples include penicillamine.

Post-renal
Retroperitoneal fibrosis with urinary tract obstruction may result from the use of methysergide.

Use of drugs in patients with impaired renal function

Many aspects of drug handling are altered in patients with renal impairment.

Absorption. This may be unpredictable in uraemia as vomiting and confusion are frequently present.

Metabolism. Oxidative metabolism of drugs by the liver may be altered in uraemia. This is rarely of clinical significance.

The rate of drug metabolism by the kidney may be reduced as a result of:
- Reduced drug catabolism, e.g. of insulin
- Reduced conversion of a precursor to a more active metabolite, e.g. the conversion of 25-hydroxycholecalciferol to the more active 1,25-dihydroxycholecalciferol.

Protein binding. Many patients with renal disease are hypoproteinaemic. Reduced protein binding of a drug potentiates its activity and increases the potential for toxic side-effects. Measurement of the total plasma concentration of such a drug can give misleading results. For example, the serum concentration of phenytoin required to produce an anti-epileptic effect is much higher in normal individuals than in those with renal failure, since in the latter proportionately more drug is present in the free form.

Hydrogen ions, which are retained in renal failure, bind to receptors for acidic drugs such as sulphonamides, penicillin and salicylates, thus enhancing their potential for causing toxicity.

Volume of distribution. Salt and water overload or depletion may occur in patients with renal disease. This affects the concentration of drug obtained from a given dose.

End organ sensitivity. The renal response to drug treatment may be reduced in renal disease. For example, mild thiazide diuretics have little diuretic effect in patients with severe renal impairment.

Renal elimination. By far the most important problem in the use of drugs in renal failure concerns the reduced elimination of many drugs normally excreted by the kidneys.

Water-soluble drugs such as gentamicin which are poorly absorbed from the gut, typically given by injection and are not metabolized by the liver give rise to far more problems than lipid-soluble drugs such as propranolol which are well-absorbed and principally metabolized by the liver. Metabolites of lipid-soluble drugs, however, may themselves be water-soluble and potentially toxic.

Drugs causing uraemia by effects upon protein anabolism and catabolism
Tetracyclines, with the exception of doxycycline, have an anti-anabolic effect and as a result the concentration of nitrogenous waste products is increased. They may also cause impairment of GFR by a direct effect. Corticosteroids have a catabolic effect and so also increase the production of nitrogenous wastes. A patient with moderate impairment of renal function may therefore become severely uraemic if given tetracyclines or corticosteroid therapy.

Drugs and toxic agents causing specific renal tubular syndromes include mercury, lead, cadmium and vitamin D intoxication.

Problem patients
Particular problems are presented by patients in whom renal function is altering rapidly, such as those with recovering acute tubular necrosis and those on regular dialysis treatment. In addition, drugs may be removed by dialysis, which will affect the dosage required.

Safe prescribing in renal disease

Safe prescribing in renal failure demands knowledge of the clinical pharmacology of the drug and its metabolites in normal individuals and in uraemia. The clinician should ask the following questions when prescribing:

1 Is treatment mandatory?
   Unless it is, it should be withheld.

2 Can the drug reach its site of action?
   For example, there is little point in prescribing the urinary antiseptic nitrofurantoin in renal failure since bacteriostatic concentrations will not be attained in the urine.

3 Is the drug's metabolism altered in uraemia?

4 Will accumulation of the drug or metabolites occur?
   Even if accumulation is a potential problem owing to the drug or its metabolites being excreted by the kidneys, it is not necessarily an indication to change the drug given. The size of the loading dose will depend upon the size of the patient and is unrelated to renal function. Avoidance of toxic levels of drug in blood and tissues subsequently requires the administration of normal doses of the drug at longer time intervals than usual or smaller doses at the usual time intervals.

5 Is the drug toxic?

6 Are the effective concentrations of the drug in biological tissues similar to the toxic concentrations?

7 Should blood levels of the drug be measured?

8 Will the drug worsen the uraemic state by means other than nephrotoxicity, e.g. steroids, tetracycline?

9 Is the drug a sodium or potassium salt?
   These are potentially hazardous in uraemia.

Not surprisingly, adverse drug reactions are more than twice as common in renal failure as in normal individuals. Careful attention to the above and careful titration of the dose of drug employed should reduce this problem.

The dose may be titrated by:
● Observation of its clinical effect, e.g. hypotensive agents
● Early detection of toxic effects
● Measurement of drug levels in the blood, e.g. gentamicin levels

Renal failure

Renal impairment describes a reduction in renal excretory or regulatory function without elevation of the blood urea or serum creatinine. *Renal failure* or *uraemia* describe more severe functional impairment when blood urea and serum creatinine are elevated. The development of 'renal hypertension' can occur early in renal disease, but disturbances of endocrine or metabolic function are usually only seen in renal failure.

Acute renal failure (ARF) is the loss of renal function developing over days or a few weeks. *Chronic renal failure (CRF)* is the loss of function developing over a period of months or years.

Acute deterioration in function may occur on a background of known or unknown chronic renal failure and is known as 'acute-on-chronic' renal failure.

Causes of renal failure

Renal failure, whether acute or chronic, may be due to pre-renal, renal or post-renal causes or some combination of these:
● *Pre-renal* causes are a reduction in renal blood flow, for a variety of reasons, increased production of waste products, or both (Table 9.17).
● *Renal* causes are intrinsic diseases of the kidneys themselves. These can be subdivided into glomerular, tubulo-interstitial or vascular disease (Table 9.18)
● *Post-renal* causes are diseases leading to obstruction to urine outflow (obstructive nephropathy; Fig. 9.29).

Table 9.17 Pre-renal causes of renal failure.

Circulatory failure
Volume depletion with inadequate replacement
  Vomiting and diarrhoea
  Fistula drainage
  Polyuria (diuretics, diabetic ketoacidosis, post-obstruction)
Shock
  Haemorrhage
  Septicaemia
  Extensive burns
Cardiac failure
Severe liver failure (hepato-renal syndrome)
Renal artery obstruction

Increased production of waste products (urea)
Infection/tissue damage ⎫
Upper gastrointestinal bleeding ⎬ Uraemia unusual unless there is also failure of excretion
Steroid therapy ⎪
Tetracyclines ⎭

Table 9.18 Renal causes of renal failure.

Glomerular
Glomerulonephritis
  Primary
  Part of a systemic vasculitis (systemic lupus
    erythematosus, polyarteritis nodosa, Wegener's
    granulomatosis)
Diabetic nephropathy
Amyloidosis

Tubulo-interstitial
Acute tubular necrosis
  Shock
  Ischaemia/hypoxia
  Drugs
  Chemical poisons
Acute cortical necrosis
Acute and chronic tubulo-interstitial nephritis
Congenital/inherited
  Medullary cystic disease
  Polycystic disease

Vascular
Hypertensive nephrosclerosis
Polyarteritis
Atheroma kidney

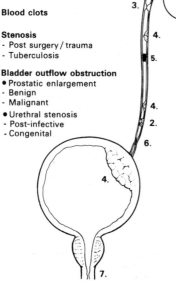

1. **Tubular blockage**
  - Hyperuricaemia
  - Myeloma protein

2. **Stones**

3. **Pelvi-ureteric obstruction**

4. **Tumour**

5. **Blood clots**

6. **Stenosis**
  - Post surgery / trauma
  - Tuberculosis

7. **Bladder outflow obstruction**
  • Prostatic enlargement
  - Benign
  - Malignant
  • Urethral stenosis
  - Post-infective
  - Congenital

Fig. 9.29 Post-renal causes of renal failure (obstructive nephropathy).

Acute or acute-on-chronic renal failure

Glomerulonephritis, acute tubulo-interstitial nephritis and obstructive nephropathy are the commonest causes of acute renal failure (ARF) in domiciliary practice, while acute volume depletion and acute tubular necrosis are more often seen in hospital practice.

The major functional and clinical sequelae of ARF are set out in Table 9.19.

In *domiciliary practice* ARF most often presents:
- As acute oliguria with or without haematuria
- With fluid retention (peripheral oedema or increasing breathlessness)
- With uraemia, giving rise to anorexia, nausea and vomiting

Occasionally the picture is dominated by symptoms of hypertension such as headaches and impaired vision. The clinical features may also be related to any systemic disease causing the renal failure. Examples include:
- The generalized rash and polyarthropathy occurring with drug hypersensitivity
- The muscle pain due to rhabdomyolysis occurring with heroin abuse
- The dyspnoea and haemoptysis occurring in Goodpasture's syndrome

In *hospital practice* ARF usually presents with increasing uraemia or with oliguria. It most often develops in a setting of severe illness in association with shock, recent major surgery or trauma, or sepsis.

Pre-renal causes are common from fluid loss due to:
- Diuretics
- Gut losses
- Polyuria following the relief of urinary obstruction

The various diseases causing *intrinsic* renal failure are discussed under their relevant sections. Special mention must at this point be made of acute tubular necrosis and acute cortical necrosis.

Acute tubular necrosis (ATN)

ATN is a condition in which there is acute tubular cell damage. It accounts for some 75% of cases of ARF seen in hospital practice. Known as the 'crush syndrome' in World War II, it was originally ascribed to a mixture of hypoxic damage to the metabolically active tubular cells during periods of shock and reduced renal blood flow plus tubular cell injury due to myoglobin released from crushed muscle. It is now known to occur in a variety of situations where there is reduced renal perfusion with or without major trauma or sepsis, as well as following the administration of certain drugs or exposure to chemical toxins.

Table 9.19 Major functional and clinical sequelae of acute renal failure.

Functional changes	Clinical sequelae
Loss of excretory function	
Retention of waste products (e.g. urea, creatinine, phosphate)	Uraemic symptoms (anorexia, nausea, vomiting) Bleeding tendency Impaired resistance to infection Reduced wound healing
Retention of drugs	Drug toxicity
Loss of regulatory function	
Retention of sodium chloride and water	Oedema (peripheral, pulmonary, cerebral) Hypertension
Retention of potassium	Cardiac arrhythmias
Retention of fixed acid	Acidotic breathing Arrhythmia in patients with ischaemic heart disease

ATN is characterized by acute, usually oliguric, potentially reversible renal failure. The oliguria is due to a variable combination of tubular cell necrosis, tubular obstruction caused by cell debris and, possibly most importantly, reduced cortical perfusion due to arteriolar vasoconstriction. Urine output decreases over 1–5 days to severe oliguria (< 300 ml urine per day). Urine osmolality is low (< 350 mosmol·kg^{-1}). There is commonly mild proteinuria on Stix testing and microscopy shows granular or tubular cell casts. The urine/plasma creatinine concentration ratio is usually less than 20 and the urinary sodium concentration more than 50 mmol·l^{-1}. Serial measurement shows a rise in blood urea and serum creatinine and, in oliguric patients with tissue injury, there may be a rapid rise in serum potassium.

Symptoms and signs of uraemia and fluid overload are often dominated by those of the causal condition, e.g. major trauma or septicaemia. Occasionally urine output is maintained (non-oliguric ATN), the dominant features being progressive moderate uraemia. Hyperkalaemia and fluid overload are less likely to occur in this situation.

Acute cortical necrosis
Acute cortical necrosis may be considered a more extreme form of ATN due to more severe and prolonged ischaemia. It mainly occurs in association with abruptio placentae, but it also occurs occasionally (1–2%) as a result of other circumstances that may cause ATN. It is characterized by extensive necrosis of the cortical tissue and acute oliguric renal failure. There is little potential for recovery; limited recovery of function, depending on subcapsular or juxtamedullary nephrons, may be achieved, but many cases require permanent renal replacement therapy. The diagnosis of acute cortical necrosis is usually suspected if there is a history of abruptio placentae or if there is failure to recover renal function after 30 days of suspected ATN. It can be confirmed by renal biopsy. Occasionally x-ray evidence of linear cortical calcification may develop after 4–8 weeks.

HISTORY

The history which may be taken from the patient or his relatives, is primarily aimed at identifying possible pre-renal (Table 9.17), renal (Table 9.18) or post-renal causes (Fig. 9.29) of renal failure. In hospital patients careful review of input–output charts and serial weight measurements can be invaluable. Intrinsic renal disease may be indicated by a history suggestive of previous renal disease, symptoms suggestive of systemic vasculitis or a history of exposure to drugs or chemicals. In the hospitalized patient ARF may be insidious and identified simply by the observation of a steadily rising blood urea. Causes such as heart failure, diuretic overdose or volume depletion due to gastrointestinal losses or polyuria should be sought. Possible causes of ATN such as severe trauma, recent surgery, or septicaemia are usually self-evident. Post-renal causes may be indicated by a history of prostatism, stone disease or haematuria, abdominal or pelvic surgery, or of cancer (Fig. 9.29).

PHYSICAL EXAMINATION

The first important aspect of examination is to define the presence or absence of circulatory failure due to volume depletion. This includes:
- Measurement of blood pressure (lying and standing if possible)
- Assessment of central venous pressure (CVP)

- Assessment of the presence or absence of oedema
- Assessment of the state of the peripheral circulation

In overt hypovolaemic shock there will be pallor, hypotension, cold peripheral parts and tachycardia. More often, circulatory failure is less obvious. Lack of a visible venous pulsation in the neck when supine indicates a low CVP and circulatory volume depletion. When in doubt, measurement of the CVP by insertion of a central venous line is immensely valuable (see p. 434). If associated with postural hypotension (a fall in standing systolic pressure of more than 20 mmHg from the recumbent value, or to less than 100 mmHg) and no oedema, a low CVP is good evidence of volume depletion. Conversely, the presence of oedema, an elevated jugular venous pressure (JVP) and evidence of pulmonary congestion indicates heart failure or primary fluid overload.

Equally important is the exclusion of bladder outflow obstruction by careful examination for a large bladder or, if doubt exists, by aseptic bladder catheterization. A self-retaining catheter with continuous closed-seal drainage is instituted if bladder outflow obstruction is confirmed. If obstruction is not confirmed, the catheter should be removed after 50 ml of 1% noxythiolin has been instilled to prevent catheter-induced infection.

Rectal examination must always be performed to assess the prostate in males for size and possible malignancy, to identify the presence of pelvic cancer in either sex, and to look for melaena.

Acute tenderness in the renal angles or over the lower poles of the kidney anteriorly suggests acute tubulo-interstitial nephritis, whether due to infection or other causes (Table 9.18). This sign may also be found with acute glomerulonephritis.

A more general examination may be helpful in making the diagnosis; for example:
- The presence of jaundice or the stigmata of liver failure suggest hepatorenal failure.
- The presence of skin lesions may suggest a systemic hypersensitivity reaction, vasculitis, septicaemia or allergy, which may have resulted in tubulo-interstitial nephritis.
- The retinal lesions of diabetes or malignant hypertension may be found.

INVESTIGATION

Chemical and microscopic examination of the urine is essential.

Proteinuria. In pure pre-renal or post-renal failure proteinuria is usually absent or slight (+) at most. Conversely, heavy proteinuria (++ or more) suggests intrinsic renal disease, most often glomerular in nature.

Haematuria. Haematuria is uncommon in pre-renal failure. It may occur with post-renal disease (tumours, stones), and is usual in intrinsic renal disease.

Urine microscopy. The presence of red cell casts on microscopy is highly suggestive of glomerulonephritis, but they may also be seen in acute tubulo-interstitial disease.

The presence of bacteriuria and pyuria suggest infection.

Urine culture. Culture of clean-catch midstream urine or catheter specimens must always be carried out.

Chemical testing of urine. With pre-renal 'circulatory' failure the *healthy* kidney responds with avid retention of salt and water. The urine is thus concentrated (osmolality > 500 mosmol·kg^{-1}), low in sodium ($<$ 20 mmol·l^{-1}), with a urine/plasma concentration ratio of more than 8:1 for urea or more than 40:1 for creatinine. Similar urinary findings may be observed in acute glomerulonephritis. In patients with acute tubulo-interstitial disease, urine concentrating ability is lost, as is the ability to conserve sodium, the urine being isosmolar with plasma and the urinary sodium usually being greater than 50 mosmol·kg^{-1}. A similar pattern is usually seen in chronic glomerular disease and obstructive nephropathy. Thus urine osmolality, sodium concentration and urine/plasma concentration ratio of creatinine or urea may be of value in distinguishing pre-renal from other forms of renal failure. However, they are seldom measured in clinical practice.

Diagnosis of pre-renal 'circulatory' ARF

If, on the basis of the history and clinical examination, pre-renal (volume depletion) circulatory failure is diagnosed or strongly suspected, the effect of volume repletion on renal function must be tested. Volume repletion should be with an appropriate fluid: blood should be used in the case of post-haemorrhagic shock (or human albumin in an emergency) and normal saline if fluid depletion is due to vomiting, diarrhoea or polyuria. Fluid replacement is most safely given with simultaneous measurement of the CVP. With pure pre-renal failure, urine output should increase with volume replacement.

Forced diuresis in 'incipient ATN'

It has been postulated that early renal damage due to ATN may be reversible ('incipient ATN') if the kidneys are subjected to a powerful diuretic stimulus. When the CVP or JVP returns to normal with fluid replacement but urine output does not increase, or in patients who are not volume depleted but have been exposed to conditions predisposing to ATN, it is usual to give a powerful diuretic combination of 20% mannitol 100 ml i.v. over 5–10 min followed by frusemide 120 mg i.v. over 5–10 min. A satisfactory response is a urine output of more than 40 ml·h^{-1}. If the response is equivocal (10–40 ml·h^{-1}), the diuretic stimulus may be repeated *once* after 2 h. If there is no increase in urine output, this procedure should not be repeated a second time. The administration of more than 40 g of mannitol per day to the oliguric patient is potentially harmful. The urine flow rate in response to forced diuresis may be monitored in the unconscious patient by bladder catheterization, but the catheter must be removed as soon as possible in diuresing patients and immediately if no diuresis occurs.

If these measures do not induce a diuresis, the diagnosis of pre-renal circulatory failure or incipient ATN has been excluded. The differential diagnosis then lies between intrinsic renal disease and obstructive nephropathy.

Distinction between renal and post-renal failure

Clues may be provided by the history and clinical examination, including urinalysis. Haematuria with red cell casts, recent trauma or sepsis with hypotension, and exposure to nephrotoxic drugs or chemicals all suggest intrinsic disease, while a previous history of stone disease or a 'frozen' or solid pelvis on rectal examination (indicating a pelvic carcinoma) suggest obstructive nephropathy. In the absence of obvious acute glomerulo-nephritis or acute tubulo-interstitial nephritis it is usually necessary to exclude obstruction by renal imaging. Anuria should always be considered to be due to obstruction until proved otherwise.

Renal imaging. This should be carried out as soon as possible both to define or exclude obstruction and to define renal size. The investigation of first choice is renal ultrasonography. Plain abdominal x-rays and renal tomography are performed to exclude radio-dense stones. Ultrasound will define or exclude obstruction and allow measurement of renal size in the majority of patients. If ultrasound is not available, or if doubt exists about the results, high-dose excretion urography should be carried out and will give the same information.

If obstruction is diagnosed by ultrasound or excretion urography, definition of the site of obstruction commonly requires antegrade or retrograde ureterography (see p. 378).

Diagnosis of renal causes of ARF

If obstruction is excluded, renal failure is due to intrinsic renal disease. Further investigation of the *nature* of the disease depends on the history, urinalysis, renal size and renal biopsy. If the kidneys are small on renal imaging, the intrinsic renal disease is long-standing and irreversible. Definition of the precise pathology will not usually influence management. If the kidneys are normal or large and the history and urinalysis, including urine culture, suggest acute glomerulonephritis, acute tubular

necrosis or bacterial pyelonephritis, further investigation is rarely necessary for management purposes. If the diagnosis is unclear, renal biopsy should be performed.

MANAGEMENT

Pre-renal causes

Diagnosis of pre-renal circulatory failure as the cause of ARF requires volume repletion to be carried out (see above), and this is also the first step in management. After this, continuing careful assessment of fluid and electrolyte requirement is necessary, especially in polyuric patients and in those with continuing gastrointestinal losses:

- The patient must be weighed daily to ensure stable fluid balance.
- The JVP must be checked regularly and the presence or absence of peripheral oedema recorded.
- Lying and standing blood pressure must be recorded at least twice daily.
- Careful fluid input–output records are essential.
- Plasma electrolytes must be measured daily to ensure adequate replacement of sodium and potassium. Measurement of the daily excretion of these cations is rarely necessary.

Fluid is always best given by mouth as water. Supplements of sodium or potassium may be required depending on dietary intake and daily measurement of plasma electrolytes.

Oral supplements are best given as Slow Sodium and effervescent potassium (bicarbonate-containing) or Slow-K (chloride-containing). Average daily excretion of these electrolytes is set out in Table 10.3 (see p. 434). If oral replacement is impossible, intravenous infusion is required. The volume of fluid needed is gauged from the urinary output, the daily clinical assessment of fluid balance and daily weighing. The nature of fluid required can be roughly predicted from Table 10.3 (see p. 434). Plasma electrolyte levels should be checked daily.

Treatment of symptomatic pre-renal uraemia caused by the administration of tetracycline or steroids includes withdrawal of these drugs.

Renal and post-renal causes

The management of renal failure due to intrinsic disease or obstructive nephropathy which cannot be immediately relieved involves the restoration of normal fluid and electrolyte balance and the control of uraemia and acidosis.

Maintaining fluid balance. The principles involved in controlling fluid balance (and uraemia and acidosis) may be summed up succinctly as 'what goes in, must come out'. Normally the kidneys keep the volume of body water constant by increasing or decreasing the urine volume in response to an increased or decreased fluid intake. In acute oliguric or polyuric renal failure this function is lost. It is then necessary to match fluid intake to urine output. Patients with ARF may, at the time of presentation, be hypovolaemic, normovolaemic or fluid overloaded. Treatment of volume depletion is discussed on p. 414.

In patients with ARF who are in normal fluid balance (i.e. who have a normal JVP and no evidence of systemic oedema or pulmonary congestion), fluid balance is maintained by a daily fluid intake of 300–500 ml plus an amount equal to the total fluid output on the previous day, i.e. urine volume plus any losses in vomit, stools, and fistula drainage. Careful records of all fluid intake and output are therefore essential. This is supported by daily weighing, the objective being to keep the patient's weight constant or with daily losses of no more than 0.5 kg in hypercatabolic patients who are losing flesh weight. Twice daily assessment of the JVP, lying and standing blood pressure, the presence or absence of systemic oedema and pulmonary congestion is mandatory. An increase in weight, a rise in JVP or the development of oedema indicates too large a fluid ration, while an excessive fall in weight or the development of postural hypotension indicates the reverse.

In patients presenting with fluid overload (i.e. who have an elevated JVP with systemic or pulmonary oedema), an attempt must be made to get rid of fluid. The effects of large doses of diuretics, e.g. frusemide 180 mg i.v. or 500–1000 mg orally, may be tested. If no diuresis occurs and the patient has clinical or radiological evidence of pulmonary congestion, fluid must be removed by dialysis or ultrafiltration. Once the fluid balance has been corrected, it must be maintained as described for patients in normal fluid balance.

Electrolyte balance. In general, patients with oliguric renal failure cannot excrete sodium or potassium. Their intake of both must therefore be reduced to a minimum compatible with an adequate diet. Satisfactory control is assessed by daily measurement of the plasma electrolytes.

In polyuric patients, e.g. those in the recovery phase of ATN or following the relief of urinary obstruction, increased amounts of sodium and potassium may be lost in the urine, as shown by falling plasma levels. Such patients need supplements of both (see above).

Hyperkalaemia leading to cardiac arrhythmias and cardiac arrest is a major hazard in oliguric renal failure, especially where there has been extensive trauma or hypoxia, both of which may lead to flooding of the extracellular fluid with potassium from the cells. Acute-onset hyperkalaemia is more dangerous than that developing over weeks or months. The immediate danger of dysrhythmia is best assessed from the ECG when typical changes (Fig. 10.6, p. 441)

indicate the need for immediate and effective control of hyperkalaemia by dialysis (see p. 417). Temporary measures to control hyperkalaemia include the use of ion-exchange resins or the intravenous infusion of glucose and insulin (see p. 441).

Control of uraemia. The retention of waste products is less immediately life-threatening than fluid overload or hyperkalaemia. In otherwise healthy patients (e.g. those with acute glomerulonephritis) the increase in blood urea and serum creatinine are usually gradual and can be controlled by dietary restriction of protein to approximately 40 g per day, 75% of which must be first class protein. Some 2000–2500 kcal must be provided in the diet made up from fats and carbohydrate, commonly supplemented by starch hydrolysates such as Caloreen or Hycal. More strict protein restriction to 30 g per day is now rarely used. Diets for such patients should also be low in sodium (< 30 mmol per day) and potassium (< 20 mmol per day).

In patients with oliguric renal failure following sepsis, trauma or major surgery, tissue catabolism is greatly increased and the accumulation of waste products is faster. Again, dietary restriction of protein, sodium, and potassium, but with adequate calories, must be introduced. Such patients commonly require dialysis to control their uraemia. There is no absolute level of blood urea or serum creatinine above which dialysis should be commenced; rather it is the *rate* of rise in urea, plus fluid overload or hyperkalaemia, which indicate the need for dialysis. Overt symptoms of uraemia (anorexia, nausea, vomiting) plus severe acidosis certainly require dialysis. In the absence of these, it is generally felt that dialysis should be used if the blood urea exceeds 40 mmol·l^{-1} or serum creatinine exceeds 800 μmol·l^{-1}. Early dialysis with a protein intake of about 70 g is favoured in surgical or post-trauma cases in the belief that it may reduce the risk of infection and promote wound healing.

Control of acidosis. Acidosis rarely requires treatment per se as its severity commonly parallels that of the uraemia, for which dialysis may be indicated. Without removal of fixed acid by dialysis, acidosis is difficult to correct in oliguric patients because of the hazard of fluid overload which is inherent in intravenous infusions of sodium bicarbonate or other buffers. If control of acidosis is essential, as for example in patients with cardiac ischaemia, it is best achieved by dialysis.

General management

Many patients with oliguric renal failure are severely ill and have infections. They require dedicated nursing care and constant supervision. Infection must be controlled, but the choice of antibiotics (and indeed of all drugs) must take account of altered drug excretion due to renal failure.

Blood purification and ultrafiltration
A variety of techniques is now available for the removal of waste products of metabolism, the 'normalization' of plasma electrolytes and the removal of plasma water (ultrafiltration).

Peritoneal dialysis. This is the usual first-line technique because it is widely available and easily instituted using a hard PVC catheter introduced into the peritoneal space using a trocar through a small scalpel skin stab. In patients who have had abdominal surgery, peritoneal dialysis may not be possible and in hypercatabolic patients it may be insufficient to control the uraemia. The principles of peritoneal dialysis are discussed on p. 422.

Temporary (acute) peritoneal dialysis

Indications
- Severe uraemia
  (a) Used in acute renal failure continuously or intermittently until renal function recovers
  (b) used in chronic renal failure for support until long-term dialysis is instituted

Insertion of catheter
Using a sterile technique:
- Local anesthetic is injected in the midline below the umbilicus.
- A small cut is made in the skin with a scalpel.
- A rigid plastic catheter is inserted through the abdominal wall into the peritoneal cavity using a trocar.
- The catheter is firmly bound to the abdomen.

The catheter can remain in situ for several days or a few weeks.

Peritoneal dialysis
- In acute renal failure, approximately 2 l of sterile dialysate solution are instilled into and drained out of the abdomen approximately hourly.
- A typical composition of the dialysate is sodium 135 mmol·l^{-1}, chloride 105 mmol·l^{-1}, potassium 0 mmol·l^{-1}, glucose 80 mmol·l^{-1} (1.5%), calcium 1.75 mmol·l^{-1}, magnesium 0.50 mmol·l^{-1}, and lactate 35 mmol·l^{-1}.
- Net fluid removal is achieved by osmosis. 1.5% glucose is approximately isotonic with plasma. Higher concentrations of glucose are used if fluid needs to be removed.

Complications
- Leakage
- Pain—usually short lasting and not severe
- Peritonitis
  (a) Uncommon with careful technique
  (b) Treated with appropriate antibiotics added to the dialysate solution or with withdrawal of the catheter

---

Haemodialysis. This is the most popular alternative to peritoneal dialysis. It is significantly more efficient than peritoneal dialysis for blood purification. It is now most commonly performed using temporary cannulation of the subclavian or femoral veins. It requires quite sophisticated equipment and special expertise in its use. It can therefore only be performed in specialist centres. The principles of haemodialysis are discussed on p. 421.

Haemofiltration. This is a third alternative which is becoming increasingly popular. In this procedure, which is less likely than haemodialysis to cause acute hypotension in patients with septicaemia or with poor myocardial function, large volumes of plasma water are removed using a porous filter and are replaced by a sterile electrolyte solution. Although, like haemodialysis, it can be carried out intermittently using a machine, it is most popularly performed as continuous 'arteriovenous' haemofiltration (CAVH). The patient's systemic arterial pressure drives blood through the extracorporeal circuit. Between 10 and 20 l of plasma water are removed daily and replaced by electrolyte solution (Fig. 9.30). Drawbacks include the need to insert cannulas into a major artery (usually the radial artery) and a draining vein to form an arteriovenous shunt and the need for very frequent assessment of fluid balance. A considerable attraction of CAVH is that the water removed creates space for intravenous feeding when this is necessary.

Recovery phase of ARF
Paradoxically the recovery phase of ARF is often the most dangerous. As glomerular filtration rate increases, large volumes of urine may be passed before the damaged tubules fully recover their ability to retain salt and water. This carries the risk of fluid depletion and hypokalaemia. This so-called 'polyuric phase' of ARF can last for several days and demands careful monitoring of plasma sodium and potassium levels to detect a negative balance of either.

PROGNOSIS

In acute tubular necrosis, the commonest renal lesion, the renal prognosis is excellent; 95% of patients recover satisfactory renal function within 6 weeks. Unfortunately acute tubular necrosis often develops in patients who have a poor chance of survival for non-renal reasons. The outlook is particularly poor in patients with severe trauma, multisystem failure and overwhelming sepsis. In those who survive, renal function usually returns to normal within a few months. In patients with cortical necrosis, only partial recovery of function, if any, can be expected.

The prognosis in patients with acute glomerulo-

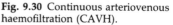

Fig. 9.30 Continuous arteriovenous haemofiltration (CAVH).

nephritis, acute tubulo-interstitial nephritis or obstructive nephropathy is discussed on pp. 386, 395 and 409.

Chronic renal failure

Although chronic renal failure (CRF) is not common, its impact in fiscal, political and ethical terms has been enormous since the introduction of long-term haemodialysis in the 1960s and increasingly successful transplantation in the 1970s. Long-term dialysis and transplantation together are often referred to as 'renal replacement'.

PREVALENCE AND CAUSES

An indication of the prevalence and causes of CRF are shown in Fig. 9.31. These data are for patients who reach end-stage renal failure (ESRF) and who are accepted for dialysis and renal transplantation.

The distribution of primary renal disease varies little between countries, except for analgesic nephropathy (see p. 396), which is particularly common in Australian women. Glomerulonephritis is the most common cause of ESRF, followed by chronic atrophic pyelonephritis (see pp. 386 and 392).

A pessimistic outlook with respect to long-term renal replacement in patients with diabetic nephropathy in the past has recently given way to a more optimistic and positive approach in these patients. Diabetics now comprise the fastest growing group of patients accepted for dialysis and transplantation in Europe. Polycystic disease of the kidney is the most common cause of inherited renal disease leading to ESRF. In ESRF a histological diagnosis is often not available as biopsy of small kidneys is not warranted. It is likely therefore that many patients in the 'uncertain' group have chronic glomerulonephritis.

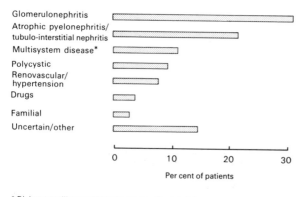

Fig. 9.31 Distribution of type of primary renal disease in patients accepted for dialysis and transplantation in the years 1980–1982. (Data from the Registry of the European Dialysis and Transplant Association—European Renal Association.)

CLINICAL FEATURES

Asymptomatic CRF may be discovered on routine health screening programmes, as a chance finding in hospitalized patients, or during follow-up of patients known to have had renal disease.

In patients with chronic renal disease, symptomatic uraemia is not uncommonly precipitated by pre-renal factors such as increased tissue catabolism associated with infection, tetracycline therapy, volume depletion due to vomiting or diarrhoea, or the development of malignant phase hypertension. A pre-renal factor must always be sought and treated if present.

Symptomatic uraemia most often presents with gastrointestinal symptoms (anorexia, nausea, vomiting) but it may manifest as symptoms of anaemia, bone disease, hypertension or hypertensive heart failure. In CRF hypertension has usually been long-standing and frequently severe. Advanced coronary artery and peripheral vascular disease may be present even in young patients.

Symptoms and signs

In severe renal failure, practically every system of the body is affected and leads to symptoms (Fig. 9.32). Minor symptoms such as lethargy, fatigue and nocturia have often gone unnoticed for many months and are only recognized when patients are specifically questioned about them. Menstrual disturbances, particularly amenorrhoea, and erectile impotence are troublesome symptoms. The accumulation of 'toxic metabolites' in uraemia sometimes causes a peripheral neuropathy which is characteristically reversible with dialysis treatment. Yellow-brown pigmentation of the skin, which is often dry and itchy, commonly occurs.

Anorexia, nausea and vomiting. These are the most typical symptoms of uraemia and are usually attributed to the formation of ammonia in the upper gastrointestinal tract from urea. They are uncommon until the blood urea exceeds 30 mmol·l^{-1}. In patients with renal disease but in whom the blood urea level is less than 20 mmol·l^{-1}, such symptoms should not be attributed to 'uraemia' and an alternative cause should be sought.

Anaemia. This is a typical feature of advanced renal disease. It is normochromic and normocytic in type. Symptoms of fatigue and shortness of breath on exertion may occur. The anaemia is primarily due to reduced erythropoietin production by the kidney, but when there is severe uraemia (i.e. blood urea > 30 mmol·l^{-1}) a shortened red cell life and toxic marrow depression also contribute.

The blood urea must always be measured in patients with unexplained normochromic, normocytic anaemia. It is not uncommon for a uraemic patient to have received courses of iron for anaemia many months before presenting with renal failure. Not surprisingly, the anaemia typically does not respond.

Renal osteodystrophy

The term renal osteodystrophy embraces the various forms of bone disease which develop in CRF, i.e. osteomalacia, secondary and tertiary hyperparathyroidism and osteosclerosis (Fig. 9.33).

Osteomalacia. The kidney is unable to produce the metabolically active 1,25-dihydroxy cholecalciferol (see p. 374), which are essential for the normal mineralization of bone and for the absorption of calcium from the gut.

Anaemia
Pallor
Lethargy
Breathlessness
on exercise

Platelet abnormality
Epistaxis
Bruising

Skin
Pigmentation
Pruritus

GI tract
Anorexia, nausea,
vomiting
Diarrhoea

Endocrine /gonads
Amenorrhoea
Erectile impotence
Infertility

Peripheral neuropathy

CNS
Confusion, coma, fits
(severe uraemia)

CVS
Uraemic pericarditis
Hypertension
Peripheral vascular disease
Heart failure

Renal
Nocturia
Polyuria
Salt and water retention

Oedema

Renal osteodystrophy
Osteomalacia
Muscle weakness
Bone pain
Hyperparathyroidism
Osteosclerosis

Fig. 9.32 Symptoms and signs of chronic renal failure. Oedema may be due to a combination of primary renal salt and water retention and heart failure.

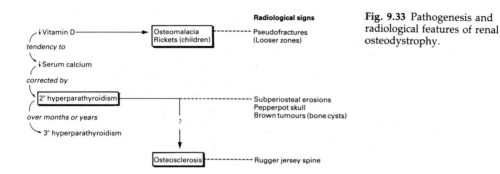

Fig. 9.33 Pathogenesis and radiological features of renal osteodystrophy.

Hyperparathyroidism. Poor absorption of dietary calcium and phosphate retention lowers the serum calcium. Parathormone is released in response to hypocalcaemia and promotes resorption of calcium from bone and increased proximal tubular reabsorption of calcium in the kidney in an attempt to correct the low serum calcium. Over months or years, this 'secondary' hyperparathyroidism can lead to severe decalcification of the skeleton associated with the classical radiological appearances listed in Fig. 9.33.

A common, but not inevitable, sequel to long-standing secondary hyperparathyroidism is hyperplasia of the glands leading to autonomous or 'tertiary' hyperparathyroidism. In this condition parathormone is released inappropriately, resulting in hypercalcaemia and severe bone disease. Hyperparathyroidism causes bone and joint pains and a high serum alkaline phosphatase. Histologically there is increased osteoclastic activity and characteristic cysts in which fibrous tissue is seen (osteitis fibrosa cystica or von Recklinghausen's disease of bone).

Osteosclerosis. The third bone lesion found in CRF is osteosclerosis (meaning literally 'hardening of bone'). It may be a direct result of excess parathormone. Alternate bands of sclerotic and porotic bone in the vertebrae produce the characteristic 'rugger-jersey spine' x-ray appearance.

INVESTIGATION

As with ARF it is critical to define renal size and to exclude treatable obstruction. When renal failure is modest (blood urea < 20 mmol·l^{-1}) high-dose excretion urography can commonly show details of the calyces and allow identification of conditions such as papillary necrosis. With more severe renal impairment calyceal detail may not be shown. In such cases plain renal tomography plus ultrasonography can identify renal size and define or exclude obstruction, eliminating the need for excretion urography. If the kidneys are not obstructed or shrunken, transcutaneous biopsy is required to exclude treatable tubulo-interstitial disease. An exception to this is where there is a long history of diabetes and evidence of diabetic retinopathy, when the diagnosis of diabetic glomerulosclerosis can be presumed. Conversely, renal failure should not be ascribed to diabetic glomerulosclerosis if there is no retinopathy. If the kidneys are found to be small, smooth and non-obstructed it is difficult to distinguish between chronic glomerulonephritis, chronic tubulo-interstitial nephritis or nephrosclerosis.

MANAGEMENT

Dietary protein restriction
Protein restriction not only reduces the rate of production of nitrogenous waste products, but there is increasing evidence that it also slows down the rate of decline of function in certain chronic renal diseases. Restricting the amount of protein in the daily diet to between 40 and 50 g strikes a balance between achieving these objectives and avoiding protein malnutrition. Protein restriction should be introduced when the creatinine clearance falls below 30 ml·min^{-1}. Potassium intake may also have to be reduced. Patients with symptomatic uraemia who cannot be controlled on a 40 g protein diet should be considered for renal replacement (see p. 424).

Blood pressure control
Hypertension should always be treated in patients with chronic renal disease since it will accelerate loss of kidney function if uncontrolled. Initial control of hypertension may be accompanied by some reduction in GFR, but this is preferable to hypertensive kidney damage. Renal hypertension usually responds to conventional treatment with a diuretic, beta-blocker, and if necessary a vasodilator drug (see p. 544). Salt intake should be reduced to 50 mmol per day.

Some patients with diseases primarily affecting the medulla (e.g. chronic pyelonephritis, papillary necrosis or post-obstructive atrophy) may be unable to conserve salt and water and saline depletion, hypotension and pre-renal failure may result. This should always be suspected in patients with a normal or low blood pressure who have a normal or low

JVP and no oedema. Postural hypotension supports a diagnosis of volume depletion. This diagnosis is confirmed if, after the cautious prescription of salt supplements (Slow Sodium 10–20 mmol three times daily) and a high fluid intake, the blood pressure rises, the postural hypotension disappears, the renal function improves and the body weight increases without the development of oedema. Enough salt is given to just avoid causing abnormal elevation of the JVP or the development of oedema. Elimination of pre-renal failure in these circumstances may result in a marked improvement in renal function.

Treatment of anaemia

There is no specific treatment for the erythropoietin-deficient anaemia of chronic renal disease. Control of severe uraemia (blood urea > 30 mmol·l^{-1}) may reduce haemolysis and marrow depression. The only other treatment available is blood transfusion. Most patients adjust to haemoglobin levels of between 6 and 9 g·dl^{-1}. A policy of minimal transfusion is adopted both to minimize the risk of transmission of viral infection and to avoid sensitization to white cell antigens which may compromise successful transplantation in the future. However, there is strong evidence that blood transfusion actually enhances the chances of a successful kidney transplant through mechanisms which are not understood. A compromise is therefore required. Potential transplant recipients are therefore given only the minimum number of transfusions needed but are electively transfused with three units of blood every 2 years. Transfusion must be given in patients with increasing exertional dyspnoea.

Treatment of renal osteodystrophy

Aluminium hydroxide preparations are used to bind dietary phosphate in the gut, which helps to reduce the serum phosphate level. Vitamin D treatment is usually withheld until there are symptoms or biochemical and/or radiological evidence of bone disease; dihydrotachysterol 0.2–0.6 mg daily or alfacalcidol (1α-hydroxycholecalciferol) 1 μg daily are most often used, with regular monthly checks on the serum calcium to avoid hypercalcaemia. Drug treatment is continued until x-rays show healing of the bones and the serum alkaline phophatase level has returned to normal. Long-term low-dose treatment or 'prophylaxis' may be employed but carries the risk of vitamin D intoxication and requires regular serum calcium measurements.

Tertiary hyperparathyroidism does not usually occur until the patients have received dialysis treatment for several years (see p. 420).

Socioeconomic aspects

Because dialysis and/or transplantation are required to replace renal function, forward planning on an individual basis is essential. This includes assessment of the patient's home, which may have to be converted to take dialysis equipment. Job prospects and economic resources need to be considered, given that a certain amount of time will be taken up with self-treatment in the future and mobility will be limited. The prospects for live donor kidney transplantation need to be carefully assessed.

For all these reasons it is customary to transfer patients with progressive kidney failure to their 'local' specialist centre after the initial diagnosis has been made and management implemented. Most centres now employ specially trained personnel to deal with these problems.

Patient education

Involvement in various aspects of treatment at an early stage often helps prepare the way for the complicated specialist training which may lie ahead. Dietary and drug treatment should be explained and the patient should be encouraged to question changes in treatment. Cannulation of forearm veins may prejudice the successful creation of vascular access for dialysis in the future (see below). The responsibility for making sure that this does not happen can largely be passed to the patient.

Replacement of renal function by dialysis

Apart from protein restriction and the control of hypertension there is little that can be done to influence the natural history of chronic renal disease. Tragically, patients all too frequently present with symptoms and signs of ESRF. Since the late 1960s increasing numbers of patients with ESRF have had 'replacement' of renal function by dialysis and transplantation. At the end of 1984 in Europe there were 70 831 patients on haemodialysis, 1812 on haemofiltration and 8168 on long-term peritoneal dialysis, and 22 833 patients were alive with a functioning graft.

Haemodialysis. Thomas Graham (1805–1869) first coined the term 'dialysis' to describe the diffusion of crystalloids from a mixture of crystalloids and colloids through a vegetable parchment membrane. The principles of haemodialysis are illustrated in Fig. 9.34. Blood is perfused in a thin film across a membrane (usually prepared from cellulose) which has a surface area of approximately 1 m^2 and is permeable to water, electrolytes and small molecules such as urea and creatinine. Dialysate solution flows on the opposite side of the membrane. Diffusion of solutes takes place in both directions. The concentration of potassium in the dialysate is chosen to allow diffusion from the blood at a rate just below that which creates hypokalaemia, and the concentration of ionized calcium is chosen such that there is slow diffusion *into* the blood. This helps to alleviate the problems of calcium balance in ESRF. Diffusion into the blood of acetate, which is rapidly metabolized to bicarbonate, compensates for the loss of regeneration of bicarbonate which normally takes place in the

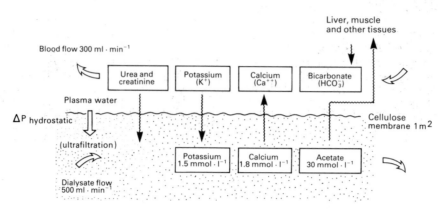

Fig. 9.34 The principles of haemodialysis.

kidney. Acetate is usually used because bicarbonate itself cannot easily be held in solution.

Ingested water and water produced by catabolism accumulates between dialysis sessions and has to be removed. Removal of plasma water on dialysis is achieved by creating a hydrostatic pressure gradient across the membrane (ultrafiltration).

Haemodialysis requires easy access to the circulation. This is most commonly achieved by creating a fistula between the radial artery and the cephalic vein at the wrist. For dialysis, needles are inserted into the high flow 'arterialized' forearm veins which result.

It has been found that patients remain well and can survive many years with between 12 and 21 h of dialysis each week. Usually this is split into three or sometimes two sessions. Hypertension is usually controlled by the gradual removal of salt and water during the first few months of dialysis, hypotensive drugs being gradually withdrawn. Dietary protein intake is increased to about 60 g per day.

Peritoneal dialysis. Although peritoneal dialysis has been used for many years in acute renal failure, its long term use in ESRF has been employed only since the late 1970s. Continuous 'ambulatory' peritoneal dialysis (CAPD) is being increasingly adopted and is now the preferred method of dialysis in some centres. Low capital costs and the necessity of only a short training period for the patient are particularly attractive in units with an active transplantation programme, when the need for dependence on dialysis for more than a few years is unlikely for the majority.

The peritoneal membrane has a surface area of approximately 2 m^2 in the average adult. CAPD requires the surgical implantation of a soft Silastic rubber catheter (Tenckhoff) into the abdominal cavity (a hard PVC catheter is usually used for peritoneal dialysis in acute renal failure). Dialysate (usually 2 l) is run from a bag into the abdomen, the

Home haemodialysis

The majority (56%) of haemodialysis patients in the UK have self-supervised home haemodialysis. The majority (90%) of patients in the rest of Europe have hospital-based dialysis.

Advantages of home haemodialysis
- Confidence in own treatment
- Reduced travelling
- Less time off work
- Dialysis times are at the patient's own choosing—more socially acceptable
- Hepatitis B infection is very rare
- Approximately one-third of the cost of hospital dialysis in the long term.

Requirements
- Suitable home available
- Home conversion—a separate room is needed with special plumbing and drains
- Several months training period in hospital
- Facility for easy telephone communication with dialysis nurses, technicians and doctor if necessary

Disadvantages
- Patient may need rehousing
- Expensive if patient is transplanted within a few months of starting home dialysis

'Minimal care' dialysis units are gaining popularity. Patients supervise their own treatment in small 'satellite' units with minimal supervision. The bed station and equipment are shared by several patients, and it is less expensive than hospital dialysis. In some cases, these units have social advantages over home dialysis.

line connecting the bag and catheter is clamped, and the bag is rolled up and placed in a belt or pocket. The fluid stays in the abdomen for several hours before being siphoned off back into the bag, which is then discarded. A fresh bag of dialysate is connected and the cycle restarts. Between three and five exchanges are usually required every day.

The principles employed in peritoneal dialysis for the diffusion of solutes and electrolytes are the same as for haemodialysis except that potassium-free dialysate is used (Fig. 9.35). Ultrafiltration is effected by osmosis: the dialysate is made hypertonic with respect to plasma by the addition of glucose. The higher the osmolality of the dialysate, the higher the ultrafiltration rate.

Outlook and complications of dialysis. Overall, the 5-year survival rate of patients on haemodialysis is approximately 70%, most of the deaths being due to cardiovascular disease. In many cases this results from hypertension present before starting dialysis. In the individual patient, haemodialysis is compatible with survival for more than 20 years and a high proportion of patients are successfully rehabilitated. Many return to their previous occupations despite the time needed to perform dialysis (which can often be performed at night).

Patients on long-term dialysis are commonly infertile. Pregnancies are few and successful pregnancy almost unknown in female dialysis patients. Only a small number of babies have been fathered by patients on dialysis. Erectile impotence is a very distressing complication which is estimated to affect approximately 30% of male patients. In general, these problems are reversed by successful transplantation.

Despite a clearer understanding of the role of the kidney in calcium metabolism, bone disease remains an important cause of morbidity in dialysis patients. The likelihood of parathyroidectomy for tertiary hyperparathyroidism increases with time on dialysis: the prevalence of parathyroidectomy in patients who have been on dialysis for less than 5 years is 2%, and 16% in those who have had dialysis for over 10 years. Either subtotal parathyroidectomy or total parathyroidectomy with or without implantation of parathyroid remnants in the forearm is performed. This latter operation in theory allows easy access to parathyroid tissue should it subsequently become overactive.

While vascular access is the 'Achilles heel' of successful haemodialysis, peritonitis is the major drawback of CAPD and half the patients who start CAPD change to some other treatment within 2 years as a result. On the other hand, very successful rehabilitation is possible using CAPD and this treatment has offered new hope to diabetic patients and elderly patients, in whom problems with vascular access and blood pressure stability on haemodialysis tend to be considerable.

Fig. 9.35 The principles of peritoneal dialysis.

Renal transplantation

Successful renal transplantation offers the potential for complete rehabilitation in ESRF. It allows freedom from dietary and fluid restriction, anaemia and infertility are corrected, and the likelihood of requiring parathyroidectomy is reduced.

Coincident with the use of lower doses of immunosuppressive drugs, patient survival has increased over the years such that the 1-year survival rate is over 95% for live donor recipients and over 85% for cadaver graft recipients. With the use of newer immunosuppressive drugs, the graft survival rate has improved, being approximately 80% at 2 years. For this reason some patients who are satisfactorily established on dialysis treatment are increasingly electing to undergo transplantation.

The likelihood of transplant rejection is less in patients who have previously had blood transfusion (see above). Tissue matching (see p. 110) of the donor kidney and the recipient improves the likelihood of a successful outcome.

The transplant operation is relatively straightforward. The donor kidney is placed in an extraperitoneal pouch in the groin (Fig. 9.36) and the renal artery and vein are anatomosed to the recipient's iliac vessels. The donor ureter is implanted into the bladder through a submucosal tunnel designed to prevent reflux. The recipient's own kidneys are left undisturbed unless there is another indication for nephrectomy.

Immunosuppressive drugs are given from the moment of transplantation. Prednisolone and azathioprine have been almost universally used until recently. Cyclosporin A, in spite of its nephrotoxicity and expense, is now being increasingly employed because of its remarkable immunosuppressive properties.

Rejection of the transplant, if it is to take place, usually occurs within the first few months. This is also the period when the patient is at greatest risk from infection. Viral infections (e.g. with cytomegalovirus) which generally produce trivial illnesses in normal people can produce life-threatening infections in immunosuppressed patients. There are also longer term complications of immunosuppressive therapy: avascular necrosis of the femoral head due to corticosteroid drugs is not uncommon, and there is an increased incidence of squamous cell carcinoma of the skin and of non-Hodgkin's lymphoma in transplant recipients, although the actual numbers who develop these complications are very small.

Despite the success of cadaveric renal transplantation, the number of patients on dialysis awaiting transplantation continues to increase. The cause of this is a shortage of cadaver organs. Since several studies indicate that throughout the country there are potentially sufficient donors to meet the needs of transplantation, it follows that donor organs are being wasted. The reasons for this are complex but include reluctance on the part of both the public and the medical profession to consider organ donation, insufficiently streamlined organizations for the recovery of donor kidneys, and continuing unjustified anxiety about the diagnosis of death.

Cystic, congenital and familial disease

CYSTIC RENAL DISEASE

Solitary or multiple renal cysts are common, especially with advancing age: 50% of those aged 50 years or more have one or more such cysts. They have no special significance except in the differential diagnosis of renal tumours (see p. 427). Such cysts are often asymptomatic and are found on excretion urography or ultrasound examination performed for some other reason. Occasionally they may cause pain and/or haematuria due to their large size or bleeding may occur into the cyst.

Adult polycystic renal disease

Adult polycystic renal disease (APCD) is an important cystic disease of the kidney which is relatively common. Inherited in an autosomal dominant manner, it is manifested in infancy as tiny cystic lesions distributed throughout both kidneys and should be distinguished from juvenile nephronophthisis (see below). The precise mechanism for cyst formation is disputed. With advancing age the cysts enlarge at a variable rate, often at the same rate within family groups but at different rates between different families. There is progressive asymmetric renal enlargement, with compression of intervening renal tissue and progressive loss of excretory function.

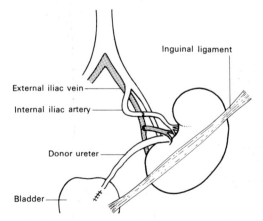

Inguinal ligament

External iliac vein

Internal iliac artery

Donor ureter

Bladder

Fig. 9.36 The anatomy of a transplant operation.

Clinical presentation may be at any age from the second decade. Presenting symptoms include:

- Acute loin pain and/or haematuria due to haemorrhage into a cyst
- Vague loin or abdominal discomfort due to the increasing size of the kidneys
- The development of hypertension or symptoms of uraemia

Increasingly APCD is diagnosed by ultrasound screening of the children of parents known to have the condition.

The natural history of the disease is one of progressive renal impairment, sometimes punctuated by acute episodes of loin pain and haematuria and commonly associated with the development of hypertension. It is popularly believed that there is an increased incidence of urinary tract infection in patients with APCD. There is little evidence to support this, but if such patients do develop infection it may be more difficult to eradicate. As mentioned earlier, the rate of progression to renal failure is variable, but tends to follow the same pattern in families. Some may reach end-stage renal failure at 40 years but others survive to 70 years or more.

Approximately 30% of patients with APCD have hepatic cysts; these rarely cause liver dysfunction. Cysts may more rarely develop in the pancreas, spleen, ovary and other organs. Berry aneurysms of the cerebral vessels are not infrequent and may result in subarachnoid or cerebral haemorrhage. Renal neoplasms may develop in polycystic kidneys and are difficult to diagnose.

Polycythaemia is a not uncommon association.

DIAGNOSIS

Physical examination commonly reveals large, irregular kidneys and possibly hepatomegaly. Definitive diagnosis was previously based on excretion urography, but is now more easily established by ultrasound examination (Fig. 9.37). However, such renal imaging techniques may be equivocal, especially in subjects under the age of 20 years. For this reason screening should not be carried out before this age. If doubt exists, CT renal scanning is more sensitive in identifying small cysts.

TREATMENT

The disease is always progressive. The most important aspect of management is regular blood pressure recording in affected patients, with control of hypertension as it develops. Uncontrolled hypertension accelerates the loss of kidney function. Some patients may develop salt and water wasting as the disease advances (see p. 420), when salt replacement with Slow Sodium can improve excretory function. Many patients will require renal replacement by dialysis and/or transplantation.

SCREENING

There is debate as to whether the children and siblings of patients with established APCD should be routinely offered screening. We believe that this should be offered to identify patients with this disorder, who must then have regular blood pressure checks and should be offered genetic counselling in respect of family planning. Screening should not be carried out before the age of 20 years, as excluding the condition may be difficult and hypertension is unusual before this age, as is the start of new families.

Medullary cystic disease ('juvenile nephronophthsis')

Developing early in childhood, this condition is commonly inherited in an autosomal recessive manner. A similar condition developing later in childhood is inherited as an autosomal dominant trait, but sporadic cases occur in both conditions. Despite its name, the dominant histological finding is interstitial inflammation and tubular atrophy, with later development of medullary cysts. Progressive glomerular failure is a secondary consequence.

The dominant features are polyuria, polydipsia

Fig. 9.37 Ultrasound scan of a polycystic kidney showing an enlarged kidney with many cysts of varying size.

and growth retardation. Diagnosis is based on the family history and renal biopsy, the cysts rarely being visualized by imaging techniques.

Medullary sponge kidney

Medullary sponge kidney is an uncommon but not rare condition which usually presents with renal colic or haematuria. Though it is most often sporadic, a few affected families have been reported. The condition is characterized by dilatation of the collecting ducts in the papillae, sometimes with cystic change. In severe cases the medullary area has a sponge-like appearance. The condition may affect one or both kidneys or only part of one kidney. Cyst formation is commonly associated with the development of small calculi within the cyst which, in some cases, may be compounded by associated hypercalciuria or renal tubular acidosis (see p. 445). Hemihypertrophy of the skeleton has been described in this condition.

Medullary sponge kidney most often presents with haematuria or ureteric colic. The diagnosis is made by excretion urography, which shows small calculi in the papillary zones with an increase in radiodensity *around* these following injection of contrast medium as the dilated or cystic collecting ducts are filled with contrast (Fig. 9.20).

The natural history is one of intermittent colic with passage of small stones or haematuria. Renal function is usually well maintained and renal failure is unusual, except where obstructive nephropathy develops due to the growth of stones in the pelvis or ureters.

CONGENITAL ABNORMALITIES

Agenesis

Bilateral agenesis is incompatible with extrauterine life. Unilateral agenesis ('a solitary kidney') occurs in 1 in 1000 of the population. It is usually associated with compensatory hypertrophy of the single kidney and normal renal function. Save for the potential hazard of trauma to this solitary kidney, it has no clinical significance.

Hypoplasia

Renal hypoplasia (failed development) of one kidney is uncommon, and hypoplasia of both kidneys is rare. It may be difficult to distinguish unilateral renal hypoplasia from a small kidney due to renal artery stenosis, obstruction or reflux nephropathy in early life. Clinical interest in the condition most often arises in patients with hypertension, where the small kidney may be considered the cause. If the small kidney is shown by radioisotope studies to contribute no useful renal function and if the hyperten-

sion has developed in a young subject or is difficult to control by medical treatment, nephrectomy should be undertaken.

Ectopic kidneys

Defects in embryological renal development may lead to ectopic or maldeveloped renal systems. At the risk of oversimplification, the kidneys may be thought of as developing in the embryo as one structure in the 'pelvic' area, migrating upwards and separating with growth. Failure in normal development may result in failure of the kidneys to migrate normally and indeed they may fail to separate. This results in a 'pelvic kidney' when one or both remain in the pelvis, a 'crossed ectopic kidney' when both have moved to the same side of the spine, a horseshoe or discoid kidney when there is partial (usually fusion of the lower poles) or total failure of separation.

In clinical practice the main problem associated with ectopic kidneys usually relates to impaired urinary drainage with secondary obstruction or stone formation. This may be compounded if infection supervenes, the poor drainage making eradication of infection difficult and predisposing to stone formation. Pelvic kidneys may interfere with parturition.

OTHER FAMILIAL RENAL DISEASE

Familial renal disease is in general rare, but there are a number of familial conditions which, among other things, can affect the kidneys.

Alport's syndrome

Alport's syndrome is a rare condition characterized by hereditary nephritis with haematuria, progressive renal failure and nerve deafness. It is principally expressed in males and an X-linked mode of inheritance has been postulated. Haematuria is the usual presenting symptom, and is often related to upper respiratory infections. Specific testing reveals a high frequency deafness in most, but not all, cases. Some 15% of cases may have ocular abnormalities such as cataract, conical cornea and dislocated small lens. The disease is progressive and accounts for some 5% of cases of end-stage renal failure in childhood or adolescence.

Congenital nephrotic syndrome

This syndrome is rare.

Renal tubular transport defects

Renal tubular transport defects include cystinuria, Hartnup's disease, adult Fanconi syndrome, galactosaemia and fructosaemia. They are discussed in more detail on p. 774.

Renal glycosuria

Renal glycosuria, in which there is glucose in the urine in subjects demonstrated to have normal blood glucose levels, who are not starved and who have no other urinary abnormality, is uncommon. Such patients have either a defect in the tubular threshold for reabsorption of glucose in the proximal tubule (a 'splayed' reabsorption curve) or a defect in the maximal tubular reabsorption of glucose. Both autosomal dominant and recessive inheritance have been postulated. It has no clinical significance except in the differential diagnosis of patients with diabetes mellitus or other tubular disorders such as the Fanconi syndrome.

Tumours of the kidney and genitourinary tract

MALIGNANT RENAL TUMOURS

These comprise 1–2% of all malignant tumours, and the male/female ratio is 2:1.

Renal cell carcinoma

Renal cell carcinomas (previously called hypernephromas or Grawitz tumours) arise from proximal tubular epithelium. They are the commonest renal tumour in adults. They rarely present before the age of 40, the average age of presentation being 55 years.

PATHOLOGY

The tumours may be solitary, multiple or occasionally bilateral. The tumour lies within the kidney but it may eventually penetrate the capsule. Macroscopically, its cut surface appears as a yellow mass, sometimes containing areas of haemorrhage and cystic degeneration. Local invasion of renal veins and spread to the opposite kidney may occur, as may metastasis to lymph nodes, liver, bone and lung (often as an apparently solitary metastasis). Renal cell carcinomas are highly vascular tumours. Microscopically the tumour is composed of large cells containing clear cytoplasm.

CLINICAL FEATURES

Patients present with haematuria, loin pain and a mass in the flank. Malaise, anorexia and weight loss may occur, and occasionally patients present with polycythaemia (see p. 288). Pyrexia is present in about one-fifth of patients and approximately one-quarter present with metastases. Rarely, a left-sided varicocele may be associated with left-sided tumours that have invaded the renal vein and caused obstruction to drainage of the left testicular vein.

DIAGNOSIS

Excretion urography will reveal a space-occupying lesion in the kidney; 10% of these show calcification.

Ultrasonography is used to demonstrate the solid lesion and to examine the patency of the renal vein and inferior vena cava. CT scanning can also be used to identify the renal lesion and involvement of the renal vein or inferior vena cava. Renal arteriography will reveal the tumour's circulation (Fig. 9.38). Urine cytology for malignant cells is of no value. The ESR is usually raised.

TREATMENT

Treatment is by nephrectomy unless bilateral tumours are present or the contralateral kidney functions poorly, in which case conservative surgery such as partial nephrectomy may be indicated. If metastases are present nephrectomy may still be warranted since regression of metastases has been reported after removal of the main tumour mass.

Fig. 9.38 Renal arteriogram in a patient with renal carcinoma. Note the abnormal tumour circulation.

Severe flank pain may also demand nephrectomy despite the presence of metastases. Radiotherapy and chemotherapy have no proven value. Medroxyprogesterone acetate is of some value in controlling metastatic disease.

PROGNOSIS

The prognosis depends upon the degree of differentiation of the tumour and whether or not metastases are present. In the absence of metastases, the 5-year survival rate exceeds 50%.

Nephroblastoma (Wilms' tumour)

This tumour is seen mainly within the first 3 years of life and may be bilateral. It presents as an abdominal mass, rarely with haematuria. Diagnosis is established by excretion urography followed by arteriography. A combination of nephrectomy, radiotherapy and chemotherapy has much improved survival rates, and the majority of children, even those with metastatic disease, are cured.

BENIGN RENAL TUMOURS

Renal adenoma

Benign adenomas are usually an incidental finding, presenting as a space-occupying lesion on excretion urography. They seldom cause symptoms. On urography they may be difficult to distinguish from a renal cell carcinoma.

Simple cysts

Simple cysts are common. They are discussed in more detail on p. 424.

Differentiation of benign renal cyst from malignant tumour
If a space-occupying lesion is a chance finding on excretion urography in a patient with no relevant symptoms and no haematuria, ultrasonography should be carried out. If the lesion is transonic with no features suggesting a tumour, no further investigation is required. If haematuria has been present, a needle should be inserted into the transonic lesion and cyst fluid aspirated and examined for malignant cells. Contrast medium may be injected to delineate the walls of the cyst. Lesions shown to be solid or non-homogeneous on ultrasonography require further investigation by CT or arteriography.

UROTHELIAL TUMOURS

The calyces, renal pelvis, ureter, bladder and urethra are lined by transitional cell epithelium. Transitional cell tumours account for about 3% of deaths from all forms of malignancy. Such tumours are uncommon below the age of 40 years, and the male/female ratio is 4:1. Bladder tumours are about 50 times as common as those of the ureter or renal pelvis.

PREDISPOSING FACTORS

These include:
- Cigarette smoking
- Exposure to industrial carcinogens such as beta-naphthylamine and benzidene. Workers in the chemical, cable and rubber industries are at particular risk.
- Exposure to drugs, e.g. phenacetin, cyclophosphamide
- Chronic inflammation, e.g. schistosomiasis (usually associated with squamous carcinoma)

PRESENTATION

Painless haematuria is the commonest presenting symptom of bladder malignancy, although pain may occur due to clot retention. Symptoms suggestive of urinary tract infection may develop in the absence of significant bacteriuria. In patients with bladder cancer, pain may also result from local nerve involvement.

Presenting symptoms may result from local metastases.

Transitional cell carcinomas in the kidney and ureter may present with haematuria. They may also give rise to flank pain, particularly if urinary tract obstruction is present.

INVESTIGATION

Investigation includes:
- Cytological examination of urine for malignant cells
- Excretion urography
- Cystoscopy if no evidence of upper urinary tract pathology has been found

Cytoscopy may be omitted in men under 20 and women under 30 years if significant bacteriuria accompanies the haematuria and both cease following control of the infection, and if urine cytology and excretion urography are normal. With these exceptions, it is essential that haematuria is always investigated.

In cases where the tumour is not clearly outlined on excretion urography, abdominal CT scanning and/or retrograde ureterography may be helpful.

TREATMENT

Pelvic and ureteric tumours
These are treated by nephroureterectomy. Radiotherapy and chemotherapy appear to be of little or no value.

Subsequently cystoscopy should be regularly carried out, since about half the patients will develop bladder tumours.

Bladder tumours

Treatment depends upon the stage of the tumour (in particular whether it has penetrated the bladder muscle) and its degree of differentiation. Treatment options include local cystodiathermy and/or resection with follow-up check cystoscopies, cystectomy, radiotherapy, or local and systemic chemotherapy.

PROGNOSIS

The prognosis ranges from a 5-year survival rate of 80% for lesions not involving bladder muscle to 5% for those presenting with metastases.

BENIGN ENLARGEMENT OF THE PROSTATE GLAND

Benign prostatic enlargement occurs most often in men over the age of 60 years. Such enlargement is much less common in black and Asian individuals. It is unknown in eunuchs. The aetiology of the condition is unknown.

Microscopically, hyperplasia affects the glandular and connective tissue elements of the prostate. Enlargement of the gland stretches and distorts the urethra, obstructing bladder outflow. The bladder musculature hypertrophies so that a higher than usual pressure is generated within the bladder in order to overcome the obstruction and to enable voiding of urine to occur. Bands of muscle fibre are seen at cystoscopy (trabeculation). Eventually the bladder becomes dilated and the muscle hypotonic. The sphincter mechanism at the vesico-ureteric junction may be impaired and reflux of urine from the bladder into the ureters and upper urinary tract may occur.

CLINICAL FEATURES

Frequency of urination, usually first noted as nocturia, is a common early symptom. Difficulty or delay in initiating urination, with variability and reduced forcefulness of the urinary stream are often present. Suprapubic pain occurs if bladder bacteriuria is present, if a bladder calculus has formed as a result of stagnation of urine within the bladder, or in acute retention of urine. Flank pain may accompany dilatation of the upper tracts. Acute retention of urine (see p. 405) or retention with overflow incontinence may occur. Occasionally, severe haematuria results from rupture of prostatic veins or as a consequence of bacteriuria or stone disease. Some patients present with severe renal failure.

Abdominal examination for bladder enlargement together with examination of the rectum are essential. A benign prostate feels smooth. An accurate impression of prostatic size cannot be obtained on rectal examination.

INVESTIGATION

This should include urine culture, assessment of renal function by measuring the blood urea or serum creatinine, a plain abdominal x-ray, and renal ultrasonography to define whether upper tract dilatation is present. Excretion urography is not usually necessary unless facilities for ultrasonography are limited. If possible, an act of urination should be watched and the flow rate of urine measured. The completeness of bladder emptying after an act of voiding can be assessed by ultrasonography or by inspection of the after-voiding radiograph carried out during excretion urography. Cystourethroscopy is essential.

MANAGEMENT AND PROGNOSIS

Patients with prostatic symptoms who do not have upper tract dilatation require surgery only if symptoms are troublesome or acute retention has occurred. Eradication of bacteriuria may relieve symptoms originally attributed to outflow obstruction.

Deterioration in renal function or the development of upper tract dilatation requires surgery. Transurethral resection is usually successful unless the gland is very large. It carries a lower morbidity and mortality with a shorter stay in hospital than open prostatectomy. Very large glands require open transvesical prostatectomy.

In acute retention or retention with overflow, the first priorities are to relieve pain and to establish urethral catheter drainage. The bladder should be decompressed slowly to prevent bleeding from the mucosa. If urethral catheterization is impossible, suprapubic catheter drainage should be carried out. The choice of further management is then between immediate prostatectomy, a period of catheter drainage followed by prostatectomy, or the acceptance of a permanent indwelling suprapubic or urethral catheter.

PROSTATIC CARCINOMA

This accounts for 7% of all cancers in men and is the fourth commonest cause of death from malignant disease in men in England and Wales. Malignant change within the prostate becomes increasingly common with advancing age. By the age of 80 years, 80% of men have malignant foci within the gland, but most of these appear to lie dormant. Histologically, the tumour is an adenocarcinoma. Hormonal factors are thought to play a role in the aetiology.

CLINICAL FEATURES

Presentation is usually with symptoms of lower urinary tract obstruction or of metastatic spread, particularly to bone. The diagnosis may be made by the incidental finding of a hard irregular gland on rectal examination or as an unexpected histological result after prostatectomy for what was believed to be benign prostatic hypertrophy.

INVESTIGATION

A histological diagnosis is essential before treatment is considered. This may be obtained:
● By cytological staining of biopsy material from the prostate
● By histological examination of biopsy material or material obtained at transurethral or open prostatectomy

If metastases are present, serum acid phosphatase may be elevated; it is a myth that elevated levels occur as a result of rectal examination.

Ultrasonography is of value in defining the size of the gland and staging any tumour present. The upper renal tracts can be examined by ultrasonography for evidence of dilatation. Bone metastases may appear as osteosclerotic lesions on x-ray or may be detected by isotopic bone scans.

TREATMENT

Treatment is by prostatectomy for disease confined to the gland, combined with bilateral orchidectomy or stilboestrol or anti-androgen therapy if metastases are present. External pelvic irradiation is used in some locally infiltrating prostatic malignancies.

PROGNOSIS

The duration of survival depends on the age of the patient and the degree of differentiation and extent of the tumour.

TESTICULAR TUMOURS

Testicular tumours, though uncommon, are the commonest malignant disease in men between the ages of 29 and 34 years. All such tumours should nowadays be regarded as curable. Patient survival depends upon early diagnosis, accurate staging of the tumour and appropriate treatment and follow-up. The expertise of a specialist centre is invaluable.

More than 96% of testicular tumours arise from germ cells. Two main types of tumour exist:
● Seminomas (about one-third)
● Teratomas (about two-thirds)

AETIOLOGY

The aetiology is unknown. The risk of malignant change is much greater in undescended testes and there is a history of orchidopexy in about 10% of patients.

CLINICAL FEATURES

Common presenting symptoms are:
● Testicular swelling, which may be painless or painful
● Symptoms from metastases

DIFFERENTIAL DIAGNOSIS

The differential diagnosis includes:
● Epididymo-orchitis
● Torsion
● Chronic infection, e.g. tuberculosis, syphilitic gumma

INVESTIGATION

Diagnosis may only be possible after surgical exploration of the testis through the groin. Scrotal exploration and scrotal testicular biopsy should be avoided owing to the high incidence of tumour implantation.

Staging of the tumour will require:
● Chest x-ray to look for metastases
● Estimation of alpha-fetoprotein and beta-human chorionic gonadotrophin concentrations (tumour markers)
● Abdominal CT scanning

TREATMENT

Seminomas are radiosensitive, so tumours confined to the testis or with metastases below the diaphragm only are treated by radiotherapy. More widespread tumours require chemotherapy.

Teratomas are treated by orchidectomy if the growth is confined to the testis. Chemotherapy is required for more widespread disease.

Further reading

Black D & Jones NF (1979) *Renal Disease*, 4th edn. Oxford: Blackwell Scientific.
Massry SG & Glassock RJ (eds) (1983) *Textbook of Nephrology*. Baltimore: Williams & Wilkins.
Wood RFM (1983) *Renal Transplantation: A Clinical Handbook*. London: Baillière Tindall.

10

Water, Electrolyte and Acid–Base Homeostasis

Water and electrolyte homeostasis

In health the volume and composition of body fluids are held remarkably constant from day to day. The end-organ primarily responsible for this is the kidney. In disease this constancy of the 'milieu interieur' can be seriously deranged as a result of:

- Extrarenal factors (e.g. vomiting or diarrhoea)
- Endocrine disturbances
- Intrinsic renal disease

The diagnosis and management of such disturbances requires a knowledge of certain physiological principles and rules for clinical assessment.

Physiological principles

It is helpful in clinical practice to distinguish between the *volume* of any body fluid and its *composition*. These may be disturbed singly or together.

Body fluid volume and distribution

Water is the chief constituent of the body, accounting for 45–80% of the body weight. This percentage varies with age, sex and body build (Table 10.1), being greater in men, in thin subjects and in infants. An average 75 kg male has about 45 l of water. Two-thirds of this is intracellular fluid (ICF). The remain-

Table 10.1 Body water as a percentage of body weight.

Build	Infants	Men	Women
Thin	80%	65%	55%
Average	70%	60%	50%
Fat	65%	55%	45%

ing 15 l is extracellular fluid (ECF) and is divided between the interstitial fluid (IF) (10 l) and the vascular compartment (VC) (5 l) (see Fig. 10.1). A fourth, 'transcellular' compartment includes cerebrospinal, synovial, pleural and pericardial fluids, plus water in the gut. Normally this is small, but in disease, e.g. in paralytic ileus or massive pleural effusion, it can become important.

Distribution of water between the extracellular and intracellular compartments depends on an osmotic equilibrium between them.

The osmolality of a solution is determined by the total concentration of dissolved or colloid particles within the solution. Thus, 1 mol of sodium chloride dissolved in 1 kg of water has an osmolality of 2 osmol·kg^{-1}, as sodium chloride freely dissociates into the two particles, sodium and chloride. One mole of urea (which does not dissociate) in 1 kg of water has an osmolality of 1 osmol·kg^{-1}. One millimole of sodium chloride in 1 kg of water gives an osmolality of 2 mosmol·kg^{-1}.

In a complex solution of several electrolytes, osmolality can be calculated by adding together the molar concentration of all the constituents, taking account of the degree of dissociation. As sodium and chloride are the dominant ECF ions, plasma osmolality is, for practical purposes:

$$\text{sodium concentration (mmol·l}^{-1}) \times 2 + 10$$

The 10 takes into account the osmolality of the glucose and urea in the plasma.

The concentration of particles, i.e. the osmolality, within the ICF and the ECF is always in equilibrium. Addition of water to the ECF reduces its osmolality,

Fig. 10.1 Distribution of body water in a 75 kg man.

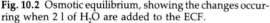

Fig. 10.2 Osmotic equilibrium, showing the changes occurring when 2 l of H₂O are added to the ECF.

causes disequilibrium in osmolality between the two compartments, and leads to water moving into cells until the osmolality equilibrium is re-established (see Fig. 10.2). Loss of water from the ECF would do the reverse.

Partitioning of water between the vascular and interstitial compartments depends on osmotic equilibrium, but is also affected by the osmotic pressure exerted by non-diffusible plasma proteins (mainly albumin). This 'oncotic pressure', equal to about 25 mmHg, is critical to the circulation of fluid between the capillaries and interstitial fluid. Fluid leaves the arteriolar end of capillary beds under the influence of capillary hydrostatic pressure and is 'recaptured' at the low pressure, venous end by the oncotic pressure of plasma proteins. In hypo-albuminaemic states, this balance is lost and oedema fluid accumulates in the tissues. Conversely, removal of water from plasma, e.g. by ultrafiltration in patients with kidney failure (see p. 417), causes a rise in plasma oncotic pressure which 'sucks' fluid into the vascular compartment. The balance of fluid between the two compartments is also dependent on the Gibbs–Donnan equilibrium (this explains the unequal distribution of diffusible ions on the two sides of a semi-permeable membrane if one side contains a poorly diffusible ion). The result of both these effects is that the osmolality of plasma is marginally greater than that of interstitial fluid and the electrolyte composition of the two compartments is also slightly different (Table 10.2).

The composition of body fluids

The composition of intracellular, interstitial and plasma fluid is set out in Table 10.2. Allowing for the plasma oncotic pressure and the Gibbs–Donnan distribution, plasma and interstitial fluid have, for practical purposes, the same electrolyte content. Intracellular fluid, which constitutes two-thirds of body fluid, is quite different. In particular, sodium and chloride ions are primarily extracellular, while potassium is the dominant intracellular cation balanced by phosphate, sulphate and bicarbonate ions and protein. This 'in–out' difference in the distribution of

Table 10.2 Electrolyte composition of intracellular and extracellular fluids.

	Plasma (mmol·l⁻¹)	Interstitial fluid (mmol·l⁻¹)	Intracellular fluid (mmol·l⁻¹)
Na⁺	142	144	10
K⁺	4	4	160
Ca²⁺	2.5	1.25	1.5
Mg²⁺	1.0	0.5	13
Cl⁻	102	114	2
HCO₃⁻	26	30	8
PO₄²⁻	1.0	1.0	57
SO₄²⁻	0.5	0.5	10
Organic acid	6	5	
Protein	16	0	55

Fig. 10.3 The effects of saline and dextrose saline on osmotic equilibrium.

sodium and potassium is a consequence of the metabolic cell pumps and is dependent on normal oxygenation and metabolism. The separation of sodium and potassium outside and inside cells has important consequences in relation to fluid distribution. Since sodium and chloride are extracellular, loss or addition of salt-containing solutions primarily affects the volume of the ECF and only affects the ICF if there is also a change in the osmolality of the ECF. Thus intravenous infusion of 'normal' (isotonic) saline (150 mmol sodium per litre) primarily affects the volume of the ECF (see Fig. 10.3), while $\frac{1}{5}$ normal dextrose saline (30 mmol sodium per litre) will distribute between both the ECF and the ICF, since the glucose but not the sodium enters the cells.

Factors controlling volume and composition

Body water homeostasis is effected by thirst and the urine-concentrating and diluting functions of the kidney. These in turn are controlled by intracellular osmoreceptors, principally in the hypothalamus, to some extent by volume receptors in capacitance vessels close to the heart, and possibly via the renin–angiotensin system. Of these, the major and best-understood control is via osmoreceptors. An increase in intracellular osmolality stimulates both thirst and the release of ADH from the posterior pituitary, while a fall has the opposite effect. Thirst stimulates increased water intake, while ADH increases the reabsorption of water from tubular fluid by its action on the distal tubules of the kidney, thus causing a reduction in the urine output.

Control of effective circulating blood volume
For the health of all tissues it is essential that there is a constant circulation of blood, both to supply oxygen and nutrients and to remove waste products. To achieve this there must be an adequate pump (the heart) and an appropriate circulating blood volume. The importance of maintaining the circulating blood volume is reflected in the variety of 'feedback' systems which exist to guard it. Apart from the

control of the circulating red cell mass, these operate primarily through the control of body sodium and the secondary control of accompanying water.

Control of body sodium and extracellular body fluid
Sodium and its accompanying anions, principally chloride and bicarbonate, are the main extracellular electrolytes. They are the main determinants of plasma osmolality and, through osmoreceptors, they control water homeostasis. It is the *amount* of sodium in the ECF, with adjustment of water balance to a normal body fluid osmolality, which determines the *volume* of the ECF; control of the volume of ECF is thus achieved by controlling the amount of sodium in the ECF.

To understand disturbance of fluid balance, it is essential clearly to distinguish between the *concentration* of sodium in the ECF (in practice, the plasma sodium) and the *amount* of sodium present (see Fig. 10.4). Concentration only tells the relative amounts of sodium to water; it tells nothing about the absolute amount or volume of either. In practice, this requires a separate clinical assessment of the volume of the ECF.

Control of the volume of ECF via control of sodium balance is dependent on a variety of volume receptors or sensors. Volume receptors are believed

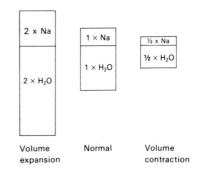

Fig. 10.4 The relationship of sodium to water in isonatraemia.

to be present in the large-capacitance vessels close to the heart and possibly in heart muscle. Receptors in the atrial mucosa control the release of a potent natriuretic hormone—atrial natriuretic peptide—which also inhibits the release of aldosterone. Receptors in the walls of the afferent glomerular arterioles respond, via the juxtaglomerular apparatus, to changes in renal perfusion, and control the activity of the renin–angiotensin–aldosterone system. Neurogenic reflexes within the kidney may also be involved, and the circulation of a natriuretic hormone, the source of which is unclear, is postulated. The final common path for such regulatory systems is to increase or decrease the renal excretion of sodium in the event of an increase or decrease in effective circulating blood volume. An increase in the reabsorption of salt, with concomitant retention of water (due to a change in osmolality), expands the vascular and interstitial compartments, while increased sodium excretion has the opposite effects.

Clinical assessment of water and electrolyte balance

HISTORY

The first essential step is a careful history to define circumstances which might lead to fluid and electrolyte imbalance. The average normal daily intakes of sodium, potassium and water are 100–250 mmol, 40–120 mmol, and 500–2500 ml, respectively. The possible losses from the gut are given in Table 10.3. Daily urinary losses vary greatly; they may be as much as 5 l or more of water, with loss of 150–200 mmol of sodium or 50–100 mmol of potassium.

PHYSICAL EXAMINATION

Except in severe dehydration, the time-honoured assessment of skin turgor, intraocular pressure and the state of the tongue is imprecise and of limited

value. Of much greater importance is careful assessment of the circulatory status and the presence or absence of oedema. Circulatory failure may be obvious, with recumbent hypotension, tachycardia and cold peripheral parts. When less obvious, particular attention must be paid to the jugular venous pressure (JVP) and to the presence or absence of postural hypotension. Usually a normal or elevated JVP can be defined, but if in doubt, and especially in oliguric patients, a central venous line must be inserted to record central venous pressure (CVP).

An elevated JVP or CVP always indicates fluid overload, except in acute heart failure. A low JVP or CVP in a setting of fluid loss or incomplete replacement must be taken as evidence of volume depletion and is an indication for the administration of fluids. A normal or low blood pressure in a previously hypertensive patient in the absence of drug treatment or evidence of acute myocardial damage is also highly suggestive of fluid depletion.

Postural hypotension (a fall of systolic blood pressure after 5 min of standing of more than 20 mmHg from the recumbent value or to less than 100 mmHg) may result from:
- Hypotensive drugs
- Autonomic neuropathy
- Volume depletion

A low JVP plus postural hypotension in an appropriate clinical setting provide very strong evidence for volume depletion.

Sacral or symmetrical peripheral oedema and, less reliably, basal lung crackles are evidence of fluid overload, whether due to oliguric renal failure, heart failure or hypoalbuminaemic states. Only very rarely, and usually in a setting of excessive diuretic therapy for heart failure or gross hypoalbuminaemic states, is it possible to have oedema associated with a *reduced* blood volume due to salt and water depletion.

Evidence of weight loss due to negative fluid balance is rarely available at the time of first presentation, except in severe cases when it has been noted by the patient or his relatives. In hospital, review of weight charts is valuable. An acute increase or

Table 10.3 Average concentrations and potential daily losses of water and electrolytes from the gut.

	Na$^+$ (mmol·l^{-1})	K$^+$ (mmol·l^{-1})	Cl$^-$ (mmol·l^{-1})	Volume (ml)
Stomach	50	10	110	2500
Small intestine:				
Recent ileostomy	120	5	110	1500
Adapted ileostomy	50	4	25	500
Bile	140	5	105	500
Pancreatic juice	140	5	60	700
Diarrhoea	130	10–50	95	1000–2000+

decrease in weight always reflects a change in water balance, and in problem cases, daily weighing is mandatory. In hospitalized patients, careful review of 'input/output' charts can also give valuable information, but these are often inaccurate.

It should be noted that the physical signs described relate primarily to changes in the ECF volume, especially the intravascular volume. In turn these relate principally to changes in body fluid balance due to salt and water—the most common clinical problem. Pure water loss or excess has much less effect on the circulation, as the altered water volume is 'shared' by all of the 45 l of body water; quite severe losses or excesses can be tolerated haemodynamically and can be difficult to detect on clinical examination (see Fig. 10.2). Net water loss or gain is more readily identified by the development of hyper- or hyponatraemia. Pure water loss is uncommon; pure water excess is usually iatrogenic.

INVESTIGATION

Haematological investigation
In an appropriate setting an abnormally high haemoglobin or haematocrit suggests fluid depletion. The clinical situation is, however, often complex. Interpretation of haemoglobin level or haematocrit is particularly difficult in patients who are anaemic or who have lost blood as a result of the underlying disease.

Biochemical investigation
Having assessed the volume of body fluid, the nature of the fluid loss or excess can be defined by measurement of plasma electrolytes, particularly the plasma sodium. It must be re-emphasized that sodium concentration does *not* of itself give information as to whether there is sodium depletion or overload. Rather, consideration of plasma sodium concentration taken in conjunction with an assessment of body fluid volume allows definition of the nature of the problem and the measures required to treat it.

The causes and nature of disturbances in water and electrolyte balance

The major causes for a disturbance in fluid and electrolyte balance are set out in Table 10.4. At the time of presentation the situation is commonly confused by partial correction of the problem by the patient, e.g. thirst and increased water intake in diarrhoea, or by partial or over-enthusiastic treatment by attending clinicians.

Table 10.4 Causes of fluid and electrolyte disturbances.

LOSSES
Gut
Vomiting
Diarrhoea
Fistula or 'ostomies'
Paralytic ileus
Kidney
Diuretic therapy
Polyuria
Post-obstructive
Post acute tubular necrosis
Severe renal failure
Hypokalaemia
Lithium therapy
Hypercalcaemia
Diabetes mellitus
Diabetes insipidus
Adrenal failure
REDUCED INTAKE
Loss of thirst mechanism
Unconscious/confused states
Hypothalamic lesion (rare)
Lack of access to water
Unconscious/confused states
Bedridden
Infants
Inappropriate/inadequate intake
Hospitalized patients, especially on i.v. regimens
FLUID RETENTION
Heart failure
Hypoproteinaemia, e.g. cirrhosis, nephrotic syndrome
Oliguric renal failure
Cirrhosis
Excessive fluid replacement
Inappropriate ADH secretion

Following a careful history, the volume of body fluid (especially the ECF) and its composition with respect to sodium and potassium concentrations should be assessed. The ECF volume may be normal, expanded or contracted (see Figs. 10.4 and 10.5). At the same time the serum sodium may be normal, increased or decreased (see Fig. 10.5).

NORMO-NATRAEMIC VOLUME OVERLOAD OR DEFICIT

This is the most common disturbance. The fluid overload or deficit is normally modest, and may be due to heart failure, oliguric renal failure, hypoalbuminic states, vomiting, diarrhoea or polyuria from whatever cause. It is identified by clinical evidence of fluid overload or deficit plus a serum sodium value within the normal range of 135–150 mmol·l^{-1}.

Hyponatraemia

Water excess	Normal	Sodium deficit
1 × Na	1 × Na	½ × Na
2 × H₂O	1 × H₂O	1 × H₂O

Hypernatraemia

Water deficit	Normal	Sodium excess
1 × Na	1 × Na	2 × Na
½ × H₂O	1 × H₂O	1 × H₂O

Fig. 10.5 The relationship of sodium to water in hypo-natraemia and hypernatraemia.

TREATMENT

Treatment may be divided into primary and secondary.

Primary treatment
This is directed at eliminating the cause of the problem, e.g.
● Improvement in cardiac function
● Correction of hypoalbuminaemia
● Arrest of vomiting and diarrhoea
● Removal of drugs causing polyuria

Secondary treatment
This is concerned with correcting the salt and water abnormality pending the response to primary treatment or alleviating the situation when primary treatment is not possible.

Salt and water overload. This requires:
● Restriction in sodium intake—a 'no added salt regimen', allowing salt only in cooking with no addition of salt at table and avoidance of salty foods (50 mmol of sodium daily)
● Diuretic (or more correctly natriuretic) treatment with thiazide diuretics (e.g. bendrofluazide 5 mg twice daily). More powerful loop diuretics (frusemide or ethacrynic acid) should only be used when a thiazide diuretic fails *or* where there is severe renal failure or life-threatening pulmonary congestion.
● Modest restriction in water intake (1000 ml per day). This is usually sufficient since, if the sodium overload is corrected, the accompanying water overload will correct itself.

Normo-natraemic volume depletion. This requires replacement of salt and water. This is best done orally if possible.

If kidney function is normal an increased water intake (2–3 l per day) accompanied by 60–80 mmol of sodium chloride (6–8 tablets Slow Sodium daily in divided doses) will suffice, as sodium retention by the kidneys will be maximal. In the presence of salt-wasting kidney disease, larger amounts of sodium chloride may be required. These are best supplied by the *cautious* infusion of normal saline.

HYPONATRAEMIA

Hyponatraemia may be due to an excess of body water with a normal amount of body sodium, a normal amount of water with reduced sodium, or some combination of the two (Fig. 10.5). Rarely it may be pseudohyponatraemia, where a high lipid content in plasma, as in diabetes or the nephrotic syndrome, results in a spuriously low measured sodium concentration, the sodium being confined to the aqueous phase but having its concentration expressed in terms of the total volume of plasma.

Salt-deficient hyponatraemia

The commonest sites of large sodium losses (see Table 10.4) are:
● *The gut.* Vomiting, diarrhoea or sequestration of fluid in paralytic ileus can lead to considerable losses of sodium and potassium as well as causing acid–base disturbance.
● *The kidney.* Renal salt loss is usually less obvious than loss from the gut, and occurs as a result of defective tubular reabsorption, whether as a result of:
  (a) Osmotic diuresis (e.g. hyperglycaemia) or severe uraemia
  (b) Excessive use of diuretics
  (c) Adrenocortical insufficiency (see p. 724)
  (d) Tubulo-interstitial renal disease

With the exception of the recovery phase of acute tubular necrosis (see p. 417), salt-wasting renal disease is most often associated with disease of the medullary area, as in:
● Atrophic pyelonephritis
● Obstructive nephropathy
● Tubulo-interstitial disease due to:
  (a) Sickle cell disease or trait
  (b) Analgesic nephropathy
  (c) Diabetes mellitus
● Medullary cystic disease

Hyponatraemia due to salt loss in excess of water initially suppresses ADH secretion via the osmo-receptors, but as fluid volume is lost, volume receptors override the osmoreceptors and stimulate both thirst and the release of ADH. With extrarenal losses and normal kidneys, the urinary excretion of sodium falls in response to the volume depletion, as does water excretion, leading to concentrated urine containing less than 10 mmol·l^{-1} of sodium. However, in salt-wasting kidney disease, renal compensation cannot occur and the only protection is increased water intake in response to thirst.

CLINICAL FEATURES

With sodium depletion the clinical picture is usually dominated by features of volume depletion. This gives rise to dehydration.

The diagnosis is usually obvious where there is a history of gut losses, diabetes mellitus or diuretic abuse. Losses due to renal or adrenocortical disease may be less easily identified and are suggested by a urinary sodium concentration of more than 20 mmol·l^{-1} in the presence of clinically evident volume depletion.

TREATMENT

This is directed at the primary cause whenever possible. Increased salt intake as Slow Sodium 60–80 mmol daily is all that is required in the relatively healthy patient who can take this by mouth. In the face of vomiting or severe volume depletion, intravenous infusion of normal saline may be required. Potassium supplements and correction of acid–base abnormalities may also be required.

Guidelines for intravenous fluid administration in fluid and electrolyte disturbances

Only use if not possible to give fluids by mouth or nasogastric tube.

If hypovolaemic, correct with:
● Normal saline
   or
● Normal saline alternating with 1.4% sodium bicarbonate if acidotic

For maintenance fluid balance:
● 'Guesstimate' daily water and salt losses (see Table 10.3).
● Identify appropriate fluid (see Table 10.5).
● Confirm replacement is appropriate by assessing daily body *fluid volume* clinically and fluid composition from plasma electrolytes

If hypervolaemic:
● Give no fluid
● Give minimum fluid required for parenteral drugs in a fluid compatible with drug (usually 5% glucose)

It cannot be overemphasized that, apart from in severe fluid overload or in life-threatening pulmon-ary congestion or severe volume depletion due to gross salt and water loss (as in infants), aggressive correction of abnormalities of salt and water balance are rarely justified, and are often dangerous. Gradual correction over 48 h is generally satisfactory. Aggressive volume repletion demands obsessional monitoring of the CVP, which is best done by a CVP line, and regular checks for evidence of pulmonary congestion or peripheral oedema.

Table 10.5 gives a list of fluids and electrolytes available for intravenous use.

Hyponatraemia due to water excess ('dilutional hyponatraemia')

This results from an intake of water in excess of the kidneys' ability to excrete it. It is uncommon with normal kidney function, requiring an intake of approximately 1 l·h^{-1}. Over-generous infusion of 5% glucose into postoperative patients is one of the commonest causes, in which situation it is exacerbated by increased ADH secretion in response to stress. Some degree of hyponatraemia is usual in acute oliguric renal failure, while in patients with chronic renal failure it is most often due to ill-advised advice to 'push' fluids.

The commonest presentation of hyponatraemia due to water excess is in patients with severe cardiac failure, hepatic cirrhosis or the nephrotic syndrome. In all these conditions there is usually an element of reduced glomerular filtration rate with avid reabsorption of sodium and chloride in the proximal tubule. This leads to reduced delivery of chloride to the 'diluting' ascending limb of Henle's loop and a reduced ability to generate 'free water', with a consequent inability to excrete dilute urine. This is commonly compounded by the administration of diuretics that block chloride reabsorption and interfere with the dilution of filtrate either in Henle's loop (loop diuretics) or distally (thiazides).

Adrenal insufficiency (see p. 724) also interferes with the renal excretion of water.

CLINICAL FEATURES

Symptoms are common with dilutional hyponatraemia when this develops acutely. They are principally neurological and are due to the movement of water into brain cells in response to the fall in extracellular osmolality. Symptoms rarely occur until the serum sodium is less than 120 mmol·l^{-1} and are more usually associated with values around 110 mmol·l^{-1} or lower. Symptoms include confusion and restlessness leading to drowsiness, myoclonic jerks, generalized convulsions and eventually coma.

TREATMENT

Most cases are simply managed by restriction in water intake with review of diuretic therapy.

Table 10.5 Intravenous fluids in general use for fluid and electrolyte disturbances.

	Na^+ (mmol·l^{-1})	K^+ (mmol·l^{-1})	HCO_3^- or equivalent (mmol·l^{-1})	Cl^- (mmol·l^{-1})	Ca^{2+} (mmol·l^{-1})	Indication (see footnotes)
Normal plasma values	142	4.5	26	103	2.5	
Sodium chloride 0.9% ('normal saline')	150	—	—	150	—	1
Sodium chloride 0.18% + glucose 4% ('1/5 normal saline')	30	—	—	30	—	2
Glucose 5%	—	—	—	—	—	3
Sodium bicarbonate 1.4%	167	—	167	—	—	4
Sodium bicarbonate 8.4%	1000	—	1000	—	—	5
Compound sodium lactate (Hartmann's)	131	5	29	111	2	6

1. Volume expansion in hypovolaemic patients. Rarely to maintain fluid balance when there are large losses of sodium in urine.

2. Maintenance of fluid balance in normo-volaemic, normo-natraemic patients.

3. To replace *water*. May be alternated with normal saline as an alternative to (2).

4. For volume expansion in hypovolaemic, *acidotic* patients alternating with (1). Occasionally for maintenance of fluid balance combined with (2) in salt-wasting, acidotic patients. To induce forced alkaline diuresis, e.g. in salicylate poisoning.

5. Small amounts (100–200 ml) used to correct acidosis following cardiac arrest.

6. Reserve for healthy (e.g. postoperative) patients. *Never* in patients with renal disease because of potassium content. Best avoided.

Hypertonic salt solutions should never be used in oedematous patients. The use of hypertonic saline should be restricted to patients with acute water intoxication and *must* be given slowly (not more than 70 mmol·h^{-1}), the aim being to increase the serum sodium to more than 125 mmol·l^{-1}. Rapid infusion of hypertonic saline carries a risk of acute heart failure due to sodium overload or brain damage due to acute fluid shifts.

In already fluid-overloaded patients, mannitol 20% 100 ml may be infused in an attempt to increase renal water excretion.

Syndrome of inappropriate ADH secretion

This is described in Chapter 16. It is manifest as hyponatraemia with normal or slight expansion of ECF volume.

HYPERNATRAEMIA

This is most often the result of a loss of water in excess of sodium. A true excess of body sodium with normal water (see Fig. 10.5) is rare and is usually iatrogenic. Loss of water from the ECF is buffered by the movement of water from the ICF to maintain osmotic equilibrium. Water losses must therefore be massive to induce a significant rise in serum sodium. Water depletion results either from inadequate intake or losses from the gut, kidneys or via the skin and lungs.

Insufficient intake is most often found in the elderly or neonates or in unconscious patients when access to water is denied or confusion or coma eliminates the normal response to thirst. Rarely it is due to hypothalamic disease with loss of normal thirst. The situation is exacerbated by increased losses of fluid.

Gastrointestinal fluids are for the most part hypotonic (see Table 10.3). Thus, unreplaced losses due to vomiting or diarrhoea result in hypernatraemia. Similarly, litres of hypotonic fluid can be lost from the skin or lungs, especially in febrile diseases and in hot, dry climates. Infants, because of their large surface area relative to volume, are at special risk. Hypernatraemia due to large water losses is also common in patients with extensive burns.

Renal losses of water in sufficient excess of sodium to induce hypernatraemia occur only in patients with diabetes insipidus or in those undergoing spontaneous osmotic diuresis as in severe hyperglycaemia or (less often) uraemia. The latter mechanism was responsible for the hypernatraemia formerly seen in neurosurgical wards when unconscious patients were tube-fed solutions high in protein and low in water.

Hypernatraemia due to salt excess is virtually always iatrogenic, as the result of a too liberal infusion of hypertonic saline or bicarbonate solution, or the accidental addition of salt rather than sugar to an infant's feed.

CLINICAL FEATURES

Water-depletion hypernatraemia is associated with signs of volume depletion and circulatory failure. If acute, hypernatraemia may lead to venous thrombosis in infants and cerebral symptoms such as lethargy, drowsiness, muscle twitching and coma secondary to brain cell dehydration.

TREATMENT

The hyperosmolality must be corrected slowly. Water should be given by mouth whenever possible, but intravenous infusion is usually necessary. If the plasma sodium is more than 170 mmol·l^{-1}, normal saline (150 mmol sodium per litre) is given to allow gradual correction. If the plasma sodium is 150 mmol·l^{-1} or less, $\frac{1}{5}$ normal dextrose saline (30 mmol sodium per litre) should be used. The aim is to correct the hypernatraemia over 48 h. Too fast correction can result in cerebral oedema or brain haemorrhage.

DISORDERS OF POTASSIUM METABOLISM

Physiological considerations
Ninety eight per cent of body potassium is intra-cellular at a concentration of approximately 160 mmol·l^{-1}, contrasting with an extracellular con-centration of 3.5–5.0 mmol·l^{-1} (see Table 10.2). This 'in–out' ratio is critical for the normal activity of all cells. Dietary intake of potassium is normally 80–150 mmol daily and balanced excretion is principally via the kidneys with a small amount (5–15 mmol) excreted in the faeces.

Control of the distribution of potassium between the ECF and the ICF is dependent on metabolic cell pumps and is influenced by:
- *pH*. Potassium moves into cells in alkalosis and out of cells in acidosis.
- *Aldosterone*. An increase or decrease in plasma potassium increases or decreases aldosterone production. It is suspected, but not proved, that aldosterone increases the uptake of potassium into cells.
- *Insulin*. An increase in plasma potassium increases insulin release. Exogenous insulin increases potassium uptake into liver and muscle cells, but the physiological role of endogenous insulin in potassium metabolism is less clear.
- *Beta-adrenergic nervous activity*. Hyperkalaemia is

seen in treatment with beta-blocking drugs and in autonomic neuropathy, suggesting a role for the beta-adrenergic nervous system in controlling 'in–out' potassium balance.

In the kidney, filtered potassium is normally totally absorbed in the proximal tubule, controlled secretion occurring in the distal tubule and collecting ducts. Several factors control potassium secretion. A high intake leads to adaptive increased potassium secre-tion. Any condition that increases delivery of sodium to the distal nephron, such as salt loading, loop diuretics or osmotic diuretics, increases potassium secretion. Mineralocorticoids enhance sodium reab-sorption and potassium secretion. Systemic alkalosis increases potassium secretion, while acidosis decreases it, probably as a result of a shift of potass-ium into or out of tubular cells, as occurs with cells generally. Finally, potassium secretion increases with urine flow rate.

Hypokalaemia

Hypokalaemia may result from a shift of potassium into cells (internal imbalance) or from the loss of potassium via the kidneys or the gut (Table 10.6). Vomit contains relatively little potassium (5–10 mmol·l^{-1}), but persistent vomiting leads to a hypochloraemic alkalosis due to loss of chloride and gastric acid, which causes severe renal wasting of potassium and movement of potassium into cells. Liquid stool contains 10–50 mmol·l^{-1} of potassium, so profuse diarrhoea can induce marked

Table 10.6 Causes of hypokalaemia.

Intracellular shifts
Alkalosis
High-dose insulin
Periodic paralysis (see p. 866)
Renal wasting
Diuresis
Drugs
Osmotic (e.g. hyperglycaemia, uraemia)
Renal tubular acidosis
Hyperaldosteronism—primary or secondary
Cushing's and adrenogenital syndromes
Bartter's syndrome
Drugs (e.g. liquorice, carbenoxolone sodium, gentamicin toxicity)
Leukaemia
Gastrointestinal loss
Vomiting and diarrhoea
Ileostomy or ureterosigmoidostomy
Purgative abuse
Anorexia nervosa with bulimia
Villous adenoma of rectum

hypokalaemia. Chronic laxative-induced purgation can also cause hypokalaemia. Much less common is loss of potassium from a villous adenoma of the colon or rectum or loss in patients with ureterosigmoidostomies.

Renal potassium wasting is most often due to diuretic drugs, being more common with large doses and in the presence of secondary hyperaldosteronism, as occurs in severe heart failure, hepatic cirrhosis or the nephrotic syndrome. Severe hypokalaemia, especially in women, may be seen as a result of self-treatment with diuretics for cosmetic reasons and in anorexia nervosa. The other important causes of renal potassium wasting are primary hyperaldosteronism (see p. 740), Cushing's syndrome (see p. 726) or adrenogenital syndromes. Liquorice in large amounts and carbenoxolone sodium (prescribed for peptic ulcer treatment) have an aldosterone-like effect which can lead to hypokalaemia. Rare causes include Bartter's syndrome, renin-secreting tumours and Liddel's syndrome.

CLINICAL FEATURES

Marked hypokalaemia (less than 2.5 mmol·l^{-1}) is associated with impaired muscle function and increased myocardial excitability, and may be immediately life-threatening because of severe cardiac dysrhythmia—a risk increased by digitalization. In skeletal muscle there is weakness, sometimes progressing to paralysis, with absent reflexes. Hypokalaemia may result in ileus of the gut. In the kidney, hypokalaemia impairs concentrating ability (nephrogenic diabetes insipidus), and may reduce the GFR and increase sodium retention. The dominant clinical feature of this renal impairment is polyuria, especially nocturia.

TREATMENT

Treatment must be directed at correcting the hypokalaemia and eliminating the cause of potassium loss. In most cases, withdrawal of oral diuretics or purgation, accompanied by the oral administration of potassium supplements in the form of slow-release potassium or effervescent potassium, is all that is required. Only in severe cases (potassium $<2.5 \text{ mmol·l}^{-1}$) is intravenous potassium replacement required, e.g. where there are cardiac arrhythmias, muscle weakness or severe diabetic ketoacidosis. When used, intravenous therapy must take account of renal function, and replacement at rates greater than 20 mmol·h^{-1} should only be used with hourly monitoring of serum potassium and ECG changes.

The treatment of adrenal disorders is described on p. 726.

Hyperkalaemia

Hyperkalaemia is much less common than hypokalaemia but is more dangerous, the commonest clinical manifestation being cardiac arrest. It occasionally presents with muscle weakness. Diagnosis depends on clinical awareness of its possible development in certain situations (Table 10.7).

Hyperkalaemia rarely occurs in healthy patients except with gross abuse of potassium-retaining diuretics or overdose with potassium supplements. It may occur in hospital practice if intravenous infusion of potassium exceeds 20 mmol·h^{-1}. It most often develops on a background of renal or adrenal disease. Haemolysed blood samples produce an 'apparent' hyperkalaemia; laboratory reports on blood samples should always indicate whether the specimen received was haemolysed.

In acute or chronic renal failure, hyperkalaemia rarely occurs spontaneously except where there is oliguria. It is more likely to occur if patients with renal disease take food rich in potassium or potassium supplements, or are treated with potassium-sparing diuretics (amiloride, triamterene or spironolactone) or angiotensin converting enzyme (ACE) inhibitors. Hyperkalaemia also occurs if there is a shift of potassium out of cells due to acidosis, crush or ischaemic injuries, burns, rhabdomyolysis from muscle injury, or massive death of tumour cells in response to treatment. Loss of potassium from cells may follow use of certain muscle relaxants, e.g. suxamethonium. Rarely, hyperkalaemia occurs spontaneously in patients with severe renal tubular disorders where there is a defect in potassium secretion.

Addison's disease and isolated hypoaldosteronism are commonly associated with modest (5.0–6.5 mmol·l^{-1}) hyperkalaemia (see p. 726); other clinical features usually suggest the diagnosis.

TREATMENT

A serum potassium of more than 7.0 mmol·l^{-1} is a medical emergency, and is associated with ECG

Table 10.7 Causes of hyperkalaemia

Excessive intake
Impaired renal excretion
Oliguric renal failure
Potassium-sparing diuretics, e.g. amiloride
Adrenal insufficiency
Renal tubulo-interstitial disease
ACE inhibitors, e.g. enalapril
Loss of potassium from cells
Acidosis
Crush injury, rhabdomyolysis, burns
Tumour therapy
Suxamethonium

Fig. 10.6 Progressive ECG changes with increasing hyperkalaemia. (a) Normal. (b) Tented T wave. (c) Reduced P wave with increased QRS complex. (d) 'Sine wave' pattern (pre-cardiac arrest).

changes (see Fig.10.6). Intravenous glucose (50 g) plus 15 units of soluble insulin will lower potassium rapidly, the effect lasting for 1–2 h. 4.2% Sodium bicarbonate 50–100 ml i.v. will also reduce the potassium level and help correct acidosis, but must be used sparingly in fluid-overloaded patients. If severe ECG changes are present, intravenous 10% calcium gluconate (10–30 ml over 5–10 min) is required; the effect is short-lived, but the dose can be repeated. These are all emergency measures which 'push' potassium back into cells. Removal of potassium from the body requires either cation exchange resins (e.g. 15–20 g of calcium resonium three times daily by mouth or retention enema) or dialysis. Hyperkalaemia is also helped by mild diarrhoea induced by oral lactulose 10–20 ml three times daily, which also avoids constipation when resins are used.

DISORDERS OF MAGNESIUM METABOLISM

Plasma magnesium levels are normally maintained within the range 0.7–1.1 mmol·l^{-1}. Like potassium, magnesium is principally an intracellular cation (Table 10.2). Regulation of magnesium balance is mainly via the kidney. Primary disturbance of magnesium balance is uncommon, hypo- or hypermagnesaemia usually developing on a background of more obvious fluid and electrolyte disturbances. Disturbance in magnesium balance should always be suspected in association with other fluid and electrolyte disturbances when the patient develops unexpected neurological signs or symptoms.

Hypomagnesaemia

This most often develops as a result of deficient intake, defective gut absorption, or excessive gut or urinary loss (see Table 10.8). It can also occur with acute pancreatitis, possibly due to the formation of magnesium soaps in the areas of fat necrosis. Calcium deficiency usually develops with hypomagnesaemia.

Table 10.8 Causes of hypomagnesaemia.

Decreased intake
Starvation
Prolonged parenteral feeding

Decreased gut absorption
Malabsorption syndrome
Extensive small gut resection

Gut losses
Prolonged nasogastric suction
Excessive purgation
Gastrointestinal/biliary fistula
Severe diarrhoea

Excessive urine losses
Diuretic states due to:
  Loop diuretics
  Postobstruction
  Recovery phase of acute tubular necrosis
  Hyperglycaemia
  Diabetic ketoacidosis
Renal tubular acidosis
Chronic alcoholism
Gentamicin toxicity
Primary aldosteronism
Hypothyroidism

Acute pancreatitis

CLINICAL FEATURES

Symptoms and signs include irritability, tremor, ataxia, carpopedal spasm, hyperreflexia, confusional and hallucinatory states and epileptiform convulsions. The serum magnesium is usually less than 0.7 mmol·l^{-1}. An ECG may show a prolonged QT interval, broad flattened T waves and occasional shortening of the ST segment.

TREATMENT

This involves the withdrawal of precipitating agents such as diuretics or purgatives and the parenteral infusion of 50 mmol of magnesium chloride in 1 l of 5% dextrose or other isotonic fluid over 12–24 h. This should be repeated daily until the plasma magnesium level is normal.

Hypermagnesaemia

This primarily occurs in patients with acute or chronic renal failure given magnesium-containing laxatives or antacids. It can also be induced by magnesium-containing enemas. Mild hypermagnesaemia may occur in patients with adrenal insufficiency.

CLINICAL FEATURES

Symptoms and signs relate to neurological and cardiovascular depression, and include weakness with hyporeflexia proceeding to narcosis, respiratory paralysis and cardiac conduction defects. Symptoms usually develop when the plasma magnesium level exceeds 2 mmol·l^{-1}.

TREATMENT

Treatment requires withdrawal of magnesium therapy and the intravenous injection of 10 ml of calcium gluconate 10% (which contains 2.25 mmol calcium), to be repeated as necessary to lower the plasma magnesium level. Dialysis may be required in patients with severe renal failure. Respiratory failure requires artificial ventilation until the plasma magnesium level returns to normal levels.

Acid–base homeostasis

The concentration of hydrogen ions ($[H^+]$) is enormously important to most cell metabolism. For this reason intracellular and extracellular $[H^+]$ is normally controlled very tightly. The negative logarithm of $[H^+]$ (known as the pH) is commonly measured, but its use may conceal large changes in the $[H^+]$ (Table 10.9); it is therefore better to use the $[H^+]$. Normal resting arterial blood $[H^+]$ is approximately 40 nmol·l^{-1} (pH 7.4). The major source of H^+ is tissue respiration ($H_2O + CO_2 = H^+ \cdot HCO_3^-$). Ten times less H^+ comes from organic acid production (lactic, hydroxybutyric, acetoacetic and free fatty acids) and ten times less again from the dietary 'fixed acids'—sulphuric and phosphoric acid. H^+ derived from cell respiration is eliminated via the lungs, organic acids are normally metabolized in liver and other tissues, and fixed acids are excreted via the kidney (Table 10.10). Between production and excretion there is an extremely efficient buffering system such that the concentration of H^+ inside and outside cells is very constant. Buffers include haemoglobin, proteins, bicarbonate and phosphate. Most important is the bicarbonate–carbonic acid buffer system expressed in the classic Henderson–Hasselbalch equation (see Fig. 10.7): as $H^+ \cdot HCO_3^-$ (which is

Table 10.9 Relationship between $[H^+]$ and pH.

$[H^+]$ (nmol·l^{-1})	pH
100 000	4
10 000	5
1 000	6
100	7
10	8
1	9
Ranges in blood	
126	6.90
100	7.00
79	7.10
63	7.20
50	7.30
40	7.40
32	7.50
25	7.60
20	7.70
16	7.80

$$pH = pK + \log \frac{[HCO_3^-]}{[H^+ \cdot HCO_3^-]}$$

Fig. 10.7 The Henderson–Hasselbalch equation.

dependent on the P_{CO_2}) increases or decreases, bicarbonate also increases or decreases (by renal conservation or secretion) to maintain constant pH.

Capacity in the buffering system is maintained by the ease with which carbonic acid can be disposed of via the lungs and by the excretion of fixed acid by the kidneys (see Fig. 10.8).

$$CO_2 + H_2O \rightleftharpoons H_2CO_3 \rightleftharpoons H^+ + HCO_3^-$$

Adjusted by lungs   Adjusted by kidneys

Fig. 10.8 The bicarbonate–carbonic acid buffering system.

Table 10.10 Source and elimination of hydrogen ions.

Nature	Daily production (moles)	Source	Elimination
CO_2 ($H_2O + CO_2 \rightarrow$ $H^+ + HCO_3^-$)	15	Tissue respiration	Lungs
Organic acids	1.5	Liver, muscle, brain	Liver and most tissues
Fixed acids	0.1	Diet	Kidneys

DIAGNOSIS OF ACID–BASE DISTURBANCES

Except in acute respiratory distress, symptoms are non-specific and are described below. The most definitive means of diagnosing acid–base disorder is by measuring the $[H^+]$ and $P_a co_2$ in arterial or arterialized venous blood plus the plasma electrolytes.

Acid–base disorders may be diagnosed using diagrams such as that shown in Fig. 10.9. In this figure the hatched area represents the normal range. The bands show the range of expected response in uncomplicated metabolic or respiratory acid–base disorders. Where results fall outside these bands (in area A, B, C or D) the patient has a mixed respiratory and metabolic acid–base disorder. In the case of areas B and D, one of the components can be compensating for the other. For example, in chronic respiratory disease with a respiratory acidosis (area B) there is retention of carbon dioxide and an increase in arterial $P co_2$, and the kidneys compensate by retaining bicarbonate. The consequence of this is to normalize the arterial $[H^+]$, but with elevation of the $P co_2$. In a metabolic acidosis (area D), the body retains fixed acids and the lungs compensate by hyperventilating and blowing off CO_2, leading to a decrease in arterial $P co_2$. Sequential measurement of $[H^+]$ and $P_a co_2$ permits assessment of response to treatment.

Calculation of 'standard bicarbonate', 'base excess' or 'base deficit' from widely used acid–base analytical equipment is inaccurate and often confus-

ing or misleading. This stems from the fact that the bicarbonate titration curve of blood measured in vitro differs from that in vivo and takes no account of interstitial and intracellular fluid buffering. It does not therefore represent the true in vivo situation. Further, an 'excess' of bicarbonate may be a desirable compensatory mechanism as, for example, in chronic respiratory acidosis and is then *not* a primary defect. Casual interpretation of these values can be misleading, and their use is best abandoned in favour of the approach outlined above.

Anion gap

The main electrolytes measured in plasma are sodium, potassium, chloride and bicarbonate. The sum of the cations sodium and potassium normally exceeds that of chloride and bicarbonate by 10–18 $mmol \cdot l^{-1}$. This is known as the anion gap. This gap is made up by negative charged proteins, phosphate and organic acids (see Fig. 10.10). Calculation of this gap is of great value in identifying and managing metabolic acidosis, in which the anion gap may be normal or increased.

Normal anion gap acidosis (hyperchloraemic acidosis)
This occurs when bicarbonate is lost via the gut or the kidneys. Rarely it is due to the ingestion of H^+ as ammonium chloride. Chloride is retained as bicarbonate is lost (see Fig. 10.10).

Increased anion gap acidosis
This results from the retention of 'fixed' or organic acids and is most often seen in uraemia, keto-acidosis, lactic acidosis and salicylate poisoning. Bicarbonate is utilized to maintain a normal $[H^+]$ and therefore decreases. Chloride may be normal or low (see Fig. 10.10).

Given a careful history and awareness of the causes of acid–base imbalance, diagnosis can be based on these measurements.

CAUSES OF ACID-BASE DISTURBANCES

As respiratory acidosis and alkalosis are dealt with in Chapter 12, only metabolic acidosis and alkalosis will be discussed in this section.

Metabolic acidosis

It is convenient to subdivide metabolic acidosis into conditions associated with increased acid production or defective excretion (high anion gap) and those primarily due to loss of bicarbonate (hypochloraemic acidosis; normal anion gap). A third iatrogenic cause is a normal anion gap associated with rapid volume repletion (dilutional acidosis) or following ingestion or infusion of acidifying agents such as ammonium

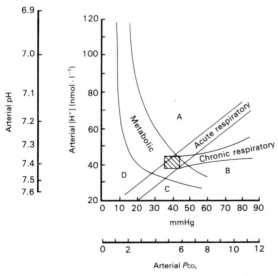

Fig. 10.9 Diagram for analysis of acid-base disturbances from measured $[H^+]$ and $P_a co_2$. The cross-hatched area shows the normal range. From Cohen RD & Woods HF (1983) Disturbances of acid–base homeostasis. In Weatherall DJ, Ledingham JGG & Warrell DA (eds) *Oxford Textbook of Medicine*, pp. 9.116–9.126. Oxford: Oxford University Press. With permission.

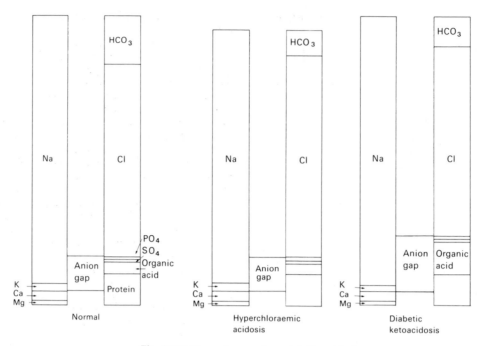

Fig. 10.10 The anion gap in metabolic acidosis.

chloride or intravenous feeds containing an excess of cationic amino acids. The commonest causes for metabolic acidosis are shown in Tables 10.11 and 10.12.

Renal excretion of H^+
H^+ is excreted by the kidney in two ways (see Fig. 10.11):
- Combined with buffer (mostly phosphate), the amount being proportional to the amount of filtered buffer and urine $[H^+]$
- As ammonium (NH_4^+), when hydrogen secreted into the urine combines with ammonia (NH_3) produced from glutamine by the renal tubular cell

Loss of bicarbonate in the urine represents 'failed' H^+ secretion, while H^+ secretion in the urine indicates regeneration of bicarbonate (see Fig. 10.11). In health, acidosis increases ammonia production and urine $[H^+]$, both facilitating H^+ excretion. In renal disease the ability to excrete the normal daily fixed acid production from dietary protein (60–100 mmol daily) or increased H^+ loads is reduced as a result of reduced glomerular filtration, tubular disease, or a combination of both.

Uraemic acidosis
Uraemia is most often due to renal disease in which there is loss of both glomeruli and tubules. As a consequence the filtered load (GFR × plasma level) of phosphate and NH_3 production are reduced, leading to failed excretion of H^+ and acidosis. As a result

Table 10.11 Causes of metabolic acidosis with a normal anion gap.

Gastrointestinal bicarbonate loss
Diarrhoea
Pancreatic fistula
Ureterosigmoidostomy

Renal tubular acidosis
'Classical', 'distal type':
  Primary
  Acquired
    Primary biliary cirrhosis
    Chronic active hepatitis
    Obstructive nephropathy
    Vitamin D intoxication
    Hypergammaglobulinaemia

Bicarbonate wastage, 'proximal type':
  Primary
    Isolated
    Part of Fanconi syndrome
  Acquired
    Hyperparathyroidism
    Hypoaldosteronism
    Heavy metal poisoning (e.g. mercury)
    Paraproteinaemia (e.g. myeloma)

Acetazolamide therapy

Ingestion/infusion
NH_4Cl
Feeding excess cationic amino acids

Dilutional acidosis
Rapid i.v. hydration

Table 10.12 Causes of metabolic acidosis with a high anion gap.

Uraemic acidosis

Drug poisoning
Salicylates
Methanol
Ethylene glycol
Paraldehyde

Ketoacidosis
Diabetes
Starvation
Alcohol poisoning

Lactic acidosis
Type A:
    Strenuous exercise
    Shock
    Severe hypoxia

Type B:
    Biguanide drugs—phenformin, metformin
    Acute liver failure
    Poisoning—ethanol, paracetamol
    Leukaemia, reticulosis
    Intravenous nutrition with fructose and sorbitol

Fig. 10.11 Renal tubular excretion of H^+.

of the secondary retention of phosphate, its plasma level rises, and there is an increase in the amount of phosphate filtered and therefore in the amount available for buffering. Acidosis is associated with acid urine, which also increases buffering. In addition, acidosis stimulates increased NH_3 production in the remaining nephrons. These compensatory mechanisms plus the buffering of H^+ by bone allow a mild to moderate acidosis to persist as a steady state for long periods in patients which chronic renal failure.

Plasma bicarbonate is reduced and the anion gap increased.

Symptoms are unusual unless the plasma bicarbonate is very low (<10 mmol·l^{-1}), leading to hyperventilation with sighing respiration (Kussmaul's respiration or air hunger).

Treatment of uraemic acidosis requires a reduction in the acid load from dietary protein. This is rarely necessary for the acidosis per se, protein usually being restricted to control symptoms of uraemia or to reduce the rate of decline in renal function (see p. 420). Treatment with sodium bicarbonate rarely works as bicarbonate is lost in the urine. It is also potentially dangerous, the sodium load exacerbating hypertension and predisposing to salt and water retention with pulmonary congestion. However, sodium bicarbonate supplements can be very effective in patients with sodium-losing chronic renal disease (see p. 420). Severe acidosis requires removal of fixed acid by dialysis.

Renal tubular acidosis
In 'distal' or 'classical' renal tubular acidosis (RTA) patients are unable to increase the urine [H^+] above 10 000 nmol·l^{-1} (i.e. pH <5) due to an inability to create a high concentration gradient of H^+ between the distal tubular cell and the tubular fluid. Patients most often present with renal stones or nephrocalcinosis, but they may occasionally present with symptoms of hypokalaemia or hypocalcaemia due to associated potassium and calcium wastage. RTA may be present at birth or may be acquired in later life (Table 10.11). There is variable hyperchloraemic acidosis (normal anion gap) with an alkaline urine, the [H^+] of which does not increase above 10 000 nmol·l^{-1} (i.e. pH <5) following oral ammonium chloride loading (100 mg·kg^{-1}).

Proximal (bicarbonate-wasting) RTA is due to a failure in proximal tubular reabsorption of bicarbonate. Serum bicarbonate falls until the 'filtered load' equals the reduced reabsorptive capacity, when urine may again become acid (bicarbonate <18 mmol·l^{-1}). It may be a primary developmental defect or may be acquired (Table 10.11). The RTA may be an isolated defect or part of the Fanconi syndrome (see p. 774). Diagnosis is usually based on plasma electrolyte measurements or is made as a result of symptoms due to hypokalaemia or hypocalcaemia.

Diabetic ketoacidosis
This is dealt with on p. 757. This is a high anion gap acidosis due to the accumulation of organic acids, acetoacetic acid and hydroxybutyric acid due to reduced peripheral utilization and increased production.

Lactic acidosis
Lactic acid (as lactate) is normally present in the venous blood in low concentrations (0.6–

1.2 mmol·l^{-1}), increasing up to 10-fold after severe exercise. Lactic acidosis should be suspected in patients with high anion gap metabolic acidosis when there is no uraemia or diabetic ketoacidosis. It most often occurs in association with circulatory failure or shock, with or without severe hypoxia, when peripheral metabolism of lactate is reduced and production is increased (type A). The potential for lactic acidosis increases where there is liver disease (reduced metabolism of lactate) or impaired renal excretion of acid.

The other major cause (type B) is as a result of various drugs or poisons (Table 10.12). With these there is variable increase in the production of lactate and reduced liver metabolism. It may occur de novo in severe liver failure. Cases may present acutely with nausea, vomiting, epigastric pain, hyperventilation and impaired consciousness. The diagnosis is based on recognizing a high anion gap acidosis in the absence of uraemia or diabetic ketoacidosis, and can be confirmed by demonstration of a high level of lactate in plasma.

Treatment of lactic acidosis involves correction of the cause. In the case of circulatory failure and hypoxia, correction of these must be pursued, but care should be taken with vasoconstrictor drugs which may increase lactate production. Causal drugs or poisons must be stopped and measures to accelerate their excretion employed. Because of the negative ionotropic effect on cardiac output, intravenous infusion of sodium bicarbonate is necessary; large amounts (500–1000 mmol) may be required. Dialysis may be used if sodium overload is a problem. Trihydroxymethylaminomethane (THAM) buffer 0.3 M solution (pH 10.2) is also an occasionally valuable adjunct to treatment.

Metabolic alkalosis

This is much less common than acidosis and is often associated with potassium or chloride depletion. The main causes are persistent vomiting, diuretic therapy or hyperaldosteronism; other causes are much less common (Table 10.13).

Vomiting

The amount of H$^+$ and chloride lost in vomitus may be considerable, especially in pyloric stenosis. Hypochloraemic alkalosis develops, leading to hypokalaemia, and considerable loss of potassium in the urine. Symptoms are those of volume depletion and hypokalaemia.

The urine contains very little chloride (<10 mmol·l^{-1}) and is acid despite a systemic alkalosis. Treatment includes intravenous normal saline with potassium supplements to correct first

Table 10.13 Causes and mechanisms of metabolic alkalosis.

Vomiting
Loss of gastric H$^+$ and Cl$^-$
Secondary renal potassium wasting with acid urine

Diuretics
Renal chloride wasting commonly associated with hypokalaemia

Hyperaldosteronism
Increased reabsorption of bicarbonate
Hypochloraemic alkalosis

Excess liquorice ingestion

Carbenoxolone sodium

Milk alkali syndrome
Excess intake of calcium and calcium antacids (rare)

Excess i.v. NaHCO$_3$
Treatment of acidosis
Treatment of salicylate/barbiturate poisoning

the chloride deficit and then the potassium deficit. The bicarbonate excess will correct itself.

Diuretic therapy

Diuretic therapy, especially with loop diuretics, may induce a hypochloraemic alkalosis, often associated with hypokalaemia, by blocking the renal reabsorption of chloride. Treatment includes review of the diuretic therapy, oral supplements of potassium chloride (Slow-K 2 tablets [16 mmol potassium] three times daily) or the use of potassium-sparing diuretics (amiloride, triamterene or spironolactone).

Hyperaldosteronism or an excessive intake of liquorice or carbenoxolone sodium, which have an aldosterone-like effect, is usually associated with a moderate hypochloraemic alkalosis with potassium depletion. The alkalosis is possibly due to increased renal bicarbonate reabsorption. Treatment is that of the primary cause.

Further reading

Cohen RD & Woods HF (1983) Disturbances of acid–base homeostasis. In Weatherall DJ, Ledingham JGG & Warrell DA (eds) *Oxford Textbook of Medicine*, pp. 9.116–9.126. Oxford: Oxford University Press.
Pitts RF (1974) *Physiology of the Kidney and Body Fluids*, 3rd edn. Chicago: Year Book Medical Publishers.

11
Cardiovascular Disease

seen in the tropics; cardiac problems associated with protein–energy malnutrition are seen in countries where famine and malnutrition occur; cardiomyopathy is seen with beriberi and myocarditis is seen with other diseases associated with the tropics, e.g. Chagas' disease, typhoid fever and diphtheria.

Congenital heart disease is important in the young and is responsible for approximately 1% of deaths in patients below 15 years of age.

Lastly, pulmonary heart disease is common in countries with a high incidence of smoking.

Essential anatomy, physiology and embryology of the heart

The cellular basis of myocardial contraction

Myocardial fibres consist of bundles of parallel myofibrils. Each myofibril is made up of a series of sarcomeres (Fig. 11.1). A sarcomere is bound by two transverse Z lines to each of which is attached a perpendicular filament of the protein actin. The actin filaments from each of the two Z bands overlap with thicker parallel protein filaments known as myosin. The molecular weight of myosin is approximately 500 000 and that of actin is about 47 000. Actin and myosin molecules are attached to each other by cross-bridges which contain ATPase.

During cardiac contraction the length of the actin and myosin molecules does not change. Rather, the actin molecules slide between the myosin molecules when a high energy bond of ATP is split by the ATPase. This interaction requires magnesium ions. Calcium ions are also required to inactivate another protein called troponin, which ordinarily inhibits the actin–myosin interaction. Calcium is made available during the plateau phase of each action potential by calcium ions entering the cell and being mobilized from the sarcoplasm.

Starling's law of the heart

The contractile function of an isolated strip of cardiac tissue can be described by the relationship between the velocity of muscle contraction, the load that may be moved by the contracting muscle, and the extent

Introduction

In the Western Hemisphere approximately 50% of deaths are related to cardiovascular disease. This is due mainly to ischaemic heart disease which could, perhaps, be significantly reduced if smoking were prohibited, lifestyle moderated (e.g. weight reduction) and the intake of cholesterol and saturated fats reduced. Whilst the incidence of rheumatic heart disease is decreasing in the West, it is still an important problem world-wide, predominantly in countries with poor sanitation, overcrowding and malnutrition. Up to one-third of all cardiac cases admitted to hospital in, for example, India, Jamaica, Egypt or the Philippines are due to rheumatic heart disease. Hypertension is another major cause of mortality, being responsible for 10% of deaths world-wide. The incidence of hypertension usually increases with age and is higher in Western countries. There is also a wide geographical variation in other cardiac diseases: endomyocardial fibrosis is

Fig. 11.1 A schematic diagram showing the structure of a myofibril. The myofibrils are made up of a series of sarcomeres joined at the Z line.

to which the muscle is stretched before contracting. As with all other types of muscle, the velocity of contraction of myocardial tissue is reduced by increasing the load against which the tissue must contract. However, in the non-failing heart, pre-stretching of cardiac muscle improves the relationship between the force and velocity of contraction (Fig. 11.2).

This phenomenon was described in the intact heart as an increase of stroke volume (ventricular performance) with an enlargement of the diastolic volume (pre-load), and is known as 'Starling's law of the heart' or the 'Frank–Starling relationship'. It has been transcribed into more clinically relevant indices. Thus, stroke work (aortic pressure × stroke volume) is increased as ventricular end-diastolic volume is raised. Alternatively, within certain limits, cardiac output rises as pulmonary capillary wedge pressure increases. This clinical relationship is described by the ventricular function curve (Fig. 11.2, which also shows the effect of sympathetic stimulation).

The conduction system of the heart

Each natural heart beat begins in the heart's pacemaker—the sinoatrial (SA) node. This is a crescent-shaped structure which is located around the medial and anterior aspect of the junction between the superior vena cava and the right atrium (Fig. 11.3). Progressive loss of the diastolic resting membrane potential is followed, when the threshold potential has been reached, by a more rapid depolarization of the sinus node tissue. This depolarization triggers depolarization of the atrial myocardium. The atrial tissue is activated like a 'forest fire', but the activation peters out when the insulating layer between the atrium and the ventricle—the annulus fibrosus—is reached.

The depolarization continues to conduct slowly through the atrioventricular (AV) node. This is a small, bean-shaped structure that lies beneath the right atrial endocardium within the lower interatrial septum. The AV node continues as the His bundle, which penetrates the annulus fibrosus and conducts

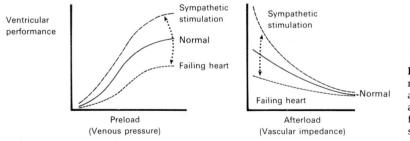

Fig. 11.2 The Frank Starling mechanism, showing the effect of alterations in preload (left) and afterload (right) in the normal and failing heart and during sympathetic stimulation.

Fig. 11.3 The normal cardiac conduction system. SA = sino-atrial; AV = atrioventricular.

the cardiac impulse rapidly towards the ventricle. The His bundle reaches the crest of the interventricular septum and divides into the right bundle branch and the main left bundle branch.

The right bundle branch continues down the right side of the interventricular septum until it reaches the right ventricular apex, from where it radiates and divides to form the Purkinje network, which spreads throughout the subendocardial surface of the right ventricle.

The main left bundle branch is a short structure which fans out into many strands on the left side of the interventricular septum. These strands can be grouped into an anterior superior division (the anterior hemibundle) and a posterior inferior division (the posterior hemibundle). The anterior hemibundle supplies the subendocardial Purkinje network of the anterior and superior surfaces of the left ventricle, and the inferior hemibundle supplies the inferior and posterior surfaces. Impulse conduction through the AV node is slow and depends on action potentials largely produced by slow transmembrane calcium flux. In the atria, ventricles and His–Purkinje system conduction is rapid and is due to action potentials generated by rapid transmembrane sodium diffusion.

The coronary circulation

The coronary arterial system (Fig. 11.4) consists of the right and left coronary arteries. The right coronary artery arises from the right coronary sinus and courses through the right side of the atrioventricular groove, giving off vessels that supply the right atrium and the right ventricle. The vessel usually continues as the posterior descending coronary artery, which runs in the posterior interventricular groove and supplies the posterior part of the inter-ventricular septum and the posterior left ventricular wall.

The left coronary artery arises from the left coronary sinus. The first part is known as the left main coronary artery, and is usually not more than 2.5 cm long. It then divides into the left anterior descending and the left circumflex arteries. The left anterior descending artery runs in the anterior interventricular groove and supplies the anterior septum and the anterior left ventricular wall. The left circumflex artery travels along the left atrioventricular groove and gives off branches to the left atrium and the left ventricle (marginal branches).

The sinus node and the AV node are supplied by the right coronary artery in 60% and 90% of people, respectively. Therefore, disease in this artery may cause sinus bradycardia and AV nodal block. The majority of the left ventricle is supplied by the left coronary artery, so that stenosis in the left main artery is extremely dangerous; total obstruction of this vessel is rarely compatible with life.

The fetal circulation

In utero, the pulmonary circulation is largely unnecessary because fetal blood is oxygenated by placental blood flow, a parallel and integral element in the systemic circulation. In the fetus, systemic

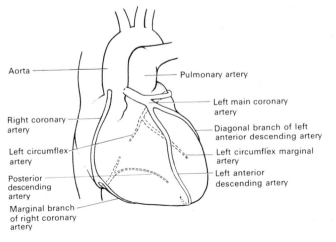

Fig. 11.4 Diagram of the normal coronary arterial anatomy.

venous blood returning to the right atrium is partly deflected through the foramen ovale to the left atrium. Blood which passes through the right ventricle is diverted away from the pulmonary arteries to the aorta through the ductus arteriosus. Thus, the systemic venous return, which is a mixture of oxygenated and deoxygenated blood, is mostly returned to the systemic arterial system.

At birth, inspiration dilates the pulmonary arterioles, resulting in a dramatic reduction of pulmonary vascular resistance. Blood therefore flows through the pulmonary circulation. The increased oxygen tension triggers closure of the ductus arteriosus, and the reduced right atrial pressure and increasing left atrial pressure tend to close the foramen ovale. Thus, the circulation is divided into two separate circuits connected in series.

In the fetus the left and right heart both propel blood from the systemic veins to the systemic arteries; thus, severe abnormalities of the heart may not compromise fetal blood flow.

The cardiac cycle (Fig. 11.5)

The first event in the cardiac cycle is atrial depolarization (a P wave on the surface ECG) followed by right atrial and then left atrial contraction. Ventricular activation (the QRS complex on the ECG) follows after a short interval (the PR interval). Left ventricular contraction starts and shortly thereafter right ventricular contraction begins. The increased ventricular pressures exceed the atrial pressures, and close first the mitral and then the tricuspid valves. Until the aortic and pulmonary valves open, the ventricles contract with no change of volume (isovolumetric contraction). When ventricular pressures rise above the aortic and pulmonary artery pressures, the pulmonary valve and then the aortic valve open and ventricular ejection occurs. As the ventricles begin to relax, their pressures fall below the aortic and pulmonary arterial pressures, and aortic valve closure is followed by pulmonary valve closure. Isovolumetric relaxation then occurs after the ventricular pressures have fallen below the right atrial and left atrial pressures and the tricuspid and mitral valves open.

The cardiac cycle determines the sequence of heart sounds. Thus:

- The *first* heart sound is produced by virtually simultaneous closure of the mitral and tricuspid valves.
- The *second* heart sound comprises the aortic valve closure sound followed by pulmonary valve closure.
- The *third* heart sound, which is due to rapid ventricular filling, occurs when the tricuspid and mitral valves open.
- The *fourth* heart sound, which is due to ventricular filling following atrial contraction, succeeds the P wave and occurs before ventricular systole.

Opening sounds of the aortic and pulmonary valves (ejection clicks) follow the first heart sound, and opening sounds (snaps) of the mitral and tricuspid valves follow the second heart sound but are earlier than the third heart sounds. Heart sounds other than the first and second heart sounds are usually abnormal (see p. 459).

Fig. 11.5 The cardiac cycle.

Symptoms of heart disease

Dyspnoea, chest pain, palpitations, syncope, fatigue and ankle swelling are the usual symptoms produced by cardiac disease. However, patients are often completely asymptomatic until a relatively late stage in their illness.

Dyspnoea

Dyspnoea is an awareness of breathlessness. It can be due to cardiac or respiratory causes. It is also a symptom during exercise in healthy people.

Breathlessness may occur only on exercise or may be present at rest. The New York Heart Association has graded this symptom (see Table 11.1) but this classification, although often used, has now been officially discontinued and is replaced by a very similar grading known as 'cardiac status' (Table 11.2).

It is also clinically valuable to grade dyspnoea by the amount of physical exertion possible before breathlessness occurs, e.g. climbing 14 stairs or walking 200 yards on the flat.

Left ventricular failure causes dyspnoea because of a rise in left atrial pressure and pulmonary capillary pressure leading to interstitial and alveolar oedema. This makes the lung stiff (less compliant) and this increases the amount of respiratory effort necessary to breathe. Usually a fast breathing rate (tachypnoea) is also present due to stimulation of the pulmonary stretch receptors.

Table 11.1 The New York Heart Association functional and therapeutic classification applied to dyspnoea.

Grade 1	No breathlessness
Grade 2	Breathlessness on severe exertion
Grade 3	Breathlessness on mild exertion
Grade 4	Breathlessness at rest

Table 11.2 The New York Heart Association grading of 'cardiac status'.

Grade 1	Uncompromised
Grade 2	Slightly compromised
Grade 3	Moderately compromised
Grade 4	Severely compromised

Orthopnoea

This is a form of breathlessness that occurs when the patient lies flat. Orthopnoea occurs because lying flat results in the redistribution of blood, leading to an increased central and pulmonary blood volume. Recumbancy also causes the abdominal contents to press up against the diaphragm. Both factors increase the difficulty of breathing. Patients usually cope with orthopnoea by propping themselves up with pillows. It is convenient to grade orthopnoea by the number of pillows used, e.g. 'three pillow orthopnoea'. However, patients may also sleep with pillows for comfort.

Paroxysmal nocturnal dyspnoea (PND)

This occurs when there is an accumulation of fluid in the lungs (pulmonary oedema) at night. The mechanism is similar to orthopnoea, but because sensory awareness is depressed during sleep, severe interstitial and alveolar oedema can accumulate. The patient is awoken from sleep fighting for breath, a dramatic and frightening experience. The breathlessness may be relieved by sitting on the side of the bed or getting up. Sometimes the patient will get up and open a window to gasp for fresh air. Wheezing, due to bronchial endothelial oedema, is common (cardiac asthma), and a cough, often productive of frothy or blood-tinged sputum, usually occurs. The patient is vasoconstricted and therefore cold and cyanosed. Initially these episodes terminate spontaneously. Episodes of 'PND', often with coughing, can occur in asthma, but conventionally the term is reserved for cardiac problems.

Cheyne–Stokes respiration (see also p. 789)

In very severe heart failure, alternate hyperventilation and apnoea known as Cheyne–Stokes respiration may occur. This may also develop in the elderly without obvious heart failure. It is related to depression of the respiratory centre, which is partly due to prolonged circulation time and cerebrovascular disease. This type of respiration is also seen after morphine administration.

Chest pain

Pain in the chest is the commonest symptom associated with ischaemic heart disease.

Angina pectoris

Angina pectoris literally means a strangling sensation (angina) in the chest (pectoris). It is a gripping or crushing central chest pain (or discomfort) that may be felt around the whole chest or deep within the chest. The pain may radiate into the neck or jaw and, rarely, into the teeth, back or abdomen. It is associated with heaviness, paraesthesia or pain in one (usually the left) or both arms. It is typically provoked by exercise and is promptly relieved by rest. A pain of similar distribution and type also occurs at rest in myocardial infarction (see p. 504). The mechanism of the pain is myocardial hypoxia secondary to inadequate coronary blood flow. Sharp pains over the heart are not usually angina. Angina should be classified according to the Canadian Cardiovascular Society grading of angina of effort (Table 11.3) although most physicians find that a verbal description is adequate.

Other causes of chest pain
The pain of pericarditis is felt in the centre of the chest and, like that of pleurisy, is aggravated by movement, posture, respiration and coughing. It is sharp and severe.

Left, submammary stabbing pain, known as 'precordial catch', is usually associated with anxiety and is sometimes known as effort (Da Costa's) syndrome. Occasionally, cardiac conditions such as mitral valve prolapse cause similar pain.

Other causes of chest pain are pulmonary embolism, pulmonary hypertension, costochondritis, pleurisy, oesophageal spasm or reflux, mediastinitis and a dissecting or enlarging aortic aneurysm.

Palpitations

A palpitation is an increased awareness of the normal heart beat or the sensation of slow or rapid heart rate or an irregular heart rhythm. The normal heart beat is sensed when the patient is anxious, excited, exercising, or lying on the left side. The most common arrhythmias to be felt as palpitations are premature ectopic beats and paroxysmal tachycardias.

Premature beats
These are usually felt as 'missed beats' because the premature beat is followed by a pause before the next normal beat, which is rather forceful because of the longer diastolic filling period. Premature beats often occur in clusters and may cause the patient much anxiety.

Paroxysmal tachycardias
These start abruptly and may terminate equally suddenly. Often, however, the tachycardia slows before terminating and therefore seems to fade away. Paroxysmal atrial fibrillation is noticeably irregular, whereas other forms of paroxysmal supraventricular or ventricular tachycardia are regular. Paroxysms of rapid tachycardia, especially when prolonged, may be associated with syncope, presyncope, dyspnoea or chest pain. Palpitations can be graded in a similar way to the grading of dyspnoea or angina (see Table 11.4). Supraventricular tachycardias, such as atrial fibrillation or junctional tachycardias, may produce polyuria.

Bradycardias
An unduly slow heart rate may be appreciated as slow, regular, 'heavy' or forceful beats. Most often bradycardias are not felt as palpitations.

Syncope

Syncope can be due to many causes (see p. 826). The commonest syncopal attacks are vasovagal in nature (simple faints) and are not due to serious disease. Vasovagal attacks are due to venous pooling (postural hypotension) or may be provoked by fright or shock. They are associated with a prodrome, which may consist of dizziness, nausea, sweating, ringing in the ears, a sinking feeling and yawning. There is peripheral vasodilatation and a bradycardia. Recovery occurs within a few seconds.

Cardiovascular syncope is usually sudden and brief. The classical variety is known as a Stokes–Adams attack and is due to a disturbance of cardiac rhythm, e.g. a profound bradycardia related to complete heart block. Without warning the patient falls to the ground, pale and deeply unconscious. The pulse is usually very slow or absent. After a few seconds the patient flushes brightly and recovers consciousness as the pulse quickens. If the period of unconsciousness is prolonged the patient may suffer a generalized convulsion but this is not usual. Often there are no sequelae but the patient may injure himself during the fall.

Table 11.3 The Canadian Cardiovascular Society grading of angina of effort.

Grade I	Ordinary physical activity does not cause angina (strenuous physical activity provokes angina)
Grade II	Slight limitations of ordinary physical activity (climbing more than one flight of stairs or walking uphill provokes angina)
Grade III	Marked limitation of ordinary physical activity (walking on the level or climbing one flight of stairs provokes angina)
Grade IV	Inability to carry on any physical activity (angina may be present at rest)

Table 11.4 Palpitations graded according to symptoms.

Grade 0	Asymptomatic
Grade 1	Non-sustained palpitations (<30 s)
Grade 2	Sustained palpitations (>30 s)
Grade 3	Palpitations plus other symptoms (e.g. dyspnoea, chest pain, dizziness)
Grade 4	Syncope

Table 11.5 Cardiac causes of syncope.

Arrhythmias
Ventricular tachycardia
Rapid supraventricular tachycardia
Sinus arrest
AV block
Artificial pacemaker failure
Obstruction
Aortic stenosis
Hypertrophic obstructive cardiomyopathy
Fallot's tetralogy
Pulmonary hypertension/embolism
Atrial myxoma
Atrial thrombus
Defective prosthetic valve

Other causes of syncope due to heart disease can be grouped as cardiac arrhythmias or valvular or vascular obstruction (see Table 11.5).

Fatigue

This symptom, which consists of tiredness and lethargy, is associated with heart failure, persistent cardiac arrhythmias and cyanotic heart disease. It is due to poor cerebral and peripheral perfusion and poor oxygenation. When severe cardiac disorders are not present, an active infection such as bacterial endocarditis may be responsible. However, disorders of most systems may produce this non-specific symptom. Drugs prescribed for angina or hypertension, particularly beta-blockers, may cause fatigue.

Oedema

Heart failure results in salt and water retention. Retained fluid accumulates in the feet and ankles of ambulant patients and over the sacrum of bed-bound patients. The oedema associated with heart failure becomes progressively worse during the day and is often absent on initial rising as the fluid is reabsorbed on lying down. When severe, the calf and thigh may become oedematous and ascites or a pleural effusion may develop.

Examination of the cardiovascular system

GENERAL EXAMINATION

General features of the patient's well-being should be noted as well as the presence of anaemia, obesity, jaundice and cachexia.

Clubbing (see also p. 562)

The most common cardiac causes of severe clubbing are subacute infective endocarditis and congenital cyanotic heart disease, particularly Fallot's tetralogy. Clubbing takes many months to develop and is therefore not seen in acute endocarditis or in neonates or infants with cyanotic heart disease. Clubbing seen in cor pulmonale is due to the underlying pulmonary disease (e.g. bronchiectasis or fibrosing alveolitis).

Splinter haemorrhages

These small, subungal linear haemorrhages are most frequently due to trauma but are also caused by infective endocarditis. Traumatic splinters are usually confined to the line where the nail meets the nail bed, and are usually rather pale and few in number. The splinter haemorrhages seen with infective endocarditis are often florid, blotchy and deep red or black. They may be multiple but more importantly they may develop without obvious traumatic cause and may occur anywhere in the nail bed.

Cyanosis

This is a dusky blue discoloration of the skin (particularly at the extremities) or of the mucous membranes. It is due to the presence of unoxygenated haemoglobin (traditionally at least 5 $g \cdot dl^{-1}$ of blood) and, occasionally, of other reduction products of haemoglobin such as sulphaemoglobin or methaemoglobin. Cyanosis is more readily provoked in the presence of polycythaemia and is uncommon when anaemia is present. Cyanosis is either central or peripheral.

Central cyanosis
This is present when the tongue is cyanosed. It is caused by cardiac failure, respiratory failure, pulmonary embolus and right-to-left intracardiac shunts. The central cyanosis of pulmonary or cardiac failure is improved by breathing oxygen if the degree of shunting is small.

Peripheral cyanosis
This is due to vasoconstriction and stasis of blood in the extremities, and increased oxygen extraction by peripheral tissues. Peripheral cyanosis occurs in congestive heart failure, shock, exposure to cold temperatures and with abnormalities of the peripheral circulation.

THE ARTERIAL PULSE

A pulse is felt by compressing an artery against a bone. The first pulse to be examined is the right radial pulse. The timing of the left radial and femoral pulses are then compared with that of the right radial pulse. Delayed pulsation occurs with stenotic lesions, particularly of the aorta (coarctation). The radial pulse is examined to reveal the pulse rate, the heart rhythm and the quality of the vessel wall. A large volume pulse will also be obvious, especially if the arm is raised and the pulse felt by gripping the wrist so that the palm of the examiner's hand is located over the radial pulse.

Rate

The pulse rate should be between 60 and 100 beats per minute (bpm) when an adult patient is lying quietly in bed. Young children may have higher pulse rates whilst athletes and elderly adults may have slower rates. Although the exact pulse rate may not be important for the purposes of a casual examination, the rate may be compared with previous or later measurements. It is therefore important that, as with other clinical measurements, the rate is accurately determined and recorded. It should be counted for at least 15 s. When the pulse is irregular, not all beats may be transmitted to the wrist and it is therefore best to count the pulse whilst at the same time listening to the heart beat with a stethoscope. A deficit between the radial pulse and the apex rate is then obvious. Such an apex–radial (pulse) deficit is common in atrial fibrillation.

Rhythm

In normal subjects the pulse is regular except for a slight quickening in early inspiration and a slowing in expiration (sinus arrhythmia). Irregularities of the pulse rhythm are usually due to premature beats, intermittent heart block or atrial fibrillation.

Premature beats occur as occasional or repeated irregularity superimposed on a regular pulse rhythm. Similarly, intermittent heart block is revealed by occasional beats dropped from an otherwise regular rhythm. A totally irregular pattern (irregularly irregular) of heart beats occurs in atrial fibrillation. This irregular pattern persists when the pulse quickens in response to exercise in contrast to pulse irregularity due to ectopic beats, which disappears on exercise. However, this is not a reliable way to distinguish ectopic beats from other causes of pulse irregularity.

Vessel wall

An obviously rigid vessel wall may be felt, but this sign of atherosclerosis is not reliable.

Carotid pulse

The amplitude and shape of the carotid pulse is examined. Usually carotid pulsation is not visible, but a very large volume pulse may be apparent as pulsation of the neck (Corrigan's sign). A large volume pulse occurs in high output states and in aortic regurgitation. The carotid pulse is also visible when the carotid artery is aneurysmal or kinked. The right carotid is palpated lightly in order to detect a thrill.

A large volume pulse with a brisk rise and fall is known as a collapsing or waterhammer pulse (Fig. 11.6). It is found in the elderly when the aorta is rigid, or when the cardiac output is high, e.g. in thyrotoxicosis, anaemia or fever. Aortic valvular regurgitation or a persistent ductus arteriosus also cause a collapsing pulse. A large volume pulse that is not collapsing in nature is associated with the large stroke volume which is necessary if bradycardia is present.

A small volume pulse is seen in cardiac failure, shock and obstructive vascular or valvular disease. It is also present when tachycardia occurs. The pulse of aortic stenosis is not only small in volume but is slow in rising to a peak (plateau pulse) and is often associated with a notch on the upstroke (anacrotic pulse) or a systolic shudder or thrill.

Fig. 11.6 Various arterial wave forms.

Other changes in arterial pulse

Paradoxical pulse (pulsus paradoxus) (Fig 11.6)
'Paradoxical pulse' is a misnomer, as it is an exaggeration of the normal pattern. During inspiration the pulse pressure (the difference between the systolic and diastolic blood pressures) falls because inspiration prevents the heart filling by splinting it between the expanding lungs and within the pericardial sheath, which is tightened by the descending diaphragm. Inspiration leads to increased systemic venous return and increased right ventricular volume, which consequently restricts left ventricular filling and reduces left ventricular stroke volume. Normally the difference in pulse pressure in inspiration and expiration is no more than 10 mmHg. This can be easily measured using the sphygmomanometer. In severe airflow limitation (especially status asthmaticus), constructive pericarditis, pericardial effusion, pericardial tamponade, restrictive cardiomyopathy or endocardial fibrosis, the pulse pressure during inspiration falls further than normal (and can be zero in deep inspiration). The difference in pulse pressure between inspiration and expiration thus increases, e.g. to 15 mmHg.

Alternating pulse (pulsus alternans)
This is characterized by alternate beats that are weak and strong but with a regular rhythm. An alternating pulse is a feature of severe myocardial failure and is due to the prolonged recovery time of damaged myocardium. It indicates a very poor prognosis. It is easily noticed when taking the blood pressure because the systolic blood pressure may vary from beat to beat by as much as 50 mmHg. Pulsus alternans may also occur when there is rapid, abnormal tachycardia. In this case it acts as a compensatory mechanism and does not indicate a poor prognosis. Pulsus alternans should be distinguished from a bigeminal pulse (see below).

Bigeminal pulse (pulsus bigeminus)
This is due to premature ectopic beats following every sinus beat. The rhythm is not regular (Fig. 11.6) because every weak pulse is premature.

Pulsus bisferiens
This is a pulse that is found in hypertrophic obstructive cardiomyopathy and in aortic regurgitation combined with aortic stenosis. The first systolic wave is the 'percussion' wave produced by the transmission of the left ventricular pressure in early systole. The second peak is the 'tidal' wave caused by recoil of the vascular bed. This normally happens in diastole (the dicrotic wave), but when the left ventricle empties rapidly or is obstructed from emptying completely, the tidal wave occurs in late systole. The result is a palpable double pulse.

BLOOD PRESSURE

The peak systemic arterial blood pressure is produced by transmission of left ventricular systolic pressure. The diastolic blood pressure is maintained by vascular tone and an intact aortic valve.

Taking the blood pressure
- The blood pressure is taken in the (right) arm with the patient relaxed and comfortable.
- The sphygmomanometer cuff is wrapped around the upper arm with the inflation bag placed over the brachial artery.
- The cuff is inflated until the pressure exceeds the arterial pressure and the radial pulse is no longer palpable.
- The diaphragm of the stethoscope is positioned over the brachial artery just below the cuff.
- The cuff pressure is slowly reduced until sounds (Korotkoff sounds) can be heard (phase 1). This is the systolic pressure.
- The pressure is allowed to fall further until the Korotkoff sounds become suddenly muffled (phase 4).
- The pressure is allowed to fall still further until they disappear (phase 5).

The diastolic pressure is usually taken as phase 5 because this phase is more reproducible and nearer to the intravascular diastolic pressure. The Korotkoff sounds may disappear (phase 2) and reappear (phase 3) between the systolic and diastolic pressures. It is important not to mistake phase 2 for the diastolic pressure or phase 3 for the systolic pressure.

The normal blood pressure

There is no single blood pressure or limited range of blood pressures that is normal in all subjects and circumstances. However:
- In a resting adult the systolic blood pressure does not usually exceed 150 mmHg and the diastolic pressure does not exceed 90 mmHg.
- In children or young adults the pressures are correspondingly less.
- In the elderly the rigidity of the arterial vessels produces an increase, predominantly in the systolic blood pressure.
- There is a diurnal variation of blood pressure, the pressure during the day being greater than at night.
- Anxiety and exertion increase the blood pressure.

Note that a cuff that is too small leads to overestimation of the pressure. For example, if a standard arm cuff size (12 cm) is used in an obese patient, the pressure measured will be too high. Similarly, if an arm cuff is used on the thigh (with the diaphragm of the stethoscope applied over the popliteal artery), the femoral pressure will be overestimated. The usual thigh cuff is 15 cm wide. Smaller cuff sizes are available for children and thin adults.

Variations in blood pressure

The systolic blood pressure varies by up to 10 mmHg between the right and left brachial arteries. Standing usually causes a slight reduction of the systolic pressure (<20 mmHg) and an increase in the diastolic blood pressure (<10 mmHg). In postural (orthostatic) hypotension, a large postural fall of both the systolic and diastolic pressures is associated with dizziness. When an irregular heart rhythm such as atrial fibrillation is present, the blood pressure is somewhat variable. Because the blood pressure is normally liable to variation it must be estimated on several occasions before it can be declared elevated.

JUGULAR VENOUS PULSE

There are no valves between the internal jugular vein and the right atrium and observation of the column of blood in the internal jugular system is therefore a good measure of right atrial pressure. The external jugular cannot be relied upon because of its valves and because it may be obstructed by the fascial and muscular layers through which it passes; it can only be used if typical venous pulsation is seen, indicating no obstruction to flow.

Measurement of the jugular pressure

- The patient is positioned at about 45° to the horizontal (between 30° and 60°, wherever the top of the venous pulsation can be seen).
- The head is supported by a pillow and the neck is slightly flexed to allow the skin and muscle overlying the vein to relax.
- The jugular venous pressure is measured as the vertical distance between the manubriosternal angle and the top of the venous column.
- The normal jugular venous pressure is usually less than 3 cm, which is equivalent to a right atrial pressure of 8 cm when measured with reference to a point midway between the anterior and posterior surfaces of the chest. The venous pulsations are not usually palpable (except for the forceful venous distension associated with tricuspid regurgitation).
- Pulsations should be looked for before touching the neck.
- Gentle pressure at the root of the neck may abolish visible venous pulsation and may make a vein visible by causing distension above the occlusion.

An abnormally low jugular venous pressure cannot be measured clinically. Causes include haemorrhage and other forms of hypovolaemia.

Elevation of the jugular venous pressure is produced by:
- Right heart failure
- Constrictive pericarditis
- Cardiac tamponade
- Over-transfusion or excessive infusion of fluids
- Superior vena caval obstruction (but in this case pulsation is absent)

In constrictive pericarditis or cardiac tamponade, ventricular filling is reduced during inspiration because the ventricles are squeezed by the pericardial fluid or non-compliant pericardium, which tightens as the diaphragm descends. Thus, the level of venous pressure increases during inspiration (Kussmaul's sign).

Other causes of an increased jugular pressure also distort the shape of the pressure wave and are considered below.

The hepatojugular (abdomino-jugular) reflex

This is a clinical test whereby abdominal compression (not necessarily over the liver) causes an increase in central and hence jugular venous pressure. This increase in venous pressure is normally reversed within a few heart beats because of a consequent increase in cardiac output. In heart failure, cardiac output cannot increase as readily and the jugular venous pressure remains elevated. This is a difficult clinical sign to elicit and to interpret. However, the hepatojugular reflex is a simple way of confirming the venous nature of a pulsation observed in the neck.

The jugular venous pressure wave

This consists of three peaks and two troughs (Fig. 11.7). The peaks are described as *a*, *c* and *v* waves and the troughs are known as *x* and *y* descents:
- The *a wave* is produced by atrial systole.
- The *x descent* occurs when the atrial contraction finishes.
- As the pressure falls there is a small transient increase that produces a positive deflection called the *c wave*. This is caused by transmission of the rapidly increasing right ventricular pressure before the tricuspid valve closes.
- The *v wave* develops as the venous return fills the right atrium during continued ventricular systole.
- The *y descent* follows the *v* wave when the tricuspid valve opens.

The *a* wave can be distinguished from the *v* wave by observing the venous pulse whilst palpating the carotid artery. The *a* wave occurs immediately before carotid pulsation and the *v* wave occurs simultaneously with carotid pulsation.

The main abnormalities of the shape of the jugular venous pressure wave are elevations of the *a*

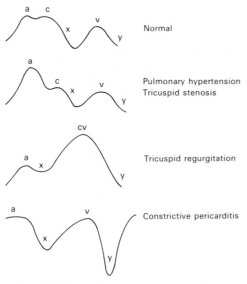

Fig. 11.7 Various jugular venous wave forms.

and *v* waves and steepness of the *y* descent (Fig. 11.7).

Large a waves
These are caused by increased resistance to ventricular filling, as seen with right ventricular hypertrophy due to pulmonary hypertension or pulmonary stenosis. They may also be caused by tricuspid stenosis, but this is unusual because patients with tricuspid stenosis are usually in atrial fibrillation and therefore do not have *a* waves.

A very large *a* wave occurs when the atrium contracts against a closed tricuspid valve. This is known as a 'cannon wave'. Cannon waves occur irregularly in complete heart block and in ventricular tachycardia. In both these situations there is atrioventricular dissociation, and by random chance there is occasional simultaneous atrial and ventricular contraction. In junctional rhythms the atria and ventricles usually contract simultaneously and regular cannon waves are produced.

Large v waves
Tricuspid regurgitation results in giant *v* waves (systolic waves), because the right ventricular pressure is transmitted directly to the right atrium and the great veins.

Steep y descent
Diastolic collapse of elevated venous pressure can occur in right ventricular failure, but is more dramatic in constrictive pericarditis and tricuspid regurgitation. At the end of the ventricular systole the elevated atrial pressure suddenly falls when the tricuspid valve opens. However, the ventricles are

stiff and cannot be distended. The venous pressure therefore rapidly rises again. This rapid fall and rise of the jugular venous pulse is known as Friedreich's sign.

EXAMINATION OF THE PRECORDIUM

Inspection

Deformities should be looked for as they can mimic cardiac abnormalities. For example, pectus excavatum (funnel chest) or kyphoscoliosis may cause an ejection systolic murmur. The position of the apex beat and other cardiac pulsations should be noted; a left ventricular aneurysm may produce an eccentric and abnormal pulsation.

Palpation

The apex beat is defined as the most inferior and most lateral point of cardiac pulsation. It is usually felt just inside the mid-clavicular line at the level of the fourth or fifth left intercostal space. Cardiac enlargement, particularly left ventricular dilatation, displaces the apex beat to the left. The apex beat may also be displaced by a pneumothorax, pulmonary collapse or skeletal abnormalities such as scoliosis. The character of the apex beat is also important. It is normally just palpable and is confined to a point that can be covered by one finger. There are several abnormal forms of pulsation:

- *Tapping apex beat*—a sudden but brief cardiac impulse felt in mitral stenosis
- *Thrusting apex beat*—vigorous but non-sustained pulsation typical of 'volume overload' due to mitral or aortic regurgitation
- *Heaving apex beat*—vigorous and sustained pulsation due to 'pressure overload' as in aortic stenosis and systemic hypertension
- *Impalpable apex beat*—occurs in emphysema, pleural effusion, obesity and pericardial effusion
- *Double apex beat*—two apical pulsations with each heart beat may be felt in hypertrophic cardiomyopathy. This may be due to a palpable atrial impulse. A double apex can also be due to accentuated outward moment in late systole in ventricular aneurysm.

A parasternal heave is elicited by pressing the outstretched hand flat against the sternum or against the costal cartilages just to the left of the sternum. It occurs because of right ventricular hypertrophy. An enlarged left atrium may also cause a parasternal heave. Left atrial pulsation can be distinguished from pulsation due to right ventricular hypertrophy because it occurs before the apex beat or carotid pulsation.

Vigorous pulmonary artery pulsation may be appreciated by palpation in the second left interspace. This is usually due to pulmonary hypertension.

Thrills are palpable murmurs which are most easily appreciated with the flat or ulnar border of the hand rather than with the fingers. A thrill implies a definite abnormality. Systolic thrills in the aortic area are usualy due to aortic stenosis, whereas at the apex a systolic thrill is due to mitral regurgitation. A diastolic thrill is usually caused by mitral stenosis; a diastolic thrill due to aortic regurgitation is uncommon.

Heart sounds that are very loud may also be palpated. In systemic hypertension the aortic second sound may be felt, and in pulmonary hypertension the pulmonary component of the second sound may be felt. Occasionally a third or fourth heart sound may be palpated.

Percussion

Percussion is not usually undertaken, but it may allow the approximate position and size of the heart to be determined.

Auscultation

The sounds best heard with the bell or the diaphragm of the stethoscope are shown in Table 11.6. Other heart sounds and murmurs are heard equally well with the bell or diaphragm; most listeners prefer the diaphragm.

Although it is important to auscultate over most of the precordium, there are four areas where the heart sounds and valvular murmurs are best heard:
- The *aortic area* is in the second intercostal interspace immediately to the right of the sternum. The aorta arches upwards and forwards from the aortic valve and the murmur of aortic stenosis is transmitted best to this area.
- The *pulmonary area* is in the second interspace just to the left of the sternum. This is the closest point to the pulmonary valve, where the murmur of pulmonary stenosis and the pulmonary component of the second heart sound are loudest.

Table 11.6 Use of the stethoscope.

Bell (for low-frequency sounds)	Diaphragm (for high-frequency sounds)
Mid-diastolic rumbles of mitral stenosis and tricuspid stenosis	Early diastolic murmurs of aortic and pulmonary regurgitation
Third and fourth heart sounds	Second heart sound
	Systolic clicks and opening snaps

- The *tricuspid area* is in the fourth interspace to the left of the sternum (left sternal edge). Not only is this close to the tricuspid valve but is also over the right ventricle. Therefore, as well as the murmurs and sounds from the tricuspid valve, the murmurs of pulmonary and aortic regurgitation and third and fourth right ventricular sounds are heard well here.
- The *mitral area or apex* is the point at which the apex beat is felt. The first heart sound and mitral murmurs are loudest here, and aortic regurgitation and third and fourth left ventricular sounds are often heard best at this point.

Each part of the cardiac cycle must be identified and listened to separately. The sequence of cardiac auscultation is summarized in Table 11.7. The identification of the sounds can only be improved by practice; if there is any difficulty, the carotid should be palpated simultaneously as the first heart sound will precede the carotid pulsation.

Apart from the heart sounds, other 'short' sounds including clicks, snaps, plops and knocks may be heard. In addition, sustained noises from within the heart (murmurs) and vascular system (bruits) and from other extra cardiac sources (e.g. the rub of pericarditis) must be identified.

Heart sounds
The first heart sound. This is caused by the closure of the mitral and tricuspid valves and is best heard at the cardiac apex. The sound is usually single but may be slightly split. If split, this 'double' sound at the

Table 11.7 Summary of the auscultation procedure.

The mitral, tricuspid, pulmonary and aortic areas should be auscultated in turn.

1 *Supine*
   First heart sound—mitral area
   Second heart sound—pulmonary and aortic areas, during respiration
   Third and fourth heart sounds—mitral and tricuspid areas
   Clicks, snaps, plops, knocks—mitral and tricuspid areas
   Systolic murmurs—all four auscultation areas, also the neck, axilla and back

2 *Sitting forward*
   Aortic diastolic murmur—tricuspid and mitral areas

3 *Lying on left side*
   Mitral diastolic murmur—mitral area (exactly over the apex beat)

4 *During inspiration and expiration*—see Table 11.9

5 *Exercise, squatting, Valsalva manoeuvres*
   Can be used to accentuate murmurs

beginning of systole must be distinguished from the combination of the first heart sound with a fourth heart sound or with an ejection click.

The first heart sound is loud when the patient is thin and when the circulation is hyperdynamic, e.g. due to anaemia or thyrotoxicosis. The sound is also loud if the valve is still open when ventricular systole begins, e.g. mitral stenosis.

A soft first heart sound occurs in patients with obesity, emphysema or pericardial effusion. It is also present when the valve leaflets are immobile, e.g. in severe calcific mitral stenosis, or when the leaflets are partly closed when systole begins, which occurs when the PR interval is long. A soft first heart sound also occurs when the valve does not close properly, as in mitral regurgitation. Heart failure and cardiogenic shock are also associated with a soft first heart sound.

The intensity of the first heart sound is variable when the relationship between atrial and ventricular systole is not constant, e.g. during ventricular tachycardia or complete heart block: when the PR interval is short the sound is loud, and when the PR interval is long the sound is soft.

The second heart sound. This is caused by the closure of the aortic and pulmonary valves and is best heard with the diaphragm of the stethoscope placed over the aortic or pulmonary area. Unless excessively loud, the pulmonary component of the second sound is only heard in the pulmonary area. Left heart emptying is usually finished just before right heart emptying; therefore the pulmonary component of the second sound closely follows the aortic component. Inspiration results in increased venous return to the right heart, which further delays right heart emptying. The pulmonary sound is therefore delayed further on inspiration and the second heart sound becomes audibly split (Fig. 11.8). Splitting of

the second heart sound on inspiration is known as normal or physiological splitting and is most commonly heard in children or young adults.

Reversed splitting of the second heart sound (when the aortic component follows the pulmonary component) may occur on expiration. It is due to a fixed delay in left heart emptying caused by aortic stenosis, left bundle branch block or left ventricular failure. Thus, when right heart emptying is delayed during inspiration, the two sounds move together, and when the right heart empties more quickly during expiration, the sounds move apart.

The fixed delay in the emptying of the right ventricle produced, for example, by right bundle branch block or pulmonary stenosis will result in wide splitting of the second heart sound. With an atrial septal defect there is usually some degree of right bundle branch block, and because of shunting of blood from the left to the right atrium the right-sided cardiac output is high and ventricular emptying is further delayed. The second heart sound is therefore widely split. Because communication at atrial level prevents differential changes of the venous return during inspiration and expiration, the wide splitting of the second heart sound is not varied by respiration. This is called fixed splitting.

The aortic second sound is louder in systemic hypertension and when a hyperdynamic circulation is present. It is soft in aortic stenosis because the valve is relatively immobile, and it is soft in cardiac failure because of low blood flow. Similarly, the pulmonary component of the second heart sound is loud in pulmonary hypertension and soft in pulmonary stenosis.

Additional heart sounds (Fig. 11.9). Third and fourth heart sounds are low frequency sounds best heard at, and between, the lower left sternal edge and the cardiac apex. They are diastolic in timing, representing ventricular filling, and are heard as soft 'thudding' noises immediately before the first sound (fourth sound) or after the second sound (third sound). The presence of a third or fourth sound produces a triple rhythm which, when associated with sinus tachycardia, sounds like a galloping horse—a gallop rhythm. The cadence of a gallop rhythm due to a third heart sound has been likened to 'Kentucky', whilst that due to a fourth heart sound resembles 'Tennessee'. When both third and fourth heart sounds occur there is usually a marked sinus tachycardia, which results in a short diastolic period so that third and fourth sounds occur simultaneously. This is known as a summation gallop.

The third sound is due to rapid ventricular filling as soon as the mitral and tricuspid valves open. It is a normal finding in children and young adults when it is heard at the apex, especially in the left lateral position. In those over 40 years it represents heart failure or volume overload, e.g. due to mitral regurgitation. It is therefore sometimes referred to as

Fig. 11.8 Variations of the second heart sound. A2 = aortic component; P2 = pulmonary component.

Fig. 11.9 Normal and additional heart sounds and the conditions in which they are found. S1 = first heart sound; A2 = aortic component of the second sound; P2 = pulmonary component of the second sound; S3 = third heart sound; S4 = fourth heart sound; EC = ejection click; OS = opening snap; MSC = mid-systolic click.

a sound of 'distress'. A right ventricular third sound is heard best at the left sternal edge, and a left ventricular third sound is heard at the apex.

The fourth sound is caused by the surge of ventricular filling that accompanies atrial systole. It therefore occurs in late diastole. It may be a normal finding in an elderly subject, but in younger patients it usually indicates increased ventricular stiffness associated with hypertension, aortic stenosis or acute myocardial infarction. It is called the sound of cardiac 'stress', and can sometimes be felt.

Abnormal heart valves may cause an audible signal when opening. An ejection click is a high frequency sound, best heard with the diaphragm of the stethoscope at the left sternal edge, and occurs immediately following the first heart sound. It is produced by the sudden opening of a deformed but mobile aortic or pulmonary valve. It is most commonly heard in association with a bicuspid aortic valve when it is easily heard throughout the respiratory cycle. A stenotic pulmonary valve also produces an ejection click, but this is best heard on expiration. A dilated aorta or pulmonary artery may also give rise to an ejection click.

A stenotic mitral or tricuspid valve may produce a high frequency opening snap that occurs just after the second heart sound. It is best heard with the diaphragm of the stethoscope at the left sternal edge or between the left sternal edge and the apex. It can be distinguished from a split second sound or a third sound by the site at which it is best heard, its higher frequency and its lack of respiratory variation.

A mid-systolic click (or clicks) is due to sudden prolapse of the mitral valve into the left atrium during ventricular systole. It occurs when the mitral valve is congenitally deformed or has undergone myxomatous degeneration, as in the mitral valve prolapse syndrome. These auscultatory features are inconsistent and wax and wane with time.

Tumour plops are low frequency sounds produced by the sudden checking of the travel of an atrial tumour when it reaches the valve. Such sounds occur after an opening snap, but before a third sound would be expected. The pericardial knock is another sound that occurs in this position in the cardiac cycle. Like a third heart sound, it is low frequency. It is heard in constrictive pericarditis and is due to rather early, sudden and marked halting of ventricular filling due to constriction.

Prosthetic sounds
Mechanical replacement heart valves produce loud clicks due to the opening and closing of the valve. These prosthetic sounds may be muffled or absent if valve movement is impeded by thrombus or vegetations.

Heart murmurs
Turbulent blood flow causes heart murmurs. Turbulence may be produced when there is high blood flow through a normal valve, or when there is normal blood flow through an abnormal valve or into a dilated chamber. Turbulence is also caused by the regurgitation of blood through a leaking valve. Murmurs produced by high velocity blood flow (e.g. the systolic murmur of mitral regurgitation) are high frequency and are often described as 'blowing' in quality. The intensity of murmurs is determined not only by the blood velocity but also by the volume of blood producing the murmur and the distance of the source of the murmur from the stethoscope. Right-sided murmurs tend to become louder on inspiration because inspiration increases the venous return to the right heart.

Heart murmurs may occur with a normal or near normal heart (innocent murmurs). They are usually soft and short and occur early in systole. Murmurs also occur in the following situations:
● Anaemia, thyrotoxicosis and other causes of a high cardiac output produce flow murmurs, which are usually brief systolic ejection murmurs heard best at the left sternal edge or in the pulmonary area. These murmurs are believed to emanate from the pulmonary or aortic valve. Similar murmurs are heard in association with skeletal abnormalities such as kyphoscoliosis or funnel chest.
● A very small ventricular septal defect may produce a short early systolic murmur, heard well at the left sternal edge. The murmur is short because contraction of the ventricle closes the small defect early in systole.

- A buzzing, twanging or vibratory murmur, called Still's murmur, may be heard at the lower left sternal edge or cardiac apex. It is thought to arise from the region below the aortic valve.

Murmurs are classified as systolic, diastolic or continuous. Another functional classification divides systolic murmurs into ejection or regurgitant. Murmurs should be carefully assessed; a summary of the auscultation procedure is shown in Table 11.7. The intensity of cardiac murmurs can be graded as indicated in Table 11.8.

Systolic murmurs (see Table 11.9). Systolic murmurs occur synchronously with carotid pulsation. There are three main varieties of pathological systolic murmur:
- *Ejection (mid-)systolic murmurs* are heard separately from the first and second heart sounds. Their intensity rises then falls, being greatest in mid-systole.
- *Pan-systolic murmurs* extend from the first to the second heart sound and tend to be of constant intensity throughout the whole of systole.
- *Late systolic murmurs* are separated from the first sound but extend up to the second sound.

Diastolic murmurs (see Table 11.9). Diastolic murmurs are always associated with cardiac disease. They are of two types:
- *Mid-diastolic murmurs* usually arise from the mitral and tricuspid valves. In aortic regurgitation the flow of blood back into the left ventricle may partially close and obstruct the mitral valve producing a mitral mid-diastolic murmur (Austin Flint murmur).
- *Early diastolic murmurs* usually result from aortic regurgitation and rarely from pulmonary regurgitation. These murmurs begin with the second

Table 11.8 The grading of murmur intensity.

Grade	Systolic murmurs	Diastolic murmurs
1	Very soft (heard only in good circumstances)	Very soft (heard only in good circumstances)
2	Soft	Soft
3	Moderate	Moderate
4	Loud	Loud or associated with palpable thrill
5	Very loud	—
6	Very loud (no stethoscope needed) or associated with palpable thrill	—

Table 11.9 Some common structural causes of murmurs.

Murmur	Position where murmur is best heard
SYSTOLIC	
Ejection (mid-) systolic	
Aortic stenosis	Aortic area and clavicles
Pulmonary stenosis ⎫	Left sternal edge on
Atrial septal defect ⎬	inspiration
Left (e.g. hypertrophic cardiomyopathy—HCM) and right (e.g. Fallot's tetralogy) outflow tract obstruction may also cause mid-systolic murmurs	
Pan-systolic	
Mitral regurgitation (blowing)	Apex to axilla
Tricuspid regurgitation (low pitched)	Left sternal edge
Ventricular septal defect (loud and rough)	Left sternal edge
Late systolic	
Dynamic outflow tract obstruction (HCM)	Accentuated on standing
Mitral valve prolapse	Apex
Coarctation of the aorta	Left sternal edge
DIASTOLIC	
Mid-diastolic	
Mitral stenosis (low frequency rumbling)	Apex, patient on left side, accentuated on exertion
Tricuspid stenosis	As for mitral stenosis
Austin Flint murmur	Apex
Early diastolic	
Aortic regurgitation (blowing, high pitched)	Left sternal edge and apex, patient sitting forward and in expiration
Pulmonary regurgitation (blowing, variable pitch)	Right of sternum, louder on inspiration
Graham Steell in pulmonary hypertension (due to mitral stenosis)	Left sternal edge

heart sound and are blowing (high pitched) in quality. Pulmonary hypertension secondary to mitral stenosis may lead to pulmonary valve regurgitation (Graham Steell murmur).

Continuous murmurs. A continuous murmur may occur because of a combination of systolic and diastolic murmurs, due to connections between the aorta and pulmonary artery (e.g. patent ductus arteriosus) or due to arteriovenous anastamoses and collateral circulations such as those associated with coarctation of the aorta. High venous flow, especially in young children, can produce a continuous venous hum in the neck. This is reduced by occluding the vein or by lying the child flat. Similarly, high mammary blood flow in pregnant or lactating women can produce a continuous murmur known as a mammary souffle.

Extra cardiac sounds

Bruits, usually due to arterial stenoses, are murmurs arising from a peripheral artery, including the distal aorta.

A pericardial friction rub is a scratching or crunching noise produced by the movement of inflamed pericardium. Since it is relatively high frequency it is best heard with the diaphragm. It is most obvious in systole but may also be heard in early diastole or synchronously with atrial contraction. It should be listened for during both held inspiration and expiration.

Cardiac investigations

Chest x-ray

This is an essential investigation. It is taken in the postero-anterior (PA) direction with the heart close to the x-ray film to minimize magnification with respect to the thorax. A left lateral and a penetrated PA film are also taken in patients with abnormal plain PA films. The cardiac structures and great vessels that can be seen on these x-rays are indicated in Fig. 11.10.

Heart size

Heart size can be assessed from the PA chest film; the maximum transverse diameter of the heart is compared with the maximum transverse diameter of the chest (see Fig. 11.10).

This cardiothoracic ratio (CTR) is usually less than 50%, except in neonates, infants, athletes and patients with skeletal abnormalities such as scoliosis and funnel chest. A transverse cardiac diameter of more than 15.5 cm is abnormal. Pericardial effusion or cardiac dilatation causes an increase in the ratio.

A pericardial effusion produces a globular, sharp-edged shadow. This enlargement may occur quite suddenly and, unlike heart failure, there is no associated change in the pulmonary vasculature. The echocardiogram is more specific than the chest x-ray for the diagnosis of pericardial effusion, particularly because at least 250 ml of fluid must accumulate before x-ray changes are apparent.

Certain patterns of specific chamber enlargement may be seen on the chest x-ray:
- *Left atrial dilatation* results in prominence of the left atrial appendage on the left heart border, a double atrial shadow to the right of the sternum, and splaying of the carina because a large left atrium elevates the left main bronchus (Fig. 11.11). On a lateral chest x-ray an enlarged left atrium bulges backwards, indenting the barium-filled oesophagus.
- *Left ventricular enlargement* results in an increase in the CTR and a smooth elongation and increased convexity of the left heart border. A left ventricular aneurysm may produce a distinct bulge or distortion of the left heart border.
- *Right atrial enlargement* results in the right border

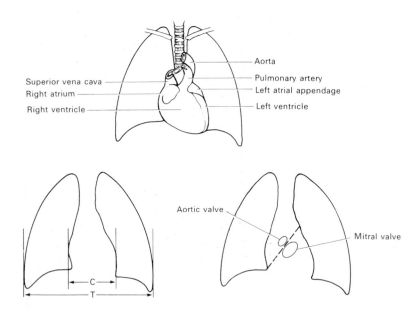

Superior vena cava
Right atrium
Right ventricle

Aorta
Pulmonary artery
Left atrial appendage
Left ventricle

Aortic valve
Mitral valve

Fig. 11.10 Diagrams to show the heart silhouette on the chest x-ray, measurement of the cardiothoracic ratio (CTR) and the location of the cardiac valves. CTR = C/T × 100%; normal CTR = < 50%.

Fig. 11.11 X-ray of mitral stenosis showing left atrial dilatation (arrow).

Fig. 11.12 X-ray showing heavy calcification of the pericardium.

of the heart projecting into the right lower lung field.
- *Right ventricular enlargement* results in an increase of the CTR and an upward displacement of the apex of the heart because the enlarging right ventricle pushes the left ventricle leftwards, upwards and eventually backwards. Differentiation of left from right ventricular enlargement may be difficult from the shape of the left heart border alone, but the lateral view shows enlargement anteriorly for the right ventricle and posteriorly for the left ventricle.
- *Ascending aortic dilatation* is seen as a prominence of the aortic shadow to the right of the mediastinum.
- *Enlargement of the pulmonary artery* in pulmonary hypertension and left-to-right shunts produces a prominent bulge on the left hand border of the mediastinum below the aortic knuckle.

Calcification
Calcification in the cardiovascular system occurs because of tissue degeneration. Calcification is visible on a lateral or a penetrated PA film, but is best studied by fluoroscopy. Various types of calcification can occur:
- *Pericardial calcification* (Fig. 11.12) may be seen as plaque-like opacities over the surface of the heart, but particularly concentrated in the AV groove. Such calcification often results from tuberculous pericarditis and may be associated with pericardial constriction.

- *Valvular calcification* may result from long-standing rheumatic or congenital heart disease. The aortic and mitral valves are most commonly affected. On the lateral film, a calcified aortic valve is seen on or above a line joining the carina to the sternophrenic angle. Mitral valvular calcification is seen below and behind this line.
- *Myocardial calcification* may occur in association with a left ventricular aneurysm.
- *Calcification of the aorta* is a common, normal finding in patients over the age of 40 years and appears as a curvi-linear opacity around the circumference of the aortic knuckle. Calcification in the ascending aorta usually denotes syphilitic aortitis whereas in the descending aorta it is due to atheroma or, in the younger patient, to nonspecific aortitis.
- *Coronary arterial calcification*, especially of the proximal left coronary artery, is associated with coronary atheroma but does not necessarily correspond to the site of maximal stenosis.

Lung fields
Pulmonary plethora results from left-to-right shunts, e.g. atrial or ventricular septal defects. It is seen as a general increase in the vascularity of the lung fields and as an increase in the diameter of the pulmonary arteries, especially the right lower lobe artery, which normally should not exceed 16 mm in diameter.

Pulmonary oligaemia is a paucity of vascular markings and a reduction in the width of the arteries. It occurs in situations where there is reduced pulmonary blood flow, such as pulmonary embolism, severe pulmonary stenosis and Fallot's tetralogy.

Pulmonary arterial hypertension may result from pulmonary embolism, chronic lung disease or chronic heart disease such as ventricular septal defect or mitral valve stenosis. In addition to x-ray features of these conditions, the pulmonary arteries are prominent close to the hili but are very reduced in size (pruned) in the peripheral lung fields. This pattern is usually symmetrical.

Pulmonary venous hypertension occurs in left ventricular failure or mitral valve disease. Normal pulmonary venous pressure is 5–14 mmHg at rest. Mild pulmonary venous hypertension (15–20 mmHg) produces isolated dilatation of the upper lobe pulmonary veins. Interstitial oedema occurs when the pressure is between 21 and 30 mmHg. This manifests as fluid collections in the interlobar fissures, interlobular septa (Kerley B lines) and pleural spaces. Alveolar oedema occurs when the pressure exceeds 30 mmHg, appearing as areas of central consolidation, indistinctness of the hilar regions, haziness and mottling of the lung fields (Fig. 11.13) and pleural effusions. Patients with long-standing elevation of the pulmonary venous pressure have reactive thickening of the pulmonary arteriolar intima, which protects the alveoli from pulmonary oedema. Thus, in these patients the pulmonary venous pressure may increase to well above 30 mmHg before frank pulmonary oedema develops.

Fluoroscopy

Image intensification allows the heart and great vessels to be viewed continuously by means of x-ray. Indications for fluoroscopy include evaluation of cardiac function by observing the pulsations of the chambers of the heart and great vessels, and the assessment of artificial heart valves, although echocardiography is better for these purposes. Cardiac fluoroscopy is useful for the detection of small areas of cardiac calcification, and is essential for the insertion of cardiac catheters and pacemaker electrodes.

Electrocardiography

The electrocardiogram (ECG) is a recording from the surface of the body of the electro-potential changes produced by the depolarization and repolarization of myocardial cells (see Fig. 11.30, p. 478). At rest, the intracellular voltage of the myocardium is polarized at -90 mV compared with that of the extracellular space. This diastolic voltage difference occurs because of the high intracellular potassium concentration, which is maintained by the sodium–potassium pump despite the free membrane permeability to potassium. Depolarization of cardiac cells occurs when there is a sudden increase in the permeability of the membrane to sodium. Sodium rushes into the cell and the negative resting voltage is lost (stage 0; see Fig. 11.30). The depolarization of a myocardial cell causes the depolarization of adjacent cells and, in the healthy heart, the entire myocardium is depolarized in a coordinated fashion. During repolarization, cellular electrolyte balance is slowly restored (stages 1, 2, and 3). Slow diastolic depolarization (stage 4) follows until the threshold potential is reached. Another action potential then follows (see Fig. 11.30).

The ECG is recorded from two or more simultaneous points of skin contact (electrodes). The conventional ECG consists of 12 'leads' of which three are bipolar and the rest are unipolar (Table 11.10 and Fig. 11.14). When cardiac activation proceeds towards the positive contact, an upward deflection is produced on the ECG. The leads may be

Fig. 11.13 X-rays showing pulmonary oedema before (left) and after treatment (right).

Table 11.10 ECG leads.

	ECG lead	Connection			Orientation
Standard leads of Einthoven (bipolar)	I	LA	v.	RA	Lateral
	II	LL	v.	RA	Inferior/lateral
	III	LL	v.	LA	Inferior/cavity
Augmented leads of Goldberger ('unipolar')	AVR	RA	v.	LA+LL	Cavity
	AVL	LA	v.	RA+LL	Lateral
	AVF	LL	v.	RA+LA	Inferior
Chest leads of Wilson (unipolar)	V_1	4th RICS PS	v.	RA+LL+LA	Cavity
	V_2	4th LICS PS	v.	RA+LL+LA	Septum/anterior
	V_3	4th/5th LICS PS-MCL	v.	RA+LL+LA	Septum/anterior
	V_4	5th LICS MCL	v.	RA+LL+LA	Anterior
	V_5	5th LICS AAL	v.	RA+LL+LA	Anterior/lateral
	V_6	5th LICS MAL	v.	RA+LL+LA	Lateral

LA = left arm
RA = right arm
LL = left leg

RA+LL+LA = Wilson's common terminal
RICS = right intercostal space

LICS = left intercostal space
PS = parasternal
MCL = mid-clavicular line
AAL = anterior axillary line
MAL = mid-axillary line
PS-MCL = midway between PS and MCL

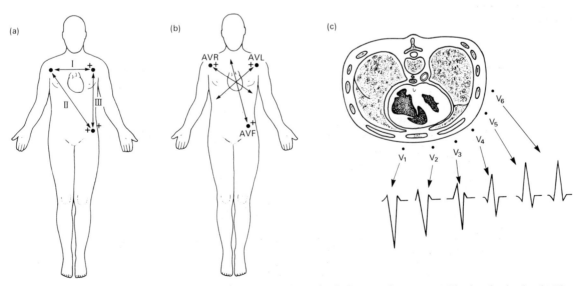

Fig. 11.14 The connections or directions which comprise the 12-lead electrocardiogram. (a) The bipolar leads. (b) The unipolar leads. (c) The chest leads.

grouped according to the part of the heart faced by the positive contact (see Fig. 11.14). Thus:

- Leads AVL, I and V_6 face the lateral wall of the left ventricle.
- Leads II, III and AVF face the inferior wall of the left ventricle.
- Leads V_1 and V_2 face the right ventricle.
- Leads V_3 and V_4 overlie the interventricular septum.
- Leads V_4 and V_5 are close to the anterior surface of the left ventricle.
- Leads V_1 and AVR look into the cavity of the ventricles.

There is some overlap between these approximate orientations.

The shape of the normal electrocardiographic wave form (Fig. 11.15) has important similarities, whatever the orientation. The first deflection is caused by atrial depolarization, and it is a low amplitude, slow deflection called a P wave. The QRS complex results from ventricular depolarization and is sharper and larger in amplitude than the P wave. The T wave is another slow and low amplitude deflection that results from ventricular repolarization.

The atrial repolarization wave is not seen in a conventional ECG because it is low in voltage and is hidden by the QRS complex.

The PR interval is the length of time from the start of the P wave to the start of the QRS complex. It is the time taken for activation to pass from the sinus node, through the atrium, AV node and the His Purkinje system to the ventricle.

The QT interval extends from the start of the QRS complex to the end of the T wave. This interval represents the time taken to depolarize and repolarize the ventricular myocardium.

The ST segment is the period between the end of the QRS complex and the start of the T wave. In the normal heart, all cells are depolarized during this phase of the ECG.

The normal values for the electrocardiographic intervals are indicated in Table 11.11. Leads that face the lateral wall of the left ventricle have predominantly positive deflections, and leads looking into the ventricular cavity are usually negative. Detailed patterns depend on the size, shape and rhythm of the heart and the characteristics of the torso.

The ECG is the most commonly used cardiac investigation. It is conventionally recorded at 25 mm·s^{-1} (England and North America) or 50 mm·s^{-1} (Europe). Standard ECG paper is illustrated in Fig. 11.15. There are bold lines drawn every 0.2 s and fine lines occur at 40 ms intervals. The usual voltage calibration is 1 mV·cm^{-1}. The normal 12-lead ECG is shown in Fig. 11.16.

Cardiac vectors
At any point in time during depolarization and repolarization, electrical potentials are being propagated in different directions. Most of these cancel each other out and only the net force is recorded. This net force in the frontal plane is known as the cardiac vector (Fig. 11.17a).

The mean QRS vector can be calculated from the standard leads (Fig. 11.17b); it normally lies between $-30°$ and $+90°$. Left axis deviation lies between $-30°$ and $-90°$ and right axis deviation between $+90°$ and $+150°$. Calculation of this vector is occasionally useful in the diagnosis of cardiac disorders.

Exercise electrocardiography (see p. 501)
This is a technique used to assess the cardiac response to exercise. The ECG is recorded *whilst* climbing stairs, riding a bicycle ergometer, or walking or running on a treadmill. Recording the ECG *after* the exercise is not an adequate form of stress test. Normally there is little change in the T wave or ST segment.

Myocardial ischaemia provoked by exertion results in ST segment depression (>1 mm) in leads facing the affected area. Although most abnormali-

Fig. 11.15 The waves and elaboration of the normal electrocardiogram. From Goldman MJ (1976) *Principles of Clinical Electrocardiography*, 9th edn. Los Altos, California: Lange.

Table 11.11 Normal ECG intervals.

P wave duration	≤0.12 s
PR interval	0.12–0.22 s
QRS complex duration	≤0.10 s
Corrected QT (QT_c)	≤0.44 s

$$QT_c = \frac{QT}{\sqrt{RR \text{ interval}}}$$

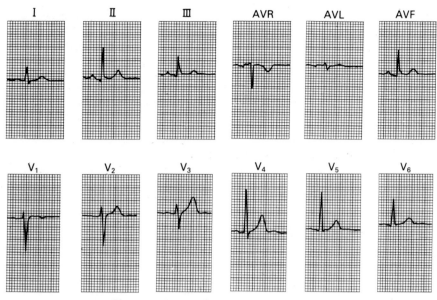

Fig. 11.16 A normal 12-lead electrocardiogram.

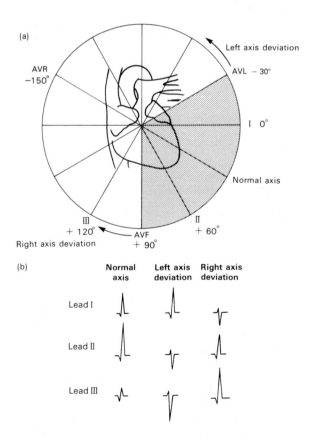

Fig. 11.17 (a) The hexaxial reference system illustrating the six leads in the frontal plane, e.g. lead I is 0°; lead II is +60° and lead III is +120°. (b) Calculating the direction of the cardiac vector. In the first column the QRS complex with zero magnitude, i.e. when the positive and negative deflections are equal, is seen in lead III. The mean QRS vector is therefore perpendicular to lead III and is either −150° or +30°. Lead I is positive, so the axis must be +30°, which is normal. In left axis deviation (second column) the main deflection is positive (R wave) in lead I and negative (S wave) in lead III. In right axis deviation (third column) the main deflection is negative (S wave) in lead I and positive (R wave) in lead III.

ties are detected in leads V_5 (anterior and lateral ischaemia) or AVF (inferior ischaemia), it is best to record a full 12-lead ECG. The form of ST segment depression provoked by ischaemia is characteristic: it is either planar or shows down-sloping depression (see Fig. 11.18). Up-sloping depression is a non-specific finding. During an exercise test the exercise tolerance, blood pressure and rhythm responses to exercise are also assessed. Exercise causes an increase in heart rate and blood pressure. A sustained fall in blood pressure indicates severe coronary artery disease.

The usual indications and contraindications for the test are shown in Table 11.12.

24-h ambulatory taped electrocardiography

This is a technique for recording transient changes such as a brief paroxysm of tachycardia, an occasional pause in the rhythm, or intermittent ST segment shifts. A conventional 12-lead ECG is recorded in less than a minute and usually samples approximately 30–50 complexes. In a 24-h period, over 100 000 complexes are recorded. Such a large amount of data must be analysed by automatic or semi-automatic methods. This technique is called 'Holter' electrocardiography after its inventor. For those patients with very intermittent symptoms, a small tape or solid state recorder can be used for several months until a symptomatic event is captured by applying the device to the skin when the symptom occurs.

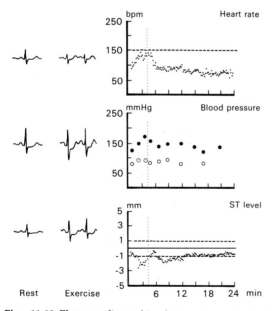

Fig. 11.18 Electrocardiographic, heart rate and blood pressure changes on exercise, showing characteristic down-sloping ST segment depression in response to 4 min of exercise in a patient with myocardial ischaemia. The end of the exercise period is indicated by the dotted line.

Table 11.12 Indications and contraindications for exercise electrocardiography.

Indications
Diagnosis of chest pain
Provocation of ischaemia
Evaluation of treatment of angina
Provocation of arrhythmia
Evaluation of treatment of arrhythmia
Risk assessment after myocardial infarction
Functional assessment in a patient with heart disease

Contraindications
Recent myocardial infarction (within 1 week); a limited test recommended within 1 month
Unstable angina
Uncompensated heart failure
Severe aortic stenosis
Malignant hypertension

NB   Provided that adequate precautions are observed (doctor and resuscitation facilities available, continuous monitoring), the mortality from exercise testing is less than 0.01%. Myocardial infarction occurs in less than 0.05%.

Phonocardiography

The application of a sensitive microphone to the chest wall allows heart sounds and murmurs to be recorded. Usually cardiac, carotid or jugular pulsations are recorded at the same time. The technique is difficult and, except for research purposes, has been largely superseded by echocardiography and other non-invasive techniques.

Echocardiography

A piezo-electric crystal is used to emit acoustic pulses at high frequency (2–3 MHz, typically 2.5 MHz). These ultrasonic signals, reflected by moving cardiac structures, are received back by the same crystal. Because soundwaves have a known velocity, the structures reflecting them can be localized. The reflected signals are displayed against time on an oscilloscope or strip chart recorder to produce an M-mode scan (Fig. 11.19). Because bone and air are relatively impervious to the transmission of sound, it is only possible to image the heart through small 'windows', such as the third left intercostal space close to the sternum, or the cardiac apex. Echocardiography can also be used to build up a two-dimensional scan of the moving heart by using multiple transducers or rapid oscillation of a single transducer (Fig. 11.20). The echocardiogram is particularly useful for investigating:
- *Pericardial effusions*. Body fluids do not reflect ultrasound. Effusions are therefore detected as echo-free zones in front or behind the heart (Fig. 11.21).

Fig. 11.19 An M-mode echocardiogram. This is a 'sweep' from the left ventricle to the aorta as shown on the inset. CW = chest wall; RVOT = right ventricular outflow tract; IVS = interventricular septum; LV = left ventricle; LA = left atrium; AMVC = anterior mitral valve cusp; PMVC = posterior mitral valve cusp; RV = right ventricle. Note the pattern of movement of the AMVC. At the onset of diastole there is a rapid anterior movement followed by a slower backward movement. It moves sharply anteriorly at the end of diastole owing to atrial contraction. The PMVC moves in the opposite direction to the AMVC.

Fig. 11.20 Normal two-dimensional echocardiogram in the parasternal 'long axis'. The diagram shows the anatomy of the area scanned and a diagrammatic representation of the echocardiogram. LV = left ventricle, LA = left atrium; RVOT = right ventricular outflow tract; IVS = interventricular septum; PMVC = posterior mitral valve cusp; AMVC = anterior mitral valve cusp.

ECG

EPICARDIUM

Electrical Alternans

EFFUSION

Fig. 11.21 Echocardiogram showing pericardial effusion. This is revealed by the echo-free space between the chest wall and the epicardium of the right ventricle. The large arrows indicate the epicardium. The ECG shows electrical alternans, which may be a feature of pericardial effusion (see p. 539). In this record the ECG trace overlies the effusion.

- *The mitral valve.* The motion of the mitral valve leaflets can be accurately measured. Thick rheumatic mitral valves produce dense reflections, and the movement of the leaflets is slow and restricted (Fig. 11.22).
- *The left ventricular muscle.* Hypertrophy of the left ventricular myocardium, particularly the septum, can be accurately measured from echocardiograms. The movement of the ventricular myocardium can also be assessed. The size of atrial and ventricular cavities can be measured.
- *An intracardiac mass.* The vegetations of endocarditis, intracardiac thrombi and tumours can be easily visualized with echocardiography, especially when displayed in two dimensions.

Because echocardiography is non-invasive, it is particularly useful for the diagnosis of congenital heart defects in neonates and children. Good echocardiograms cannot be obtained in obese or uncooperative subjects and in those with chronic lung disease or chest wall deformities.

Ultrasonic signals (Doppler sonography) can also be used to assess the direction and velocity of blood flow. Aortic or mitral stenosis or regurgitation can be evaluated using this valuable technique.

Nuclear imaging

Nuclear imaging techniques are primarily used in ischaemic heart disease. Myocardial structure and function can be assessed by radionuclide-imaging techniques.

Thallium-201 imaging

This is used to detect myocardial ischaemia and infarction. Thallium, which behaves like potassium, is taken up by healthy myocardium. Ischaemia or infarction produces a nuclear image with a 'cold' spot (Fig. 11.23). The isotope is usually administered during exercise and an image is taken soon after the exercise. Three or four hours later the heart is scanned again to obtain a redistribution image. The disappearance of the cold spot on the redistribution image implies ischaemia provoked by exertion and reversed by rest, whereas a persistent cold spot indicates infarction.

Pyrophosphate scan

Pyrophosphate labelled with technetium-99m concentrates in bone and acutely infarcted myocardium. The isotope should be injected intravenously between 1 and 5 days (best on the second or third day) following a myocardial infarction. Imaging a few hours later detects a 'hot spot' (Fig. 11.24) in the region of the infarction. Scans are difficult to interpret because calcified costal cartilage and breast tissue may both concentrate the isotope. On the other hand, infarction may not result in the expected hot spot because the isotope is prevented from reaching the infarct due to complete occlusion of coronary

Fig. 11.22 An M-mode echocardiogram of a patient with mitral stenosis. CW = chest wall; IVS = interventricular septum; MV = mitral valve; AMVC = anterior mitral valve cusp; PMVC = posterior mitral valve cusp; LV = left ventricle; RV = right ventricle; LA = left atrium. Note the thickened mitral valve cusps (AMVC and PMVC) and the abnormal pattern of restricted movements of the AMVC. The PMVC moves anteriorly during diastole so that the valve opening is severely restricted.

Fig. 11.23 Thallium myocardial perfusion scans using a grey scale (increased activity being whiter). The exercise scan (right) shows a defect at the top (between 10 and 12 o'clock) which fills in after 4 h rest (left). This suggests reversible myocardial ischaemia.

Fig. 11.24 Infarct-avid scans using technetium-labelled pyrophosphate. A negative scan (left) shows bone uptake in the ribs and sternum; the darker circles are position markers. A positive scan (right) shows myocardial uptake with a density greater than the ribs but slightly less than the sternum. AP = anterior–posterior.

vessels to the infarcted myocardium. False-positive scans may occur in unstable angina.

Radionuclide ventriculography

Two methods are used to obtain blood pool images:

- A *MUGA* (multi-gated acquisition) or equilibrium image is obtained by intravenous injection of technetium-99m attached to the patient's own red cells in vivo and which is therefore retained in the vascular space. Over 200 heart beats are imaged. Comparison of the study with the ECG allows systolic and diastolic points of the cycle to be identified.
- A *first pass study* images the heart as a bolus of isotope makes a single pass through the circulation.

These techniques are complementary, but both outline the cardiac chambers, particularly the left ventricle, by imaging the isotope within the central circulation during systole and diastole. The percentage of the left ventricular volume ejected with each systole (the ejection fraction) can be accurately measured, and any section of the left ventricular wall that contracts abnormally (a wall motion defect) can be visualized (Fig. 11.25). Radionuclide studies may be performed at rest and during exercise to assess changes in cardiac function. A deterioration on exercise suggests coronary disease or myocardial abnormality.

Cardiac catheterization

Cardiac catheterization is the introduction of a thin radiopaque tube (catheter) into the circulation.

The right heart is catheterized by introducing the catheter into a peripheral vein and advancing it through the right atrium and ventricle into the pulmonary artery. The left heart is reached by way of a peripheral artery. The catheter is manipulated through the aortic valve into the left ventricle.

The pressures in the right heart chambers, left ventricle, aorta and pulmonary artery can be measured directly. An indirect measure of left atrial pressure can be obtained by 'wedging' a catheter into

	rest	exercise
baseline	EF .65 HR 82	EF .41 HR 136
nifedipine	EF .65 HR 110	EF .85 HR 143

Fig. 11.25 First-pass radionuclide angiograms. The images show the diastolic perimeter surrounding the systolic image. The ejection fraction (EF)—the proportion of diastolic blood ejected during systole—and the heart rate (HR) are shown. These two rest and exercise studies show a control test (top), repeated after nifedipine (bottom). Note the improved exercise EF after nifedipine, suggesting amelioration of ischaemia.

the distal pulmonary artery (see also p. 477). In this position the pressure from the right ventricle is obstructed by the catheter and only the pulmonary venous and left atrial pressures are recorded. Pressure measurements are used to quantify stenoses or measure contractile function.

During cardiac catheterization, blood samples may be withdrawn to measure the concentration of ischaemic metabolites, e.g. lactate, and the oxygen content. These estimations are used to gauge ischaemia, quantify intracardiac shunts, and measure cardiac output.

Contrast cine-angiograms are also taken during catheterization. Radiopaque contrast material is injected into the cardiac chambers (Fig. 11.26), arterial trunks or coronary arteries. Fig. 11.27 shows

(a)   (b)

Fig. 11.26 Left ventricular angiogram. (a) End-systolic and (b) end-diastolic cine angiogram frames.

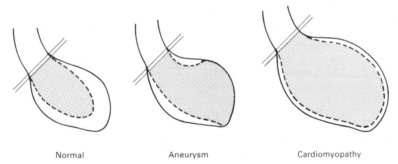

Normal   Aneurysm   Cardiomyopathy

Fig. 11.27 Diagrams showing left ventricular angiograms. A normal picture is compared with those showing an aneurysm and cardiomyopathy. The solid line represents the end-diastolic perimeter and the dotted line the end-systolic perimeter of the left ventricle. The double line marks the plane of the aortic valve.

a normal angiogram compared with angiograms in patients with aneurysm and cardiomyopathy.

Magnetic resonance imaging

This non-invasive imaging technique does not involve harmful radiation. A powerful magnetic field is used to line up the protons in the hydrogen atoms of the body, each of which can be thought of as a tiny magnet. A radio-frequency emission distorts this line-up, but when the radio waves are turned off, the atoms return to their previous position and give off energy. This energy can be reconstituted as an image. Magnetic resonance imaging of the heart is complicated because the heart is a moving structure, but the technique is already finding clinical application for imaging vascular structures.

Therapeutic procedures

Cardiac resuscitation

No matter where cardiac arrest occurs it is essential that someone close to the victim institutes basic life support. The longer the period of respiratory and circulatory arrest, the less the possibility of restoring healthy life. After 3 min there will be permanent cerebral dysfunction. Because sudden unexpected cardiac arrest is relatively common in the hospital, medical students and all doctors must know what to do. A cardiac arrest usually causes a great deal of excitement and some panic. Therefore, it is very important that the basic procedure is well known. A standard procedure must be used in order that a variety of personnel may work easily together. The scheme that follows is recommended by the UK Resuscitation Council. It should be practised on a resuscitation dummy at least every 6 months.

Basic life support
The first step is to establish if the victim is unconscious (shake and shout at the patient) and whether there is a pulse. It is best to feel the carotid pulse by pressing backwards just to the side of the thyroid cartilage. If there is no pulse, immediately call for help. Quickly place the victim in an accessible position with firm underlying support (e.g. on his back on the floor), and begin basic life support. This can be remembered as A (airway) and B (breathing) and C (circulation).

Airway. Any loose obstruction (e.g. blood and mucus) in the mouth and pharynx should be quickly removed. Unless already detached, leave false teeth in place because they give form and support to the oral cavity. Open the airway by flexing the neck and extending the head ('sniffing the morning air' position).

Breathing. Look for the rise and fall of the chest and abdomen. If there is no respiration, begin expired air respiration. With the head of the victim tilted backwards and the chin pulled forward the rescuer takes a deep breath and seals his lips around the mouth or nose of the victim. Four quick puffs are given. Expired air respiration is the only method of artificial respiration that successfully ventilates the patient. The mechanical methods of Holger and Neilson, Shaeffer and Sylvester are completely useless because they result in the movement of less air than is required to fill the dead space.

If the airway is obstructed, the head, neck and jaw are readjusted and another check is made for debris in the mouth. If obstruction persists, any foreign body stuck in the larynx or upper airway should be removed by a firm thrust to the epigastrium (the *Heimlich manoeuvre*, see p. 576).

Circulation. Circulation is achieved by external chest compression. The heel of one hand is placed over the lower half of the victim's sternum and the heel of the second hand is placed over the first with the fingers interlocked. The arms are kept straight and the sternum is rhythmically depressed by 1½–2 inches. Chest compression does not massage the heart. The thorax acts as a pump and the heart provides a system of one-way valves to ensure forward circulation.

Respiration and compression is now continued as follows:
● *Single rescuer* — compression at a rate of 80 beats per minute with two respirations after 15 compressions.
● *Two rescuers* — continuous compressions at a rate of 60 beats per minute and one respiration given after every 5 compressions.

If possible, it is better to give compressions without interruption. This maintains adequate cerebral and coronary perfusion pressures. Ventilation can easily be achieved despite continued chest compression.

Advanced cardiac life support
By the time effective life support has been established, more help should have arrived and advanced cardiac life support can begin. This consists of ECG monitoring, endotracheal intubation and setting up an intravenous infusion in a large peripheral vein or a central vein. Immediate therapy includes defibrillation, oxygen and cardioactive drugs. It is not possible to recommend an exact sequence of management because it will depend on the arrival of skilled personnel and equipment and the nature of the cardiac arrest. However, as soon as possible the ECG should be connected. At first this is easily achieved by monitoring the ECG through the paddles of a defibrillator. Later, electrodes, leads and specific ECG scopes can be set up. If the ECG shows ventricular fibrillation, no time should be lost before defibrillating the patient. If initial defibrillation attempts are unsuccessful, time can then be spent intubating the patient and setting up an intravenous infusion whilst the circulation is supported by external chest compression. If there is any difficulty in intubating the patient, ventilation should be continued by means of an airway, a ventilating bag and oxygen.

There are three main mechanisms of sudden unexpected cardiac arrest:
● Ventricular fibrillation
● Asystole
● Electromechanical dissociation

Three quarters of arrests are due to ventricular fibrillation. Only a very small proportion are due to electromechanical dissociation, and the remainder are due to asystole. In patients dying of other causes, such as terminal pneumonia, the heart rhythm is described as being agonal. This is characterized by an inexorable slowing and widening of the QRS complexes associated with falling blood pressure and cardiac output. This type of arrhythmia is very difficult to reverse and usually no attempt should be made because it is the result rather than the cause of death.

Arrests are treated in the following ways:
● *Ventricular fibrillation* is readily treated with defibrillation, anti-arrhythmic drugs and cardiac stimulants.
● *Asystole* is more difficult to treat but the heart may respond to atropine or adrenaline. If there is any

Sudden death

Each year in the UK there are approximately 100 000 unexpected deaths occurring within 24 h of the development of cardiac symptoms. About half of these deaths are almost instantaneous. There are several causes:
- Cardiac arrhythmias (e.g. ventricular fibrillation)
- Sudden pump failure (e.g. acute myocardial infarction)
- Acute circulatory obstruction (e.g. pulmonary embolism)
- Cardiovascular rupture (e.g. dissecting aneurysm of the aorta, myocardial rupture)
- Vasomotor collapse (e.g. pulmonary hypertension)

Most deaths are due to ventricular fibrillation, and a small proportion are due to severe bradyarrhythmias. Although coronary disease is frequent in these victims, acute coronary occlusion and myocardial infarction is relatively uncommon (~40%).

sign of electrocardiographic activity, emergency pacing should be used.
- *Electromechanical dissociation* is often due to a severe mechanical problem such as pericardial tamponade or massive pulmonary embolism.

These conditions should be treated urgently. Toxic levels of cardiodepressant drugs, such as beta blockers, may also cause electromechanical dissociation. If there is an antidote, such as adrenaline, it should be administered.

Fig. 11.28 shows the treatments recommended by the UK Resuscitation Council.

Defibrillation
This technique is used for the conversion of ventricular fibrillation to sinus rhythm. Electrical energy is discharged through two paddles placed on the chest wall. Either 200 J (or Watt-seconds) or 400 J charges are used for defibrillation.
    The paddles are placed in one of two positions:
- One paddle is placed to the right of the upper sternum and the other over the cardiac apex.
- One paddle is placed under the tip of the left scapula and the other is placed over the anterior wall of the left chest.

Electrode jelly or electrolyte gel pads should be used to ensure good contact between the electrode paddles and the skin. Jelly smeared carelessly across the chest may cause short circuits and arcing of the charge. All personnel should stand clear of the patient.

Fig. 11.28 Schema for management of the three common forms of cardiac arrest: ventricular fibrillation, ventricular asystole and electromechanical dissociation. (Based on recommendations of the UK Resuscitation Council.)

When the defibrillator is discharged, a high voltage field envelops the heart. This depolarizes the whole heart and allows an organized heart rhythm to emerge.

DC-cardioversion

Tachyarrhythmias that do not respond to medical treatment or that are associated with severe haemodynamic disturbance may be converted to sinus rhythm by the use of a transthoracic electric shock. A short-acting general anaesthetic is used. Muscle relaxants are not usually given. When the arrhythmia has definite QRS complexes, the delivery of the shock should be timed to occur with the downstroke of the QRS complex (synchronization) (Fig. 11.29). This is the major difference between defibrillation and cardioversion, since a non-synchronized shock is used to defibrillate.

Indications for cardioversion are atrial fibrillation and atrial flutter of recent onset (less than 1 year), and ventricular tachycardia. Very occasionally, sustained junctional tachycardias may have to be DC-cardioverted to sinus rhythm.

If the arrhythmia, especially atrial fibrillation, has been present for more than a few days, it is wise to anticoagulate the patient for several weeks before elective cardioversion. This reduces the risk of embolization.

Digoxin toxicity may lead to ventricular arrhythmias or asystole following cardioversion. Therapeutic digitalization does not increase the risks of cardioversion, but it is conventional to omit digoxin several days prior to elective cardioversion in order to be sure that toxicity is not present.

Repeated cardioversion leads to an enzyme rise because of damage to the muscles of the chest wall. Specific cardiac enzymes may increase slightly because of myocardial damage produced by the shock.

Temporary pacing

Symptomatic bradycardias unresponsive to atropine are treated with a cardiac pacemaker. A temporary pacemaker (external unit) may be connected to the myocardium by a thin (French gauge 5 or 6), bipolar pacing electrode wire inserted via a subclavian or internal jugular vein and manipulated into the right ventricular apex using cardiac fluoroscopy. The energy needed for successful pacing (the pacing threshold) is assessed by reducing the energy until the pacemaker fails to stimulate the tissue (loss of capture). The output energy is then set at three times its threshold value to prevent inadvertent loss of capture. If the threshold increases above 5 V, the pacemaker wire should be resited. A temporary pacemaker unit is almost always set to work 'on demand', i.e. to fire only when a spontaneous beat has not occurred. The rate of temporary pacing is usually 60–80 beats per minute.

Permanent pacing

Permanent pacemakers are fully implanted in the body and connected to the heart by one or two electrode leads. The pacemaker is powered by solid state lithium batteries which usually last from 5–10 years. Modern pacemakers are often 'programmable'. This means that their operating characteristics (e.g. the pacing rate) can be changed by a programmer which transmits specific electromagnetic signals through the skin. The pacemaker leads are passed transvenously to the right heart chambers. Most pacemakers are designed to pace and sense the ventricles. Occasionally, e.g. in symptomatic sinus bradycardia, an atrial pacemaker may be implanted. Pacemakers that are connected to both the right atrium and ventricle ('dual chamber' pacemaker) are now increasingly being used in order to simulate the natural pacemaker and activation sequence of the heart. Another form of 'physiological' pacemaker is the 'rate responsive' system which, by measuring activity, respiration, biochemical or electrical indicators, changes its rate of pacing so that it is appropriate to the level of exertion.

Permanent pacemakers are inserted under local anaesthetic using fluoroscopy to guide the insertion of the electrode leads. Antibiotics may be prescribed prophylactically.

Complications are few but include:

- *Infection.* When a pacemaker system is infected, antibiotic treatment is not sufficient and the pacemaker must usually be removed before antibiotics will subdue the infection. Another pacemaker is fitted later.

Tachycardia   Sinus rhythm

↑
Synchronized DC shock

Fig. 11.29 DC cardioversion of a supraventricular tachycardia to sinus rhythm. The direct current shock is delivered synchronously with the QRS complex.

- *Erosion*. The pacemaker may erode through the skin. This is usually due to a low grade infection. Mechanical factors may also be responsible.
- *Lead displacement*. In most cases the pacing lead is securely wedged into the trabeculae of the right ventricle. It rarely displaces but when it does it may lead to sudden loss of pacing and a recurrence of pre-pacing symptoms.
- *Pacemaker malfunction*. This is now a very uncommon complication but requires the replacement of the pacemaker.

Pericardiocentesis

A pericardial effusion is an accumulation of fluid between the parietal and visceral layers of pericardium. Fluid is removed to relieve symptoms due to haemodynamic embarrassment or for diagnostic purposes. Pericardial aspiration or pericardiocentesis is performed by inserting a needle into the pericardial space, usually via a subxiphisternal route under ultrasound imaging. If a large volume of fluid is to be removed, a wide bore needle and cannula are inserted. The needle may be removed and the cannula left in situ to drain the fluid. Fluid that is removed is sent for chemical analysis, microscopy, including cytology, and culture. If a reaccumulation of pericardial fluid is anticipated, the cannula may be left in place for several days or an operation can be performed to cut a window in the parietal pericardium (fenestration) or to remove a large section of the pericardium.

Right heart bedside catheterization

Bedside catheterization of the pulmonary artery with a Swan–Ganz catheter is performed in patients with:

- Cardiac failure
- Cardiogenic shock
- Doubtful fluid status

The catheter is used to measure cardiac output, pulmonary artery pressure, right atrial pressure and the pulmonary artery wedge pressure (an indirect measurement of left atrial pressure). The measurement of these pressures and the cardiac output allows appropriate therapy to be prescribed and the effects of that therapy to be monitored. The catheter also provides a route for the delivery of drugs to the central circulation (see Fig. 13.14, p. 634).

Intra-aortic balloon pumping

This is a technique used to assist temporarily the failing left ventricle. A catheter with a long sausage-shaped balloon at its tip is introduced percutaneously into the femoral artery and manipulated under x-ray control so that the balloon lies in the descending aorta just below the aortic arch. The balloon is rhythmically deflated and inflated with carbon dioxide gas. Using the ECG or intra-aortic pressure changes, the inflation is timed to occur during ventricular diastole to increase diastolic aortic pressure and consequently to improve coronary and cerebral blood flow. During systole the balloon is deflated, resulting in a reduction in the resistance to left ventricular emptying.

Balloon pumping is used:

- To improve cardiac output when there is a transient or reversible depression of left ventricular function, e.g. in a patient with severe mitral valve regurgitation who is awaiting surgical replacement of the mitral valve or in a patient with a ventricular septal defect due to septal infarction
- To treat unstable angina pectoris by improving coronary flow and decreasing myocardial oxygen consumption by reducing the 'afterload'. This technique may be successful, even when medical therapy has failed. It is followed by early arteriography and appropriate definitive therapy such as surgery or coronary angioplasty.

Balloon pumping should not be used when there is no remediable cause of cardiac dysfunction. It is also unsuitable in patients with aortic valve regurgitation or dissection of the aorta.

Complications of balloon pumping occur in about 20% of cases and include aortic dissection, leg ischaemia, emboli from the balloon, and balloon rupture. Embolic complications are reduced by anticoagulation with heparin.

Cardiac arrhythmias

An abnormality of the cardiac rhythm is called a cardiac arrhythmia. Such a disturbance of rhythm may cause sudden death, syncope, dizziness, palpitations or no symptoms at all. There are two main types of arrhythmia:

- *Bradycardia*, where the heart rate is slow (<60 beats per minute). The slower the heart rate the more likely the arrhythmia will be symptomatic.
- *Tachycardia*, where the heart rate is fast (>100 beats per minute). Tachycardias are more symptomatic when the arrhythmia is fast and sustained. Tachycardias are subdivided into *supraventricular tachycardias*, which arise from the atrium or the atrioventricular junction, and *ventricular tachycardias*, which arise from the ventricles.

Ventricular tachyarrhythmias tend to be more symptomatic than supraventricular tachycardias. Some arrhythmias occur in patients with apparently normal hearts, and in others arrhythmias reflect underlying cardiac abnormalities. When myocardial function is poor, arrhythmias tend to be more symptomatic and are potentially life threatening.

Mechanisms of arrhythmia production

There are four main mechanisms of tachycardia production:
- Two are abnormalities of automaticity, which might theoretically arise from a single disordered cell.
- Two are abnormalities of conduction, which require abnormal interaction between cells.

Fig. 11.30 shows the mechanisms of arrhythmias.

Accelerated automaticity

The normal mechanism of cardiac rhythmicity is slow depolarization of the transmembrane voltage during diastole until the threshold potential is reached and the pacemaker fires. This mechanism may be accelerated by increasing the rate of diastolic depolarization or changing the threshold potential. Such changes are thought to produce sinus tachycardia and accelerated AV nodal rhythms.

Triggered automaticity

Myocardial damage can result in oscillations of the end of the action potential. These oscillations may reach threshold potential and produce an arrhythmia. The abnormal oscillations can be exaggerated by pacing and by catecholamines and these stimuli can be used to trigger this abnormal form of automaticity. Some of the arrhythmias produced by digoxin toxicity are due to triggered automaticity.

Reflection

If adjacent cells repolarize at different rates, the cells that repolarize more quickly may be restimulated by those cells that have not yet repolarized. The ventricular tachyarrhythmias associated with the long QT syndrome may result from this mechanism.

Re-entry (or circus movement)

A wave of depolarization may be forced to travel in one direction around a ring of cardiac tissue. If the time to conduct around the ring is longer than the recovery of any tissue within the ring, circus movement will result, producing a tachycardia. The majority of regular paroxysmal tachycardias are thought to be produced by this mechanism.

SINUS RHYTHMS

The normal cardiac pacemaker is the sinus node and, like most cardiac tissue, it depolarizes spontaneously (see Fig. 11.3). Its rate of discharge is controlled by the autonomic nervous system. Normally the parasympathetic system predominates, resulting in slowing of the spontaneous discharge rate from approximately 100 to 70 beats per minute. A reduction of parasympathetic tone or an increase in sym-

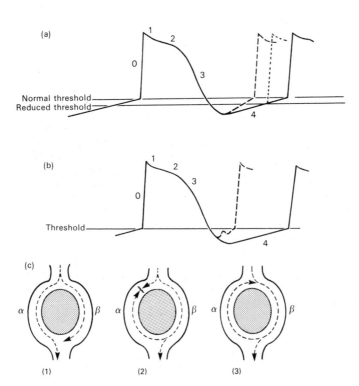

Fig. 11.30 Mechanisms of arrhythmogenesis. (a) and (b) show action potentials (i.e. the potential difference between intra- and extracellular fluid) of ventricular myocardium after stimulation. (a) shows increased automaticity due to a reduced threshold potential or an increased slope of phase 4 depolarization (see p. 464). (b) shows abnormal automaticity due to 'after' depolarizations reaching threshold potential. (c) shows the mechanism of circus movement or re-entry. In panel (1) the impulse passes down both limbs of the potential tachycardia circuit. In panel (2) the impulse is blocked in the alpha pathway but proceeds slowly down the beta pathway and returns along the alpha pathway. In panel (3) the impulse travels so slowly along the beta pathway that when it returns along the alpha pathway to its starting point it is able to travel again down the beta pathway, producing a circus movement tachycardia.

pathetic stimulation leads to tachycardia; conversely, increased parasympathetic tone and decreased sympathetic stimulation produces bradycardia. The sinus rate in women is slightly faster than in men. Normal sinus rhythm is characterized by P waves which are upright in leads I and II of the ECG (Fig. 11.16), but are inverted in the cavity leads (Fig. 11.31).

Sinus arrhythmia

Fluctuations of autonomic tone result in phasic changes of the sinus discharge rate. Thus, during inspiration parasympathetic tone falls and the heart rate quickens, and on expiration the heart rate falls. This variation is normal, particularly in children and young adults.

Sinus bradycardia

A sinus rate of less than 60 beats per minute during the day or less than 50 beats per minute at night is known as sinus bradycardia. It is usually asymptomatic unless the rate is very slow. It is normal in athletes and in elderly patients. Causes include:
- Hypothermia, hypothyroidism, cholestatic jaundice and raised intracranial pressure
- Drug therapy with beta blockers, digitalis and other anti-arrhythmic drugs
- Acute ischaemia and infarction of the sinus node
- Chronic degenerative changes such as fibrosis of the atrium and sinus node

TREATMENT

Treatment of acute symptomatic sinus bradycardia is atropine 600 µg i.v. If the symptomatic arrhythmia persists, a cardiac pacemaker is required.

Sinus tachycardia

Sinus rate acceleration to more than 100 beats per minute is known as sinus tachycardia. Causes include:
- Fever
- Exercise
- Emotion
- Pregnancy
- Anaemia
- Cardiac failure with compensatory sinus tachycardia
- Thyrotoxicosis
- Catecholamine excess
- Primary sinus tachycardia (rare)

TREATMENT

This involves correction of the condition causing the tachycardia. If necessary, beta-blockers may be used to slow the sinus rate, but not in heart failure.

PATHOLOGICAL BRADYCARDIAS

There are two main forms of severe bradycardia: sinus node disease and atrioventricular block.

Sinus node disease (sick sinus syndrome)

Sinus node disease is caused by ischaemia, infarction or degenerative disease of the sinus node. It is characterized by long intervals between consecutive P waves (>2 s) on the ECG (see Fig. 11.31). These sinus pauses may be an exact multiple of the basic sinus interval (sinoatrial exit block) or not (sinus arrest). Both conditions have a similar prognosis.

Fig. 11.31 (a) An ECG showing normal sinus rhythm. (b) An ECG from a patient with sick sinus syndrome. This shows sinus arrest (only occasional sinus P waves) and junctional escape beats (J). P waves are inverted in these cavity leads.

Sinus pauses and sinus bradycardia may allow cardiac tachyarrhythmias to emerge. A combination of fast and slow supraventricular rhythms is known as the tachycardia–bradycardia (tachy-brady) syndrome.

TREATMENT

Treatment of chronic symptomatic sick sinus syndrome requires permanent pacing, with additional anti-arrhythmic drugs to manage any tachycardia element. Thromboembolism is common in sick sinus syndrome and patients should be anticoagulated unless there is a contraindication.

Atrioventricular (AV) block

There are three forms: first degree block, second degree (partial) block and third degree (complete) block.

First degree AV block
This is simple prolongation of the PR interval to more than 0.22 s. Every atrial depolarization is followed by conduction to the ventricles but with delay (Fig. 11.32).

Fig. 11.32 An ECG showing first degree atrioventricular block with a prolonged PR interval. In this trace ST depression is also present.

Second degree (partial) AV block
This occurs when some P waves conduct and others do not. There are several forms of second degree AV block (Fig. 11.33):
- Mobitz I block (Wenckebach phenomenon) is progressive PR interval prolongation until a P wave fails to conduct. The PR interval before the blocked P wave is much longer than the PR interval after the blocked P wave.
- Mobitz II block occurs when a dropped QRS complex is not preceded by progressive PR interval prolongation.

(a)

(b)

(c)

Fig. 11.33 Three varieties of second degree atrioventricular (AV) block. (a) Wenckebach (Mobitz type I) AV block. The PR interval gradually prolongs until the P wave does not conduct to the ventricles (arrows). (b) Mobitz type II AV block. The P waves which do not conduct to the ventricles (arrows) are not preceded by gradual PR interval prolongation. (c) Two P waves to each QRS complex. The PR interval prior to the dropped P wave is always the same. It is not possible to define this type of AV block as type I or type II Mobitz block and it is, therefore, a third variety of second degree AV block.

- *2 : 1 or 3 : 1 block* occurs when every second or third P wave conducts to the ventricles. This form of second degree block is neither Mobitz I nor II. 4 : 1 block, 5 : 1 block, etc. can also occur.

Traditionally, Wenckebach block is said to be more benign than other forms of second degree block, but recent evidence suggests that all forms of second degree AV block have a similar prognosis. Patients with this conduction problem are usually asymptomatic. A close watch should be kept on them although no treatment is necessary unless more serious or symptomatic heart block develops.

Third degree (complete) AV block
This occurs when no P waves conduct to the ventricles (Fig. 11.34). In this situation life is maintained by a spontaneous escape rhythm that has either broad (>0.1 s) or narrow (≤0.1 s) QRS complexes.

Narrow complex (Fig. 11.34a). This is due to disease in the AV node or the proximal His bundle. The escape rhythm occurs with an adequate rate (50–60 beats per minute) and is relatively reliable. It occurs in association with:
- Congenital heart disease (such as transposition of the great arteries)
- An isolated congenital problem (congenital heart block)
- Inferior wall myocardial infarction
- Diphtheria
- Rheumatic fever
- Toxic concentrations of drugs such as digitalis, verapamil or beta-blockers

Treatment is often unnecessary except for the eradication of toxic causes. Recent onset narrow complex AV block due to acute myocardial infarction may respond to intravenous atropine but a temporary pacemaker may be necessary. Chronic narrow com-

(a)

(b)

(c)

Fig. 11.34 Three examples of complete heart block. (a) Congenital complete heart block. The QRS complex is narrow (0.08 s) and the QRS rate is relatively rapid (52 beats per minute). (b) Acquired complete heart block. The QRS complex is broad (0.13 s) and the QRS rate is relatively slow (38 beats per minute). (c) Drug-induced complete heart block in a patient with atrial fibrillation rather than sinus rhythm (note the undulating baseline but the regular and slow ventricular rate).

plex AV block requires permanent pacing if it is symptomatic or associated with heart disease.

Occasionally, permanent pacing is advocated for asymptomatic, isolated, congenital AV block.

Broad complex (Fig. 11.34b). This occurs because of disease in the Purkinje system. The escape pacemaker arises from the distal Purkinje network or the ventricular myocardium. The resulting rhythm is slow (15–40 beats per minute) and relatively unreliable. Dizziness and blackouts (Stokes–Adams attacks) often occur. In the elderly it is usually caused by degenerative fibrosis and calcification of the distal conduction system (Lenegre's disease) or the more proximal conduction system (Lev's disease). In younger patients broad complex AV block may be caused by ischaemic heart disease.

A permanent pacemaker should always be inserted, as the mortality from the condition, even when asymptomatic, is considerably reduced by pacing.

Intraventricular conduction disturbances

The intraventricular conduction system consists of the His bundle, the right and left bundle branches and the antero-superior and postero-inferior divisions of the left bundle branch. Various conduction disturbances can occur:

- *His bundle delay* may produce a long PR interval but it is often too small a delay to be noticed on the surface ECG.
- *Blocked His bundle conduction* produces AV block.
- *Bundle branch conduction delay* produces trivial widening of the QRS complex (up to 0.11 s). This is known as incomplete bundle branch block.
- *Complete block of a bundle branch* is associated with a wider QRS complex (0.12 s or more). The shape of the QRS depends on whether the right or the left bundle is blocked. *Right bundle branch block* (an example is shown in Fig. 11.56, p. 509) produces late activation of the right ventricle. This is seen as deep S waves in leads I and V_6 and as a tall late R wave in lead V_1 (see Fig. 11.74) (late activation moving towards right- and away from left-sided leads). *Left bundle branch block* (Fig. 11.35) produces the opposite, i.e. a deep S wave in lead V_1 and a tall late R wave in leads I and V_6. Because left bundle branch conduction is normally responsible for the initial ventricular activation, left bundle branch block also produces abnormal Q waves.

  Delay or block in the divisions of the left bundle branch produces a swing in the direction of depolarization (electrical axis) of the heart. When the antero-superior division is blocked, the left ventricle is activated from inferior to superior. This produces a superior (leftwards) movement of the axis. Delay or block in the postero-inferior division swings the QRS axis inferiorly.
- *Bifascicular block* (see Fig. 11.56) is a combination of

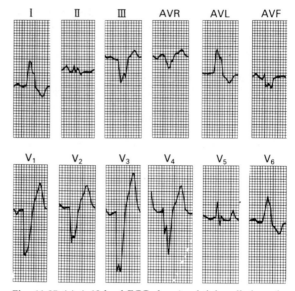

Fig. 11.35 (a) A 12-lead ECG showing left bundle branch block. The QRS duration is greater than 0.12 s. Note the broad notched R waves with ST depression in leads I, AVL and V_6 and the broad QS waves in V_1–V_3.

a block of any two of the following: the right bundle branch, the left antero-superior division and the left postero-inferior division. Block of the remaining fascicle will result in complete AV block.

CLINICAL FEATURES

Intraventricular conduction disturbances other than complete block of the His bundle are usually asymptomatic. Sometimes left bundle branch block actually seems to provoke chest pain.

Right bundle branch block causes wide but physiological splitting of the second heart sound. Left bundle branch block may cause reverse splitting of the second sound. Patients with intraventricular conduction disturbances may complain of syncope. This is due to intermittent complete heart block or to ventricular tachyarrhythmias. ECG monitoring and electrophysiological study is needed to determine the cause of syncope in these patients.

CAUSES

Right bundle branch block (Table 11.13) occurs as an isolated congenital anomaly or is associated with right ventricular volume overload. Left bundle branch block (Table 11.14) is almost always caused by disease of the left ventricle. All forms of intraventricular conduction disturbance may be caused by ischaemic heart disease and cardiomyopathy.

Conduction system fibrosis and calcification (Lenegre's disease and Lev's disease, see above) are progressive conditions which may present with bun-

Table 11.13 Causes of right bundle branch block. It is also a normal finding in 1% of young adults and 5% of elderly adults.

Congenital heart disease
Atrial septal defect
Fallot's tetralogy
Pulmonary stenosis
Ventricular septal defect
Pulmonary disease
Cor pulmonale
Recurrent pulmonary embolism
Acute pulmonary embolism (transient)
Myocardial disease
Acute myocardial infarction
Cardiomyopathy
Conduction system fibrosis
Drugs and electrolytes
Hyperkalaemia
Class Ia drugs (see p. 491)
Right ventriculotomy

Table 11.14 Causes of left bundle branch block.

Left ventricular outflow obstruction
Aortic stenosis
Hypertension
Coronary artery disease
Acute myocardial infarction
Severe coronary disease (two- to three-vessel disease)
Cardiomyopathy
Conduction system fibrosis

dle branch block or bifascicular block and eventually lead to complete heart block, when a pacemaker will be required.

PATHOLOGICAL TACHYCARDIAS

Atrial tachyarrhythmias

Ectopic beats, tachycardia, flutter and fibrillation may all arise from the atrial myocardium. They share common aetiologies, which are listed in Table 11.15.

Atrial ectopic beats
These often cause no symptoms although they may be sensed as an irregularity or heaviness of the heart beat. On the ECG they appear as early and abnormal P waves, and are usually, but not always, followed by normal QRS complexes (see Fig. 11.37a).

Treatment is not normally required unless the ectopic beats provoke more significant arrhythmias, when beta-blockade is usually effective.

Table 11.15 Causes of atrial arrhythmias.

Ischaemic heart disease
Rheumatic heart disease
Thyrotoxicosis
Cardiomyopathy
Lone atrial fibrillation (i.e. no cause discovered)
Wolff–Parkinson–White syndrome
Pneumonia
Atrial septal defect
Carcinoma of the bronchus
Pericarditis
Pulmonary embolus
Acute and chronic alcohol abuse

Atrial tachycardia
This is an uncommon arrhythmia. (Previously, arrhythmias arising from the AV junction were wrongly called 'atrial tachycardias'.) There are three varieties of true atrial tachycardia:
- Paroxysmal tachycardia
- Chronic tachycardia
- Atrial tachycardia with block

All are usually associated with heart disease, but chronic atrial tachycardia may occur in young children with no obvious heart disease. Atrial tachycardia with block is often a result of digitalis poisoning.

Fig. 11.36 demonstrates an atrial tachycardia at an atrial rate of 150 beats per minute. The P waves are abnormally shaped and occur in front of the QRS complexes. Carotid sinus massage may increase AV block during tachycardia but does not usually terminate the arrhythmia. Treatment with class Ia, Ic or III drugs (see p. 493) is usually successful.

Fig. 11.36 Atrial tachycardia with second degree atrioventricular block. Note the fast atrial (P wave) rate of 150 per minute and the slower ventricular (R wave) rate of 75 per minute. This arrhythmia is most commonly due to digoxin toxicity.

Atrial flutter

This is a rhythm disturbance that is almost always associated with organic heart disease. The atrial rate varies between 280 and 350 beats per minute but is usually around 300 beats per minute.

Symptoms are largely related to the degree of AV block. Most often, every second flutter beat conducts, giving a ventricular rate of 150 beats per minute. Occasionally, every beat conducts, producing a heart rate of 300 beats per minute. More often, especially when patients are receiving treatment, AV conduction block reduces the heart rate to approximately 75 beats per minute.

The ECG shows regular sawtooth-like atrial flutter waves (F waves) between QRST complexes (Fig. 11.37b and c). If they are not clearly visible, AV conduction may be transiently impaired by carotid sinus massage or by the administration of AV nodal blocking drugs such as verapamil.

Treatment of an acute paroxysm is electrical cardioversion. Prophylaxis is achieved with class Ia, Ic or III drugs (see p. 491). If the arrhythmia is chronic, AV nodal blocking drugs (classes II or IV, or digitalis) are used.

Atrial fibrillation

This is a common arrhythmia, occurring in between 5 and 10% of patients over 65 years of age. It also occurs, particularly in a paroxysmal form, in younger patients. It is caused by a raised atrial pressure, increased atrial muscle mass, atrial fibrosis, or inflammation and infiltration of the atrium.

Atrial fibrillation is continuous, rapid (400 or more beats per minute) activation of the atria. The

Fig. 11.37 ECGs of a variety of atrial arrhythmias. (a) Atrial premature beats (arrows). The premature P wave is different to the sinus P wave and conducts to the ventricle with a slightly prolonged PR interval. (b) Atrial flutter. The flutter waves are marked with an F. In this case the flutter frequency is 270 per minute. Every second flutter wave is transmitted to the ventricles, and the ventricular rate is therefore 135 per minute. (c) Atrial flutter at a frequency of 305 per minute. The ventricular rate is approximately 38 per minute. Therefore, only one in eight flutter waves is transmitted to the ventricles. (d) Irregular ventricular response. This is typical of rapidly conducted atrial fibrillation. (e) Moderate conduction of atrial fibrillation. The underlying baseline undulations can now be appreciated. (f) So-called 'slow' atrial fibrillation. The ventricular response rate is slow and the underlying atrial fibrillation is seen as minor fluctuations of the baseline.

atria respond electrically at this rate but there is practically no mechanical action and only a proportion of the impulses are conducted.

The aetiology (see Table 11.15) includes most cardiac disorders, but in some patients no cause can be found — 'lone atrial fibrillation'. Thyrotoxicosis may provoke atrial fibrillation, sometimes as virtually the only feature of the disease (apathetic hyperthyroidism). Thyroid function tests are mandatory in any patient with unaccounted atrial fibrillation. Particularly when caused by rheumatic mitral stenosis, the onset of atrial fibrillation results in considerable worsening of cardiac failure.

Clinically the patient has a totally irregular pulse, as opposed to a basically regular pulse with an occasional irregularity (e.g. extra-systoles) or recurring irregular patterns (e.g. Wenckebach block). The irregular nature of the pulse in atrial fibrillation is maintained during exercise.

The ECG shows fine oscillations of the baseline (so-called fibrillation or 'f' waves) and no clear P waves. The QRS rhythm is rapid and irregular. Untreated, the ventricular rate is usually 120–180 beats per minute, but it slows with treatment (Fig. 11.37d, e and f).

When atrial fibrillation is due to an acute precipitating event such as alcohol toxicity, chest infection or thyrotoxicosis, the provoking cause should be treated before attempting to convert the arrhythmia. Conversion to sinus rhythm can then be achieved by electrical DC-cardioversion (see p. 476) in about 80% of patients.

Intravenous infusion of some anti-arrhythmic drugs, e.g. classes Ia, Ib and III drugs, is often used to restore sinus rhythm. This is known as medical cardioversion. Electrical cardioversion is often also necessary. Recurrent paroxysms may be prevented by oral medication with class Ia, Ic or III drugs.

If the arrhythmia is chronic and cannot be converted to sinus rhythm, AV nodal blocking drugs should be used to control the ventricular response rate. The most usual drug for this purpose is digoxin.

Anticoagulation is advised for patients with established (chronic) atrial fibrillation or for recurrent paroxysms of atrial fibrillation if the cause is mitral valve disease, alcoholic heart disease (unless the patient is still drinking), thyrotoxicosis or sick sinus syndrome, because of the risk of atrial thrombosis and embolism.

Junctional tachycardia

Almost all junctional tachycardia is paroxysmal in nature. There is usually no associated structural heart disease but there may be demonstrable electrophysiological or electrocardiographic abnormalities such as the Wolff–Parkinson–White syndrome (Fig. 11.38) (see p. 487) or the Lown–Ganong–Levine syndrome (in which there is an additional anomalous

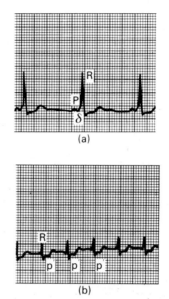

Fig. 11.38 An ECG showing Wolff–Parkinson–White syndrome. (a) A trace taken during sinus rhythm demonstrating a short PR interval (0.09 s) and broad QRS complex (0.12 s). (b) A trace demonstrating the paroxysmal junctional tachycardia associated with this syndrome. Notice the tachycardia p' waves which closely follow each QRS complex. δ = delta wave.

connection between the atrium and the bundle of His).

There are two main varieties of junctional tachycardia:
- Intra-AV nodal tachycardia
- Atrioventricular tachycardia

Both tachycardias are re-entry in type. In the intra-AV nodal re-entry tachycardia the entire tachycardia circuit is confined to the AV node and its surrounding myocardium. In atrioventricular re-entry tachycardia there is a large circuit comprising the AV node, the His bundle, the ventricle, an abnormal connection and the atrium. The abnormal connection linking the ventricle to the atrium completes the circuit necessary to sustain the tachycardia.

Typically, the tachycardia strikes suddenly without obvious provocation, but exertion, coffee, tea and alcohol may aggravate or induce the arrhythmia. The rhythm is rapid (140–280 beats per minute) and regular. An attack may stop spontaneously or may continue indefinitely until medical intervention. The predominant symptom is palpitations, but chest pain, dyspnoea and polyuria may develop. The polyuria occurs because tachycardia leads to an elevated atrial pressure and the release of atrial natriuretic peptide and other hormones.

The rhythm is recognized by normal QRS complexes at a rate of 140–280 beats per minute.

Sometimes the QRS complexes will show typical bundle branch block (aberration). The P waves may occur simultaneously with the QRS complex (AV nodal tachycardia) or just after the QRS in the ST segment or the T wave (atrioventricular tachycardia).

TREATMENT

An acute paroxysm of tachycardia is easy to treat.

Vagotonic manoeuvres

Most supraventricular arrhythmias require conduction through the AV node for their continuation or their expression at ventricular level. An intense efferent vagal discharge increases AV nodal conduction time and the AV nodal recovery time. Thus atrial arrhythmias may be revealed by vagotonic stimulation, which blocks the transmission of these arrhythmias to the ventricles, and junctional tachycardias that involve continuous circulation (circus movement or re-entry) involving the AV node may be terminated by these manoeuvres.

Carotid sinus massage, ocular pressure, immersion of the face in water (diving reflex) and the Valsalva manoeuvre may be used to stimulate the vagal efferent discharge. Of these techniques the Valsalva manoeuvre is the best. It should be performed when the patient is resting in the supine position (thus avoiding elevated background sympathetic tone). Several seconds after the release of strain, the resulting intense vagal effect may terminate a junctional re-entry tachycardia or may produce sufficient AV block to reveal an underlying atrial tachyarrhythmia.

Carotid sinus massage

Carotid sinus massage is performed for three reasons:
- To break supraventricular tachycardia by blocking AV nodal conduction
- To reveal on the ECG the P wave pattern of an atrial arrhythmia by reducing the frequency of AV nodal conduction during the tachycardia so that the QRS complexes do not mask the atrial activity
- To test for carotid sinus hypersensitivity, which is a severe fall in blood pressure or heart rate in response to carotid sinus stimulation

Carotid sinus massage is performed by locating the carotid pulse, ensuring that no bruit is present, and rubbing the carotid with a circular motion for 5–10 s.

Each carotid should be tried in turn. In general, right carotid pressure tends to slow the sinus rate and left carotid pressure tends to impair AV nodal conduction.

Drug treatment

If physical manoeuvres are not successful, verapamil 10 mg i.v. over 5–10 min is given. Within a few minutes of such treatment, 90% of tachycardias will terminate (Fig. 11.39). It is important not to give verapamil if the patient has already been given intravenous or oral beta-blockade. In such a case an additional dose of beta-blocker should be considered.

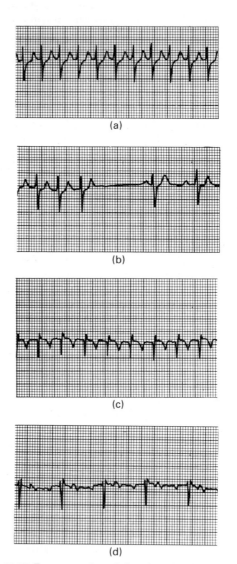

(a)

(b)

(c)

(d)

Fig. 11.39 Two examples of the slowing of tachycardia following the administration of anti-arrhythmic drugs. (a) A supraventricular tachycardia (rate = 205 beats per minute) before treatment with verapamil. (b) The result 60 s later. The tachycardia slows to 130 beats per minute before terminating abruptly and revealing sinus rhythm. (c) Atrial tachycardia at a rate of 170 beats per minute. It is difficult to discern the atrial tachycardia waves. Verapamil is administered and the result is shown in (d). Now the atrial tachycardia is easily seen. The proportion of atrial tachycardia beats transmitted to the ventricles has been reduced following the administration of verapamil.

Other treatments

Rarely, medical therapy fails to terminate a tachycardia and rapid atrial pacing (directly or via the oesophagus) or DC-cardioversion may be considered.

Prophylaxis

To prevent recurrences, drugs may be used to impair AV nodal conduction (classes II and IV and digoxin), impair abnormal connection conduction (classes Ia and III) or suppress the ectopic beats which initiate the arrhythmia (classes I, II and III) (see p. 491).

Wolff–Parkinson–White (WPW) syndrome

This is a congenital condition caused by an abnormal myocardial connection between atrium and ventricle (bundle of Kent). During sinus rhythm the electrical impulse can conduct quickly over this abnormal connection to depolarize the ventricles abnormally. This results in the typical ECG pattern of WPW syndrome—a short PR interval and a wide QRS complex that begins as a slurred part known as the delta wave (see Fig. 11.38). About half of those with WPW pattern on the ECG have tachycardias (see Fig. 11.38b). The tachycardias are of two sorts:

- *Atrioventricular re-entry.* This is a circus movement tachycardia in which a depolarization wave travels from the atrium to the ventricle, usually through the AV node, and from the ventricle to the atrium through the abnormal pathway. Intravenous verapamil will terminate most of these tachycardias.
- *Atrial fibrillation.* During atrial fibrillation the ventricles may be depolarized by impulses travelling over both the abnormal and the normal pathways. The conduction ability of the abnormal pathway is depressed by drugs that affect the atrium (e.g. disopyramide and amiodarone) but not by verapamil and digoxin which, paradoxically, may improve conduction over the abnormal pathway. Therefore, neither verapamil nor digoxin should be used to treat atrial fibrillation associated with the WPW syndrome.

Patients with frequent tachyarrhythmias should have appropriate prophylactic therapy as above, but some require surgery. The operation is designed to locate and destroy the accessory pathway.

Ventricular tachyarrhythmias

There are four main types of ventricular tachyarrhythmia:
- Ventricular premature beats
- Ventricular tachycardia
- Ventricular fibrillation
- Torsades de pointes (twisting of points)

Except for torsades de pointes, most ventricular arrhythmias are caused by coronary heart disease, hypertension or cardiomyopathy. Torsades de pointes arises when ventricular repolarization is greatly prolonged (long QT interval). The causes of QT prolongation and torsades de pointes are listed in Table 11.16. Congenital QT prolongation may be associated with syncope, and torsades de pointes may cause sudden death. Torsades de pointes may (Jervell–Lange-Nielsen syndrome) or may not (Romano–Ward syndrome) be associated with congenital deafness.

Ventricular premature beats

These may be uncomfortable, especially when frequent. The patient may complain of extra beats, missed beats or heavy beats because it may be the premature beat, the post-ectopic pause or the next sinus beat that is noticed by the patient. The pulse is irregular due to the premature beats. Some early beats may not be felt at the wrist. When a premature beat occurs regularly after every normal beat, 'pulsus bigeminus' may occur.

On the ECG (Fig. 11.40) the premature beat has a broad (>0.12 s) and bizarre QRS complex because it arises from an abnormal (ectopic) site in the ventricular myocardium. Following the premature beat there is usually a complete compensatory pause because the timing of sinus rhythm is not influenced by the premature beat.

Ventricular premature beats have been graded in order of severity. The 'Lown Classification' (Table 11.17) is designed for premature beats occurring in the setting of acute myocardial infarction, but has been wrongly applied to other situations. This is

Table 11.16 Causes of long QT interval and torsades de pointes tachycardia.

Congenital syndromes
Jervell–Lange-Nielsen (autosomal recessive)
Romano–Ward (autosomal dominant)

Electrolyte abnormalities
Hypokalaemia
Hypomagnesaemia
Hypocalcaemia

Drugs
Quinidine (and other class 1a anti-arrhythmic drugs)
Amiodarone (and other class III anti-arrhythmic drugs)
Amitriptyline (and other tricyclic antidepressants)
Chlorpromazine (and other phenothiazine drugs)

Poisons
Organophosphate insecticides

Miscellaneous
Bradycardia
Mitral valve prolapse
Acute myocardial infarction
Prolonged fasting and liquid protein diets (long term)
Central nervous system diseases

Fig. 11.40 Varieties of ventricular ectopic activity. (a) Two ventricular ectopic beats of different morphology (multi-morphological). (b) Two ventricular premature beats (VPBs) occurring one after the other (a pair or couplet of VPBs). (c) Frequently repetitive ventricular ectopic activity of a single morphology. (d) A brief run of ventricular tachycardia (non-sustained ventricular tachycardia) which follows previous ectopic activity.

Table 11.17 Grading system for ventricular premature beats (VPBs) following acute myocardial infarction, as proposed by Lown.

Grade	Description
0	No VPBs
1	Occasionally VPBs (<30/h, 1/min)
2	Frequent VPBs (≥30/h)
3	Multiform VPBs
4A	Couplets (two consecutive VPBs)
4B	Repetitive VPBs (3 or more)
5	Early VPBs (R-on-T)

particularly true of R-on-T ventricular premature beats (occurring simultaneously with the upstroke or peak of the T wave of the previous beat). Following myocardial infarction, such premature beats may induce ventricular fibrillation. This is extremely uncommon in other circumstances.

Treatment of ventricular ectopics may be advised because of symptoms or because they may provoke or threaten to provoke more serious arrhythmias. If structural heart disease is present and premature beats are frequent or run together (three or more beats at a time), treatment is offered. Drugs from classes I, II or III (see p. 491) are used. In the absence of heart disease, ventricular premature beats may be safely ignored.

Ventricular tachycardia

This is defined as three or more ventricular beats occurring at a rate of 120 beats per minute or more. Often the patient will be hypotensive and ill but some ventricular tachycardias are well tolerated.

Examination reveals a pulse rate of 120–220 beats per minute. Usually there are clinical signs of atrio-ventricular dissociation, i.e. intermittent cannon 'a' waves and variable intensity of the first heart sound.

The ECG shows a rapid ventricular rhythm with broad (often 140 msec or more), abnormal QRS complexes. Dissociated P wave activity may be seen (Fig. 11.41). Supraventricular tachycardia with bundle branch block (aberration) may resemble ventricular tachycardia on the ECG; the diagnostic features are indicated in Table 11.18. In all cases of doubt, a ventricular tachycardia should be diagnosed.

Table 11.18 ECG distinction between supraventricular tachycardia (SVT) with bundle branch block and ventricular tachycardia (VT).

VT is more likely than SVT with bundle branch block when there is:
1 A very broad QRS (>0.14 s)
2 AV dissociation
3 A bifid, upright QRS with a taller first peak in V_1
4 A deep S wave in V_6
5 A concordant (same polarity) QRS direction (V_1–V_6)

Treatment may be urgent depending on the haemodynamic situation. If the cardiac output and the blood pressure are very depressed, emergency DC-cardioversion must be considered. On the other hand, if the blood pressure and cardiac output are well maintained, intravenous therapy with class I (see p. 491) drugs is usually advised. First line drug treatment consists of lignocaine (50–100 mg i.v. over 5 min) followed by a lignocaine infusion (2–4 mg·min^{-1} i.v.). DC-cardioversion may be necessary if medical therapy is unsuccessful. The administration of multiple anti-arrhythmic drugs should be avoided.

Prophylaxis against relapse is extremely important. If possible, the likely success of therapy should be judged by Holter monitoring, exercise testing or other provocative techniques. Initial therapy is usually with a beta-blocker if exercise induces the arrhythmia, or a class I drug (see p. 491) if exercise is not responsible. If these drugs fail, a class III drug such as amiodarone or sotalol is tried. When severe left ventricular dysfunction is present, most anti-arrhythmic drugs cannot be used because they cause further depression of myocardial function (negative inotropic effect). In such cases amiodarone or mexiletine may be the agent of choice.

Ventricular fibrillation

This is very rapid and irregular ventricular activation with no mechanical effect. The patient is pulseless, becomes rapidly unconscious, and respiration ceases. The ECG shows shapeless, rapid oscillations and there is no hint of organized complexes (Fig. 11.42). It is usually provoked by a ventricular ectopic

Fig. 11.41 ECG rhythm strip. Ventricular tachycardia at a rate of 140 beats per minute following three sinus beats at a rate of 92 beats per minute.

Fig. 11.42 A rhythm strip demonstrating four beats of sinus rhythm followed by a ventricular ectopic beat which initiates ventricular fibrillation. The ST segment during sinus rhythm is elevated owing to acute myocardial infarction.

beat (especially in acute myocardial infarction), ventricular tachyardia or torsades de pointes. Ventricular fibrillation rarely reverses spontaneously. The only effective treatment is electrical defibrillation or, on rare occasions, intravenous bretylium 5–10 mg·kg^{-1} over 5 min. Basic and advanced cardiac life support is needed (see p. 474).

If the attack of ventricular fibrillation occurs during the first day or two of an acute myocardial infarction, it is probable that prophylactic therapy will be unnecessary. If the ventricular fibrillation was not related to an acute infarction, prophylaxis with anti-arrhythmic drugs, especially amiodarone or beta-blockers, and possibly an implantable defibrillator (see p. 492) may be necessary.

Torsades de pointes (see Table 11.16)
This arrhythmia is usually short in duration and spontaneously reverts to sinus rhythm. It does, however, give rise to presyncope or syncope and occasionally converts to ventricular fibrillation, and sudden death may occur. It is characterized on the ECG by rapid, irregular, sharp complexes which change from an upright to an inverted position (Fig. 11.43). Between spells of tachycardia the ECG shows a prolonged QT interval: the corrected QT (see Table 11.11) is equal to or greater than 440 ms. Fig. 11.44 shows a further example of a prolonged QT interval. The arrhythmia is treated as follows:
● Any electrolyte disturbance is corrected.
● Causative drugs are stopped.
● The heart rate is maintained with atrial or ventricular pacing.
● Intravenous isoprenaline may be effective when QT prolongation is acquired.

● Beta-blockade or left stellectomy is advised if the QT prolongation is congenital. (Isoprenaline is contraindicated for congenital long QT syndrome.)

MANAGEMENT OF ARRHYTHMIAS

Many cardiac arrhythmias are symptomatic, and some are life-threatening. Treatment is directed towards relieving symptoms and removing the threat to life. Usually arrhythmias can only be suppressed, but occasionally, for example with surgical treatment, a complete cure can be effected.

Arrhythmias such as ventricular tachycardia must be terminated, but others, such as atrial fibrillation, may not easily convert to sinus rhythm. In this case, control of the ventricular rate response is the best treatment available.

Arrhythmias can be managed by a wide variety of means (Table 11.19), ranging from simple techniques that increase vagal tone to expensive and sophisticated treatments such as surgery or implantable electronic devices. Because of the large numbers of patients who suffer from arrhythmias, anti-arrhythmic drugs remain the most important form of treatment.

Anti-arrhythmic drugs

Drugs that modify the rhythm and conduction of the heart may be used to prevent cardiac arrhythmias. It is important to realize that all such drugs may aggravate or produce arrhythmias. They may also depress ventricular contractibility and must there-

Fig. 11.43 An ECG demonstrating a supraventricular rhythm with a long QT interval giving way to atypical ventricular tachycardia (torsades de pointes). The tachycardia is short lived and is followed by a brief period of idioventricular rhythm.

Fig. 11.44 A 12-lead ECG from an 11-year-old child with a history of syncope demonstrating sinus bradycardia with a long QT interval (560 ms). The ECG is typical of the hereditary long QT syndrome.

fore be used with caution. There are more than 30 anti-arrhythmic drugs. They are classified according to their effect on the action potential (Vaughan Williams' classification; see Table 11.20 and Fig. 11.45).

Table 11.19 Management of arrhythmias.

Aims
Cure
Prevention (suppression)
Termination
Reduction of ventricular rate

Techniques available
Vagotonic methods (see p. 486)
DC cardioversion (see p. 476)
Anti-arrhythmic drugs (see p. 490)
Pacemakers and other electronic devices (see p. 492)
Surgery and other ablation methods (see p. 492)

Table 11.20 Vaughan Williams' classification of anti-arrhythmic drugs.

Class I	
Ia	Quinidine, procainamide, disopyramide
Ib	Lignocaine, mexiletine, tocainide
Ic	Flecainide
Class II	Beta-adrenergic blocking drugs
Class III	Amiodarone, sotalol, bretylium
Class IV	Verapamil, diltiazem

All class I agents inhibit the fast sodium channel and reduce maximal rate of rise of phase O

Class Ia agents:
Lengthen action
potential

Class Ib agents:
Shorten action
potential

Class Ic agents:
No effect on duration
of action potential

Class II agents
(beta-blocking agents):
Predominant action
on sinus node

Class III agents:
Widen duration
of action potential

Class IV agents
(calcium channel
blocking agents):
Predominant action
on AV node

Fig. 11.45 Vaughan Williams' classification of anti-arrhythmic drugs based on their effect on cardiac action potentials. 0 = 0 mV. The dotted curves indicate the effects of the drugs.

Class I drugs
These are membrane-depressant drugs which reduce the rate of entry of sodium into the cell. They may slow conduction, delay recovery or reduce the spontaneous discharge rate of myocardial cells.

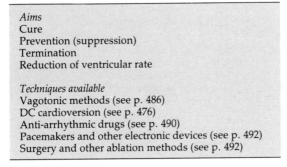

Class Ia drugs (e.g. disopyramide) lengthen the action potential, Class Ib drugs (e.g. lignocaine) shorten the action potential, and Class Ic (flecainide) do not affect the duration of the action potential.

Class II drugs

These anti-sympathetic drugs prevent the effects of catecholamines on the action potential. Most are beta-adrenergic antagonists. Cardioselective beta-blockers (beta-1) include metoprolol, atenolol and acebutolol.

Class III drugs

These prolong the action potential and do not affect sodium transport through the membrane. There are two major drugs in this class: amiodarone and sotalol. Sotalol is also a beta-blocker.

Class IV drugs

These are calcium antagonists which reduce the plateau phase of the action potential. They are particularly effective at slowing conduction in nodal tissue. Verapamil is the most important drug in this group. Nifedipine is also a calcium antagonist but has less effect on nodal tissue. Diltiazem has important anti-arrhythmic effects.

Another, clinically important classification is based on the part of the heart that is affected by the anti-arrhythmic drug (Fig. 11.46).

Important features of the major anti-arrhythmic drugs are given in Table 11.21.

Other management techniques

Although anti-arrhythmic drugs are the mainstay of tachycardia treatment, other techniques are sometimes necessary. Surgical division of the anomalous connections responsible for the WPW syndrome is now possible with virtually no surgical mortality and very little morbidity. Ventricular tachycardia can be eradicated by surgical removal of the focus of the arrhythmia, but this operation carries considerable risk and is reserved for very serious problems. It is now possible to destroy the AV node or His bundle by electrical energy delivered through a catheter electrode and discharged close to the AV conduction system. This procedure effectively prevents the conduction of atrial arrhythmias or interrupts the circuit responsible for the arrhythmias. In any case a ventricular pacemaker is then needed to prevent ventricular bradycardia. Pacemakers of another sort can also be used to interrupt repetitive paroxysms of tachycardia.

Implantable automatic cardioverter–defibrillator

Serious ventricular arrhythmias (ventricular fibrillation or rapid ventricular tachycardia with hypotension) carry a mortality within 1 year of up to 40%. Anti-arrhythmic drug therapy, particularly with amiodarone, may reduce the mortality. An important alternative therapy is the implantable, automatic cardioverter–defibrillator (IACD), which can recognize ventricular tachycardia or fibrillation and auto-

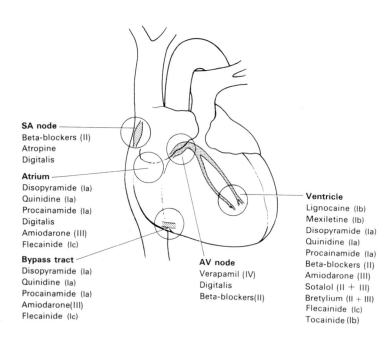

Fig. 11.46 Drugs which affect different parts of the heart. The Vaughan Williams' class is given in parentheses.

Table 11.21 Details of anti-arrhythmic drugs. (For class II drugs (beta blockers) see Table 11.36.)

	Quinidine	Disopyramide	Lignocaine	Mexiletine	Flecainide	Amiodarone	Sotalol	Verapamil	Diltiazem	Digoxin
Class:	Ia	Ia	Ib	Ib	Ic	III	III	IV	IV	N/A
Daily dose:	250–500 mg orally	100–250 mg ×3 orally	1–4 mg·min⁻¹ (50–150 mg i.v. loading dose)	400–800 mg orally loading 150–300 mg maintenance	100 mg ×2 orally	200 mg ×1–2 orally	80–160 mg ×2–3 orally	0.1 mg·kg⁻¹ i.v. 40–160 mg ×3–4 orally	60–120 mg ×3–4 orally	0.25 mg ×1 orally
Protein binding:	75%	40–90%	50–80%	70%	50%	98%	<10%	90%	80%	25%
Half-life:	6 h	5 h	1½ h	15 h	18 h	50 days +	24 h	6 h	2–8 h	36 h
Plasma therapeutic range:	2–5 µg·ml⁻¹	3–6 µg·ml⁻¹	2–6 µg·ml⁻¹	0.5–2.0 µg·ml⁻¹	0.2–0.8 µg·ml⁻¹	0.2–5.0 µg·ml⁻¹	0.3–1.5 µg·ml⁻¹	0.1–0.3 µg·ml⁻¹	0.02–0.16 µg·ml⁻¹	0.5–2.5 ng·ml⁻¹
Indications:	AF PSVT VT VPBs WPW	AF PSVT VT VPBs WPW	VPBs VT/VF associated with myocardial infarction	VPBs VT, especially after myocardial infarction	VPBs VT PSVT WPW	VT/VF WPW PSVT AF	VT WPW PSVT	PSVT	PSVT	AF/AFL PSVT
Side-effects:	Nausea Diarrhoea Rash Fever Cinchonism Syncope Blood dyscrasia	Hypotension Anticholinergic effects Dry mouth Urinary hesitancy Blurred vision Heart failure AV block	Confusion Convulsions	Confusion Tremor Bradycardia Hypotension	Dizziness Visual disturbance	Corneal deposits Photosensitivity Skin pigmentation Thyroid disturbance Pulmonary alveolitis Nightmares Liver disease	Ventricular arrhythmias Bradycardia Heart failure Bronchospasm	Nausea Vomiting Constipation Flushing Headache Bradycardia Fluid retention	Nausea Vomiting Constipation Flushing Headache Bradycardia Fluid retention	Nausea Anorexia Vomiting Visual disturbance Bradycardia

AF = atrial fibrillation
PSVT = paroxysmal supraventricular tachycardia
VT = ventricular tachycardia
VF = ventricular fibrillation
WPW = Wolff-Parkinson–White syndrome
AFL = atrial flutter
VPBs = ventricular premature beats
N/A = not applicable

matically deliver a defibrillating shock to the heart. It is relatively small (250 ml) and is powered by lithium batteries sufficient to provide energy for about 100 shocks each of 25–30 J. The device is usually implanted behind the rectus abdominis muscle and is connected to the heart by several wires and electrodes. When an arrhythmia develops that requires treatment, the device takes about 15 s to recognize the arrhythmia and charge its capacitors. It then delivers the defibrillating discharge. The shock may be painful, particularly if the patient is still fully conscious.

The use of this device has cut the sudden death rate in patients with serious ventricular arrhythmias to between 5 and 10% in the first year. However, because of its expense it is not widely available.

Cardiac failure

Cardiac failure occurs when, despite normal venous pressures, the heart cannot maintain sufficient cardiac output to meet the needs of the body. The causes of myocardial failure include:
- Myocardial dysfunction, e.g. cardiomyopathy, ischaemic heart disease
- Volume overload, e.g. valvular regurgitation —aortic or mitral
- Obstruction to cardiac output—aortic stenosis or hypertension
- Obligatory high cardiac output, e.g. Paget's disease, beriberi, anaemia, thyrotoxicosis, systemic-to-pulmonary shunts
- Prevention of ventricular filling, e.g. constrictive pericarditis, pericardial tamponade, restrictive cardiomyopathy
- Mechanical disadvantage, such as a large left ventricular aneurysm
- Change of rhythm, e.g. atrial fibrillation

Haemodynamic effects of myocardial failure

When the myocardium begins to fail, its velocity of contraction and the active tension that it is capable of developing are reduced. Factors involved are the venous return, the outflow resistance, the contractility of the myocardium, and salt and water retention.

Venous return (pre-load). In the intact heart, myocardial failure leads to a reduction of the volume of blood ejected with each heart beat and an increase in the volume of blood remaining after systole. This increased diastolic volume stretches the myocardial fibres and, as Starling's law of the heart would suggest, myocardial contraction is restored. However, the failing myocardium results in depres-

sion of the ventricular function curve (cardiac output plotted against the ventricular diastolic volume) (see Fig. 11.2, p. 448).

Slight myocardial depression is not associated with a reduction in cardiac output because it is maintained by an increase in venous pressure (and hence diastolic volume). However, the volume of blood ejected with each heart beat (ejection fraction) is reduced early in heart failure. Sinus tachycardia also ensures that any reduction of stroke volume is compensated for by the increase in heart rate; cardiac output (stroke volume × heart rate) is therefore maintained.

When there is more severe myocardial dysfunction, cardiac output can only be maintained by a large increase in venous pressure and/or marked sinus tachycardia. This eventually results in further depression of the ventricular function curve and reduced contractility. The resultant increased venous pressure contributes to the development of dyspnoea, due to the accumulation of interstitial and alveolar fluid, and to the occurrence of hepatic enlargement, ascites and dependent oedema, due to increased systemic venous pressure. Despite symptoms due to increased venous pressure, the cardiac output at rest may not be much depressed, but myocardial and haemodynamic reserve is so compromised that a normal increase in cardiac output cannot be produced by exercise.

In very severe heart failure the cardiac output at rest is depressed, despite high venous pressures. The inadequate cardiac output is redistributed to maintain perfusion of vital organs, such as the heart, brain and kidneys, at the expense of the skin and muscle.

Outflow resistance (after-load) (see Fig. 13.2, p. 625 and Fig. 13.4, p. 626). This is the load or resistance against which the ventricle contracts. It is formed by the:
- Pulmonary and systemic resistance
- Physical characteristics of the vessel walls
- Volume of blood that is ejected

An increase in afterload decreases the cardiac output. This decrease in function with further increase of end-diastolic volume and dilatation of the ventricle itself further exacerbates the problem of afterload. This is expressed by Laplace's law: the tension of the myocardium (T) is proportional to the intraventricular pressure (P) multiplied by the radius of the ventricular chamber (R), i.e. $T \propto PR$.

Myocardial contractility (inotropic state). The state of the myocardium also influences performance. Increased contractility (positive inotropism) can result from increased sympathetic drive, and this is a normal part of the Frank–Starling relationship (see Fig. 11.2). Conversely, myocardial depressants (e.g. hypoxia) decrease myocardial contractility (negative inotropism).

Salt and water retention. The increase in venous pressure that occurs when the ventricles fail leads to the retention of salt and water and their accumulation in the interstitial space. Reduced cardiac output leads to the diversion of blood away from the renal cortex, glomerular filtration falls, and salt and water excretion is impaired under the control of the renin–aldosterone system (see p. 739).

Thus, both increased venous pressure ('backward' heart failure) and reduced cardiac output ('forward' heart failure) contribute to salt and water retention. The increased salt and water loads further increase venous pressures, which, in the early stages of heart failure, improves cardiac output by the operation of the Starling mechanism. In severe heart failure the ventricular function curve is so flat or has plateaued such that further increases in venous pressure do not stimulate an increased cardiac output.

Clinical syndromes of heart failure

The division of heart failure into the syndromes of right, left, and congestive (biventricular) cardiac failure is clinically useful, but it is rare for any part of the heart to fail in isolation.

Right heart failure
This syndrome usually occurs in:
- Chronic lung disease (cor pulmonale)
- Pulmonary embolism or pulmonary hypertension
- Rheumatic tricuspid valve disease
- Pulmonary stenosis
- Left-to-right shunts due to atrial or ventricular septal defects

Right ventricular infarction and pre-existing left heart failure, and mitral stenosis with pulmonary hypertension are also causes of right heart failure.

Symptoms include breathlessness, ankle oedema and fatigue. The physical signs are more obvious than the symptoms. High systemic venous pressure leads to:
- Distension of the jugular veins
- Tender and smooth enlargement of the liver
- The development of ascites
- Dependent pitting oedema

Dilatation of the right ventricle produces cardiac enlargement and may give rise to functional tricuspid valve regurgitation with a pan-systolic murmur. A tachycardia with a right ventricular third or fourth heart sound is usual.

Left heart failure
Causes include:
- Ischaemic heart disease (commonest cause)
- Systemic hypertension
- Cardiomyopathies
- Mitral and aortic valve disease

A persistent ductus arteriosus increases the left ventricular output and may cause left ventricular failure. Mitral stenosis causes left atrial hypertension and left heart failure but does not itself cause failure of the left ventricle.

Symptoms consist predominantly of fatigue, weakness, dyspnoea, orthopnoea and paroxysmal nocturnal dyspnoea.

Physical signs are few and not very impressive until the failure is severe. Some cardiac enlargement may be demonstrable. Auscultation may reveal a left ventricular third or fourth heart sound. Basal pulmonary crackles may be heard. In severe left ventricular failure the patient has severe pulmonary oedema (see p. 497). The chest x-ray is the most useful investigation (see p. 464).

Congestive (biventricular) cardiac failure
This term is used variously but is best confined to the development of right heart failure consequent to previous left heart failure. The clinical presentation is thus a combination of the above signs and symptoms. There is continued congestion of the lungs and oedema of dependent parts with a large heart.

Acute heart failure
Acute failure of the heart may occur when a valve suddenly becomes regurgitant, the interventricular septum ruptures to form a ventricular septal defect (VSD) or the circulation is obstructed. The most common examples are papillary muscle or chordal rupture giving rise to mitral regurgitation, sudden aortic valve regurgitation due to infective endocarditis, acute pulmonary embolus and cardiac tamponade. In each case severe cardiac failure can occur without noticeable cardiac enlargement.

High output heart failure
The heart may not be able to circulate the high cardiac output found in conditions such as Paget's disease, beriberi, thyrotoxicosis, gram-negative septicaemia, and systemic arteriovenous fistula. This form of heart failure is characterized by cardiac enlargement, a tachycardia, and an additional third or fourth heart sound (gallop rhythm). Unlike low output heart failure, the oxygen content of systemic venous blood is high because there is a large volume of systemic arterial blood that is not delivered to or necessary for metabolizing tissue.

Factors aggravating or precipitating heart failure

Any factor that increases the burden on the heart may aggravate existing heart failure or initiate failure. These factors should be carefully considered in patients who present with heart failure. The most common are arrhythmias, anaemia, thyrotoxicosis, pregnancy, infective endocarditis, pulmonary infection, and adjustment of heart failure therapy.

The treatment of heart failure

The management of heart failure requires that any factor aggravating the failure should be identified and treated. Similarly, the cause of heart failure should be elucidated and, if possible, should be corrected. Heart failure may be directly treated by reduction of physical activity, dietary modifications and drug management.

Reduction of physical activity

The development of heart failure requires that the patient rests in bed for some days. The reduced physical activity usually leads to an improved cardiac status. Deep venous thrombosis should be avoided by regular leg exercises, low dose subcutaneous heparin treatment (see below) and elastic support stockings.

Dietary modifications

Large meals should be avoided and, if necessary, weight reduction should be undertaken. The most important dietary modification is salt reduction. A low-sodium diet (see Appendices) is unpalatable and is rarely necessary. Foods rich in salt, the use of salt in cooking, and the addition of salt at the table should be avoided.

Drug management

The pharmacological management of heart failure relies on three categories of drug: diuretics, digitalis glycosides and vasodilators.

Diuretics. These act by increasing salt and water excretion by the kidneys by blocking tubular reabsorption of sodium and chloride. The reduction in the circulatory volume lowers both the systemic (e.g. the jugular venous pressure) and the pulmonary venous pressure. The ventricular filling pressure (pre-load) is thereby reduced. Because the ventricular function curve (relationship between pre-load and cardiac output) is rather flat in heart failure, this does not significantly decrease cardiac output but decreases peripheral oedema and relieves dyspnoea due to decreased pulmonary congestion. The peripheral arteriolar dilatation caused by diuretics such as frusemide produces a reduction in left ventricular after-load, thereby improving cardiac function.

Diuretics can act in different ways:
- Frusemide (20–200 mg daily) and bumetanide (1–20 mg daily) are 'loop diuretics' which act by reducing the reabsorption of sodium and chloride in the ascending limb of the loop of Henle (see p. 372). This causes a potent diuresis as the concentrating power of the kidneys is reduced. There is also increased potassium loss.
- Spironolactone (100–200 mg daily) is a specific competitive antagonist to aldosterone and has a potassium-sparing effect in addition to its diuretic action. It should not be used in renal failure.

- Amiloride (5–20 mg daily) and triamterene (200 mg daily) act by inhibiting both the absorption of sodium and the secretion of potassium in the distal tubule.
- Thiazides such as bendrofluazide (5–10 mg) act on the distal convoluted tubule by decreasing sodium and chloride absorption. Potassium excretion is enhanced.

Severe heart failure requires treatment with powerful loop diuretics such as frusemide (80–120 mg i.v.), bumetanide (2 mg i.v.) and ethacrynic acid (50 mg i.v.). When the patient is in severe heart failure, the diuretic must be given intravenously because it may not be absorbed when administered orally.

Less severe heart failure may be satisfactorily treated with oral diuretics such as frusemide or bumetanide, which may be much more effective when combined with an aldosterone antagonist such as spironolactone, or a thiazide diuretic, especially chlorthalidone (50 mg daily) or metolazone (5–10 mg daily).

Mild heart failure is usually treated with an oral thiazide, e.g. bendrofluazide. Hypokalaemia must be avoided by adding potassium supplements or preferably by combining thiazides with potassium-conserving diuretics such as amiloride or triamterene. Too vigorous a diuresis may produce hypovolaemia, hyponatraemia or dilutional hyponatraemia (when proportionately more sodium is lost than water).

Digitalis glycosides. Digitalis glycosides are still the only commonly used orally active drugs that effectively increase the force of cardiac contraction (i.e. the inotropic state). The most common glycoside is digoxin, which has a half-life of approximately 1.5 days; 90% is excreted unchanged in the urine. Digoxin improves cardiac contraction when given to patients with congestive cardiac failure and is particularly valuable when atrial fibrillation is present because it also reduces the ventricular response rate.

Digoxin has a positive inotropic effect because it inhibits the sodium–potassium pump which normally maintains a high intracellular potassium concentration. In the presence of digoxin, a relatively high intracellular sodium concentration occurs, allowing intracellular sodium to be exchanged for extracellular calcium. Thus, intracellular calcium is increased and by inhibiting troponin this allows myosin and actin to bind far more readily. Thus a positive inotropic effect, i.e. upward movement of the ventricular function curve, is produced.

Digoxin is usually administered orally (1 mg and then 0.25–0.5 mg daily thereafter); if a more rapid effect is needed, the first dose may be given intravenously (5–75 $\mu g \cdot kg^{-1}$ body weight over approximately 30 min). The daily maintenance dose for elderly patients may be as little as 62.5 μg.

Digoxin is not given intramuscularly because it is painful when given in this way.

Digitalis toxicity was very common when the bioavailability of digoxin tablets was so variable. It is now less common, but still occurs when hypokalaemia, hypoxaemia (particularly due to chronic lung disease) or renal impairment is also present. In addition, patients with myxoedema are particularly sensitive to digoxin. Concurrent treatment with quinidine reduces the renal elimination of digoxin and may also lead to digoxin toxicity. The most common features of digoxin toxicity are:

- Anorexia, nausea and vomiting
- Cardiac arrhythmias, e.g. ventricular premature beats, ventricular tachycardia and AV block
- Digoxin blood levels above $2.5 \text{ ng} \cdot \text{ml}^{-1}$ ($3 \text{ nmol} \cdot \text{l}^{-1}$)

Digoxin toxicity is treated by discontinuation of the drug, restoration of the serum potassium and specific management of arrhythmia complications. Digoxin antibodies (Fab fragments) are a specific antidote which may be useful.

Vasodilators (see also pp. 544 and 638). Heart failure results in high venous pressures which significantly contribute to the production of pulmonary and dependent oedema. In severe heart failure the increase in venous pressure does not elevate cardiac output because the ventricular function curve is virtually flat (see Fig. 13.3, p. 626). It is therefore appropriate to reduce the venous pressure. If diuretics are not sufficiently effective, dilatation of the venous vascular bed with nitrates such as glyceryl trinitrate and isosorbide mono- or dinitrate is usually very helpful in reducing the pre-load.

Arteriolar constriction also occurs in heart failure from a variety of neural and humoral reactions. It is initially helpful in maintaining blood pressure and redistributing blood flow, but in the later stages of heart failure the constricted arterial bed prevents blood flow. The administration of arterial vasodilators such as alpha-adrenergic blockers (e.g. prazosin), angiotensin-converting enzyme inhibitors (e.g. captopril and enalapril) and direct smooth muscle relaxants (e.g. hydralazine) leads to an increased cardiac output and little or no fall in blood pressure because the decrease in peripheral resistance (after-load) is compensated for by the increased cardiac output. Arterial vasodilatation results in upward movement of the ventricular function curve (see Fig. 13.4, p. 626).

Some of these agents (e.g. prazosin, captopril) act on both the venous and the arterial vessels, thereby reducing pre- and after-load.

Pulmonary oedema

This is a very frightening, life-threatening emergency characterized by extreme breathlessness. The dyspnoea may first occur at night in the form of paroxysmal dyspnoea, when the reabsorption of dependent oedema when lying flat and the relative insensitivity of the respiratory centre at night allow pulmonary congestion to develop. In more severe cases the patient is severely breathless at all times of the day.

PATHOPHYSIOLOGY

Left ventricular failure and mitral valve disease cause pulmonary oedema because of increased pulmonary capillary pressure. A pressure above 20 mmHg causes increased filtration of fluid out of the capillaries into the interstitial space (interstitial oedema). Further accumulation of fluid disrupts intercellular membranes, leading to the collection of fluid in the alveolar spaces (alveolar oedema). Alveolar oedema occurs when the capillary pressure exceeds the total oncotic pressures (approximately 30 mmHg).

CLINICAL FEATURES

Interstitial oedema presents with dyspnoea and tachypnoea.

Patients with alveolar oedema are acutely breathless, wheezing, anxious and perspire profusely. In addition, they usually have a cough productive of frothy, blood-tinged (pink) sputum, which can be copious. The patient is tachypnoeic with peripheral circulatory shutdown. There is a tachycardia, a raised venous pressure and a gallop rhythm. Crackles and wheeze are heard throughout the chest. The arterial Po_2 falls and initially the $P_a\text{co}_2$ also falls due to overbreathing. Later, however, the $P_a\text{co}_2$ increases because of impaired gas exchange. The chest x-ray shows diffuse haziness due to alveolar fluid and the Kerley B lines of interstitial oedema (see Fig. 11.13, p. 464). The abnormality can be unilateral, giving the appearance of a tumour which disappears on treatment (a pseudotumour).

TREATMENT

- The patient should be placed in the sitting position.
- High concentration oxygen (60% via a variable performance mask) is given unless it is suspected that there is a co-existing chronic hypercapnia due to long-standing respiratory failure. In severe cases it may be necessary to ventilate the patient using positive pressure techniques (see p. 642).
- Intravenous diuretic treatment with frusemide, bumetanide or ethacrynic acid is given. These diuretics produce *immediate* vasodilatation in addition to the more delayed diuretic response.
- Morphine (10–20 mg i.v. depending on the size of the patient) together with an antiemetic such as metoclopramide (10 mg i.v.) or cyclizine (50 mg i.v.) is given. Morphine sedates the patient and

causes systemic vasodilatation; it must be avoided if the systemic arterial pressure is less than 90 mmHg. Respiratory depression occurs with large doses of morphine.

- Venous vasodilators, such as glyceryl trinitrate, may produce prompt relief by reducing the preload. Cardiac output may be increased by using arterial vasodilatation, such as occurs with hydralazine (Table 11.22).
- Aminophylline (250–500 mg or 5 mg·kg^{-1} i.v.) is infused over 10 min. Aminophylline is a phosphodiesterase inhibitor which causes bronchodilatation, vasodilatation and increased cardiac contractility. It must be given slowly because of the risk of precipitating ventricular arrhythmias. It is particularly useful when bronchospasm is present.
- Venesection and mechanical methods of reducing venous return (e.g. sphygmomanometer cuffs inflated to 10 mmHg below diastolic blood pressure and placed around the thighs) are rarely used and are usually inefficient.

In a severe case, after the acute emergency is controlled a pulmonary artery balloon catheter may be inserted to monitor progress and treatment. Any factor that precipitated the heart failure, such as cardiac arrhythmias or chest infection, should be corrected. The underlying cardiac problem should be diagnosed and treated.

Cardiogenic shock

Shock is a severe failure of tissue perfusion, usually characterized by hypotension, a low cardiac output and signs of poor tissue perfusion such as oliguria, cold extremities and poor cerebral function. Cardiogenic shock is an extreme type of cardiac failure with a high mortality of approximately 90%. Its most common cause is myocardial infarction.

Cardiogenic shock must be differentiated from other forms of shock. Cardiogenic shock is diagnosed when the shock syndrome occurs despite an adequate or elevated pulmonary capillary wedge

pressure and in the absence of mechanical circulatory obstruction. An essential element in this diagnosis is the measurement of the pulmonary capillary wedge pressure (see p. 634). In situations where the vascular capacity has expanded or the circulatory fluid volume has decreased, the wedge pressure will be low. In cardiogenic shock the wedge pressure is normal or elevated.

The mortality rate in cardiogenic shock is so high because of the vicious downward spiral that occurs: hypotension due to pump failure results in a reduction of coronary flow, which results in further impairment of pump function, and so on.

TREATMENT (see also p. 635)

- Patients require intensive care (see Chapter 13).
- General measures such as complete rest, continuous 100% oxygen administration and pain relief are essential.
- The infusion of fluid is necessary if the pulmonary capillary wedge pressure is below 18 mmHg, which is probably the optimal 'filling pressure' with which to prime a failing heart.
- Short-acting venous dilators such as glyceryl trinitrate or sodium nitroprusside should be administered intravenously if the wedge pressure is 25 mmHg or more. Aortic diastolic pressure (coronary perfusion pressure) may be increased with vasopressor medications such as adrenaline or high dose dopamine.
- Cardiac inotropes such as dobutamine and dopamine may be used. Dopamine also selectively increases renal perfusion.
- Mechanical assist devices such as an intra-aortic balloon pump may be used (see p. 477). Although leading to a temporary improvement, long-term prognosis is not improved unless there is a surgically correctable cause, such as a ruptured interventricular septum or acute mitral regurgitation.

Ischaemic heart disease

An imbalance between the supply of oxygen (and other essential myocardial nutrients) and the myocardial demand for these substances results in myocardial ischaemia. The causes are as follows:
1 The coronary blood flow to a region of the myocardium may be reduced by an obstruction due to:
- Atheroma
- Thrombosis
- Spasm
- Embolus
- Coronary ostial stenosis (e.g. syphilis)
- Coronary arteritis (e.g. polyarteritis)

Table 11.22 The effects of vasodilator drugs.

| | Effect | |
	Preload	Afterload
Nitroprusside	↓	0
Glyceryl trinitrate	↓	0
Isosorbide	↓	↓
Prazosin	↓	↓
Captopril/enalapril	↓	↓
Hydralazine	0	↓

2 There can be a decrease in the flow of oxygenated blood to the myocardium due to:
- Anaemia
- Carboxyhaemoglobinaemia
- Hypotension causing decreased coronary perfusion pressure

3 An increased demand for oxygen may occur due to an increase in cardiac output, e.g. during exercise or in thyrotoxicosis, or myocardial hypertrophy, e.g. from aortic stenosis or hypertension.

In types 2 and 3, ischaemia may occur despite normal coronary arteries. In a small number of cases, ischaemia develops despite normal coronary arteries and a normal demand for oxygen. This condition is known as syndrome X and is possibly caused by an inability to transport oxygen across the myocardial cell membrane.

The most common cause of ischaemic heart disease is coronary atheroma, which causes a fixed obstruction to coronary blood flow. Variations in the tone of smooth muscle in the wall of a coronary artery may add an important element of dynamic or variable obstruction. Sometimes an extreme increase in coronary tone may produce coronary spasm and severely reduced coronary blood flow in the absence of any underlying coronary atheroma.

Atheroma

The word 'atheroma' comes from the Greek word *athere* meaning 'porridge'. It is a condition that affects medium-sized arteries and is characterized by the development of atherosclerotic plaques. Such a plaque consists of a necrotic core, rich in cholesterol and other lipids, surrounded by smooth muscle cells and fibrous tissue. There are two main theories of plaque development:
- Insudation may be due to the accumulation of plasma constituents such as cholesterol in the intima of the arterial wall because of low grade inflammation. This theory was suggested by Virchow.
- Platelet thrombi may develop on areas of damaged intima. Rokitansky suggested that the organization of these thrombi could lead to atheroma.

AETIOLOGY OF CORONARY ATHEROMA

The immediate cause of this condition is not known. However, a number of 'risk' factors are known to predispose to coronary atherosclerosis. Some of these, such as age, sex and family history, cannot be modified, whereas other major risk factors, such as serum cholesterol, smoking habits and hypertension, can be changed. There are a number of other factors, such as lack of exercise, personality type and stress, that may be implicated in the causation of atherosclerosis (see Table 11.23).

Table 11.23 Risk factors for coronary disease.

Fixed
Age
Male sex
Positive family history
Changeable with treatment
Strong association
Hyperlipidaemia
Cigarette smoking
Hypertension
Diabetes mellitus
Weak association
Personality
Obesity
Gout
Soft water
Lack of exercise
Contraceptive pill
Heavy alcohol consumption

Age

Atherosclerosis develops progressively as age advances. It is rarely present in early childhood, except in familial hyperlipidaemia, but it is often detectable in post-mortem specimens of young men between 20 and 30 years. It is almost universal in the elderly in the Western World.

Sex

Men are more affected than pre-menopausal women. However, after the menopause the incidence of atheroma in women becomes similar to that in men. The cause of this difference in incidence is not clearly understood.

Family history

Coronary artery disease is often found in several members of the same family. Because the disease is so prevalent and because other risk factors are familial, it is uncertain whether family history is an independent risk factor.

Hyperlipidaemia (see p. 771)

Atherosclerotic plaques contain cholesterol. A high serum cholesterol, especially when associated with low values of high density lipoproteins, is strongly associated with coronary atheroma. High triglyceride levels are less definitely linked with coronary atheroma. Types IIa and IIb, III and IV hyperlipoproteinaemia, as classified by the World Health Organization, are associated with an increased risk of coronary atherosclerosis. Vigorous treatment of children with these familial conditions may retard the development of atherosclerosis. There is little definite evidence that dietary modification to reduce serum cholesterol and triglycerides will significantly reduce the risk of developing atherosclerosis in adults. However, reduced carbohydrate intake (to lower serum triglycerides) and the avoidance of animal fat and dietary cholesterol (to reduce serum cholesterol) are usually advised. The advantages of drug-induced changes in serum lipids must be judged against any side-effects that these drugs may cause.

Smoking

In men, the risk of developing coronary artery disease is directly related to the number of cigarettes smoked. This relationship is less certain, but still important, in women and in cigar and pipe smokers. The risk from smoking declines to almost normal after 10 years of abstention.

Hypertension

Both systolic and diastolic hypertension are associated with an increased risk of coronary artery disease. The risk is the same for men and women. Reduction of blood pressure with hypotensive therapy reduces the risks of a cerebrovascular accident and of cardiac events such as myocardial infarction.

Other factors

Lack of exercise increases the risk of coronary artery disease, and regular exercise probably protects against its development. Diabetes mellitus, or even just an abnormal glucose tolerance test, is associated with vascular disease. Obesity is certainly associated with coronary artery disease, but it is not certain whether obesity itself is independently linked with the condition.

A certain kind of personality type known as 'type A', which is characterized by largely unsuccessful aggression, ambition, compulsion and competitiveness, is said to be associated twice as frequently with coronary artery disease than is 'type B' (the converse of type A). Gout, oral contraceptives, alcohol and soft water have also been suggested as risk factors for coronary atheroma.

It is clear that many factors influence the development of coronary atheroma. It is not certain that modification of any of these can substantially reverse the established atherosclerotic process.

Angina (see p. 451)

Angina ranges from a mild ache to a most severe pain which provokes sweating and fear. It is generally described as 'heavy', 'crushing' or 'gripping', and the patient may indicate the type of pain by clenching his fist or gripping his hands together. Occasionally these symptoms may occur in the arms without any chest pain.

There are several types of angina; these are described below.

Classical or exertional angina

Physical exertion, especially after a meal, in cold weather or walking against the wind, provokes this pain. It is also aggravated by anger or excitement. The pain usually fades quickly (in less than 3 min) when the patient ceases to exert himself. Sometimes the pain will disappear even though exertion continues ('walking through the pain'); the exertion threshold for the development of pain is very variable. Usually, pain is more easily provoked in the early morning than later in the day. This type of angina can be graded as in Table 11.3 (see p. 452).

Decubitus angina

This is angina that occurs when the patient lies down. It usually occurs in association with heart failure because of the increased central blood volume and consequent myocardial tensions which develop in the recumbent position.

Nocturnal angina

This is angina that wakes the patient from sleep. It may be due to heart failure, coronary spasm or vivid dreams.

Variant (Prinzmetal's) angina

A classical attack of variant angina, as described by Prinzmetal, has no obvious provocation. It occurs at rest, especially at night or in the early morning, and is rarely induced by exertion. It occurs more frequently in women and the pain is usually more severe and more prolonged than in classical angina. It produces a characteristic electrocardiographic feature of ST segment elevation developing during the pain. Arrhythmias—both heart block and ventricular tachycardia—are common in the ischaemic episode.

Prinzmetal's angina is caused by spasm of a coronary artery. More often, variant angina is not classical Prinzmetal's angina but is due to variation in coronary arterial tone rather than frank coronary arterial spasm. Such patients have a varying exercise threshold for the provocation of angina.

Unstable angina

Unstable angina includes angina of very recent onset, worsening angina or angina at rest. A number of terms, such as crescendo angina, pre-infarction angina and intermediate chest pain syndrome, have been used to describe angina which is provoked more easily and persists for a longer duration than ordinary angina or which fails to respond readily to therapy. Whilst the pain is present, myocardial infarction must be considered, but with angina the ECG changes (T wave inversion or ST segment depression) are only transient and cardiac enzyme levels are not elevated. Unless vigorously treated, a large proportion of patients with unstable angina will proceed to develop a myocardial infarction within weeks.

EXAMINATION

There are usually no abnormal findings in angina, although a fourth heart sound may be heard. Any factor responsible for angina (e.g. thyrotoxicosis) or risk factors may lead to physical signs such as nicotine staining, hypertension or xanthelasma.

DIAGNOSIS

The primary diagnosis rests on the description of the chest pain as investigations may be normal.

INVESTIGATION

Resting ECG

This is usually normal between attacks, although an old myocardial infarction, left ventricular hypertrophy or myopathic changes may be present. During an attack, transient ST segment depression, symmetrical T wave inversion or tall, pointed, upright T waves may appear.

A normal ECG between attacks or even during an attack cannot definitely exclude angina pectoris. Typical ECG changes during an attack are strong pointers to the diagnosis of angina.

Exercise ECG (see p. 466)

When angina is provoked by exertion, an exercise stress ECG should be performed. ST segment depression greater than or equal to 1 mm suggests myocardial ischaemia, especially if typical chest pain occurs at the same time. The severity of the electrocardiographic changes indicates the extent of the coronary artery disease. Approximately 75% of patients with severe coronary artery disease will give a positive test. Stress testing is less reliable in women and is confused by electrolyte abnormalities, therapy with digoxin, and intraventricular conduction disturbances. A normal stress test does not definitely exclude coronary disease.

Cardiac scintigraphy

Uptake of thallium-201 (see p. 470). This is useful:
● When the exercise test is equivocal
● In deciding whether stenotic vessels on angiography are giving rise to ischaemic areas on exercise

A normal perfusion scan after exercise makes significant coronary artery disease unlikely.

Radionuclide ventriculography (see p. 472). This can be used to outline the left venticle. When part of the left ventricular wall is ischaemic it does not contract normally, producing an abnormal image. This test can be performed at rest and during exertion. The ejection fraction is a good index of ventricular function and is useful in the assessment of patients for coronary artery bypass surgery.

Echocardiography (see p. 468)

This can be used to assess ventricular wall involvement and ventricular function.

Coronary angiography

This is occasionally useful in patients with chest pain when the cause is unclear. More often, the test is performed to delineate the exact coronary anatomy (Fig. 11.47) prior to coronary grafting or coronary angioplasty. Coronary angiography should only be performed when the benefit in terms of diagnosis and potential treatment outweighs the small risk associated with the procedure (a mortality of less than 1 in 1000 cases) (see Table 11.24).

A coronary angiogram may not reveal coronary spasm unless an intracoronary injection of dihydroergotamine has been given. This test is not often performed because the induction of coronary spasm may prove difficult to reverse and its clinical relevance is uncertain.

TREATMENT

Management of an acute attack

An acute attack is treated by stopping exercise (exertional angina) or by getting up (decubitus angina) and dissolving a fresh glyceryl trinitrate tablet

Fig. 11.47 Coronary angiogram demonstrating a tight stenosis in the left main coronary artery.

Table 11.24 Indications for coronary angiography.

Angina refractory to medical therapy
Unstable angina
Angina occurring after myocardial infarction
Subendocardial myocardial infarction (non-Q-wave infarction)
Prior to valve surgery in a patient with possible coronary disease
Severely abnormal exercise ECG
Angina or myocardial infarction in a young (<50 years) patient

(0.5 mg) under the tongue. After 2–3 min the angina usually recedes. When the pain is relieved the glyceryl trinitrate tablet is spat out or swallowed to inactivate it. This minimizes the main side-effect which is a severe pounding headache. Some prefer to use an aerosol formulation of glyceryl trinitrate which, unlike the tablets, is stable for a long period. If glyceryl trinitrate cannot be tolerated, a capsule of nifedipine may be chewed or sucked. However, this has similar side-effects to glyceryl trinitrate.

General management
Patients should be reassured that their condition is not uniformly or rapidly fatal. Many have a good prognosis—30% survive for more than 10 years and spontaneous remission does occur. Any underlying problems such as obesity, thyrotoxicosis, anaemia or aortic stenosis should be treated. Risk factors should be evaluated and steps made to correct them. Smoking must be stopped. Patients must be encouraged not to do things that they know provoke their angina, but this must not lead to a severe restriction of lifestyle. Regular exercise sufficient to improve the fitness of the patient will tend to increase the threshold to angina. Exercise is not recommended unless the cardiovascular response to exertion (treadmill ECG test) has been documented. Emotional crises and overexcitement must be minimized.

Medical treatment
Patients should be told to suck a tablet of glyceryl trinitrate before exertion rather than waiting for the pain to commence. They must be specifically encouraged to do this, because many prefer to believe that it is better to suffer the pain than to take more tablets. When angina occurs frequently, or with only modest exertion, regular prophylactic therapy should be advised. This consists of nitrates, beta-adrenergic blocking drugs or calcium antagonists.

Nitrates such as glyceryl trinitrate are available in a variety of slow release formulations, particularly infiltrated skin plasters and buccal pellets. Alternatively, tablets of long-acting nitrate preparations such as isosorbide dinitrate or isosorbide mononitrate may be used. Nitrates are successful in the treatment of angina pectoris because they reduce venous and hence intracardiac diastolic pressures, they reduce the impedance to the emptying of the left ventricle, and they relax the tone of the coronary arteries.

Beta-adrenergic blocking drugs reduce heart rate (negative chronotropic effect) and the force of ventricular contraction (negative inotropic effect), both of which reduce myocardial oxygen demand, especially on exercise. Sufficient beta-blocker to reduce the resting heart rate to about 60 beats per minute is usually necessary to achieve relief from angina. Very high doses of beta-blockers are no longer used because of side-effects and the possibility of infarction or arrhythmia on withdrawal, and because many alternative therapies are available. Propranolol 40–80 mg three times daily is the drug most widely used.

Relatively cardioselective beta-blockers (beta-1-antagonists) such as atenolol (100 mg daily) or metoprolol (50 mg three times daily) are often preferred because they have fewer side-effects.

Calcium antagonists such as nifedipine, verapamil and diltiazem block calcium flux into the cell and the utilization of calcium within the cell. They relax coronary arteries and other vascular systems and also reduce the force of left ventricular contraction, reducing the oxygen demand and improving the angina. Nifedipine 20–30 mg daily is the calcium antagonist most commonly used in angina.

Coronary angioplasty
This is a technique of dilating coronary atheromatous obstructions by inflating a balloon against the obstruction (Fig. 11.48). The balloon, which is mounted on the tip of a very thin catheter, is inserted through the obstruction using x-ray fluoroscopy, and it is then inflated with dilute contrast material. Multiple inflations of the balloon using a pressure of several atmospheres will squash and crack the atheroma and relieve the obstruction. This technique is widely applied for the treatment of angina due to isolated, proximal, non-calcified, atheromatous plaques, usually in patients with a relatively short history of coronary ischaemia. Multiple lesions may be treated and repeat procedures can be undertaken.

Surgical management
When angina worsens or persists despite general measures and optimal medical treatment, the option of surgery should be considered. The patient should be assessed using exercise testing and angiography. Symptomatic patients with left main stem obstructions, two- or three-vessel involvement and good ventricular function should be treated surgically.

There are three operations currently used for the relief of myocardial ischaemia:
● Coronary artery vein bypass grafting (CAVBG) (Fig. 11.49) involves taking a vein, usually from the leg (saphenous) and bypassing the coronary obstruction by suturing the vein (reversed because of the venous valves) between the aorta and the coronary artery distal to the obstruction.
● An internal mammary artery may be mobilized and implanted into the left anterior descending coronary artery distal to an obstruction (Fig. 11.49).
● Endarterectomy (removal of an atheromatous obstruction) can sometimes be successful when combined with bypass or internal mammary artery grafting.

Surgery provides dramatic relief from angina in

(a)

(b)

(c)

Fig. 11.48 (a) Stenosis in right coronary artery (arrow). (b) Dilatation of the stenosis using an angioplasty baloon. (c) Postdilatation—the obstruction is no longer seen.

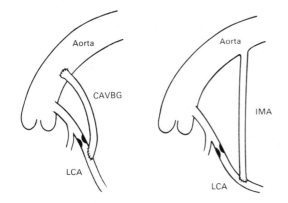

Fig. 11.49 The relief of coronary obstruction by surgical techniques: coronary artery vein bypass grafting (CAVBG) or internal mammary arterial implantation (IMA). In both of these examples the graft bypasses a coronary obstruction in the left coronary artery (LCA).

about 90% of those operated on. When surgery is performed for left main stem obstruction or for three-vessel disease involvement, an improved life span and quality of life can be expected. Surgical mortality should be weil below 1% in patients with normal left ventricular function. Progressive slow occlusion of grafts with atheroma occurs in a significant number of cases (5–10% a year).

Treatment of variant angina
The treatment of variant angina is slightly different. Nitrates and calcium antagonists are useful, but beta-blockers may increase coronary tone and exacerbate the angina, so should not be used. It may be necessary to treat the arrhythmias provoked by the spasm. Surgical relief is rarely necessary or possible.

Treatment of unstable angina.
Unstable angina should be managed vigorously by bed rest, sedation, oxygen and sometimes anticoa-

gulation plus medical therapy for the angina. Calcium antagonists are particularly valuable for the treatment of this condition but usually beta-blockers, nitrates and calcium antagonists are all used in combination. Aspirin decreases both death and myocardial infarction. Intra-aortic balloon pumping may be needed (see p. 477) if medical therapy fails.

Irrespective of the immediate success of treatment, early coronary angiography and, depending on the results, urgent referral for surgery is usually advised. There is a high incidence of myocardial infarction following unstable angina pectoris.

Myocardial infarction

Myocardial infarction is now the most common cause of death in the UK and other developed countries, but it was hardly known before 1910. It almost always occurs in patients with coronary atheroma because of sudden coronary thrombosis due to stasis and intimal injury resulting from haemorrhage into a plaque or spasm around the plaque. About 6 h after the onset of infarction the myocardium is pale and swollen, and at 24 h the necrotic tissue appears deep red due to haemorrhage. In the next weeks an inflammatory reaction develops, lymphocytes infiltrate and the infarcted tissue turns grey. Necrotic tissue is replaced by mononuclear cells, and gradually a thin fibrous scar develops.

CLINICAL PRESENTATION

Myocardial infarction presents with chest pain, similar in character to exertional angina pectoris, but usually occurring at rest and lasting for some hours. The pain may be so severe that the patient may fear imminent death ('angor animi'), but it may be less severe and mistaken for indigestion. It is usually sudden in onset, but it may develop gradually. The pain of myocardial infarction is often associated with restlessness and the patients usually cannot remain still. Sweating, nausea and vomiting are often associated with myocardial infarction.

About 20% of patients with myocardial infarction have no pain. Diabetics and elderly patients often have 'silent' myocardial infarctions. In these cases the myocardial infarction may go unnoticed or may produce hypotension, breathlessness or arrhythmias.

Physical signs

Usually there are no abnormal physical signs unless complications develop. Hypotension, which may first occur several hours after the onset of infarction and may increase over the following 3–4 days, abnormal precordial pulsation due to the systolic bulging of the infarcted myocardium, an additional heart sound (particularly a fourth heart sound), and sinus tachycardia may be noted in some patients. A raised venous pressure and basal crackles are common. As the infarction progresses, a modest fever (up to 38°C) due to muscle necrosis and lasting for up to 7 days occurs. A pericardial friction rub may develop.

INVESTIGATION

Non-specific tests

Non-specific abnormalities such as an increased ESR (up to 70 mm in the first hour) and a polymorphonuclear leucocytosis (up to 20×10^9/l) may occur in the first few days following myocardial infarction.

Cardiac enzymes (Fig. 11.50)

Necrotic cardiac tissue releases cellular enzymes; three of these are commonly assayed.

- *Lactic dehydrogenase* (LDH) peaks at 3–4 days and remains elevated for 10–14 days. LDH is not only present in cardiac muscle but is also released from damaged liver, skeletal muscle and red blood cells. There are five isoenzymes, and cardiac necrosis causes a predominant increase of LDH 1, which can also be measured as hydroxybutyrate dehydrogenase (HBD).

- *Aspartate aminotransferase* (AST), which was formerly called serum glutamic oxaloacetic transaminase (SGOT), peaks at 24–48 h and may fall to normal by 72 h. AST is also released by damaged red blood cells, kidney, liver and lungs.

- *Creatine kinase* (CK) is released by infarcted myocardium and peaks within 24 h. It is usually back to normal before 48 h. It is also produced by damaged skeletal muscle and brain. The myocardial-bound (MB) isoenzyme fraction of CK is specific for heart muscle damage. A several-fold increase in total CK, but not in MB CK, can be produced by an intramuscular injection. Cardioversion can increase both the total CK and the MB isoenzyme fraction of CK. The size of the infarction determines the total enzyme release. Large infarcts tend to produce high serum levels of enzymes.

Fig. 11.50 The enzyme profile in acute myocardial infarction. CK = creatine kinase; AST = aspartate aminotransferase; LDH = lactic dehydrogenase.

Enzymes are usually estimated for the first 3 days following a suspected myocardial infarction. The first assay is often normal and subsequent assays will show a three-fold or more increase in the majority of cases.

The ECG
The ECG is particularly valuable for the diagnosis of myocardial infarction. In the majority of cases the development of a full thickness myocardial infarction is associated with evolving electrocardiographic features.

A Q wave (Fig. 11.51) is a broad (>1 mm) and deep (>2 mm or more than 25% of the amplitude of the following R wave) negative deflection which starts the QRS complex. It may occur normally in leads AVR and V_1 (and sometimes in lead III), but in other leads it is abnormal. Abnormal Q waves are produced by several abnormalities such as left bundle branch block, ventricular tachycardia and the Wolff–Parkinson–White syndrome. The gradual development of Q waves over minutes or hours suggests the occurrence of a full thickness (as opposed to a subendocardial) myocardial infarction. They develop because the electrical silence of infarcted cardiac tissue results in a so-called 'window' through which the normal endocardial to epicardial activation of the opposite non-infarcted ventricular wall is 'seen' resulting in an unopposed depolarization front moving away from an electrode situated over the epicardial surface of the infarct (Fig. 11.51). Q waves are usually permanent electrocardiographic features following full-thickness myocardial infarction.

T wave and ST segment changes result from ischaemia and injury. They are therefore often transient, occurring only during the acute attack. The progressive changes or evolution of the ECG during the course of a full-thickness myocardial infarction are illustrated in Fig. 11.52.

With subendocardial infarction (Fig. 11.53) only the endocardial surface is infarcted and Q waves do not develop. ST segment and T wave changes are

Q ≥ 1 mm wide (0.04 s)
and/or
≥2 mm deep (0.2 mV)

Fig. 11.51 The electrocardiographic features of myocardial infarction, showing a Q wave, ST elevation and T wave inversion.

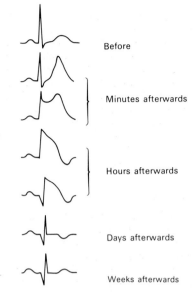

Before

Minutes afterwards

Hours afterwards

Days afterwards

Weeks afterwards

Fig. 11.52 Electrocardiographic evolution of myocardial infarction. After the first few minutes the T waves become tall, pointed and upright and there is ST segment elevation. After the first few hours the T waves invert, the R wave voltage is decreased and Q waves develop. After a few days the ST segment returns to normal. After weeks or months the T wave may return to upright but the Q wave remains.

therefore the only ECG features of a subendocardial infarction. Because the injury is endocardial rather than predominantly epicardial, ST segment depression rather than elevation is usual.

Typically ECG changes (Table 11.25) are usually confined to the ECG leads that 'face' the infarction. Therefore, an inferior wall myocardial infarction is diagnosed when the ECG findings are seen in leads II, III and AVF (Fig. 11.54). Lateral infarction produces changes in leads I, II and AVL. In anterior infarction, leads V_2–V_5 may be affected (Table 11.25). Changes seen in an anterolateral infarction are shown in Fig 11.55. Because there are no posterior leads, a true posterior wall infarct is usually diagnosed by the appearance of mirror image or reciprocal changes in leads V_1 and V_2, i.e. the development of a tall initial R wave, ST segment depression and tall, upright T waves. These reciprocal changes can also be seen in association with other infarctions. For example, in an inferior wall myocardial infarction, anterior ST segment depression may be seen.

A normal ECG, especially early in the presentation, does not exclude myocardial infarction.

Pyrophosphate scanning (see p. 470)
This test is particularly useful when the ECG is unhelpful because of pre-existing abnormalities such as left bundle branch block. Imaging is performed about 2 h after the injection of the isotope to detect the infarcted area.

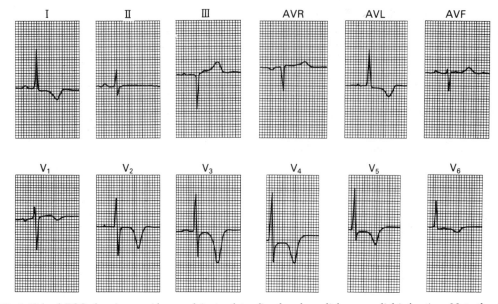

Fig. 11.53 A 12-lead ECG showing a widespread (anterolateral) subendocardial myocardial infarction. Note the deeply inverted, symmetrical T waves in addition to ST depression.

Table 11.25 ECG leads showing changes following different infarcts.

Infarct site	Leads showing main changes
Anterior:	
Small	V_3–V_4
Extensive	V_2–V_5
Inferior	II, III, AVF
Lateral	I, II, AVL
Posterior	V_1, V_2 (reciprocal)
Anteroseptal	V_1–V_3
Anterolateral	V_4–V_6, I, AVL
Subendocardial	Any lead

MANAGEMENT

During an acute myocardial infarction, lethal arrhythmias may occur. Patients should therefore be admitted to the coronary care unit as soon as possible. Here, the ECG should be monitored continuously for the first 48 h to allow the detection of arrhythmias such as 'R-on-T' ventricular ectopic beats, which may precipitate ventricular fibrillation. Even if these potentially provocative arrhythmias are not seen, it is important that ventricular fibrillation is recognized promptly and that resuscitation is started immediately. Therefore, patients should not be kept in casualty departments waiting for ECGs and chest x-rays but should be admitted immediately to the coronary care unit.

The pain of a myocardial infarction should be treated promptly with powerful analgesics such as morphine (10–20 mg i.v. or s.c.) or diamorphine (5–10 mg i.v. or s.c.) combined with antiemetics such as cyclizine (50 mg i.v.) or metoclopramide (10 mg i.v.). Pain should also be treated with nitrates. If there is no hypotension, sublingual glyceryl trinitrate should be given. Alternatively, especially if the haemodynamic situation is not stable, continuous intravenous infusion of isosorbide dinitrate should be considered.

Sedation is important. Anxious patients should be reassured and mild sedation, in addition to analgesia, may be necessary. A quiet atmosphere should reduce anxiety.

Bedrest is advised for the first 24–48 h, after which the patient is progressively mobilized. Smoking is not allowed.

Oxygen is usually given routinely because during an acute myocardial infarction the arterial Po_2 is reduced. Oxygen at 60% is usually administered by face mask or nasal cannulae for several hours following myocardial infarction.

Anticoagulation is useful for patients who are immobilized for long periods. Usually, heparin (5000 units 8-hourly s.c.) is sufficient. Patients with severe cardiac failure or cardiogenic shock are particularly vulnerable to thromboembolism. In these cases intravenous heparinization by continuous infusion (10 000 units in 6 h) is appropriate. Early mobiliza-

Fig. 11.54 A 12-lead ECG showing an acute inferior wall myocardial infarction. Notice the raised ST segment and Q waves in the inferior leads (II, III and AVF). The additional T wave inversion in V_4 and V_5 probably represents anterior wall ischaemia.

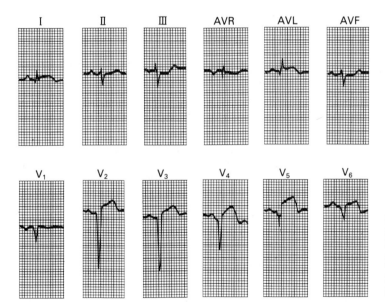

Fig. 11.55 A 12-lead ECG showing an acute anterolateral myocardial infarction. Notice the ST segment elevation in leads I, AVL and V_2 to V_6. The T wave is inverted in leads I, AVL and V_3 to V_6. Pathological Q waves are seen in leads V_2 to V_6.

tion policies have reduced the need for anticoagulation except in high risk cases.

An intravenous cannula is always inserted so that emergency intravenous medication can be administered.

Both streptokinase (1.5 megaunits over several hours) and activated tissue plasminogen can be given intravenously to patients who present early in the course of their myocardial infarction (within 4–6 h of the onset of pain). Such therapy is intended to dissolve the thrombus that initiates the infarct, thereby limiting the extent of the infarction. This therapy is now being increasingly used because initial trials of its efficacy have demonstrated a reduction in early mortality of up to 25%.

Home versus hospital care of myocardial infarction victims
Coronary care units were developed to facilitate the detection and treatment of arrhythmias occurring in the immediate post-infarction period. However, it

has been suggested that the coronary care ward is a frightening environment which may itself increase the incidence of these arrhythmias. There have been several studies comparing home care and coronary ward care of patients with myocardial infarction. The conclusions have been controversial but home care can be considered if:

- The patient has suffered a myocardial infarction 24 h or more previously
- There are no complications such as shock or arrhythmia
- The patient is 70 years or older

However, most patients suffering from myocardial infarction should be cared for in the coronary care ward of a hospital where sudden and perhaps fatal complications can be promptly recognized and effectively treated.

Mobile coronary care units

Because a large proportion of deaths from myocardial infarction are due to arrhythmias that occur in the first few minutes of the infarction, it is logical to train ambulance-men in methods of advanced cardiac life support and to provide them with the equipment to perform these techniques (intravenous infusion, endotracheal intubation and ventilation, and ECG monitoring and defibrillation). Ambulances manned and equipped in this way are called mobile coronary care units (CCUs), coronary rescue vehicles or cardiac resuscitation vehicles. This kind of ambulance is sent to those patients who have severe chest pain or who have collapsed unconscious. Together with the training in basic life support of a significant proportion (at least one-third) of the general public, mobile CCUs have reduced the incidence of sudden unexpected cardiac death, whether due to myocardial infarction or to arrhythmias unrelated to acute myocardial infarction. The provision of such vehicles is still patchy, but this service is becoming increasingly available in the UK.

COMPLICATIONS

In the acute phase, i.e. the first 2 to 3 days following a myocardial infarction, cardiac arrhythmias, cardiac failure and pericarditis are the most common complications. Later, recurrent infarction, angina, thromboembolism, mitral valve regurgitation, and ventricular septal or free wall rupture may occur. Late complications include the post-myocardial infarction syndrome (Dressler's syndrome), shoulder–hand syndrome, ventricular aneurysm and recurrent cardiac arrhythmias.

Cardiac arrhythmias

These are described in detail on pp. 477–494.

Ventricular extrasystoles. These commonly occur after myocardial infarction. Their occurrence may precede the development of ventricular fibrillation. If they are frequent (more than five per minute), multiform (different shapes) or R-on-T (falling on the upstroke or peak of the preceding T wave), they are usually treated with lignocaine 50–100 mg i.v. over 5 min followed by 1–4 mg·min^{-1} by continuous infusion, which is slowly reduced and discontinued over 24 h.

Ventricular tachycardia. This may degenerate into ventricular fibrillation or may itself produce serious haemodynamic consequences. It is treated with intravenous lignocaine. If haemodynamic deterioration occurs, the tachycardia is immediately treated with synchronized cardioversion (initially 200 J).

Ventricular fibrillation. This may occur in the first few hours or days following a myocardial infarction in the absence of severe cardiac failure or cardiogenic shock. This is known as primary ventricular fibrillation. It is treated with prompt defibrillation (200–400 J). Intravenous lignocaine is usually prescribed in an attempt to prevent recurrences of ventricular fibrillation. The prognosis is usually very good because the electrical derangement is only transient.

When ventricular fibrillation occurs in the setting of heart failure, shock or aneurysm, it is called secondary ventricular fibrillation. It is treated in a similar way to primary ventricular fibrillation, but the prognosis is very poor unless the underlying haemodynamic or mechanical cause can be corrected.

Atrial fibrillation. This occurs in about 10% of patients with myocardial infarction. It is due to atrial irritation caused by heart failure, pericarditis and atrial ischaemia or infarction. It may be managed with intravenous digoxin or intravenous amiodarone and by treatment of the underlying pathology.

Sinus bradycardia. This is especially associated with acute inferior wall myocardial infarction. Symptoms emerge only when the bradycardia is severe. When symptomatic, treatment consists of elevating the foot of the bed and giving intravenous atropine 600 µg if necessary. When sinus bradycardia occurs, an escape rhythm such as idioventricular rhythm (wide QRS complexes with a regular rhythm at 50–100 beats per minute) or idiojunctional rhythm (narrow QRS complexes) may occur. Usually no specific treatment is required.

It has been suggested that sinus bradycardia following myocardial infarction may predispose to the emergence of ventricular fibrillation. Severe sinus bradycardia associated with symptoms or the emergence of unstable rhythms may need treatment with temporary pacing.

Sinus tachycardia. This is produced by heart failure,

fever and anxiety. Usually no specific treatment is needed.

Conduction disturbances. These are common following myocardial infarction. AV nodal delay (first degree AV block) or higher degrees of block may occur during acute myocardial infarction, especially of the inferior wall. First degree block does not need treatment, but progressive or complete block may need treatment with atropine or an artificial temporary pacemaker. Such blocks may last for only a few minutes but frequently persist for days or several weeks; they are rarely permanent.

Acute anterior wall myocardial infarction may produce damage to the distal conduction system (the His bundle or the bundle branches). The development of complete heart block usually implies a large myocardial infarction and a poor prognosis. The ventricular escape rhythm is slow and unreliable and a temporary pacemaker is necessary. This form of block is often permanent.

The development of complete AV block (Table 11.26) can be expected in 20–30% of cases where progressive bundle branch block (right bundle branch block and then right bundle branch block with a QRS axis shift) has already occurred (see Fig. 11.56).

Cardiac failure and cardiogenic shock

Heart failure after acute myocardial infarction is graded according to a clinical classification (Table 11.27).

Mild left heart failure (a few basal crackles which

Table 11.26 Progression from different types of fascicular block to complete heart block in patients with acute myocardial infarction.

Type of fascicular block	% progressing to complete heart block
LAH	4
LPH	8
Long PR interval	10
LBBB	10
RBBB	20
RBBB + LAH	30
RBBB + LPH	40
RBBB + (LPH *or* LAH) + Long PR interval	40

LAH = left anterior hemiblock
LPH = left posterior hemiblock
LBBB = left bundle branch block
RBBB = right bundle branch block

persist after coughing, an extra heart sound and upper lobe blood diversion on the chest x-ray) occurs in about 40% of patients with acute myocardial infarction. Treatment for a few days with a mild diuretic such as a thiazide is usually all that is needed.

A large myocardial infarction may lead to severe

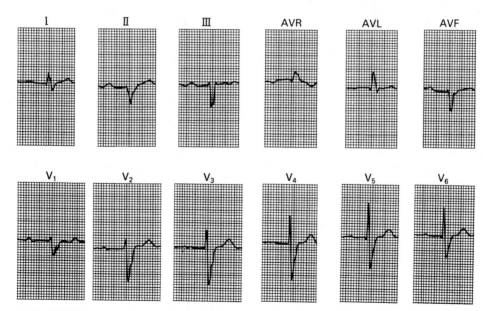

Fig. 11.56 A 12-lead ECG demonstrating a prolonged PR interval (0.32 s), a broad QRS complex with a deep S wave in leads I and V_6 (right bundle branch block) and left axis deviation (−75°). This electrocardiographic picture is consistent with bifascicular block.

Table 11.27 Killip (clinical) classification of heart failure in patients with acute myocardial infarction.

Class	Description	Incidence (%)	Mortality (%)
I	No heart failure	40	5
II	Mild left ventricular failure	40	20
III	Pulmonary oedema	10	40
IV	Cardiogenic shock	10	90

heart failure and pulmonary oedema. In such cases more prolonged and powerful diuretics and vasodilator treatment may be necessary.

In very severe cases a pulmonary artery balloon catheter is used to measure the pulmonary artery and 'left atrial' pressures and the cardiac output. Treatment is with loop diuretics, vasodilators (see p. 496) and, occasionally, digoxin.

Severe heart failure may also follow ventricular septal rupture or mitral valve papillary muscle rupture. Both of these conditions present with worsening heart failure, a systolic thrill and a loud pansystolic murmur, widely heard over the precordium. Often, echocardiography and right heart catheterization with a balloon catheter is needed to differentiate between these two conditions. Both are associated with a poor prognosis, but vigorous treatment including early surgical correction may be successful.

Ventricular asynergy and papillary muscle dysfunction (not rupture) may produce mild mitral regurgitation in association with heart failure. This causes a transient, soft, pan-systolic murmur in up to half of those with acute myocardial infarction. In these cases no specific treatment is necessary for the mitral regurgitation.

Cardiac rupture results in almost immediate cardiac tamponade and is usually fatal within a few minutes. Electromechanical dissociation, i.e. no pulse or cardiac output but a persistently normal rhythm on the ECG, is the classical presentation. Treatment is rarely successful.

Cardiogenic shock is an extreme form of cardiac failure or circulatory collapse. Its features and management are described on p. 498. The mortality from this condition is about 90%. The majority of those rescued have a complication that can be treated surgically (e.g. left ventricular aneurysm, torrential mitral regurgitation or ventricular septal perforation).

Thromboembolism
Bedrest and cardiac failure contribute to the common occurrence of thrombosis and embolism associated with myocardial infarction. Only 10% of patients have clinical features of thromboembolism, but in almost 50% of patients who die there is evidence of emboli. Deep venous thrombosis (see p. 549) is the most common manifestation, and pulmonary embolism may result from this. A left ventricular mural thrombus may form on the endocardial surface of the infarcted region. Such a thrombus is dislodged, forming a systemic embolus, in 15% of cases. Prophylactic anticoagulation with subcutaneous heparin probably reduces the risk of this complication.

Other complications
The shoulder–hand syndrome. This consists of pain and immobility of the left arm in the weeks and months following an acute myocardial infarction. Early mobilization reduces the incidence of this symptom and physiotherapy improves those symptoms that do occur.

Pericarditis. This is characterized by sharp chest pain and a pericardial rub. It frequently occurs in the first few days after an acute myocardial infarction, especially following anterior wall infarction. Anticoagulation should be avoided in these patients and anti-inflammatory medication is usually a successful treatment.

The post-myocardial infarction syndrome (Dressler's syndrome). This occurs weeks to months after an acute myocardial infarction, and consists of a combination of pericarditis, fever and a pericardial effusion. It is caused by an autoimmune response to damaged cardiac tissue and is more common after a second or subsequent myocardial infarction. Anti-inflammatory medication, including systemic corticosteroids, may be necessary. Anticoagulation should be avoided.

Left ventricular aneurysm. This is a late complication. Patients present with heart failure, arrhythmias or emboli. It is characterized by ventricular asynergy, often palpable as a double impulse, a fourth heart sound, persistent ST segment elevation on the ECG and sometimes a visible bulge on the chest x-ray. Treatment includes suitable anti-arrhythmic drugs, anticoagulants and medication for heart failure. Surgical removal of the aneurysm (aneurysmectomy) may be necessary if arrhythmias or embolic or haemodynamic complications occur.

REHABILITATION

If possible, full mobilization should be achieved within 1 week to 10 days to reduce the degree of physical and mental debility inflicted by this illness. Strong reassurance and constant encouragement is very important. Prior to discharge it is ideal to assess:
- The heart size (chest x-ray)
- The cardiovascular response to stress (limited or sub-maximal exercise test)

- An arrhythmia profile (24-h taped ECG)
- Ventricular function (echocardiogram or nuclear angiogram)

Any abnormalities that are detected should be treated appropriately.

In patients with recurrent angina, multiple infarctions or a positive stress test and in those under 40 years of age, early angiography is usually advised. Surgery is indicated for left main coronary artery occlusion and multiple vessel involvement.

Structured psychological and physical rehabilitation schemes are valuable but are only available in a few centres. Six to eight weeks following the myocardial infarction, the patient will probably be able to return to full-time employment and car driving. By this time the infarcted area will have been replaced by fibrous tissue.

Follow-up treatment
The patient may be discharged taking regular beta-blockade (e.g. propranolol 80 mg twice daily), which has been shown to reduce the incidence of sudden death in the 6 months following acute myocardial infarction. Timolol and metoprolol are similarly effective. There is a suggestion that long-term aspirin (75 mg daily) further reduces cardiac events following myocardial infarction, but there is little similar evidence for other antithrombotic and anticoagulant medications. Routine treatment with other anti-arrhythmic drugs has not proved beneficial in reducing the incidence of sudden death following myocardial infarction.

PROGNOSIS

Statistics concerning sudden death from acute myocardial infarction and from other cardiac causes are so often combined that it is difficult to accurately assess the mortality specifically from myocardial infarction. Assuming that all sudden unexpected cardiac death is due to myocardial infarction, then about 50% of those who die do so within the first 2–3 h, and 75% of the deaths occur within 24 h. Of those who leave hospital alive, about 15–25% die in the first year, and thereafter the annual mortality is 5–10%. Fifty per cent of myocardial infarction victims survive for 10 years. Factors suggesting an unfavourable prognosis include a large myocardial infarction, heart failure, a large heart on chest x-ray, ventricular arrhythmias, multiple infarctions and recurrent angina.

Rheumatic fever

Rheumatic fever is an inflammatory disease that occurs in children and young adults (the first attack usually occurs between 5 and 15 years of age) as a result of infection with group A *Streptococcus*. It affects the heart, skin, joints and central nervous system. It is common in the Middle East, Far East, eastern Europe and South America, but it is now rare in the UK, western Europe and North America. This decline in the incidence of rheumatic fever (from 10% of children in the 1920s to 0.01% today) parallels the reduction in all streptococcal infections and is largely due to improved sanitation and also to the use of antibiotics.

Pharyngeal infection with group A *Streptococcus* may be followed by the clinical syndrome of rheumatic fever. This is thought to develop because of an autoimmune reaction triggered by the infecting *Streptococcus*. The condition is not due to direct infection of the heart or to the production of a toxin.

PATHOLOGY

All three layers of the heart may be affected. The characteristic lesion of rheumatic carditis is the Aschoff nodule, which is a granulomatous lesion with a central necrotic area occurring in the myocardium, particularly in the subendocardium of the left ventricle. Small, warty vegetations may develop on the endocardium, particularly on the heart valves. This leads to some degree of valvular regurgitation. A serofibrinous effusion characterizes the acute pericarditis that occurs.

The synovial membranes are acutely inflamed during rheumatic fever, and subcutaneous nodules (which are also granulomatous lesions) are seen in the acute stage of the disease.

CLINICAL FEATURES

The disease presents suddenly, with fever, joint pains, malaise and loss of appetite. The clinical features depend on the organs that are involved. Diagnosis relies on the presence of two or more major clinical manifestations or one major manifestation plus two or more minor features. These are known as the Duckett–Jones criteria (see Table 11.28).

Carditis manifests as:
- New or changed heart murmurs
- The development of cardiac enlargement or cardiac failure
- The appearance of a pericardial effusion and ECG changes of pericarditis (raised ST segments) or myocarditis (inverted or flattened T waves, first

Table 11.28 Revised Duckett–Jones criteria for the diagnosis of rheumatic fever. The diagnosis is made on the basis of two or more major criteria, or one major plus two or more minor criteria.

Major criteria
Carditis
Polyarthritis
Chorea
Erythema marginatum
Subcutaneous nodules

Minor criteria
Fever
Arthralgia
Previous rheumatic fever
Raised ESR
Leucocytosis
Prolonged PR interval on ECG

Plus evidence of antecedent streptococcal infection, e.g. positive throat cultures for group A streptococcus, elevated ASO titre (>250 units) or other streptococcal antibodies, or a history of recent scarlet fever

degree or greater AV block or other cardiac arrhythmias
- A transient diastolic mitral (Carey–Coombs) murmur due to mitral valvulitis

Non-cardiac features include the following:
- A fever with an apparently excessive tachycardia is usually present.
- The arthritis associated with rheumatic fever is classically a fleeting polyarthritis affecting large joints such as the knees, elbows, ankles and wrists. The joints are swollen, red and tender. As the inflammation in one joint recedes, another becomes affected. Once the acute inflammation disappears, the rheumatic process leaves the joints normal.
- Sydenham's chorea (or St Vitus' dance) (see p. 832) is involvement of the central nervous system which develops late after a streptococcal infection. Sufferers are noticeably 'fidgety' and display spasmodic, unintentional movements. Speech is often affected.
- Skin manifestations include erythema marginatum, a transient pink rash with slightly raised edges, which occurs in 20% of cases. The erythematous areas found mostly on the trunk and limbs coalesce into crescent- or ring-shaped patches. Subcutaneous nodules, which are painless, pea-sized, hard nodules beneath the skin, may also occur, particularly over tendons, joints and bony prominences.

INVESTIGATION

- Throat swabs are cultured for the group A *Streptococcus*.

- Serological changes may indicate a recent streptoccocal infection. The antistreptolysin O titre, and sometimes others such as the anti-streptokinase titre, are performed.
- Non-specific indicators of inflammation such as the ESR and the C-reactive protein levels are usually elevated.

TREATMENT

Patients with fever, active arthritis or active carditis should be completely rested in bed. When the clinical syndrome has subsided (e.g. no pyrexia, normal pulse rate, normal ESR, normal white count) the patient may be mobilized.

Residual streptococcal infections should be eradicated with a single intramuscular injection of 916 mg of benzathine penicillin or oral phenoxymethyl penicillin 500 mg four times daily for 1 week. This therapy should be administered even if nasal or pharyngeal swabs do not culture the *Streptococcus*.

High-dose salicylate (preferably acetyl salicylate, i.e. aspirin) therapy is given to the limit of tolerance determined by the development of tinnitus. If carditis is present, systemic corticosteroids may be given. Prednisolone 60–120 mg in four divided doses each day is administered until the clinical syndrome is improved and the ESR has fallen to normal. Steroids are then tapered off over 2–4 weeks. However, the efficacy of steroids is in doubt.

Recurrences are most common when persistent cardiac damage is present, and are prevented by the continued administration of oral phenoxymethyl penicillin 250 mg daily or by monthly injections of 916 mg of benzathine penicillin until the age of 20 or for 5 years after the latest attack (see p. 12). A sulphonamide (e.g. sulphadimidine) may be used if the patient is allergic to penicillin. Any streptococcal infection that does develop should be very promptly treated.

Chronic rheumatic heart disease

More than 50% of those who suffer acute rheumatic fever *with carditis* will later (after 10–20 years) develop chronic rheumatic valvular disease, predominantly affecting the mitral and aortic valves (see Table 11.29).

Table 11.29 Rheumatic valvular lesions.

Valves involved	% of cases
Mitral valve alone	50
Mitral and aortic valves	40
Mitral, aortic and tricuspid	5
Aortic valve alone	2
All other combinations	3

Valvular heart disease

MITRAL STENOSIS

Almost all mitral stenosis is due to rheumatic heart disease:

- At least 50% of sufferers have a history of rheumatic fever or chorea.
- The single most common valve lesion due to rheumatic fever is pure mitral stenosis (50%)
- The mitral valve is affected in over 90% of those with rheumatic valvular heart disease
- Rheumatic mitral stenosis is much more common in women.
- The pathological process results after some years in valve thickening, cusp fusion, calcium deposition, a narrowed (stenotic) valve orifice and progressive immobility of the valve cusps.

Other causes

- Lutembacher's syndrome is the combination of acquired mitral stenosis and an atrial septal defect.
- A rare form of congenital mitral stenosis can occur.
- In the elderly a syndrome similar to mitral stenosis can develop because of calcification and fibrosis of the valve, valve ring and subvalvular apparatus (chordae tendineae).

PATHOPHYSIOLOGY

When the normal valve orifice area of 5 cm^2 is reduced to approximately 1 cm^2, severe mitral stenosis is present. In order that sufficient cardiac output will be maintained, the left atrial pressure increases and left atrial hypertrophy and dilatation occurs. Consequently, pulmonary venous, pulmonary arterial and right heart pressures also increase. The increase in pulmonary capillary pressure is followed by the development of pulmonary oedema. This is partially prevented by alveolar and capillary thickening and pulmonary arterial vasoconstriction (reactive pulmonary hypertension). Pulmonary hypertension leads to right ventricular hypertrophy, dilatation and failure. Right ventricular dilatation results in tricuspid regurgitation. The complications of mitral stenosis (see Table 11.30) are frequent.

SYMPTOMS

Usually there are no symptoms until the valve orifice is moderately stenosed, i.e. has an area of 2 cm^2. In Europe this does not usually occur until several decades after the first attack of rheumatic fever, but in the Middle or Far East, children of 10–20 years of age may have severe calcific mitral stenosis.

Table 11.30 Complications of mitral stenosis.

Atrial fibrillation
Systemic embolization
Pulmonary hypertension
Pulmonary infarction
Chest infections
Infective endocarditis (rare)
Tricuspid regurgitation
Right ventricular failure

Because of pulmonary venous hypertension and recurrent bronchitis, progressively severe dyspnoea develops. A cough productive of blood-tinged, frothy sputum is quite common, and occasionally frank haemoptysis may occur. The development of pulmonary hypertension eventually leads to right heart failure and its symptoms of weakness, fatigue and abdominal or lower limb swelling.

The large left atrium favours atrial fibrillation, giving rise to symptoms such as palpitations. Atrial fibrillation may result in systemic and pulmonary emboli, which give rise to cerebral, mesenteric, renal and pulmonary infarcts.

SIGNS

Face
Severe mitral stenosis with pulmonary hypertension is associated with the so-called mitral facies or malar flush. This is a bilateral, cyanotic or dusky pink discoloration over the upper cheeks which is due to arteriovenous anastamoses and vascular stasis.

Pulse
At first the pulse is regular (sinus rhythm) but later the irregular pulse of atrial fibrillation usually develops. The onset of atrial fibrillation often causes a dramatic clinical deterioration.

Jugular veins
If right heart failure develops there is obvious distension of the jugular veins. If pulmonary hypertension or tricuspid stenosis is present, the *a* wave will be prominent provided that atrial fibrillation has not supervened.

Apex beat
The apex beat is 'tapping' in quality. This is the result of a palpable first heart sound combined with left ventricular backward displacement produced by an enlarging right ventricle. A diastolic thrill may be felt at the apex. If pulmonary hypertension is present the closure of the pulmonary valve may be felt in the second left intercostal space to the side of the

Mitral regurgitation

Mitral stenosis

Murmurs heard best with patient on left side

Fig. 11.57 Auscultatory features associated with mitral regurgitation and mitral stenosis. S_1 = first heart sound; S_2 = second heart sound; S_3 = third heart sound; OS = opening snap; A_2 = aortic component of the second heart sound; P_2 = pulmonary component of the second heart sound; PSM = pansystolic murmur; MDM = mid-diastolic murmur; PSA = presystolic accentuation.

sternum. A parasternal heave due to right ventricular hypertrophy may also be felt.

Auscultation

Auscultation (see Fig. 11.57) reveals a loud first heart sound because the cusps are kept open until the beginning of ventricular systole. In early diastole a sound is produced when the mitral valve opens (opening snap). This is followed by a diastolic rumbling murmur, usually localized to the apex and best heard with the patient inclined towards the left. The murmur is due to turbulent blood flow through the narrowed valve. If the patient is in sinus rhythm the murmur becomes louder when atrial systole occurs. This is called pre-systolic accentuation.

The severity of mitral stenosis is judged by the closeness of the opening snap and the following diastolic murmur to the second heart sound. In severe mitral stenosis the very high left atrial pressure opens the mitral valve earlier in diastole.

As the valve cusps become immobile, the loud first heart sound softens and the opening snap disappears. When pulmonary hypertension occurs, the pulmonary component of the second sound is increased in intensity and the mitral diastolic murmur may become quieter because of the reduction of cardiac output.

INVESTIGATION

Chest x-ray

The chest x-ray usually shows a generally small heart with an enlarged left atrium (see Fig. 11.11 and p. 462). Pulmonary venous hypertension (see p. 464) is usually also present. Late in the course of the disease a calcified mitral valve may be seen on a penetrated or lateral view. The signs of pulmonary oedema or pulmonary hypertension may also be apparent when the disease is severe.

ECG

In sinus rhythm the ECG shows a bifid P wave due to delayed left atrial activation (Fig. 11.58). This double-humped P wave is best seen in leads II, V_3 and V_4. A biphasic P wave with a large late negative component is seen in lead V_1 (Fig. 11.59). However, atrial fibrillation is frequently present. As the disease pro-

	Lead II	Lead V_1
Normal P wave		
P mitrale (left atrial hypertrophy)		
P pulmonale (right atrial hypertrophy)		
Retrograde P wave		

Fig. 11.58 A bifid P wave as seen on the ECG in mitral stenosis (P mitrale). Also shown for comparison are other P wave abnormalities.

gresses, the ECG features of right ventricular hypertrophy (right axis deviation and perhaps tall R waves in lead V_1) may develop (Fig. 11.59).

Echocardiogram

The echocardiogram is very useful for the diagnosis and assessment of mitral stenosis. The movement of the valve cusps and the rate of diastolic filling of the left ventricle may be measured—severe mitral stenosis produces immobility of the valve cusps and slow filling of the ventricles (see Fig. 11.22, p. 471). The echocardiogram appearances are usually sufficiently accurate to allow surgical management to be considered.

Cardiac catheterization

This is only required if an adequate echocardiogram is impossible to obtain or if coexisting cardiac problems (e.g. mitral regurgitation or coronary artery disease) are suspected. The typical findings in mitral stenosis are a diastolic pressure that is higher in the left atrium than in the left ventricle (Fig. 11.60). This gradient of pressure is usually proportional to the degree of the stenosis.

TREATMENT

Mild mitral stenosis may need no treatment other than prompt therapy of attacks of bronchitis. Although infective endocarditis in pure mitral stenosis is uncommon, antibiotic prophylaxis is

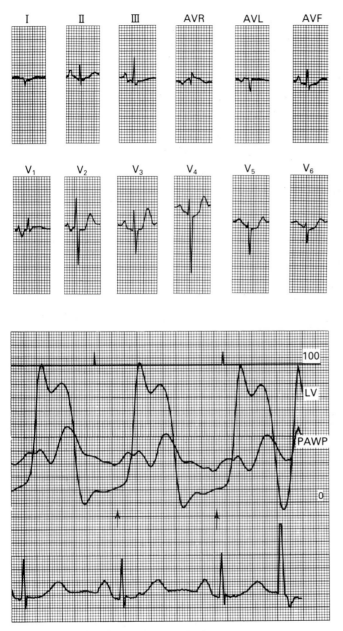

I   II   III   AVR   AVL   AVF

Fig. 11.59 A 12-lead ECG of a patient with severe mitral stenosis. Note the right axis deviation (frontal plane axis = +120°), the left atrial conduction abnormality (large terminal negative component of the P wave in V_1) and the right ventricular hypertrophy (R wave in V_1 and right axis deviation).

V_1 V_2 V_3 V_4 V_5 V_6

100

LV

PAWP

0

Fig. 11.60 Simultaneous recordings of the ECG, the left ventricular (LV) and the pulmonary arterial wedge pressure (PAWP). The PAWP is almost equivalent to the left atrial pressure. Thus at end-diastole (the onset of the QRS complex) the PAWP is significantly higher than the left ventricular pressure (arrows). The pressure gradient is due to mitral valve stenosis.

advised (see p. 527). Early symptoms of mitral stenosis such as mild dyspnoea can usually be treated with low doses of diuretics. The onset of atrial fibrillation requires treatment with digoxin and anticoagulation to prevent atrial thrombus and systemic embolization. If pulmonary hypertension develops or the symptoms of pulmonary congestion persist despite therapy, surgical relief of the mitral stenosis is advised. There are three types of operation: closed valvotomy, open valvotomy and mitral valve replacement.

Closed valvotomy

This operation is advised for patients with mobile, non-calcified and non-regurgitant mitral valves. The fused cusps are forced apart by a dilator introduced through the apex of the left ventricle and guided into position by the surgeon's finger inserted via the left atrial appendage. Cardiopulmonary bypass is not needed for this operation. Closed valvotomy may produce a good result for 10 or more years. The valve cusps often re-fuse and eventually another operation may be necessary.

Open valvotomy

This operation is often preferred to closed valvotomy. The cusps are carefully dissected apart under direct vision. Cardiopulmonary bypass is required. Open dissection reduces the likelihood of causing traumatic mitral regurgitation.

Mitral valve replacement

Replacement of the mitral valve is necessary:
- If mitral regurgitation is also present
- If there is a badly diseased or badly calcified stenotic valve (which cannot be reopened without producing significant regurgitation)

Artificial valves may work successfully for more than 20 years. Anticoagulants are generally necessary to prevent the formation of thrombus, which might obstruct the valve or embolize.

MITRAL REGURGITATION

Of the many causes of mitral valve regurgitation, rheumatic heart disease (50%) and the prolapsing mitral valve are the most common. Any disease that causes dilatation of the left ventricle may cause mild mitral regurgitation, e.g.:
- Aortic valve disease
- Acute rheumatic fever
- Myocarditis
- Cardiomyopathy
- Hypertensive heart disease
- Ischaemic heart disease

Other causes
- In hypertrophic cardiomyopathy, left ventricular contraction is disorganized and mitral regurgitation often results.
- It may follow myocardial infarction or infective endocarditis.
- It may occur in connective tissue disorders such as systemic lupus erythematosus.
- Collagen abnormalities such as Marfan's syndrome and Ehlers–Danlos syndrome may be associated with mitral regurgitation.
- Degeneration of the valve cusps or mitral annular calcification may result in regurgitation.
- Rupture of the chordae tendineae (due to myocardial infarction or trauma) and infective endocarditis may cause very sudden mitral regurgitation.

PATHOPHYSIOLOGY

Regurgitation into the left atrium produces left atrial dilatation but little increase in left atrial pressure if the regurgitation is long standing as the regurgitant flow is accommodated by the large left atrium. With acute mitral regurgitation the normal compliance of the left atrium does not allow much dilatation and the left atrial pressure rises. Thus, in acute mitral regurgitation the left atrial *v* wave is greatly increased and pulmonary venous pressure rises to produce pulmonary oedema.

Since a proportion of the stroke volume is regurgitated, the stroke volume increases to maintain the forward cardiac output and the left ventricle therefore enlarges.

SYMPTOMS

Mitral regurgitation can be present for many years and the cardiac dimensions may be greatly increased before any symptoms occur. The increased stroke volume may be sensed as a 'palpitation'. Dyspnoea and orthopnoea may develop due to pulmonary venous hypertension occurring as a direct result of the mitral regurgitation and secondarily to left ventricular failure. Fatigue and lethargy develop because of the reduced cardiac output. In the late stages of the disease the symptoms of right heart failure also occur and eventually congestive cardiac failure. Cardiac cachexia may develop. Thromboembolism is less common than in mitral stenosis, but subacute infective endocarditis is much more common.

SIGNS

The physical signs (Fig. 11.57) of uncomplicated mitral regurgitation are:
- A laterally displaced, thrusting, diffuse apex beat and a systolic thrill
- A soft first heart sound because of the incomplete apposition of the valve cusps and their partial closure by the time ventricular systole begins
- A pan-systolic murmur due to regurgitation occurring throughout the whole of systole, which is loudest at the apex but radiates widely over the precordium and into the axilla
- A prominent third heart sound occurs because of the sudden rush of blood back into the dilated left ventricle in early diastole. Sometimes a short mid-diastolic flow murmur may follow the third heart sound.

The signs related to atrial fibrillation, pulmonary hypertension, and left and right heart failure may develop later in the disease. The onset of atrial fibrillation has a much less dramatic effect on symptoms than in mitral stenosis.

INVESTIGATION

Chest x-ray

The chest x-ray may show left atrial and left ventricular enlargement. There is an increase in the cardiothoracic ratio, and valve calcification may be seen.

ECG

The ECG shows the features of left atrial delay (bifid P waves) and left ventricular hypertrophy (see Fig. 11.61) as manifest by tall R waves in the left lateral leads, e.g. leads I, AVL and V_6, and deep S waves in the right-sided precordial leads, e.g. leads V_1 and V_2. (SV_1 plus RV_5 or RV_6 >35 mm indicates left ventricular hypertrophy.) Left ventricular hypertrophy occurs in about 50% of patients with mitral regurgitation. Atrial fibrillation may be present.

Echocardiogram

The echocardiogram shows a dilated left atrium and left ventricle. There may be specific features of chordal or papillary muscle rupture.

Cardiac catheterization

This demonstrates a prominent left atrial systolic pressure wave, and when contrast is injected into the left ventricle it may be seen regurgitating into an enlarged left atrium during systole.

TREATMENT

The development of symptoms usually dictates the need for treatment. Mild mitral regurgitation can usually be managed medically with diuretics for pulmonary congestion, and with digoxin, and possibly anticoagulation, for atrial fibrillation. Antibiotic prophylaxis against bacterial endocarditis is mandatory (see p. 12).

More severe symptoms that are unresponsive to medical therapy require mitral valve replacement or, occasionally, operative repair of the mitral valve. Rarely, progressive left ventricular enlargement in a relatively asymptomatic patient may indicate that surgery is necessary. Sudden torrential mitral regurgitation, as seen with chordal or papillary rupture or infective endocarditis, may necessitate emergency mitral valve replacement.

Prolapsing (billowing) mitral valve

This is also known as Barlow's syndrome or floppy mitral valve. It is due to excessively large mitral valve leaflets, an enlarged mitral annulus, abnormally long chordae or disordered papillary muscle contraction. Histology may demonstrate myxomatous degeneration of the mitral valve leaflets. It is more commonly seen in young women than in men or older women and it has a familial incidence. Its cause is usually unknown but it may be due to Marfan's syndrome, thyrotoxicosis, or rheumatic or ischaemic heart disease. It also occurs in association with atrial septal defect and as part of hypertrophic cardiomyopathy. Mild mitral valve prolapse is so common that it should be regarded as a normal variant.

PATHOPHYSIOLOGY

During ventricular systole, a mitral valve leaflet (most commonly the posterior leaflet) prolapses into the left atrium. This may result in abnormal ventricular contraction, papillary muscle strain and some mitral regurgitation. Usually the syndrome is not haemodynamically serious. Thromboembolism may occur.

SYMPTOMS

Atypical chest pain is the most common symptom. Usually the pain is left submammary and stabbing in

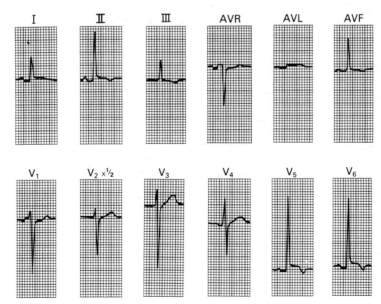

Fig. 11.61 A 12-lead ECG showing features of left ventricular hypertrophy. Note the size of the S wave in V_1 (26 mm).

quality. Sometimes it is substernal, aching and severe. Rarely it is similar to typical angina pectoris. Palpitations may be experienced because of the abnormal ventricular contraction or because of the atrial and ventricular arrhythmias that are commonly associated with mitral valve prolapse.

SIGNS

The most common sign is a mid-systolic click, which is produced by the sudden prolapse of the valve and the tensing of the chordae tendineae that occurs during systole. This may be followed by a late systolic murmur due to some regurgitation. Sometimes, pan-systolic mitral regurgitation occurs. The signs typically fade quickly but return later.

INVESTIGATION

Chest x-ray
The chest x-ray is usually normal unless significant mitral regurgitation is present.

ECG
The ECG is often abnormal with inverted or biphasic T waves in the inferior leads (leads II, III and AVF) and in the left lateral precordial leads (leads V_5 and V_6). The ST segment may also be slightly depressed in these leads.

Echocardiogram
The echocardiogram typically shows posterior movement of one or both mitral valve cusps into the left atrium during systole.

Cardiac catheterization
Contrast angiograms performed during cardiac catheterization reveal the systolic prolapse of the mitral valve into the left atrium, and mitral regurgitation, if present, is seen.

TREATMENT

Usually, beta-blockade is effective for the treatment of the atypical chest pain and palpitations. Sometimes more specific anti-arrhythmic drug treatment is necessary. When a prolapsing mitral valve is associated with significant mitral regurgitation and atrial fibrillation, anticoagulation is advised to prevent thromboembolism. Very occasionally, mitral valve replacement may be necessary for severe regurgitation. Prophylaxis against endocarditis (see p. 12) is advised if there is significant mitral valve regurgitation.

AORTIC STENOSIS

There are three causes of aortic valve stenosis:
- Congenital aortic valve stenosis develops pro-

gressively because of turbulent blood flow through a congenitally abnormal (usually bicuspid) aortic valve. Most congenitally abnormal aortic valves occur in men.
- Rheumatic fever results in progressive fusion, thickening and calcification of a previously normal three-cusped aortic valve. In rheumatic heart disease the aortic valve is affected in about 45% of cases. Usually there is associated mitral valve disease.
- The wear and tear of age may lead to arteriosclerotic degeneration and calcification of the aortic valve. It is not usually severely stenotic and symptoms are not usually present.

Valvular aortic stenosis should be distinguished from other causes of obstruction to left ventricular emptying (Fig. 11.62), which include:
- Supravalvular obstruction—a congenital fibrous diaphragm above the aortic valve
- Hypertrophic cardiomyopathy—septal muscle hypertrophy obstructs left ventricular outflow
- Subvalvular aortic stenosis—a congenital condition in which a fibrous ridge or diaphragm is situated immediately below the aortic valve

PATHOPHYSIOLOGY

Obstructed left ventricular emptying leads to increased left ventricular pressure and compensatory left ventricular hypertrophy. In turn, this results in relative ischaemia of the left ventricular myocardium, and consequent angina, arrhythmias and left ventricular failure. The obstruction to left ventricular emptying is relatively more severe on exercise. Normally, exercise causes a many-fold increase in cardiac output, but when there is severe narrowing of

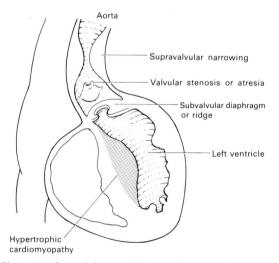

Fig. 11.62 Several forms of left ventricular outflow tract obstruction.

the aortic valve orifice the cardiac output can hardly increase. Thus, the blood pressure falls, coronary ischaemia worsens, the myocardium fails and cardiac arrhythmias develop particularly on exercise.

SYMPTOMS

There are usually no symptoms until aortic stenosis is moderately severe (when the aortic orifice is reduced to one-third of its normal size). At this stage, exercise-induced syncope, angina and dyspnoea may develop. When symptoms occur, the prognosis is poor—on average, death occurs within 2–3 years if there has been no surgical intervention.

SIGNS

Aortic stenosis is characterized by abnormalities of the pulse, precordial pulsation and auscultation.

Pulse
The carotid pulse is slow rising or plateau in nature (see p. 454).

Precordial palpation
The apex beat is not usually displaced because hypertrophy (as opposed to dilatation) does not produce noticeable cardiomegaly. However, the pulsation is sustained and obvious—a *heaving apex beat*. A double impulse is sometimes felt because the fourth heart sound or atrial contraction ('kick') may be palpable. A systolic thrill may be felt in the aortic area.

Auscultation (see Fig. 11.63)
The most obvious auscultatory finding in aortic stenosis is a mid-systolic ejection murmur that is usually 'diamond' shaped (crescendo–decrescendo). The murmur is usually longer when the disease is more severe, as a longer left ventricular ejection time is needed. The intensity of the murmur is not a good guide to the severity of the condition because it is lessened by a reduced cardiac output. The murmur is usually rough in quality and best heard in the aortic area. It radiates widely and is usually easily heard over the clavicles and the carotid arteries.

Other findings
- A systolic ejection click (see p. 460), unless the valve has become immobile and calcified
- Soft or inaudible aortic second heart sound when the aortic valve becomes immobile
- Reversed splitting of the second heart sound (splitting on expiration) (see p. 459)
- A prominent fourth heart sound (see p. 459), unless coexisting mitral stenosis prevents this

Degenerative disease of the aortic valve (aortic sclerosis) results in a loud mid-systolic murmur but, because there is little stenosis, there are no signs of left ventricular hypertrophy or of a slow rising pulse. This murmur can be ignored.

INVESTIGATION

Chest x-ray
The chest x-ray usually reveals a relatively small heart with a prominent, dilated, ascending aorta. This occurs because turbulent blood flow above the stenosed aortic valve produces so-called 'post-stenotic dilatation'. The aortic valve may be calcified. When heart failure occurs, the cardiothoracic ratio increases.

ECG
The ECG shows left ventricular hypertrophy and left atrial delay. A left ventricular 'strain' pattern due to 'pressure overload' (depressed ST segments and T wave inversion in leads orientated towards the left ventricle, i.e. leads I, AVL, V_5 and V_6) is common when the disease is severe. Usually, sinus rhythm is present, but ventricular arrhythmias may be recorded.

Echocardiogram
The echocardiogram readily demonstrates the thickened, calcified and immobile aortic valve cusps (see Fig. 11.64). Left ventricular hypertrophy may also be seen.

Cardiac catheterization
Cardiac catheterization is used to document the systolic pressure difference (gradient) between the

Fig. **11.63** Auscultatory features of aortic stenosis and aortic regurgitation. S_1 = first heart sound; S_2 = second heart sound; EC = ejection click; MSM = mid-systolic murmur; EDM = early diastolic murmur.

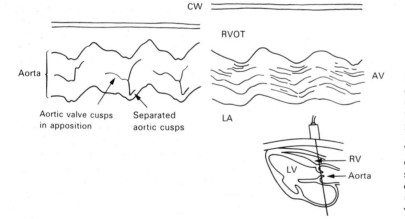

Fig. 11.64 An M-mode echocardiogram showing a normal (left) and stenotic (right) aortic valve. CW = chest wall; RVOT = right ventricular outflow tract; AV = aortic valve; LA = left atrium. There are multiple dense linear echoes in the aortic root. The inset shows the anatomical path of the echo beam through the chest. RV = right ventricle; LV = left ventricle.

aorta and the left ventricle (Fig. 11.65). A gradient of 50 mmHg or more is usually sufficient to advise surgery. A trivial degree of aortic regurgitation which is undetectable clinically is often demonstrated by contrast aortography. Coronary angiography is important before recommending surgery.

TREATMENT

Patients with aortic stenosis should not overly exert themselves, and in particular they should not compete in strenuous physical games. Angina is best treated with beta-blockade because vasodilators such as glyceryl trinitrate or isosorbide dinitrate may aggravate exertional syncope. Antibiotic prophylaxis against infective endocarditis is essential (see p. 12).

Irrespective of symptoms, aortic valve replacement with a prosthetic or tissue valve is recommended when aortic stenosis is severe. Cardiopulmonary bypass is necessary to achieve this. Provided that the valve is not severely deformed or heavily calcified, critical aortic stenosis in childhood or adolescence can be treated by valvotomy (performed under direct vision by the surgeon or by balloon dilatation using x-ray visualization). This produces temporary relief from the obstruction. Aortic valve replacement will usually be needed a few years later.

Fig. 11.65 ECG and pressure trace as a cardiac catheter is withdrawn from the left ventricle (LV) to the aorta (AO). Note that the peak systolic pressure changes from 250 to 130 mmHg (arrow). The 120 mmHg peak-to-peak systolic gradient indicates severe aortic valvular stenosis.

AORTIC REGURGITATION

The most common causes of aortic regurgitation are rheumatic fever and infective endocarditis complicating a previously damaged valve. This can be a congenitally abnormal valve (e.g. a bicuspid valve) or one damaged by rheumatic fever. There are numerous other causes and associations (see Table 11.31). The majority of patients with aortic regurgitation are men (75%), but rheumatic aortic regurgitation occurs more commonly in women.

Table 11.31 Causes and associations of aortic regurgitation.

Acute aortic regurgitation
Acute rheumatic fever
Infective endocarditis
Dissection of the aorta
Ruptured sinus of Valsalva aneurysm
Failure of prosthetic heart valve
Chronic aortic regurgitation
Rheumatic heart disease
Syphilis
Arthritides
Reiter's syndrome
Ankylosing spondylitis
Rheumatoid arthritis
Hypertension (severe)
Bicuspid aortic valve
Aortic endocarditis
Marfan's syndrome
Osteogenesis imperfecta

PATHOPHYSIOLOGY

Aortic regurgitation is reflux of blood from the aorta through the aortic valve into the left ventricle during diastole. If net cardiac output is to be maintained, the total volume of blood pumped into the aorta must increase, and consequently the left ventricular size must enlarge. Because of the aortic run-off during diastole, diastolic blood pressure falls and coronary perfusion is decreased. In addition, the larger left ventricular size is mechanically less efficient so that the demand for oxygen is more, and cardiac ischaemia develops.

SYMPTOMS

In aortic regurgitation significant symptoms occur late and do not develop until left ventricular failure occurs. As with mitral regurgitation, a common symptom is 'pounding of the heart' because of the increased left ventricular size and its vigorous pulsation. Angina pectoris is a frequent complaint. Varying grades of dyspnoea occur depending on the extent of left ventricular dilatation and dysfunction. Arrhythmias are relatively uncommon.

SIGNS

The signs of aortic regurgitation are many and are due to the hyperdynamic circulation, reflux of blood into the left ventricle and the increased left ventricular size.

The pulse is bounding or collapsing (see p. 454). The following signs, which are rare, also indicate a hyperdynamic circulation:

- Quincke's sign—capillary pulsation in the nail beds
- De Musset's sign—head nodding with each heart beat

- Durozier's sign—systolic bruit over the femoral arteries when the stethoscope is lightly applied
- Pistol shot femorals—a sharp bang heard on auscultation over the femoral arteries in time with each heart beat

The apex beat is displaced laterally and downwards and is thrusting in quality.

On auscultation there is a high-pitched diastolic murmur running from the aortic component of the second heart sound (Fig. 11.63). It is loudest in early diastole and is heard best at the lower left sternal edge or the cardiac apex.

INVESTIGATION

Chest x-ray
The chest x-ray features are those of left ventricular enlargement and possibly of dilatation of the ascending aorta. The ascending aortic wall may be calcified in syphilis and the aortic valve may be calcified if valvular disease is responsible for the regurgitation.

ECG
The ECG appearances are those of left ventricular hypertrophy due to 'volume overload', i.e. tall R waves and deeply inverted T waves in the left-sided leads, and deep S waves in the right-sided leads. Normally, sinus rhythm is present.

Echocardiogram
The echocardiogram demonstrates vigorous cardiac contraction and a dilated left ventricle. The aortic root may also be enlarged. Diastolic fluttering of the mitral leaflets or septum occurs in severe aortic regurgitation (producing the Austin Flint murmur, see p. 461).

Cardiac catheterization
During cardiac catheterization, injection of contrast medium into the aorta (aortography) will outline aortic valvular abnormalities and allow assessment of the degree of regurgitation.

TREATMENT

The underlying cause of aortic regurgitation (e.g. syphilitic aortitis or infective endocarditis) may require specific treatment. The treatment of aortic regurgitation usually requires aortic valve replacement but the timing of surgery is important.

Because symptoms do not develop until the myocardium fails and because the myocardium does not recover fully after surgery, it is important to operate before significant symptoms occur. The timing of the operation is best determined according to haemodynamic, echocardiographic or nuclear angiographic criteria.

Both mechanical prostheses and tissue valves are used. Tissue valves are preferred in the elderly and when anticoagulants must be avoided, but are contraindicated in children and young adults because of the rapid calcification and degeneration of the valves.

Antibiotic prophylaxis against infective endocarditis (see p. 12) is necessary even if a prosthetic valve replacement has been performed.

TRICUSPID STENOSIS

This uncommon valve lesion, which is seen much more often in women than in men, is usually due to rheumatic heart disease and is frequently associated with mitral and/or aortic valve disease. Tricuspid stenosis is also seen in the carcinoid syndrome.

PATHOPHYSIOLOGY

Tricuspid valve stenosis results in a reduced cardiac output, which is restored towards normal when the right atrial pressure increases. The resulting systemic venous congestion produces hepatomegaly, ascites and dependent oedema.

SYMPTOMS

Usually, patients with tricuspid stenosis complain of symptoms due to the associated left-sided rheumatic valve lesions. The abdominal pain (due to hepatomegaly) and swelling (due to ascites) and peripheral oedema which occur are relatively severe when compared with the degree of dyspnoea.

SIGNS

If the patient remains in sinus rhythm, which is unusual, there is a prominent jugular venous 'a' wave. This presystolic pulsation may also be felt over the liver. There is usually a rumbling mid-diastolic murmur, which is heard best at the lower left sternal edge and is louder on inspiration. It may be missed because of the murmur of coexisting mitral stenosis. A tricuspid opening snap may occasionally be heard.

Hepatomegaly, abdominal ascites and dependent oedema may be present.

INVESTIGATION

Chest x-ray
On the chest x-ray there may be a prominent right atrial bulge.

ECG
The enlarged right atrium may be manifest on the ECG by peaked, tall P waves (≥3 mm) in lead 2.

Echocardiogram
The echocardiogram may show a thickened and

immobile tricuspid valve, but this is not so clearly seen as an abnormal mitral valve.

Cardiac catheterization
This demonstrates a diastolic pressure gradient between the right atrium and the right ventricle. Contrast injection will demonstrate a large right atrium.

TREATMENT

Medical management consists of diuretic therapy and salt restriction. Tricuspid valvotomy is occasionally possible, but tricuspid valve replacement is often necessary. Other valves usually also need replacement because tricuspid valve stenosis is rarely an isolated lesion.

TRICUSPID REGURGITATION

Functional tricuspid regurgitation may occur whenever the right ventricle dilates, e.g. in cor pulmonale, myocardial infarction or pulmonary hypertension.

Organic tricuspid regurgitation may occur with rheumatic heart disease, infective endocarditis, carcinoid syndrome, Ebstein's anomaly (a congenitally malpositioned tricuspid valve) and other congenital abnormalities of the atrioventricular valves.

SYMPTOMS AND SIGNS

The valvular regurgitation gives rise to high right atrial and systemic venous pressure. Patients may complain of the symptoms of right heart failure.

Physical signs include a large jugular venous *cv* wave and a palpable liver that pulsates in systole. Usually a right ventricular impulse may be felt at the left sternal edge, and there is a blowing pan-systolic murmur, best heard on inspiration at the lower left sternal edge. Atrial fibrillation is common.

TREATMENT

Functional tricuspid regurgitation usually disappears with medical management. Severe organic tricuspid regurgitation may require operative repair of the tricuspid valve (annuloplasty or plication). Very occasionally, tricuspid valve replacement may be necessary. In drug addicts with infective endocarditis of the tricuspid valve, surgical removal of the valve is recommended to eradicate the infection. This is usually well tolerated in the short term. The insertion of prosthetic valves for this condition is considered later.

PULMONARY STENOSIS

This is usually a congenital lesion, but it may rarely result from rheumatic fever or from the carcinoid syndrome. Congenital pulmonary stenosis may be associated with an intact ventricular septum or with a ventricular septal defect (Fallot's tetralogy).

Pulmonary stenosis may be valvular, subvalvular or supravalvular. Multiple congenital pulmonary arterial stenoses are usually due to infection with rubella during pregnancy.

SYMPTOMS AND SIGNS

The obstruction to right ventricular emptying results in right ventricular hypertrophy which in turn leads to right atrial hypertrophy. Severe pulmonary obstruction may be incompatible with life, but lesser degrees of obstruction give rise to fatigue, syncope and the symptoms of right heart failure. Mild pulmonary stenosis may be asymptomatic.

The physical signs are characterized by a harsh mid-systolic ejection murmur, best heard on inspiration to the left of the sternum in the second intercostal space. This murmur is often associated with a thrill. The pulmonary closure sound is usually delayed and soft. There may be a pulmonary ejection sound if the obstruction is valvular. A right ventricular fourth sound and a prominent jugular venous 'a' wave are present when the stenosis is moderately severe. A right ventricular heave may be felt.

INVESTIGATION

Chest x-ray
The chest x-ray usually shows a prominent pulmonary artery due to post-stenotic dilatation.

ECG
The ECG demonstrates both right atrial and right ventricular hypertrophy, although it may sometimes be normal even in severe pulmonary stenosis.

Cardiac catheterization
The passage of a catheter through the right heart allows the level and degree of the stenosis to be established by measuring the systolic pressure gradient.

TREATMENT

Treatment of severe pulmonary stenosis requires pulmonary valvotomy (balloon valvotomy or direct surgery).

PULMONARY REGURGITATION

This is the most common acquired lesion of the pulmonary valve. It results from dilatation of the pulmonary valve ring, which occurs with pulmonary hypertension. It is characterized by a decrescendo diastolic murmur beginning with the pulmonary component of the second sound (Graham Steell murmur) which is difficult to distinguish from the murmur of aortic regurgitation. Pulmonary regurgitation usually causes no symptoms and treatment is rarely necessary.

Infective endocarditis

Infective endocarditis is an infection of the endocardium or vascular endothelium. The disease may occasionally occur as a fulminating or acute infection, but more commonly runs an insidious course and is known as subacute (bacterial) endocarditis (SBE). Endocarditis occurs most commonly on rheumatic or congenitally abnormal valves as well as in mitral valve prolapse and calcified aortic valve disease. It also occurs in association with congenital lesions such as ventricular septal defect or persistent ductus arteriosus. A very similar disease may occur from infection of arteriovenous fistulas. Prosthetic valves or prosthetic vascular material may be similarly infected. The organisms are often non-virulent.

Virulent organisms may infect normal valves, especially when the victim is generally debilitated or immunologically incompetent.

The term 'infective endocarditis' is preferred because not all the infecting organisms are bacteria.

AETIOLOGY

Many organisms cause infective endocarditis. At the present time the most common organisms are:

- *Streptococcus viridans* (e.g. *S. mitis* and *S. sanguis*). These organisms are part of the bacterial flora of the pharynx and upper respiratory tract, and the infection may follow dental extraction or cleaning, tonsillectomy or bronchoscopy.
- *Streptococcus faecalis* (found in perineal and faecal bacterial flora). Infections with this organism are more usual in older men with prostatic disease, in women with genitourinary infections, or following pelvic surgery.
- *Staphylococcus aureus*. This organism may cause subacute endocarditis and is responsible for 50% of the acute forms. Patients with central venous catheters used for parenteral feeding, temporary pacemaker electrode catheters or pulmonary artery (Swan–Ganz) catheters are prone to this infection. Cellulitis or skin abscesses are often the origin of the infection, particularly in drug addicts who 'mainline'.

Infective endocarditis can also be caused by:

- *Staphylococcus epidermidis, Histoplasma, Brucella, Candida* and *Aspergillus*. Infections with these organisms are particularly common in intravenous drug addicts, alcoholics and patients with prosthetic heart valves.
- *Coxiella burnetii* (the causative organism of Q fever, see p. 50). This may cause a subacute infection.

PATHOLOGY

Infection occurs along the edges of the heart valves. It is more common on the left side, with mitral and aortic regurgitation being the commonest valve lesions complicated by endocarditis. In drug addicts the valves in the right heart are usually affected.

The endocardium on the low pressure side of a shunt such as a ventricular septal defect is infected and it is the pulmonary artery that is infected when a persistent ductus arteriosus is present; in both instances the lesions are 'jet lesions' produced on the wall opposite the shunt (Fig. 11.66).

Hypertrophic cardiomyopathy, syphilitic aortic regurgitation, prolapsing mitral valve and arteriosclerotic valve lesions may also be rarely complicated by endocarditis.

The lesion of infective endocarditis is a mass of fibrous tissue, platelets and infecting organisms known as a vegetation. The chance of an organism sticking to a vegetation is increased because of the clumping together of bacteria caused by agglutinating antibodies. These can develop because of

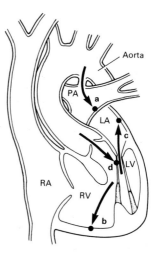

Fig. 11.66 Diagram of jet lesions produced in infective endocarditis. **a** = a lesion in the pulmonary artery (PA) because of a ductus arteriosus. **b** = a lesion in the right ventricle (RV) due to a ventricular septal defect. **c** = a lesion in the left atrium (LA) due to mitral regurgitation. **d** = a lesion in the left ventricle (LV) and on the mitral valve chordae tendineae due to aortic regurgitation. RA = right atrium.

repeated infection with the bacterium over a period of years. In acute endocarditis, vegetations may be very large and may embolize. Virulent microorganisms may rapidly destroy the valve cusp, producing ulceration and regurgitation.

The extracardiac manifestations result either from embolization or from the deposition of immune complexes. The latter is thought to be responsible for arthralgia, Roth spots and Janeway lesions, focal glomerulonephritis and acute vasculitis (see below).

Splenic and renal infarcts are produced by emboli. Myocardial infarction can result from coronary emboli, and pulmonary infarction may occur if right-sided lesions embolize.

PRESENTATIONS

Subacute endocarditis
The patient presents with fever, night sweats, weight loss, weakness and symptoms due to cardiac failure or embolism. Another important presentation is the combination of renal failure and a heart murmur. It is not usually possible to date the onset of the illness.

Acute endocarditis
Following an acute suppurative illness such as pneumonia or meningitis, the development of acute endocarditis is suggested by the persistence of fever and the development of heart murmurs, vasculitis (with petechial haemorrhage) and emboli, including metastatic abscesses. The onset of severe heart failure may indicate chordal rupture or acute valvular destruction.

Prosthetic endocarditis
There are two varieties: the first develops soon after surgery and is due to infection of the prosthesis at surgery, and the second occurs late and follows a bacteraemia. In both cases it is the valve ring that is infected. This produces myocardial abscesses and damage, for example to the conduction system. Vegetations in the valve may prevent it from opening and closing properly. Emboli are common.

CLINICAL FEATURES (see Table 11.32)

The patients are often elderly. They appear pale (often anaemic) and ill, are intermittently pyrexial and may complain of myalgia and arthralgia. Some of the following signs and symptoms may be present.

Cardiac findings
The signs of any underlying heart disease should be obvious, but occasionally only trivial lesions such as mild aortic regurgitation or a bicuspid aortic valve are present. The development of a new murmur or a

Table 11.32 Clinical features of infective endocarditis.

	Approximate %
General systems:	
Malaise	95
Clubbing	10
Cardiac:	
Murmurs	90
Cardiac failure	50
Arthralgia	25
Pyrexia	90
Skin lesions:	
Osler's nodes	15
Splinter haemorrhages	10
Janeway lesions	5
Petechiae	50
Eyes:	
Roth spots	5
Conjunctival splinter haemorrhages	Rare
Splenomegaly	40
Neurological:	
Cerebral emboli	20
Mycotic aneurysm	10
Renal:	
Haematuria	70

change in the character of an existing murmur may warn of the presence of endocarditis.

Vascular lesions
Small petechial or mucosal haemorrhages occur because of vasculitis. They are usually small and red, usually with a pale centre. They frequently appear on the mucosa of the pharynx and conjunctivae. Sometimes they are seen on the retinae (Roth spots). Small, flat, erythematous, non-tender macules are seen mainly on the thenar and hypothenar eminences (Janeway lesions); these blanch with pressure. Splinter haemorrhages may develop.

Embolic lesions such as hard, painful, tender, subcutaneous swellings occur in the fingers, toes, palms and soles (Osler's nodes).

Clubbing of the fingers
Mild clubbing of the fingers and toes appears late in the disease, and thus it only occurs in subacute endocarditis. It is rare nowadays because of relatively rapid diagnosis and treatment of the endocarditis.

Splenomegaly
Slight splenomegaly is common. If a splenic infarct has occurred, the spleen may be painful and tender and a friction rub may be heard over it.

Renal lesions
Haematuria is common, usually due to infarction as a result of emboli. Renal abscesses and acute glomerulonephritis also occur.

Arthritis
Arthritis of the major joints is frequently seen.

Other embolic phenomena
Cerebral emboli can occur, usually to the middle cerebral artery or its branches. Mycotic infected aneurysms are seen and may present after the endocarditis has healed. Peripheral arterial, pulmonary and coronary infarcts may also occur.

INVESTIGATION

- A normochromic normocytic anaemia is usual and the ESR is increased. A polymorphonuclear leucocytosis is common and thrombocytopenia can occasionally occur.
- Liver function tests are often mildly disturbed with, in particular, an increased serum alkaline phosphatase.
- Serum immunoglobulins are increased, but total complement and C3 complement are decreased due to immune complex disease. Circulating immune complexes are present in more than 70% of cases but are not routinely measured.
- Proteinuria may occur and microscopic haematuria is nearly always present.

Blood cultures are positive in about three-quarters of cases. At least six sets of samples are usually taken and cultured in aerobic and anaerobic conditions. Special culture techniques may be necessary for unusual microorganisms such as *Brucella* and *Histoplasma*. Serological tests are needed to incriminate *Coxiella* and *Chlamydia*, and may be helpful for *Candida* and *Brucella*.

Echocardiography is used to visualize vegetations (Fig. 11.67), but small vegetations typical of the subacute disease can be missed. Echocardiography is useful to document valvular dysfunction and to identify patients in need of urgent surgery. Vegetations may persist despite treatment.

TREATMENT

Drug therapy
Any underlying infection should be treated (e.g. a dental abscess should be drained). The endocarditis is treated with bactericidal antibiotics chosen on the basis of the results of the blood culture and antibiotic sensitivity assessment. The treatment should continue for 4–6 weeks and at least the first 2 weeks of therapy should be parenteral, usually intravenous. Serum levels are measured and 'back titration' is performed to ensure that sufficient bactericidal antibiotic activity is present to inhibit growth of the organism.

Streptococcus viridans is usually treated with benzylpenicillin 12 g daily, with added probenecid. Gentamicin 40 mg 8-hourly by slow intravenous infusion should be added for the first 2 weeks because of the additive effects of gentamicin and penicillin against *S. viridans*.

Streptococcus faecalis is managed with penicillin and gentamicin (3 mg·kg^{-1} in divided 8-hourly doses). The exact dose of gentamicin depends on renal function and efficacy, and blood levels should be measured at least twice each week. The dosage of penicillin should be somewhat higher (up to 24 g daily) than for *S. viridans* because *S. faecalis* is relatively insensitive to penicillin. Amoxycillin 6 g daily is often substituted.

It is more difficult to choose antibiotics when the infecting organism has not been isolated. However, in the acute form of the disease this is likely to be *Staphylococcus*, and treatment should include flucloxacillin and fusidic acid. In the subacute form, unless it is highly likely that the infecting organism is *Streptococcus viridans*, it is usual to begin treatment with a broad-spectrum combination of antibiotics

Fig. 11.67 Two-dimensional and M-mode echocardiograms of the mitral valve demonstrating mitral valve vegetations. veg = vegetation; CW = chest wall; RV = right ventricle; IVS = interventricular septum; MV = mitral valve.

such as gentamicin and amoxycillin. The treatment is adjusted if it is not successful.

The recurrence of fever may suggest that the antibiotic therapy is inadequate, but may also signal a drug reaction. The antibiotics may be omitted for 24–72 h to test this.

Surgery
There are several situations when surgery is necessary:
- Extensive damage to a valve
- Infection of prosthetic material
- Worsening renal failure
- Persistent infection but failure to culture an organism
- Embolization
- Large vegetations

The timing of surgery is important. On the one hand the infection should, if possible, be eradicated before surgery is undertaken, but on the other hand the heart should not be left in a badly compromised haemodynamic state. In general, early surgery is preferable.

PROGNOSIS

The prognosis is worse when the organism cannot be isolated, when cardiac failure is present, when infection occurs on a prosthetic valve, and when the microorganisms found are resistant to therapy. In general, 70% of those affected are effectively treated, but greater awareness of the subacute form of the disease will improve the success rate.

PROPHYLAXIS (see p. 12)

Those at risk of developing endocarditis should receive antibiotic therapy before undergoing a procedure likely to result in a bacteraemia. The form of the prophylaxis depends on the procedure and on the likelihood of endocarditis. High risk patients are those with a prosthetic heart valve or a previous history of endocarditis.

Congenital heart disease

A congenital cardiac malformation occurs in about 1% of live births. There is an overall male predominance, although some individual lesions (e.g. atrial septal defect and persistent ductus arteriosus) occur more commonly in females. The aetiology of congenital cardiac disease is often unknown but involves:
- Maternal rubella infection (persistent ductus

arteriosus, and pulmonary valvular and arterial stenosis)
- Maternal alcohol abuse (septal defects)
- Maternal drug treatment and radiation
- Genetic abnormalities, e.g. the familial form of atrial septal defect and congenital heart block
- Chromosomal abnormalities, e.g. septal defects and mitral and tricuspid valve defects associated with Down's syndrome (trisomy 21) or coarctation of the aorta in Turner's syndrome (45, XO).

Some symptoms and signs are common in congenital heart disease:
- *Central cyanosis* occurs because of right-to-left shunting of blood or because of complete mixing of systemic and pulmonary blood flow.
- *Pulmonary hypertension* results from large left-to-right shunts. The persistently raised pulmonary flow leads to the development of increased pulmonary artery vascular resistance and consequent pulmonary hypertension. This is known as the Eisenmenger reaction (or the Eisenmenger syndrome when due specifically to a ventricular septal defect). The development of pulmonary hypertension significantly worsens the prognosis.
- *Clubbing of the fingers* may occur in congenital cardiac conditions associated with prolonged cyanosis.
- *Paradoxical embolism* of thrombus from the systemic veins to the systemic arterial system may occur when a communication exists between the right and left heart.
- *Reduced growth* is common in children with cyanotic heart disease.
- *Syncope* is common when severe right or left ventricular outflow tract obstruction is present. Exertional syncope, associated with deepening central cyanosis, may occur in Fallot's tetralogy. Exercise results in increased resistance to pulmonary blood flow but reduced systemic vascular resistance. Thus, the right-to-left shunt increases and cerebral oxygenation falls.
- *Squatting* is the posture adopted by children with Fallot's tetralogy. It results in obstruction of venous return of desaturated blood and an increase in the peripheral systemic vascular resistance. This leads to a reduced right-to-left shunt and improved cerebral oxygenation.

The most common congenital lesions are shown in Table 11.33.

Ventricular septal defect (VSD)

VSD is the most common congenital cardiac malformation (1 in 500 live births). It may occur as an isolated abnormality or in association with other anomalies. Left ventricular pressure is higher than right ventricular pressure; blood therefore moves

Table 11.33 Common congenital lesions.

	% of all congenital lesions
Ventricular septal defect	39
Atrial septal defect	10
Persistent ductus arteriosus	10
Pulmonary stenosis	7
Coarctation of the aorta	7
Aortic stenosis	6
Fallot's tetralogy	6
Others	15

from left to right and pulmonary blood flow increases. When pulmonary blood flow is very large, obliterative pulmonary vascular changes may cause the pulmonary arterial pressure to equal the systemic pressure (Eisenmenger's syndrome). Consequently, the shunt is reduced or reversed (becoming right-to-left) and central cyanosis may develop.

CLINICAL FEATURES

A small VSD (maladie de Roger) presents with a loud and sometimes long systolic murmur in an asymptomatic patient. Such VSDs usually close spontaneously. Moderate VSDs produce some fatigue and dyspnoea. Physical signs include cardiac enlargement and a prominent apex beat. There is often a palpable systolic thrill at the lower left sternal edge. A loud 'tearing' pan-systolic murmur is heard at the same position.

Large VSDs are associated with increasing pulmonary hypertension (right ventricular parasternal heave and a loud, pulmonary component of the second heart sound). The murmur may be soft because the increased right ventricular pressure may be nearly equal to the left ventricular pressure such that flow across the VSD is small.

INVESTIGATION

A small VSD produces no abnormal x-ray or ECG findings. On the chest x-ray, larger defects show a prominent pulmonary artery due to increased pulmonary blood flow. In Eisenmenger's syndrome the radiological signs of pulmonary hypertension (i.e. 'pruned' pulmonary arteries) can be seen. Cardiomegaly occurs when a moderate or a large VSD is present. The ECG shows features of both left and right ventricular hypertrophy. The size and location of the VSD, and its haemodynamic consequences, can be assessed by echocardiography. The diagnosis can be proved by cardiac catheterization.

TREATMENT

Moderate and large VSDs should be surgically repaired before the development of severe pulmonary hypertension. Bacterial endocarditis prophylaxis (see p. 12) should be advised.

Atrial septal defect (ASD)

This congenital condition is often first diagnosed in adults. It is more common in women than in men. There are two types of ASD—ostium secundum and ostium primum. The common form of ASD is ostium secundum. Communication at the level of the atria allows left-to-right shunting of blood. Because the pulmonary vascular resistance is low and the right ventricle is easily distended (i.e. it is compliant), there is a considerable increase in right heart output. Above the age of 30 years there may be an increase in pulmonary vascular resistance, which gives rise to pulmonary hypertension. Atrial arrhythmias, particularly atrial fibrillation, are common at this stage.

CLINICAL FEATURES

Most children with ASDs are asymptomatic, although they are prone to pulmonary infection. Some complain of dyspnoea and weakness. Palpitations due to atrial arrhythmias are not uncommon. Right heart failure may develop in later life.

The physical signs of ASD reflect the volume overloading of the right ventricle. Therefore, the splitting of the second sound is wide and fixed (see p. 459). The increased flow through the right heart produces a loud ejection systolic pulmonary flow murmur, and sometimes a diastolic tricuspid flow murmur may be heard. A right ventricular impulse can usually be felt.

INVESTIGATION

- The chest x-ray shows a prominent pulmonary artery and pulmonary plethora (Fig. 11.68). Fig. 11.69 shows a more severe case with pulmonary hypertension. There may be noticeable right ventricular enlargement.
- The ECG usually shows some degree of right bundle branch block (because of dilatation of the right ventricle) and right axis deviation. The echocardiogram demonstrates right ventricular and pulmonary arterial dilatation. The interventricular septum moves abnormally. Sometimes the ASD is part of a major developmental abnormality that may also involve the ventricular septum and the mitral and tricuspid valves. In this case there is left axis deviation on the ECG.
- Cardiac catheterization allows the type of ASD to be determined.

Fig. 11.68 Chest x-ray of a patient with an atrial septal defect. Notice the prominent pulmonary artery (arrow) and the plethoric lung fields.

Fig. 11.69 Chest x-ray from a patient with pulmonary hypertension secondary to an atrial septal defect. It shows enlargement of the heart and a prominent pulmonary artery with greatly enlarged proximal branches.

TREATMENT

A significant ASD (i.e. a pulmonary flow that is more than 50% increased when compared with systemic flow) should be repaired before the age of 10 years or as soon as possible if first diagnosed in adulthood. There is a good result from surgery unless pulmonary hypertension has developed.

Persistent ductus arteriosus (PDA)

The ductus arteriosus connects the pulmonary artery at its bifurcation to the descending aorta immediately distal to the subclavian artery. In fetal life the ductus diverts blood away from the unexpanded, and hence high resistance, pulmonary circulation into the systemic circulation, where the blood is reoxygenated as it passes through the placenta. At birth, the high oxygen in the lungs and the reduced pulmonary vascular resistance triggers closure of the duct. If the duct is malformed, i.e. it does not contain sufficient elastic tissue, it will not close. This is more common in females and is sometimes associated with maternal rubella. Premature babies are often born with persistent ducts which are anatomically normal but are immature in that they lack the mechanism to close.

Because aortic pressure exceeds pulmonary artery pressure throughout the cardiac cycle, a persistent duct produces continuous aorta-to-pulmonary artery shunting. This leads to an increased pulmonary venous return to the left heart and an increased left ventricular volume load.

CLINICAL FEATURES

If the shunt is large, the left heart volume overload results in severe left heart failure. However, there are often no symptoms until later in life when heart failure or infective endocarditis develops.

The characteristic physical sign is a continuous 'machinery' murmur (due to turbulent aortic-to-pulmonary artery shunting in both systole and diastole), best heard below the left clavicle in the first interspace or over the first rib. A thrill may often be felt. The peripheral pulse is large in volume ('bounding') because of the increased left heart blood flow and the decompression of the aorta into the pulmonary artery.

INVESTIGATION

The aorta and pulmonary arterial system are prominent radiologically. There is both a left atrial abnor-

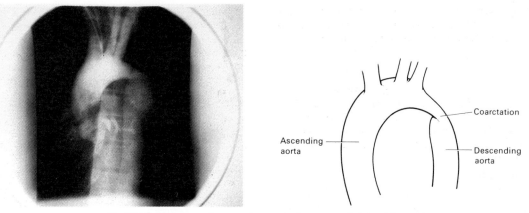

Fig. 11.70 An arch aortogram demonstrating a coarctation of the aorta.

mality and left ventricular hypertrophy on the ECG. The echocardiogram shows a dilated left atrium and left ventricle.

TREATMENT

Premature infants with a persistent duct may be treated medically with indomethacin, which inhibits prostaglandin production and stimulates duct closure. In other cases the duct can be ligated surgically with very little risk. Surgery should be performed as soon as possible and not later than 5 years.

Coarctation of the aorta

Coarctation of the aorta occurs twice as commonly in men as in women. However, it is also associated with Turner's syndrome. The coarctation is a narrowing of the aorta at, or just distal to, the insertion of the ductus arteriosus (Fig. 11.70). In 80% of cases coarctation of the aorta is associated with a bicuspid (and potentially stenotic) aortic valve.

Severe narrowing of the aorta encourages the formation of a collateral arterial circulation involving the periscapular and intercostal arteries. Decreased renal perfusion can lead to the development of systemic hypertension which persists even after surgical correction.

CLINICAL FEATURES

Coarctation of the aorta is often asymptomatic for many years. Headaches and nose bleeds (due to hypertension) and claudication and cold legs (due to poor blood flow in the lower limbs) may be present.

Physical examination reveals hypertension in the upper limbs, and weak, delayed (radio-femoral delay) pulses in the legs.

A mid-to-late systolic murmur due to turbulent flow through the coarctation may be heard over the upper precordium or the back. Vascular bruits from the collateral circulation may also be heard.

INVESTIGATION

The chest x-ray may reveal a dilated aorta indented at the site of the coarctation. This is manifested by an aorta (seen in the upper right mediastinum) shaped like a figure 3. In adults, tortuous and dilated collateral intercostal arteries may erode the undersurfaces of the ribs ('rib notching') (Fig. 11.71). The ECG

Fig. 11.71 An x-ray from a patient with coarctation of the aorta. Notice the notching of the underside of the upper ribs.

demonstrates left ventricular hypertrophy. Digital vascular imaging allows the coarctation to be visualized after the intravenous injection of contrast.

TREATMENT

The treatment is surgical excision of the coarctation and end-to-end anastomosis of the aorta. If the coarctation is extensive, prosthetic vascular grafts may be needed. Hypertension may not resolve after successful surgery because of previous damage to the kidneys.

Fallot's tetralogy

This is the most common cyanotic congenital heart abnormality in children who survive beyond the neonatal period. It consists of the following (Fig. 11.72):

- A ventricular septal defect (VSD)
- Right ventricular outflow obstruction. The level of the obstruction may be subvalvular, valvular or supravalvular. The commonest obstruction is subvalvular, either alone (50%) or in combination with valvular stenosis (25%).
- Positioning of the aorta above the VSD ('overriding aorta').
- Right ventricular hypertrophy

This combination of lesions leads to a high right ventricular pressure and right-to-left shunting of blood through the VSD. Thus the patient is centrally cyanosed.

CLINICAL FEATURES

Children with this condition may present with dyspnoea or fatigue or with hypoxic episodes (Fallot's spells), i.e. deep cyanosis and possible syncope, on exertion. Squatting is common (see p. 527).

Physical signs include a parasternal heave and a systolic ejection murmur, often associated with a thrill in the second left interspace close to the

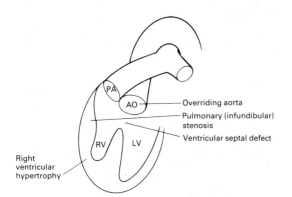

Fig. 11.72 The four features of Fallot's tetralogy.

sternum. The second heart sound is usually single because the pulmonary component is too soft to be heard. Central cyanosis is commonly present from birth, and finger clubbing and polycythaemia are obvious after about 1 year. Growth may be retarded.

INVESTIGATION

The chest x-ray shows a large right ventricle and a small pulmonary artery. The ECG reveals right ventricular hypertrophy and the echocardiogram demonstrates discontinuity between the aorta and the anterior wall of the ventricular septum. Cardiac catheterization is essential to evaluate the size and degree of the right ventricular outflow obstruction.

TREATMENT

Complete surgical correction of this combination of lesions is possible even in infancy. Often a palliative procedure—an anastomosis between a subclavian artery and a pulmonary artery (Blalock shunt)—is performed on very young infants.

This operation results in an increased blood supply to the lungs. Fallot's spells may need treatment with beta-blockade, or when severe, with diamorphine to relax the right ventricular outflow obstruction.

Pulmonary heart disease

Pulmonary hypertension

An elevated pulmonary arterial pressure, known as pulmonary hypertension, has numerous causes:

- Chronic lung disease, which is diagnosed clinically and by abnormalities of lung function
- Increased pulmonary blood flow because of left-to-right shunting through a ventricular septal defect, atrial septal defect or persistent ductus arteriosus
- Left ventricular failure, mitral valve disease, left atrial tumour or thrombus, or pulmonary veno-occlusive disease, which cause an elevation in the pulmonary arterial pressure secondary to an elevation of the pulmonary venous and pulmonary capillary pressure; the pulmonary wedge pressure is elevated in these cases
- Pulmonary thromboembolic disease
- Primary pulmonary hypertension, a rare condition seen predominantly in young women. Its aetiology is unknown but recurrent small pulmonary emboli, pulmonary vasoconstriction due to neural, humoral factors or drugs (e.g. oral contraceptives, crotalaria teas and the appetite suppressant fenfluramine), connective tissue

disease and familial causes have all been suggested.

Pulmonary hypertension leads to enlarged proximal pulmonary arteries, right ventricular hypertrophy and right atrial dilatation. The pulmonary arterial changes depend on the aetiology of the pulmonary hypertension.

Multiple peripheral pulmonary arterial stenoses can produce a syndrome that is similar to pulmonary hypertension, but the pressure in the distal pulmonary bed is normal or low.

CLINICAL FEATURES

Chest pain, exertional dyspnoea, syncope and fatigue are common symptoms, and sudden death may occur. Other symptoms are due to the cause of the pulmonary hypertension.

On physical examination there is a prominent *a* wave in the jugular venous pulse, a right ventricular (parasternal) heave and a loud pulmonary component to the second heart sound. Other findings include a right ventricular fourth heart sound, a systolic pulmonary ejection click, a mid-systolic ejection murmur and an early diastolic murmur due to pulmonary regurgitation (Graham Steell murmur). If tricuspid regurgitation develops, there is a pansystolic murmur and a large jugular *v* wave.

INVESTIGATION

The chest x-ray may show right ventricular enlargement and right atrial dilatation. The pulmonary artery is usually prominent and the enlarged proximal pulmonary arteries taper rapidly. Peripheral lung fields are oligaemic.

The ECG demonstrates right ventricular hypertrophy (right axis deviation, possibly a predominant R wave in lead V_1, and inverted T waves in right precordial leads) and a right atrial abnormality (tall peaked P waves in lead II) (Fig. 11.73).

Other investigations are performed to evaluate the cause of pulmonary hypertension. It is particularly important to look for treatable conditions such as left-to-right shunts, mitral stenosis or left atrial tumours. Radioisotope lung scans and sometimes open lung biopsy are performed, e.g. in young patients with severe pulmonary hypertension of unknown cause. Pulmonary angiography is dangerous and is rarely necessary.

TREATMENT

Treatment is determined by the condition underlying pulmonary hypertension. Primary pulmonary hypertension is treated with anticoagulation (because of the possibility of recurrent thromboembolism). Diuretic treatment may be used for right ventricular failure, but care should be taken to avoid reduction of the left ventricular filling pressure. Hypoxia is avoided by the use of oxygen therapy when necessary. Vasodilators including calcium antagonists such as verapamil have been tried, but with little long-term success. Usually there is a progressive downhill course. Heart and lung transplantation is now possible for young patients with this condition.

Pulmonary embolism (acute cor pulmonale)

Thrombus, usually formed in the systemic veins or rarely in the right heart, may dislodge and embolize

Fig. 11.73 A 12-lead ECG demonstrating pulmonary hypertension. There is right axis deviation (+120°), right ventricular hypertrophy (dominant secondary R wave [R'] in V_1) and a combination of left and right atrial conduction abnormalities.

into the pulmonary arterial system. Post-mortem studies indicate that this is a very common condition (microemboli are found in up to 60% of autopsies) but it is not usually diagnosed this frequently in life. Ten per cent of clinical pulmonary emboli are fatal.

Conditions leading to the formation of clot in the systemic veins (and hence predisposing to pulmonary emboli) include prolonged bedrest, pelvic and lower limb fractures, pelvic or abdominal surgery, cardiac failure, pregnancy and childbirth, oral contraceptive drugs, malignant disease, chronic pulmonary disease and hypercoagulable states.

Atrial fibrillation may allow thrombus formation in the right atrium, and septal or right ventricular infarction may favour thrombosis in the right ventricle. A small proportion (less than 10%) of pulmonary emboli are due to these cardiac causes.

After pulmonary embolism, lung tissue is ventilated but not perfused, resulting in impaired gas exchange. After some hours surfactant is no longer produced by the non-perfused lung, alveolar collapse occurs and hypoxaemia is the result. The haemodynamic consequence of pulmonary embolism is an elevation of pulmonary arterial pressure and a reduction in cardiac output. The zone of lung that is no longer perfused by the pulmonary artery may infarct but often does not do so because oxygen continues to be supplied by the bronchial circulation and the airways.

CLINICAL FEATURES

A small embolus may present with effort dyspnoea, tiredness, syncope and, occasionally, cardiac arrhythmias.

A medium-sized embolus leading to pulmonary infarction can present with sudden onset of pleuritic pain, cough with haemoptysis, and dyspnoea.

A massive pulmonary embolus presents as a medical emergency: the patient has severe central chest pain and suddenly becomes shocked, pale and sweaty, with marked tachypnoea and tachycardia. Syncope may result if the cardiac output is transiently but dramatically reduced. Death may rapidly follow.

Physical signs vary according to the size of the embolus and the occurrence of pulmonary infarction:

- A small embolus may reveal no abnormal signs apart from a few basal crackles.
- Large emboli lead to a right ventricular heave, a gallop rhythm, tachycardia and a prominent 'a' wave in the jugular venous pulse. The second heart sound may be loud because of pulmonary hypertension or soft if the cardiac output is very reduced. Continuous (systolic and diastolic) murmurs may be generated by turbulent blood flow around the embolic obstructions.
- With pulmonary infarction, a pleural rub and pyrexia may also be present.

- In about 50% of cases there is evidence of deep venous thrombosis, especially in the lower limbs or pelvic veins.

INVESTIGATION

The chest x-ray is often normal but the abrupt cut-off of a pulmonary artery or a translucency of an underperfused distal zone is occasionally seen. Later, atelectasis leads to opacities. An infarction may be visualized as a wedge-shaped opacity adjacent to the pleural edge, a pleural effusion and a raised hemidiaphragm. Past infarcts may be seen as opaque linear scars.

The ECG is usually normal except for sinus tachycardia. In relatively severe cases, however, right atrial dilatation produces tall, peaked P waves in lead II, and right ventricular hypertrophy and dilatation give rise to right axis deviation, some degree of right bundle branch block and T wave inversion in the right precordial leads (Fig. 11.74). The classical pattern of an S wave in lead I and a Q wave and inverted T waves in lead III (S1, Q3, T3), which reflects right ventricular 'strain', is not usually present.

If pulmonary infarction has occurred there will be a polymorphonuclear leucocytosis, an elevated ESR and increased lactate dehydrogenase levels.

Pulmonary embolism usually results in arterial hypoxaemia and hypocapnia.

A pulmonary technetium-99m scintigram may demonstrate underperfused areas (Fig. 11.75). The specificity of this technique is greatly improved when combined with a ventilation scintigram performed after inhalation of radioactive xenon gas (p. 565). The finding of a non-perfused but ventilated zone is more suggestive of pulmonary embolism.

Pulmonary angiography is sometimes undertaken if surgery is considered in acute massive embolism. The test is performed by injecting contrast material through a catheter inserted into the main pulmonary artery. Filling defects or obstructed vessels can be delineated (Fig. 11.76). Angiography is hazardous but the risk may be reduced if contrast is injected into each pulmonary artery separately. If the patient is in extremis and the diagnosis is obvious, surgery should proceed without prior angiography.

TREATMENT

Prevention of further emboli
The basis of therapy is intravenous heparin, starting with a bolus of 5000 units and followed by the continuous infusion of 10 000 units every 6 h. Oral anticoagulants are usually begun after 48 h and the heparin is tapered off as the oral anticoagulant becomes effective. Oral anticoagulants are continued for 6 weeks to 6 months, depending on the likelihood of recurrence of venous thrombosis or embolism.

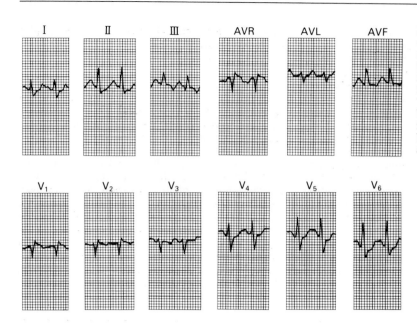

Fig. 11.74 A 12-lead ECG demonstrating some features of acute pulmonary embolism. There is an S wave in lead I, a Q wave in lead III and an inverted T wave in lead III (the S1, Q3, T3 pattern). There is sinus tachycardia (160 beats per minute) and an incomplete right bundle branch block pattern (an R wave in AVR and V_1 and an S wave in V_6).

Fig. 11.75 Perfusion lung scan using technetium-labelled macroaggregates. Multiple perfusion defects are seen, the most prominent in the right mid-zone (left). This is suggestive of multiple pulmonary emboli.

(a)   (b)

Fig. 11.76 Pulmonary arteriogram (subtraction film). (a) Many parts of the lungs are under-perfused. An embolus is particularly well seen as filling defects in the vessel to the right upper lobe. (b) Repeat angiogram after treatment with streptokinase.

Dissolution of the thrombus

Fibrinolytic therapy such as streptokinase (600 000 iu stat i.v. with hydrocortisone cover, followed by streptokinase 100 000 i.v. hourly) is often used following a major embolism. It may also be given into the pulmonary artery.

Surgical embolectomy

This is rarely necessary but when the haemodynamic circumstances are very severe there may be no alternative. Inferior vena caval interruption or plication, or the insertion of a filter into the inferior vena cava, may occasionally be necessary if anticoagulant or fibrinolytic therapy is contraindicated or fails to prevent recurrences of pulmonary embolism.

Chronic cor pulmonale

Cor pulmonale is the commonest variety of pulmonary hypertensive heart disease.

CAUSES

These are listed in Table 11.34.

PATHOPHYSIOLOGY

Pulmonary vascular resistance is increased because of effective loss of pulmonary tissue and because of pulmonary vasoconstriction caused by hypoxia and acidosis. The increased pulmonary vascular resistance leads to pulmonary hypertension, which initially occurs only during an acute respiratory infection. Eventually, the pulmonary hypertension becomes persistent and progressively more severe. The pulmonary vascular bed is gradually obliterated by muscular hypertrophy of the arterioles and thrombus formation. Right ventricular function is progressively compromised because of the increased pressure load. Hypoxia further impairs right ventricular function, and as it develops, left ventricular function is also depressed.

CLINICAL FEATURES

The clinical features are those of pulmonary hypertension and right ventricular failure occurring in patients with chronic chest disease. The dominant clinical picture depends on the type of lung disease.

TREATMENT

Vigorous therapy of the pulmonary condition may lead to marked improvement of blood gases and consequent improvement of the heart failure. Acute chest infections must be treated promptly. Oxygen therapy over a long period may reduce established pulmonary hypertension, with improvement in overall prognosis (see p. 583). Any heart failure should be treated (see p. 496).

Atrial myxoma

This is the commonest primary cardiac tumour. A myxoma usually develops in the left atrium and is a polypoid, gelatinous structure attached by a pedicle to the atrial septum. The tumour may obstruct the mitral valve or may be a site of thrombi which then embolize. It is also associated with constitutional symptoms: the patient may present with dyspnoea, syncope or a mild fever. The most important physical signs are a loud first heart sound, a tumour 'plop' (a loud third heart sound produced as the pedunculated tumour comes to an abrupt halt), a mid-diastolic murmur, and signs due to embolization. A raised ESR is usually present.

The diagnosis is easily made by echocardiography because the tumour is demonstrated as a dense space-occupying lesion. Surgical removal usually results in a complete cure.

Myxomas may also occur in the right atrium or in the ventricles. Other primary cardiac tumours include rhabdomyomas and sarcomas.

Myocardial disease

Myocardial disease that is *not* due to hypertension, ischaemic heart disease, rheumatic heart disease, congenital heart disease or cor pulmonale may be caused by:

- An acute inflammatory pathology (myocarditis)
- Chronic myocardial pathology (cardiomyopathy)

Table 11.34 Causes of cor pulmonale.

Intrinsic lung disease, e.g.
Chronic bronchitis and emphysema
Asthma
Pulmonary fibrosis
Recurrent pulmonary emboli
Skeletal abnormalities, e.g.
Kyphoscoliosis
Hypoventilation, e.g.
Morbid obesity (Pickwickian syndrome)
Neuromuscular disease, e.g.
Poliomyelitis
Myasthenia gravis
Obstruction, e.g.
Sleep-apnoea syndrome

MYOCARDITIS

Acute myocarditis usually follows an infectious process. Causative factors include:
- Viruses, particularly coxsackie, influenza, rubella, polio, adeno- and echoviruses
- *Rickettsia, Chlamydia, Coxiella* (the causative agent of Q fever)
- *Toxoplasma gondii*—a common cause of myocarditis in the newborn or in immunologically compromised adults
- Protozoa, e.g. *Trypanosoma cruzi*, which causes Chagas' disease and is endemic in central and south America
- Radiation, chemicals and drugs, e.g. lead poisoning, emetine and chloroquine
- Bacterial infection, e.g. diphtheria, which is due to an exotoxin produced by *Corynebacterium*

Idiopathic myocarditis also occurs.

CLINICAL FEATURES

Patients present with an acute illness, often characterized by fever and cardiac failure. There may be a history of previous respiratory or febrile illness. Physical examination reveals soft heart sounds, a prominent third sound and tachycardia (gallop rhythm). Often, a pericardial friction rub may be heard.

INVESTIGATION

The chest x-ray may show some cardiac enlargement, depending on the stage and virulence of the disease
- The ECG demonstrates ST and T wave abnormalities and arrhythmias. Diphtheritic myocarditis may induce heart block, and Chagas' disease produces both heart block and ventricular tachyarrhythmias.
- Cardiac enzymes are elevated.
- Cardiac biopsy shows acute inflammation.

TREATMENT

General management includes bedrest and the eradication of any acute infection. Therapy is directed towards the management of cardiac failure and the treatment of cardiac arrhythmias. Depending on the aetiology, the prognosis is usually good, although a chronic cardiomyopathy may occasionally ensue.

CARDIOMYOPATHY

These chronic conditions are classified according to their clinical presentation as:
- Dilated cardiomyopathy—ventricular dilatation
- Hypertrophic cardiomyopathy—myocardial hypertrophy
- Restrictive cardiomyopathy—impaired ventricular filling

Dilated cardiomyopathy

The majority of cardiomyopathies are of the dilated (congestive) variety. Many cases have no known aetiology, but causes include:
- Generalized disease, e.g. haemochromatosis, sarcoidosis
- Connective tissue disorders, e.g. systemic lupus erythematosus, systemic sclerosis
- Neuromuscular disease, e.g. muscular dystrophy, Friedreich's ataxia
- Glycogen storage disease, e.g. Pompe's disease
- Primary heart muscle disease e.g. amyloidosis
- Alcohol excess
- Cytotoxic drug therapy, e.g. doxorubicin, daunorubicin, cyclophosphamide
- Postpartum cardiomyopathy

CLINICAL FEATURES

Symptoms depend on the relative degree of right and left heart failure and the incidence of cardiac arrhythmias and emboli.

Physical signs reflect heart failure, i.e. cardiomegaly, tachycardia, jugular venous pressure elevation, third or fourth heart sounds and basal crackles. Ventricular dilatation leads to functional mitral or tricuspid valvular regurgitation.

INVESTIGATION

- Generalized cardiac enlargement is demonstrable on the chest x-ray
- Diffuse non-specific ST segment and T wave changes are seen on the ECG. Conduction disturbances, sinus tachycardia, and arrhythmias (such as atrial fibrillation, ventricular premature contractions or ventricular tachycardia) may also be seen.
- The echocardiogram reveals ventricular dilatation and poor ventricular contraction (Fig. 11.77).
- Cardiac biopsy shows variable fibrosis.

TREATMENT

Management involves the conventional treatment of heart failure and arrhythmias. A history of embolization is an indication for anticoagulant treatment. Prolonged bedrest, corticosteroid therapy, the avoidance of alcohol, and nutritional supplements may be indicated in special cases. Severe congestive cardiomyopathy in relatively young adults may be treated with cardiac transplantation.

Hypertrophic cardiomyopathy (HCM)

Also known as hypertrophic obstructive cardiomyopathy (HOCM), this is characterized by marked

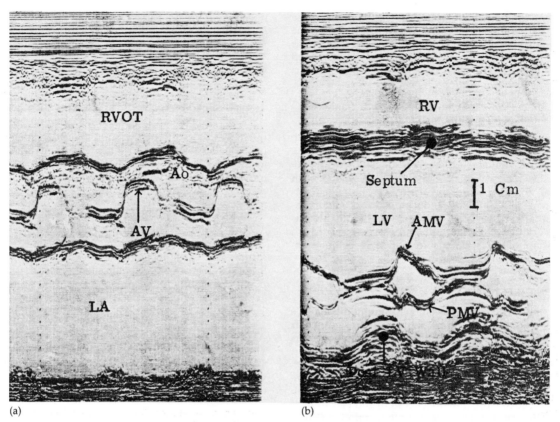

Fig. 11.77 M-mode echocardiogram from a patient with congestive cardiomyopathy. The left atrium (LA) and left ventricle (LV) are enlarged. Also seen are the anterior (AMV) and posterior (PMV) leaflets of the mitral valve, the right ventricle (RV) and the right ventricular outflow tract (RVOT). (a) Section through the RVOT, aortic valve and left atrium (for a diagrammatic representation see Fig. 11.64, p. 520). (b) Section through the right and left ventricles and mitral valve (for a diagrammatic representation see Fig. 11.22, p. 471).

hypertrophy of the left ventricle, particularly the interventricular septum. The hypertrophied muscle results in distorted left ventricular contraction and abnormal mitral valve movement during systole. Some degree of mitral regurgitation may develop. Apposition of the anterior cusp of the mitral valve to the hypertrophied septum may cause some obstruction to left ventricular emptying. About half the cases of hypertrophic cardiomyopathy are familial (inherited in an autosomal dominant manner), but the sporadic cases are of unknown aetiology.

CLINICAL FEATURES

Patients with this condition may present with syncope or pre-syncope (typically exertional), angina, cardiac arrhythmias or sudden death. As with other cardiomyopathies, dyspnoea due to left ventricular failure is a common but late presentation. In this case left ventricular failure is not due to the failing contractile function of the myocardium; instead, it is due to the inability of the heart muscle to relax. Thus, left ventricular filling and therefore left ventricular emptying is impaired.

The classical physical findings are:

- A double apical pulse (due to a palpable fourth heart sound)
- A jerky carotid pulse because of sudden obstruction to left ventricular outflow during systole
- A late systolic murmur because of left ventricular outflow obstruction late in systole
- A pan-systolic murmur due to mitral regurgitation
- A fourth heart sound

INVESTIGATION

- The chest x-ray is usually unremarkable.
- The ECG demonstrates left ventricular hypertrophy (see Fig. 11.61, p. 517.)
- The echocardiogram is diagnostic because it shows septal hypertrophy (often greater than the hypertrophy of the posterior wall), abnormal mitral valve movement and a very vigorously contracting ventricle.

TREATMENT

Firstly, sudden death must be avoided by anti-arrhythmic treatment. Long-term amiodarone treatment is effective. Syncope or chest pain may be treated with beta-blockade. Vasodilators should be avoided because they may aggravate left ventricular outflow obstruction due to peripheral venous blood pooling. Occasionally, resection of septal myocardium may be indicated.

Restrictive cardiomyopathy

Some cardiomyopathies do not present with muscular hypertrophy or ventricular dilatation. Instead, ventricular filling is restricted (as with constrictive pericarditis). Conditions associated with this form of cardiomyopathy are amyloidosis, sarcoidosis, Löffler's endocarditis and endomyocardial fibrosis; in the latter two conditions there is myocardial and endocardial fibrosis associated with eosinophilia. Thrombus formation is common in restrictive cardiomyopathy.

CLINICAL FEATURES

Dyspnoea, fatigue and embolic symptoms may be the presenting features. Restriction to ventricular filling also results in persistently elevated venous pressures and consequent hepatic enlargement, ascites and dependent oedema.

Physical signs are similar to those of constrictive pericarditis, i.e. a high jugular venous pressure with diastolic collapse (Friedreich's sign) and elevation of the jugular venous pressure with inspiration (Kussmaul's sign). Cardiac enlargement with a third or fourth heart sound is common.

INVESTIGATION

- The chest x-ray confirms the cardiac enlargement.
- The ECG usually has generally low voltage and ST segment and T wave abnormalities.
- The echocardiogram shows symmetrical myocardial thickening and a normal systolic ejection fraction, but impaired ventricular filling.
- Transvenous endocardial biopsy may be useful for more detailed diagnosis.

TREATMENT

There is no specific treatment. Cardiac failure and embolic problems should be treated. Cardiac transplantation should be considered in some severe cases.

Pericardial disease

The normal pericardium lubricates the surface of the heart, prevents sudden deformation or dislocation of the heart, and acts as a barrier to the spread of infection. There are three common presentations of pericardial disease:
- Acute pericarditis
- Pericardial effusion
- Constrictive pericarditis

ACUTE PERICARDITIS

Inflammation of the pericardium gives rise to chest pain that is substernal and sharp. It may be referred to the neck or shoulders. It is relieved by sitting forward and made worse by lying down and, like pleurisy, is aggravated by movement and respiration.

Acute pericarditis has numerous aetiologies, but coxsackie viral infections and myocardial infarction are the commonest causes in the UK. Viral pericarditis can occur in epidemics. Other aetiologies include uraemia, connective tissue disease, trauma, post-pericardiotomy, rheumatic fever, tuberculosis and malignancy.

CLINICAL FEATURES

The cardinal clinical sign is a pericardial friction rub. There is usually a fever when pericarditis is due to viral or bacterial infection, rheumatic fever or myocardial infarction.

INVESTIGATION

During the first week of the illness the ECG shows ST segment elevation, concave upwards, in all leads facing the epicardial surface, i.e. the anterior, lateral and inferior leads (Fig. 11.78). ST segment depression is only seen in the cavity leads (AVR and V_1). Later, the ST segment falls and T wave inversion develops. As the illness improves the T waves become normal.

Cardiac enzymes may be elevated if there is associated myocarditis.

TREATMENT

Treatment consists of anti-inflammatory medication such as oral aspirin, naproxen or indomethacin. Occasionally, if pericarditis is severe or recurrent, systemic corticosteroids may be needed.

Varieties of pericarditis

Viral pericarditis
This tends to affect young adults and is sudden in onset. Usually, the illness lasts for only a few weeks and the prognosis is good. However, recurrences do occur.

Bacterial pericarditis
Septicaemia or pneumonia may rarely be compli-

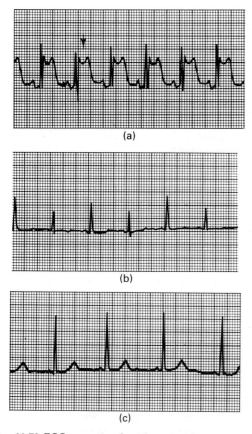

Fig. 11.78 ECGs associated with pericarditis. (a) Acute pericarditis. Note the raised ST segment, concave upwards (arrow). (b) Chronic phase of pericarditis associated with a pericardial effusion. Note the T wave flattening and inversion and the alternation of the QRS amplitude (QRS alternans). (c) The same patient after evacuation of the pericardial fluid. Note that the QRS voltage has increased and the T waves have returned to normal.

cated by purulent pericarditis. *Staphylococcus* and *Haemophilus influenzae* account for two-thirds of such cases.

Antibiotics and surgical drainage may be required. This form of pericarditis, especially when due to *Staphylococcus*, can be fatal.

Tuberculous pericarditis

This is typified by a chronic low grade fever, especially in the evening, associated with signs and symptoms of acute pericarditis, malaise and weight loss. Pericardial aspiration may be required to make the diagnosis. The pericardial effusion is usually serous but may be blood-stained. Specific antituberculous chemotherapy is needed.

Uraemic pericarditis

This is uncommon and is often asymptomatic. It usually develops in the terminal stages of uraemia.

Pericarditis following myocardial infarction

A pericardial friction rub and the recurrence of chest pain and fever occurs in about 20% of patients during the first few days after myocardial infarction, especially anterior wall infarction.

Dressler's syndrome

This is pericarditis occurring 1 month to 1 year after an acute myocardial infarction (see p. 510).

Malignant pericarditis

Carcinoma of the bronchus, carcinoma of the breast and Hodgkin's disease are the most common tumours to infiltrate the pericardium. Leukaemia and malignant melanoma are also associated with pericarditis. Pericardiocentesis may be useful in diagnosing the malignancy.

PERICARDIAL EFFUSION

Although acute pericarditis is initially dry and fibrinous, almost all aetiologies of this inflammatory reaction also induce the formation of a pericardial effusion. The effusion collects in the closed pericardium. When the pericardium can distend no more, it may produce mechanical embarrassment to the circulation by preventing ventricular filling; this is called cardiac tamponade.

CLINICAL FEATURES

The clinical features include a raised jugular venous pressure, with sharp diastolic collapse (Friedreich's sign), a paradoxical pulse (the blood pressure falls during inspiration), increased neck vein distension during inspiration (Kussmaul's sign) and reduced cardiac output. Because of the effusion, the apex beat may not be palpable and heart sounds are soft. Although a friction rub is often heard, it may be quieter than before the fluid accumulated as the effusion separates the visceral from the parietal pericardium.

INVESTIGATION

The ECG shows reduced voltages, and the chest x-ray may demonstrate an increasingly large globular heart with sharp outlines. The pulmonary veins are typically not distended.

Echocardiography is the most useful technique for demonstrating a pericardial effusion (see Fig. 11.21, p. 470).

TREATMENT

When the effusion collects rapidly and the circulation is embarrassed, the effusion must be tapped. Pericardiocentesis is also indicated when a malignant, tuberculous or a purulent effusion is suspected. Reaccumulation may require pericardial fenestration, i.e. the surgical creation of a window in the pericardium.

CONSTRICTIVE PERICARDITIS

Following tuberculous pericarditis, haemopericardium, or acute pericarditis due to viral infection, bacterial infection or rheumatic heart disease, the pericardium may become thick, fibrous and calcified. The heart is then encased in a solid shell and cannot fill properly.

CLINICAL FEATURES

There are signs of systemic venous congestion, i.e. ascites, dependent oedema, hepatomegaly and jugular venous distension, without much breathlessness or pulmonary venous distension. There are also signs of impaired ventricular filling, i.e. Kussmaul's sign, Friedreich's sign and pulsus paradoxus.

Atrial fibrillation is common (30%) and a loud heart sound called a pericardial knock due to rapid ventricular filling may be heard. This is an early third heart sound.

Other causes of ascites must be excluded (see p. 235).

INVESTIGATION

The chest x-ray shows a relatively small heart with obvious calcification seen on the lateral film and using fluoroscopy.

The ECG shows low QRS voltages and T wave inversion, and the echocardiogram may demonstrate the thickened pericardium and the relative immobility of the heart.

TREATMENT

Treatment involves the surgical removal of a substantial proportion of the pericardium. About half the patients do well, but in the others persistent constriction, atrial fibrillation and myocardial disease prevent full recovery.

The cardiovascular system in systemic disease

The heart can be involved in many diseases (see Table 11.35).

Table 11.35 Cardiac involvement in systemic disease.

Disease	Cardiac involvement
Syphilis	Aortic regurgitation Coronary arterial stenosis (ostial) Ascending aortic aneurysm
Endocrine disease	
Diabetes mellitus	Coronary artery disease
Thyrotoxicosis	Atrial fibrillation Cardiomyopathy
Hypothyroidism	Bradycardia Heart failure Coronary disease Pericardial effusion
Acromegaly	Cardiomegaly Hypertension Cardiac arrhythmias
Cushing's syndrome	Hypertension
Conn's syndrome	Hypertension
Phaeochromocytoma	Hypertension
Connective tissue disorders	
Systemic lupus erythematosus	Non-infective endocarditis (Libman Sachs) Myocarditis Pericarditis
Systemic sclerosis	Myocarditis Pericarditis Arrhythmias
Polyarteritis nodosa	Hypertension Pericarditis Arrhythmias
Rheumatoid disease	Aortic and mitral regurgitation Pericarditis
Renal failure	Hypertension Heart failure Pericarditis Infective endocarditis
Morbid obesity	Hypertension Cardiomegaly Associated with atherosclerotic coronary artery disease
Gout	Hypertension
Carcinoid syndrome	Pulmonary stenosis Tricuspid stenosis
Alcohol	Cardiomyopathy Atrial arrhythmias

Systemic hypertension

No particular level of blood pressure can be used to distinguish hypertensive patients from normotensive subjects. The blood pressure is a continuous variable, with a more or less Poisson distribution in the population. There is no evidence of a bimodal distribution. The level of blood pressure can be said to be abnormal when it is associated with a clear increase in morbidity and mortality. This level varies with age, sex, race and country. For life insurance reasons and for simple clinical purposes, a diastolic blood pressure in a young adult above 105 mmHg is taken as definitely hypertensive and a pressure above 95 mmHg is regarded as probably hypertensive. The World Health Organization have used a definition of 160/95 mmHg, and in Framingham, a small town in Massachusetts, USA, where a very detailed population study is being carried out, 160/95 mmHg was deemed abnormal and 140/90 to 160/95 mmHg was regarded as borderline. The significance of a single elevated reading is unclear and for a firm diagnosis the blood pressure should be elevated on more than one examination.

CAUSES

In the large majority of cases no cause can be identified, and this form of hypertension is known as primary or essential. A cause of hypertension can be discovered in less than 10% of cases; such cases are known as secondary hypertension.

Essential hypertension
No single factor has been found to explain essential hypertension; many factors are probably responsible. The blood pressure is determined by the product of the cardiac output and the peripheral vascular resistance.

In the early stages of essential hypertension the increase of blood pressure is due to a small increase in cardiac output. This could be due to sympathetic overactivity. Later in the disease, the cardiac output is normal but the peripheral resistance is increased. It is possible that the initial increase in cardiac output induces vascular changes which then sustain and increase the blood pressure.

The baroreceptor reflexes operate at a higher pressure in hypertension. An increased blood pressure should stimulate a bradycardia via the carotid sinus baroreceptor mechanism. This does not happen in essential hypertension. This abnormal reflex may be due to the hypertension rather than be its cause.

In a small proportion of patients with essential hypertension, catecholamine levels are slightly increased, and in others the plasma renin is higher than normal. The relevance of these humoral factors is not known.

As yet unidentified dietary factors may induce essential hypertension. Obesity is associated with hypertension and a low salt intake protects against hypertension.

Genetic factors are also certainly relevant because there are racial and familial tendencies to hypertension. It is likely that many genes are involved.

Secondary hypertension
This should always be considered in patients with hypertension. In particular, a careful search should be made in hypertensive patients presenting under the age of 35 years. The causes of secondary hypertension can be divided into renal, endocrine, cardiovascular, pregnancy and drugs.

Renal causes (see p. 397). Renal diseases are the most common causes of secondary hypertension, accounting for over 80% of cases. Chronic glomerulonephritis, chronic atrophic pyelonephritis and congenital polycystic kidneys are the conditions usually involved. It may be difficult to determine whether renal disease has caused hypertension or whether the hypertension has produced the renal disease.

The mechanism by which renal disease causes hypertension is probably related to salt and water retention. Occasionally, renal artery stenosis due to fibromuscular hyperplasia or atheroma may cause hypertension (renovascular hypertension) due to excess renin production (see p. 398).

Endocrine causes (see Table 16.49, p. 739). These include:
- Conn's syndrome
- Phaeochromocytoma
- Cushing's syndrome
- Acromegaly

Cardiovascular causes. Renovascular hypertension is discussed above.

Coarctation of the aorta (see p. 530) should be considered in young patients with hypertension and a late systolic murmur.

Pregnancy. Hypertension in the early stages of pregnancy is usually essential hypertension or due to renal disease.

Pre-eclampsia or toxaemia of pregnancy is diagnosed when hypertension develops in the last 3 months of pregnancy and is associated with oedema and proteinuria. The cause of pre-eclampsia is unknown but the treatment involves bedrest and antihypertensive drugs known to be safe in pregnancy. Methyldopa is usually recommended.

Pre-eclampsia may worsen, with the development of severe hypertension, nausea, vomiting, pulmonary oedema and fits. This condition, known as eclampsia, needs urgent treatment. If the high pressure cannot be reduced, the pregnancy may need to be terminated.

Drugs. Oestrogen-containing contraceptives, other steroids, carbenoxolone, liquorice and vasopressin may all cause hypertension. Paroxysms of severe hypertension may occur in patients taking monoamine oxidase inhibitors who eat cheese or other tyramine-containing foods and wines.

PATHOPHYSIOLOGY

An increase in vascular tone initially accounts for the increased peripheral vascular resistance. As the disease progresses, the walls of small arteries thicken and atheroma develops in larger arteries. Malignant hypertension is characterized by fibrinoid necrosis of the vascular wall.

The increased peripheral vascular resistance leads to a greater impedance to left ventricular emptying. Consequently, left ventricular hypertrophy develops.

A reduction in renal perfusion pressure can occur, leading to decreased glomerular filtration and reduced sodium and water excretion. The renal changes are described in more detail on p. 397. The decreased renal perfusion leads to the production of renin, which converts angiotensinogen to angiotensin I. This is changed to angiotensin II, which stimulates the secretion of aldosterone and further contributes to salt and water retention (see Fig. 16.31, p. 740).

Secondary aldosteronism, which occurs with severe or accelerated hypertension and with the use of diuretics, is characterized by high serum levels of aldosterone and renin. In primary aldosteronism (Conn's syndrome), only the aldosterone is raised. About 10% of patients with essential hypertension have a high plasma renin level, and 25% have a low renin level.

In some cases the pressure rises rapidly and these patients are said to have 'accelerated' or 'malignant' hypertension. Without treatment death occurs within 1–2 years.

The accelerated rise in blood pressure produces cerebral oedema, left ventricular failure and severe renal impairment, with proteinuria and microscopic haematuria. Retinal haemorrhages, exudates and papilloedema are also seen.

COMPLICATIONS

Hypertension is a risk factor for developing atheroma and patients may therefore develop thrombotic cerebral vascular disease, coronary artery disease and peripheral vascular disease. The increased pressure in the circulation can result in heart failure, cerebral haemorrhage, renal disease and dissecting aortic aneurysms.

ASSESSMENT OF PATIENTS

The possible causes and consequences of hypertension are assessed. In uncomplicated or essential hypertension, apart from the high blood pressure there are usually no signs, symptoms or abnormal investigations.

History
The patient with mild hypertension is usually asymptomatic. Nose bleeds and headaches have been traditionally regarded as possible symptoms, but are probably no commoner than in the general population. There may be a past history of renal disease or a family history of hypertension.

Secondary causes of hypertension are suggested by a specific history, such as attacks of sweating and tachycardia in phaeochromocytoma.

Angina may occur either because of associated coronary artery disease or because of the high oxygen demand from hypertrophied muscle. If cardiac failure develops, breathlessness occurs.

Accelerated or malignant hypertension presents with visual impairment, nausea and vomiting, fits, transient paralysis, severe headaches, impairment of consciousness, or symptoms of acute cardiac failure.

Examination
In the majority of patients the only sign is the high blood pressure, but in others, features of the cause of hypertension may be noted. For example, there may be an abdominal bruit due to renovascular obstruction, or delayed femoral pulses due to coarctation of the aorta.

Hypertensive heart disease presents with a loud aortic second sound, a prominent left ventricular apical heave and a fourth heart sound. Sinus tachycardia and a third heart sound develop if cardiac failure occurs.

Examination of the retina may reveal various abnormalities which are known as Keith–Wagener retinal changes. They are graded as follows:

- *Grade 1*—increased tortuosity of retinal arteries and increased reflectiveness (silver wiring)
- *Grade 2*—grade 1 plus the appearance of arteriovenous (AV) nipping produced when thickened retinal arteries pass over the retinal veins
- *Grade 3*—grade 2 plus flame-shaped haemorrhages and soft 'cotton wool' exudates
- *Grade 4*—grade 3 plus papilloedema (bulging and blurring of the edges of the optic disc)

INVESTIGATION (see also p. 739)

Routine investigation of a hypertensive patient should always include:
- A chest x-ray

- An ECG
- Urinalysis
- Fasting blood lipids
- Urea and electrolytes

If the blood urea is abnormal, the creatinine level, creatinine clearance, intravenous excretion urography, renal ultrasound and other tests of renal function are necessary. If the tests of renal function or an abnormal bruit suggest a renovascular cause, renal angiography is essential.

If coarctation of the aorta is suspected, digital vascular imaging with intravenous contrast injection will usually demonstrate the lesion.

If the patient is not taking diuretics, a low serum potassium should suggest an endocrine problem, and aldosterone, cortisol and renin measurements should be performed. A history suggestive of phaeochromocytoma can be investigated with serum catecholamines or urinary catecholamine metabolites such as vanillylmandelic acid (VMA).

The chest x-ray may show a large heart and pulmonary congestion if heart failure has developed, or rib notching in coarctation of the aorta.

The ECG may show left ventricular hypertrophy or signs of myocardial infarction or ischaemia. Very rarely, ECG features of hyperkalaemia (see Fig. 10.6, p. 441) (e.g. with renal failure) or hypokalaemia may be detected.

TREATMENT

In the young, the secondary causes of hypertension should be excluded before treatment is commenced. When the blood pressure is only mildly or moderately elevated, it may be difficult to persuade an asymptomatic patient that treatment is necessary. However, there are definite advantages from treating diastolic blood pressures in excess of 105 mmHg. If the diastolic blood pressure is between 95 and 105 mmHg it should be carefully reassessed on several occasions with the patient in a comfortable, relaxed position. If it is truly elevated (above 95 mmHg) it should be actively treated, especially in young men, and particularly so if there is any evidence of hypertensive retinal, cardiac or renal changes. In elderly patients it is probably unnecessary, and possibly unwise, to attempt to treat mild hypertension, but more severe hypertension (diastolic pressures greater than 105 mmHg) should be cautiously reduced. The Framingham studies have shown that the systolic blood pressure is as important as the diastolic blood pressure and is the best guide to the risk of peripheral arterial disease. Thus, a man with a systolic pressure of 170 mmHg has twice the risk of dying compared with a man with a systolic pressure of 120 mmHg. Borderline or labile hypertension, where the blood pressure readings are occasionally above normal, was also shown to have

an increased mortality of one-and-a-half to two times in this study.

General measures
A review of the patient's lifestyle and diet may suggest modifications that could lead to some reduction of blood pressure, such as:
- *Weight reduction.* Obese patients should lose weight. This leads to a true fall in blood pressure as well as to a reduction of artifactually increased cuff measurements.
- *Reduction of heavy alcohol consumption.* This also leads to a small reduction in blood pressure.
- *Salt restriction.* This may be an effective method of reducing blood pressure. Usually, the patient is advised not to add salt at the table.
- *Regular exercise, meditation and biofeedback.* These are all techniques that have been claimed to lead to blood pressure reduction. An attempt should be made to reduce stress and anxiety.

Patients should also be told to stop smoking to reduce their overall coronary risk. It is doubtful whether cessation of smoking reduces the blood pressure except in malignant hypertension. Hyperlipidaemia should also be corrected (see p. 773) to reduce the risk of atheroma.

Drug treatment
A large number of drugs are used to treat hypertension. This reflects the difficulty in finding a single drug that effectively lowers blood pressure without producing side-effects, which may be more troublesome or more dangerous than the hypertension itself. Compliance is a problem as the side-effects of drug therapy are frequent and the immediate benefits of treatment are not obvious to the patient.

Diuretics. Loop diuretics (e.g. frusemide 40 mg daily or bumetanide 1–2 mg daily) and thiazide diuretics (e.g. bendrofluazide 5 mg daily or cyclopenthiazide 0.5 mg daily) are equally effective at lowering the blood pressure. Thiazides are usually preferred because the duration of action is longer, the diuresis is not so severe, and they cost less. Loop diuretics are restricted to those with cardiac or renal impairment for whom an additional diuretic effect is required.

Although diuretics may lower blood pressure transiently by sodium and water excretion, they also act by directly dilating arterioles. Oral potassium supplements are often not required. Occasionally, hypokalaemia occurs and this is most effectively treated with a potassium-sparing diuretic.

Potassium-sparing diuretics (e.g. triamterene 150–250 mg daily, spironolactone 50–200 mg and amiloride 5–10 mg daily), are not effective hypotensive agents, with the exception of spironolactone, in primary or secondary aldosteronism. These diuretics are combined with others to treat hypokalaemia, which very occasionally occurs in hypertensive patients on diuretics.

Thiazide diuretics may cause hyperuricaemia and may precipitate gout or provoke or worsen glucose intolerance. Thiazide diuretics increase the serum renin level. Unlike other hypotensives, their effect is not postural.

Beta-adrenergic antagonists (see Table 11.36). The mechanism by which beta-blockers reduce hypertension is unclear. Although they reduce the force of cardiac contraction and renin production, they probably act predominantly via the central nervous system. Beta-blockers also reduce anxiety. Propranolol 80 mg twice daily, atenolol 50–100 mg daily and oxprenolol 80 mg twice daily have been most widely used for the treatment of blood pressure, but there is a wide range of beta-blockers with different properties:

- Cardioselectivity implies a greater effect on beta-1-receptors (cardiac receptors) than on beta-2-receptors. Such a selective effect is preferred when bronchospasm, intermittent claudication or diabetes is present. Metoprolol, atenolol and acebutolol are cardioselective beta-blockers.
- Intrinsic sympathomimetic activity (ISA) is necessary if bradycardia complicates therapy with beta-blockade. Pindolol has the largest degree of ISA.
- Poor lipid solubility (e.g. sotalol) is an advantage if central nervous system side-effects are prominent.

The complications of beta-blockade include aggravation of ventricular failure, bradycardia, cold extremities, aching muscles, fatigue, weakness, bad dreams and hallucinations. Non-selective beta-blockade may lead to elevation of serum potassium and may mask or prolong the effects of hypoglycaemia.

Vasodilators. Dilatation of the peripheral arterioles leads to a fall in blood pressure. There are many mechanisms by which vasodilatation can be achieved.

- Calcium antagonists such as nifedipine (20 mg twice daily), diltiazem (60 mg three times daily) and verapamil (120–240 mg daily in divided doses) reduce blood pressure predominantly by arteriolar dilatation, but also by reducing the force of cardiac contraction. They have proven to be effective antihypertensive agents with only a few side-effects; those which do occur include bradycardia and conduction defects (verapamil and diltiazem), headaches, constipation and fluid retention.
- Alpha-1 adrenergic antagonists such as prazosin (500 µg to a maximum of 20 mg daily) and indoramin (25 mg twice daily) are post-synaptic alpha-blockers which produce vasodilatation and are very effective hypotensive drugs. Their main complication is marked hypotension following the first dose, especially when the patient is salt-depleted because of previous diuretic therapy.

Pre-synaptic (alpha-2 adrenergic) antagonists such as phentolamine are now only used in combination with beta-blockers in the treatment of phaeochromocytoma.

Labetolol (300–600 mg daily in divided doses)—a combined beta- and alpha-blocker—is used for the treatment of phaeochromocytoma and for essential and malignant hypertension. It must be given three or four times each day.

- Angiotensin-converting enzyme (ACE) inhibitors such as captopril (50–150 mg daily in divided doses) and enalapril (10–20 mg daily) block the conversion of angiotensin I to angiotensin II, which is a more powerful vasoconstrictor. ACE inhibitors also block the degradation of bradykinin, which is a vasodilator. Their side-

Table 11.36 Main properties of beta-blockers.

	Cardiac selectivity	Partial agonist activity	Lipid solubility	Plasma half-life
Acebutalol	+	+	0	5 h
Atenolol	+	0	0	6 h
Metoprolol	+	0	+	4 h
Nadolol	0	0	0	20 h
Oxprenolol	0	++	+	1.5 h
Pindolol	0	+++	+	4 h
Propranolol	0	0	++	5 h
Sotalol	0	0	0	10 h
Timolol	0	0	+	5 h

effects include first-dose hypotension, a metallic taste, proteinuria, skin rashes and leucopenia.

- Non-diuretic thiazides, including indapamide (2.5 mg daily in the morning) and diazoxide (250–600 mg i.v. in divided doses), produce vasodilatation and are used as hypotensive agents. They produce fluid retention and may provoke glucose intolerance.
- Hydralazine (up to 150 mg daily in divided doses) and minoxidil (10 mg or more daily; maximum 50 mg) directly dilate the peripheral arterioles, leading to a fall in blood pressure. Hydralazine, when given in doses greater than 200 mg daily, may provoke a lupus erythematosus-like syndrome, and minoxidil produces fluid retention and an increase in facial and body hair (hypertrichosis) which renders it unsuitable for women. Both drugs are complicated by sinus tachycardia, which may cause uncomfortable palpitations. They are therefore often combined with beta-blockade.
- Sodium nitroprusside is effective as an arterial and venous dilator when given intravenously. However, it is inconvenient to use because it must be protected from light to prevent degradation. It is useful for the treatment of hypertensive emergencies.
- Centrally acting drugs such as methyldopa (a false adrenergic transmitter) (750 mg daily in divided doses) and clonidine (an alpha-2-agonist) (0.1–0.3 mg daily in divided doses) reduce the degree of vasomotor tone. Both drugs are complicated by tiredness, fluid retention and mild postural hypotension. Methyldopa may also cause a dry mouth, impotence, pyrexia and a positive Coombs' test. Very rarely, a haemolytic anaemia may be produced. It can also rarely cause chronic active hepatitis. Clonidine may cause depression and it is important that it is not stopped suddenly because severe rebound hypertension may occur.
- Debrisoquine, bethanidine and guanethidine block post-synaptic adrenergic neurones and are powerful hypotensive drugs. They are not often used nowadays because of their side-effects, which include marked postural hypotension, bradycardia, diarrhoea, nasal congestion, salivary gland pain and inability to ejaculate.

Stepped care for the control of hypertension
The majority of patients with mild or moderate hypertension can be treated as outpatients. The usual practice is to attempt to reduce the blood pressure to about 150/95 mmHg. If general adjustment to lifestyle and diet have not led to an adequate fall in the blood pressure, it is conventional to prescribe either a beta-blocker or a diuretic. Diuretics (e.g. bendrofluazide 5–10 mg daily) are preferred if heart failure or peripheral vascular disease is present, but beta-blockers (e.g. propranolol 80 mg twice daily or atenolol 100 mg daily) are more suitable if the patient complains of angina. Recently, calcium antagonists such as nifedipine 10 mg twice daily have also been used as a first-line therapy.

If single drug treatment is unsuccessful, it is appropriate to prescribe both a beta-blocker or a calcium antagonist in combination with a diuretic. The combination of beta-blockers and diuretics is particularly attractive because some of their side-effects are partially antagonistic. For example, beta-blockers lead to potassium retention, aggravation of heart failure and decreased renin secretion, whilst thiazide diuretics induce the opposite changes. If these combined therapies are insufficient, more powerful vasodilators such as hydralazine, captopril, enalapril or prazosin are added to the regimen. Centrally acting compounds and adrenergic blockers may be used if these prove inadequate.

It is essential that the patient understands that high blood pressure does not go away after a single course of treatment. It is necessary to continue treatment for many years or for life. In addition, the patient's blood pressure must be checked at regular intervals.

Hypertension that is unresponsive to treatment is usually due to the patient not taking the drugs prescribed or to the presence of an underlying primary cause such as coarctation or renal artery stenosis. Such underlying causes must be discovered and corrected before therapy will succeed.

The management of severe or malignant hypertension
Patients with severe hypertension should be admitted to hospital for urgent treatment under close supervision, and frequent blood pressure measurements should be taken. Hypertensive emergencies should be treated by bringing the blood pressure quickly back to about 110 mmHg diastolic. It is wise to reduce the pressure over about 1 h. This can normally be achieved with oral hydralazine 25 mg or a beta-blocker. Parenteral treatment is seldom necessary. Oral nifedipine (chewed) or captopril may also be effective. In resistant cases, intravenous nitroprusside, labetalol or diazoxide can be used. Too rapid a reduction in blood pressure may lead to cerebral or coronary thrombosis.

The management of hypertension during pregnancy
Mild hypertension in pregnancy is usual, but more severe hypertension (>140/90 mmHg), associated with proteinuria and peripheral oedema, may be a prelude to eclampsia. Pre-eclampsia is treated with bedrest and hypotensive drugs known to be safe in pregnancy. Methyldopa, propranolol and hydralazine are usually used. Full-blown eclampsia, consisting of fits, gross hypertension, proteinuria and fluid retention, is treated as a hypertensive emergency with intravenous hydralazine.

PROGNOSIS

Patients with untreated malignant or accelerated hypertension have a very poor prognosis—more than 90% will die within the first year. Effective reduction in the blood pressure leads to a dramatic improvement of prognosis. In general, the risk from hypertension depends on:

- The level of blood pressure
- The presence of retinal changes
- The presence of cardiac or renal complications
- The sex of the patient (men are more at risk than women)
- The coexistence of coronary disease and risk factors for coronary disease such as high plasma lipids, diabetes and smoking
- The age of the patient (young patients fare worse than the old)

The cause of death in hypertensive patients is usually myocardial infarction, cardiac failure, renal failure or cerebrovascular accident. Effective treatment of moderate hypertension clearly improves the prognosis for each of these causes of death. The treatment of even mild hypertension reduces the likelihood of stroke or cardiac failure.

The heart in pregnancy

In pregnancy the cardiac output and blood volume increase from the second month up to the thirtieth week to 30–50% above the normal levels. This, along with the increased metabolic work, produces the physical signs of warm extremities, a tachycardia with a large volume pulse and a slight rise in venous pressure. The apex beat is displaced, due partly to cardiomegaly and partly to a raised diaphragm. The increased blood flow produces a pulmonary systolic murmur and a third heart sound. The diastolic blood pressure is lower due to vasodilatation.

The added burden of pregnancy on the cardiovascular system can make underlying, otherwise latent, disease clinically apparent. Ten per cent of maternal deaths in England and Wales are due to heart disease. This is usually rheumatic or congenital in origin, but any heart disease can be seen in pregnancy. Moderate to severe mitral stenosis can cause breathlessness early in pregnancy and may lead to pulmonary oedema later in pregnancy. Pregnancy should be avoided in severe mitral stenosis or delayed until after valvotomy. Termination may be necessary in a severe case occurring before the sixteenth week. Most cases of congenital heart disease have been corrected by the time women reach the reproductive age. However, patients with small and uncomplicated septal defects usually tolerate pregnancy well. Patients with prosthetic valves are usually on anticoagulant therapy. This may require a change to heparin as warfarin can cause fetal abnormalities. Patients with pulmonary hypertension of any aetiology have an extremely high mortality (up to 50%) either during or immediately after delivery, and termination should be considered.

Postpartum or late in pregnancy, a cardiomyopathy of uncertain aetiology is sometimes seen. There is also a rise in thromboembolic complications of cardiac disease due to the hypercoagulability which exists postpartum. Sepsis is a risk during delivery, and patients with heart disease may be at risk of developing infective endocarditis.

Peripheral vascular disease

ARTERIAL DISEASE

This can be due to a number of pathological processes.

Arteriosclerosis
This is the term applied to generalized, age-related arterial changes, which are exaggerated in hypertension. In arteries down to 1 mm in diameter these changes initially take the form of compensatory muscular hypertrophy of the media, which is followed by fibrosis and dilatation of the lumen. In hypertensive vessels of this size, atheroma is often superadded.

Smaller arteries show different changes that are usually most marked in the viscera, especially in the kidneys. Here, though there is medial hypertrophy, the predominant change is intimal thickening by concentric layers of connective tissue, with luminal narrowing.

Arterioles undergo hyaline thickening of their walls and luminal narrowing. The narrowing of small vessels in the kidney due to hypertension causes renal ischaemia, which further promotes hypertension.

In malignant hypertension arterioles also show fibrinoid necrosis of their walls.

Mönckeberg's sclerosis
This is a degenerative disease of unknown cause, characterized by dystrophic calcification of the media. It is especially common in the major lower limb arteries of the elderly, and there is an increased incidence of this degeneration in diabetics.

Cystic medial necrosis or degeneration
This describes mucoid degeneration of the collagen and elastic tissue of the media, often with cystic

changes. It occurs mainly in elderly hypertensives. Dissecting aneurysms of the thoracic aorta are often due to this process. Cystic medial degeneration also occurs in inherited defects of collagen tissue formation (e.g. Marfan's syndrome, Ehlers–Danlos syndrome), again resulting in dissecting aneurysms.

Atheroma

The pathogenesis of this condition is described on p. 499. The different vessels which may be involved are shown in Table 11.37. Atheroma seldom involves arteries of less than 2 mm in diameter.

Chronic ischaemia of the legs

This is due to atheromatous disease involving the aorta, iliac and/or any other peripheral vessels. It consequently occurs over the age of 50 years, chiefly in men who are smokers.

SYMPTOMS

- Ischaemic, cramp-like pain, usually in the calves during exercise and relieved by rest (intermittent claudication)
- Rest pain
- Non-healing leg ulcers or gangrene

Both limbs are often affected, but usually one is more severely affected than the other.

SIGNS

- Cold limb with dry skin and lack of hair
- Absent pulses to diseased areas
- Ulceration or gangrene

INVESTIGATION

- X-rays may show calcification of the arteries of the leg.
- Doppler ultrasound is of some help in defining the severity of the lesion.
- Aortography by direct injection of contrast medium into the aorta is used. Angiography is also performed via a percutaneous catheter inserted into the brachial artery, and recently, digital vascular imaging with an intravenous

injection has been used. These investigations show narrowing and stenosis of the arteries.

MANAGEMENT

General

- Risk factors should be reduced (e.g. smoking should be stopped, diabetes should be treated, and weight should be reduced).
- The limbs should be kept warm but local heat should not be applied.
- Care should be taken to avoid infection, trauma, etc. of the feet. Elderly patients often need regular visits to a chiropodist.
- Regular exercise should be taken to encourage the development of anastomotic vessels.
- Vasodilators should not be used.
- Anticoagulants are of no benefit.

Surgery

- Surgery should not be considered for 3 months after symptoms have developed, to allow time for collaterals to develop.
- Aorto-iliac bypass grafts give good results, but reconstruction surgery for blockages below the inguinal ligament is less successful.
- Balloon dilatation via a catheter inserted into the artery is useful for local iliac or femoral stenoses.
- Amputation is necessary for severely ischaemic limbs, usually those with gangrene. Rehabilitation may take months in the elderly and is often unsuccessful.

Many of the patients have generalized atheromatous conditions so that the overall prognosis often dictates the outcome of localized disease.

Acute ischaemia of the legs

Like chronic ischaemia of the legs, this is mainly due to atheromatous disease with thrombosis, but it can also occur due to embolism from the heart (e.g. in atrial fibrillation) or from an atheromatous central vessel.

The clinical picture is of an acutely painful, pale, paralysed, pulseless limb.

Treatment is surgical, with removal of the clot. If gangrene develops, amputation is necessary.

Aortic aneurysms

Abdominal aneurysms

The commonest aortic aneurysms are abdominal. These are usually due to atheroma.

Asymptomatic aneurysms may be found as a pulsatile mass on examination or as calcification on an x-ray. A CT scan or ultrasound of the abdomen will demonstrate the size of the aneurysm, the thickness of the aortic wall and whether any leak has occurred. An expanding aneurysm may cause epigastric or back pain. Rupture presents with epi-

Table 11.37 Common sites of clinically significant atherosclerosis in order of frequency.

Abdominal aorta and iliac arteries
Proximal coronary arteries
Femoral and popliteal arteries, and thoracic aorta
Internal carotid arteries
Vertebrobasilar system

gastric pain radiating through to the back. A pulsatile mass is felt and the patient is shocked.

Treatment of symptomatic aneurysms is surgical. A ruptured aneurysm requires emergency surgery, but even then the mortality is high. Large, asymptomatic aneurysms should also be treated surgically (except in the very old) because those larger than 6 cm in diameter have a high risk of rupture.

Thoracic aneurysms

Most thoracic aneurysms in the past were due to syphilis, but now many are due to atheromatous disease. The aneurysms may affect all parts of the thoracic aorta—the ascending aorta, the arch and the descending aorta.

Most are asymptomatic, but when large they can give rise to chest pain or to evidence of pressure on other organs such as the superior vena cava or the oesophagus. They can rupture.

Dissecting aortic aneurysms

In the majority of cases, the dissection starts in the ascending aorta. Pain, which is severe and central, often radiating to the back, is the major symptom. The pain radiates down the arms and into the neck and can be difficult to distinguish from myocardial infarction.

On examination, the patient is usually shocked and there may be neurological signs due to the involvement of the spinal vessels. The peripheral pulses may be absent, but this is not invariable.

The diagnosis is suggested by the presence of back pain with no ECG or enzyme changes of myocardial infarction. The chest x-ray may show a wide mediastinum and CT scanning and ultrasonography are helpful. Aortography may be necessary to confirm the diagnosis.

Half of the patients are hypertensive and this should be controlled immediately. Emergency surgery is necessary for many dissections.

There is an increased risk of dissection in pregnancy.

Thromboangiitis obliterans (Buerger's disease)

Although this was once thought to be a separate entity, it is now known that it occurs in young men who smoke and is indistinguishable from atheromatous disease.

Takayasu's syndrome

This is rare, except in Japan. It is known as 'pulseless disease' or the aortic arch syndrome. It is of unknown aetiology and occurs in young females. There is a vasculitis involving the aortic arch as well as other major arteries. There is also a systemic illness, with pain and tenderness over the affected arteries. Absent peripheral pulses and hypertension are usually found. Corticosteroids help the constitu-

tional symptoms. Heart failure and cerebrovascular accidents eventually occur, but most patients survive for at least 5 years.

Cardiovascular syphilis

This gives rise to
- Uncomplicated aortitis
- Aortic aneurysms, usually in the ascending part
- Aortic valvulitis with regurgitation
- Stenosis of the coronary ostia

The diagnosis is confirmed by serology. Treatment is with penicillin. Aneurysms and valvular disease are treated as necessary by the usual methods.

Connective tissue disorders

These cause vasculitis and can give rise to peripheral vascular disease. They are discussed on p. 339.

Raynaud's phenomenon

Raynaud's phenomenon consists of spasm of the arteries supplying the fingers or toes and is usually precipitated by cold and relieved by heat. When Raynaud's phenomenon occurs without any underlying disorder, it is then known as Raynaud's disease. This is a common disease affecting 5% of the population and occurring predominantly in young women. The disorder is usually bilateral and fingers are affected more commonly than toes. There is an initial pallor of the skin resulting from vasoconstriction and this is followed by cyanosis due to sluggish blood flow. Redness finally occurs due to hyperaemia. The duration of the attacks can be variable and can sometimes last for hours. Numbness and burning of the fingers usually occurs and pain can be severe, particularly in the re-warming phase.

Between the attacks the pulses and the digits appear normal, but trophic changes with small areas of gangrene can occur in severe and persistent cases.

DIAGNOSIS

Primary Raynaud's disease must be differentiated from secondary causes of Raynaud's phenomenon, which are chiefly disorders of connective tissue, particularly systemic sclerosis. It can also occur in cryoglobulinaemia and as a side-effect of drug treatment, especially with beta-blocking agents.

TREATMENT

No treatment is usually required for the attacks but any underlying disease must be looked for. The hands and feet should be kept warm, and smoking should be avoided. Beta-blockers should be stopped. Nifedipine 10 mg three times daily may be helpful.

VENOUS DISEASE

Varicose veins

Varicose veins are a common problem, sometimes giving rise to pain. They are treated by injection or surgery.

Venous thrombosis

Thrombosis can occur in any vein, but the veins of the leg and the pelvis are the commonest sites.

Superficial thrombophlebitis
This commonly involves the saphenous veins and is often associated with varicosities. Occasionally the axillary vein is involved, usually as a result of trauma. There is local superficial inflammation of the vein wall, with secondary thrombosis.

The clinical picture is of a painful, tender, cord-like structure with associated redness and swelling.

The condition usually responds to symptomatic treatment with rest, elevation of the limb and analgesics (e.g. non-steroidal anti-inflammatory drugs). Anticoagulants are not necessary as embolism does not occur from superficial thrombophlebitis.

Deep vein thrombosis
A thrombus forms in the vein, and any inflammation of the vein wall is secondary to this.

Thrombosis commonly occurs after periods of immobilization, but it can occur in normal individuals for no obvious reasons. The precipitating factors are discussed on p. 300.

Deep-vein thrombosis occurs in 50% of patients after prostatectomy or following a cerebral vascular accident. In addition, one-third of patients with a myocardial infarct have a deep-vein thrombosis.

Thrombosis can occur in any vein of the leg, but is particularly found in the veins of the calf. It is often undetected; autopsy figures give an incidence of over 60% in hospitalized patients.

Clinical features. The major presenting features are:
- Asymptomatic, presenting with clinical features of pulmonary embolism (see p. 533)
- Pain in the calf, often presenting with swelling, redness and engorged superficial veins. The affected calf is often warmer and there may be ankle oedema. Homans' sign (pain in the calf on dorsiflexion of the foot) is often present, but is not diagnostic and occurs with all lesions of the calf.

Thrombosis in the iliofemoral region can present with severe pain, but there are often few physical signs apart from occasional swelling of the thigh and/or ankle oedema.

Complete occlusion, particularly of a large vein, can lead to a cyanotic discoloration of the limb and severe oedema, which can very rarely lead to venous gangrene.

Pulmonary embolism can occur with any deep vein thrombosis but is more frequent from an iliofemoral thrombosis and is rare with thrombosis confined to veins below the knee. Spread of thrombosis can occur proximally without clinical evidence, so the extent of the thrombosis must be assessed by venography.

Investigation. Clinical diagnosis is unreliable and venography is the investigation of choice. It should always be performed in any patient in whom anticoagulation therapy is contemplated. It is a reliable technique and can detect virtually all thrombi that are present. A vein in the foot is injected with contrast, and most veins of the leg and thigh can be visualized. Percutaneous iliofemoral venography is sometimes required to detect venous thrombosis in the pelvis.

Examination by the Doppler technique, ^{131}I-labelled fibrinogen and plethysmography are unreliable and have largely been superseded by venography which, although invasive and more painful than the other techniques, is much more dependable.

Treatment. The aim of treatment is to prevent propagation of the thrombus, destruction of the venous valves and pulmonary embolism. This is achieved with anticoagulation (see p. 300) and bedrest until the patient is fully anticoagulated. The patient should then be mobilized, with an elastic stocking giving graduated pressure over the leg.

Heparin is given normally for 48 h but how long warfarin should be given is debatable—3 months is the usual recommended period. Anticoagulants do not affect the thrombus that is already present.

Thrombolytic therapy (see p. 300) is used for patients with a large iliofemoral thrombosis.

Prognosis. Destruction of the deep vein valves produces a clinically painful, swollen limb which is made worse by standing and which is accompanied by oedema and sometimes venous eczema. It occurs in approximately half of the patients with a clinically symptomatic deep vein thrombosis, and it means that elastic support stockings are then required for life.

Prevention. Subcutaneous low dose heparin (see p. 300) should be given to patients with cardiac failure, a myocardial infarct or surgery to the leg or pelvis.

Early ambulation is indicated as most thromboses occur within the first 72 h following surgery. Leg exercises should be encouraged and patients should not sit in a chair with their legs immobilized on a stool. An elastic support stocking should be given to patients at high risk, e.g. those with a history of thrombosis or with obesity.

Further reading

Braunwald E (1984) *Heart Disease*, 2nd edn. Philadelphia: WB Saunders.

Chesler E (1981) *Schrire's Clinical Cardiology*, 4th edn. Bristol: John Wright.

Fleming JS & Braimbridge MV (1974) *Lecture Notes On Cardiology*, 2nd edn. Oxford: Blackwell Scientific.

Hampton JR (1986) *The ECG Made Easy*, 3rd edn. Edinburgh: Churchill Livingstone.

Hurst JW (1986) *The Heart*, 6th edn. New York: McGraw-Hill.

Julian DG (1983) *Cardiology*, 4th edn. London: Baillière Tindall.

Sokolow M & McIlroy MB (1984) *Clinical Cardiology*, 4th edn. New York: Lange.

A glossary of terms and abbreviations used in this chapter is given in the Appendices on p. 963.

Diseases of the respiratory system are a major cause of morbidity and mortality throughout the world. In the UK respiratory diseases account for approximately one-fifth of all deaths, exceeded only by heart disease. Respiratory disorders are the single biggest cause of days lost from work and generate the largest number of visits to general practitioners. While some diseases such as tuberculosis are clearly in decline, the prevalence of others, such as asthma, is probably increasing; chronic bronchitis and emphysema continue to remain a major problem in the UK.

New problems are appearing such as the outbreaks of legionnaires' disease and infections with microorganisms normally considered to have low pathogenicity, such as *Mycobacterium avium*, *Mycobacterium intracellulare* and *Pneumocystis carinii*, in patients suffering from acquired immunodeficiency syndrome (AIDS). There is still no cure for the common cold, and in spite of intense efforts to discourage cigarette smoking, carcinoma of the bronchus remains the commonest cancer.

Structure of the respiratory system

The nose

The anterior one-third of the nasal cavity is divided into right and left halves by the nasal septum (Fig. 12.1). The nasal vestibule leads to the internal ostium

(a) which is the narrowest part of the nasal cavity. This causes a resistance to airflow which is 50% greater when breathing through the nose than through the mouth. The respiratory region (b) is divided by three folds arising from the lateral wall, termed the superior turbinate (ST), middle turbinate (MT) and inferior turbinate (IT). Behind these turbinates are situated the openings of the nasolacrymal duct and the frontal, ethmoidal and maxillary sinuses. The olfactory region for smell is found above the superior turbinate. The nasal cavities communicate with the nasopharynx via the posterior nasal apertures [the choanae (c)], and the eustachian tube opens into this area just above the soft palate.

The pharynx and larynx

The pharynx is divided by the soft palate into an upper nasopharyngeal and lower oropharyngeal region. There are numerous collections of lymphoid tissue arranged in a circular fashion around the nasopharynx; these include the adenoids. The tonsils lie between the anterior and posterior fauces, separating the mouth from the oropharynx.

The larynx consists of a number of articulated cartilages, vocal cords, muscles and ligaments, all of which serve to keep the airway open during breathing and occlude it during swallowing.

The main motor nerve to the larynx is the recurrent laryngeal nerve. The left recurrent laryngeal nerve leaves the vagus at the level of the aortic arch, hooking round it to run upwards through the mediastinum between the trachea and the oesophagus; it can be affected by disease in these areas. The principal tensor of the vocal cords is the external branch of the superior laryngeal nerve, which can be injured during thyroidectomy.

The trachea, bronchi and bronchioles

The trachea is 10–12 cm in length. It lies slightly to the right of the midline and divides at the carina into right and left main bronchi. The carina lies under the junction of the manubrium sternum and the second right costal cartilage.

The right main bronchus is more vertical than the left and, hence, inhaled material is more likely to pass into it.

The right main bronchus divides into the upper lobe bronchus and the intermediate bronchus, which

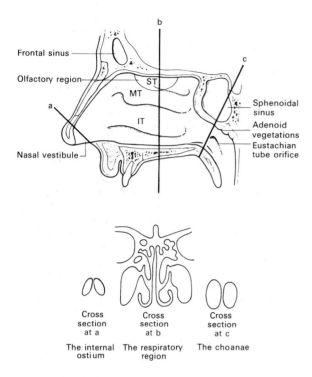

Frontal sinus

Olfactory region

ST

MT

a

IT

Nasal vestibule

Sphenoidal sinus

Adenoid vegetations

Eustachian tube orifice

Cross section at a

Cross section at b

Cross section at c

The internal ostium

The respiratory region

The choanae

Fig. 12.1 The anatomy of the nose. *Top* Longitudinal section. *Bottom* Cross sections. ST = superior turbinate; MT = middle turbinate; IT = inferior turbinate.

further subdivides into the middle and lower lobe bronchi. On the left the main bronchus divides into upper and lower lobe bronchi only. Each lobar bronchus further divides into segmental and subsegmental bronchi.

There are about 25 divisions in all between the trachea and the alveoli. In the first seven divisions the bronchi have:

- Walls consisting of cartilage and smooth muscle
- Epithelial lining with cilia and goblet cells
- Submucosal mucus-secreting glands

In the next 16–18 divisions the bronchioles have:

- No cartilage and a muscular layer which progressively becomes thinner
- A single layer of ciliated cells, but very few goblet cells
- Granulated Clara cells which produce a surfactant-like substance

The ciliated epithelium is an important defence mechanism. Each cell contains approximately 200 cilia beating at 1000 times per minute in organized waves of contraction. Mucus, which contains macrophages, cell debris, inhaled particles and bacteria, is moved by the cilia towards the larynx at about 1.5 cm per minute—the 'mucociliary escalator' (see below).

The bronchioles finally divide within the acinus into smaller respiratory bronchioles which have alveoli arising from the surface (Fig. 12.2). Each

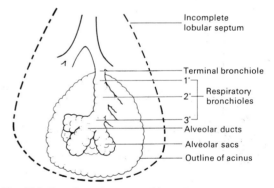

Incomplete lobular septum

Terminal bronchiole

1°

Respiratory bronchioles

2°

3°

Alveolar ducts

Alveolar sacs

Outline of acinus

Fig. 12.2 Branches of a terminal bronchiole ending in the alveolar sacs.

respiratory bronchiole supplies approximately 200 alveoli via alveolar ducts. The term 'small airways' refers to bronchioles of less than 2 mm; there are 30 000 of these in the average lung.

The alveoli

There are approximately 300 million alveoli in each lung. Their total surface area is 40–80 m^2. The epithelial lining consists largely of type I pneumocytes (Fig. 12.3). These cells have an extremely attenuated cytoplasm, and thus provide only a thin barrier to gas exchange.

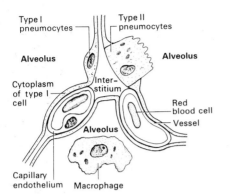

Fig. 12.3 The structure of alveoli, showing the pneumocytes and capillaries.

Type II pneumocytes are slightly more numerous than type I cells but cover less of the epithelial lining. They are found generally in the borders of the alveolus and contain distinctive lamellar vacuoles, thought to be the source of surfactant. Type II cells are fixed to type I cells by tight junctions which limit the fluid movements in and out of the alveoli. Macrophages are also present in the alveoli and are involved in the defence mechanisms of the lung.

The pores of Kohn are holes in the alveolar wall allowing communication beween alveoli of adjoining lobules.

The lungs

The lungs are separated into lobes by invaginations of the pleura which are often incomplete. The right lung has three lobes, whereas the left lung has two. These are shown with their surface anatomy in Fig. 12.4.

The position of the oblique fissures and the right horizontal fissure is shown in Fig. 12.4. The upper lobe lies mainly in front of the lower lobe and therefore signs on the right side in the front of the chest found on physical examination are due to lesions mainly of the upper lobe or part of the middle lobe.

Each lobe is further subdivided into bronchopulmonary segments by fibrous septa which extend inwards from the pleural surface. Each segment receives its own segmental bronchus.

The bronchopulmonary segment is further divided into individual lobules approximately 1 cm in diameter and generally pyramidal in shape, the apex lying towards the bronchioles supplying them. Within each lobule a terminal bronchus supplies an acinus and within this structure further divisions of the bronchioles eventually give rise to the alveoli.

The pleura

This is a layer of connective tissue covered by a simple squamous epithelium. The visceral pleura covers the surface of the lung, lines the interlobar fissures, and is continuous at the hilum with the parietal pleura, which lines the inside of the hemithorax. At the hilum the visceral pleura continues alongside the branching bronchial tree for some distance before reflecting back to join the parietal pleura. The pleurae are in apposition apart from a small quantity of lubricating fluid, so the pleural cavity is only a potential space.

Pulmonary vasculature and lymphatics

The pulmonary artery divides to accompany the bronchi. The arterioles accompanying the respiratory bronchioles are thin-walled and contain little smooth muscle. The pulmonary venules drain laterally to the periphery of the lobules, pass centrally in the interlobular and intersegmental septa, and eventually join to form the four main pulmonary veins.

In addition, a further bronchial circulation arises from the descending aorta. These bronchial arteries supply tissues down to the level of the respiratory bronchiole. The bronchial veins drain into the pulmonary vein, forming part of the physiological shunt observed in normal individuals.

Lymphatic channels lie in the potential interstitial space between the alveolar cells and the capillary endothelium of the pulmonary arterioles.

Physiology of the respiratory system

The nose

The major functions of nasal breathing are:
- To heat and moisten the air
- To remove particulate matter

About 10 000 l of particle-laden air are inhaled daily. Deposited particles are removed from the nasal mucosa within 15 minutes compared with 60–120 days from the alveolus. The relatively low flow rates and turbulence of inspired air is ideal for particle deposition, and few particles greater than 10 μm pass through the nose. For this reason nasal secretion contains many protective proteins in the form of antibodies, lysozymes and interferon. In addition, the cilia of the nasal epithelium move the mucous gel layer rapidly back to the oropharynx where it is swallowed. Bacteria have little chance of settling in the nose. Mucociliary protection against viral infections is more difficult since viruses appear to possess a special affinity for receptors on cilia.

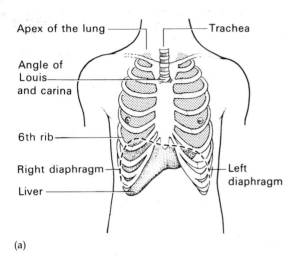

Apex of the lung

Trachea

Angle of
Louis
and carina

6th rib

Right diaphragm

Liver

Left
diaphragm

(a)

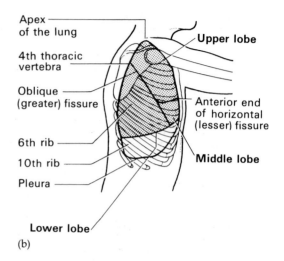

Apex
of the lung

Upper lobe

4th thoracic
vertebra

Oblique
(greater) fissure

Anterior end
of horizontal
(lesser) fissure

6th rib

10th rib

Pleura

Middle lobe

Lower lobe

(b)

(c)

Posterior ends
of ribs

Clavicle

Aortic knuckle

Lungs

Hilum (pulmonary
arteries)

Right atrial
border

Border of
left ventricle

Right diaphragm

Left diaphragm

(d)

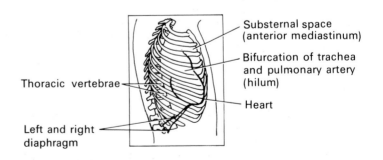

Substernal space
(anterior mediastinum)

Bifurcation of trachea
and pulmonary artery
(hilum)

Thoracic vertebrae

Heart

Left and right
diaphragm

Fig. 12.4 Surface anatomy and divisions of the lung. (a) Anterior. (b) Lateral. (c) PA x-ray. (d) Lateral x-ray.

Breathing

Lung ventilation can be considered in two parts:
- The mechanical process of inspiration and expiration
- The control of respiration to a level appropriate for the metabolic needs

Mechanical process

Inspiration is an active process and results from the descent of the diaphragm and movement of the ribs upwards and outwards under the influence of the intercostal muscles.

Expiration follows passively as a result of gradual lessening of contraction of the intercostal muscles, allowing the lungs to collapse under the influence of their own elastic forces.

Inspiration against increased resistance may require the use of the accessory muscles of ventilation, such as the sternomastoid and scalene muscles. Forced expiration is also accomplished with the aid of accessory muscles, chiefly those of the abdominal wall, which help to push up the diaphragm.

The lungs have an inherent elastic property which causes them to tend to collapse away from the thoracic wall, generating a negative pressure within the pleural space. The strength of this retractive force relates to the volume of the lung; for example, at higher lung volumes the lung is stretched more, and a greater negative intrapleural pressure is generated.

Lung compliance is a measure of the relationship between this retractive force and lung volume. It is defined as the change in lung volume brought about by unit change in transpulmonary (intrapleural) pressure and is measured in litres per kilopascal ($l \cdot kPa^{-1}$). At the end of a quiet expiration, the retractive force exerted by the lungs is balanced by the tendency of the thoracic wall to spring outwards. At this point respiratory muscles are resting and the volume of the lung is known as the *functional residual capacity* (FRC) (see p. 568).

Diseases which can affect the movement of the thoracic cage and diaphragm can have a profound effect on ventilation. These include diseases of the thoracic spine such as ankylosing spondylitis and kyphoscoliosis, neuropathies (e.g. the Guillain–Barré syndrome), injury to the phrenic nerves, and myasthenia gravis.

The control of respiration

Coordinated respiratory movements result from rhythmical discharges arising in an anatomically ill-defined group of interconnected neurones in the reticular substance of the brain stem known as the respiratory centre. Motor discharges from the respiratory centre travel via the phrenic and intercostal nerves to the respiratory musculature.

The pressures of oxygen and carbon dioxide in arterial blood are closely controlled. In a typical normal adult at rest:

- The pulmonary blood flow of 5 $l \cdot min^{-1}$ carries 11 $mmol \cdot min^{-1}$ (250 $ml \cdot min^{-1}$) of oxygen from the lungs to the tissues.
- Ventilation at about 6 $l \cdot min^{-1}$ carries 9 $mmol \cdot min^{-1}$ (200 $ml \cdot min^{-1}$) of carbon dioxide out of the body.
- The normal pressure of oxygen in arterial blood (P_aO_2) is between 11 and 13 kPa (83 and 98 mmHg).
- The normal pressure of carbon dioxide in arterial blood (P_aCO_2) is 4.8–6.0 kPa (36–45 mmHg).

Neurogenic and chemical factors are involved in the control of ventilation.

Neurogenic factors. Neural stimuli include:
- Consciously induced changes in rate and depth of breathing
- Impulses from limb receptors, as in exercise, which causes respiratory stimulation
- Impulses arising from pulmonary receptors sensitive to stretch and bronchial irritation
- Juxtapulmonary capillary receptors (J receptors) stimulated by pulmonary congestion
- Impulses arising from receptors in muscles and joints of the chest wall

Abnormal stimuli include:
- Lesions in the pons and midbrain, which give rise to central neurogenic hyper- or hypoventilation
- Medullary compression, which leads to respiratory depression

Chemical stimuli. Peripheral and central (in the respiratory centre) chemoreceptors cause an increase in ventilation when they are stimulated by:
- *Carbon dioxide.* The strongest respiratory stimulant to breathing is a rise in P_aCO_2. Sensitivity to this may be lost in chronic bronchitis so that in these patients hypoxaemia is the chief stimulus to respiratory drive; treatment with oxygen may therefore reduce respiratory drive and produce a further rise in P_aCO_2.
- *Hydrogen ion concentration of arterial blood.* An increase in [H^+] owing to metabolic acidosis will increase ventilation with a fall in P_aCO_2. In respiratory disease, [H^+] and P_aCO_2 rise together.
- *Oxygen.* Peripheral chemoreceptors in the carotid and aortic bodies respond to reduced P_aO_2. The stimulus is not strong unless the P_aO_2 is below 8 kPa. These chemoreceptors also respond to increases in [H^+].

The respiratory centre is depressed by severe hypoxaemia and sedatives (e.g. opiates), and stimulated by large doses of aspirin or by pyrexia.

In certain common conditions such as mild asthma, pulmonary embolism and pneumonia there is an increase in ventilation leading to a reduction in the P_aCO_2. These conditions probably cause this effect through stimulation of irritant receptors in the bronchioles and J receptors stimulated deep in the parenchyma of the lung.

Anxiety or hysteria cause hyperventilation, and increased ventilation is also a prominent feature of metabolic acidosis.

The airways of the lungs

The sites of greatest resistance to airflow are the larynx, trachea and main bronchi, but the principal diseases causing chronic airflow limitation generally affect the smaller airways.

The airways can be divided into an intrapulmonary component supported by the elastic recoil of the surrounding alveoli and the largely extrapulmonary (but intrathoracic) cartilaginous bronchi.

Movement of air through the airways results from a difference between the pressure in the alveoli and the atmospheric pressure; a positive alveolar pressure occurs in expiration and a negative alveolar pressure occurs in inspiration.

Alveolar pressure is equal to the elastic recoil pressure of the lung (P_{el}) plus the pleural pressure (P_{pl}). P_{el} is always positive, and during normal tidal respiration P_{pl} is always negative, even during expiration, when it acts as a brake to the normal lung recoil. This 'relaxed' expiration can be enhanced by increasing the pleural pressure above atmospheric pressure by using the expiratory muscles, but once pleural pressure rises a little above atmospheric pressure, flow limitation occurs and the speed of expiration cannot be further increased.

As air flows from the alveoli towards the mouth there is a gradual loss of pressure owing to flow resistance (see Fig. 12.5). When the outside of the intrathoracic airways is exposed to a positive pleural pressure there is a tendency for the collapsible airways to narrow at the point where the intraluminal pressure falls below the pleural pressure. At this stage further expiratory effort causes further airway collapse.

The determinant of the maximal achievable expiratory flow is the elastic recoil pressure, which approximates to the pressure drop from the alveoli to the point of narrowing. Loss of the elastic recoil of the lung as occurs in emphysema thus leads to severe limitation of airflow. Since the elastic recoil pressure of the lung depends upon how greatly it is stretched, it follows that high expiratory flow rates can be obtained at high lung volumes. As volume decreases through expiration, the maximum flow rate becomes progressively reduced.

On inspiration the intrapleural pressure is always less than the intraluminal pressure within the intrathoracic airways, so there is no limitation to airflow with increasing effort. Inspiratory flow is limited only by the power of the inspiratory muscles.

The relationship between maximal flow rates on expiration and inspiration is demonstrated by the

$$\text{Alveolar pressure} = \text{elastic recoil pressure of lung} + \text{pleural pressure}$$

Fig. 12.5 Schematic diagram showing the ventilatory forces during expiration in normal people and patients with chronic bronchitis and emphysema. The respiratory system is represented by a single alveolus and airway in a box and the pressures given are illustrative. In expiratory airflow limitation there is a decrease in elastic recoil (a), a decrease in the number of peripheral airways, and a reduction in calibre of these airways (b). The resistance of the peripheral airways is therefore increased and the pressure drop from the alveoli to the mouth is more rapid. Thus in expiration the collapsibility of these airways is enhanced and patients with airflow limitation need to purse their lips (c) in order to maintain an intra-airway pressure so that their peripheral airways do not collapse.

maximal flow volume (MFV) loops shown in Fig. 12.6.

The measurement of the volume that can be forced in from residual volume in 1 s (FIV_1) will always be greater than that which can be forced out from TLC in one second (FEV_1). Thus the ratio of FEV_1 to FIV_1 is below 1. The only exception to this occurs when there is significant obstruction to the airways outside the thorax, e.g. a tumour mass in the upper part of the trachea. Under these circumstances expiratory airway narrowing is prevented by the tracheal resistance (a situation similar to pursing the lips) and expiratory airflow becomes more effort-dependent. During forced inspiration this same resistance causes such negative intraluminal pressure that the trachea is compressed by the surround-

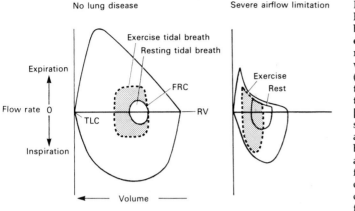

Fig. 12.6 Maximal flow volume loops showing the relationship between maximal flow rates on expiration and inspiration in a normal subject (left) and a patient with severe airflow limitation (right). Flow volume loops during tidal breathing at rest (starting from the functional residual capacity [FRC]) and during exercise are also shown. The highest flow rates are achieved when forced expiration begins at total lung capacity (TLC) and represent the peak expiratory flow rate (PEFR). As air is blown out of the lung, so the flow rate decreases until no more air can be forced out, a point known as the residual volume (RV). Because inspiratory airflow is only dependent on effort, the shape of the maximal inspiratory flow volume loop is quite different, and inspiratory flow remains at a high rate throughout the manoeuvre.

ing atmospheric pressure. Inspiratory flow thus becomes less effort-dependent, and the ratio of FEV_1 to FIV_1 becomes greater than 1. This phenomenon, and the characteristic flow volume loops, is used to diagnose upper airways obstruction.

In subjects with healthy lungs the clinical importance of flow limitation will not be apparent since maximal flow rates are rarely achieved even during vigorous exercise. However, in patients with severe chronic bronchitis and emphysema, limitation of expiratory flow occurs even during tidal breathing at rest (see Fig. 12.6). To increase ventilation these patients have to breathe at higher lung volumes and also allow more time for expiration by increasing flow rates during inspiration, where there is proportionately much less flow limitation. This explains the clinical phenomenon of a prolonged expiratory time in patients with severe airflow limitation.

Ventilation and perfusion relationships

For efficient gas exchange it is important that there is a match between ventilation of the alveoli ($\dot{V}_A$) and their perfusion ($\dot{Q}$). There is a wide variation in the $\dot{V}_A/\dot{Q}$ ratio throughout both normal and diseased lung. In the normal lung the extreme relationships between alveolar ventilation and perfusion are:

- Ventilation but no perfusion (physiological dead space)
- Perfusion but no ventilation (physiological shunting)

These and the 'ideal' match are illustrated in Fig. 12.7. In normal lungs there is a tendency for ventila-

tion not to be matched by perfusion towards the apices, with the reverse occurring at the bases.

An increased physiological shunt results in arterial hypoxaemia. The effects of an increased physiological dead space can usually be overcome by a compensatory increase in the ventilation of normally perfused alveoli. In advanced disease this compensation cannot occur, leading to increased alveolar and arterial P_{CO_2}, together with hypoxaemia.

Hypoxaemia occurs more readily than hypercapnoea because of the different ways in which oxygen and carbon dioxide are carried in the blood. Carbon dioxide can be considered to be in simple solution in the plasma, the volume carried being proportional to the partial pressure. Oxygen is carried in chemical combination with haemoglobin in the red blood cell, and the relationship between the volume carried and the partial pressure is not linear (see Fig. 13.5, p. 626). Alveolar hyperventilation resulting in a low alveolar P_{CO_2} and a high alveolar P_{O_2} will therefore lead to a marked reduction in the carbon dioxide content of the resulting blood but no increase in the oxygen content. The hypoxaemia of even a small amount of physiological shunting cannot therefore be compensated for by hyperventilation.

The P_aO_2 and P_aCO_2 of some individuals who have mild disease of the lung causing slight $\dot{V}/\dot{Q}$ mismatch may still be normal. Increasing the requirements for gas exchange by exercise will widen the $\dot{V}/\dot{Q}$ mismatch and the P_aO_2 will fall.

$\dot{V}/\dot{Q}$ mismatch is by far the commonest cause of arterial hypoxaemia.

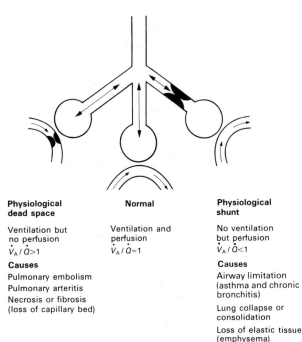

Physiological dead space

Ventilation but no perfusion
$\dot{V}_A / \dot{Q} > 1$

Causes
Pulmonary embolism
Pulmonary arteritis
Necrosis or fibrosis (loss of capillary bed)

Normal

Ventilation and perfusion
$\dot{V}_A / \dot{Q} = 1$

Physiological shunt

No ventilation but perfusion
$\dot{V}_A / \dot{Q} < 1$

Causes
Airway limitation (asthma and chronic bronchitis)

Lung collapse or consolidation

Loss of elastic tissue (emphysema)

Diseases of the chest wall

Fig. 12.7 Relationships between ventilation and perfusion: a schematic diagram showing the alveolar/capillary interface. The centre shows normal ventilation and perfusion. On the left there is a block in perfusion (physiological dead space), whilst on the right there is reduced ventilation (physiological shunting).

Alveolar stability

The alveoli of the lung are essentially hollow spheres. Surface tension acting at the curved internal surface tends to cause the sphere to decrease in size. The surface tension within the alveoli would make the lungs extremely difficult to distend were it not for the presence of surfactant. The type II cells within the alveolus secrete an insoluble lipoprotein largely consisting of dipalmitoyl lecithin, which forms a thin mono-molecular layer at the air–fluid interface. Surfactant reduces surface tension so that alveoli remain stable.

Fluid surfaces covered with surfactant exhibit a phenomenon known as hysteresis, i.e. the surface-tension-lowering effect of surfactant can be improved by a transient increase in the size of the surface area of the alveoli. During quiet breathing, small areas of the lung undergo collapse, but it is possible to re-expand these rapidly by a deep breath, hence the importance of sighs or deep breaths as a feature of normal breathing. Failure of such a mechanism, which can occur, for example, in patients with fractured ribs, gives rise to patchy basal lung collapse. Surfactant levels may be reduced in a number of diseases which cause damage to the lung (e.g. pneumonia), and may play a central role in the respiratory distress syndrome of the newborn. Severe reduction in perfusion of the lung causes impairment of surfactant activity and may well account for the characteristic areas of collapse associated with pulmonary embolism.

Defence mechanisms of the respiratory tract

Pulmonary disease often results from a failure of the many defence mechanisms which usually protect the lung in a healthy individual (Fig. 12.8). These mechanisms can be divided into physical and physiological or humoral and cellular mechanisms.

Physical and physiological mechanisms

The following mechanisms are important:
- *Humidification*—prevents dehydration of the epithelium
- *Particle removal*—over 90% of particles greater than 10 μm in diameter are removed in the nostril or nasopharynx. Of the remainder, 5–10 μm particles become impacted in the carina and 1–2 μm particles are deposited in the distal lungs. Most pollen grains (>20 μm) are deposited in the nose and conjunctiva
- *Particle expulsion*—by coughing, sneezing or gagging
- *Respiratory tract secretions*

The mucus of the respiratory tract is a gelatinous substance consisting chiefly of acid and neutral polysaccharides. The mucus consists of a 5 μm thick gel which is relatively impermeable to water. This

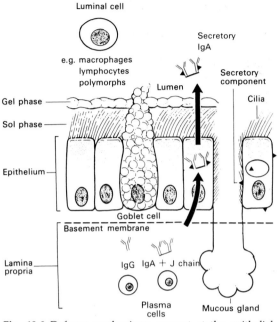

Luminal cell

e.g. macrophages
lymphocytes
polymorphs

Secretory
IgA

Secretory
component

Lumen

Gel phase

Sol phase

Epithelium

Cilia

Goblet cell

Basement membrane

Lamina
propria

IgG   IgA + J chain

Plasma
cells

Mucous gland

Fig. 12.8 Defence mechanisms present at the epithelial surface.

floats on a liquid or sol layer which is present around the cilia of the epithelial cells. The gel layer is secreted from goblet cells and mucous glands as distinct globules that coalesce increasingly in the central airways to form a more or less continuous mucus blanket. Under normal conditions the tips of the cilia are in contact with the undersurface of the gel phase and coordinate their movement to push the mucus blanket upwards. Whilst it may only take 30 to 60 minutes for mucus to be cleared from the large bronchi, there may be a delay of several days before clearance is achieved from respiratory bronchioles. One of the major long-term effects of cigarette smoking is a reduction in mucociliary transport. This contributes to recurrent infection and in the larger airways it prolongs contact with carcinogens.

Congenital defects in mucociliary transport occur. In the 'immotile cilia' syndrome there is an absence of the dynein arms in the cilia themselves, and in cystic fibrosis an abnormal mucus is associated with ciliary dyskinesia. Both diseases are characterized by recurrent infections and eventually with the development of bronchiectasis.

Humoral and cellular mechanisms

Non-specific soluble factors
- *Alpha-1-antitrypsin* is present in lung secretions. It inhibits chymotrypsin and trypsin and neutralizes proteases and elastase.

- *Lysozyme* is an enzyme found in granulocytes which has bacteriocidal properties.
- *Lactoferrin* is synthesized from epithelial cells and neutrophil granulocytes and has bacteriocidal properties.
- *Interferon* is produced by most cells in response to viral infection. It is a potent suppressor of lymphocyte function and lowers the threshold for mast cell histamine release. It renders other cells resistant to infection by other viruses.
- *Complement* is present in secretions. In association with antibodies, it plays an important cytotoxic role.

Alveolar macrophages

These are derived from precursors in the bone marrow and migrate to the lungs via the bloodstream. They phagocytose particles, including bacteria, and are removed by the mucociliary escalator, lymphatics and bloodstream. They are the dominant cell in the airways and comprise 90% of all cells obtained by bronchoalveolar lavage.

Macrophages process antigens and, in combination with their own HLA antigens, present them to T lymphocytes (see Fig. 2.9, p. 109). This is the trigger for the complex interaction between cells which results in the development of both cellular and humoral immunity.

Lymphoid tissue (see p. 111)

The bronchus-associated lymphoid tissue consists of lymphocytes present either in aggregates (tonsils and adenoids) or scattered. It forms an important immunological defence mechanism. Lymphocytes become sensitized to antigens, resulting in local production of secretory IgA. IgG and IgE are also present in secretions derived from B lymphocytes in the lamina propria.

Respiratory symptoms

Runny, blocked nose and sneezing

Nasal symptoms are extremely common. The differentiation between the common cold or allergic rhinitis as a cause of 'runny nose' (rhinorrhoea), nasal blockage and attacks of sneezing is difficult. In allergic rhinitis, symptoms may be seasonal, following contact with grass pollen, or perennial when the house-dust mite is the important allergen. Colds are frequent during the winter, but if more than three occur the patient is probably suffering from perennial rhinitis rather than from infection due to a virus. Patients may be able to identify the cause of their symptoms if, for example, they sneeze whilst walking in the park in summer or after making beds.

Nasal secretions are usually thin and runny in rhinitis but thicker and yellow-green in the common cold. Nose bleeds and blood-stained nasal discharge are common occurrences and are not as serious as haemoptysis. Nevertheless, a blood-stained nasal discharge associated with nasal obstruction and pain may be the presenting feature of a nasal tumour. Total nasal blockage with loss of smell is often a feature of nasal polyps.

Cough

Cough is the commonest manifestation of lower respiratory tract disease. Smokers often have a morning cough with little sputum. Cough is the cardinal feature of chronic bronchitis, while sputum production and coughing, particularly at night, can be symptoms of asthma. Cough also occurs in asthmatics after mild exertion or following a forced expiration. A cough can also occur for psychological reasons.

A worsening cough is the commonest presenting symptom of a bronchial carcinoma and should not be overlooked. The explosive character of a normal cough is lost when laryngeal paralysis is present—a bovine cough—usually resulting from carcinoma of the bronchus infiltrating the left recurrent laryngeal nerve. Cough may be accompanied by stridor in whooping cough and in the presence of laryngeal or tracheal obstruction.

Despite the popularity of cough mixtures, the correct treatment of this symptom is to identify and treat the underlying cause. Cough may persist in some individuals for many weeks following a respiratory tract infection, perhaps as the result of persisting bronchial inflammation, a process which may settle with inhaled corticosteroid treatment.

Sputum

Approximately 100 ml of mucus is produced daily in a healthy, non-smoking individual. This flows at a regular pace up the airways, through the larynx, and is swallowed. Excess mucus is expectorated as sputum. The commonest cause of excess mucus production is cigarette smoking.

Mucoid sputum is clear and white but can contain black specks resulting from the inhalation of carbon. Yellow or green sputum is due to the presence of cellular material, including bronchial epithelial cells, or neutrophil or eosinophil granulocytes. Yellow sputum is not necessarily due to infection, as eosinophils in the sputum, as seen in asthma, can give the same appearance. The production of large quantities of yellow or green sputum is characteristic of bronchiectasis.

Blood-stained sputum (haemoptysis) varies from small streaks of blood to massive bleeding. It requires thorough investigation. The following should be borne in mind:

- The commonest cause of haemoptysis is acute infection. It should not be attributed to chronic bronchitis without investigation.
- Other common causes are pulmonary infarction, bronchial carcinoma and tuberculosis.
- In lobar pneumonia, the sputum is rusty in appearance when blood is present.
- Pink, frothy sputum is seen in pulmonary oedema.
- In bronchiectasis, the blood is often mixed with purulent sputum.
- Large haemoptyses are usually due to bronchiectasis or tuberculosis.
- Uncommon causes of haemoptyses are idiopathic pulmonary haemosiderosis, Goodpasture's syndrome, trauma, blood disorders and benign tumours.

Haemoptysis should always be investigated. Often, the diagnosis can be made from a chest x-ray.

Firm plugs of sputum may be coughed up by patients suffering from an exacerbation of allergic bronchopulmonary aspergillosis; sometimes such sputum may appear as firm threads representing casts from inflamed bronchi.

Breathlessness

Breathlessness should be assessed in relation to the patient's lifestyle. For example, a moderate degree of breathlessness may be totally disabling if the patient has to climb many flights of stairs to reach home. A grading for breathlessness is given on p. 451.

The term *dyspnoea* should be used to describe a sense of awareness of increased respiratory effort which is unpleasant and which is recognized by the patient as being inappropriate. It is highly unlikely that a patient will use this term himself. Patients may complain of tightness in the chest; this must be differentiated from angina.

Orthopnoea (see p. 451) is breathlessness on lying down and is partly due to the weight of the abdominal contents pushing the diaphragm further into the thorax. Such patients are also made uncomfortable by bending over.

The terms *tachypnoea* and *hyperpnoea* refer respectively to an increased rate of breathing and an increased level of ventilation which may be appropriate to the situation (e.g. during exercise). *Hyperventilation* is overbreathing and results in a lowering of the alveolar and arterial P_{CO_2}.

Paroxysmal nocturnal dyspnoea is described on p. 451.

Wheezing

Wheezing is a common complaint and can be the result of airflow limitation due to any cause. The symptom of wheezing is *not* diagnostic of asthma; it may be absent in the early stages of this disease, and may also occur in patients with chronic bronchitis and emphysema.

Chest pain

The commonest type of chest pain encountered in respiratory disease is a localized sharp pain, often referred to as pleuritic. It is made worse by deep breathing or coughing and can be precisely localized by the patient. Localized anterior chest pain may be accompanied by tenderness of a costochondral junction due to costochondritis. Pain in the shoulder tips suggests irritation of the diaphragmatic pleura, whereas central chest pain radiating to the neck and arms is typically of cardiac origin. Retrosternal soreness may occur in patients with tracheitis, and a constant, severe, dull pain may be the result of invasion of the thoracic wall by carcinoma.

Examination of the respiratory system

The nose

The anterior part of the nose can be examined using a nasal speculum and light source. In allergic rhinitis the mucosa lining the nasal septum and inferior turbinate appears swollen and a dark red or plum colour. Nasal polyps can also be identified, as can a frequent site of nasal haemorrhage (Little's area).

The chest (Table 12.1)

Radiology has become an essential part of examination of the chest. Diseases such as tuberculosis or lung cancer may not be detectable on clinical examination but are obvious on the chest x-ray. Conversely, the abnormal physical signs in asthma or chronic bronchitis may be associated with a normal chest x-ray.

Inspection

The patient should be observed carefully, paying particular attention to mental alertness, cyanosis, breathlessness at rest, use of accessory muscles and any deformity or scars on the chest. A coarse tremor or flap of the outstretched hands indicates CO_2 intoxication. Prominant veins on the chest may imply obstruction of the superior vena cava. The jugular venous pressure should be assessed.

Central cyanosis (see p. 453) is assessed on the colour of the tongue and lips, and indicates a P_aO_2 of below 6 kPa. *Peripheral cyanosis* is noted on the fingernails and skin of the extremities, and in the

Table 12.1 Physical signs of respiratory infection.

Pathological process	Chest wall movement	Mediastinal displacement	Percussion note	Breath sounds	Vocal resonance	Added sounds
Consolidation (i.e. lobar pneumonia)	Reduced on affected side	None	Dull	Bronchial	Increased	Fine crackles
Collapse						
Major bronchus	Reduced on affected side	Towards lesion	Dull	Diminished or absent	Reduced or absent	None
Peripheral bronchus	Reduced on affected side	Towards lesion	Dull	Bronchial	Increased	Coarse crackles
Fibrosis						
Localized	Reduced on affected side	Towards lesion	Dull	Bronchial	Increased	Coarse crackles
Generalized (i.e. cryptogenic fibrosing alveolitis)	Reduced on both sides	None	Normal	Vesicular	Increased	Coarse crackles
Pleural effusion (>500 ml)	Reduced on affected side	Away from lesion (in massive effusion)	Stony dull	Vesicular reduced or absent	Reduced or absent	None
Large pneumothorax	Reduced on affected side	Away from lesion	Normal or hyper-resonant	Reduced or absent	Reduced or absent	None
Asthma	Reduced on both sides	None	Normal	Vesicular Prolonged expiration	Normal	Expiratory polyphonic wheeze
Chronic bronchitis and emphysema	Reduced on both sides	None	Normal	Vesicular Prolonged expiration	Normal	Expiratory polyphonic wheeze and coarse crackles

absence of central cyanosis is due to a reduced peripheral circulation.

Finger clubbing is present when the normal angle between the base of the nail and the nail fold is lost. The base of the nail is fluctuant owing to increased vascularity, and there is an increased curvature of the nail in all directions, with expansion of the end of the digit. Some causes of clubbing are given in Table 12.2. Clubbing is not seen in chronic bronchitis.

Palpation

The position of the mediastinum should be ascertained by checking to see if the trachea is central and if the cardiac apex is in the fifth intercostal space. The supraclavicular fossa is examined for enlarged lymph nodes. The distance between the sternal notch and the cricoid cartilage (three to four finger breadths in full expiration) is reduced in patients with severe airflow limitation. Movement of the upper and lower parts of the chest should be assessed. Compression of the chest laterally and antero-posteriorly may produce a localized pain suggestive of a rib fracture.

Percussion

This should be performed symmetrically on both sides for comparison. Liver dullness is usually detected anteriorly at the level of the sixth rib. Liver and cardiac dullness are lost with over-inflated lungs. The percussion note is dull over consolidation and stony dull over a pleural effusion.

Auscultation

The diaphragm of the stethoscope should be used. The patient is asked to take deep breaths through the mouth. Inspiration sounds more prolonged than expiration. Healthy lungs filter off most of the high-frequency component, mainly due to turbulent flow in the larynx. Normal breath sounds are harsher anteriorly over the upper lobes (particularly on the right) and described as vesicular. Vesicular sounds may be loud in a thin healthy subject or soft in patients with emphysema. Breath sounds are reduced or absent in a pneumothorax, over a pleural effusion or when the bronchus to a lobe is obstructed by a carcinoma.

Bronchial breathing. These abnormal breath sounds are heard best over consolidated or collapsed lung and sometimes over areas of localized fibrosis or bronchiectasis. Such areas conduct the high frequency hissing component of breath sounds well. Characteristically, the noise heard during inspiration and expiration is equally long, but separated by a short silent phase. Bronchial breathing can be imitated by listening over the larynx, particularly if the subject breathes with the vocal cords in a position to sound a whispered 'eee'.

Whispering pectoriloquy (whispered sounds heard distinctly) invariably accompanies bronchial breathing.

Added sounds. Many terms are still used to describe additional sounds heard over the lung fields. The terms rhonchi, râles and crepitations are best discarded and replaced with the simple terms wheezes and crackles.

Wheeze is usually heard during expiration and results from vibrations in the collapsible part of the airways when apposition occurs as a result of the flow-limiting mechanisms. Wheezes are heard in asthma and in chronic bronchitis and emphysema, but are not invariably present. In the most severe cases of asthma a wheeze may not be heard as the airflow may be insufficient to generate the sound. Wheezes may be monophonic (single large airway obstruction) or polyphonic (narrowing of many small airways).

Crackles. These brief crackling sounds are probably produced by opening of previously closed bronchioles, and their timing during breathing is of significance—early inspiratory crackles are associated with diffuse airflow limitation, whereas late inspiratory crackles are characteristically heard in pulmonary oedema, fibrosis of the lung and bronchiectasis. They may be described as fine or coarse but this is of no significance.

Pleural rub. This is a creaking or groaning sound which is usually well-localized. It is indicative of inflammation and roughening of the pleural surfaces, which normally glide silently over one another.

Vocal resonance and fremitus. Healthy lung attenuates high frequency notes, leaving the booming low-pitched components of speech. Consolidated lung has the reverse effect, transmitting the high

Table 12.2 Some causes of finger clubbing.

Respiratory
Bronchial carcinoma, especially epidermoid (squamous cell) type—major cause
Chronic suppurative lung disease
    Bronchiectasis
    Lung abscess
    Empyema
Pulmonary fibrosis (e.g. cryptogenic fibrosing alveolitis)
Pleural and mediastinal tumours (e.g. mesothelioma)

Cardiovascular
Cyanotic heart disease
Subacute bacterial endocarditis

Miscellaneous
Congenital—no disease
Cirrhosis
Inflammatory bowel disease

frequencies; the spoken word then takes on a bleating quality. Whispered speech can barely be heard over healthy lung, whereas consolidation allows its clear transmission. Sonorous sounds such as '99' are well-transmitted across healthy lung to produce vibration which can be felt over the chest wall. Consolidated lung transmits these low frequency noises less well, and pleural fluid severely dampens or obliterates the vibrations altogether.

Additional bedside tests

Since so many patients with respiratory disease have airflow limitation, airflow should be routinely measured at the bedside using a peak flow meter (see p. 566). This will provide a much more accurate assessment than any physical sign.

If signs and chest x-ray suggest pleural fluid, this can be readily confirmed by aspiration using a fine needle and a 20 ml syringe. The nature of the pleural fluid can be assessed (blood-stained, purulent or clear) and specimens sent immediately for bacterial culture and cytological examination for malignant cells (see below).

Investigation of respiratory disease

Routine haematological and biochemical tests

These should include tests for:
● Haemoglobin, to detect the presence of anaemia
● PCV (secondary polycythaemia occurs with chronic bronchitis and emphysema)

Other blood investigations sometimes required include alpha-1-antitrypsin levels, autoantibodies, and, in asthma, IgE to specific allergens (RAST; see p. 124) and *Aspergillus* antibodies.

Sputum

Sputum should be inspected for:
● Colour—yellow-green indicates inflammation (infection or allergy)
—presence of blood suggests neoplasm or pulmonary infarct

Microbiological studies (Gram stain and culture) are not helpful in upper respiratory tract infections or in acute or chronic bronchitis. They are of value in:
● Pneumonia
● Diagnosis of tuberculosis (Ziehl–Neelsen stain)
● Unusual clinical problems
● *Aspergillus* lung disease

Cytology

This is extremely useful in the diagnosis of bronchial carcinoma. Advantages are:
● Quick result
● Cheap
● Non-invasive

However, its value depends on the presence of a reliable cytologist.

Transtracheal aspiration
This technique involves pushing a needle through the cricothyroid membrane through which a catheter is threaded to a position just above the carina. This procedure induces coughing, and specimens are collected by aspiration or by the introduction and subsequent aspiration of sterile saline. It is an excellent technique (although not often required) for assessing infection in the lower respiratory tract because it obviates any possibility of contamination of the specimen with bacteria from the pharynx and mouth.

Chest x-ray

The following must be taken into account when viewing films:
● Centring of the film. The distance between each clavicular head and the spinal processes must be equal.
● Penetration
● The view. Postero-anterior (PA) is the routine film. Antero-posterior (AP) films are only taken in very ill patients who are unable to stand up or be taken to the radiology department; the cardiac outline appears bigger and the scapulae cannot be moved out of the way.

The following should be noted:
● The shape and bony structure of the chest wall
● Whether the trachea is central
● Whether the diaphragm is elevated or flat
● The shape, size and position of the heart
● The shape and size of the hilar shadows
● The vascular shadowing and the size and shape of any abnormalities of the lungs

X-ray abnormalities
Collapse and consolidation. The x-ray changes in collapse of a whole lung or lobe are illustrated in Figs. 12.9 and 12.10. Note that with middle lobe collapse all that may be detected is a loss of the clear outline of the right atrium, which distinguishes it from collapse of the right lower lobe. In consolidation the segments or lobes of the lung are opaque but the bronchi are patent, producing an air bronchogram. Causes of collapse are shown in Table 12.3.

Pleural effusion. Pleural effusions need to be more

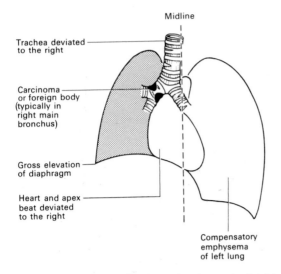

Fig. 12.9 Collapse of the right lung, showing a raised right diaphragm and compensatory emphysema of the left lung.

Table 12.3 Causes of collapse of the lung.

Tumours

Enlarged tracheobronchial lymph nodes due to:
  Malignant disease
  Tuberculosis

Inhaled foreign bodies (e.g. peanut) in children, usually in the right main bronchus

Bronchial casts or plugs (e.g. allergic bronchopulmonary aspergillosis)

Retained secretions—postoperatively and in debilitated patients

than 500 ml to cause much more than blunting of the costophrenic angle. On an erect film they produce a characteristic shadow with a curved upper edge rising into the axilla. If very large, the whole of one side of the thorax may be opaque, with shift of the mediastinum to the opposite side.

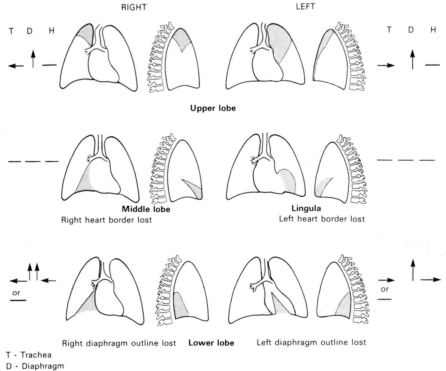

Fig. 12.10 Chest x-ray appearances of lobar collapse.

Fibrosis. Localized fibrosis causes streaky shadowing, and the accompanying loss of lung volume causes mediastinal structures to move to the same side. More generalized fibrosis in the lung can lead to a honeycomb appearance (see p. 610), seen as diffuse shadows containing multiple circular translucences a few millimetres in diameter.

Round shadows. The causes of round shadows are shown in Table 12.4.

Miliary mottling. This term describes numerous minute opacities, 1–3 mm in size, which are caused by many pathological processes. The commoner causes are miliary tuberculosis, pneumoconiosis, sarcoidosis, fibrosing alveolitis and pulmonary oedema, though the latter is usually peri-hilar and accompanied by larger, fluffy shadows. A rare but striking cause of miliary mottling is pulmonary microlithiasis.

Computed tomography

This technique shows lesions that are too small to be seen on a chest x-ray. It gives a much clearer indication of the extent of the disease and correlates better with clinical symptoms and pulmonary function tests. It is of particular value in:
- Assessing intrathoracic spread of carcinoma of the bronchus
- Detecting pulmonary involvement in diseases such as sarcoidosis and lymphoma
- Detecting pulmonary lesions in individuals exposed to industrial dusts

Table 12.4 Causes of round shadows in the lung.

Carcinoma
Metastatic tumours (usually multiple shadows)
Tuberculoma (may be calcification within the lesion)
Lung abscess (usually with fluid level)
Encysted interlobar effusion (usually in horizontal fissure)
Hydatid cysts (rare and often with a fluid level)
Arteriovenous malformations (usually adjacent to a vascular shadow)
Aspergilloma
Rheumatoid nodules

Rare causes
  Bronchial carcinoid
  Cylindroma
  Chondroma
  Lipoma

Other shadows related to mediastinum
  Pericardium
  Oesophagus } Seen on lateral chest x-ray
  Spinal cord

Radioisotope lung scanning

This technique has been widely used for the detection of pulmonary emboli.

Perfusion scan
Macro-aggregated human albumin labelled with technetium-99m is injected intravenously. The particles are of such a size that they impact in pulmonary capillaries, where they remain for a few hours. A gamma camera is then used to detect the position of the macro-aggregated human albumin. The resultant pattern indicates the distribution of pulmonary blood flow; cold areas occur where there is defective blood flow (e.g. in pulmonary emboli).

Disadvantages. Areas of lung with diminished perfusion caused by pulmonary emboli cannot be distinguished from those in which pulmonary blood flow has been closed down by poor ventilation of the adjacent lung. For example, mild asthma can cause a patchy appearance. (NB Peak flow should always be measured before a scan.)

In addition, in patients with an obvious radiological abnormality, a scan cannot differentiate pulmonary embolism from other causes of defective perfusion.

Value. Radioisotope scanning is particularly of value in patients whose chest x-ray is normal and in whom pulmonary embolism is suspected. Multiple cold areas on the scan with only a single abnormality on the x-ray support the diagnosis of pulmonary embolism.

Ventilation–perfusion scan
Xenon-133 gas is inhaled into the lung and its distribution detected at the same time as a perfusion scan is carried out. Using the two scans, a pulmonary embolus causes a striking diminution of perfusion relative to ventilation. Other lung diseases (e.g. asthma or pneumonia) impair both ventilation and perfusion. Unfortunately, however, a pulmonary embolus often produces substantial changes in the lung substance (e.g. atelectasis) so that such a clear distinction is not always obvious. Nevertheless, this is a better technique than perfusion scan alone.

Disadvantages. Xenon-133 has only a short half-life and most laboratories do not have the necessary equipment for its measurement.

Respiratory function tests

In practice, airflow limitation can be assessed by use of relatively simple tests which have good intra-subject repeatability. Normal values are required for their interpretation as these tests vary considerably, not only with sex, age and height, but also within individuals of the same age, sex and height. The standard deviation about the mean for a group of individuals is therefore very high; for example, the standard deviation for the peak expiratory flow rate is approximately 50 l·min^{-1} and for the forced expiratory volume in one second it is approximately 0.4 l·min^{-1}. Repeated measurements of lung function are required for assessing the progression of disease in an individual patient.

Tests of ventilatory function
These tests are mainly used to assess the degree of airflow limitation present during expiration.

Peak expiratory flow rate (PEFR). This is an extremely simple and cheap test. Subjects are asked to take a full inspiration to total lung capacity and then blow out forcefully into the Wright peak flow meter (shown in Fig. 12.11), which is held horizontally; the lips must be placed tightly around the mouthpiece. The best of three tests is recorded.

This peak flow meter records the maximum expiratory flow rate within the first 2 ms of expiration. It is a reasonable measure of airflow limitation, and the intra-subject reliability is good. Regular measurements of peak flow rates on waking, during the afternoon, and before bed demonstrate the wide diurnal variations in airflow limitation which characterize asthma and allow an objective assessment of treatment to be made (see Fig. 12.12).

Fig. 12.11 Peak flow measurements. (a) Peak flow meter. The lips should be tight around the mouthpiece. (b) Graph of normal readings for men and women.

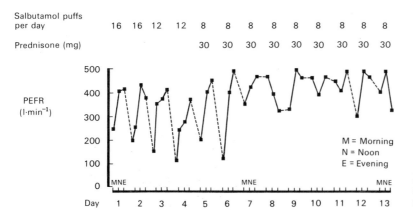

Fig. 12.12 Diurnal variability in airflow limitation showing the effect of steroids.

Spirometry. The Vitalograph spirometer measures the forced expiratory volume in one second (FEV_1) and the forced vital capacity (FVC). Both the FEV_1 and FVC are related to height, age and sex. The instrument used is shown in Fig 12.13a. The technique involves a maximum inspiration followed by a forced expiration (for as long as possible) into the dry bellows spirometer. The act of expiration triggers the moving record chart, which measures volume against time. The record chart moves for a total of 5 s, but expiration should continue until all the air has been expelled from the lungs, as patients with severe airflow limitation may have a very prolonged forced expiratory time. This is demonstrated on the record chart in Fig. 12.13.

The FEV_1 expressed as a percentage of the FVC is an excellent measure of airflow limitation. In normal subjects it is around 75%. With increasing *airflow limitation* the FEV_1 falls proportionately more than the FVC, so that the FEV_1/FVC is reduced. With *restrictive lung disease* the FEV_1 and the FVC are reduced in the same proportion and the FEV_1/FVC remains normal or may even increase because of the enhanced elastic recoil.

It is important to realize that in chronic airflow limitation (particularly in emphysema and asthma) the total lung capacity is usually increased, yet there is nearly always some reduction in the FVC. This is the result of disease in the small airways causing obstruction to airflow before the normal residual volume is reached. This trapping of air within the lung (giving an increased residual volume) is a characteristic feature of these diseases.

Other tests. Tests such as the measurement of airways resistance in a body plethysmograph are more sensitive, but the equipment is expensive and the necessary manoeuvres are too exhausting for many patients with chronic airflow limitation.

Flow volume loops (see p. 556). The ability to measure flow rates against volume (flow volume loops; see

Fig. 12.13 Spirometry. (a) Diagram of a patient using a spirometer. (b) Graph showing restrictive pattern (FEV_1 and FVC reduced). (c) Graph showing airflow limitation (FEV_1 only reduced). (d) Graph showing normal patterns for age and sex.

Fig. 12.6, p. 557) enables a more sophisticated analysis to be made of the site of airflow limitation within the lung. At the start of expiration from total lung capacity, the site of maximum resistance is the large airways, and this accounts for the flow reduction in the first 25% of the curve. As the lung volume reduces further, so the elastic pressures within the lung holding open the smaller airways reduce, and disease either of the lung parenchyma or the small airways themselves becomes readily apparent. For example, in diseases such as chronic bronchitis and emphysema, where the brunt of the disease falls upon the smaller airways, flow rates at 50% or 25% of the vital capacity may be disproportionately reduced when compared with flow rates at larger lung volumes.

Lung volume. The subdivisions of the lung volume are shown in Fig. 12.14. Tidal volume and vital capacity can be measured using a simple spirometer, but the total lung capacity (TLC) and the residual volume needs to be measured by an alternative technique. TLC is measured by connecting the lungs to a reservoir containing a known amount of non-absorbable gas (helium) which can readily be measured. If the concentration of the gas in the reservoir is known at the start of the test and is measured after equilibration of the gas has occurred (when the patient has breathed in and out of the reservoir) the dilution of the gas will reflect the TLC, this technique is known as *helium dilution*. Residual volume can be calculated by subtracting the vital capacity from the TLC.

The TLC measured using this technique is inaccurate if large cystic spaces are present in the lung because the helium cannot diffuse into them. Under these circumstances the thoracic gas volume can be measured more accurately using a body plethysmograph. The difference between the two measurements can be used to define the extent of non-communicating air space within the lungs.

Measurement of blood gases
This technique is described on p. 640.

The measurement of the partial pressure of both oxygen and carbon dioxide within arterial blood is an extremely useful test in diseases of the respiratory and circulatory systems. It is essential in the manage-ment of cases of respiratory failure and severe asthma, when repeated measurements are often the best guide to therapy.

Transfer factor. This measures the transfer of gas across the alveolar–capillary membrane and reflects the uptake of oxygen from the alveolus into the red cell. A low concentration of carbon monoxide is inhaled and is avidly taken up in a linear fashion by circulating haemoglobin, the amount of which must be known when the test is performed. In normal lungs the transfer factor is a true measure of the diffusing capacity of the lungs for oxygen and depends on the thickness of the alveolar–capillary membrane. In lung disease the diffusing capacity (D_{co}) also depends on the $\dot{V}_A/\dot{Q}$ relationship as well as on the area and thickness of the alveolar membrane. To control for differences in lung volume the uptake of carbon monoxide is related to the lung volume; this is known as the transfer coefficient (K_{co}).

Gas transfer is usually reduced in patients with severe degrees of emphysema and fibrosis. Overall gas transfer can be thought of as a relatively non-specific test of lung function but one which can be particularly used in the early detection and assessment of progress of diseases affecting the lung parenchyma (e.g. cryptogenic pulmonary fibrosis, sarcoidosis and asbestosis).

Exercise tests

The predominant symptom in respiratory medicine is that of breathlessness. The degree of disability produced by breathlessness can be assessed before and after treatment by asking the patient to walk for 6 min along a measured track. This has been shown to be a reproducible and useful test.

Pleural aspiration

This should always be performed when fluid is present. An ordinary needle attached to a 20 ml syringe is used. The needle is inserted through an intercostal space over an area of dullness. Fluid is withdrawn and the presence of any blood noted. Samples are sent for protein estimation, cytology and bacteriological examination, including culture

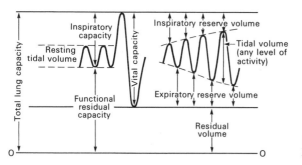

Fig. 12.14 The subdivisions of the lung volume.

and Ziehl-Neelsen stain for tuberculosis. Large amounts of fluid can be aspirated through a large needle to help relieve extreme breathlessness.

Pleural biopsy

Experienced operators obtain tissue in nearly all patients and, provided multiple specimens are taken, positive results may be expected in up to 80% of cases of tuberculosis and in 60% of cases of malignancy. The technique is illustrated in Fig. 12.15.

Pleural biopsy

- Pleural biopsy is usually performed at the end of the aspiration of fluid.
- A small skin incision is made, as the end of the Abrams' pleural biopsy needle is fairly blunt.
- Once in place through the pleura, the back part of the needle is rotated to open the notch; this is kept pointing forward.
- With lateral pressure the needle is withdrawn so that the notch will snag against the pleura.
- The needle is held firmly and the hexagonal grip twisted clockwise to cut the biopsy. To avoid damage to the intercostal vessel or nerve the notch should never be directed upwards when the biopsy is taken.
- Several biopsies should be taken at different angles by repeated insertion of the needle.
- Specimens should be put in sterile saline for culture for tuberculosis and put in 10% formol saline for histological examination.

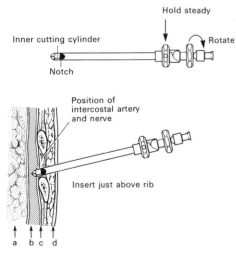

Fig. 12.15 Technique of pleural biopsy. The biopsy needle is shown penetrating the chest wall. a = lung parenchyma; b = pleural space; c = muscle; d = skin and subcutaneous tissue.

Mediastinoscopy and scalene node biopsy

This techique involves inspection of the mediastinal structures using a mediastinoscope inserted by blunt dissection downwards from behind the proximal end of the clavicle. Subsequent biopsy of tissue may be performed.

Fibreoptic bronchoscopy

The introduction of this technique has transformed the investigation of pulmonary disease. Central bronchial lesions can be biopsied readily. Washings can be taken from lobes containing more peripheral lesions for cytological examination for malignant cells, and appropriate staining and culture for bacteria including *Mycobacterium* and *Pneumocystis carinii*.

Fibreoptic bronchoscopy

This enables the direct visualization of the bronchial tree as far as the subsegmental bronchi under a local anaesthetic.

Indications
- Lesions requiring biopsy seen on chest x-ray
- Haemoptysis
- Stridor
- Positive sputum cytology for malignant cells with no chest x-ray abnormality
- Collection of bronchial secretions for bacteriology, especially tuberculosis
- Recurrent laryngeal nerve paralysis of unknown aetiology
- Infiltrative lung disease (to obtain a transbronchial biopsy)
- Investigation of collapsed lobes or segments and aspiration of mucus plugs

Procedure
- The patient is starved overnight.
- Atropine 0.6 mg i.m. is given 30 min before the procedure.
- Topical anaesthesia (xylocaine 4% spray) is applied to the nose, nasopharynx and pharynx.
- Intravenous sedation (e.g. diazepam 10 mg) is given.
- The bronchoscope is passed through the nose, nasopharynx and pharynx under direct vision to minimize trauma.
- Xylocaine (2 ml of 4%) is dropped through the instrument onto the vocal cords.
- The bronchoscope is passed through the cords into the trachea.
- All segmental and subsegmental orifices should be identified.
- Biopsies and brushings should be taken of macroscopic abnormalities or occasionally from peripheral lesions under radiographic control.

Diffuse parenchymal lung disease can be investigated using transbronchial biopsy. The biopsy forceps are pushed as far as possible to the periphery of the lung, the patient is asked to breathe in, and the jaws of the forceps are closed, removing a small piece of peripheral airway and surrounding lung parenchyma. Biplanar screening allows isolated peripheral lesions to be biopsied in the same way. A histological diagnosis can be made in 95% of central lung cancers but only in 50–75% of peripheral lesions biopsied during fibreoptic bronchoscopy.

Peripheral lesions can also be biopsied directly percutaneously using a fine needle.

Broncho-alveolar lavage

This technique can also be used both in patients who have disease confined to one lobe and in those with more diffuse lung disease. The tip of the fibreoptic bronchoscope is lodged in the segmental orifice and 20 ml of 0.9% sterile saline is squirted down the suction port of the bronchoscope and immediately aspirated. This is repeated five times; about 40–60% of the total volume is recovered. Fluid is strained through two layers of surgical gauze and the volume noted. The cells are then spun down and resuspended at a concentration of 1×10^7 cells per millilitre for differential counting. The changes seen in different diseases of the lung are shown in Table 12.5. Since there is a considerable overlap in the distribution of cells seen in broncho-alveolar wash specimens in different diseases, this technique has no value in diagnosis. However, it can be used to monitor progression of disease since improvement is characterized by a reduction in the number of cells and a return towards the normal proportions of different cell types.

Skin prick tests (Fig. 12.16)

The tip of a fine needle is placed through a drop of allergen solution on the volar surface of the forearm

Table 12.5 Broncho-alveolar lavage—changes in cell numbers and proportions in different diseases.

Disease	Number of cells ($\times 10^6$/ml)	Alveolar macrophages	Lymphocytes T	B	Null	Neutrophils	Granulocytes Eosinophils	Mast cells/basophils
None	14	90	5	1	2	<1	<1	<1
Smokers	→	→	→	→	→	↑	→	→
Sarcoidosis	↑↑	↓↓	↑↑	↑	↑	→	→	→
Cryptogenic fibrosing alveolitis	↑↑	↓	→	→	→	↑↑	→	→
Extrinsic allergic bronchiolar alveolitis	↑↑	↓	↑	→	→	↑	↑	→

→ = no change from normal; ↑ = increased from normal; ↑↑ = greatly increased from normal; ↓ = decreased from normal; ↓↓ = greatly decreased from normal

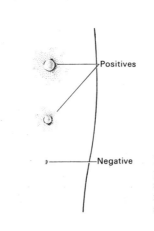

Fig. 12.16 The technique of skin-prick testing with allergen solutions, showing positive reactions with induration and surrounding erythema.

into the epidermis, which is gently pricked with an upward lifting motion. A separate needle should be used for each allergen. If the patient is sensitive to the allergen, a weal develops and the diameter of the induration (not the erythema) should be measured after 15 min. A weal of at least 2 mm in diameter and greater than the reaction to the control solution is a positive test.

Skin tests can be inhibited by concurrent administration of antihistamines, so these should be stopped 48 h before testing. It is not inhibited by bronchodilators or corticosteroids.

With most allergens there is a good correlation between the diameter of the weal and levels of specific IgE antibody in the serum. The results should be interpreted in the light of the history (see p. 590).

A *late reaction* is the development of a larger, 1–5 cm, oedematous skin reaction 2–3 h after pricking. This occurs with allergens from *Aspergillus fumigatus*, but also follows large, immediate skin reactions induced by allergens from other common inhalant allergens.

Smoking

Epidemiology

In 1980 the General Household Survey in the UK showed a continuing decline to 42% in the prevalence of cigarette smoking amongst British men, whilst the prevalence in women remained unchanged at 37%. In young people aged 16–19 years, the proportion of smokers fell from 43% to 32% between 1972 and 1980, and in men over 60 years from 47% to 36%. A greater proportion of professional workers than manual workers have given up smoking. In the USA the proportion of adult males who smoke is now only 36% and in women the prevalence is now 29%.

Dangers

Cigarette smoking is addictive. Smoking nearly always begins in adolescence for psychosocial reasons and, once it is a regular habit, the pharmacological properties of nicotine play an important part in persistence, conferring some advantage to the smoker's mood. Very few cigarette smokers (less than 2%) can limit themselves to occasional or intermittent smoking. The dangers are listed in Table 12.6.

There is a significant dose–response relationship between the smoking of 0–40 cigarettes daily and lung cancer mortality. Sputum production and airflow limitation increase with daily cigarette con-

Table 12.6 The dangers of cigarette smoking.

Lung cancer
Chronic bronchitis and emphysema
Carcinoma of the oesophagus
Ischaemic heart disease
Peripheral vascular disease
Bladder cancer
An increase in abnormal spermatozoa
Memory problems

Maternal smoking
A decrease in birthweight of the infant
An increase in fetal and neonatal mortality

Passive smoking
Risk of pneumonia and bronchitis in infants of smoking parents
An increase in cough and breathlessness in smokers and non-smokers with chronic bronchitis, emphysema and asthma
Increased cancer risk

sumption, and effort tolerance decreases, partly due to high levels of carboxyhaemoglobin in bronchitic patients. Smoking and asbestos exposure are synergystic in producing bronchial carcinoma, increasing the risk in asbestos workers by up to five to eight times that of non-smokers exposed to asbestos.

Cigarette smokers who change to other forms of tobacco are unlikely to reduce the risk, as they continue to inhale, and some of the highest levels of carboxyhaemoglobin have been found in cigar smokers.

Toxic effects

Cigarette smoke contains polycyclic aromatic hydrocarbons and nitrosamines, which are potent carcinogens and mutagens in animals. It causes release of enzymes from neutrophil granulocytes and macrophages that are capable of destroying elastin and leading to lung damage. Pulmonary epithelial permeability increases even in symptomless cigarette smokers, and correlates with the concentation of carboxyhaemoglobin in blood. This altered permeability possibly allows easier access to carcinogens.

Stopping smoking

If the entire population could be persuaded to stop smoking, the effect on health care in the Western World would be enormous. National campaigns run by central government linked to bans on advertisement and a substantial increase in the cost of cigarettes are the most certain ways of achieving this. Only 15% of general practitioners surveyed in 1982 actually encouraged their patients to give up smoking, yet simple advice and follow-up can motivate some

5% of their patients to stop. In smoking withdrawal clinics, success rates of 80% can be achieved in the first month, though only 15–20% of patients remain abstinent in the long term. Nicotine chewing gum has been advocated, but is probably no better than verbal advice. Chest symptoms usually have to be severe to stop patients from smoking.

Diseases of the upper respiratory tract

The common cold (acute coryza)

This highly infectious illness comprises a mild systemic upset and prominent nasal symptoms. It is due to infection by rhinoviruses, the majority of which belong to the picornavirus group and exist in at least 100 different antigenic strains. Infectivity from close personal contact (nasal mucus on hands) or droplets is high in the early stages of the infection, and spread is facilitated by overcrowding and poor ventilation. On average, individuals suffer 2–3 colds per year, but the incidence lessens with age, presumably as a result of accumulating immunity to the causative virus strains. The incubation is from 12 h to an upper limit of 5 days. The clinical features are tiredness, slight pyrexia, malaise, and a sore nose and pharynx. Profuse, watery nasal discharge, eventually becoming thick and mucopurulent, persists for up to a week. Sneezing is present in the early stage. Secondary bacterial infection occurs only in a minority.

Sinusitis

Sinusitis is an infection of the paranasal sinuses which often complicates upper respiratory tract infections, e.g. coryza or allergic rhinitis. Acute infections are usually caused by *Streptococcus pneumoniae* and *Haemophilus influenzae*. Symptoms include frontal headache and facial pain and tenderness, usually with nasal discharge, but are often difficult to differentiate from symptoms of the common cold.

Treatment is with antibiotics, e.g. amoxycillin. Rare complications include local and cerebral abscesses. Chronic sinusitis can be a cause of headaches, but often these headaches are due to tension.

Rhinitis

Rhinitis is present if sneezing attacks, nasal discharge or blockage occur for more than an hour on most days for:
- A limited period of the year (seasonal rhinitis)
- Throughout the whole year (perennial rhinitis)

Seasonal rhinitis

This is often called hay fever and is the most common of all allergic diseases. The term hay fever is inappropriate since fever rarely occurs and hay is not the cause. It is better described as seasonal allergic rhinitis. World-wide prevalence rates vary from 2 to 20%. Prevalence is maximum in the second decade, when up to 20% of young people suffer symptoms in June and July.

Nasal irritation, sneezing and watery rhinorrhoea are the most troublesome symptoms, but many also suffer from itching of the eyes and soft palate and occasionally even itching of the ears due to the common innervation of the pharyngeal mucosa and the ear. In addition, approximately 20% suffer from attacks of asthma.

Symptoms in March, April or May are due to allergy to pollens from hazel, elder and birch trees (see Fig. 12.17). In London, symptoms occur in:
- April and May due to plane tree pollen
- The first or second week of June due to grass pollen, as pollen counts then exceed 50 grains per m³ of air
- August and September due to moulds, particularly those from *Alternaria tenuis*, which grows on a variety of cultivated plants including wheat, and as 'early blight' on potatoes. *Cladosporium herbarum* grows around the roots of grass and its

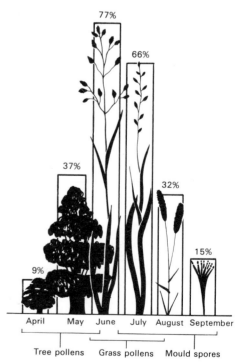

Fig. 12.17 Seasonal allergic rhinitis, giving the proportion of patients whose symptoms are worse in the month indicated. The causative allergens are also shown.

spores become airborne during lawn mowing. It causes allergic rhinitis throughout the summer months and may be identified in patients whose symptoms are not related to pollen counts.

● The autumn, when symptoms may develop from allergy to the spores of *Aspergillus fumigatus* which readily grows on decaying plant material such as compost heaps and piles of leaves.

Figure 12.17 shows the proportion of patients with seasonal allergic rhinitis whose symptoms are worst in each month in relation to the common allergen.

Perennial rhinitis
Patients with perennial rhinitis rarely have symptoms that affect the eyes or throat. Half have symptoms predominantly of sneezing and watery rhinorrhoea, whilst the other half complain mostly of nasal blockage. The patient may lose the sense of smell and taste. A swollen mucosa can obstruct drainage from the sinuses, causing sinusitis in half of the patients. Perennial rhinitis is most frequent in the second and third decade, decreasing with age, and can be divided into three main types:

Perennial allergic rhinitis. The major cause of this is an allergen called P1 contained in the faecal particles of the house-dust mite; these particles are approximately 20 µm in diameter (Fig. 12.18), not dissimilar in size to pollen grains. The house-dust mite itself is about 0.5 mm in size, invisible to the naked eye (Fig. 12.18), and is found in dust throughout the house, particularly in older, damp dwellings. They depend for nourishment upon desquamated human skin scales and are found in abundance (4000 mites per gram of surface dust) in human bedding.

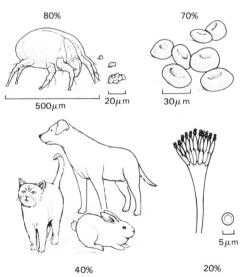

Fig. 12.18 Common allergens causing allergic rhinitis and asthma—the house dust mite, faeces of house dust mites, pollen grains, domestic pets, and moulds.

The next most common allergens come from domestic pets and are proteins derived from urine or saliva spread over the surface of the animal as well as skin protein. Allergy to urinary protein from small mammals is a major cause of morbidity amongst laboratory workers.

Industrial dust, vapours and fumes are more likely to cause occupationally related perennial rhinitis than asthma.

The presence of perennial rhinitis makes the nose more reactive to non-specific stimuli such as cigarette smoke, washing powders, household detergents, strong perfumes and traffic fumes; these are *not* acting as allergens.

Perennial non-allergic rhinitis with eosinophilia. No extrinsic allergic cause can be identified in these patients, either from the history or on skin testing, but like patients with perennial allergic rhinitis, eosinophilic granulocytes are present in nasal secretions.

Vasomotor rhinitis. These patients with perennial rhinitis have no demonstrable allergy or eosinophilia in nasal secretions. They may be suffering from non-specific nasal hyper-reactivity due to an imbalance of the autonomic nervous system innervating the erectile tissue (sinusoids) in the nasal mucosa.

Nasal polyps. These are round, smooth, soft, semi-translucent, pale or yellow, glistening structures attached to the nasal or sinus mucosa by a relatively narrow stalk or pedicle and occur in patients with both allergic and vasomotor rhinitis. They cause nasal obstruction, loss of smell and taste and mouth breathing, but rarely sneezing, since the mucosa of the polyp is largely denervated.

PATHOGENESIS

Sneezing, increased secretion and changes in mucosal blood flow are mediated by efferent nerve fibres. Mucus production results largely from parasympathetic stimulation, whilst blood vessels are under both sympathetic and parasympathetic control. Sympathetic fibres maintain tonic contraction of blood vessels, keeping the sinusoids of the nose partially constricted with good nasal patency. Stimulation of the parasympathetic system dilates these blood vessels. This stimulation varies spontaneously in a cyclical fashion so that air intake alternates slowly over several hours from one nostril to the other. The erectile cavernous nasal sinusoids can be influenced by emotion which, in turn, can effect nasal patency. It is thought that vasomotor rhinitis results from an imbalance in stimulation of the sympathetic and parasympathetic systems, with a preponderance of parasympathetic effects leading to nasal blockage.

Allergic rhinitis develops as a result of interaction between the inhaled allergen and adjacent molecules of IgE antibody. This is present on the surface of basophils and/or mast cells which are found in nasal secretions and within the nasal epithelium. Release of preformed mediators, in particular histamine, causes an increase in permeability of the epithelium, allowing allergen to reach IgE-primed mast cells in the lamina propria. Sneezing results from stimulation of afferent nerve endings and begins within minutes of the allergen entering the nose. This is followed by nasal secretion and eventually nasal blockage at a maximum of 15–20 min after contact with the allergen.

Although the mast cell contains or can generate many other potent vasomotor and chemotactic factors, the exact role for each of these has still to be evaluated (Fig. 12.29, p. 589). It is likely that histamine plays a more important role in the development of allergic rhinitis than of asthma, since anti-histamines are a useful and effective treatment for allergic rhinitis but are of little value in the everyday management of asthma. More mast cells are present in the nasal mucosa of individuals with rhinitis compared with those without rhinitis, and probably increase as allergen stimulation continues, accounting for the increasing responsiveness of the nose to lower amounts of grass pollen as the season continues. The mechanisms for recruitment of mast cells under these circumstances may involve the release of interleukin-3 from T lymphocytes.

DIAGNOSIS AND INVESTIGATION

- A detailed history is mandatory for the diagnosis of allergic factors in rhinitis.
- Skin prick testing (see Fig. 12.16) indicates that the mechanisms leading to allergic rhinitis (or asthma) are present in human skin. It does not necessarily mean that the particular allergen producing the weal causes the respiratory disease. However, if there is a positive clinical history for that allergen, a causative role is likely.
- The total amount of IgE in serum is normal in patients who suffer solely from allergic rhinitis. Specific serum IgE antibody against the particular allergen provides no more information than the skin prick test.
- The production of nasal secretions and sneezing can be compared after administration of allergen and saline. Such nasal provocation tests are rarely required to make the diagnosis.
- Stained smears of nasal secretion are of value in the following ways:
  - (a) Eosinophilia (>25% of total cells) indicates the presence of allergic rhinitis or non-allergic rhinitis with nasal eosinophilia.
  - (b) Neutrophil granulocytes are seen in rhinovirus infection. In vasomotor rhinitis there are a few cells, but eosinophil granulocytes are infrequent.

TREATMENT

Allergen avoidance
Removal of a household pet or total enclosure of industrial processes releasing sensitizing agents can lead to cure of rhinitis and, indeed, asthma.

Pollen avoidance is impossible. Contact may be diminished by wearing sunglasses, driving with the car windows shut, avoiding walks in the countryside (particularly in the late afternoon when the number of pollen grains is highest at ground level), and keeping the bedroom window shut at night. These measures are rarely sufficient in themselves to control symptoms. Exposure to pollen is generally lower at the seaside where sea breezes keep pollen grains inland. Patients can be advised to avoid trouble by taking holidays in Northern climates where pollen counts are lower or at times when the pollen season is over.

The house-dust mite infests most areas of the house, and is not confined to the bedroom. Mite counts are extremely low in hospitals where carpets are absent, floors are cleaned frequently and mattresses and pillows are covered in plastic sheeting that can be wiped down. Such conditions need to be reproduced in the home if mite counts are to be reduced to levels that would diminish symptoms. Anti-fungal agents (natamycin spray) have been used to kill fungi such as *Aspergillus* spp. (which help to break down human keratin for mite consumption), and acaricides, which directly kill mites, are currently under trial, but these methods require long-term evaluation.

Antihistamines
Antihistamines remain the commonest therapy for rhinitis, and many can be purchased directly over the counter in the UK. They are particularly effective against sneezing, but are less effective against rhinorrhoea and have little influence on nasal blockage. Many antihistamines, e.g. chlorpheniramine (4 mg three times daily) or clemastine (1 mg twice daily), have sedative effects. Newer drugs such as astemizole (10 mg daily) and terfenadine (60 mg twice daily) are water-soluble, do not cross the blood–brain barrier and are therefore not associated with sedation. Although rarely sufficient for the treatment of rhinitis, antihistamines will control itching in the eyes and palate.

Decongestants
Drugs with sympathomimetic activity are widely used for the treatment of nasal obstruction. They may be taken orally or more commonly as nasal drops or sprays (e.g. ephedrine nasal drops). Xylometazoline and oxymetazoline are widely used since they have a prolonged action and

tachyphylaxis does not develop. Secondary nasal hyperaemia can occur some hours later as a rebound effect and rhinitis medicamentosa can develop if patients subsequently take increasing quantities of the local decongestant to overcome this phenomenon. Local decongestants may be the only effective treatment for vasomotor rhinitis, but patients must be warned about rebound nasal obstruction and must use the drug carefully. Usually, such preparations should only be prescribed for a limited period to open the nasal airways for administration of other therapy, particularly topical corticosteroids.

Anti-allergic drugs
These drugs are thought to prevent release of mediators from mast cells, which are activated by combination of allergen with surface-bound IgE antibody. Sodium cromoglycate applied topically in spray or powder form is of limited value in the treatment of allergic rhinitis, though is very effective in the management of allergic conjunctivitis. Ketotifen, an oral preparation considered to have potent antihistaminic and some anti-allergic activity, can be effective in both children and adults at a dose of 1 mg twice daily. Sedation is a problem initially in 20% of patients treated, though, as with other drugs with antihistaminic properties, many patients acclimatize to this and only 5% remain substantially sedated.

Corticosteroids
The most effective treatment for rhinitis is the use of small doses of topically administered corticosteroid preparations (e.g. beclomethasone spray twice daily). The amount used is insufficient to cause systemic effects and the effect is primarily anti-inflammatory. Preparations should be taken prior to the start of seasonal symptoms. The combination of a topical corticosteroid with a non-sedative antihistamine taken regularly is particularly effective.

Seasonal and perennial rhinitis respond readily to treatment with oral prednisolone 5–10 mg daily if other therapy has failed. Some patients with severe perennial rhinitis may require continuous small doses (2.5–5 mg) of daily prednisolone. Nasal polyps respond well to such oral doses of corticosteroids and their recurrence may be prevented by continuous application of topical corticosteroids.

Hyposensitization
The principle of hyposensitization is to inject gradually increasing amounts of the allergen that causes the patient's rhinitis to the point where symptoms begin to occur. This means that courses of hyposensitization must be tailored for each individual. Although its mode of action remains unknown, improvements in isolation of relevant allergens, better standardization and more stable preparations may make the technique more efficacious. In general, hyposensitization should be reserved for patients with allergic rhinitis caused by grass pollen or the house-dust mite, and it should be remembered that even in these cases symptomatic treatment is often more effective. Anaphylaxis can occur and suitable precautions should be taken (see p. 651).

Pharyngitis

Only about one-third of sore throats are due to infection with a haemolytic streptococcus and this proportion appears to be falling. The commonest viruses causing pharyngitis are those of the adenovirus group, which consists of about 32 serotypes. Endemic adenovirus infection causes the common sore throat, in which the oropharynx and soft palate are reddened and the tonsils are inflamed and swollen. Within one or two days the tonsillar lymph nodes enlarge. Occasionally, localized epidemics occur, particularly in schools in the summertime, with episodes of fever, conjunctivitis, pharyngitis and lymphadenitis of the neck glands; these are due to adenovirus serotype 8. These diseases are self-limiting, and symptomatic treatment is all that is required.

Acute laryngotracheobronchitis

Acute laryngitis is an occasional but striking complication of upper respiratory tract infections, particularly those caused by viruses of the para-influenza group and the measles virus. Inflammatory oedema extends to the vocal cords and the epiglottis, causing considerable narrowing of the airway; in addition, there may be associated tracheitis or tracheobronchitis. Children under the age of 3 years are most severely affected. The voice becomes hoarse, the cough assumes a barking quality (croup) and there is audible laryngeal stridor. Progressive airway obstruction may occur, with recession of the soft tissue of the neck and abdomen during inspiration, and in severe cases central cyanosis may occur. Inhalation of steam may be helpful; in severe cases bronchoscopy and endotracheal intubation may be necessary. Oxygen and adequate fluids should be given. Rarely, a tracheostomy may be required.

Acute epiglottitis

Haemophilus influenzae type B can cause life-threatening infection of the epiglottis, a condition that is rare over the age of 5 years. The young child becomes extremely ill with a high fever, and severe airflow obstruction may rapidly occur. This is a life-threatening emergency and requires urgent endotracheal intubation and intravenous ampicillin. The epiglottis, which is red and swollen, should not be inspected until facilities to maintain the airways are available.

Influenza (see p. 59)

The influenza virus belongs to the orthomyxovirus group and exists in two main forms—A and B. Influenza B is associated with localized outbreaks of milder nature, whereas influenza A is the cause of world-wide pandemics. Influenza A has a capacity to develop new antigenic variants at irregular intervals. Human immunity develops against the haemagglutinin (H) antigen and the neuraminidase (N) antigen on the viral surface. Major shifts in the antigenic make-up of influenza A viruses provide the necessary conditions for major pandemics, whereas minor antigenic drifts give rise to less severe epidemics since immunity in the population is blunted.

The most serious pandemic of influenza occurred in 1918, and was associated with more than 20 million deaths world-wide. More recently, in 1957, a major shift in the antigenic make-up of the virus led to the appearance of influenza A2 type H2-N2, which caused a world-wide pandemic. There were 15 million cases in Britain, mainly in young people; the 5000 deaths were mostly due to secondary pneumonia. A further pandemic occurred in 1968 due to the emergence of Hong Kong influenza type H3-N2, and minor antigenic drifts have caused outbreaks around the world ever since.

CLINICAL FEATURES

The incubation period of influenza is usually 1–3 days. The illness starts abruptly with a fever, shivering and generalized aching in the limbs. This is associated with severe headache, soreness of the throat and a persistent dry cough which can last for several weeks. Influenza viruses can cause a prolonged period of debility and depression which may take weeks or months to clear; this is known as the post viral syndrome.

COMPLICATIONS

Secondary bacterial infection, particularly with *Streptococcus pneumoniae* and *Haemophilus influenzae*, is common following influenza virus infection. Rarer, but more serious, is the development of pneumonia caused by *Staphylococcus aureus*, which has a mortality of up to 20%. Post-infectious encephalomyelitis rarely occurs after infection with influenza virus.

DIAGNOSIS

Laboratory diagnosis of all cases is not necessary. Definitive diagnosis can be established by demonstrating a fourfold increase in the complement-fixing antibody or the haemagglutinin antibody when measured before and after an interval of 1–2 weeks. Viral cultures are still a research procedure.

TREATMENT

Treatment is bedrest and aspirin, together with antibiotics for individuals with chronic bronchitis, or heart or renal disease.

PROPHYLYAXIS

Protection by influenza vaccines is only effective in up to 70% of people and is of short duration, usually lasting for only 1 year. Vaccines are prepared from formalin or ultraviolet-irradiated virus grown in chick embryo, and are given parenterally. More recently vaccines have become more purified and have less side-effects since they are now being made of antigens from disrupted viruses. Influenza vaccine should not be given to individuals who are allergic to egg protein. New vaccines have to be prepared to cover each change in viral antigenicity and are therefore in limited supply at the start of an epidemic. Routine vaccination is reserved for susceptible people with chronic heart, lung or kidney disease, the elderly, and key hospital and health service personnel.

Amantadine hydrochloride 100–200 mg daily may attenuate influenza A infection and should be reserved for individuals with chronic respiratory or cardiovascular disease who have not been previously immunized.

Inhalation of foreign bodies

Children inhale foreign bodies, frequently peanuts, more commonly than adults. In the adult, inhalation often occurs after an excess of alcohol or under general anaesthesia (loose dentures).

When the foreign body is large it may impact in the trachea. The person chokes and then becomes silent; death occurs unless the material is quickly removed.

Impaction usually occurs in the right main bronchus and produces:
● Choking
● Persistent monophonic wheeze
● Later, persistent suppurative pneumonia
● Lung abscess (common)

Treatment of inhaled foreign bodies

Emergency
The Heimlich manoeuvre is used to expel the obstructing object:
● Stand behind patient.
● Encircle your arms around the upper part of the abdomen just below the patient's rib cage.
● Give a sharp, forceful squeeze, forcing the diaphragm sharply into the thorax. This should expel sufficient air from the lungs to force the foreign body out of the trachea.

Non-emergency
Fibreoptic bronchoscopy should be performed.

Diseases of the lower respiratory tract

Acute bronchitis

Acute bronchitis in previously healthy subjects is often viral. Bacterial infection with organisms such as *Streptococcus pneumoniae* and *Haemophilus influenzae* is a common sequel to viral infections, and is more likely to occur in individuals who are cigarette smokers and in those with chronic bronchitis and emphysema.

The illness begins with an irritating, unproductive cough, together with discomfort behind the sternum. This may be associated with tightness in the chest, wheezing and shortness of breath. The cough becomes productive, the sputum being yellow or green. There is a mild fever and a neutrophil leucocytosis; wheeze with occasional crackles can be heard on auscultation. In otherwise healthy adults the disease improves spontaneously in 4–8 days without the patient becoming seriously ill. Treatment with antibiotics may be given, e.g. amoxycillin 250 mg three times daily, though it is not known whether this hastens recovery in otherwise healthy individuals.

Chronic bronchitis and emphysema

Definitions
Chronic bronchitis is defined on the basis of the *history* as:
- Cough productive of sputum on most days for at least three months of the year for more than one year

Emphysema on the other hand is defined *pathologically* as:
- Dilatation and destruction of the lung tissue distal to the terminal bronchioles

Clinical observations led to the suggestion that there were two distinct types of patient:
- The *type A* fighter is *pink and puffing* in that, although he is very breathless, arterial tensions of oxygen and carbon dioxide are relatively normal and there is no cor pulmonale. These individuals were thought to be suffering predominantly from emphysema with little bronchitis.
- The *type B* non-fighter, on the other hand, is *blue and bloated*. He does not appear to be breathless, but has marked arterial hypoxaemia, carbon dioxide retention, secondary polycythaemia and cor pulmonale. These patients were thought to be suffering predominantly from chronic bronchitis.

Although this is an attractive concept and has some clinical usefulness, it is not supported by post mortem studies which have shown no difference in the degree of mucous gland hyperplasia (i.e. bronchitis) or in the amount of emphysema in patients with type A compared with type B disease.

Autopsy studies have also shown that substantial numbers of centri-acinar emphysematous spaces are found in the lungs of 50% of British smokers over the age of 60 years and are unrelated to the diagnosis of significant respiratory disease before death.

Because of the difficulty of making a clear diagnosis between chronic bronchitis and emphysema during life, alternative terms such as chronic obstructive pulmonary disease (COPD), chronic obstructive lung disease (COLD) or chronic obstructive airways disease (COAD) were introduced to cover both of these conditions. These terms are unhelpful and should be replaced by the term 'chronic bronchitis and emphysema', as both these conditions co-exist to a greater or lesser degree in each patient.

It is now recognized that the common tests for 'airway obstruction', the FEV_1 and PEFR, actually measure airflow limitation caused by both loss of elastic recoil and/or narrowing of airways. This has led to the introduction of the term 'chronic airflow limitation', which is the preferred terminology to describe the functional and physiological problem in chronic bronchitis and emphysema.

EPIDEMIOLOGY AND AETIOLOGY

Chronic bronchitis and emphysema (often referred to as the English disease) were always considered to be a particular problem in the UK, with a prevalence diagnosed on history of 17% in men and 8% in women in the age group 40–64 years. However, in the USA similar prevalence figures have been obtained and many Third World countries are also showing an increased prevalence.

There is no doubt that cigarette smoking is a major factor in the development of chronic bronchitis and emphysema. Not only are these diseases virtually confined to cigarette smokers, they are also related to the number of cigarettes smoked per day. The risk of death from chronic bronchitis and emphysema in patients smoking 30 cigarettes daily is 20 times that of a non-smoker. The bronchitis mortality amongst male doctors in relation to the number of cigarettes smoked is shown in Fig. 12.19.

Climate and air pollution are of less importance; nevertheless, there is a great increase in mortality from chronic bronchitis and emphysema during periods of heavy atmospheric pollution. The effect of urbanization, social class and occupation may also play a part in aetiology, but these effects are difficult to separate from that of smoking.

The socioeconomic burden of chronic bronchitis and emphysema is considerable. Between 1976 and 1977 in the UK chronic bronchitis and emphysema were certified as causing 26 million lost working days

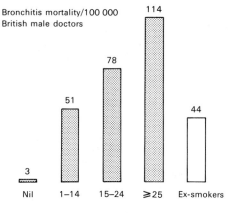

Bronchitis mortality/100 000
British male doctors

Cigarettes/day

Fig. 12.19 Bronchitis death rates per 100 000 British male doctors according to their smoking habits. From Doll R & Peto R (1976) *British Medical Journal* ii: 1525.

for men and 2.6 million lost working days for women, accounting for some 10% of all days of sickness absence from work, much the highest of any defined disease entity. Nevertheless, the number of patients discharged from hospitals in the UK with this disease has been steadily falling; the death rate has also fallen in the last 20 years from 30 000 to 20 000 per year.

PATHOPHYSIOLOGY (Fig. 12.20)

Chronic bronchitis
The most consistent pathological finding in chronic bronchitis is hypertrophy of the mucus-secreting glands of the bronchial tree. The hypertrophy of these mucous glands is evenly distributed throughout the lung, and is mainly seen in the larger bronchi. In addition, the number of mucus-secreting goblet cells increases. This leads to increased mucus production and the regular expectoration of sputum.

In more advanced cases the bronchi themselves are obviously inflamed and pus is seen in the lumen. Microscopically there is infiltration of the walls of the bronchi and bronchioles with acute and chronic inflammatory cells. The epithelial layer may become ulcerated and when the ulcers heal, squamous epithelium may replace the columnar cells. The inflammation leads to widespread narrowing in the peripheral airways.

There is increasing evidence that the small airways are particularly affected early on in the disease, initially without the development of any significant breathlessness. This initial inflammation of the small airways is reversible and accounts for the improvement in airway function if smoking is stopped in the early stages of the disease.

Further progression of the disease leads to progressive squamous cell metaplasia, and fibrosis of the bronchial walls. The physiological consequences of these changes is the development of airflow limitation. If the airway narrowing is combined with emphysema (causing loss of the elastic recoil of the lung) the resulting airflow limitation is even more severe.

Emphysema
Emphysema can be classified according to the site of damage:
- In *centri-acinar emphysema* distension and damage of lung tissue is concentrated around the respiratory bronchioles, whilst the more distal alveolar ducts and alveoli tend to be well preserved. This form of emphysema is extremely common; when of modest extent, it is not necessarily associated with disability. Severe centri-acinar emphysema is associated with substantial airflow limitation.
- *Pan-acinar emphysema* is less common. Here, distension and destruction appear to involve the whole of the acinus, and in the extreme form, the lung becomes a mass of bullae. Severe airflow limitation and $\dot{V}_A/\dot{Q}$ mismatch occur.
- In *irregular emphysema* there is scarring and damage affecting the lung parenchyma patchily without particular regard for acinar structure.

Emphysema can lead to expiratory airflow limitation (see p. 556) and air trapping. The loss of lung elastic recoil results in an increase in total lung capacity,

Stenosis

Narrowing of small airways
in chronic bronchitis

Centri-acinar
emphysema

Pan-acinar emphysema

Fig. 12.20 The pathological features of chronic bronchitis and emphysema.

while the loss of alveoli with emphysema results in decreased gas transfer.

$\dot{V}_A/\dot{Q}$ mismatch occurs partly because of the damage by mucus plugs to the intrinsic airways from chronic bronchitis and also because of the rapid expiratory closure of the smaller airways owing to loss of elastic recoil from emphysema. This leads to a fall in P_aO_2 and a subsequent rise in P_aCO_2.

CO_2 is normally the major stimulant of the respiratory centre. In the face of a prolonged high P_aCO_2, this sensitivity is diminished and hypoxaemia becomes the chief drive to respiration. In this situation an attempt to abolish hypoxaemia by administration of oxygen can result in an increase in P_aCO_2 by decreasing the respiratory drive.

PATHOGENESIS

Cigarette smoking
Broncho-alveolar washes have shown that smokers have neutrophil granulocytes present within the lumen of the lung which are absent in non-smokers. Additionally, the small airways of smokers are infiltrated by granulocytes. These granulocytes are capable of releasing elastases and proteases, which possibly help to produce emphysema.

The hypertrophy of mucous glands in the larger airways is thought to be a direct response to persistent irritation resulting from the inhalation of cigarette smoke. The smoke has an adverse effect on surfactant, favouring over-distension of the lungs.

Infections
Infections are frequent and are often the precipitating cause of acute exacerbations of the disease. However, the role of infection in the development of the progressive airflow limitation that characterizes disabling chronic bronchitis and emphysema is far less clear. Nevertheless, release of enzymes from the excess neutrophil granulocytes found in infections probably adds to the lung damage.

Alpha-1-antitrypsin deficiency
This was first discovered in the 1960s in a family with early-onset emphysema. Many different phenotypes of alpha-1-antitrypsin deficiency have been recognized and these are also associated with liver disease (see p. 241). The three main types are MM (normal), MZ (heterozygous deficiency) and ZZ (homozygous deficiency) groups; these are defined by the serum level of antitrypsin. About 1 in 5000 children in Britain is born with the homozygous deficiency, but not all develop chest disease. Those that do develop breathlessness under the age of 40 years have radiographic evidence of basal emphysema and are usually, but not always, cigarette smokers. Purulent sputum contains enzymes (elastases and proteases) that are normally inhibited by alpha-1-antitrypsin, and lack of this compound allows lung breakdown to proceed unchecked. This led to an attractive hypothesis for the mechanism of tissue damage in chronic bronchitis and emphysema, but no decrease in other forms of enzyme inhibition has been demonstrated.

CLINICAL FEATURES

Symptoms
The characteristic symptoms of chronic bronchitis and emphysema are cough with the production of sputum, wheeze and breathlessness following many years of a smoker's cough. Colds seem to 'go down to the chest' and frequent infective exacerbations occur, giving purulent sputum. Symptoms can be worsened by non-specific factors such as cold, foggy weather and atmospheric pollution. With advanced disease, breathlessness becomes severe even after mild exercise such as dressing.

Signs
In mild disease there are no signs apart from 'wheeze' throughout the chest. In severe disease, the patient is tachypoenic, with prolonged expiration. The accessory muscles of respiration are used and there may be intercostal indrawing on inspiration and pursing of the lips on expiration (see Fig. 12.5). Chest expansion is poor, the lungs are hyperinflated, and there is loss of the normal cardiac and liver dullness.

The 'pink puffer' is always breathless and is not usually cyanosed. Rarely oedema or heart failure may be seen.

The 'blue bloater' is oedematous, deeply cyanosed, with hypoventilation and often little respiratory effort. These patients are likely to have hypercapnoea which gives the following physical findings:
- Peripheral vasodilatation
- A bounding pulse
- Later, a coarse flapping tremor of the outstretched hands

More severe hypercapnoea leads to:
- Confusion
- Progressive drowsiness and coma with papilloedema

There is often considerable overlap between these two clinical patterns.

COMPLICATIONS

Respiratory failure
The latter stages of chronic bronchitis and emphysema are characterized by the development of respiratory failure. For practical purposes this is said to occur when there is either a P_aO_2 of less than 8 kPa (60 mmHg) or a P_aCO_2 of more than 7 kPa (55 mmHg) (see Chapter 13).

The persistence of chronic alveolar hypoxia and hypercapnoea leads to constriction of the pulmonary arterioles and subsequent pulmonary arterial hypertension.

Cor pulmonale

Patients may develop cor pulmonale (see p. 535), which is defined as heart disease secondary to disease of the lung. It is characterized by pulmonary hypertension, right ventricular hypertrophy, and eventually right heart failure. On examination the patient is centrally cyanosed (due to the lung disease) and, when heart failure develops, breathlessness and ankle oedema occur. Initially a prominent parasternal heave may be felt due to right ventricular hypertrophy and a loud pulmonary second sound may be heard. In very severe pulmonary hypertension there is incompetence of the pulmonary valve. With right heart failure tricuspid incompetence may develop with a greatly elevated JVP, ascites and upper abdominal pain due to swelling of the liver.

DIAGNOSIS

This is usually clinical. There is a history of breathlessness and sputum production in a lifetime smoker. It is unwise to make a diagnosis of chronic bronchitis and emphysema in the absence of cigarette smoking unless there is a family history of lung disease suggestive of a deficiency of alpha-1-antitrypsin.

In clinical practice emphysema is often incorrectly diagnosed on signs of over-inflation of the lungs (e.g. loss of liver dullness on percussion), but this may occur with other diseases such as asthma. Furthermore, centri-acinar emphysema may be present without signs of over-inflation. Some elderly men develop a barrel-shaped chest due to osteoporosis of the spine and a consequent decrease in height. This should not be attributed to emphysema.

In a number of patients the airflow limitation is reversible and the distinction between asthma and chronic bronchitis and emphysema can be difficult.

INVESTIGATION

- *Lung function tests* show evidence of airflow limitation (see Figs. 12.6 and 12.13). The ratio of the FEV_1 to the FVC is reduced and the PEFR is low. Lung volumes may be normal or increased, and the gas transfer coefficient of carbon monoxide is low when significant emphysema is present.
- On *chest x-ray* the diagnosis of chronic bronchitis and emphysema is not always possible, even when the disease is advanced. The classic features are the presence of bullae, severe over-inflation of the lungs with low, flattened diaphragms, and a large retrosternal air space on the lateral film. There may also be a deficiency of blood vessels in the peripheral half of the lung fields compared with relatively easily visible proximal vessels.

  The chest x-ray can be normal even with advanced disease.
- The *haemoglobin level* and *PCV* may be elevated.
- *Blood gases* are often normal. In the advanced case there is evidence of hypoxia and hypercapnoea.
- *Sputum examination* is unnecessary in the ordinary case as *Streptococcus pneumoniae* or *Haemophilus influenzae* are the only common organisms to produce acute exacerbations.
- *Electrocardiogram.* In cor pulmonale the P wave is taller (P pulmonale) and there may be right bundle branch block (rSR' complex) and the changes of right ventricular hypertrophy.

TREATMENT

The single most important aspect in the management of chronic bronchitis and emphysema is to persuade the patient to stop smoking. Even at a late stage of the disease this may slow down the rate of deterioration and prolong the time before disability and death occur (see Fig. 12.21). Accompanying heart failure should be treated (see p. 496).

Drug therapy

Drug therapy is used both for the short-term management of exacerbations and for the long-term relief of symptoms. In some cases the therapy is similar to that used in asthma (see p. 591).

Bronchodilators. Many patients feel less breathless following the inhalation of a beta-adrenoceptor agonist such as salbutamol (two puffs of inhaler 4–6 hourly). Objective evidence of improvement in the peak flow or FEV_1 may be small, but with severe disability it may be of considerable help.

Corticosteroids. In symptomatic patients with chronic bronchitis and emphysema, a trial of corticosteroids is always indicated since a proportion of patients have a large, unsuspected, asthmatic element to their disease and airway function may improve considerably. Prednisolone 30 mg daily should be given for 2 weeks, with measurements of lung function before and after the treatment period. If there is objective evidence of a substantial degree of improvement in airflow limitation ($\geq 15\%$), prednisolone should be gradually reduced and replaced by inhaled corticosteroids (beclomethasone, two puffs four times daily).

Antibiotics. Prompt antibiotic treatment shortens exacerbations and should always be given in acute episodes as they may prevent subsequent further lung damage. Patients can be given a supply of antibiotics to keep at home to start as soon as their sputum turns yellow or green. Treatment should

Fig. 12.21 Influence of smoking on airflow limitation. From Fletcher CM & Peto R (1977) *British Medical Journal* i: 1645

be with amoxycillin 500 mg three times daily or erythromycin 500 mg three times daily. Recently, amoxycillin-resistant *Haemophilus influenzae* has been identified, but it rarely accounts for more than 2–5% of the positive cultures.

Long-term treatment with antibiotics remains controversial. They were once thought to be of no value, but eradication of infection and keeping the lower respiratory tract free of bacteria may help to prevent deterioration in lung function.

Mucolytics and vaccines. There is little evidence that mucolytics are of any benefit, though it is vital that patients are encouraged to cough up sputum. Symptomatic treatment with steam inhalations may help to liquefy the sputum so that it can be more easily coughed up. Influenza vaccines should be given yearly to patients with disabling chronic bronchitis and emphysema.

Treatment of respiratory failure
There are many causes of respiratory failure (see Fig. 12.22), but by far the most common is chronic bronchitis and emphysema. In this type II respiratory failure the $P_a\text{co}_2$ is elevated and the $P_a\text{o}_2$ is reduced. It is important to realize that whereas hypercapnoea is intoxicating, hypoxaemia is potentially lethal. The primary aim of the management of respiratory failure is to improve the $P_a\text{o}_2$ by continuous controlled oxygen therapy. This nearly always also leads to a rise in the $P_a\text{co}_2$ (see p. 555). Small increases in $P_a\text{co}_2$ can be tolerated, but not if the pH falls dramatically. The pH should not be allowed to fall below 7.25; under such circumstances, increased ventilation must be achieved either by the use of a respiratory stimulant or by artificial ventilation.

Fig. 12.23 shows a fixed performance mask (Venturi mask) for the administration of oxygen. This style of mask is used when only low concentrations of oxygen can be given. It should be compared with

the variable performance face mask (see Fig. 13.15, p. 641).

Initially, 24% oxygen is given, which is only slightly greater than the concentration of oxygen in air but, because of the shape of the oxygen–haemoglobin dissociation curve, this small increase in oxygen is valuable. Gradually, the concentration of inspired oxygen can be increased if there is no dramatic rise in the $P_a\text{co}_2$.

Additional measures. These include:
● *Removal* of *retained secretions.* The patient should be encouraged to cough to remove secretions. If this fails, bronchoscopy and/or aspiration via an endotracheal tube may be necessary. A tracheostomy is only rarely required.
● *Respiratory stimulants.* Doxapram, 0.5–4 mg·min^{-1} by slow i.v. infusion, given intravenously may help in the short term to arouse the patient and to stimulate coughing, with clearance of some secretions.
● *Assisted ventilation* (see p. 642). This is occasionally used in patients with chronic bronchitis and emphysema with severe respiratory failure when there is a definite precipitating factor, and the overall prognosis is reasonable. This can be a difficult ethical problem.

Corticosteroids, antibiotics and bronchodilators should also be administered (see above).

Long-term oxygen therapy
Two controlled trials (chiefly in men) have indicated that the continuous administration of 2 l of oxygen per minute via nasal prongs to achieve an oxygen saturation of greater than 90% for large proportions of the day can prolong life. Survival curves from these two studies are shown in Fig. 12.24. Only 30% of those not receiving long-term oxygen therapy survived for more than 5 years. A fall in pulmonary

Fig. 12.22 Algorithm for the treatment of respiratory failure. LVF = left ventricular failure.

Fig. 12.23 'Fixed performance' device for administration of oxygen to spontaneously breathing patients (Venturi mask). Oxygen is delivered through the injector of the Venturi mask at a given flow rate. A fixed amount of air is entrapped and the inspired oxygen can be accurately predicted. Masks are available to deliver 24%, 28% and 34% oxygen.

Fig. 12.24 Cumulative survival curves for patients receiving oxygen.

artery pressure was achieved if oxygen was given for 15 h daily, but substantial improvement in mortality was only achieved by the administration of oxygen for 19 h daily. These results suggest that long-term continuous domiciliary oxygen therapy will benefit patients who have:

- Chronic bronchitis and emphysema with an FEV_1 of less than 1.2 l
- A P_aO_2 on air of less than 9 kPa (68 mmHg)
- Carboxyhaemoglobin of less than 3%, i.e. patients who have stopped smoking

The provision of 19 h of oxygen daily at a flow rate of $1-3 \, l \cdot min^{-1}$ to increase the arterial oxygen saturation to over 90% needs 20 oxygen cylinders per week. This is extremely expensive. Oxygen concentrators are cheaper and are now available through the health service in the UK.

Additional therapy
Pulmonary hypertension can be partially relieved by the use of oral beta-adrenoceptor stimulants such as salbutamol (4 mg three times daily), but whether this is useful in the long term is unknown.

The sensation of breathlessness can be reduced by the use of either promethazine 125 mg daily or dihydrocodeine $1 \, mg \cdot kg^{-1}$ by mouth. Reduced breathlessness and increased exercise tolerance also result from the combined administration of dihydrocodeine and oxygen delivered from a portable cylinder.

PROGNOSIS

In general, 50% of patients with severe breathlessness die within 5 years (Fig. 12.24), but even in this severe group, stopping smoking helps the prognosis.

Nocturnal hypoxia

Recently it has been shown that patients with chronic bronchitis and emphysema who show severe arterial hypoxaemia also suffer from profound nocturnal hypoxaemia with a P_aO_2 as low as 2.5 kPa (19 mmHg), particularly during the rapid eye movement (REM) phase of sleep.

Because patients with chronic bronchitis and emphysema are already hypoxic, the fall in P_aO_2 produces a much larger fall in oxygen saturation (owing to the steepness of the oxyhaemoglobin dissociation curve) and desaturation of up to 50% occurs. The mechanism is alveolar hypoventilation owing to:

- Inhibition of intercostal and accessory muscles in REM sleep
- Shallow breathing in REM sleep, which reduces ventilation, particularly in severe chronic airway disease
- An increase in upper airway resistance owing to a reduction in muscle tone

These nocturnal hypoxaemic episodes are associated with a further rise in pulmonary arterial pressure, and the majority of deaths in patients with chronic bronchitis and emphysema occur during the night, possibly due to cardiac arrhythmias. These patients additionally show severe secondary polycythaemia, partly as a result of the severe nocturnal hypoxaemia.

Each episode of desaturation is usually terminated by arousal from sleep, so that normal sleep is reduced and the patient suffers from daytime sleepiness. Treatment is with nocturnal administration of oxygen.

Patients with arterial hypoxaemia should never be given sleeping tablets, which will further depress respiratory drive.

Obstructive sleep apnoea

This can also occur in patients with chronic bronchitis and emphysema and, again, because these patients are already hypoxic, the effect on oxygen saturation is more profound.

Obstructive sleep apnoea is, however, common in normal individuals, particularly after alcohol or sedatives which decrease upper airway muscle activity. In addition, many subjects who are obese have small oropharyngeal lumens and nasal obstruction. Usually in a period of REM sleep, apposition of the tongue and palate to the posterior pharyngeal wall results in obstruction to airflow and the patients become asphyxiated, with arousal from sleep occurring as a result of apnoea. This sequence of events may be repeated many times during the night.

This condition should be suspected in patients who complain of daytime sleepiness and morning headache. At night, snoring is common, with recurrent awakenings. Obstructive sleep apnoea can lead to cardiac arrhythmias or sudden death.

Treatment includes avoidance of alcohol and sedatives, and weight reduction in the obese. Continuous positive airway pressure applied through the nose may be required.

Bronchiectasis

Bronchiectasis may simply be defined as dilatation of the bronchi. Bronchial walls become inflamed, thickened and irreversibly damaged. The mucociliary transport mechanism is impaired and frequent bacterial infections ensue. Clinically, the disease is characterized by cough productive of large amounts of sputum.

EPIDEMIOLOGY

Prior to the discovery and clinical use of antibiotics, bronchiectasis was a frequent outcome of slowly resolving pneumonia. Most cases now arise in childhood and even the incidence in this age group has dropped. Both sexes can develop bronchiectasis, but an increased male preponderance over 45 years has been noted.

AETIOLOGY

The aetiology is uncertain, but bronchial obstruction followed by infection plays a major role.

Bronchiectasis is a rare complication of whooping cough and measles in the Western World. Localized bronchiectasis is also rarely seen in tuberculous enlargement of lymph nodes at the hilum of the lung, particularly around the origin of the middle lobe bronchus. Bronchial obstruction in children from other causes (e.g. inhaled peanuts) can give rise to gross suppurative lung disease and residual bronchiectasis.

Recently progressive bronchiectasis has been described in non-smoking patients of both sexes, with no other underlying cause. This syndrome is known as chronic bronchial sepsis.

Cystic fibrosis (p. 585) also leads to bronchiectasis as over 75% of children with cystic fibrosis now survive to adult life. Bronchiectasis can also be associated with other congenital abnormalities, e.g. Kartagener's syndrome, which is characterized by sinusitis and transposition of viscera with bronchiectasis, and is associated with 'immotile cilia'.

CLINICAL FEATURES

Patients with mild bronchiectasis only suffer from production of yellow or green sputum after viral infections. Localized areas of the lung may be particularly affected, when sputum production will depend on position. As the condition worsens the patient suffers from persistent halitosis, recurrent febrile episodes with malaise, and episodes of pneumonia. Clubbing occurs, and coarse crackles can be heard over the affected areas, usually the bases of the lungs. When the condition is severe there is continuous production of foul-smelling, thick, khaki-coloured sputum. Haemoptysis, either as blood-stained sputum or as a massive haemorrhage, can occur. Breathlessness may result from airflow limitation.

INVESTIGATION

● The *chest x-ray* may be quite normal or may show dilated bronchi with thickened bronchial walls and sometimes multiple cysts containing fluid.
● *CT scanning* can show bronchial wall thickening.
● *Bronchograms* are required to confirm the diagnosis. This investigation is uncomfortable for the patient and is only required if the diagnosis is in doubt or where there is reason to believe that the disease may be localized and therefore amenable to surgical treatment. Typical patterns of bronchography are shown in Fig. 12.25. The left lower lobe and lingula are the commonest sites for localized disease.
● *Sputum examination* with culture and sensitivity of the organisms is essential for adequate treatment. The major pathogens are *Staphylococcus aureus, Pseudomonas aeruginosa* and *Haemophilus influenzae*. Other pathogens include *Streptococcus pneumoniae* and *Klebsiella pneumoniae*. *Aspergillus fumigatus* can be isolated from 10% of sputum specimens in cystic fibrosis, but the role of this organism is uncertain.

TREATMENT

Postural drainage
Postural drainage is of vital importance, and patients must be trained to tip themselves into appropriate positions at least three times daily for 10–20 min. Most patients find that lying over the side of the bed with head and thorax down is the most effective position.

Antibiotics
Experience from the treatment of cystic fibrosis suggests that bronchopulmonary infections should be eradicated if progression of the disease is to be halted. In mild cases, intermittent chemotherapy with amoxycillin 500 mg 8-hourly may be the only therapy needed. Flucloxacillin 500 mg 6-hourly is the best treatment if *Staphylococcus aureus* is isolated. Chloramphenicol is a useful drug in persistent infection.

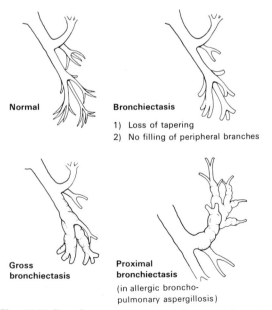

Fig. 12.25 Bronchograms in normal lung and bronchiectasis.

If the sputum remains yellow or green despite regular physiotherapy and intermittent chemotherapy, or if lung function deteriorates despite treatment with bronchodilators, continuous oral chemotherapy should be considered.

A major problem is infection with *Pseudomonas aeruginosa*, for which only parenteral or aerosol chemotherapy is effective. Drug regimens involving tobramycin or gentamicin together with carbenicillin or azlocillin are often required. High sputum levels of antibiotics can be achieved by inhalation. A treatment regimen of carbenicillin 1g and gentamicin 80 mg given by a compressor-driven nebulizer twice daily has been found to be of benefit in young adult patients with chronic *Pseudomonas* infection.

Bronchodilators

Bronchodilators may be useful in patients with demonstrable airflow limitation.

Surgery

Unfortunately, bronchiectasis is rarely sufficiently localized for surgery to be of any value.

COMPLICATIONS

The incidence of complications has fallen with antibiotic therapy. Pneumonia, pneumothorax, empyema and metastatic cerebral abscess can occur. Severe, life-threatening haemoptysis can also occur, particularly in patients with cystic fibrosis.

Cystic fibrosis

Cystic fibrosis (CF) is due to a dysfunction of all exocrine glands resulting in abnormal mucus production. The classical form of the syndrome includes bronchopulmonary infection and pancreatic insufficiency, with a high sweat sodium concentration. It is a recessively inherited disorder (abnormality of chromosome 7) with a carrier frequency in caucasians of 1 in 20–25. In America, western Europe and Australasia, 1 in 2000 births are homozygotes for the CF gene, but the carrier frequency in mongoloid races is considerably less and CF is unknown in blacks. The heterozygous state cannot be reliably detected at present and does not carry with it any predisposition to respiratory disease.

The basic defect in CF remains unknown, but there is a generalized abnormality of membrane transport.

CLINICAL FEATURES

Although the lungs of babies born with CF are structurally normal at birth, respiratory symptoms are usually the presenting feature. CF is now the commonest cause of recurrent bronchopulmonary infection in childhood, and is an important cause in early adult life. Finger clubbing is almost universal, haemoptysis is frequent, and breathlessness occurs in the later stages as airflow limitation develops. Older children may also develop nasal polyps.

Puberty and skeletal maturity are delayed in most patients with the disease. Males are almost always infertile due to failure of development of the vas deferens and epididymis. Females are able to conceive, but often develop secondary amenorrhoea as the disease progresses.

About 85% of patients have symptomatic steatorrhoea owing to pancreatic dysfunction (see p. 257). Children may be born with meconium ileus due to the viscoid consistency of meconium in CF, and later in life develop the meconium ileus equivalent (MIE) syndrome, an important cause of small intestinal obstruction unique to CF.

Cholesterol gallstones appear to occur with increased frequency, and cirrhosis develops in about 5% of older patients.

DIAGNOSIS

The diagnosis of CF in older children and adults may be difficult. It depends on the clinical history together with:
- A family history of the disease
- A high sweat sodium concentration over 60 mmol·l^{-1}. (Meticulous technique by laboratories performing regular sweat analysis is essential, but the test is still difficult to interpret in adults.)
- Absent vas deferens and epididymis.

TREATMENT

Treatment for the respiratory disease is described under bronchiectasis on p. 584. The treatment of pancreatic insufficiency is described on p. 258.

PROGNOSIS

The prognosis has consistently improved; most children now survive into their teens. The long-term outlook is uncertain, but progressive respiratory failure almost inevitably occurs. Genetic advice can only be given in general terms as there is no exact way of detecting carriers. However 1 in 4 children of two carriers is likely to be affected. The diagnosis can now be made in utero (see p. 105).

Asthma

Asthma is defined as partial obstruction to airflow in the intrathoracic airways that varies in severity over short periods of time, either spontaneously or as a result of treatment. The diagnosis of asthma depends upon showing these changes objectively using lung function tests.

PREVALENCE

Until recently it was considered that asthma affected approximately 5% of the population at some stage during their life. Increasing recognition of the disease (and possibly an increasing incidence) suggests that the prevalence, particularly in the second decade of life, may be as high as 10–15%. There is also a geographical variation, with asthma being common in, for example, New Zealand, but being much rarer in Far Eastern countries such as China and Malaysia. Long-term follow-up of Third World countries suggests that the disease may become more frequent as individuals become more 'Westernized'. Studies of occupational asthma suggest that a high percentage of the workforce, perhaps up to 20%, may become asthmatic if exposed to potent sensitizers.

AETIOLOGY AND PATHOGENESIS

There are two major factors involved in the development of extrinsic asthma and many other stimuli which can precipitate attacks (Fig. 12.26).

Atopy and allergy
The term 'atopy' was used by clinicians at the beginning of the century to describe a group of disorders, including asthma and hay fever, that appeared:
- To run in families
- To have characteristic wealing skin reactions to common allergens in the environment
- To have circulating antibody in their serum which could be transferred to the skin of non-sensitized individuals.

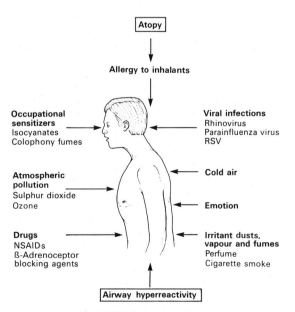

Fig. 12.26 Causes of asthma.

The term is now best used to describe those individuals who readily develop antibodies of immunoglobulin E (IgE) class against common materials present in the environment. Such antibodies are present in 30–40% of the population, the proportion being greatest in the third and fourth decades of life and reducing with age.

Increased responsiveness of the airways of the lung (bronchial hyper-reactivity)
The definition of asthma used in North America incorporates a well-known feature of the disease —an increased responsiveness of the airways to non-specific stimuli (i.e. bronchial hyper-reactivity). Bronchial reactivity can be demonstrated by asking the patient to inhale gradually increasing concentrations either of histamine or methacholine (*bronchial provocation tests*). This induces a transient episode of airflow limitation in susceptible individuals (approximately 30% of the population); the dose of the agonist (provocation dose) necessary to produce a 20% fall in FEV_1 is known as the $PD_{20}FEV_1$. Patients with clinical symptoms of asthma respond to very low doses of methacholine, i.e. they have a low $PD_{20}FEV_1$. In general, the greater the degree of hyper-reactivity, the more persistent the symptoms and the greater the need for treatment.

In another group of subjects, the lungs react to methacholine but at a higher concentration. These include patients with:
- Attacks of asthma only on extreme exertion
- A viral infection
- Problems with asthma in the grass pollen season
- Allergic rhinitis who do not complain of any lower respiratory tract symptoms until specifically questioned

Although the degree of hyper-reactivity can itself be influenced by allergic mechanisms (see p. 588 and Fig. 12.29), its pathogenesis and mode of inheritance remain to be elucidated.

Allergens
The allergens involved are similar to those in rhinitis, though the particle size of pollens (>20 μm) means that they are much more likely to cause conjunctivitis, rhinitis and pharyngitis than asthma. Allergens from the faecal particles of the house-dust mite are the most important extrinsic cause of asthma worldwide. The fungal spores from *Aspergillus fumigatus* give rise to a complex series of lung diseases, including asthma (see p. 608).

PATHOGENESIS AND PRECIPITATING FACTORS

Occupational sensitizers
Over 200 materials encountered at the work place are known to give rise to occupational asthma. The seven most important causes are recognized occupational diseases in the UK and patients in insurable

employment are therefore eligible for statutory compensation provided they apply within 10 years of leaving the occupation where the asthma developed (Table 12.7). The development of asthma following exposure to some of these materials is linked to the development of specific IgE antibody in serum in some cases, whilst in others the cause has yet to be determined.

The proportion of employees developing occupational asthma depends primarily upon the level of exposure. Proper enclosure of industrial processes or appropriate ventilation can greatly reduce the risk. Atopic individuals develop occupational asthma more rapidly when exposed to agents causing the development of specific IgE antibody. Non-atopic individuals can also develop asthma when exposed to such agents, but usually after a longer period.

Non-specific factors

The characteristic feature of bronchial hyper-reactivity in asthmatics means that as well as reacting to specific antigens their airways will also respond to a wide variety of non-specific stimuli.

Cold air and exercise. Most asthmatics experience an attack of wheezing after prolonged and continuous exercise. Typically, the attack does not occur during the exercise period, but at its conclusion. The inhalation of cold, dry air will also precipitate an attack. In both cases the wheezing is thought to be precipitated by the cooling and drying of the epithelial lining of the bronchi. Exercise and cold air provocation tests can be performed.

Table 12.7 Occupational asthma in the UK.

Cause	Source
Non-IgE related	
Isocyanates	Polyurethane varnishes Industrial coatings
Colophony fumes	Soldering Electronics industry
IgE related	
Allergens from animals and insects	Laboratories
Allergens from flour and grain	Farmers Millers Grain handlers
Proteolytic enzymes	Manufacture (but not use) of 'biological' washing powders
Complex salts of platinum	Metal refining
Acid anhydrides and polyamine hardening agents	Industrial coatings

Atmospheric pollution and irritant dusts, vapours and fumes. Many patients with asthma experience worsening of symptoms on contact with cigarette smoke, car exhaust fumes, strong perfumes or high concentrations of dust in the atmosphere. Further minor epidemics of the disease have occurred during periods of heavy atmospheric pollution in industrial areas, caused by the presence of high concentrations of sulphur dioxide and ozone in the air.

Emotion. It is well known that emotional factors may influence asthma, but there is no evidence that patients with the disease are any more psychologically disturbed than their non-asthmatic peers.

Drugs. Non-steroidal anti-inflammatory drugs (NSAIDs), particularly aspirin, have an important role in the development and precipitation of attacks in approximately 5% of patients with asthma. This effect is almost universal in those individuals who have both nasal polyps and asthma. The precise mechanism involved is unknown, but it is thought that treatment with these drugs leads to an imbalance in the metabolism of arachidonic acid. NSAIDs inhibit arachidonic acid metabolism via the cyclo-oxygenase pathway, preventing the synthesis of prostaglandins. It is suggested that under these circumstances arachidonic acid is preferentially metabolized via the lipoxygenase pathway, resulting in the production of leukotrienes, previously known as the slow-reacting substances for anaphylaxis (see Fig. 12.27).

The airways of the lung have a direct parasympathetic innervation which tends to produce bronchoconstriction. There is no direct sympathetic innervation of the smooth muscle of the bronchi, and antagonism of parasympathetically induced bronchoconstriction is critically dependent upon circulating adrenaline acting through beta-2 receptors on the surface of smooth muscle cells. Inhibition of this effect by beta-adrenoreceptor-blocking drugs such as propranolol leads to bronchoconstriction and airflow limitation, but only in asthmatic subjects. The so-called selective beta-1-adrenoceptor-blocking drugs such as atenolol may still induce attacks of asthma; their use in asthmatic patients for hypertension or angina should be questioned and calcium antagonists such as nifedipine used if appropriate.

Allergen-induced asthma

The experimental inhalation of allergen by atopic asthmatic individuals leads to the development of four types of reaction, as illustrated in Fig. 12.28.

The commonest reaction is *immediate asthma*, in which airflow limitation begins within minutes of contact with the allergen, reaches its maximum in 15–20 min and subsides by 1 h.

Many asthmatics subsequently develop a more prolonged and sustained attack of airflow limitation which responds poorly to inhalation of bronchodil-

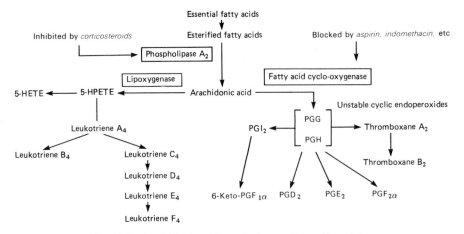

Fig. 12.27 Arachidonic acid metabolism and the effect of drugs.

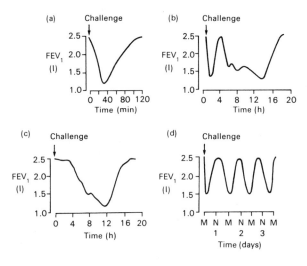

Fig. 12.28 Different types of asthmatic reactions following challenge with allergen. (a) Immediate asthma. (b) Dual asthmatic response. (c) Isolated late reaction. (d) Recurrent asthmatic reactions. M = midnight; N = noon.

ator drugs such as salbutamol—the *late-phase reaction*.

The combination of an immediate reaction followed by a late reaction is known as a *dual asthmatic response*.

The inhalation of some materials, particularly occupational sensitizers such as the isocyanates, usually causes the development of an *isolated late reaction* with no preceding immediate response.

The development of the late-phase reaction is associated with an increase in the underlying level of bronchial hyper-reactivity such that individuals may show continuing episodes of asthma on subsequent days—*recurrent asthmatic reactions*.

In allergen-induced asthma mast cells are found free in the lumen of the airways where they interact with inhaled allergen through surface-bound IgE molecules. Release of histamine causes increased permeability of the epithelium, allowing subsequent interaction of the allergen with mast cells in the epithelium itself and the lamina propria. The subsequent sequence of events is shown in Fig. 12.29.

Early phase (immediate asthma) is thought to develop from the action of histamine and the slow-releasing substances of anaphylaxis (the leukotrienes) on the smooth muscle of the airways.

Mast cells contain important preformed factors:
- Histamine
- Neutrophil chemotactic factor (NCF)
- Eosinophilic chemotactic factors (ECFs)

Neutrophils and eosinophils enter affected tissues within 1–8 h and are followed by infiltration of macrophages. These cells contain large quantities of powerful mediators:
- *Leukotrienes* (LT) cause continuing constriction of

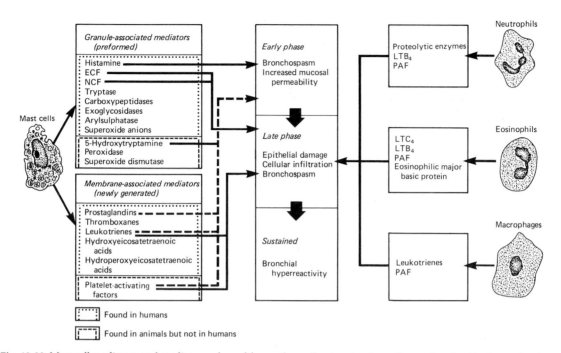

Fig. 12.29 Mast cell mediators and mediators released from other cells, showing the pathways involved in the production of inflammation, bronchospasm and bronchial hyperreactivity.

smooth muscles. LTB is chemotactic for neutrophils and eosinophils and attracts these to the site of the lesion.
- *Platelet activating factor* (PAF) causes continuing inflammation leading to bronchial hyperreactivity.
- *Eosinophilic major basic protein* causes shedding of the epithelium.

All the above result in a self-generating inflammatory reaction which causes the late phase asthmatic reaction and subsequent sustained bronchial hyperreactivity (see Fig. 12.29).

Asthma is now considered to be an inflammatory disease. Post-mortem studies show that there is marked infiltration of the tissues with eosinophils, macrophages and lymphocytes, with shedding of the epithelium, thickening of the basement membrane and some hypertrophy of smooth muscle. The small bronchi may be obstructed by viscid sputum containing eosinophils and Charcot–Leyden crystals, which represent accumulation of secretions from eosinophils including major basic protein.

CLASSIFICATION

Traditionally, asthma has been divided into:
- Extrinsic—implying a definite external cause
- Intrinsic or cryptogenic—when no causative agent can be identified

Typically, *extrinsic asthma* occurs in atopic individuals who show positive skin prick reactions to common inhaled allergens. Positive skin tests to inhalant allergens are shown in 90% of children, whereas only 50% of adults show this phenomenon. Eczema is often seen in childhood (see p. 904).

Intrinsic asthma often starts in middle age. Nevertheless, many show positive skin tests and on close questioning give a history of respiratory symptoms compatible with childhood asthma.

This classification is of little value in clinical practice. Non-atopic individuals may develop asthma in middle age from extrinsic causes such as sensitization to occupational agents or aspirin intolerance, or because they were given beta-adrenoceptor-blocking agents for concurrent hypertension or angina. Extrinsic causes must be considered in all cases of asthma and, where possible, avoided.

CLINICAL FEATURES

Patients suffering from asthma exhibit virtually identical symptoms to those suffering from airflow limitation caused by chronic bronchitis and emphysema. Wheezing attacks and episodic shortness of breath are almost universal. There is an initial tendency for symptoms to be worst during the night. Cough is a frequent symptom which sometimes predominates and is often misdiagnosed as being due to bronchitis. Nocturnal cough can be a presenting feature.

There is a tremendous variation in the frequency and duration of the attacks. Some patients may have only one or two attacks a year which last for a few hours, whilst others may have attacks lasting for weeks. Some patients can have chronic symptoms. Attacks may be precipitated by all the factors illustrated in Fig. 12.26; the signs of asthma are illustrated in Table 12.1.

INVESTIGATION

There is no single satisfactory diagnostic test for all asthmatic patients.

Lung function tests

Traditionally, the diagnosis of asthma is based on the demonstration of a greater than 15% improvement in FEV_1 or PEFR following the inhalation of a bronchodilator. However, this is often not present if the asthma is in remission or in very severe chronic disease when little reversibility can be demonstrated.

Peak flow charts

Measurements of PEFR on waking, in the middle of the day, and before bed are particularly useful in demonstrating the variable airflow limitation which characterizes the disease. An example is shown in Fig. 12.12. This technique is also of help in the longer-term assessment of the patient's disease and its response to treatment. Peak flows need to be measured over several days and preferably over a weekend or short holiday if the effect of work exposure is also being studied.

Exercise tests

These have been widely used in the diagnosis of asthma in children. Ideally, the child should run for 6 min on a treadmill at a workload sufficient to increase the heart rate above 160 beats·m^{-1}. A negative test does not rule out asthma.

Histamine or methacholine bronchial provocation tests (see p. 586)

This test indicates the presence of bronchial hyper-reactivity, a feature found in all asthmatics, and can be particularly useful in investigating those patients whose main symptom is cough. The test should not be performed on individuals who have poor lung function ($FEV_1 < 1.5$ l).

Trial of corticosteroids

Prednisolone 30 mg orally should be given daily for 2 weeks to all patients who present with severe airflow limitation. A substantial improvement (>15%) confirms the presence of an asthmatic element and that the administration of steroids will prove beneficial to the patient. The dose is slowly reduced over several weeks and is replaced by inhaled corticosteroids in those who will benefit.

Blood and sputum tests

Patients with asthma may have an increase in the number of eosinophil granulocytes in peripheral blood ($>0.4 \times 10^9$/l). This is rarely helpful in the diagnosis. The presence of large numbers of eosinophil granulocytes, particularly when present in clumps in sputum, is helpful in the differential diagnosis of asthma from chronic bronchitis and emphysema.

Chest x-ray

There are no diagnostic features of asthma on the chest x-ray. A chest x-ray may be helpful in excluding a pneumothorax, which can occur as a complication, or in detecting the pulmonary shadows associated with allergic bronchopulmonary aspergillosis.

Skin tests (see p. 570)

Skin prick tests should be performed in all cases of asthma to help identify extrinsic causes. Experimentally, the inhalation of an allergen which gives rise to a large weal on skin testing will almost always produce an attack of asthma in patients with the disease, but whether or not this occurs in everyday life depends on the concentrations encountered in the atmosphere.

Allergen provocation tests

These are seldom, if ever, required in the clinical investigation of patients. An exception is the investigation of food allergy causing asthma. This diagnosis is difficult; blind oral challenges with the food disguised in opaque gelatine capsules are necessary to confirm or refute a causative link (see p. 146).

MANAGEMENT

Asthma is an extremely common disease producing considerable morbidity. The aim of treatment must be to allow the asthmatic patient to lead as normal a life as possible. Sufficient therapy should be administered to enable the patient to keep fit and take part in sporting activities. Children should not be prevented from taking part in games because of their asthma. Since it is a chronic disease, patients must understand the purpose of each treatment and be able to take part in the management of their own disease. Many asthmatics belong to self-help groups whose aim is to further their understanding of the disease and to foster self-confidence and fitness.

Control of extrinsic factors

Avoidance of exposure to extrinsic agents remains difficult and is described in detail in the management of allergic rhinitis (p. 574).

Avoidance of major allergens (e.g. the house-dust mite) can be helpful, but is difficult to achieve, short of living at high altitude where mites cannot survive, or in hospital where the environment is too hostile (see p. 574). The development of an effective acaricide harmless to man could prove valuable in the management of asthma.

Individuals intolerant to aspirin may benefit, though are rarely cured, by avoiding salicylates. Other agents, e.g. preservatives and colouring materials such as tartrazine, should be avoided if shown to be a causative factor. Fifty per cent of individuals sensitized to occupational agents may be cured if they are kept permanently away from exposure. The remaining 50% continue to have symptoms as severe as when exposed to materials at work. This is particularly so if they had been symptomatic for a long time before the diagnosis was made.

This underlines two points:
- The importance of the rapid identification of extrinsic cases of asthma and their removal wherever possible (e.g. the family pet)
- Once extrinsic asthma is initiated, it may become self-perpetuating.

Hyposensitization
This form of treatment is not as effective for allergic asthma as for allergic rhinitis and is rarely advised for the management of asthma alone.

Drug treatment
The mainstay of asthma therapy is the use of therapeutic agents delivered as aerosols or powders direct into the lungs. The advantages of this method of administration are obvious. Drugs are delivered direct to the lung and the first-pass metabolism in the liver is avoided; both these factors mean that much lower doses are necessary and unwanted effects are slight.

Inhaled therapy

Use of an inhaler
- The canister is shaken.
- The patient exhales to functional residual capacity (not residual volume), i.e. normal expiration.
- The aerosol nozzle is placed to the open mouth.
- The patient simultaneously inhales rapidly and activates the aerosol.
- Inhalation is completed.
- The breath is held for 10 s if possible.
- Even with good technique only 15% of the contents is inhaled and 85% is deposited on the wall of the pharynx and ultimately swallowed.

Spacers
These are plastic spheres inserted between the patient's mouth and the inhaler. They are designed to reduce particle velocity so that less drug is deposited in the mouth. Spacers also diminish the need for coordination between aerosol activation and inhalation. They are useful in children and in the elderly.

The effective use of inhaled therapy depends upon careful instruction and training of the patient. At best only 15% of the aerosolized material will enter the respiratory tract. Many patients and doctors remain frightened to use aerosols because in the early 1960s there was a parallel between an increase in sudden deaths from asthma and sales of isoprenaline (a non-selective beta-adrenoceptor agonist) aerosols. In fact this was largely due to insufficient treatment of asthmatic patients with corticosteroids such that they took increasing doses of isoprenaline, but died of asthma.

Beta-2-adrenoceptor agonists. The newer bronchodilator preparations contain beta-adrenoceptor agonists which, unlike isoprenaline, are selective for the beta-2-adrenoceptors of the respiratory tract and do not stimulate the beta-1-adrenoceptors of the myocardium. These drugs are potent bronchodilators in that they cause relaxation of bronchial smooth muscle. Such treatment is very effective in relieving symptoms but does little for the underlying inflammatory nature of the disease. Inhalants such as salbutamol or terbutaline should be prescribed as two puffs four times daily, but only the mildest asthmatics with intermittent attacks should rely upon this treatment alone. Some patients use nebulizers at home for self-administration of salbutamol.

Other inhalants such as anti-cholinergic agents (e.g. ipratropium bromide one to two puffs three or four times daily) may be helpful.

Anti-allergic drugs. The exact mode of action of sodium cromoglycate remains unknown, but it is postulated that it prevents release of mediators from mast cells. This drug is particularly effective in younger patients with mild but frequent asthma. It must be taken regularly either in the form of a Spincap containing 20 mg or in aerosol form from a metered dose inhaler delivering 1 mg per puff. The dose should be two puffs four times daily from an inhaler, or one Spincap three or four times daily.

Ketotifen is a potent antihistamine which is also considered to have mast cell stabilizing properties. The indications for its use are identical to those for sodium cromoglycate. Its advantage is that it can be given as one 1 mg tablet twice daily and therefore can be given to small children who find it difficult to use a Spinhaler or a metered dose inhaler, and it may be effective against allergic disease affecting the eyes, nose and lungs.

Inhaled corticosteroids. All patients who have regular persisting symptoms in spite of treatment with a beta-2-adrenoceptor agonist and sodium cromoglycate or ketotifen need regular treatment with inhaled corticosteroids. Beclomethasone dispropionate is available in doses of 50 and 250 μg per puff, and budesonide is available in doses of 200 μg per metered inhalation. High-dose beclomethasone and budesonide should be reserved for patients who have not responded to beclomethasone 50 μg per puff. The unwanted effects of inhaled corticosteroids are oral candidiasis, which may develop in 5% of patients, and hoarseness due to the effect of corticosteroids on the laryngeal muscles. Inhaled corticosteroids have now been widely used for 15 years and no significant long-term unwanted effects have been detected.

Oral corticosteroids. Use of oral corticosteroids is necessary for those individuals not controlled on inhaled corticosteroids. The dose should be kept as low as possible to avoid side-effects. The effect of short-term treatment with prednisolone 30 mg daily is shown in Fig. 12.12.

Antibiotics. There is no evidence that antibiotics are helpful in the management of patients who suffer from properly diagnosed asthma. However, wheezing frequently occurs in exacerbations of chronic bronchitis and emphysema associated with infected sputum.

Yellow or green sputum containing eosinophils and bronchial epithelial cells may be coughed up in acute exacerbations of asthma. This is not due to bacterial infection and antibiotics are not required.

Management of severe asthma

Although this condition is often called 'status asthmaticus', it is better considered as severe asthma which has not been controlled by the patient's use of medication. Patients with severe asthma have:

- Tachycardia
- Pulsus paradoxicus (>20 mmHg). In very severe asthma no paradoxicus is detected.
- Wheezing. The chest may be silent in severe asthma due to insufficient airflow.

Patients seen with this severe form of the disease require intensive treatment and should almost always be admitted to hospital. The PEFR should be measured in all patients presenting with severe asthma, and if below 150 l·min^{-1} (in adults), the patient should be admitted.

Before giving aminophylline, the patient is asked whether he has previously been taking theophylline preparations as part of routine treatment; if so, toxic levels may result from intravenous administration of aminophylline and the drug is best avoided. Instead, slow intravenous injections of salbutamol or terbutaline at a dose of 250 μg can be administered. If aminophylline is given, it should be administered slowly over 10–15 min and only after oxygen has been administered. This drug stimulates cardiac muscle, increasing output and blood flow through poorly ventilated lungs such that the $P_a O_2$ may fall unless the inspired concentrations of oxygen are increased. The combination of stimulation of the myocardium and increasing hypoxaemia may lead to

---

Treatment of severe asthma

At home
- The patient is assessed. Tachycardia with pulsus paradoxicus and cyanosis indicate a severe attack.
- If the PEFR is less than 150 l·min^{-1} (in adults), an ambulance should be called. All doctors should carry peak flow meters.
- Aminophylline 250–500 mg i.v. is given slowly (see text).
- Hydrocortisone sodium succinate 200 mg i.v. is given.
- Oxygen is given if available.

In hospital
- The patient is reassessed.
- Oxygen is given via a variable performance mask.
- The PEFR is measured using a low-reading peak flow meter, as an ordinary meter only measures from 60 l·min^{-1} upwards.
- Nebulized salbutamol or terbutaline 5 mg is given initially.
- Hydrocortisone 200 mg i.v. is given 4-hourly for 24 h, followed by prednisolone 30 mg orally daily for 2 weeks.
- Arterial blood gases are measured; if the $P_a CO_2$ is greater than 7 kPa, ventilation should be considered.
- A chest x-ray is performed to exclude pneumothorax.
- Nebulized salbutamol or terbutaline 5 mg is administered 4-hourly.
- One of the following intravenous infusions is given if no improvement is seen:
    Aminophylline 500 mg·kg·h^{-1}
    Or salbutamol 3–20 mg·min^{-1}
    Or terbutaline 1.5–5 mg·min^{-1}

---

cardiac dysrhythmias. Hydrocortisone 200 mg i.v. should be administered 4-hourly for 24 h and 30 mg of prednisolone given orally daily. Patients who do not respond to this regimen may require ventilation.

Patients should be kept in hospital for at least 1 week since the majority of sudden deaths occur 2–5 days after admission. Oral corticosteroids should be gradually reduced on an outpatient basis until an appropriate maintenance dose or substitution by inhaled corticosteroid aerosols can be achieved.

If the patient's PEFR is greater than 150 l·min^{-1} patients may improve dramatically on intravenous drug administration of aminophylline and/or hydrocortisone, and may not need to be admitted to hospital. Their regular treatment should be increased, probably to include treatment for two weeks with 15–30 mg of prednisolone followed by a gradual reduction in the oral dose and substitution by an inhaled corticosteroid preparation.

PROGNOSIS

Although asthma often improves in children as they reach their teens, it is now realized that the disease frequently returns in the second, third and fourth decades. Overall, in adults, there is a tendency for asthma to improve with age.

Diseases of the lung parenchyma

PNEUMONIAS

Pneumonia may be defined as an inflammation of the substance of the lung, usually caused by bacteria. Clinically it presents as an acute illness characterized in the majority of cases by the presence of cough, purulent sputum and fever together with physical signs or radiological changes compatible with consolidation of the lung.

The advent of antibiotics might have been expected to decrease dramatically the mortality from pneumonia. However, mortality statistics obtained from death certificates show the reverse. This is because the dramatic decrease in deaths from pneumonia in children under 10 years has been counterbalanced by an increase in deaths from pneumonia in individuals over the age of 70 years.

CLASSIFICATION

Pneumonia can be classified both anatomically and on the basis of the aetiology.

Site
Pneumonias are either localized, e.g. affecting the whole of one lobe, or diffuse, when they primarily affect the lobules of the lung, often in association with the bronchi and bronchioles, a condition referred to as 'bronchopneumonia'.

Aetiology
An aetiological factor can be discovered in approximately 70% of patients. The term 'atypical pneumonias' was used to describe pneumonia caused by agents such as *Mycoplasma*, influenza A virus, *Chlamydia* and *Coxiella burnetii*. These types of pneumonia alone account for almost one-third of the cases of pneumonia (see Table 12.8) and the term 'atypical' should be dropped. Pneumonias may also result from:
- Chemical causes, e.g. aspiration of vomit (see p. 597)
- Radiotherapy (see p. 613)
- Allergic mechanisms (see p. 608)

Mycobacterium tuberculosis is an important cause of pneumonia; it is considered separately since both its mode of presentation and its treatment are very different from the infective agents shown in Table 12.8.

Precipitating factors
- *Streptococcus pneumoniae*—often follows influenza or para-influenza viral infection
- Hospitalized 'ill' patients—often infected with gram-negative organisms
- Cigarette smoking
- Alcohol
- Bronchiectasis (e.g. in cystic fibrosis)
- Bronchial obstruction (e.g. carcinoma)—occasionally associated with infection with 'non-pathogenic' organisms
- Immunosuppression (e.g. AIDS or treatment with cytotoxic agents)—organisms include *Pneumocystis carinii*, *Mycobacterium avium*, cytomegalovirus
- Intravenous drug abuse—frequently associated with *Staphylococcus aureus* infection
- Inhalation from oesophageal obstruction—often associated with infection with anaerobes

CLINICAL PRESENTATION

The clinical presentation varies according to the immune state of the patient and the infecting agent. In the commonest type of pneumonia—caused by *Streptococcus pneumoniae*—there is often a preceding history of a viral infection. The patient rapidly becomes more ill with a high temperature (up to 39.5°C), pleuritic pain and a dry cough. A day or two later, rusty-coloured sputum is produced and at about the same time the patient may develop labial herpes simplex. The patient breathes rapidly and shallowly, the affected side of the chest moves less, and signs of consolidation may be present together with a pleural rub.

INVESTIGATION

Chest x-ray confirms the area of consolidation, but radiological changes lag behind the clinical course so that x-ray changes may be minimal at the start of illness. Conversely, consolidation may remain on the chest x-ray for several weeks after the patient is clinically cured. The chest x-ray should always return to normal by 6 weeks, except in patients with severe airflow limitation. Persistent changes on the chest x-ray after this time suggest a bronchial abnormality, usually a carcinoma, with persisting secondary pneumonia. Chest x-rays should rarely be repeated more frequently than at weekly intervals during the acute illness and then at 6 weeks after discharge from hospital.

In *Streptococcus pneumoniae* pneumonia, there is often a white blood cell count which is greater than $15 \times 10^9/l$ (90% polymorphonuclear leucocytosis) and an ESR greater than 100 mm·h^{-1}.

The individual features of different pneumonias

Table 12.8 The aetiology of pneumonia in the UK.

Infecting agent	Frequency as a cause of pneumonia (%)	Clinical circumstance
Streptococcus pneumoniae	35	Community pneumonia, patients usually previously fit
Mycoplasma pneumoniae	18	As above
Influenza A virus (usually with a bacterial component)	7	As above
Haemophilus influenzae	5	Pre-existing lung disease chronic bronchitis and emphysema
Chlamydia psittaci	3	Contact with birds (though not inevitable)
Staphylococcus aureus	2	Children, intravenous drug abusers, associated with influenza virus infections
Legionella pneumophila	2	Institutional outbreaks (hospitals and hotels), sporadic, endemic
Coxiella burnetii	1	Abattoir and animal hide workers
Pseudomonas aeruginosa	<1	Cystic fibrosis
Pneumocystis carinii *Actinomyces israelii* *Nocardia asteroides* Cytomegalovirus *Aspergillus fumigatus*	<1	AIDS, lymphomas, leukaemias, use of cytotoxic drugs and corticosteroids
Anaerobic organisms	<1	Inhalation pneumonia, alcoholism, postoperative
None isolated	30	—

are given below. The overall investigation and management is shown in Fig. 12.30 and discussed on pp. 598–599.

Mycoplasma pneumonia

This is a common cause of pneumonia. It often occurs in patients in their teens and twenties, frequently amongst those living in boarding institutions. Generalized features such as headaches and malaise often precede the chest symptoms by 1–5 days. Cough may not be obvious initially and physical signs in the chest may be scanty.

On chest x-ray, usually only one of the lower lobes is involved, but sometimes there may be dramatic shadowing in both lower lobes. There is frequently no correlation between the x-ray appearances and the clinical state of the patient.

The white blood count is not raised. Cold agglutinins occur in half of the cases. The diagnosis is confirmed by a rising antibody titre. Treatment with erythromycin or tetracycline is effective.

Although most patients recover in 10–14 days, the disease can be protracted, with cough and x-ray appearance lasting for weeks and relapses occurring. Lung abscesses and pleural effusions are rare.

Extrapulmonary complications can occur at any time during the illness and occasionally dominate the clinical picture. Most are rare but they include:
- Myocarditis and pericarditis
- Rashes and erythema multiforme
- Haemolytic anaemia and thrombocytopenia
- Myalgia and arthralgia
- Meningo-encephalitis and other neurological abnormalities
- Gastrointestinal symptoms (e.g. vomiting, diarrhoea)

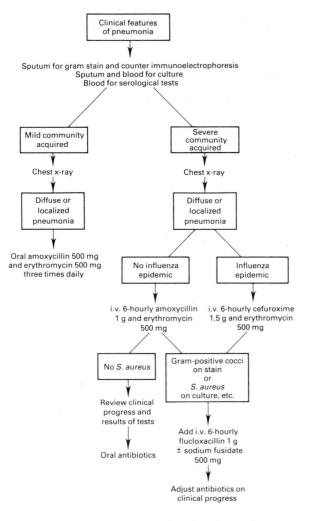

Fig. 12.30 Algorithm for the management of pneumonia (see also p. 598).

Viral pneumonia

Viral pneumonia is uncommon in adults, bacteria being the usual cause of the pneumonia per se. Rarely, influenza A virus or adenovirus infection can produce pneumonia.

Bacterial pneumonia

Haemophilus influenzae

H. influenzae is frequently identified in the yellow-green sputum produced during exacerbations of chronic bronchitis. It is therefore not surprising that this organism may be the cause of pneumonia in people suffering from chronic bronchitis and emphysema. The pneumonia can be diffuse or confined to one lobe. There are no special features to separate it from other bacterial causes of pneumonia. It responds well to treatment with amoxycillin.

Chlamydia psittaci (see p. 51)

Typically the individual has been working with infected birds, especially parrots, but a history of contact is not always elicited. The incubation period is 1–2 weeks and the disease may pursue a very low-grade course over several months. Symptoms include malaise, high fever, cough and muscular pains. The liver and spleen are occasionally enlarged and scanty 'rose spots' may be seen on the abdomen. The chest x-ray shows segmental or a diffuse pneumonia. Occasionally the illness presents with a high swinging fever and dramatic prostration with photophobia and neck stiffness which can be confused with meningitis. The diagnosis is confirmed by the demonstration of a rising titre of complement-fixing antibody. Tetracycline or erythromycin are the antibiotics of choice.

Staphylococci

Staphylococcus aureus normally only causes a

pneumonia after a preceding influenzal viral illness. The infection starts in the bronchi, leading to patchy areas of consolidation in one or more lobes which break down to form abscesses. These may appear as cysts on the chest x-ray.

Pneumothorax, effusion and empyemas are frequent. Septicaemia develops with metastatic abscesses in other organs.

Fulminating staphylococcal pneumonia occurring in influenza epidemics can lead to death in hours. All patients with this type of pneumonia are very ill; intravenous antibiotics must be administered promptly, but are not always effective.

Areas of pneumonia (septic infarcts) are also seen in staphylococcal septicaemia. This is frequently seen in intravenous drug abusers and also in patients with central catheters being used for parenteral nutrition. The infected puncture site is the source of the *Staphylococcus*. Pulmonary symptoms are often few, but breathlessness and cough occur and the chest x-ray reveals areas of consolidation. Abscess formation is frequent. Diagnosis and treatment are shown in Fig. 12.30.

Coxiella burnetii (Q-fever) (see p. 50)

The patient develops systemic symptoms of fever, malaise and headache, often associated with multiple lesions on the chest x-ray. The illness may run a chronic course and is occasionally associated with endocarditis. Diagnosis is made by an increase in the titre of complement-fixing antibody, and erythromycin or tetracycline is the usual treatment.

Legionella pneumophila (see p. 36)

Legionnaires' disease derives its name from an outbreak of serious respiratory infection amongst members of the American Legion attending the Bel Vue Stratford Hotel, Philadelphia, in the summer of 1976. Two hundred cases occurred, with a mortality of 15%. In retrospect, antibody studies showed that this organism was the cause of a number of previous outbreaks of pneumonia stretching back to 1946.

The epidemiological patterns recognized are:
- Outbreaks amongst previously fit individuals staying in hotels, institutions or hospitals where the shower facilities or cooling systems have been contaminated with the organism
- Sporadic cases occurring in many parts of the world where the source of the infection is unknown
- Outbreaks occurring in immunocompromised patients and in middle-aged and elderly male smokers

Legionella grows well in water over 25°C in temperature, and the infection is almost certainly spread by the aerosol route. Adequate chlorination and temperature control are important factors in the prevention of the disease.

The incubation period is 2–10 days. Males are affected twice as commonly as females. The infection may be mild, but the characteristic picture is of malaise, myalgia, headache and a fever with rigors and a pyrexia of up to 40°C. Half of the patients have gastrointestinal symptoms, with nausea, vomiting, diarrhoea and abdominal pain. Patients may be acutely ill, with mental confusion and other neurological signs. Haematuria occurs and occasionally renal failure.

The patient is tachypnoeic with initially a dry cough which later may become productive and purulent. The chest x-ray usually shows unilateral lobar and then multi-lobar shadowing, sometimes with a small pleural effusion. Cavitation is rare.

A strong presumptive diagnosis of *Legionella pneumophila* infection is possible in the majority of patients if they have three of the four following features:
- A prodromal virus-like illness
- A dry cough, confusion or diarrhoea
- Lymphopenia without marked leucocytosis
- Hyponatraemia

Hypoalbuminaemia and abnormal levels of liver enzymes are common in this disease. The diagnosis is confirmed by a change in antibody titre, but the quickest way is by the direct immunofluorescent staining of the organism in the pleural fluid, sputum or bronchial washings. A Gram stain does not detect the organism. Culture is possible but takes up to 3 weeks.

The organism is sensitive to erythromycin and rifampicin, which are the antibiotics of choice. Mortality can be up to 30% in elderly patients, but most patients recover spontaneously.

Gram-negative bacteria

These are the cause of many hospital-acquired pneumonias but they are occasionally responsible for cases in the community.

Klebsiella pneumoniae. Pneumonia due to *Klebsiella* usually occurs in the elderly with a history of heart or lung disease, diabetes, alcohol excess or malignancy. The onset is often sudden, with severe systemic upset. The sputum is purulent, gelatinous or blood-stained. The upper lobes are more commonly affected and the consolidation is often extensive. There is often swelling of the infected lobe so that on the lateral chest x-ray there is bulging of the fissures. The organism can be found in the sputum or in the blood. Treatment is dependent on the sensitivity of the organism, but a cephalosporin or chloramphenicol is usually required. The mortality is high, partly due to the presence of an underlying condition.

Pseudomonas aeruginosa. Pneumonia due to this organism is of considerable significance in patients with cystic fibrosis since it correlates with a worsening clinical condition and mortality. It is also seen in patients with neutropenia following cytotoxic chemotherapy. The isolation of *Pseudomonas aeruginosa* must be interpreted with care since the organism grows well on bacterial culture medium and may simply represent contamination from the upper airways. *Pseudomonas aeruginosa* infection requires combination treatment with tobramycin 3–5 mg·kg^{-1} i.v. or i.m. daily in 8-hourly doses together with carbenicillin 5 g i.v. 4- to 6-hourly. These antibiotics can be inhaled direct into the lung via nebulizers by patients with cystic fibrosis (see p. 585).

Pseudomonal infection should respond to the above regimen, but modifications may have to be made in the light of sensitivity testing. Tobramycin is nephrotoxic and produces vestibular damage so the blood levels should be monitored. Recently, two new antipseudomonal penicillins have been introduced—azlocillin and ticarcillin—both of which have greater activity than carbenicillin against these organisms.

Branhamella catarrhalis. This organism, previously known as *Neisseria catarrhalis*, has been found to be associated with exacerbations of chronic bronchitis and occasionally with fatal pneumonia. An important point about this organism is that some strains produce a beta-lactamase capable of destroying ampicillin. The exact role of this organism in bronchopulmonary infection remains to be determined.

Anaerobic bacteria
Infections with these organisms usually occur in those with an underlying condition, e.g. diabetes, and are often associated with aspiration. Bacteroides is the commonest organism and is sensitive to metronidazole. The prognosis depends largely on the precipitating cause.

Pneumonias due to opportunistic infections
These are commonly becoming recognized in the immunocompromised patient.

Pneumocystis carinii. Until recently, infection with this sporozoan was chiefly confined to patients receiving immunosuppressive treatment. In the poorer parts of the world, however, *Pneumocystis* pneumonia is not infrequently found in malnourished children. It is by far the commonest opportunistic infection, accounting for 85% of the cases of pneumonia in patients with acquired immunodeficiency syndrome (AIDS) (see p. 62).

It is likely that infection with the organism occurs by inhalation, perhaps in childhood, and the organism may remain latent for many years, being reactivated when immunosuppression occurs. Clinically the pneumonia is associated with a high fever, breathlessness and dry cough. In patients with AIDS, however, the clinical features are different, with a much more insidious onset, though fever,

dyspnoea, dry cough, weight loss and diarrhoea do occur.

The typical radiographic appearance is of diffuse bilateral alveolar and interstitial shadowing beginning in the peri-hilar regions and spreading out in a butterfly pattern.

Investigation includes fibreoptic bronchoscopy with transbronchial biopsies and bronchial washing and aspiration; the diagnosis can be made in 95% of cases by this method.

Treatment is with co-trimoxazole 1.44 g 12-hourly. The mortality partly depends on the underlying condition; with treatment it is approximately 25%.

Actinomyces israeli (see p. 36). The clinical picture is that of severe pneumonia, lung abscess or empyema.

Nocardia asteroides. This produces a similar picture to *Actinomyces*, though of greater severity. The chest x-ray often shows irregular opacities in one or both lungs, particularly in the mid-zones.

Cytomegalovirus (see p. 53). Bronchitis and pneumonia may occur but these are usually a more minor part of the generalized systemic illness.

Aspergillus fumigatus (see p. 608). This fungus gives rise to a widespread invasion of lung tissue in patients who are immunocompromised. It is a serious pneumonia which is usually rapidly fatal.

Rare infective causes of pneumonia

Pneumonia may be seen in the course of infection by *Bordetella pertussis*, typhoid and paratyphoid bacillus, brucellosis, leptospirosis and a number of viral infections including measles, chickenpox and glandular fever. It is not usually a major feature. Details of these infections are described in Chapter 1.

Aspiration pneumonia

The aspiration of gastric contents into the lungs can produce an extremely severe and sometimes fatal illness due to the intense destructiveness of gastric acid—the Mendelson syndrome. It can complicate anaesthesia, particularly during pregnancy.

In the absence of a tracheo-oesophageal fistula, aspiration only occurs during periods of impaired consciousness (e.g. during sleep), in reflux oesophagitis or oesophageal stricture, or in bulbar palsy. Because of the bronchial anatomy, the most usual site for spillage is the posterior segment of the right lower lobe. The persistent pneumonia is often due to anaerobes and it may progress to lung abscess or even bronchiectasis. It is vital to identify any underlying problem since appropriate corrective measures can lead to resolution of the pulmonary problems.

Diffuse pneumonia (bronchopneumonia)

Diffuse pneumonia is very common. It is differentiated from severe bronchitis by signs of bronchial breathing or patchy shadows on the chest x-ray.

Widespread diffuse pneumonia is a common terminal event, largely resulting from an inability of patients dying from other conditions (e.g. cancer) to cough up retained secretions, allowing infection to develop throughout the lungs. Treatment in this situation is rarely appropriate.

Complications of pneumonia

Lung abscess

This term is used to describe severe localized suppuration in the lung associated with cavity formation on the chest x-ray, often with the presence of a fluid level, and not due to tuberculosis.

Causes of lung abscesses are many but the commonest is aspiration, particularly amongst alcoholics following aspiration pneumonia. Lung abscesses also frequently follow the inhalation of a foreign body into a bronchus and occasionally occur when the bronchus is obstructed by a bronchial carcinoma.

Abscesses may develop during the course of specific pneumonias, particularly when the infecting agent is *Staphylococcus pyogenes* or *Klebsiella pneumoniae*. Septic emboli, usually staphylococci, result in multiple lung abscesses. Infarcted areas of lung may occasionally cavitate and rarely become infected. Amoebic abscesses may occasionally develop in the right lower lobe following transdiaphragmatic spread from an amoebic liver abscess.

The clinical features are those of persisting and worsening pneumonia associated with the production of large quantities of sputum which is often foul-smelling owing to the growth of anaerobic organisms. There is usually a swinging fever. Chronic or subacute lung abscesses follow an inadequately treated pneumonia. Fever, malaise and weight loss occur. The chest signs may be few, but clubbing often develops. The patient is often anaemic with a high ESR.

Empyema

Empyema means the presence of pus within the pleural cavity. This usually arises after the rupture of a lung abscess into the pleural space or from bacterial spread from a severe pneumonia. Typically an empyema cavity becomes infected with anaerobic organisms and the patient is severely ill with a high fever and a neutrophil granulocytosis.

Investigation

Bacteriological investigation of lung abscess and empyema is best conducted on specimens obtained either by transtracheal aspiration (p. 563), broncho-scopy (p. 569) or percutaneous transthoracic aspiration.

Treatment

Although anaerobic organisms are found in up to 70% of lung abscesses and empyemas, there is usually a mixed flora, often with aerobes, particularly *Streptococcus milleri*. Anaerobic cocci, black-pigmented bacteroids and fusobacterium are the commonest anaerobes found.

Antibiotics should be given to cover both aerobic and anaerobic organisms; prolonged courses are often necessary. Treatment should be amoxycillin 1 g i.v. 6-hourly, erythromycin 500 mg i.v. 8-hourly and metronidazole 500 mg i.v. 8-hourly for 5 days, followed by oral amoxycillin and metronidazole for a prolonged period. Abscesses occasionally require surgery.

Empyemas should be treated by prompt rib resection and drainage of the empyema cavity followed by appropriate antibiotic treatment for up to 6 weeks.

Management of pneumonia

This is shown in the algorithm given in Fig. 12.30.

Sputum should always be sent for culture, but in mild cases treatment can be started immediately with oral amoxycillin and erythromycin.

More severe cases need to be admitted to hospital and a chest x-ray performed. Other investigations required are:

- Sputum—Gram stain and culture
- White blood cell count and ESR
- Blood culture

Treatment should be started immediately (without waiting for the result of these investigations). In more than 20% of cases, more than one organism is involved.

Further investigations may be necessary for the diagnosis of certain types of pneumonia:

- Mycoplasma antibodies (IgM and IgG)—in acute and convalescent samples
- Legionella antibodies—immunofluorescent tests
- Pneumococcal antigen—counterimmunoelectrophoresis (CIE) of sputum, urine and serum (three to four times more sensitive than sputum or blood cultures)

A high percentage of organisms causing pneumonia (e.g. *Mycoplasma pneumoniae* and *Haemophilus influenzae*) will not respond to penicillin. This drug should no longer be prescribed and should be replaced by a combination of bactericidal antibiotics which cover the commonest organisms. Treatment is commenced with amoxycillin 1 g i.v. 6-hourly together with erythromycin 500 mg i.v. 6-hourly. The purpose of this programme is to treat pneumonia with sufficient doses of appropriate antibiotics at the earliest stage. The treatment can always be modified and reduced in the light of clinical progress and subsequent bacteriological and serological findings.

The chances of identifying a causative organism are greatly decreased in individuals who have received antibiotics in the week prior to their admission to hospital.

The overall mortality for pneumonia is currently 5%, but for pneumonia due to *Staphylococcus aureus* it is in excess of 25%. Patients who die from pneumonia usually have not received the appropriate antibiotics in sufficient doses before or during the early stages of hospital admission.

Penicillin allergy

This often poses a difficult problem. Only about 1 in 10 individuals who claim to have developed an allergic response to penicillins actually show such a reaction on further exposure. Nevertheless, a history of penicillin allergy cannot be overlooked and a cephalosporin, e.g. oral cefaclor 250 mg 8-hourly or i.v. cefuroxime 1.5 g 6- to 8-hourly, should be given instead of amoxycillin despite a 10% cross-reactivity between the two groups. If the patient has a definite history of severe reaction, then erythromycin and chloramphenicol should be used, depending on the severity of the disease.

General measures

These include care of the mouth and skin. Fluid should be encouraged to avoid dehydration. The patient is normally nursed sitting up or in the most comfortable position. Cough should normally be encouraged but if unproductive and distressing, suppressants such as codeine linctus can be given.

Pleuritic pain may require analgesia but powerful analgesia (e.g. opiates) should be used with care because they cause respiratory depression.

In severe hypoxia oxygen therapy should be given; however, since the hypoxia is often due to a physiological shunt (see p. 558), it may make little difference to the hypoxaemia.

Severe hospital-acquired pneumonias

These should be treated in the same way as severe community-acquired pneumonias. However, as anaerobic organisms may be involved, the treatment should include metronidazole if the clinical state does not improve. Immunosuppressed patients may require very high dose broad-spectrum antibiotics as well as antifungal and antiviral agents.

TUBERCULOSIS (see also p. 37)

Tuberculosis is a disease of great antiquity; for example, it has been found in Egyptian mummies. It remains a major disease of mankind on a world-wide basis. Indeed, until 50 years ago virtually everyone throughout the world was infected at some time in their lives. Fortunately, effective adequate host defence mechanisms and the small number of infecting bacilli meant that most people overcame the primary infection, and it was only when host defences were poor or the infecting dose was large that clinical disease occurred. In Western countries, better nutrition and improved social conditions have meant that the disease is now rarely encountered in the indigenous population; however, it may still be seen in conditions of social deprivation, where immunosuppressive drugs have altered the host defence mechanisms, or in acquired immunodeficiency syndrome (AIDS). Nevertheless, estimates suggest that, world-wide, ten million people develop clinical tuberculosis annually, with three million dying from the disease.

The risk of developing tuberculosis is between 20 and 50 times greater in the Third World than in the Western World.

EPIDEMIOLOGY

In the UK the incidence of tuberculosis in immigrants from the Asian subcontinent and West Indies is 40 and four times as common respectively as in the native white population. This has led to great variation in the frequency of the disease in different areas of the UK.

Mortality from tuberculosis in the UK has fallen dramatically from 150 per 100 000 at the turn of the century to less than 5 per 100 000 in the 1980s. This steady decline was occurring long before the advent of antituberculous treatment, though this did cause an accelerated decrease in death rates. The fall in mortality is particularly marked in the younger age group and is less prominent in older people.

PATHOLOGY

The first infection with *Mycobacterium tuberculosis* is known as primary tuberculosis. It is usually subpleural, often in the mid to upper zones. Within an hour of reaching the lung, tubercle bacilli reach the draining lymph nodes at the hilum of the lung and a few escape into the bloodstream.

The initial reaction comprises exudation and infiltration with neutrophil granulocytes. These are rapidly replaced by macrophages which ingest the bacilli. These interact with T lymphocytes, with the development of cellular immunity which can be demonstrated 3–8 weeks after the initial infection by the development of a positive reaction in the skin to an intradermal injection of protein from tubercle bacilli (tuberculin).

At this stage the classical pathology of tuberculosis can be seen. Granulomatous lesions consist of a central area of necrotic material of a cheesy nature, called caseation, surrounded by epithelioid cells and Langhans' giant cells with multiple nuclei, both cells being derived from the macrophage. Lymphocytes are present and there is a varying degree of fibrosis. Subsequently the caseated areas heal completely and many become calcified. It is now known that at least 20% of these calcified primary lesions contain tubercle bacilli, initially lying dormant but capable of being activated by depression of the host defence system. Reactivation leads to typical post-primary pulmonary tuberculosis with cavitation, usually in the apex or upper zone of the lung. 'Post-primary tuberculosis' refers to all forms of tuberculosis that occur after the first few weeks of the primary infection when immunity to the mycobacterium has developed.

CLINICAL FEATURES AND INVESTIGATION

Primary tuberculosis is symptomless in the great majority of individuals. Occasionally there may be a vague illness, sometimes associated with cough and wheeze. A small transient pleural effusion or erythema nodosum may occasionally occur, both representing allergic manifestations of the infective process.

Enlargement of lymph nodes compressing the bronchi can give rise to collapse of segments or lobes of the lung. Apart from cough and a monophonic wheeze, the individual remains remarkably well and the collapse disappears as the primary complex heals. Occasionally, persistent collapse can give rise to subsequent bronchiectasis, often in the middle lobe (Brock's syndrome).

The manifestations of primary and post-primary tuberculosis are shown in Fig. 12.31, together with the times when they usually occur. Extrapulmonary manifestations are summarized on p. 37. Miliary tuberculosis can occur within 3 years of the primary infection or can occur much later as a manifestation of reactivation or, rarely, reinfection with tubercle bacillus.

Reactivation in the lung or indeed in any extrapulmonary location can occur as immunity wanes, usually with age and chronic ill health (see Fig. 12.31).

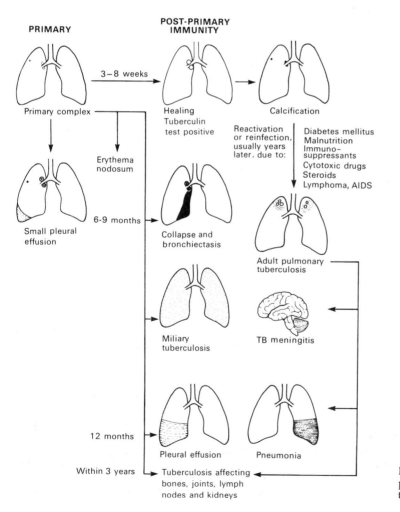

Fig. 12.31 The manifestations of primary and post-primary tuberculosis.

Miliary tuberculosis

This disease is the result of acute diffuse dissemination of tubercule bacilli via the bloodstream. It can be a difficult diagnosis to make, particularly in older people where it is particularly covert. This form of disseminated tuberculosis is universally fatal without treatment.

It may present in an entirely non-specific manner with the gradual onset of vague ill health, loss of weight and then fever. Occasionally the disease presents as tuberculous meningitis. Usually there are no abnormal physical signs in the early stages, though eventually the spleen and liver become enlarged. Choroidal tubercules are seen in the eyes. These lesions are about a quarter of the diameter of the optic disc and are yellowish and slightly shiny and raised in nature, later becoming white in the centre. There may be one or many in each eye.

The chest x-ray may be entirely normal in miliary tuberculosis as the tubercles are not visible until the miliary shadows are 1 or 2 mm in diameter; they have a hard outline. The lesions can increase in size up to 5–10 mm. Sarcoidosis and staphylococcal or mycoplasma pneumonia may mimic the chest x-ray appearance of miliary tuberculosis.

The Mantoux test is positive but may occasionally be negative in people with very severe disease. Transbronchial biopsies may frequently be positive before any abnormality is visible on the chest x-ray. CT scanning may reveal lung parenchymal abnormalities at an earlier stage.

Biopsy and culture of liver and bone marrow may be necessary in patients presenting with a pyrexia of unknown origin (PUO). In the past, a trial of antituberculous therapy was often used in individuals with a PUO. The fever should settle within 2 weeks of starting chemotherapy if it is due to tuberculosis. This approach is still occasionally used in susceptible individuals where a diagnosis cannot be confirmed.

Pulmonary tuberculosis

Typically there is gradual onset of symptoms over weeks or months. Tiredness, malaise, anorexia and loss of weight together with a fever and cough remain the outstanding features of pulmonary tuberculosis. Drenching night sweats are now rather uncommon and are more usually due to anxiety. Sputum in tuberculosis may be mucoid, purulent or blood-stained. Many patients suffer a dull ache in the chest and it is not uncommon for patients to complain of recurrent colds.

A pleural effusion or pneumonia can be the presenting feature of tuberculosis. Physical examination is of little value. Finger clubbing is only present if the disease is advanced and associated with considerable production of purulent sputum. There are often no physical signs in the chest even in the presence of extensive radiological changes, though occasionally persistent crackles may be heard. Physi-

cal signs of an associated effusion, pneumonia or fibrosis may be present.

An abnormal chest x-ray is often found with no symptoms, but the reverse is extremely rare—pulmonary tuberculosis is unlikely in the absence of any radiographic abnormality. The chest x-ray typically shows patchy or nodular shadows in the upper zones, loss of volume, and fibrosis with or without cavitation. Calcification may be present. The x-ray appearances alone may strongly suggest tuberculosis, but every effort must be made to obtain microbiological evidence. The x-rays do not give an indication of the activity of the disease. Very similar chest x-ray appearances occur in histoplasmosis and other fungal infections of the lung, including cryptococcosis, coccidioidomycosis and aspergillosis.

Lymph node tuberculosis manifestations

The patient presents with a tender lump, usually supraclavicularly or in the anterior triangle of the neck. This form of tuberculosis is discussed on p. 38.

DIAGNOSIS

- The sputum is stained with Ziehl–Neelsen (ZN) stain for acid- and alcohol-fast bacilli (AAFB).
- The sputum is cultured on Dover's or Lowenstein–Jensen medium. The bacilli may not be visualized but may grow in 4–8 weeks when cultured. Cultures to determine the sensitivity of the bacillus to antibiotics take a further 3–4 weeks.
- Fibreoptic bronchoscopy with washings from the affected lobes is useful if no sputum is available. This has replaced techniques such as gastric washings.
- Biopsies of the pleura, lymph nodes and solid lesions within the lung (tuberculomas) may be required to make the diagnosis.

PREVENTION

BCG vaccination

Vaccination with BCG (bacille Calmette–Guérin) has been given to schoolchildren in the UK since 1954. BCG is a bovine strain of *Mycobacterium tuberculosis* which lost its virulence after growth in the laboratory for many years. Early trials showed that it decreases the risk of developing tuberculosis by about 70%. With the continuing decrease in the incidence of tuberculosis it is becoming less cost-effective to administer this vaccine, and the procedure is being stopped in certain areas of the UK. However, in other areas with a high immigrant population, the vaccine is being administered 6 weeks after birth rather than at the traditional age of 13 years. This is to prevent the disease from developing in young children where it can progress extremely rapidly and in whom any delay in diagnosis can be fatal. BCG is only given to individuals who are tuberculin–negative; those with positive tests are further screened by a chest x-ray. BCG should be given at a dose of 0.1 ml intradermally to children and adults, but at a dose of 0.05 ml to infants. The practice of BCG vaccination in the UK, thereby producing cellular immunity and a positive tuberculin test, is an important reason why the Mantoux test is of little value in clinical practice for subsequent diagnosis of active disease.

Tuberculin testing

Mainly used for:
- Contact tracing
- BCG vaccination programmes

It is rarely of any value in the diagnosis of TB.

Patients are tested with:
- Purified protein derivative (PPD) of *Mycobacterium tuberculosis* OR
- Old tuberculin (OT)

The test is based on cell-mediated immunity with the development of induration and inflammation at the site of injection due to infiltration with mainly T lymphocytes.

The Mantoux test
This is used for individual patients.
- 0.1 ml of a 1:1000 strength PPD (equivalent to 10 tuberculin units) is injected intradermally.
- The induration is measured (not the erythema) after 72 h. The test is positive if the induration is 10 mm or more in diameter.

The Tine test
This is a simple test used for large-scale screening.
- Four pointed needles mounted on a plastic base are used.
- The tips of the needles are covered with OT and are pressed firmly into the skin once.
- The presence of papules which are confluent with each other after 72 h indicates a positive result.

Contact tracing
Tuberculosis is spread from person to person, and effective tracing of close contacts has helped to limit spread of the disease as well as to identify diseased individuals at an early stage. Screening procedures involve screening all close family members or other individuals who share the same kitchen and bathroom facilities. Occasionally, close contacts at work or school may also be screened. Contacts who are ill should be thoroughly investigated for tuberculosis. If well, a chest x-ray is taken and a tuberculin test performed.

In adults, provided the chest x-ray is negative and the tuberculin test is positive, nothing more need be done. In children, a positive tuberculin test is usually taken as evidence of infection, and treatment is

instituted. If the tuberculin test is negative in children and young adults (<35 years) it is repeated at 6 weeks, and if it remains negative then BCG is administered. If it has become positive (without BCG), this is again taken as an indication of active disease and the individual is treated.

Children under the age of 1 year who have a family member with tuberculosis are given chemoprophylaxis with a daily dose of isoniazid 5–10 mg·kg^{-1} together with immunization with a strain of BCG which is resistant to isoniazid.

In general, much greater emphasis is placed on contact tracing and investigation of those under the age of 35 years and in some immigrant groups (Irish and Asian) in whom the disease is more virulent and prevalent.

TREATMENT

Bed rest does not affect the outcome of the disease. Some patients will require hospitalization for a brief period; these include ill patients, those in whom the diagnosis is uncertain and, most importantly, those individuals in whom it is essential to gain cooperation. The most important factor in the successful treatment of tuberculosis lies in the continual self-administration of drugs for 6–9 months; lack of patient compliance is a major reason why 5% of patients do not respond to treatment. In vitro resistance to one or more of the antituberculous drugs occurs in less than 1% of patients in the UK.

Long-stay in hospital is now only required for persistently uncooperative patients, many of whom are homeless and alcoholics. With modern drugs the time required for treatment can be reduced.

Nine-month regimens
These have now become standard practice, with 9 months of daily administration of rifampicin 600 mg and isoniazid 300 mg. (For those whose body weight is below 55 kg, rifampicin is reduced to 450 mg daily.) These are given as combination tablets and are taken 30 min before breakfast since the absorption of rifampicin is influenced by food. This is supplemented for the first 2 months by pyrazinamide at a dose of 1.5 g (body weight <55 kg) or 2.0 g daily. Recent studies have indicated that pyrazinamide may be of particular value in treating mycobacteria present within macrophages and for this reason it may have a very valuable effect on preventing subsequent relapse.

Six-month regimens
It now seems highly likely that the use of rifampicin, isoniazid and pyrazinamide will lead to regimens that need only to be administered for 6 months. At the present time rifampicin and isoniazid are given for 6 months, with two additional drugs— pyrazinamide and streptomycin (given at a dose of 0.75–1.0 g daily depending on body weight, age and

renal function)—given for the first 2 months. It may well be that streptomycin can be omitted from such treatments, but this still has to be evaluated fully.

Unwanted effects of drug treatment
Rifampicin. This drug induces liver enzymes, which may be transiently elevated in many patients. The drug should only be stopped if the serum bilirubin becomes elevated; which is extremely rare. Thrombocytopenia has been reported. Rifampicin stains body secretions pink and the patients should be warned of the change in colour of their urine, tears and faeces. Induction of liver enzymes means that concomitant drug treatment may be made less effective (see Chapter 14) and oral contraception should not be used.

Isoniazid. This gives rise to very few unwanted effects. At high doses it may produce a peripheral neuritis, but this is extremely rare when the normal dose of 200–300 mg is given daily. Nevertheless, it is customary to prescribe pyridoxine 10 mg daily to prevent this effect. Occasionally, isoniazid gives rise to allergic reactions in the form of a skin rash and fever, and hepatitis occurs in less than 1%.

Ethambutol. This drug can cause a dose-related retrobulbar neuritis which presents with colour blindness for green, reduction in visual acuity and a central scotoma. It usually reverses provided that the drug is stopped when symptoms develop; patients should therefore be warned of its effects. Because of this problem ethambutol is rarely used.

All patients should be seen by an ophthalmologist prior to treatment.

Pyrazinamide. The main unwanted effect of this drug is severe hepatic toxicity, though recent experience suggests that this is much rarer than initially thought using present dosage schedules. Gout due to hyperuricaemia may occur.

Streptomycin. The main unwanted effect of streptomycin is irreversible damage to the vestibular nerve. It is more likely to occur in the elderly and in those with renal impairment. Allergic reactions to streptomycin are more common than to rifampicin, isoniazid and pyrazinamide.

Follow-up
Patients should be seen regularly for the duration of chemotherapy and once more after 6 months since relapse, though very unlikely, usually occurs within this period of time.

Chemoprophylaxis
Patients who have any chest x-ray changes compatible with previous tuberculosis, and who are about to undergo long-term treatment that has an immunosuppressive effect such as renal dialysis or treatment with corticosteroids, should receive chemoprophylaxis with isoniazid 200–300 mg daily.

Non-tuberculous mycobacteria

Mycobacterium kansasii occurs in water and milk, though not in soil. Disease caused by this mycobacteria has mainly been described in Europe and the USA. It rarely causes a relatively benign type of human pulmonary disease, usually in middle-aged males. Men working in dusty jobs (e.g. miners) appear to be especially at risk, as are those who have underlying chronic bronchitis and emphysema.

GRANULOMATOUS LUNG DISEASE

A granuloma is a mass or nodule composed of chronically inflamed tissue formed by the response of the mononuclear phagocyte system (macrophage/histiocyte) to a slowly soluble antigen or irritant. If the foreign substance is inert (e.g. an inhaled dust), the phagocytes turn over slowly; if the substance is toxic or reproducing, the cells turn over faster, producing a granuloma.

A granuloma is characterized by epithelioid multinucleate giant cells, as seen in tuberculosis. Granulomas may be caused by:
- Tuberculosis (see p. 599)
- Fungal and helminthic infections
- Hypersensitivity reactions
- Neoplasms

They are also found in disorders with no known cause, such as sarcoidosis.

Sarcoidosis

Sarcoidosis is a multi-system granulomatous disorder, commonly affecting young adults and usually presenting with bilateral hilar lymphadenopathy, pulmonary infiltration and skin or eye lesions. The diagnosis is often made clinically. It is confirmed when necessary on the histological evidence of widespread, non-caseating, epithelioid granulomas in more than one organ. However, poisoning with beryllium can rarely produce a clinical and histological picture identical to sarcoidosis, though contact with this element is now strictly controlled.

EPIDEMIOLOGY AND AETIOLOGY

Sarcoidosis is a common disease that is often diagnosed by mass x-ray studies. There is great geographical variation. The prevalence in Britain is approximately 19 in 100 000 of the population. It is common in the USA but is uncommon in Japan. The course of the disease is much more severe in American blacks than in whites. There is no relation with any histocompatibility antigen, but cases of sarcoidosis are seen within families, possibly suggesting an environmental factor. Other aetiological factors suggested are an atypical mycobacterium or fungus, the Epstein–Barr virus, pine pollen (because of the increased incidence of sarcoidosis in the southeastern states of the USA) and occupational, genetic, social or other environmental factors (a higher incidence occurs in rural rather than in urban populations); none have been substantiated.

IMMUNOPATHOLOGY

- The typical sarcoid granuloma consists of focal accumulation of epithelioid cells, macrophages and lymphocytes, mainly T cells.
- There is a depressed cell-mediated reactivity to tuberculin and other antigens such as *Candida albicans*.
- There is an overall lymphopenia; circulating T lymphocytes are low but B cells are slightly increased.
- Broncho-alveolar lavage shows a great increase in the number of cells; lymphocytes (particularly T lymphocytes) are greatly increased (see Table 12.5, p. 570).
- The number of alveolar macrophages is increased but they represent a reduced percentage of the total number of cells.
- Transbronchial biopsies show infiltration of the alveolar walls and interstitial spaces with mononuclear cells, mainly T cells, prior to granuloma formation.

It now seems likely that the decrease in circulating T lymphocytes and changes in delayed hypersensitivity responses are the result of sequestration of lymphocytes within the lung. There is no evidence to suggest that patients with sarcoidosis suffer from an overall defect in cellular immunity since the frequency of fungal, viral and bacterial infections is not increased and there is no substantiated evidence of a greater risk of developing malignant neoplasms.

CLINICAL FEATURES

The peak incidence is in the third and fourth decades, with a female preponderance. Sarcoidosis can affect many different organs of the body. The commonest presentation is with respiratory symptoms or abnormalities found on chest x-rays (50%). Fatigue or weight loss occurs in 5%, peripheral lymphadenopathy in 5% and a fever in 4%. A chest x-ray may be negative in up to 20% of non-respiratory cases, though lesions may be detected later.

Bilateral hilar lymphadenopathy is a characteristic feature of sarcoidosis. It is often symptomless and simply detected on a routine chest x-ray. Occasionally, the bilateral hilar lymphadenopathy is associ-

ated with a dull ache in the chest, malaise and a mild fever.

Although the chest x-ray may not show any evidence of infiltration in the lung fields, evidence from CT scanning, transbronchial biopsies and broncho-alveolar lavage indicate that the lung parenchyma is nearly always involved.

The differential diagnosis of the bilateral hilar lymphadenopathy includes:

- Malignant lymphoma—though it is rare for this only to affect the hilar lymph nodes
- Pulmonary tuberculosis—though it is rare for the hilar lymph nodes to be symmetrically enlarged
- Carcinoma of the bronchus with malignant spread to the contralateral hilar lymph nodes—again it is rare for this to give rise to a typical symmetrical picture

In the early stages it may be difficult to distinguish enlarged lymph nodes on the chest x-ray from the pulmonary arteries, and lymph node enlargement is not always symmetrical. It is for these reasons that in the absence of additional erythema nodosum (see below), histological confirmation of the disease process is advisable.

Pulmonary infiltration

This type of sarcoidosis may be progressive and may lead to increasing effort dyspnoea and eventually cor pulmonale and death. The chest x-ray shows a mottling in the mid-zones proceeding to generalized fine nodular shadows. Eventually, widespread pulmonary line shadows develop, reflecting the underlying fibrosis. A honeycomb appearance can occasionally occur. Pulmonary function tests show a typical restrictive lung defect (see below).

It is possible to have a normal chest x-ray with abnormal lung function tests, and conversely, lung infiltration may be present on the x-ray with lung function tests in the normal range.

Extrapulmonary manifestations

Skin and ocular sarcoidosis are the commonest extrapulmonary presentations.

Skin sarcoidosis. This is seen in 10% of cases; apart from erythema nodosum, a chilblain-like lesion known as lupus pernio is seen, as are nodules (see p. 934). Sarcoidosis is the commonest cause of erythema nodosum (see p. 916). The association of bilateral symmetrical hilar lymphadenopathy with erythema nodosum only occurs in sarcoidosis.

Anterior uveitis. This is common and may present with misting of vision, pain and a red eye, but posterior uveitis may simply present as progressive loss of vision. Although ocular sarcoidosis accounts for about 5% of uveitis presenting to ophthalmologists, evidence of asymptomatic uveitis may be found in up to 25% of patients with sarcoidosis.

Conjunctivitis may occur and retinal lesions have been recognized recently.

Keratoconjunctivitis sicca and lacrymal gland enlargement may also occur. Uveoparotid fever is a syndrome of bilateral uveitis and parotid gland enlargement together with occasional development of facial nerve palsy and is sometimes seen with sarcoidosis.

Metabolic. It is rare for sarcoidosis to present with problems of calcium metabolism, though hyper-calcaemia is found in 10% of established cases. Hypercalcaemia and hypercalciuria are important complications since they can lead to the develop-ment of renal calculi and nephrocalcinosis. The cause of the hypercalcaemia has recently been shown to be the high circulating 1, 25-dihydroxy vitamin D_3, 1α-hydroxylation occurring in sarcoid macrophages in the lung in addition to that taking place in the kidney.

The central nervous system. Involvement of the CNS is rare (2%), but can lead to severe neurological disease including epilepsy (see p. 840).

Bone involvement. Arthralgia without erythema nodosum is seen in 5% of cases. Bone cysts are found, particularly in the digits, with associated swelling. In the absence of swelling, routine x-rays of the hands are unnecessary.

Hepatosplenomegaly. Sarcoidosis is a cause of hepato-splenomegaly, though it is rarely of any clinical consequence.

Cardiac involvement. Cardiac involvement is rare (3%). Ventricular dysrhythmias, conduction defects and cardiomyopathy with congestive cardiac failure may be seen.

INVESTIGATION

Transbronchial biopsy is the most useful investiga-tion. Positive results are seen in 90% of cases of pulmonary sarcoidosis with or without x-ray evidence of lung involvement. The test provides positive histological evidence of a granuloma in approximately one-half of patients with clinically extrapulmonary sarcoidosis in whom the chest x-ray is normal.

The Kveim test, which involved an intradermal injection of sarcoid tissue, was regularly used for confirmation of the diagnosis. It should not now be used because of the risk of transmission of infection. It is less sensitive than, less specific than and has been superseded by the transbronchial biopsy.

The tuberculin test is negative in 80% of patients with sarcoidosis; it is of no diagnostic value.

The serum level of angiotensin-converting enzyme (ACE) is two standard deviations above the normal mean value in over 75% of patients with untreated sarcoid. Raised (but lower) levels are also seen in patients with lymphoma, pulmonary tuberculosis, asbestosis and silicosis, rendering the test of no diagnostic value. However, it is a simple test and is of use in assessing the activity of the disease and therefore as a guide to treatment with corticosteroids. Reduction of serum ACE during treatment with corticosteroids has not, however, yet been proven to reflect resolution of the disease.

Lung function tests show a restrictive lung defect with pulmonary infiltration. There is:
- A decrease in total lung capacity
- A decrease in both FEV_1 and FVC
- A decrease in gas transfer

PROGNOSIS

It is now clear that sarcoidosis is a much more severe disease in certain racial groups, particularly Ameri-can blacks, where death rates of up to 10% have been recorded. It is probable that the disease is fatal in less than 1 in 20 individuals in the UK, most often as a result of respiratory failure and cor pulmonale but, rarely, from myocardial sarcoidosis and renal damage.

The chest x-ray provides a guide to prognosis. The disease remits by 2 years in over two-thirds of patients with hilar lymphadenopathy alone, in approximately one-half with hilar lymphadenopathy plus chest x-ray evidence of pulmonary infiltration, but in only one-third of patients with x-ray evidence of infiltration without any demonstrable lymph-adenopathy.

TREATMENT

Both the need to treat and the value of corticosteroid therapy are contested in many aspects of this disease.

Hilar lymphadenopathy on its own with no evidence of chest x-ray involvement of the lungs or decrease in lung function tests does not require treatment. Persisting infiltration on the chest x-ray or abnormal lung function tests are unlikely to improve without corticosteroid treatment. If the disease is not improving spontaneously 6 months after diagnosis, treatment should be started with prednisolone 30 mg for 6 weeks, reducing to alternate day treatment with prednisolone 15 mg for 6–12 months. Although there are no controlled trials which have proved the effi-cacy of such treatment, it is difficult to withhold corticosteroids when there is continuing deteriora-tion of the disease.

Topical or systemic prednisolone should be given for patients suffering from involvement of the eyes or the presence of persistent hypercalcaemia. The erythema nodosum of sarcoidosis will respond rapidly to a short course of prednisolone 5–15 mg for 2 weeks.

Myocardial sarcoidosis and neurological manifestations are also treated with prednisolone, and uveoparotid fever responds rapidly to steroids.

Histiocytosis X

There are three variants of this disease, all characterized by the presence of granulomas consisting predominantly of characteristic histiocytes intermingled with eosinophilic and neutrophilic granulocytes, giant cells and lymphocytes. Fibrosis may occur early, with the development of multiple small cysts producing a honeycomb appearance.

Eosinophilic granuloma
This is the commonest variant in adults. It presents with increasing effort dyspnoea and cough. The chest x-ray shows diffuse bilateral mottling with translucencies with thick walls, and gas transfer is decreased. Recurrent pneumothorax occurs. The granulomas can also be found in bones.

Letterer–Siwe disease
This is usually a fatal disease of infancy which occurs under the age of 3 years. It is a widespread disease with skin lesions, lymphadenopathy, hepatosplenomegaly and bone lesions.

Hand–Schüller–Christian disease
This usually begins under the age of 5 years. It is characterized by defects in bone, exophthalmos and diabetes insipidus. Pulmonary lesions show diffuse nodular shadows with hilar lymphadenopathy simulating sarcoidosis.

Both Hand–Schüller–Christian disease and eosinophilic granuloma may recover spontaneously; survival for 20 years has been reported for both conditions.

Treatment is with corticosteroids and cyclophosphamide, though there is no evidence as yet that this treatment substantially alters the outcome.

Wegener's granulomatosis

This disease of unknown aetiology is characterized by lesions involving the upper respiratory tract, the lungs and the kidneys. Often the disease starts with severe rhinorrhoea with subsequent nasal mucosal ulceration followed by cough, haemoptysis and pleuritic pain. Occasionally there may be involvement of the skin and nervous system. A chest x-ray usually shows single or multiple nodular masses or pneumonic infiltrates with cavitation. The most remarkable radiographic feature is the migratory pattern, with large lesions clearing in one area and new lesions appearing in another.

The typical histological changes are usually best seen in the kidneys, where there is a necrotizing glomerulonephritis.

This disease was once invariably fatal but responds well to treatment with cyclophosphamide 150–200 mg daily. A variant of Wegener's granulomatosis called 'mid-line granuloma' particularly affects the nose and paranasal sinuses and is particularly mutilating; it has a poor prognosis.

RESPIRATORY MANIFESTATIONS OF SYSTEMIC CONNECTIVE TISSUE DISEASE

Rheumatoid disease (see p. 333)

The manifestations of rheumatoid disease of the lung are illustrated in Fig. 12.32.

Pleural adhesions, thickening and effusion are the commonest lesions. The effusion is often unilateral and tends to be chronic. It has a low glucose content, but this can occur in any chronic pleural effusion.

Rheumatoid diffuse fibrosing alveolitis can be considered as a variant of the cryptogenic form of the disease (see p. 610). The clinical features and gross

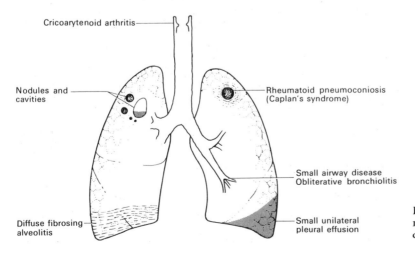

Fig. 12.32 The respiratory manifestations of rheumatoid disease.

Cricoarytenoid arthritis

Nodules and cavities

Rheumatoid pneumoconiosis (Caplan's syndrome)

Small airway disease
Obliterative bronchiolitis

Diffuse fibrosing alveolitis

Small unilateral pleural effusion

appearance are the same but the disease is often more chronic.

Rheumatoid nodules showing the typical histological appearances are rare in the lung. On the chest x-ray these appear as single or multiple nodules ranging in size from a few millimetres to a few centimetres. The nodules frequently cavitate. They usually produce no symptoms but can give rise to a pneumothorax or pleural effusion.

Obliterative disease of the small bronchioles is rare. It is characterized by progressive breathlessness and irreversible airflow limitation. Corticosteroids may prevent progression.

Involvement of the cricoarytenoid joints gives rise to dyspnoea, stridor, hoarseness and occasionally severe obstruction necessitating tracheostomy.

Caplan's syndrome is due to a combination of dust inhalation and the disturbed immunity of rheumatoid arthritis. It occurs particularly in coal worker's pneumoconiosis but it can occur in individuals exposed to other dusts, such as silica and asbestos. Typically the lesions appear as rounded nodules 0.5–5 cm in diameter, though sometimes they become incorporated into large areas of fibrosis that are indistinguishable radiologically from progressive massive fibrosis. There may be little evidence of simple pneumoconiosis prior to the development of the nodule.

These lesions may precede the development of the arthritis. Rheumatoid factor is always present in the serum.

Systemic lupus erythematosus (see p. 340)

The commonest respiratory manifestation of this disease, occurring in up to two-thirds of cases, is the development of pleurisy, with or without an effusion. Effusions are usually small and bilateral. Basal pneumonitis is often present, perhaps as a result of poor movement of the diaphragm, or restriction of chest movements due to pleural pain. Pneumonia also occurs, either due to infection or to the disease process itself. Unlike rheumatoid arthritis, diffuse pulmonary fibrosis is rare.

Systemic sclerosis

Autopsy studies have indicated that there is almost always some evidence of diffuse fibrosis of alveolar walls and obliteration of capillaries and the alveolar space. Severe changes result in nodular then streaky shadowing on the chest x-ray, followed by cystic changes, ending up with a honeycomb lung. Function tests indicate a restrictive lesion and poor gas transfer.

Pneumonia may occur due to inhalation from the dilated oesophagus. Breathlessness may be worsened by restriction of chest wall movement due to thickening and contraction of the skin and trunk.

PULMONARY INFILTRATION WITH EOSINOPHILIA (PIE)

The common types and characteristics of these diseases are shown in Table 12.9. They range from very mild, simple, pulmonary eosinophilias to the usually fatal polyarteritis nodosa.

Simple and prolonged pulmonary eosinophilia

Simple pulmonary eosinophilia is a relatively mild illness with a slight fever and cough and usually lasting for less than 2 weeks. It is probably due to a transient allergic reaction in the alveolus. Many allergens have been implicated, including *Ascaris lumbricoides*, *Ankylostoma braziliense* and *Trichuris trichiura* as well as drugs such as para-aminosalicylic acid, aspirin, penicillin, nitrofurantoin and sulphonamides. Often, no allergen is identified. No treatment is required and the disease is self-limiting. Occasionally, however, the disease becomes more prolonged, with a high fever lasting for over a month. There is usually an eosinophilia in the blood and this condition is called 'prolonged pulmonary eosinophilia'. Similar allergens are thought to be involved, with the addition of *Strongyloides stercoralis*. In both conditions the chest x-ray shows either localized or diffuse opacities. Corticosteroid

Table 12.9 Common types and characteristics of pulmonary infiltration with eosinophilia.

Disease	Symptoms	Blood eosinophils (%)	Multi-system involvement	Duration	Outcome
Simple pulmonary eosinophilia (Löffler's syndrome)	Mild	10	None	<1 month	Good
Prolonged pulmonary eosinophilia	Mild/moderate	>20	None	>1 month	Good
Asthmatic bronchopulmonary eosinophilia	Moderate/severe	5–20	None	Years	Fair
Tropical pulmonary eosinophilia	Moderate/severe	>20	None	Years	Fair
Hyper-eosinophilic syndrome	Severe	>20	Always	Months/years	Poor
Polyarteritis nodosa	Severe	>20	Always	Months/years	Poor/fair

therapy is indicated, with resolution of the disease over the ensuing weeks.

Asthmatic bronchopulmonary eosinophilia

This is characterized by the presence of asthma, transient fleeting shadows on the chest x-ray, and blood or sputum eosinophilia. By far the commonest cause world-wide is allergy to *Aspergillus fumigatus* (see below), though *Candida albicans* may be an allergen in a small number of patients. In many, the appropriate allergen has still to be identified.

Diseases caused by *Aspergillus fumigatus*

The various types of lung disease caused by *Aspergillus fumigatus* are illustrated in Fig. 12.33.

The spores of *Aspergillus fumigatus* (5 μm in

diameter) are readily inhaled and are present in the atmosphere throughout the year, though they are at their highest concentration in the late autumn. They can be grown from the sputum in up to 15% of patients with chronic lung disease in whom they do not produce disease. They are an important cause of extrinsic asthma in atopic individuals.

Allergic bronchopulmonary aspergillosis (Fig. 12.33)
In allergic bronchopulmonary aspergillosis the *Aspergillus* actually grows in the walls of the bronchi and eventually produces proximal bronchiectasis. There are episodes of eosinophilic pneumonia throughout the year, particularly in late autumn and winter. The episodes present with a wheeze, cough, fever and malaise. They are associated with expectoration of firm sputum plugs containing the fungal mycelium, which results in the clearing of the

Fig. 12.33 Diseases caused by *Aspergillus fumigatus*.

pulmonary infiltrates on the chest x-ray. Occasionally the large mucus plugs obliterate the bronchial lumen, causing collapse of the lung.

Repeated episodes of eosinophilic pneumonia left untreated can result in progressive pulmonary fibrosis which is often seen in the upper zones and can give rise to a similar chest x-ray appearance to that produced by tuberculosis.

The peripheral blood eosinophil count is usually raised, and total levels of IgE are extremely high (both that specific to *Aspergillus* and non-specific). Skin prick testing with protein allergens from *Aspergillus fumigatus* gives rise to positive immediate skin tests. Sputum may show eosinophils and mycelia, and precipitating antibodies are usually found in the serum.

Lung function tests show a decrease in lung volumes and gas transfer in more chronic cases, but in all cases evidence of reversible airflow limitation can be demonstrated.

Treatment for this allergic pneumonia is with prednisolone 30 mg daily, which readily causes clearing of the pulmonary infiltrates. Frequent episodes of the disease can be prevented by long-term treatment with prednisolone, but doses as high as 10–15 mg daily are usually required. Moderately severe asthma itself requires continuous treatment with oral corticosteroids. Inhaled corticosteroids do not influence the occurrence of pulmonary infiltrates but are useful for the asthmatic element of the disease.

Aspergilloma (Fig. 12.33)
This is a totally separate disease from allergic bronchopulmonary aspergillosis. It simply represents the growth within previously damaged lung tissue of *Aspergillus fumigatus*, which forms a ball of mycelium within lung cavities. The typical appearance on the chest x-ray is of a round lesion with an air 'halo' above it. The continuing antigenic stimulation gives rise to large quantities of precipitating antibody in the serum. The aspergilloma itself causes little trouble though occasionally massive haemoptysis may occur, requiring resection of the damaged area of lung containing the aspergilloma. Although treatment with antifungal agents such as amphotericin has been tested in both allergic bronchopulmonary aspergillosis and aspergilloma, this has had little success, though it remains the only treatment for invasive aspergillosis.

Tropical pulmonary eosinophilia

This condition presents with cough and wheeze together with fever, lassitude and weight loss. The typical appearance of the chest x-ray is of bilateral hazy mottling which is frequently uniformly distributed in both lung fields. The individual shadows may be as large as 5 mm or may become more confluent, giving the appearance of pneumonia. It is found in many tropical countries, but particularly in the Asian subcontinent, and it now seems fairly certain that the disease represents an allergic reaction to microfilaria, probably from *Wuchereria bancrofti*.

The disease is characterized by a very high eosinophil count in peripheral blood. The filarial complement fixation test is positive in almost every case. The treatment of choice is diethylcarbamazine at a dose of 5 mg·kg^{-1} body weight for 10–14 days; this usually produces a good response.

The hyper-eosinophilic syndrome

This disease is characterized by eosinophilic infiltration in various organs, sometimes associated with an eosinophilic arteritis. The heart muscle is particularly involved, but pulmonary involvement in the form of pleural effusion or interstitial lung disease occurs in about 40% of cases. Typical features are fever, weight loss, recurrent abdominal pain, persistent non-productive cough and congestive cardiac failure. Corticosteroid treatment may be of value in some cases.

Polyarteritis nodosa (see p. 345)

This is a rare disease characterized by foci of necrotizing arteritis that sooner or later affect many organs in the body. The lungs are rarely involved, except in the variant of polyarteritis nodosa known as the Churg–Strauss syndrome (see below).

The upper respiratory tract may be involved, with nasal obstruction and rhinorrhoea. The chest x-ray may show consolidation which is ill-defined and transgresses anatomical boundaries. These shadows may disappear and reappear over periods of 2–12 weeks, and some may represent intra-alveolar haemorrhage or pulmonary infarcts. The overall 5-year survival for polyarteritis nodosa is 80% with corticosteroids and immunosuppressive therapy.

Allergic granulomatosis (Churg–Strauss syndrome)
This is a more limited form of generalized polyarteritis nodosa which produces asthma. It is characterized by a high blood eosinophil count, vasculitis of small arteries and veins, and extravascular granulomas. The lungs, peripheral nerves and skin are most often affected and renal failure is much less common than in generalized polyarteritis nodosa. Transient patchy pneumonia-like shadows may occur as in polyarteritis nodosa, but sometimes these can be massive and bilateral. Skin lesions include tender subcutaneous nodules as well as petechial or purpuric lesions. The asthma in this disease responds well to corticosteroids.

GOODPASTURE'S SYNDROME AND IDIOPATHIC PULMONARY HAEMOSIDEROSIS

Goodpasture's syndrome (see also p. 386)

This disease, like polyarteritis nodosa, affects the lung and the kidneys. The disease often starts with an upper respiratory tract infection followed by cough and intermittent haemoptysis, tiredness and eventually anaemia, though massive bleeding may occur. The chest x-ray shows transient blotchy shadows due to intrapulmonary haemorrhage. These features usually precede the development of an acute glomerulonephritis by several weeks or months. The course of the disease is variable; some spontaneously improve whilst others proceed to renal failure. The disease usually occurs in individuals over 16 years of age. It is thought to be due to a type II cytotoxic hypersensitivity reaction, the hypothesis being that there may be a shared antigen between a virus and the basement membrane of both kidney and lung. Antiglomerular basement membrane antibodies are found in the serum. An association with influenza A2 virus has been reported. Treatment is with corticosteroids, but plasmapheresis to remove the antibodies has led to dramatic improvement in some cases.

Idiopathic pulmonary haemosiderosis

This is a similar disease to Goodpasture's syndrome, but the kidneys are less frequently involved. Most cases occur in children under 7 years of age. Characteristically, haemosiderin-containing macrophages are found in the sputum. The child develops a chronic cough and anaemia and the chest x-ray shows diffuse shadows due to intrapulmonary bleeding, and eventually miliary nodulation. There is an association with a sensitivity to cows' milk, and an appropriate diet is usually tried. The prognosis in general is poor and treatment with corticosteroids or azathioprine is usually given.

PULMONARY FIBROSIS AND HONEYCOMB LUNG

Pulmonary fibrosis is the end result of many diseases of the respiratory tract. It may be:
- Localized, e.g. following unresolved pneumonia
- Bilateral, e.g. in tuberculosis
- Widespread, e.g. in cryptogenic fibrosing alveolitis, due to drugs (busulphan, bleomycin and cyclophosphamide) or in industrial lung disease

Sometimes with widespread fibrosis a typical radiological appearance is seen which is known as honeycomb lung. This refers to the presence, often diffusely in both lungs, of cysts between 0.5 and 2 cm in

Table 12.10 The main causes of honeycomb lung.

Localized
Systemic sclerosis
Sarcoidosis
Tuberculosis
Asbestosis
Berylliosis
Diffuse
Cryptogenic fibrosing alveolitis
Rheumatoid lung
Histiocytosis X
Tuberose sclerosis
Neurofibromatosis

diameter which are thick-walled and do not fill with opaque material on bronchography. The cystic air spaces probably represent dilated and thickened terminal and respiratory bronchioles. The main causes are shown in Table 12.10.

Cryptogenic fibrosing alveolitis (CFA)

This relatively rare disorder of unknown aetiology causes diffuse fibrosis throughout the lung fields, usually in late middle age. The cardinal features are progressive breathlessness and cyanosis, which eventually lead to respiratory failure, pulmonary hypertension and cor pulmonale. Gross clubbing occurs in two-thirds of cases and bilateral fine end-inspiratory crackles are heard on auscultation. Rarely, an acute form known as the Hamman–Rich syndrome occurs. The chest x-ray appearance initially is of ground-glass appearance, progressing to obvious small nodular shadows with streaky fibrosis and finally a honeycomb lung.

A number of autoimmune diseases are seen in association with this condition. For example, chronic active hepatitis occurs in 5–10% of cases.

Similar lung changes are also seen in rheumatoid arthritis, systemic sclerosis and Sjögren's syndrome, often associated with Raynaud's phenomenon.

CFA has also been reported in association with coeliac disease, ulcerative colitis and renal tubular acidosis.

PATHOGENESIS

Histologically there are two main features:
- Cellular infiltration and thickening and fibrosis of the alveolar walls
- Increased cells within the alveolar space (mainly shed type II pneumocytes and macrophages)

The pathogenesis of damage and fibrosis is complex and several factors are involved (see Fig. 12.34).

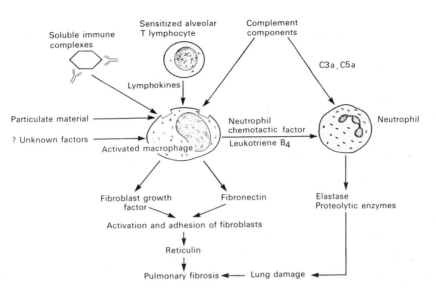

Fig. 12.34 Possible mechanisms involved in the activation of a macrophage and leading to the production of fibrosis.

INVESTIGATION

- Respiratory function tests show a restrictive ventilatory defect—the lung volumes are reduced, the FEV_1 to FVC ratio is normal to high (with both values being reduced) and gas transfer is reduced.
- Blood gases show an arterial hypoxaemia.
- The ESR is high.
- Broncho-alveolar lavage (Table 12.5, p. 570) shows increased numbers of cells (particularly neutrophils).
- Antinuclear factor is positive in one-third of patients.
- Rheumatoid factor is positive in 50% of patients.
- In younger patients histological confirmation may be necessary, requiring a transbronchial lung biopsy or even an open lung biopsy to obtain a larger specimen.

DIFFERENTIAL DIAGNOSIS

The diagnosis of CFA can be made in an elderly person presenting with the above signs and laboratory test results. In younger people the differential diagnosis includes extrinsic allergic alveolitis, bronchiectasis, chronic left heart failure, sarcoidosis, industrial lung disease and lymphangitis carcinomatosa.

PROGNOSIS AND TREATMENT

The median survival time for patients with CFA is approximately 5 years. Treatment with large doses of prednisolone (30 mg daily) is usually prescribed for disabling disease, though its benefit has still to be proved by appropriate controlled trials. Azathioprine or cyclophosphamide may also be used. Supportive treatment includes oxygen therapy.

Extrinsic allergic bronchiolar alveolitis

In this disease there is a widespread diffuse inflammatory reaction in all the small airways of the lung and alveoli. It is due to the inhalation of a number of different antigens, as illustrated in Table 12.11. By far the commonest of these diseases world-wide is

Table 12.11 Extrinsic allergic bronchiolar alveolitis.

Disease	Situation	Antigens
Farmer's lung	Forking mouldy hay or any other mouldy vegetable material	Thermophilic actinomycetes and *Micropolyspora faeni*
Bird fancier's lung	Handling pigeons, cleaning lofts or budgerigar cages	Proteins present in the 'bloom' on the feathers and in excreta
Maltworker's lung	Turning germinating barley	*Aspergillus clavatus*
Humidifier fever	Contaminated humidifying systems in air conditioners or humidifiers in factories (especially printing works)	Possibly a variety of bacteria or amoebae (e.g. *Naegleria gruberi*)

Farmer's lung, which affects up to 1 in 10 of the farming community in poor, wet, areas around the world. In Western countries the incidence is almost certainly declining as more mechanized farming procedures are introduced.

PATHOGENESIS

Histologically there is an initial infiltration of the small airways and alveolar walls with neutrophils followed by lymphocytes and macrophages, leading to the development of non-caseating granulomas. These comprise multinucleated giant cells, occasionally containing the inhaled antigenic material. The major allergic response to the inhaled antigens is through cellular immunity, though there is evidence in some cases of an additional immediate hypersensitivity reaction involving specific IgE antibody and the deposition of immune complexes. All these mechanisms can attract and activate alveolar macrophages so that continued antigenic exposure results in the development of pulmonary fibrosis.

CLINICAL FEATURES

The typical history is that of the onset of fever, malaise, cough and shortness of breath several hours after exposure to the causative antigen. For example, a farmer forking hay in the morning may only notice symptoms during the late afternoon and evening which resolve by the following morning. On examination the patient may have a fever, tachypnoea and coarse end-inspiratory crackles and wheezes throughout the chest. Cyanosis may be severe even at rest. Continuing exposure leads to a chronic illness characterized by severe weight loss, effort dyspnoea and cough, and the features of fibrosing alveolitis (see p. 610).

The chest x-ray shows fluffy nodular shadowing with the subsequent development of streaky shadows and, in very advanced cases, honeycomb lung.

INVESTIGATION

- The polymorphonuclear leucocyte count is raised in acute cases.
- Precipitating antibodies are present in the serum. A quarter of pigeon fanciers have precipitating antibody against pigeon protein and droppings in their serum but only a small proportion have lung disease. Precipitating antibodies are evidence of *exposure*, not disease.
- Lung function tests show a restrictive ventilatory defect with a decrease in gas transfer.
- Broncho-alveolar lavage (Table 12.5, p. 570) shows increased cells (lymphocytes and granulocytes).

DIFFERENTIAL DIAGNOSIS

Although an extrinsic allergic bronchiolar alveolitis due to inhalation of the spores of *Micropolyspora faeni* is common amongst farmers, it is probably more common for these individuals to suffer from asthma related to inhalation of antigens from a variety of mites which infest stored grain and other vegetable material. The common ones are *Glyciphagus domesticus*, *G. destructor* and *Acarus Siro*. Symptoms of asthma resulting from inhalation of these allergens are often mistaken for farmer's lung.

Pigeon fancier's lung is quite common, but allergy from budgerigars is very rare.

MANAGEMENT

Prevention is the aim. This can be achieved by change in work practice, with the use of silage for animal fodder and the drier storage of hay and grain. It is difficult to control pigeon fancier's lung since individuals remain addicted to their hobby.

Prednisolone, initially in large doses of 30–60 mg daily, is necessary to cause regression of the early stages of the disease. Established fibrosis will not resolve and in some patients the disease may progress inexorably to respiratory failure in spite of intensive therapy. Farmer's lung is a recognized occupational disease in the UK and sufferers are entitled to compensation depending on their degree of disability.

Humidifier fever

Humidifier fever may present with the typical features of extrinsic allergic bronchiolar alveolitis without any radiographic changes. This disease has occurred in outbreaks in factories in the UK, particularly in printing works. In North America it is more commonly found in office blocks with contaminated air conditioning systems. The cause remains unknown but probably involves several bacteria or even amoebae.

Humidifier fever can be prevented by sterilization of the recirculating water used in the very large humidifying plants in industry.

Drug-induced lung disease

Drugs may produce a wide variety of disorders of the respiratory tract. Pulmonary infiltrates with fibrosis may result from the use of a number of cytotoxic drugs used in the treatment of cancer. The commonest cause of these reactions is bleomycin. The pulmonary damage is dose related, occurring when the total dosage is greater than 450 mg, but will regress in some cases if the drug is stopped. The most sensitive test is a decrease in gas transfer and therefore gas transfer should be measured

Table 12.12 Drug-induced respiratory disease.

Disease	Drugs
Asthma ± rhinitis	Penicillins
	Sulphonamides
	Cephalosporins
	Aspirin
	NSAIDs
	Tartrazine
	Iodine-containing contrast media
	Amiodarone
	Non-selective beta-adrenoceptor-blocking drugs (e.g. propranolol)
	Suxamethonium
	Thiopentone
Pulmonary infiltrates ± fibrosis	Bleomycin
	Nitrosoureas, e.g. carmustine
	Busulphan
	Cyclophosphamide
	Procarbazine
	Chlorambucil
	Methotrexate
	Nitrofurantoin
	Paraquat
Opportunistic pulmonary infections	Corticosteroids
	Azathioprine
	Other cytotoxic drugs
Respiratory depression	Sedatives
	Opiates
SLE-like syndrome including pulmonary infiltrates, effusions and fibrosis	Hydralazine
	Procainamide
	Isoniazid
	Para-aminosalicylic acid

repeatedly during treatment with the drug. The use of corticosteroids may help resolution.

Some of the most important drugs affecting the respiratory tract are shown in Table 12.12, together with the types of reaction they produce. The list is not exhaustive; for example, over 20 different drugs are known to produce a systemic lupus erythematosus-like syndrome, sometimes complicated by pulmonary infiltrates and fibrosis. Paraquat ingestion (see p. 667) can cause severe pulmonary oedema and death, and fibrosis develops in many of those who survive.

RADIATION DAMAGE

Radiation to the lung during radiotherapy can cause a radiation pneumonitis. Patients complain of breathlessness and a dry cough. Radiation pneumonia results in a restrictive lung defect. Corticosteroids should be given in the acute stage.

OCCUPATIONAL LUNG DISEASE

Exposure to dusts, gases, vapours and fumes at work can lead to the development of the following types of lung disease:
- Acute bronchitis and even pulmonary oedema, from irritants such as sulphur dioxide, chlorine, ammonia or the oxides of nitrogen
- Pulmonary fibrosis due to mineral dust
- Occupational asthma (see Table 12.7)
- Extrinsic allergic bronchiolar alveolitis (see Table 12.11)
- Bronchial carcinoma due to industrial agents (e.g. asbestos, polycyclic hydrocarbons, radon in mines)

The degree of fibrosis that follows inhalation of mineral dust varies. Whilst iron (siderosis), barium (baritosis) and tin (stannosis) lead to dramatic dense nodular shadowing on the chest x-ray, their effect on lung function and symptoms is minimal. Exposure to silica or asbestos, on the other hand, leads to extensive fibrosis and disability. Coal dust has an intermediate fibrogenic effect but accounts for 90% of all compensated industrial lung diseases. The term pneumoconiosis means the accumulation of dust in the lungs and the reaction of the tissue to its presence. The term is not wide enough to encompass all occupational lung disease and is now generally used in relation to coal dust and its effects on the lung.

Coal worker's pneumoconiosis

Improved conditions in the coal industry have led to a considerable reduction in the number of cases of pneumoconiosis to about 2 per 1000 wage earners. The disease is caused by dust particles of approximately 2–5 μm in diameter which are retained in the small airways and alveoli of the lung. The incidence of the disease is related to total dust exposure, which is highest at the coal face, particularly if ventilation and dust suppression is poor. Two very different syndromes result from the inhalation of coal.

Simple pneumoconiosis
This simply reflects the deposition of coal dust in the lung. It produces a fine micronodular shadow on the chest x-ray and is by far the commonest type of pneumoconiosis. It is graded on the chest x-ray appearance according to standards set by the International Labour Office (see below). Considerable dispute remains about the effects of simple pneumoconiosis on respiratory function and symptoms, many arguing that the development of the latter is largely due to chronic bronchitis and emphysema, commonly related to cigarette smoking.

Categories of simple pneumoconiosis are as follows:
1 Small round opacities are definitely present but are few in number.

2 Small round opacities are numerous but normal lung markings are still visible.
3 Small round opacities are very numerous and normal lung markings are partly or totally obscured.

The importance of simple pneumoconiosis is that it may lead to the development of progressive massive fibrosis (see below). This virtually never occurs on a background of category 1 simple pneumoconiosis but occurs in 30% of those with category 3. Usually category 2 simple pneumoconiosis, which carries a 7% risk of developing PMF, must be present before benefit may be awarded for disability.

Progressive massive fibrosis (PMF)
The lesions in this disease are round fibrotic masses several centimetres in diameter, almost invariably in the upper lobes and sometimes having necrotic central cavities. The pathogenesis of PMF is still not understood, though it now seems clear that some fibrogenic promoting factor is present in individuals developing the disease. This was thought to be *Mycobacterium tuberculosis*, but is now thought to be immune complexes, analogous to the development of large fibrotic nodules in coal miners with rheumatoid arthritis (Caplan's syndrome). The development of both rheumatoid factor and antinuclear factor in the serum of patients with PMF is common, as it is in those suffering from asbestosis and silicosis. Pathologically there is apical destruction and disruption of the lung, resulting in emphysema and airway damage. Lung function tests show a mixed restrictive and obstructive ventilatory defect with loss of lung volume, irreversible airflow limitation and reduced gas transfer.

The patient with PMF suffers considerable effort dyspnoea, usually with a cough. The sputum can be black. The disease can progress (or even develop) after exposure to coal dust has ceased. Eventually respiratory failure may intervene.

Silicosis
This disease is now relatively uncommon though it may still be encountered in workers in foundries where sand used in moulds has to be removed from the metal casts (fettling), in sand blasting, and amongst stone masons and pottery and ceramic workers.

Silicosis is caused by the inhalation of silica (silicon dioxide). This dust is highly fibrogenic. For example, a coal miner can remain healthy with 30 g of coal dust in his lungs, but would be dead if he had inhaled 3 g of silica. Silica seems particularly toxic to alveolar macrophages and readily initiates the fibrogenic mechanism (see Fig. 12.34). The chest x-ray appearances and clinical features of the disease are similar to PMF. The chest x-ray appearance is distinctive: thin streaks of calcification are seen around the hilar lymph nodes ('eggshell' calcification).

Asbestosis (Table 12.13)

Asbestos is a mixture of silicates of iron, magnesium, nickel, cadmium and aluminium, and has the unique property of occurring naturally as a fibre. It pos-

Table 12.13 The effects of asbestos on the lung.

	Exposure	Chest x-ray	Lung function	Symptoms	Outcome
Asbestos bodies	Light	Normal	Normal	None	Evidence of asbestos exposure only
Pleural plaques	Light	Pleural thickening and calcification (also in diaphragmatic pleura)	Mild restriction	Rare, occasional mild effort dyspnoea	No other sequelae
Mesothelioma	Light (20–40 year interval from light exposure to disease)	Pleural effusion, usually unilateral	Restrictive ventilatory defect	Pleuritic pain, increasing dyspnoea	Median survival 2 years
Asbestosis	Heavy (5–20 year interval from exposure to disease)	Diffuse bilateral streaky shadows, honeycomb lung	Severe restrictive ventilatory defect and reduced gas transfer	Progressive dyspnoea	Poor, progression in some cases after exposure ceases
Asbestosis and carcinoma of the bronchus		The features of asbestosis plus those of bronchial carcinoma			Invariably fatal

sesses remarkable resistant properties to heat, acid and alkali, hence its widespread use. Asbestos is mined in southern Africa, Canada and the USSR. World production is still five million tons, of which 90% is chrysotile, 6% crocidolite and 4% amosite in type.

Chrysotile or white asbestos is the softest asbestos fibre. Each fibre is often as long as 2 cm but only a few micrometres thick. It is less fibrogenic than crocidolite.

Crocidolite (blue asbestos) is particularly resistant to chemical destruction. It exists in straight fibres up to 50 μm in length and 1–2 μm in width. It is now known that this type of asbestos is by far the most important in the development of all types of asbestosis and particularly of mesothelioma. This may be due to the fact that it is readily trapped in the lung. Its long, thin shape means that it can be inhaled, but subsequent rotation against the long axis of the smaller airways, particularly in turbulent airflow during expiration, causes the fibres to impact. Crocidolite is also particularly resistant to macrophage and neutrophil enzymic destruction. Exposure to asbestos occurred particularly in naval shipbuilding yards and in power stations, but its ubiquitous use meant that light exposure was common. Up to 50% of urban dwellers had evidence of asbestos bodies (asbestos fibre covered in protein secretions) in their lungs at post mortem. New regulations in the UK prevent the use of crocidolite and severely restrict the use of chrysotile, and enforce careful dust control measures. These changes should eventually abolish the problem.

There is an important synergistic relationship between asbestosis and cigarette smoking and the development of bronchial carcinoma, usually adenocarcinoma; the risk is increased fivefold. There is also an increased risk in non-smokers and it may also be present in workers exposed to asbestos who do not have clinically recognized asbestosis. It is important to remember that workers will continue to be exposed to blue asbestos in the course of demolition or in the replacement of insulation, and that there is a considerable time lag between exposure and development of the disease, particularly mesothelioma (20–40 years). Asbestos-related diseases are eligible for compensation under the Industrial Injuries Act, but they account for only one-quarter of the number of cases of compensation compared with coal worker's pneumoconiosis.

Byssinosis

This disease occurs world-wide but is declining rapidly in areas where the numbers of people employed in cotton mills are falling. In the UK the disease is confined to areas of Lancashire and Northern Ireland. The symptoms start on the first day back at work after a break (Monday sickness) with improvement as the week progresses. Tightness in the chest, cough and breathlessness occur within the first hour in dusty areas of the mill, particularly in the blowing and carding rooms where raw cotton is cleaned and the fibres straightened.

The exact nature of the disease and its aetiology remain disputed. Two important features are that pure cotton does *not* cause the disease, and that cotton dust has some effect on airflow limitation in all those exposed. Individuals with asthma are particularly badly affected and byssinosis may be classified as a form of occupational asthma. The most likely aetiology is endotoxins from bacteria present in the raw cotton causing constriction of the airways of the lung. There are no changes on the chest x-ray and there is considerable dispute as to whether the progressive airflow limitation seen in some patients with the disease is due to the cotton dust or to other effects such as cigarette smoking or co-existent asthma.

Berylliosis

Beryllium–copper alloy has a high tensile strength and is resistant to metal fatigue, high temperature and corrosion. It is used in the aerospace industry, in atomic reactors and in many electrical devices.

Although beryllium is inhaled into the lungs, it causes a systemic poisoning which gives rise to a clinical picture similar to sarcoidosis. The major chronic problem is that of progressive dyspnoea with pulmonary fibrosis. However, strict control of levels in the working atmosphere have made the disease a rarity.

Tumours of the lung

Bronchial carcinoma accounts for 95% of all primary tumours of the lung. Alveolar cell carcinoma accounts for 2% of lung tumours, and other less malignant or benign tumours account for the remaining 3%.

Benign tumours

Pulmonary hamartoma
This is the most common benign tumour of the lung and is usually seen as a very well-defined round lesion 1–2 cm in diameter in the periphery of the lung. Growth is extremely slow, but the tumour may reach several centimetres diameter. Rarely, it arises from a major bronchus and causes obstruction.

Bronchial carcinoid
This rare tumour resembles intestinal carcinoid tumour and is locally invasive, eventually spreading to mediastinal lymph nodes and finally to distant organs. It is a highly vascular tumour that projects

into the lumen of a major bronchus causing recurrent haemoptysis. It grows slowly and eventually blocks the bronchus, leading to lobar collapse. Rarely, it gives rise to the carcinoid syndrome.

Cylindroma, chondroma and lipoma
These are extremely rare tumours which may grow in the bronchus or trachea, causing obstruction.

DIAGNOSIS AND TREATMENT

These tumours are diagnosed in the same way as bronchial carcinoma (see p. 618). Treatment is surgical and should not be delayed when collapse of a lobe is imminent or when obstruction is increasing.

Lung cysts

These may be congenital, bronchogenic cysts, or may result from a sequestrated pulmonary segment. Hydatid disease causes fluid-filled cysts. Thin-walled cysts are due to lung abscesses, which are particularly found in staphylococcal pneumonia, tuberculous cavities, septic pulmonary infarction, primary bronchogenic carcinoma, cavitating metastatic neoplasm, or paragonimiasis caused by the lung fluke *Paragonimus westermani*.

MALIGNANT TUMOURS

Bronchial carcinoma

This is the most common malignant tumour in the Western World and is now the third most common cause of death in the UK after heart disease and pneumonia. Mortality rates world-wide are highest in Scotland, closely followed by England and Wales. In the UK, 35 000 people die each year from bronchial carcinoma, with a male to female ratio of 3.5 : 1. Although the rising mortality from this disease has levelled off in men, it continues to rise in women, accounting for 1 in 8 of all deaths from malignant disease in women, second only to carcinoma of the breast.

The strength of the association between cigarette smoking and bronchial carcinoma totally overshadows any other aetiological factors, but there is a higher incidence of bronchial carcinoma in urban compared with rural areas, even when allowance is made for cigarette smoking. Occupational factors include exposure to asbestos, and an association is also claimed for workers in contact with arsenic, chromium, iron oxide, petroleum products and oils, coal tar, products of coal combustion, and radiation. Tumours associated with occupational factors are mostly adenocarcinomas and appear to be less related to cigarette smoking.

Cell types
Bronchial carcinoma has now been divided into small cell carcinoma and non-small cell carcinoma, a division based on the characteristics of the disease and its response to treatment. Studies of mean doubling times of carcinomas indicate that development from the initial malignant change to presentation takes many years; for adenocarcinoma it takes approximately 15 years, for squamous carcinoma 8 years, and for small cell carcinoma 3 years.

Non-small cell carcinoma. The commonest carcinoma in this group is the *squamous* or *epidermoid carcinoma*, accounting for approximately 40% of all carcinomas. It occasionally cavitates, and widespread metastases occur relatively late.

Large cell carcinoma represents a less well-differentiated tumour which metastasizes early. It accounts for 25% of all tumours.

Adenocarcinoma arises peripherally from mucous glands in the small bronchi and often produces a subpleural mass. Invasion of the pleura and the mediastinal lymph nodes is common, as are metastases in the brain and bones. Adenocarcinoma accounts for approximately 10% of all bronchial carcinomas and frequently arises in or around scar tissue. It is the commonest bronchial carcinoma associated with asbestosis and is proportionally more common in non-smokers, in women, in the elderly, and in the Far East.

Alveolar cell carcinoma (bronchiolar carcinoma) accounts for only 1–2% of lung tumours and occurs either as a peripheral solitary nodule or as diffuse nodular lesions of multicentric origin. Occasionally this tumour is associated with expectoration of very large volumes of mucoid sputum.

Small cell carcinoma. This tumour, often called oat cell carcinoma, accounts for 20–30% of all lung cancers. It arises from endocrine cells (Kulchitsky cells). These cells are members of the APUD (amine precursors and uptake decarboxylation) system, which explains why many polypeptide hormones are secreted by these tumours. Small cell carcinoma is now considered to be a systemic disease. Although the tumour is rapidly growing and highly malignant, it is the only one of the bronchial carcinomas that responds to chemotherapy.

CLINICAL FEATURES

The frequency of the common symptoms of lung cancer on presentation is shown in Table 12.14. Chest pain and discomfort are often described as fullness and pressure in the chest. Sometimes the pain may be pleuritic due to invasion of the pleura or ribs.

Commonly there are no abnormal physical signs. Enlarged supraclavicular lymph nodes are frequently found with small cell carcinoma. There

Table 12.14 The frequency of the common presenting symptoms of bronchial carcinoma.

Symptom	Frequency
Cough	42%
Chest pain	22%
Cough and pain	15%
Coughing blood	7%
Chest infection, Malaise, Weight loss, Shortness of breath, Hoarseness, Distant spread, No symptoms	<5% each

may be signs of a pleural effusion or of lobar collapse. Signs of an unresolved pneumonia or of associated underlying disease (e.g. diffuse pulmonary fibrosis in asbestosis) may be present.

Direct spread

The tumour may directly involve the pleura and ribs. Carcinoma in the apex of the lung can erode the ribs and involve the lower part of the bronchial plexus (C8, T1 and T2), causing severe pain in the shoulder and down the inner surface of the arm (Pancoast's tumour). The sympathetic ganglion may also be involved, producing Horner's syndrome (see p. 796). Further extension may involve the recurrent laryngeal nerve as it passes down the aortic arch, causing unilateral vocal cord paresis with hoarseness and a bovine cough and rarely the tumour may cause spinal cord compression.

Bronchial carcinoma can also directly invade the phrenic nerve, causing paralysis of the diaphragm. It can involve the oesophagus, producing progressive dysphagia, and the pericardium, producing pericardial effusion and malignant dysrhythmias. It can also involve the superior vena cava, producing superior vena caval obstruction leading to early morning headache, facial congestion and oedema involving the upper limbs; the jugular veins are

Table 12.15 Non-metastatic extrapulmonary manifestations of bronchial carcinoma (percentage of all cases).

Metabolic (universal at some stage)
Loss of weight
Lassitude
Anorexia

Endocrine (10%)
Ectopic adrenocorticotrophin syndrome
Syndrome of inappropriate secretion of antidiuretic hormone (SIADH)   } Usually small cell carcinoma
Hypercalcaemia (usually squamous cell carcinoma)
Rarer—hypoglycaemia, thyrotoxicosis, gynaecomastia

Neurological (2–16%)
Encephalopathies—including subacute cerebellar degeneration
Myelopathies—motor neurone disease
Neuropathies—peripheral sensory motor neuropathy
Muscular disorders—polymyopathy, myasthenic syndrome

Vascular and haematological (rare)
Thrombophlebitis migrans
Non-bacterial thrombotic endocarditis
Microcytic and normocytic anaemia
Disseminated intravascular coagulopathy
Thrombotic thrombocytopenic purpura
Haemolytic anaemia

Skeletal
Clubbing (30%)
Hypertrophic osteoarthropathy (± gynaecomastia) (3%)

Cutaneous (rare)
Dermatomyositis
Acanthosis nigricans
Herpes zoster

distended, as are the veins on the chest that form a collateral circulation with veins arising from the abdomen.

Metastatic complications

Bony metastases are common, giving rise to severe pain and pathological fractures. There is frequent involvement of the liver. Secondary deposits in the brain present as a change in personality, epilepsy or a focal neurological lesion. Carcinoma of the bronchus is a cause of secondary deposits in the adrenal gland.

Non-metastatic extrapulmonary manifestations

Although approximately 10% of small cell tumours are thought to produce ectopic hormones at some stage, clinically important extrapulmonary manifestations are relatively rare apart from finger clubbing (Table 12.15).

Hypertrophic pulmonary osteoarthropathy (HPOA) (see also p. 355) occurs in approximately 3% of all bronchial carcinomas, particularly epidermoid (squamous) cell carcinomas and adenocarcinomas. Symptoms include joint stiffness and severe pain in the wrists and ankles, sometimes associated with gynaecomastia. X-rays show the characteristic proliferative periostitis at the distal ends of long bones, which have an onion skin appearance. HPOA is invariably associated with clubbing of the fingers. It may regress after resection of the lung tumour or as a result of vagotomy at thoracotomy.

INVESTIGATION

Chest x-ray

This is the most valuable screening test for bronchial carcinoma. It is a relatively insensitive test, however, since the tumour mass needs to be between 1 and 2 cm in size to be reliably recognized. CT scanning can identify smaller tumour masses, but is at present too time-consuming and expensive to replace the chest x-ray.

About one-half of all bronchial carcinomas arise centrally, and the other half peripherally (particularly adenocarcinomas). At the time of clinical presentation the chest x-ray will demonstrate over 90% of carcinomas. A small proportion arise within the main bronchus or trachea or else present with metastatic or non-metastatic complications but with no detectable mass on the chest x-ray.

Bronchial carcinoma can appear as round shadows on a chest x-ray (see p. 565). Characteristically the edge of the tumour has a fluffy or spiked appearance, though sometimes it may be entirely smooth with cavitation, particularly when the tumour is epidermoid in type. Carcinoma can also cause collapse of the lung.

Carcinoma causing partial obstruction of a bronchus interrupts the mucociliary escalator, and bacteria are retained within the affected lobe. This gives rise to the so-called secondary pneumonia that is commonly seen on a chest x-ray of a patient presenting with bronchial carcinoma.

The hilar lymph nodes on the side of the tumour are frequently involved in carcinoma of the lung. A large pleural effusion may also be present.

Carcinoma can spread through the lymphatic channels of the lung to give rise to lymphangitis carcinomatosa; this is usually unilateral and associated with striking dyspnoea. The chest x-ray shows streaky shadowing throughout the lung. This appearance may be seen in both lungs, particularly when it is due to metastatic spread, usually from tumours below the diaphragm (the stomach and colon) and from the breast.

Computed tomography

CT is particularly useful for identifying pathological changes in the mediastinum (e.g. enlarged lymph nodes, local spread of the tumour) and for identifying secondary spread of carcinoma to the opposite lung by detecting masses too small to be seen on the chest x-ray. For this reason CT scans should be performed on all patients prior to surgery for removal of a bronchial carcinoma.

Fibreoptic bronchoscopy (see p. 569)

This technique is used to obtain cytological specimens from peripheral lesions as well as to obtain biopsy evidence of any tumours seen. If the carcinoma involves the first 5 cm of the left main bronchus or 2 cm of the right main bronchus, the tumour is inoperable. Widening and loss of the sharp angle of the carina indicates the presence of enlarged mediastinal lymph nodes, either malignant or reactive. They can be biopsied by passage of a needle through the bronchial wall. Vocal cord paresis on the left indicates involvement of the recurrent laryngeal nerve and inoperability.

Transthoracic fine-needle aspiration biopsy

This involves the direct aspiration through the chest wall of peripheral lung lesions under appropriate x-ray or CT screening. Specimens can be obtained from 75% of peripheral lesions which could not be biopsied transbronchially. Pneumothorax occurs in 25% of patients, occasionally requiring drainage. Mild haemoptysis occurs in 5%. Implantation metastases do not occur.

TREATMENT

Surgery

The only treatment of any value for non-small cell cancer of the lung is surgery. Only 20% of all cases are suitable for resection and only 25–30% survive for 5 years, giving an overall 5-year survival of 4–8%. The mortality of thoracotomy in patients over 65 years with metastatic disease exceeds the expected 5-year survival rate and should therefore be avoided.

Preoperative assessment. Radionuclide scanning for detection of metastatic disease in liver and bone is rarely positive in the absence of symptoms or abnormal enzyme tests (alkaline phosphatase) and is therefore unnecessary. A normal CT scan indicates no mediastinal spread of the tumour and favours curative resection. An abnormal CT scan is not a definite indicator of malignant spread, since slightly enlarged mediastinal lymph nodes may result from reactive hyperplasia.

Because of their common aetiology, chronic bronchitis and emphysema are frequently present. An FEV_1 of less than 1.5 l is not compatible with an active life following pneumonectomy, although the surgery itself can be successfully accomplished. This also applies when the gas transfer test is reduced by 50%.

Radiation therapy for cure
High dose radiotherapy (6500 rad; 65 Gy) can produce results which are as good as those of surgery in patients who are fit and who have slowly growing epidermoid carcinoma. It is the treatment of choice if the tumour is inoperable for reasons such as poor lung function.

Radiation pneumonitis (defined as an acute infiltrate precisely confined to the radiation area occurring within 3 months of radiotherapy) develops in 10–15%. Radiation fibrosis, a fibrotic change occurring within a year or so of radiotherapy and not precisely confined to the radiation area, occurs to some degree in all cases. These complications are usually of little importance.

Symptomatic radiation treatment
Bone pain, haemoptysis and the superior vena cava syndrome respond favourably to irradiation in the short term.

Chemotherapy
This is not effective for the treatment of non-small cell cancer of the lung. The reverse is true for small cell cancer, where combination chemotherapy has resulted in a fivefold increase in median survival. A small number of patients enjoy several years of remission. The best results are achieved by simultaneous use of three or four of the following drugs: vincristine, cyclophosphamide, doxorubicin, lomustine, methotrexate and etoposide (see p. 305).

Terminal care (see p. 325)
Patients dying of cancer of the lung need attention to their overall well-being. They must not be ignored simply because he or she cannot be cured. A lot can be done to make the patient's remaining life symptom-free and as active as possible.

Daily treatment with prednisolone (up to 15 mg daily) may improve appetite. Morphine or diamorphine must be given regularly for pain, either in the form of a sustained–release morphine sulphate tablet twice daily or else as regular elixirs or injections. Many patients find benefit from a continuous subcutaneous injection of opiates given by a pump. Candidiasis and other infections in the mouth are common and must be looked for and treated. Patients taking opiates are frequently constipated, so regular laxatives should be prescribed. Short courses of palliative radiotherapy for bone pain, severe cough or haemoptysis are helpful.

Both the patient and the relatives require counselling, a task that should be shared between nurses, social workers, hospital chaplains and doctors.

SCREENING FOR LUNG CANCER

Lung cancer screening programmes for high risk populations have been developed in an attempt to make the diagnosis earlier and to improve survival. Two such schemes based on yearly chest x-rays and 4-monthly sputum cytology have failed to show any statistical benefit in survival, underlying the need for prevention.

Secondary tumours

Metastases in the lung are very common and usually present as round shadows 1.5–3 cm in diameter. They may be detected on chest x-ray in patients already diagnosed as having carcinoma. The primary is usually in the
- Kidney
- Prostate
- Breast
- Bone
- Gastrointestinal tract
- Cervix or ovary

They nearly always develop in the parenchyma and are often relatively asymptomatic even when the chest x-ray shows extensive pulmonary metastases. It is rare for metastases to develop in the bronchi, when they may present with haemoptysis.

Carcinoma, particularly of the stomach, pancreas and breast, can involve mediastinal glands and spread along the lymphatics of both lungs (lymphangitis carcinomatosa), which can lead to progressive and severe breathlessness. On the chest x-ray bilateral lymphadenopathy is seen together with streaky basal shadowing fanning out over both lung fields.

Occasionally a pulmonary metastasis may be detected as a solitary round shadow on chest x-ray in an asymptomatic patient. The commonest primary tumour to do this is a renal carcinoma. The differential diagnosis includes:
- Primary bronchial carcinoma
- Tuberculoma

- Benign tumour of the lung
- Hydatid cyst

Single pulmonary metastases can be removed surgically, but CT scans usually show the presence of small metastases undetected on chest x-ray.

Disorders of the chest wall and pleura

Trauma

Trauma to the thoracic wall can be due to penetrating wounds and can lead to pneumo- or haemothoraces.

Rib fractures

Rib fractures can be caused by trauma or coughing (particularly in the elderly), and can occur in patients with osteoporosis. Pathological rib fractures may be due to metastatic spread from carcinoma of the bronchus, breast, kidney, prostate and thyroid. Ribs can also become involved by a mesothelioma. Fractures may not be readily visible on a postero-anterior chest x-ray, and lateral x-rays and oblique views may be necessary.

Pain may prevent adequate chest expansion and coughing and this can lead to pneumonia.

Treatment is with adequate analgesia using oral agents or by local infiltration or an intercostal nerve block.

More than one fracture in one rib can lead to a flail segment with paradoxical movement, i.e. part of the chest wall moves inwards during inspiration. This can produce inefficient ventilation and may require intermittent positive pressure ventilation.

Rupture of the trachea or a major bronchus

Rupture of the trachea or even a major bronchus can occur during deceleration injuries, leading to pneumothorax, surgical emphysema, pneumo-mediastinum and haemoptysis. Surgical emphysema is caused by air leaking into the subcutaneous connective tissue; this also occur after the insertion of an intercostal drainage tube. A pneumomediastinum occurs when air leaks from the lung inside the parietal pleura and extending along the bronchial walls.

Rupture of the oesophagus

Rupture of the oesophagus from external injury, endoscopic procedures, bougienage or necrotic carcinoma may lead to the serious complication of mediastinitis. This requires vigorous antibacterial chemotherapy.

Lung contusion

This causes widespread fluffy shadows on the chest x-ray due to intrapulmonary haemorrhage. This may give rise to adult respiratory distress syndrome or shock lung (see p. 647).

Kyphoscoliosis

Kyphoscoliosis may be congenital, idiopathic, due to disease of the vertebrae such as TB or osteomalacia, or due to neuromuscular disease such as Friedreich's ataxia or poliomyelitis. The respiratory effects of severe kyphoscoliosis are often more pronounced than might be expected and respiratory failure and death often occur in the fourth or fifth decade. The abnormality should be corrected at an early stage if possible.

Ankylosing spondylitis

Limitation of chest wall movement is often well compensated by diaphragmatic movement, and the respiratory effects of this disease are relatively mild. It is associated with upper lobe fibrosis of unknown aetiology.

Pectus excavatum and carinatum

Pectus excavatum causes few problems other than embarrassment due to the deep vertical furrow in the chest, which can be corrected surgically. The heart is seen to lie well to the left on the chest x-ray. Pectus carinatum (pigeon chest) is often the result of rickets. No treatment is required.

Dry pleurisy

'Dry pleurisy' is the term used to describe pleurisy when there is inflammation but no appreciable effusion. The localized inflammation produces sharp localized pain, made worse on deep inspiration, coughing and occasionally on twisting and bending movements. Common causes are pneumonia, pulmonary infarct and carcinoma. Rarer causes are rheumatoid arthritis and systemic lupus erythematosus.

Epidemic myalgia (Bornholm disease) is due to infection by coxsackie B virus. This illness is common in young adults in the late summer and autumn and is characterized by an upper respiratory tract illness followed by pleuritic pain in the chest and upper abdomen with tender muscles. The chest x-ray remains normal and the illness clears within 1 week.

Pleural effusion

A pleural effusion is an excessive accumulation of fluid in the pleural space. It can be detected on x-ray when 300 ml or more of fluid is present and clinically when 500 ml or more is present. The chest x-ray appearances range from the obliteration of the costophrenic angle to dense homogeneous shadows occupying part or all of the hemithorax. Fluid below the lung (a subpulmonary effusion) can simulate a raised hemidiaphragm. Fluid in the fissures may resemble an intrapulmonary mass. The physical signs are shown in Table 12.1 (see p. 561).

Diagnosis is by pleural aspiration (see p. 568). The fluid which accumulates may be a transudate or an exudate.

Transudates. Effusions which are transudates can be bilateral. The protein content is less than 30 g·l^{-1} and the lactic dehydrogenase is less than 200 iu·l^{-1}. Causes include:
- Heart failure
- Hypoproteinaemia (e.g. nephrotic syndrome)
- Constrictive pericarditis
- Hypothyroidism
- Ovarian tumours producing right-sided pleural effusion—Meigs' syndrome

Exudates. The protein content of exudates is greater than 30 g·l^{-1} and the lactic dehydrogenase is greater than 200 iu·l^{-1}. Causes include:
- Bacterial pneumonia (common)
- Carcinoma of the bronchus (common)   } Fluid may be bloodstained
- Pulmonary infarction (common)
- Tuberculosis
- Connective tissue disease
- Post-myocardial infarction syndrome (rare)
- Acute pancreatitis (high amylase content) (rare)
- Mesothelioma (rare)
- Sarcoidosis (very rare)
- Yellow nail syndrome (effusion due to lymphoedema) (rare)
- Familial mediterranean fever (rare)

Pleural biopsy (see p. 569) may be necessary to diagnose the cause of the effusion. Treatment is of the underlying condition.

Malignant pleural effusions

Malignant pleural effusions which reaccumulate and are symptomatic can be aspirated to *dryness* followed by the instillation of a sclerosing agent such as tetracycline or bleomycin. Effusions should be drained slowly since rapid shift of the mediastinum causes severe pain and occasionally shock. This treatment produces only temporary relief.

Chylothorax

This is due to the accumulation of lymph in the pleural space, usually resulting from leakage from the thoracic duct due to infiltration by carcinoma.

Empyema

This is the presence of pus in the pleural space and can be a complication of pneumonia (see p. 598).

Pneumothorax

'Pneumothorax' means air in the pleural space. It may occur due to trauma to the chest or may be spontaneous. Pneumothoraces may be localized if the visceral pleura has previously undergone adhesion to the parietal pleura, or generalized if the whole hemithorax contains air. Normally the pressure in the pleural space is negative, but this is lost once a communication is made with atmospheric pressure; the elastic recoil pressure of the lung then causes it to partially deflate. If the communication between the airways and the pleural space remains (an open pneumothorax), a bronchopleural fistula is created. Once the communication between the lung and the pleural space is obliterated, air will be reabsorbed at a rate of 1.25% of the total radiographic volume of the hemithorax per day. Thus, a 50% collapse of the lung would take 40 days to reabsorb completely once the pneumothorax is closed.

Tension pneumothorax. A valvular mechanism may develop through which air can be sucked during inspiration but not expelled during expiration. The intrapleural pressure remains positive throughout breathing, the lung deflates further, the mediastinum shifts, and venous return to the heart decreases, with increasing respiratory and cardiac embarrassment.

Spontaneous pneumothorax

This usually occurs in young males, the male to female ratio being 6 : 1. It is caused by the rupture of a pleural bleb, usually apical, and is thought to be due to congenital defects in the connective tissue of the alveolar walls. Both lungs are affected with equal frequency. Often these patients are tall and thin.

In patients over 40 years of age, the usual cause is underlying chronic bronchitis and emphysema. Rarer causes include bronchial asthma, carcinoma, a lung abscess breaking down and leading to a bronchopleural fistula, and severe pulmonary fibrosis with cyst formation.

The sudden onset of unilateral pleuritic pain or increasing breathlessness are the usual presenting features. If the pneumothorax enlarges or a tension pneumothorax develops (very rare), the patient becomes more breathless and may develop pallor and tachycardia. There may be few physical signs if the pneumothorax is small. The characteristic features and management are shown in Fig. 12.35.

There is no universally accepted way of treating a large pneumothorax. The main aim is to get the patient back to active life as soon as possible.

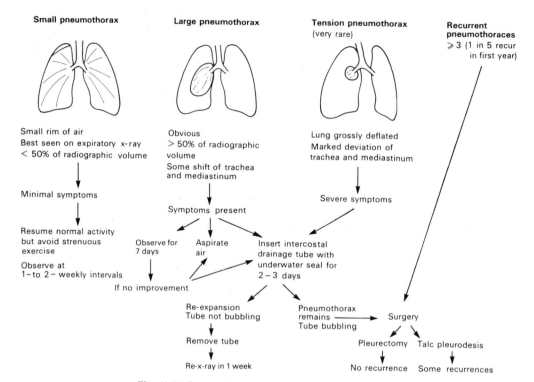

| Small pneumothorax | Large pneumothorax | Tension pneumothorax (very rare) | Recurrent pneumothoraces ⩾ 3 (1 in 5 recur in first year) |

Small rim of air
Best seen on expiratory x-ray
< 50% of radiographic volume

Obvious
> 50% of radiographic volume
Some shift of trachea and mediastinum

Lung grossly deflated
Marked deviation of trachea and mediastinum

Minimal symptoms

Symptoms present

Severe symptoms

Resume normal activity but avoid strenuous exercise

Observe at 1- to 2-weekly intervals

Observe for 7 days

Aspirate air

Insert intercostal drainage tube with underwater seal for 2–3 days

If no improvement

Re-expansion
Tube not bubbling

Pneumothorax remains ——→ Surgery
Tube bubbling

Remove tube

Pleurectomy   Talc pleurodesis

Re-x-ray in 1 week

No recurrence   Some recurrences

Fig. 12.35 Pneumothorax: an algorithm for management.

Mediastinal tumours

The mediastinum is defined as the region between the pleural sacs. It is additionally divided as shown in Fig. 12.36. Tumours affecting the mediastinum are rare.

Retrosternal or intrathoracic thyroid

The commonest mediastinal tumour is a retrosternal or intrathoracic thyroid, which is nearly always an extension of the thyroid present in the neck. Enlargement of the thyroid by a colloid goitre or malignant disease and, rarely, in thyrotoxicosis causes displacement of the trachea and oesophagus to the opposite side. Symptoms of compression develop

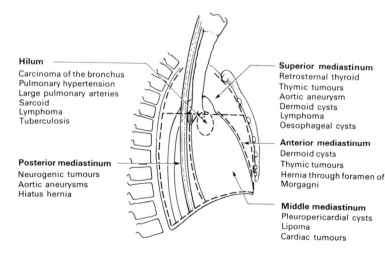

Hilum
Carcinoma of the bronchus
Pulmonary hypertension
Large pulmonary arteries
Sarcoid
Lymphoma
Tuberculosis

Posterior mediastinum
Neurogenic tumours
Aortic aneurysms
Hiatus hernia

Superior mediastinum
Retrosternal thyroid
Thymic tumours
Aortic aneurysm
Dermoid cysts
Lymphoma
Oesophageal cysts

Anterior mediastinum
Dermoid cysts
Thymic tumours
Hernia through foramen of Morgagni

Middle mediastinum
Pleuropericardial cysts
Lipoma
Cardiac tumours

Fig. 12.36 Subdivisions of the mediastinum and their tumours.

insidiously before producing the cardinal feature of dyspnoea. Very occasionally an intrathoracic thyroid may be the cause of dysphagia and, rarely, of hoarseness of the voice and vocal cord paralysis from stretching of the recurrent laryngeal nerve. The treatment is surgical removal.

Thymic tumours

The thymus is large in childhood and occupies the superior and anterior mediastinum. It involutes with age but may be enlarged both by cysts, which are rarely symptomatic, or tumours, which may cause the symptoms of myasthenia gravis or may lead to compression of the trachea or, rarely, the oesophagus. Surgery is the treatment of choice. Approximately half of the patients presenting with a thymic tumour have myasthenia gravis.

Pleuro-pericardial cysts

These cysts, which may be up to 10 cm in diameter, are filled with clear fluid and are usually situated anteriorly in the cardiophrenic angle on the right in 70% of cases. Infection only rarely occurs; malignant change does not occur. The diagnosis is usually made by needle aspiration. No treatment is required, but these patients should be followed-up as any increase in cyst size suggests an alternative pathology; surgical excision is then advisable.

Further reading

Clark T J H & Godfrey S (eds) (1983) *Asthma*, 2nd edn. London: Chapman and Hall.

Crofton J & Douglas AL (ed) (1981) *Respiratory Diseases*, 3rd edn. Oxford: Blackwell Scientific.

Flenley DC & Petty TL (eds) (1983) *Recent Advances in Respiratory Medicine* series. Edinburgh: Churchill Livingstone.

Lessof MH (ed.) (1984) *Allergy: Immunology and Clinical Aspects*. Chichester: Wiley.

Mygind N (ed.) (1986) *Essential Allergy*. Oxford: Blackwell Scientific

Sterling GM (ed.) (1983) *Respiratory Disease*. London: Heinemann.

Intensive Care

Introduction

A glossary of terms and abbreviations used in this chapter is given in the Appendices on p. 963.

Intensive care medicine (or 'critical care medicine') is concerned predominantly with the management of patients with acute life-threatening conditions ('the critically ill') in a specialized unit. It also encompasses the resuscitation and transport of those who become acutely ill, or are injured, either elsewhere in the hospital or in the community.

The development of intensive care medicine was initially stimulated by the treatment of respiratory failure with intermittent positive pressure ventilation (IPPV) and this still remains an important aspect of the specialty. Subsequently, intensive care medicine has expanded to include the management of patients with a wide variety of underlying medical and surgical disorders, as well as the care of high-risk postoperative cases. A coordinated, multidisciplinary approach is therefore essential for optimal patient care.

An intensive care ward is fully equipped with monitoring and technical facilities. Patients can receive intensive nursing care and the constant attention of appropriately trained medical staff. These conditions and facilities are not available on a busy general ward.

In all critically ill patients, the immediate objective is to preserve life and prevent, reverse or minimize damage to vital organs such as the brain and the kidneys. This is achieved by optimizing cardiovascular and respiratory function in order to maximize delivery of oxygen to the tissues.

In this chapter only cardiovascular and respiratory problems are discussed. Many patients have failure of other organs such as the kidney and liver as well; treatment of these is dealt with in the appropriate chapters. Feeding the critically ill patient is discussed in Chapter 3.

Oxygen delivery

The concept of oxygen flux (see text)

Oxygen flux = Cardiac output × Arterial oxygen content

Oxygen flux = Cardiac output × [(Hb × So_2 × 1.34) + (P_ao_2 × 0.003)]

For representative values in a normal adult, and ignoring the small amount of dissolved oxygen:

1000 ml·min^{-1} = 5000 ml × $\frac{15}{100}$ g·ml^{-1} × $\frac{99}{100}$ × 1.34

Since oxygen consumption is normally approximately 250 ml·min^{-1}, there is an excess of supply over demand which provides a margin of safety if oxygen consumption increases or oxygen delivery falls.

Oxygen delivery (oxygen flux) is defined as the total amount of oxygen delivered to the tissues per unit time. It is dependent on the volume of blood flowing through the microcirculation per minute (i.e. the total cardiac output—$\dot{Q}_t$) and the amount of oxygen contained in that blood (i.e. the arterial oxygen content—C_ao_2). Oxygen is transported in combination with haemoglobin or dissolved in plasma. The amount combined with haemoglobin is determined by the oxygen capacity of the haemoglobin (usually taken as 1.34 ml O_2 per gram of haemoglobin) and its percentage saturation with oxygen (So_2), while the volume dissolved in plasma depends on the partial pressure of oxygen (Po_2). Except when hyperbaric oxygen is administered, the amount of dissolved oxygen in plasma is sufficiently small to be ignored for most practical purposes.

There is, however, an important limitation to the application of the concept of oxygen flux in clinical practice—it does not provide any information regarding the relative flow to individual organs. Thus, for example, isoprenaline reduces the total peripheral resistance but does so mainly by increasing skin and muscle blood flow at the expense of more vital organs such as the kidneys. Moreover, some organs, notably the heart, have a very high oxygen requirement relative to their blood flow and may, therefore, become hypoxic even when overall oxygen flux is apparently adequate.

CARDIAC OUTPUT

Maintenance of an adequate cardiac output depends on the heart rate and the stroke volume (Fig. 13.1).

Cardiac output = Stroke volume x Heart rate

Pre-load Contractility After-load

Fig. 13.1 The determinants of cardiac output.

Heart rate

Extreme bradycardias and tachycardias can both cause reductions in cardiac output.

Increased heart rate
When heart rate increases, the duration of systole remains essentially unchanged, whereas diastole, and thus the time available for ventricular filling, becomes progressively shorter, and the stroke volume eventually falls. In the normal heart this occurs at rates greater than about 160 beats per minute, but in those with cardiac pathology, especially when this restricts ventricular filling (e.g. mitral stenosis), stroke volume may fall at much lower heart rates. Furthermore, tachycardias also cause a marked increase in myocardial oxygen consumption and this may precipitate ischaemia in areas of the myocardium which have reduced coronary perfusion.

Decreased heart rate
When the heart rate falls, a point is reached at which the increase in stroke volume is insufficient to com-

pensate for the bradycardia and again cardiac output falls.

Alterations in heart rate are often caused by disturbances of rhythm (e.g. atrial fibrillation, complete heart block or junctional arrhythmias), in which ventricular filling is not augmented by atrial contraction and stroke volume therefore falls.

Stroke volume

Three factors determine the stroke volume: pre-load, myocardial contractility and after-load (see p. 494).

Pre-load
This is defined as the tension of the myocardial fibres at the end of diastole, just before the onset of ventricular contraction, and is therefore related to the degree of stretch of the fibres (Fig. 13.2). The main factor influencing pre-load is the venous return. As the end-diastolic volume of the ventricle increases, stroke volume rises (Fig. 13.3).

Fig. 13.2 The relationship between myocardial tension and contraction. 'Pre-load' is the tension of the myocardial fibres prior to the onset of systole and depends on the degree to which they are passively stretched. During isometric contraction the tension in the contractile elements increases. The tension required to open the aortic valve and eject blood from the ventricle is the 'after-load'.

Myocardial oxygen consumption ($\dot{V}_m O_2$) increases only slightly with an increase in pre-load and this is therefore the most efficient way of improving cardiac output.

Myocardial contractility
The state of myocardial contractility determines the response of the ventricles to changes in pre-load and after-load. Unfortunately, contractility is often reduced in intensive-care patients, either as a result of pre-existing myocardial damage, e.g. ischaemic heart disease, or the acute disease process itself. Changes in myocardial contractility alter the slope and position of the Starling curve; the resulting worsening ventricular performance is manifested as a depressed, flattened curve (Fig. 13.3).

Fig. 13.3 Ventricular function (Starling) curve. As pre-load is increased, stroke volume rises. If the ventricle is over-stretched, stroke volume will fall (x). In myocardial failure the curve is depressed and flattened (y). Increasing contractility shifts the curve upwards and to the left (z).

After-load

This is defined as the myocardial wall tension developed during systolic ejection (Fig. 13.2). In the case of the left ventricle it is determined by the resistance imposed by the aortic valve and the peripheral vasculature and is a significant determinant of left ventricular performance. After-load is also influenced by the elasticity of the major blood vessels. Decreasing the after-load can increase the stroke volume achieved at a given pre-load (Fig. 13.4), whilst also reducing the ventricular wall tension and the myocardial oxygen consumption. The reduction in wall tension may lead to an increase in coronary blood flow, thereby improving the myocardial oxygen supply-demand ratio. An increase in after-load, on the other hand, can cause a fall in stroke volume and is a potent cause of increased $\dot{V}_mO_2$. Right ventricular after-load is normally negligible since the resistance of the pulmonary circulation is very low.

and its percentage saturation with oxygen. For this reason, maintenance of an 'adequate' haemoglobin concentration is essential in critically ill patients. However, tissue oxygenation is also dependent on blood flow. This is in turn determined not only by the cardiac output and its distribution, but also by the viscosity of the blood. The latter depends largely on the packed cell volume (PCV) and it is generally considered that the optimal balance between oxygen-carrying capacity and tissue flow is achieved at a PCV of approximately 30%.

Oxyhaemoglobin dissociation curve (Fig. 13.5)

The saturation of haemoglobin with oxygen is determined by the partial pressure of oxygen (Po_2) in the blood, the relationship between the two being described by the oxyhaemoglobin dissociation curve (Fig. 13.5). The sigmoid shape of this curve is important clinically for a number of reasons. First, falls in P_aO_2 may be tolerated provided that the percentage saturation remains above 90%. Second, increasing the P_aO_2 to above normal has only a minimal effect on oxygen content unless hyperbaric oxygen is administered (when the amount of oxygen in solution in plasma becomes significant). Third, once on the steep 'slippery slope' of the curve, a small decrease in P_aO_2 can cause large falls in oxygen content, while increasing P_aO_2 only slightly (e.g. by administering 28% oxygen to a patient with chronic bronchitis) can lead to useful increases in oxygen saturation.

The P_aO_2 is in turn influenced by the alveolar oxygen tension (P_AO_2), the efficiency of pulmonary gas exchange, and the partial pressure of oxygen in mixed venous blood ($P_{\bar{v}}O_2$).

Fig. 13.4 The effect of changes in after-load on the ventricular function curve.

OXYGENATION

The oxygen content of the arterial blood (C_aO_2), in conjunction with the cardiac output, determines oxygen delivery. As discussed above, oxygen content is dependent on the amount of haemoglobin present per unit volume of blood, its oxygen capacity

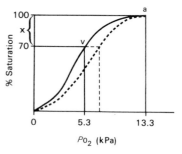

Po_2 (kPa)

Fig. 13.5 The oxyhaemoglobin dissociation curve.
a = arterial point; v = venous point;
x = arteriovenous oxygen content difference.
   The curve will move to the right (dotted line) in the presence of acidosis (metabolic or respiratory), pyrexia or an increased red cell 2,3-DPG concentration. For a given arteriovenous oxygen content difference, the mixed venous Po_2 will then be higher. Furthermore if the mixed venous Po_2 is unchanged, the arteriovenous oxygen content difference increases and more oxygen is off-loaded to the tissues.

Alveolar oxygen tension (Fig. 13.6)
Room air contains 20.93% oxygen, so that, given a normal barometric pressure of 101 kPa (760 mmHg), the inspired partial pressure of oxygen P_IO_2 is 21.2 kPa (159 mmHg). Because there is virtually no CO_2 in inspired air, and the amount of water vapour is relatively small, the remainder is largely nitrogen. However, by the time the inspired gases reach the alveoli they are fully saturated with water vapour at body temperature (37°C), which has a partial pressure of 6.3 kPa (47 mmHg), and CO_2 has been added at a partial pressure of approximately 5.3 kPa (40 mmHg). The P_AO_2 is thereby reduced to approximately 13.4 kPa (100 mmHg).

The clinician can influence P_AO_2 by administering oxygen or increasing the barometric pressure (i.e. administering hyperbaric oxygen). Because of the reciprocal relationship between the partial pressures of oxygen and carbon dioxide in the alveoli, a small increase in P_AO_2 can be produced by lowering the P_ACO_2 (e.g. using IPPV).

Pulmonary gas exchange
If lung function were perfect, alveolar gas would equilibrate completely with arterial blood and the P_aO_2 would equal the P_AO_2. Even in normal individuals, however, a small pressure gradient exists between the oxygen in the alveoli and that in the arterial blood: the alveolar—arterial oxygen difference ($P_{A-a}O_2$). This difference increases with age. Any disease of the lung parenchyma will interfere with oxygen transfer and cause an abnormal increase in $P_{A-a}O_2$. Three causes of the $P_{A-a}O_2$ can be identified.

Diffusion defects. A very small (0.133 kPa, 1 mmHg) pressure gradient probably exists between oxygen in the alveoli and that in the pulmonary capillary blood. This rarely causes hypoxaemia, even in diseases such as fibrosing alveolitis in which the alveolar capillary membrane is considerably thickened, except possibly during exercise (when pulmonary capillary transit time is markedly increased) or when the P_AO_2 is very low (e.g. at high altitudes). Because carbon dioxide is so much more soluble than oxygen its excretion is not influenced by diffusion defects.

Right-to-left shunts. Normally a small amount of venous blood bypasses the lungs via the bronchial and thebesian veins and desaturated blood from the bronchial circulation drains into the pulmonary veins. Although this amounts to only 2% of the total cardiac output, it is one cause of the $P_{A-a}O_2$ in normal subjects. In some diseases of the lung, such as lobar pneumonia, and in certain cardiac lesions, such as Fallot's tetralogy, a much larger proportion of the cardiac output passes to the left side of the heart without taking part in gas exchange, thereby causing significant arterial hypoxaemia. This hypoxaemia cannot be corrected by administering oxygen to increase the P_AO_2, because blood leaving normal alveoli is already fully saturated and further increases in P_{O_2} will not significantly affect its oxygen content. When this fully saturated blood is mixed with the shunted blood, the arterial oxygen content and therefore the P_aO_2 fall proportionately. On the other hand, because of the shape of the carbon dioxide dissociation curve (Fig. 13.7) the high P_{CO_2} of the shunted blood can be compensated for by overventilating patent alveoli, thus lowering the CO_2 content of the effluent blood. Indeed, many patients with acute right-to-left shunts hyperventilate in response to the stimulus of hypoxia or stimulation of stretch receptors in the lung, so that the P_aCO_2 is normal or low.

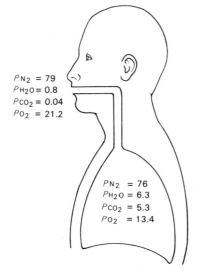

$P_{N_2} = 79$
$P_{H_2O} = 0.8$
$P_{CO_2} = 0.04$
$P_{O_2} = 21.2$

$P_{N_2} = 76$
$P_{H_2O} = 6.3$
$P_{CO_2} = 5.3$
$P_{O_2} = 13.4$

Fig. 13.6 The partial pressures of inspired and alveolar gas (values given in kilopascals).

CO$_2$ content

2.6   5.3   10

P_{CO_2} (kPa)

Fig. 13.7 The carbon dioxide dissociation curve. Note that in the physiological range the curve is essentially linear.

Ventilation/perfusion ($\dot{V}/\dot{Q}$) mismatch. This is discussed in more detail in Chapter 12.

Diseases of the lung parenchyma result in a $\dot{V}/\dot{Q}$ mismatch, producing an increase in alveolar dead space and hypoxaemia. The former can be compensated for by increasing overall ventilation. In contrast to the hypoxia resulting from a true right-to-left shunt (see above), that due to areas of low $\dot{V}/\dot{Q}$ can be partially corrected by administering oxygen and thereby increasing the $P_{A}O_2$, even in poorly ventilated areas of lung.

Mixed venous Po_2

If the $P_{\bar{v}}O_2$ (i.e. the Po_2 of pulmonary arterial blood, where the blood has been thoroughly mixed during its passage through the heart) and thus the mixed venous oxygen content falls, the effect of a given degree of pulmonary shunting on arterial oxygenation will be exacerbated. If the $P_{a}O_2$ remains constant, the $P_{\bar{v}}O_2$ will fall if more oxygen has to be extracted from each unit volume of blood arriving at the tissues. This will occur if the cardiac output, and thus oxygen delivery, falls and/or oxygen requirements of the tissues increase. Thus, worsening arterial hypoxaemia does not necessarily indicate a deterioration in pulmonary function but may instead reflect a fall in cardiac output and/or a rise in oxygen consumption.

The $P_{\bar{v}}O_2$ is also influenced by the position of the oxyhaemoglobin dissociation curve (Fig. 13.5), a factor not incorporated in the concept of oxygen flux. Thus, if the arteriovenous oxygen content difference remains constant, a shift of the curve to the right, which occurs with acidosis, hypercarbia, pyrexia and a rise in red cell 2,3-diphosphoglycerate (2,3-DPG) levels, may cause the $P_{\bar{v}}O_2$ to rise. Moreover, if the $P_{\bar{v}}O_2$ remains unchanged, more oxygen will be unloaded at tissue level. A shift of the curve to the left, on the other hand, will cause a fall in the $P_{\bar{v}}O_2$. It might be argued, then, that under certain circumstances an acidosis may be beneficial in terms of tissue oxygenation, provided that it is not severe enough to interfere with cardiac function. It is probable though, that shifts of the dissociation curve are of little clinical significance.

Acute disturbances of haemodynamic function (shock)

Shock is difficult to define. The term is used to describe acute circulatory failure resulting in generalized cellular hypoxia due to inadequate or inappropriate tissue perfusion.

CAUSES

The causes are shown in Table 13.1. Very often shock can result from a combination of these factors.

Table 13.1 Aetiology of shock.

Cardiogenic
Obstructive (i.e. obstruction to outflow), e.g. pulmonary embolus or restricted cardiac filling such as tamponade
Peripheral circulation
Hypovolaemic:
Exogenous losses
Endogenous losses
Normovolaemic:
Dilatation
Sequestration
Arteriovenous shunting

PATHOPHYSIOLOGY

Sympatho-adrenal response to shock (Fig. 13.8)

Hypotension stimulates the baroreceptors, and to a lesser extent the chemoreceptors, causing increased sympathetic nervous activity. Later this is augmented by the release of catecholamines from the adrenal medulla. The resulting vasoconstriction, together with positive inotropic and chronotropic effects, helps to restore blood pressure and cardiac output. Opioid peptides containing the enkephalin sequence have been identified within the same chromaffin cells as catecholamines and are also released into the circulation in shock.

Reduction in perfusion of the renal cortex stimulates the juxtaglomerular apparatus to release renin. This converts angiotensinogen to angiotensin I, which is in turn converted in the lungs to the potent vasoconstrictor, angiotensin II. Angiotensin II also stimulates secretion of aldosterone by the adrenal cortex, causing sodium and water retention. This helps to restore the circulating volume.

Neuroendocrine response to shock

- Release of pituitary hormones: adrenocorticotrophic hormone (ACTH), growth hormone (GH), vasopressin (antidiuretic hormone, ADH) and β-endorphin. (Endogenous opioid peptides such as β-endorphin, dynorphin and the enkephalins may also be partly responsible for some of the cardiovascular changes.)
- Release of cortisol, which causes fluid retention and antagonizes insulin
- Release of glucagon, which produces hyperglycaemia

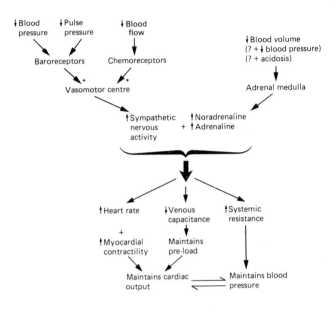

Fig. 13.8 The sympatho-adrenal response to shock.

Release of vasoactive substances

Prostaglandins (see Fig. 12.27, p. 588)
Those currently considered to be of particular importance in shock are:

- Prostacyclin, which is a vasodilator and inhibits platelet aggregation
- Thromboxane A_2, which causes pulmonary vasoconstriction and activates platelets
- $PGF_{2\alpha}$, which may be responsible for the early phase of pulmonary hypertension commonly seen in experimental septic shock

Lysosomal enzymes
These are released in response to hypoxia, ischaemia, sepsis and acidosis. As well as being directly cytotoxic, they can cause myocardial depression and coronary vasoconstriction. Furthermore, lysosomal enzymes can convert inactive kininogens, which are usually combined with alpha-2-globulin, to vasoactive kinins such as bradykinin. These substances can cause vasodilatation and increased capillary permeability, as well as myocardial depression. They can also activate clotting mechanisms.

Endotoxin
This is a complex lipopolysaccharide derived from bacterial cell walls which is released in septic shock. Its toxic effects are mediated by the phospholipid portion of the molecule known as lipid A. Endotoxin is cytotoxic, damages endothelium, uncouples oxidative phosphorylation and activates complement through both the alternate and the classical pathways.

All the above vasoactive substances are of particular importance in the pathogenesis of septic shock.

Microcirculatory changes

Since shock is a syndrome caused by inadequate tissue perfusion, the final common pathway for the pathophysiological changes is the microcirculation.

In the early stages of septic shock there is vasodilatation, opening of arteriovenous shunts, increased capillary permeability and a defect of oxygen utilization by the tissues. Initially, before hypovolaemia supervenes, or when therapeutic replacement of circulating volume has been adequate, cardiac output is usually high and peripheral resistance low. Vasodilatation and increased capillary permeability also occur in anaphylactic shock.

In the initial stages of other forms of shock, and when hypovolaemia supervenes in sepsis and anaphylaxis, increased sympathetic activity causes constriction of both pre-capillary arterioles and, to a lesser extent, the post-capillary venules. This helps to maintain the systemic blood pressure. In addition, the hydrostatic pressure within the capillaries falls and fluid is mobilized from the extravascular space into the intravascular compartment. If shock persists, the accumulation of metabolites, such as lactic acid and carbon dioxide, combined with the release of vasoactive substances, causes relaxation of the pre-capillary sphincters, while the post-capillary venules, which are more sensitive to hypoxic damage, become relatively unresponsive to these substances and remain constricted. Blood is therefore sequestered within the dilated capillary bed and fluid is forced into the extravascular spaces, causing interstitial oedema, haemoconcentration, and an increase in viscosity.

This reduction in flow through the microcirculation, combined with the increase in viscosity, makes the blood highly coagulable. Platelet aggregation and clot formation occur within the capillary bed. Plasminogen is converted to plasmin, which breaks down these clots, liberating fibrin/fibrinogen degradation products (FDPs). The cells which are supplied by capillaries blocked by this process of disseminated intravascular coagulation (DIC) inevitably become hypoxic and eventually die. Tissue ischaemia is further exacerbated as capillaries are compressed by interstitial oedema. In this way vital organs may suffer serious damage. Finally, because clotting factors and platelets are consumed in DIC (see p. 301), they are unavailable for haemostasis elsewhere and a coagulation defect results—hence the alternative name for DIC of 'consumption coagulopathy'. This process occurs earlier and is more severe in septicaemic shock.

The capillary endothelium can be damaged by a number of factors, particularly in septic shock, including DIC, microemboli, release of vasoactive compounds, complement, and leucocyte aggregation. Capillary permeability is thereby increased and fluid is lost into the interstitial space, causing further hypovolaemia, interstitial oedema and organ dysfunction.

Metabolic changes

Once the supply of oxygen to the cells is insufficient for continuation of the tricarboxylic acid (TCA) cycle, production of energy in the form of ATP becomes dependent on anaerobic metabolism. Under these circumstances glucose is metabolized in the normal way to pyruvate but is then converted to lactate instead of entering the Krebs cycle. The H^+ ions released cause a metabolic acidosis. This pathway is relatively inefficient in terms of energy production. Despite the increased cellular permeability to glucose that is induced by hypoxia, shocked patients are often hyperglycaemic because of the elevated circulating levels of insulin antagonists such as cortisol, growth hormone and catecholamines, as well as catecholamine-induced glycogen breakdown. Blood levels of fatty acids and amino acids also rise. Eventually, because of the reduced availability of ATP, the sodium pump fails, cells swell due to accumulation of salt and water, and potassium losses increase. In the final stages, release of lysosomal enzymes may contribute to cell death.

CLINICAL SIGNS

Although many clinical features are common to all types of shock there are certain important respects in which they differ:

Hypovolaemic shock
- Inadequate tissue perfusion:
  (a) Skin—cold, pale, blue, slow capillary refill

  (b) Kidneys—oliguria, anuria
  (c) Brain—confusion and restlessness
- Increased sympathetic tone:
  (a) Tachycardia
  (b) Sweating
  (c) Blood pressure—may be maintained initially (despite up to a 25% reduction in circulating volume if the patient is young and fit), but later hypotension supervenes
- Metabolic acidosis and tachypnoea

Additional clinical features may occur in the following types of shock:

Cardiogenic shock
- Signs of myocardial failure—e.g. raised JVP, pulsus alternans, 'gallop' rhythm, basal crackles

Obstructive shock
- Elevated JVP
- Pulsus paradoxus in cardiac tamponade

Anaphylactic shock (see p. 651)
- Signs of profound vasodilatation:
  (a) Warm peripheries
  (b) Low blood pressure
- Urticaria
- Bronchospasm
- Oedema of the face, pharynx and larynx
- Hypovolaemia due to capillary leak

Septic shock
- Pyrexia and rigors
- Early signs (warm normotensive or warm hypotensive):
  (a) Vasodilatation, warm peripheries
  (b) Bounding pulse
  (c) Rapid capillary refill
- Late signs (cold hypotensive):
  (a) Hypovolaemia and signs as for hypovolaemic shock (see above)
  (b) Myocardial depression
- Other signs:
  (a) Jaundice
  (b) Coma (rare)
  (c) Signs of DIC

The diagnosis of septic shock can be difficult and the clinician must have a high index of suspicion. In the elderly the classical signs may not be present and, for example, mild confusion, tachycardia and tachypnoea may be the only clues, sometimes associated with unexplained hypotension.

MONITORING

Invasive monitoring is unnecessary in straightforward cases, such as a fit young man with moderate traumatic haemorrhage, but will be required in the more seriously ill patients and in those who fail to respond to initial treatment (see later). Clinical assessment must never be neglected in favour of invasive monitoring.

Clinical indices of tissue perfusion

A patient with warm peripheries, e.g. nose and fingers, has an adequate cardiac output. Conversely, pale, cold skin indicates poor perfusion. Skin temperature measurements can help clinical evaluation as vasoconstriction is an early compensatory response.

Urinary flow is a sensitive indicator of renal perfusion and haemodynamic performance.

Blood pressure

This reflects the adequacy of the cardiac output. However, if there is vasoconstriction with a high peripheral resistance, the blood pressure may be normal, even when the cardiac output is reduced.

The absolute level of blood pressure is also important since hypotension may jeopardize perfusion of vital organs.

Blood pressure is usually measured with a sphygmomanometer, but automated instruments are now available which use a microphone to detect Korotkoff sounds. Continuous monitoring, using an intra-arterial cannula, is also possible and this has the advantage that samples can be easily obtained for blood-gas analysis. The radial artery is usually used and is punctured percutaneously (Fig. 13.9). If cannulation of the radial artery proves impossible, other larger arteries, e.g. brachial or femoral, can be used.

Radial artery cannulation

Technique
- The arm is supported, with the wrist extended, by an assistant.
- The radial artery is palpated where it arches over the head of the radius.
- In conscious patients, local anaesthetic is injected to raise a weal over the artery, taking care not to puncture the vessel or obscure its pulsation.
- A small skin incision is made over the proposed puncture site.
- A small parallel-sided cannula (20 gauge for adults, 22 gauge for children) is used in order to allow blood to flow past the cannula. Teflon is less irritant.
- The cannula is inserted over the point of maximal pulsation and advanced in line with the direction of the vessel at an angle of approximately 30°.
- 'Flashback' of blood into the cannula indicates that the radial artery has been punctured.
- The cannula is threaded off the needle into the vessel and the needle withdrawn.
- The cannula is connected to a non-compliant manometer line filled with heparinized saline. This is then connected via a transducer and continuous flush device to an oscilloscope, which records the arterial pressure.

Complications
- Thrombosis
- Loss of arterial pulsation
- Distal ischaemia, e.g. digital necrosis (rare)
- Accidental injection of drugs—can produce vascular occlusion
- Disconnection—leading to hypovolaemia

'Flashback' of arterial blood

Fig. 13.9 Percutaneous cannulation of the radial artery.

Central venous pressure (CVP)

This provides a fairly simple method of assessing the adequacy of a patient's circulating volume and the contractile state of the myocardium. The absolute value of the CVP is not as important as its response to a fluid challenge of 200–500 ml (Fig. 13.10). The hypovolaemic patient will initially respond to transfusion with little or no change in CVP, together with some improvement in cardiovascular status (falling heart rate, rising blood pressure and increased peripheral temperature). As the normovolaemic state is approached the CVP usually rises slightly and stabilizes, while other cardiovascular values normalize. At this stage, volume replacement should be slowed, or even stopped, in order to avoid

Fig. 13.10 The effects of rapid administration of a 'fluid challenge' to patients with a central venous pressure within the normal range. From Sykes MK (1963) Venous pressure as a clinical indication of adequacy of transfusion. *Annals of the Royal College of Surgeons of England* **33**: 185–197. With permission.

over-transfusion. Over-transfusion is indicated by an abrupt and sustained rise in CVP, usually accompanied by some deterioration in the patient's condition.

The CVP may be read intermittently using a manometer system (Fig. 13.11) or continuously using a transducer connected to an oscilloscope, similar to that used for intra-arterial monitoring.

Common pitfalls in interpreting CVP results are:
- Blocked catheter. This results in a sustained high reading.
- Manometer or transducer wrongly positioned. Failure to re-zero the CVP after changing the patient's position is a common cause of erroneous readings.
- Incorrect calibration. If an electronic transducer and oscilloscope is used, the system should be zeroed and calibrated prior to use.
- One or more infusions in progress through the CVP catheter. The CVP catheter may be used for other infusions and the pressure measured intermittently. A falsely high reading will result if these fluids continue to be administered by an infusion pump while the pressure is recorded.
- Catheter tip in right ventricle. If the catheter is advanced too far an unexpectedly high pressure is recorded.

The catheter should be positioned in the superior vena cava or the right atrium. It is usually inserted via a percutaneous puncture of a subclavian or internal jugular vein (Fig. 13.12).

Fig. 13.11 Central venous pressure measurement using a manometer system. The reading must be referred to the level of the right atrium (indicated by the axillary fold or, provided the patient is supine, the sternal notch) using a spirit level.

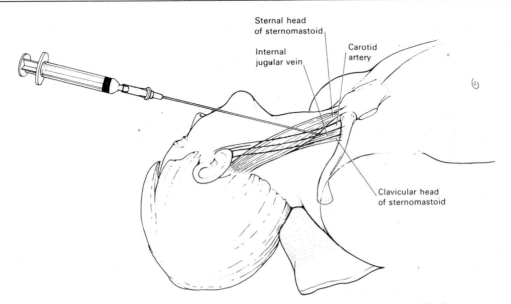

Fig. 13.12 Cannulation of the right internal jugular vein with a catheter-over-needle device.

Procedure for insertion of a central venous catheter

- The procedure is explained to the patient.
- The patient is placed head-down to distend the central veins (this facilitates cannulation and minimizes the risk of air embolism).
- The skin is cleaned. Sterile precautions are taken throughout the procedure.
- Local anaesthetic (1% plain lignocaine) is injected intradermally to raise a weal at the apex of a triangle formed by the two heads of sternomastoid with the clavicle at its base.
- A small incision is made through the weal.
- The cannula is inserted through the incision and directed laterally downwards and backwards until the vein is punctured just beneath the skin and deep to the lateral head of sternomastoid.
- It is checked that venous blood is easily aspirated using a syringe attached to the cannula.
- The cannula is threaded off the needle into the vein.
- The CVP manometer line is connected.
- If the catheter is in a large vein, venous blood will flow back when the giving-set tap is open and the infusion bottle is on the floor.
- The CVP is measured. The fluid level in the manometer should then fall rapidly and fluctuate with respiration.
- A chest x-ray should be taken to verify that the tip of the catheter is centrally placed and to exclude pneumothorax.

Possible complications

- Accidental arterial puncture (carotid or subclavian)
- Damage to thoracic duct on left
- Air embolism
- Pneumothorax
- Thrombosis
- Catheter-related sepsis

Left atrial pressure

Under most circumstances the CVP is an adequate guide to the filling pressures of both sides of the heart. However, in many critically ill patients this is not the case and there is a disparity in function between the two ventricles. Most commonly, left ventricular performance is worst, so that the left ventricular function curve is displaced downward and to the right (Fig. 13.13). This situation is encountered in some patients with clinically significant ischaemic heart disease and has also been reported in multi-system trauma, sepsis, peritonitis, hepatic failure and valvular heart disease, and after cardiac surgery. High right ventricular filling press-

Fig. 13.13 Left ventricular (LV) and right ventricular (RV) function curves in a patient with left ventricular dysfunction. Since the stroke volume of the two ventricles must be the same (except perhaps for a few beats during a period of circulatory adjustment), left atrial pressure (LAP) must be higher than right atrial pressure (RAP). Moreover, an increase in stroke volume (x) produced by a small rise in RAP (y) will be associated with a marked increase in LAP (z).

ures, with normal or low left atrial pressures, are less common but may occur in right ventricular ischaemia and in situations where the pulmonary vascular resistance (i.e. right ventricular after-load) is raised, such as acute respiratory failure.

These discrepancies between right and left ventricular performance can be exacerbated by the use of inotropic and vasoactive drugs. If there is a disparity in ventricular function after cardiac surgery then the left atrium can be cannulated directly. However, if the thorax is not open, some other means of determining left ventricular filling pressure must be devised.

Pulmonary artery pressure

A 'balloon flotation catheter' enables prompt and reliable catheterization of the pulmonary artery, without the need for screening, and minimizes the incidence of dysrhythmias.

These Swan–Ganz catheters can be inserted centrally, through the femoral vein or via a vein in the antecubital fossa. Passage of the catheter from the major veins, through the chambers of the heart, into the pulmonary artery and into the wedge position is monitored and guided by the pressure waveforms recorded from the distal lumen (Fig. 13.14). A chest x-ray should always be obtained to check the final position of the catheter. Once in place, the balloon is deflated and the pulmonary artery end-diastolic (PAEDP) and mean (PAP) pressures can be recorded. The pulmonary capillary wedge pressure (PCWP) is measured by re-inflating the balloon, thereby propelling the catheter distally until it impacts in a medium-sized pulmonary artery. In this position there is a continuous column of fluid between the distal lumen of the catheter and the left atrium, so that PCWP is usually a reflection of left atrial pressure.

The technique is generally safe—the majority of complications are related to user inexperience. Pulmonary artery catheters should preferably be removed within 48 h, since the incidence of complications then increases progressively (Table 13.2).

Cardiac output

The only quantitatively accurate methods for measuring cardiac output are invasive. Of these, the thermodilution technique is most commonly used clinically. This uses a modified Swan–Ganz catheter with a lumen opening in the right atrium and a thermistor located a few centimetres from its tip. A known volume (usually 10 ml) of ice cold 5% dextrose is injected as a bolus into the right atrium. This mixes with, and cools, the blood passing through the heart and the transient fall in temperature is continuously recorded by the thermistor in the pulmonary artery. The cardiac output is computed from the total amount of indicator (i.e. cold) injected, divided by the average concentration and the time taken to pass the thermistor.

Fig. 13.14 Passage of a Swan–Ganz catheter through the chambers of the heart into the 'wedge' position. (a) Once in the thorax, marked respiratory oscillations are seen. The catheter should be advanced further towards the lower superior vena cava/right atrium, where oscillations become more pronounced. The balloon should then be inflated and the catheter advanced. (b) When the catheter is in the right ventricle there is no dicrotic notch and the diastolic pressure is close to zero. The patient should be returned to the horizontal, or slightly head-up, position before advancing the catheter further. (c) When the catheter reaches the pulmonary artery a dicrotic notch appears and there is elevation of the diastolic pressure. The catheter should be advanced further with the balloon inflated. (d) Reappearance of a venous waveform indicates that the catheter is 'wedged'. The catheter is not advanced further. The balloon is deflated to obtain the pulmonary artery pressure. The balloon is inflated intermittently to obtain the pulmonary capillary wedge pressure.

Table 13.2 Some complications of Swan–Ganz catheters.

Complication	Comments
Dysrhythmias	May occur during passage of catheter through right ventricle Usually benign Can often be prevented with lignocaine
Sepsis	May occur at insertion site Septicaemia or endocarditis may develop
Knotting	May occur when catheter coils in right ventricle
Valve trauma	Occurs if catheter withdrawn with balloon inflated or due to valves repeatedly closing on catheter
Thrombosis/embolism	
Pulmonary infarction	May occur if catheter remains in 'wedge' position
Pulmonary artery rupture	Usually fatal May occur if balloon is inflated when catheter already 'wedged'
Balloon rupture/leak/embolism	

MANAGEMENT

A patent airway must be maintained and oxygen is given. If necessary, an oropharyngeal airway or an endotracheal tube is inserted. The latter has the advantage of preventing aspiration of gastric contents. *Very rarely* emergency tracheostomy is indicated (see below).

Pain relief is usually required. Because muscle blood flow is reduced, an opiate should be administered intravenously in small, divided doses (e.g. papaveretum 5 mg i.v.).

The underlying cause of shock should be corrected, e.g. haemorrhage should be controlled or infection eradicated.

Whatever the aetiology of the haemodynamic abnormality, tissue blood flow must be restored by achieving and maintaining an adequate cardiac output, as well as ensuring that arterial blood pressure is sufficient to maintain perfusion of vital organs.

Pre-load and volume replacement

Optimizing pre-load is the most efficient way of increasing cardiac output. Volume replacement is obviously essential in hypovolaemic shock but it is also required in anaphylactic and septic shock because of vasodilatation, sequestration of blood and loss of circulating volume due to capillary leak. Low-output, high-resistance septic shock is usually the result of hypovolaemia; rarely, myocardial failure occurs later in the course of septicaemia. Thus,

patients with sepsis will often respond well to expansion of the circulating volume, and are thereby frequently converted to a high-output, low-resistance state.

In obstructive shock, high filling pressures may be required to maintain an adequate stroke volume. Even in cardiogenic shock, careful volume expansion may, on occasions, lead to a useful increase in cardiac output. On the other hand, patients with severe cardiac failure in whom ventricular filling pressures may be markedly elevated may benefit from measures to reduce pre-load (and after-load) such as the administration of diuretics and vasodilators (see below).

The circulating volume must be replaced quickly (in minutes not hours) to reduce tissue damage and prevent acute renal failure. Fluid is administered via wide-bore intravenous cannulas to allow large volumes to be given quickly.

Care must be taken to prevent volume overload, which leads to cardiac dilatation, a reduction in stroke volume, and a rise in left atrial pressure with a risk of pulmonary oedema. Pulmonary oedema is more likely in very ill patients because of a low colloid osmotic pressure (usually due to a low serum albumin) and disruption of the pulmonary capillary endothelium (e.g. in adult respiratory distress syndrome; see p. 647). The development of pulmonary oedema can also be influenced by other unquantifiable factors, such as the hydrostatic and oncotic pressures within the interstitial spaces. Since the pulmonary lymphatics remove excess fluid, pulmonary oedema will only occur when this mechanism is overwhelmed or impaired. Left ventricular filling pressures should therefore not be allowed to rise to more than 15–18 mmHg in the critically ill. In general, however, many more patients are under-rather than over-transfused.

Choice of fluid for volume replacement
Blood. This is conventionally given for haemorrhagic shock as soon as it is available. In extreme emergencies, uncross-matched group O negative blood can be used, but an emergency cross-match can be performed in about 30 min and is as safe as the standard procedure. Donor blood is often separated into its various components for storage, necessitating the transfusion of packed red cells to maintain haemoglobin and plasma, or a plasma substitute, for volume replacement.

Complications of blood transfusion are discussed on p. 292. Special problems arise when large volumes of stored blood are transfused rapidly. These include:

- *Temperature changes.* Bank blood is stored at 4°C and transfusion may result in: hypothermia, peripheral venoconstriction, which slows the rate of the infusion, and dysrhythmias. Therefore blood should be warmed if possible prior to the transfusion.
- *Coagulopathy.* Stored blood has essentially no effective platelets and is deficient in clotting factors. Large transfusions can therefore produce a coagulation defect. This should be treated by replacing clotting factors with fresh frozen plasma and the administration of platelet concentrates.
- *Metabolic acidosis/alkalosis.* Stored blood is now preserved in citrate/phosphate/dextrose (CPD) solution, which is less acidic than the acid/citrate/dextrose (ACD) solution used previously. Metabolic acidosis attributable solely to blood transfusion is rare. A metabolic alkalosis often develops 24–48 h after a large blood transfusion, probably mainly due to metabolism of the citrate; this will be exacerbated if the preceding acidosis has been corrected with intravenous sodium bicarbonate.
- *Hypocalcaemia.* Stored blood is anticoagulated with citrate, which binds calcium ions. This can reduce total body ionized calcium levels and cause myocardial depression. This is uncommon in practice, but if necessary can be corrected by administering 10 ml of 10% calcium chloride intravenously.
- *Increased oxygen affinity.* In stored blood, the red cell 2,3-DPG content is reduced, so that the oxyhaemoglobin dissociation curve is shifted to the left. The oxygen affinity of haemoglobin is therefore increased and oxygen delivery is impaired. This effect is less marked with blood stored in CPD. Red cell levels of 2,3-DPG are

substantially restored within 12 h of transfusion.
- *Hyperkalaemia.* Potassium in the plasma rises progressively as blood is stored. However, hyperkalaemia is rarely a problem as pre-warming of the blood increases red cell metabolism —the sodium pump becomes active and potassium levels fall.
- *Microembolism.* Microaggregates in stored blood may be filtered out by the pulmonary capillaries. This process is thought by some to contribute to the adult respiratory distress syndrome.

Because of these problems, the use of crystalloid solutions, plasma, plasma substitutes and oxygen-carrying solutions for volume replacement is assuming greater importance.

Crystalloid solutions. Although crystalloid solutions, e.g. saline, are cheap, convenient to use and free of side-effects, the administration of large volumes of these fluids to critically ill patients should, in general, be avoided. They are rapidly lost from the circulation into the extravascular spaces and volumes of crystalloid two to four times that of colloid are required to achieve an equivalent haemodynamic response.

Colloidal solutions. These produce a greater, and more sustained increase in plasma volume, with associated improvements in cardiovascular function and oxygen transport. They also increase colloid osmotic pressure.

Plasma protein fraction (PPF), a natural colloid which is isotonic with plasma, is now widely available, although expensive. In normal subjects it will expand the circulating volume by an amount roughly equivalent to the volume infused. It has a half-life in the circulation of 15–17 days, although this is considerably reduced in those with increased capillary permeability. It has the same sodium content as plasma. Anaphylactoid reactions are rare (< 1% of cases). PPF should not generally be used for routine volume replacement since other cheaper solutions are equally effective in the short term.

Dextrans are polymolecular polysaccharides in either 5% dextrose or normal saline. Low molecular weight dextran (dextran 40; mol.wt 40 000) has a powerful osmotic effect, so that fluid moves from the extravascular to the intravascular compartment, thereby expanding the circulating volume by approximately twice the volume infused. Although viscosity is reduced, this may be counterbalanced by a decrease in the flexibility of the red cells. The disadvantages of dextran 40 are that it is rapidly excreted by the kidneys, it forms a complex with fibrinogen, thereby inducing a coagulopathy, and it coats the red cell membrane so that blood must be taken for cross-matching before administering dextran.

Dextran 70 (mol.wt 70 000) is also hyperoncotic,

although less so than dextran 40, and also interferes with cross-matching. However, it has a longer half-life and is probably the most suitable dextran for routine use.

There is a small risk of allergic reactions (occur in 0.07–1.1% of cases). Normally a dose of 1.5 g dextran per kg body weight should not be exceeded because of the risk of renal damage.

Haemaccel is a gelatin solution with an average molecular weight of 35 000 which is iso-osmotic with plasma. It is cheap. Large volumes of Haemaccel can be administered since coagulation defects do not occur and it does not impair renal function. However, because it readily crosses the glomerular basement membrane, its half-life in the circulation is only 2–3 h and it can promote an osmotic diuresis. Allergic reactions occur in up to 10% of cases.

Hydroxyethyl starch (HES) has a mean molecular weight of approximately 450 000 and a half-life of about 6 h. Volume expansion is equivalent to, or slightly greater than, the volume infused. The incidence of allergic reactions is approximately 0.1%. Although more expensive than gelatins, HES is likely to prove to be a most valuable volume expander.

Oxygen-carrying blood substitutes. The ideal solution for volume replacement should have:
- An oncotic pressure similar to plasma
- A long half-life
- No adverse side-effects
- No requirement for cross-matching
- A long shelf life at room temperature
- Oxygen-carrying properties

Some progress has been made towards attaining these objectives with the development of *fluorocarbon emulsions* (e.g. Fluosol-DA); these contain HES, electrolytes and an emulsifying agent. Although they are excellent volume expanders, the disadvantage is that they have a linear oxygen dissociation curve and they therefore only contribute significantly to oxygen delivery when alveolar oxygen tension is high. A number of serious adverse reactions to Fluosol-DA have been reported.

Haemoglobin solutions also have potential as oxygen-delivering resuscitation fluids, but their use is limited by their short intravascular retention time and their high affinity for oxygen.

Myocardial contractility and inotropic agents

Myocardial contractility is impaired by hypoxaemia, severe acidosis and hypocalcaemia, as well as by some drugs (e.g. beta-blockers, antidysrhythmics and sedatives). Acidosis should only be corrected when it is severe (pH < 7.2) and is thought to be impairing cardiovascular performance. Sodium bicarbonate 8.4% should then be administered in small (50 ml) aliquots, guided by frequent acid–base measurements, until the pH is returned to a safe level. Sodium overload, marked alkalosis and a shift in the oxyhaemoglobin curve to the left are potential hazards.

If there is still no improvement in cardiac output, a myocardial stimulant may be necessary. It must be remembered, however, that all inotropes increase myocardial oxygen consumption, particularly if a tachycardia develops, and that this can lead to an imbalance between myocardial oxygen supply and demand, with the development or extension of ischaemic areas. For this reason such agents should be used with extreme caution, particularly in cardiogenic shock following myocardial infarction.

In patients with septic shock and a high cardiac output, the use of inotropic agents to increase myocardial contractility is often unnecessary and illogical. Nevertheless, when severe hypotension jeopardizes perfusion of vital organs despite adequate volume replacement, inotropic agents may be used to increase blood pressure and/or redistribute blood flow (e.g. dopamine may be used to increase renal perfusion—see below).

All inotropic agents should be administered via a large central vein and their effects carefully monitored.

The most popular of the currently available inotropes are considered here (see also p. 496).

Adrenaline

Adrenaline stimulates both alpha and beta adrenergic receptors, but at low doses beta effects seem to predominate. This produces a tachycardia, with an increase in cardiac index and a fall in peripheral resistance. At higher doses, alpha-mediated vasoconstriction develops. If this produces a useful increase in perfusion pressure, urine output may increase and renal failure may be avoided. However, as the dose is further increased, cardiac output may actually fall, accompanied by marked vasoconstriction, tachycardia and a metabolic acidosis. A reduction in renal blood flow then occurs, with oliguria and a risk of acute renal failure. Prolonged high-dose administration may eventually cause peripheral gangrene. For these reasons the minimum effective dose should be used for as short a time as possible. The addition of low-dose dopamine to the regimen may help to preserve renal function (see below). Despite its disadvantages, adrenaline remains a useful potent inotrope and is used when other agents have failed.

Noradrenaline

This is predominantly an alpha adrenergic agonist and is therefore rarely used. It is of limited value in severe hypotension associated with a low peripheral resistance. It increases after-load with dangerous consequences (see below).

Isoprenaline

This beta adrenergic stimulant has both inotropic and chronotropic effects. It reduces peripheral resistance by dilating skin and muscle blood vessels and diverts flow away from vital organs such as the kidneys. The increase in cardiac output produced by isoprenaline is mainly due to the tachycardia, and this, together with the development of dysrhythmias, seriously limits its value. There are now few indications for isoprenaline in the critically ill adult.

Dopamine

Compared with isoprenaline, this agent:

● Causes less tachycardia
● Is less dysrhythmogenic
● Has a relatively greater effect on stroke volume.

When used in low doses, the peripheral resistance falls, largely due to dilatation of the splanchnic and renal vasculature. Renal and hepatic blood flow increase, urine output and renal function are improved, and it is possible that failure of these organs is thereby prevented. At higher doses, however, dopamine causes the release of noradrenaline, and vasoconstriction occurs, causing an increased after-load and raising ventricular filling pressures. This is particularly dangerous in those with cardiac failure in whom left atrial pressure is already dangerously high. This peripheral vasoconstriction can be avoided by combining high-dose dopamine with a vasodilator such as sodium nitroprusside (see below).

Dobutamine

Dobutamine is closely related to dopamine. It:

● Has no specific effect on the renal vasculature, although urine output often increases as cardiac output and blood pressure improve
● Reduces systemic resistance and improves cardiac performance, thereby decreasing both after-load and ventricular filling pressures
● Produces a greater improvement in cardiac output than dopamine for a given increase in myocardial oxygen consumption.

For these reasons dobutamine is probably the agent of choice in patients with cardiogenic shock and cardiac failure.

Opiate antagonists

Administration of the opiate antagonist, naloxone, can improve cardiovascular function in experimental shock of various aetiologies. The beneficial haemodynamic effects of naloxone are thought to be due to antagonism of the endogenous opioid systems known to be activated in shock, resulting in an increase in sympathomedullary activity. The clinical use of naloxone is, however, seriously limited by its reversal of analgesia and arousing effects. Some of the newer opiate agonist/antagonist analgesic agents, such as nalbuphine, have been shown to improve cardiovascular performance in experimental shock.

Summary

Dopamine is the inotrope of choice in most instances, but dobutamine may be used as an alternative in patients in whom the vasoconstriction produced by higher doses of dopamine might cause potentially dangerous increases in pre-load and after-load (i.e. patients with cardiac disease and septic patients with fluid overload or myocardial failure).

Adrenaline, because of its potency, remains a useful agent in those patients unresponsive to all other measures, particularly after cardiac surgery.

Diuretic therapy (see p. 496)

Diuretics increase salt and water excretion by the kidneys, thereby decreasing ventricular filling pressure (pre-load). This is the major form of therapy in sodium retention with fluid overload.

Vasodilator therapy (see also p. 496)

In selected cases, after-load reduction may be used to increase stroke volume and decrease myocardial oxygen requirements by reducing the systolic ventricular wall tension and increasing stroke volume. Vasodilatation also decreases heart size and the diastolic ventricular wall tension so that coronary blood flow is improved. The relative magnitude of the falls in pre-load and after-load depends on the pre-existing haemodynamic disturbance, concurrent volume replacement and the agent selected (see below).

Vasodilator therapy is most beneficial in patients with cardiac failure in whom the ventricular function curve is flat (see Fig. 13.4) and falls in pre-load have only a limited effect on stroke volume. This form of treatment may therefore sometimes be useful in cardiogenic shock and in the management of patients with pulmonary oedema associated with low cardiac output. They may also be valuable in shocked patients who remain vasoconstricted and oliguric.

Such therapy is potentially dangerous and should be guided by continuous haemodynamic monitoring, including pulmonary artery catheterization or direct measurement of left atrial pressure. The circulating volume must be adequate before treatment is started. Falls in pre-load should be prevented, except in those with cardiac failure, in order to avoid serious reductions in cardiac output and blood pressure. If diastolic pressure is allowed to fall, coronary blood flow may be jeopardized and, particularly if a reflex tachycardia develops in response to the hypotension, myocardial ischaemia may be precipitated.

Alpha-adrenergic antagonists
These predominantly dilate arterioles and therefore mainly influence after-load.

Phenoxybenzamine is unsuitable for use in the critically ill because of its slow onset (1–2 h to maximum effect) and prolonged duration of action (2–3 days).

Phentolamine is very potent with a rapid onset and short duration of action (15–20 min). It can be used for short-term control of blood pressure in a hypertensive crisis, but can produce a marked tachycardia.

Vasodilators acting directly on the vessel wall
These agents are those most commonly used to achieve vasodilatation in the critically ill.

Hydrallazine. This predominantly affects arterial resistance vessels. It therefore reduces after-load and blood pressure, while cardiac output and heart rate usually increase. Hydrallazine is usually given as an intravenous bolus to control acute increases in blood pressure, particularly after cardiac surgery.

Sodium nitroprusside (SNP). This dilates arterioles and venous capacitance vessels, as well as the pulmonary vasculature. This agent therefore reduces the after-load and pre-load of both ventricles and can improve cardiac output and the myocardial oxygen supply/demand ratio. It has been suggested that SNP can exacerbate myocardial ischaemia by producing a 'steal' phenomenon in the coronary circulation.

The effects of SNP are rapid in onset and spontaneously reversible within a few minutes of discontinuing the infusion.

A large overdose of SNP can cause cyanide poisoning, with intracellular hypoxia caused by inhibition of cytochrome oxidase, the terminal enzyme of the respiratory chain. This is manifested as a metabolic acidosis and a fall in the arteriovenous oxygen content difference.

Nitroglycerine (NTG) and isosorbide dinitrate (ISDN). These are both predominantly venodilators. They can therefore cause marked reductions in pre-load, which may be associated with falls in cardiac output and compensatory vasoconstriction. For the reasons discussed above, they are of most value in those with cardiac failure in whom pre-load reduction may reduce ventricular wall tension and improve coronary perfusion without adversely affecting cardiac performance. Furthermore, these agents may reverse myocardial ischaemia by increasing and redistributing coronary blood flow. They are therefore often used in preference to SNP in patients with cardiac failure and/or myocardial ischaemia. Both NTG and ISDN reduce pulmonary vascular resistance, an effect which can occasionally be exploited in patients with a low cardiac output secondary to pulmonary hypertension.

Mechanical support of the myocardium

Intra-aortic balloon counterpulsation (IABCP) is the most widely used technique for mechanical support of the failing myocardium. It is discussed on p. 477.

The use of steroids in shock

In animal studies huge doses of steroids (e.g. methylprednisolone 30 mg·kg^{-1}) given early reduce the mortality in septic shock, possibly by inhibiting complement-induced granulocyte activation and thereby limiting damage to vital organs, especially the lungs (see adult respiratory distress syndrome, p. 647).

However the clinical use of these agents is not currently recommended.

Respiratory failure

TYPES AND CAUSES

Respiratory failure occurs when pulmonary gas exchange is sufficiently impaired to cause hypoxaemia with or without hypercarbia. In practical terms respiratory failure is present when the P_aO_2 is < 8 kPa (60 mmHg) or the P_aCO_2 is > 7 kPa (55 mmHg). It can be divided into:

- Type I respiratory failure, in which the P_aO_2 is low and the P_aCO_2 is normal or low
- Type II respiratory failure, in which the P_aO_2 is low and the P_aCO_2 is high

Type I or 'acute hypoxaemia' respiratory failure occurs with diseases which damage lung tissue, with hypoxaemia due to right to left shunts or $\dot{V}/\dot{Q}$ mismatch. Common causes include pulmonary oedema, pneumonia, adult respiratory distress syndrome and, in the chronic situation, pulmonary fibrosing alveolitis.

Type II or 'ventilatory failure' occurs when alveolar ventilation is insufficient to excrete the volume of carbon dioxide being produced by tissue metabolism. Inadequate alveolar ventilation is due to reduced ventilatory effort, inability to overcome an increased resistance to ventilation, failure to compensate for an increase in dead space and/or carbon dioxide production, or a combination of these factors. The most common cause is chronic bronchitis. Other causes include chest wall deformities, respiratory muscle weakness, e.g. Guillain–Barré syndrome, and depression of the respiratory centre.

MONITORING

A clinical assessment of respiratory distress should be made on the following criteria:
- The use of accessory muscles of respiration
- Tachypnoea
- Tachycardia
- Sweating
- Pulsus paradoxus
- Inability to speak
- Signs of carbon dioxide retention (see p. 579)

This can be supplemented by measuring tidal volume and vital capacity. Blood gas analysis should be performed to guide oxygen therapy and to provide an objective assessment of respiratory function.

The most sensitive clinical indicator of increasing respiratory difficulty is a rising respiratory rate. Tidal volume is a less sensitive indicator.

Minute ventilation rises initially in acute respiratory failure and falls precipitously only at a late stage when the patient is exhausted. Vital capacity is often a better guide to deterioration and is particularly useful in patients with respiratory inadequacy due to neuromuscular problems, e.g. the Guillain–Barré syndrome, in which the vital capacity decreases as weakness increases.

Blood gas analysis

Modern automated analysers and the ease of arterial puncture have made blood gas analysis one of the most commonly performed objective tests of respiratory function.

Automation of measurements gives a false impression of reliability and accuracy and may lead to an uncritical acceptance of the results. Errors can result from malfunction of the analyser or incorrect sampling techniques. Care must be taken over the following:
- The sample should be analysed immediately or the syringe should be immersed in iced water (the end having first been sealed with a plastic cap) to prevent the continuing metabolism of white cells causing a reduction in Po_2 and a rise in Pco_2.
- The sample must be adequately anticoagulated to prevent clot formation within the analyser. However, excessive dilution of the blood with heparin, which is acidic, will significantly reduce its pH. Heparin ($1000 \ iu \cdot ml^{-1}$) should just fill the dead space of the syringe, i.e. approximately 0.1 ml. This will adequately anticoagulate a 2 ml sample.
- Air almost inevitably enters the sample. The gas tensions within these air bubbles will equilibrate with those in the blood, thereby lowering the Pco_2 and, usually, raising the Po_2 of the sample. However, provided they are ejected immediately by inverting the syringe so that the needle is pointing upwards and expelling the air that rises

to the top of the sample, their effect is insignificant.

It is unnecessary to use glass syringes since diffusion of gases into the walls of plastic syringes is not a significant problem.

Normal values of blood gas analysis are shown in Table 13.3.

The interpretation of the results of blood gas analysis can be considered in two separate parts:
- Disturbances of acid–base balance
- Alterations in oxygenation

Interpretation of results requires a knowledge of the history, the age of the patient, the inspired oxygen concentration and any other relevant treatment (e.g. the administration of sodium bicarbonate, and the ventilator settings for those on mechanical ventilation).

Disturbances of acid–base balance
The physiology of acid–base control is discussed on pp. 442–446. Acid–base disturbances can be described in relation to the diagram illustrated in Fig. 10.9 (see p. 443) which shows arterial Pco_2 plotted against hydrogen ion concentration.

Both acidosis and alkalosis can occur, each of which may be either metabolic (primarily affecting the bicarbonate component of the system) or respiratory (primarily affecting Pco_2). Compensatory changes may also be apparent. In clinical practice arterial $[H^+]$ values outside the range 18–$126 \ nmol \cdot l^{-1}$ (pH 6.9–7.7) are very rarely encountered.

Respiratory acidosis. This is caused by retention of carbon dioxide. The P_aco_2 and $[H^+]$ rise. A chronically raised P_aco_2 is compensated for by renal retention of bicarbonate and the $[H^+]$ returns towards normal. A constant arterial bicarbonate concentration is then usually established within 2–5 days. This represents a primary respiratory acidosis with a compensatory metabolic alkalosis (see p. 446). Common causes of respiratory acidosis include ventilatory failure and chronic bronchitis and emphysema (type II respiratory failure where there is a high P_aco_2 and a low P_ao_2—see Chapter 12).

Respiratory alkalosis. In this case the reverse occurs

Table 13.3 Normal values for measurements obtained when blood gas analysis is performed.

H^+	35–$45 \ nmol \cdot l^{-1}$	(pH 7.35–7.45)
Po_2	10–$13.3 \ kPa$	(75–100 mmHg)
Pco_2	4.8–$6.1 \ kPa$	(36–46 mmHg)
Plasma HCO_3^-	22–$26 \ mmol \cdot l^{-1}$	
O_2 saturation	95–100%	

and there is a fall in $P_a\text{CO}_2$ and $[\text{H}^+]$, often with a small reduction in bicarbonate concentration. If hypocarbia persists, some degree of renal compensation may occur, producing a metabolic acidosis, although in practice this is unusual. A respiratory alkalosis is often produced, intentionally or unintentionally, when patients are artificially ventilated; it may also be seen with hypoxaemic (type I) respiratory failure (see Chapter 12) and in those living at high altitudes.

Metabolic acidosis. This may be due to excessive acid production, most commonly lactic acid during an episode of shock or following cardiac arrest. Another common cause is diabetic ketoacidosis. A metabolic acidosis may also develop in chronic renal failure and following the loss of large amounts of alkali, e.g. from the lower gastrointestinal tract or in renal tubular acidosis.

Respiratory compensation for a metabolic acidosis is usually slightly delayed because the blood/brain barrier initially prevents the respiratory centre from sensing the increased blood $[\text{H}^+]$. Following this short delay, however, the patient hyperventilates and 'blows off' carbon dioxide to produce a compensatory respiratory alkalosis. There is a limit to this respiratory compensation since values for $P_a\text{CO}_2$ less than about 1.5 kPa (11 mmHg) are, in practice, never achieved. It should also be noted that respiratory compensation cannot occur if the patient's ventilation is controlled.

Metabolic alkalosis. This can be caused by loss of acid, e.g. from the stomach with nasogastric suction or in high intestinal obstruction, or excessive administration of absorbable alkali. Over-zealous treatment with intravenous sodium bicarbonate is frequently implicated. Some less common causes of metabolic alkalosis include hyperaldosteronism, Cushing's syndrome, ingestion of liquorice and severe potassium deficiency.

Respiratory compensation for a metabolic alkalosis is often slight and it is rare to encounter a $P_a\text{CO}_2 > 6.5$ kPa (50 mmHg), even with severe alkalosis.

Alterations in oxygenation
When interpreting the P_O_2 it is important to remember that it is the oxygen content of the arterial blood that matters and that this is determined by the percentage saturation of haemoglobin with oxygen. The relationship between the latter and the P_O_2 is determined by the oxyhaemoglobin dissociation curve. In general, if the saturation is greater than 90%, oxygenation can be considered to be adequate. However, it must be remembered that on the steep portion of the oxygen dissociation curve, small falls in $P_a\text{O}_2$ will cause significant reductions in oxygen content. $P_a\text{O}_2$ is also influenced by factors other than pulmonary function, including alterations in $P_{\bar{v}}\text{O}_2$ caused by changes in the metabolic rate and/or cardiac output.

MANAGEMENT OF RESPIRATORY FAILURE

Conventional management of patients with respiratory failure includes the administration of supplemental oxygen, the control of secretions, the treatment of pulmonary infection, the control of bronchospasm and measures to limit pulmonary oedema.

Oxygen therapy

Methods of oxygen administration
Oxygen is initially given via a face mask. In the majority of patients (except patients with chronic bronchitis and chronically elevated $P_a\text{CO}_2$) the concentration of oxygen given is not important and oxygen can therefore be given by a simple face mask or nasal cannula (Fig. 13.15). With these devices the inspired oxygen concentration varies from about 35% to 55%, with oxygen flow rates of between 6 and 10 $\text{l}\cdot\text{min}^{-1}$. Nasal cannulas are often preferred

Fig. 13.15 Methods of administering supplemental oxygen to the unintubated patient. (a) Simple face-mask. (b) Nasal cannulas.

because they are less claustrophobic and do not interfere with feeding or speaking, but they can cause ulceration of the nasal or pharyngeal mucosa. Fig. 13.15 should be compared with the fixed performance mask shown in Fig. 12. 23 (see p. 582) with which the oxygen concentration can be controlled. It is vital to use this latter type of mask in patients with chronic bronchitis and emphysema with chronic type II failure.

Oxygen toxicity

Experimentally, mammalian lungs have been shown to be damaged by continuous exposure to high concentrations of oxygen; oxygen toxicity in humans is less well proven. Nevertheless, it is reasonable to assume that high concentrations of oxygen might damage the lungs and so the lowest inspired oxygen concentration compatible with adequate arterial oxygenation should be used. Long-term administration of 50% oxygen or less, or of 100% oxygen for less than 24 h, is probably safe. *Dangerous hypoxia should never be tolerated through a fear of oxygen toxicity.*

Respiratory support

If despite the above measures the patient continues to deteriorate or fails to improve, the institution of some form of respiratory support should be considered.

The various techniques of respiratory support currently available are shown in Table 13.4.

Negative pressure ventilation

'Tank' ventilators were at one time widely used for the treatment of ventilatory failure complicating polio, and are still occasionally employed for long-term ventilation of patients with chronic respiratory failure due to neuromuscular disease or skeletal deformity. The patient's body is enclosed in an airtight 'tank' within which a negative pressure is created intermittently by a separate pump. Cuirass ventilators encase only the thorax.

Intermittent positive pressure ventilation (IPPV)

IPPV has a number of important advantages over negative pressure ventilation. In particular the air-way is secured and protected and secretions can be aspirated more easily. In addition, IPPV can be used more successfully in those with diseases involving the lung parenchyma. Furthermore, access to and movement of the patient is relatively unrestricted.

In recent years a number of refinements and modifications of IPPV have been described, including intermittent mandatory ventilation (IMV), and IPPV with positive end-expiratory pressure (PEEP) (sometimes known as continuous positive pressure ventilation; CPPV). These will be discussed later in this chapter.

The rational use of IPPV depends on a clear understanding of its potential beneficial effects, as well as its dangers.

Beneficial effects. These include:
- *Improved carbon dioxide elimination.* By adjusting the volume of ventilation, the $P_a\text{CO}_2$ can be returned to within normal limits.
- *Relief from exhaustion.* Artificial ventilation removes the work of breathing and relieves the extreme exhaustion which may be present in patients with respiratory failure. In some cases, if ventilation is not instituted, this exhaustion may culminate in respiratory arrest.
- *Effects on oxygenation.* In those with severe pulmonary parenchymal disease the lungs may be very stiff and the work of breathing is therefore greatly increased. Under these circumstances the institution of IPPV may significantly reduce total body oxygen consumption; consequently $P_{\bar{v}}\text{O}_2$, and thus $P_a\text{O}_2$, may improve. Because ventilated patients are connected to a leak-free circuit it is possible to administer high concentrations of oxygen (up to 100%) accurately and to apply a positive end-expiratory pressure. In selected cases the latter may reduce shunting and increase $P_a\text{O}_2$ (see below).

Indications. IPPV is instituted in acute hypoxaemic respiratory failure if the clinical signs of severe respiratory distress (e.g. respiratory rate > 40 per minute, inability to speak) persist despite maximal treatment and the patient appears exhausted. If there is confusion, a decreased conscious level, and a

Table 13.4 Techniques for respiratory support.

Technique	Comments
Negative pressure ventilation	Performed using a tank or cuirass ventilator
Intermittent positive pressure ventilation (IPPV)	Given with: zero end-expiratory pressure (ZEEP), negative end-expiratory pressure (NEEP), or positive end-expiratory pressure (PEEP)
Intermittent mandatory ventilation (IMV)	Given with ZEEP or PEEP
Continuous positive airway pressure (CPAP)	Given via an endotracheal tube or mask
High frequency jet ventilation (HFJV)	

rising $P_a\text{co}_2$ and/or extreme hypoxaemia ($P_a\text{o}_2 <$ 8 kPa) despite oxygen therapy, artificial ventilation is indicated. By this stage bedside tests of ventilation are rarely helpful.

Similar criteria for instituting IPPV are used in patients with acute exacerbations of chronic bronchitis and emphysema, combined with an assessment of the severity and nature of the underlying chronic lung disease. The patient's previous exercise tolerance and ability to lead an independent existence are perhaps the most important considerations. Those who were severely incapacitated before the acute episode will be extremely difficult to wean from the ventilator, and even if this is achieved they are unlikely to recover sufficiently to attain a reasonable lifestyle; early relapse is then to be expected. On the other hand, artificial ventilation is clearly indicated when a patient who was previously leading an active life deteriorates as a result of a potentially reversible process (e.g. infection with sputum retention or bronchospasm).

In contrast, with ventilatory failure, due for example to myasthenia gravis or Guillain–Barré syndrome, the need for artificial ventilation is influenced more by the results of bedside tests of ventilation, in particular the vital capacity, than by clinical assessment. Normally, artificial ventilation should be instituted in these patients when the vital capacity has fallen to less than 10–15 ml·kg^{-1}, since this may reduce the incidence of complications such as atelectasis and infection, as well as preventing unexpected respiratory arrest. Tidal volume and respiratory rate, on the other hand, are relatively insensitive indicators of the need for artificial ventilation in those with ventilatory failure because they change only late in the course of the disease. A high $P\text{co}_2$, particularly if it is rising, is generally an indication for urgent artificial ventilation.

Artificial ventilation may also be used to prevent deterioration to respiratory failure in susceptible patients. For example, prophylactic postoperative IPPV is now a well-established practice in poor-risk patients in whom some degree of respiratory failure is likely.

In patients with acute brain swelling, e.g. following severe head injury, it is most important to avoid hypercarbia and/or hypoxia, since both will increase intracranial blood volume, exacerbate cerebral oedema and cause a rise in intracranial pressure. Furthermore, elective hyperventilation, even in the absence of respiratory failure, can temporarily decrease cerebral blood flow and, secondarily, intracranial pressure. The value of such treatment, however, remains uncertain.

Institution. IPPV requires endotracheal intubation. If the patient is conscious the procedure must be fully explained before anaesthesia is induced. Intubating patients in severe respiratory failure is an extremely hazardous undertaking and *should only be performed by experienced staff.* In extreme emergencies it may be preferable to ventilate the patient by hand using an oropharyngeal airway, a face mask and a self-inflating bag until experienced help arrives. The patient is usually hypoxic and hypercarbic, with increased sympathetic activity, and the stimulus of laryngoscopy and intubation can precipitate dangerous arrhythmias and even cardiac arrest. If possible, therefore, the ECG should be monitored, and the patient pre-oxygenated with 100% oxygen before intubation. In some deeply comatose patients, no sedation will be required, but in the majority of patients a short-acting intravenous anaesthetic agent followed by muscle relaxation will be necessary.

The complications of endotracheal intubation are given in Table 13.5.

Endotracheal tubes can now be safely left in place for several weeks and tracheostomy is therefore less often performed. Tracheostomy may be required for the long-term control of excessive bronchial secretions, particularly in those with a reduced conscious level, and/or to maintain an airway and protect the lungs in those with impaired pharyngeal and laryngeal reflexes.

The only indication for immediate tracheostomy is a life-threatening obstruction of the upper respiratory tract which cannot be bypassed with an endotracheal tube. However, tracheostomy performed under these circumstances can be extremely hazardous. Other indications are patients with head and neck injuries, including burns to the face and upper airway.

Tracheostomy has a mortality rate of up to 3%. Complications of tracheostomy are shown in Table 13.6.

Dangers of IPPV. General dangers include:
- Complications inherent in endotracheal intubation or tracheostomy
- Disconnection or mechanical failure. These are unusual but dangerous. A method of manual ventilation, e.g. a self-inflating bag, must always be available by the bedside.
- Barotrauma. Overdistension of the lungs during IPPV can rupture alveoli and cause air to dissect centrally along the perivascular sheaths. This pulmonary interstitial air can sometimes be seen on chest x-ray as linear or circular perivascular collections or subpleural blebs. Other complications are pneumothorax, pneumomediastinum, pneumoperitoneum and subcutaneous emphysema. Intra-abdominal air originating from the alveoli is probably always associated with pneumomediastinum.

The incidence of barotrauma is greatest in those patients who require high inflation pressures, with or without a positive end-expiratory pressure, and the risk of pneumothorax is increased in those with destructive lung disease (e.g. staphylococcal

Table 13.5 Complications of endotracheal intubation.

Complication	Comments
Immediate	
Tube in one or other bronchi (usually the right)	Avoid by checking both lungs are being inflated, i.e. both sides of the chest move and air entry is heard on auscultation. X-ray to check position of tube and to exclude lung collapse.
Tube in oesophagus	Gives rise to hypoxia and abdominal distension.
Early	
Migration of the tube out of trachea	
Leaks around the tube	
Obstruction of tube due to kinking or secretions	A dangerous complication. The patient becomes distressed, cyanosed and has poor chest expansion. The following should be performed immediately:
	— Manual inflation with 100% oxygen
	— Endotracheal suction
	— Check position of tube
	— Deflate cuff
	— Check tube for 'kinks'
	If no improvement, change the endotracheal tube.
Late	
Mucosal oedema and ulceration	
Damage to the cricoarytenoid cartilages	
Tracheal narrowing and fibrosis	

Table 13.6 Complications of tracheostomy.

As for endotracheal intubation (Table 13.5), plus:

Early
Surgical complications
    Pneumothorax
    Haemorrhage
Tube misplaced in pretracheal subcutaneous tissues
Subcutaneous emphysema

Intermediate
Erosion of tracheal cartilages, leading to fatal
    haemorrhage from the innominate artery or to a
    tracheo-oesophageal fistula
Infection

Late
Tracheal stenosis at level of stoma, cuff or tube tip
Collapse of tracheal rings at level of stoma

pneumonia, emphysema), asthma or fractured ribs.

A tension pneumothorax can be rapidly fatal in ventilated patients with respiratory failure. Suggestive signs include the development or worsening of hypoxia, fighting the ventilator, an unexplained increase in inflation pressure, and hypotension and tachycardia, sometimes accompanied by a rising CVP. Examination may reveal unequal chest expansion, mediastinal shift (deviated trachea, displaced apex beat) and a hyperresonant hemithorax. Although, traditionally, breath sounds are diminished over the pneumothorax, this sign can be extremely misleading in ventilated patients. If there is time, the diagnosis can be confirmed by chest x-ray.

Other dangers of IPPV include:
- *Respiratory complications.* Patients ventilated with small tidal volumes become progressively more

hypoxic. This is probably due to collapse of peripheral alveoli and can be largely prevented by using large tidal volumes ($10–15$ ml·kg^{-1}) and reducing the respiratory rate to avoid hypocarbia.

Secondary pulmonary infection is a common and ominous complication of IPPV.

- *Cardiovascular complications.* The intermittent application of positive pressure to the lungs and thoracic wall impedes venous return and distends alveoli, thereby 'stretching' the pulmonary capillaries and causing a rise in pulmonary vascular resistance. Both these mechanisms can produce a fall in cardiac output. Recently it has been suggested that this may be exacerbated by a reduction in myocardial contractility caused by humoral or reflex mechanisms and possibly impaired coronary perfusion.

In normal subjects, the fall in cardiac output is prevented by the constriction of capacitance vessels which restores venous return. Hypovolaemia, pre-existing pulmonary hypertension, right ventricular failure and autonomic dysfunction (as may be present in those with Guillain–Barré syndrome, acute spinal cord injury or diabetes) will exacerbate the haemodynamic disturbance. Expansion of the circulating volume, on the other hand, can often restore cardiac output.

In patients with heart failure, a paradoxical rise in blood pressure and cardiac output may occur in response to positive pressure ventilation. This may be due to reversal of hypoxia and a reduction in oxygen consumption, both of which will reduce the burden on a failing heart. A further possible benefit in those with cardiac failure is that a reduction in pre-load will reduce ventricular wall tension, allowing increased coronary blood flow and improved myocardial function. Moreover, when the ventricular function curve is flat, the fall in pre-load has little effect on stroke volume, whilst stiff lungs limit the transmission of high inflation pressures to the great veins and pulmonary capillaries. Therefore IPPV should be used without hesitation in patients with cardiogenic pulmonary oedema who have severe respiratory distress and exhaustion.

- *Gastrointestinal complications.* Initially many artificially ventilated patients will develop abdominal distension associated with an ileus. The cause is unknown, although the use of non-depolarizing neuromuscular blocking agents may be in part responsible.

- *Salt and water retention.* IPPV, particularly with positive end-expiratory pressure, causes increased ADH secretion and this, combined with a fall in cardiac output and a reduction in renal cortical blood flow, can cause salt and water retention leading to interstitial oedema. This fluid retention is often particularly noticeable in the lungs, possibly because IPPV interferes with pulmonary lymphatic drainage.

Selection of the pattern of ventilation. The aim is to achieve optimal gas exchange while minimizing adverse effects on the cardiovascular system.

The duration of the inspiratory phase must be sufficient to allow adequate gas distribution to all distal lung segments; inspiration should therefore last for between 1.5 and 2.0 s. In order to minimize the fall in cardiac output, expiration should take at least twice as long as inspiration and both inflation and deflation should be relatively rapid. The influence of the shape of the inspiratory waveform on the efficiency of gas exchange is less certain.

In order to minimize the fall in cardiac output which occurs with IPPV it was suggested that the application of a *negative end-expiratory pressure* (NEEP) might increase venous return and restore cardiac output. Although this is in fact the case, NEEP also causes progressive alveolar collapse and hypoxaemia and so is rarely indicated.

IPPV with *zero end-expiratory pressure* (ZEEP) may improve oxygenation by re-expanding collapsed alveoli, improving gas distribution and reducing oxygen requirements. In order to prevent progressive alveolar collapse, large tidal volumes of $10–15$ ml·kg^{-1} should be used (see above).

IPPV with *positive end-expiratory pressure* (PEEP) should be considered if it proves impossible to achieve adequate oxygenation of arterial blood (more than 90% saturation) using conventional positive pressure ventilation without raising the inspired oxygen concentration to potentially dangerous levels (conventionally $> 50\%$). PEEP is not, however, a panacea for all patients who are hypoxic and indeed it may often be detrimental, not least because the use of levels of PEEP in excess of 5 cmH$_2$O is associated with an increased risk of barotrauma.

The primary effect of PEEP is to re-expand underventilated lung units. Provided that hypoxaemia is due to airway closure, this will reduce the shunt and increase the $P_a\text{O}_2$.

Unfortunately, the inevitable rise in mean intrathoracic pressure which follows the application of PEEP may further impede venous return, increase pulmonary vascular resistance and thus reduce cardiac output. This effect is probably least when the lungs are stiff. Moreover, the rise in pulmonary vascular resistance may be associated with dilatation of the right ventricle and distortion of the left ventricular cavity by the displaced interventricular septum. This is thought to restrict left ventricular filling and reduce stroke volume. The fall in cardiac output can be ameliorated by expanding the circulating volume, and in some cases inotropic support may be required. Thus, although arterial oxygenation is often improved by the application of PEEP, a simultaneous fall in cardiac output can lead to a reduction in total oxygen delivery.

The net effect of PEEP in an individual patient is therefore often unpredictable and is dependent on a balance of several factors. The most beneficial effects occur in those patients with large shunts due to alveolar collapse, stiff lungs, and good cardiovascular function, e.g. a young, fit patient with the adult respiratory distress syndrome (see p. 647). However, in patients with normal or high lung volumes, compliant lungs and only a modest degree of shunting, any improvement in P_aO_2 may be negated by the fall in cardiac output, particularly in those with poor cardiovascular function. Thus, PEEP should not be used in patients with emphysema or asthma and is usually of little benefit in those with fibrotic lung disease or bacterial pneumonia. Furthermore, in patients with only localized areas of diseased lung (e.g. unilateral aspiration pneumonia), PEEP may adversely affect oxygenation by overexpanding normal lung tissue and diverting blood to underventilated lung units.

Other techniques for respiratory support

Continuous positive airway pressure (CPAP). The application of CPAP achieves for the spontaneously breathing patient what PEEP does for the ventilated patient. Oxygen and air are delivered under pressure via an endotracheal tube or occasionally via a tightly fitted face-mask. Not only can it improve oxygenation but the lungs become less stiff, breathing becomes easier and vital capacity improves.

Intermittent mandatory ventilation (IMV). This technique allows the patient to breathe spontaneously between the 'mandatory' tidal volumes delivered by the ventilator. Most modern ventilators will time these mandatory breaths to coincide with the patient's own inspiratory effort (synchronized IMV; SIMV). IMV can be used with or without PEEP or CPAP. It was originally introduced as a technique for weaning patients from artificial ventilation but is increasingly being used as an alternative to conventional IPPV.

High frequency jet ventilation (HFJV). Adequate oxygenation and CO_2 elimination can be achieved by injecting gas into the trachea at rates of up to several thousand breaths per minute. In clinical practice rates of between 60 and 300 breaths per minute are usually employed.

Potential advantages of HFJV are largely related to the low peak airway pressures; thus cardiac output is maintained and the risk of barotrauma is negligible. Moreover, HFJV can be used to ventilate patients with large air leaks due, for example, to a bronchopleural fistula or lung lacerations. The place of HFJV in the management of patients with acute respiratory failure is less clear.

Weaning

It is important to discontinue artificial ventilation, and, if possible, to extubate the patient as soon as possible. On the other hand, premature attempts at weaning may be dangerous and can adversely affect the morale of conscious patients.

Because they perform no work during conventional mechanical ventilation, the respiratory muscles eventually become weak and uncoordinated. Moreover, there is usually some persisting abnormality of lung function. Thus, in patients who have been artificially ventilated for any length of time, spontaneous respiration usually has to be resumed gradually.

Criteria for weaning patients from artificial ventilation. Clinical assessment is of paramount importance when deciding whether a patient can be weaned from the ventilator. The patient's conscious level, psychological state, metabolic function, the effects of drugs, cardiovascular performance, and mechanical factors must all be taken into account. Objective criteria are based on an assessment of pulmonary gas exchange (blood gas analysis), lung mechanics and muscular strength.

Techniques for weaning. Patients who have received artificial ventilation for less than 24 h, e.g. elective IPPV after major surgery, can usually resume spontaneous respiration immediately and no weaning process is required. This procedure can also be adopted for those who have been ventilated for longer periods but who clearly fulfil the criteria for weaning outlined above.

The traditional method of weaning in difficult cases is to allow the patient to breathe entirely spontaneously for a short time, following which IPPV is reinstituted. The periods of spontaneous breathing are gradually increased and the periods of IPPV are reduced. Initially it is usually advisable to ventilate the patient throughout the night. This method has several practical disadvantages: during the period of spontaneous respiration the patient may develop progressive hypoxia and/or hypercarbia as well as an increasing sympathetic drive, resulting in tachycardia and hypertension. After a predetermined period, or earlier if tachypnoea and exhaustion develop, the patient is reconnected to IPPV. At this time, respiratory drive is high, synchronization with the ventilator is difficult and heavy sedation may be required. It is then necessary to wait until the effects of these drugs have worn off before trying another period of spontaneous respiration. This method is stressful and tiring both for patients and staff. However, some patients do not tolerate IMV (see below) and this method of weaning may then be necessary.

The above disadvantages may be overcome by using IMV. This provides a smoother, more controlled method of weaning; it may also enable weaning to commence at an earlier stage than is possible using the conventional method. There is no evidence, however, that IMV enables patients who could not be weaned using conventional methods to resume spontaneous respiration, and in some cases the weaning process may be unnecessarily prolonged.

The application of CPAP can prevent the alveolar collapse, hypoxaemia and fall in compliance which may otherwise occur when patients start to breathe spontaneously. It is therefore often used during weaning with IMV and in spontaneously breathing patients prior to extubation, particularly when they were previously receiving IPPV with PEEP.

Extubation. This should not be considered until the patient can cough, swallow, protect his own airway and is sufficiently alert to be cooperative. Patients who fulfil these criteria can be extubated provided their respiratory function has improved sufficiently to sustain spontaneous ventilation indefinitely. This is often difficult to assess and is usually largely based on the patient's ability to breathe spontaneously via the endotracheal tube over a period of time. In those who have undergone prolonged artificial ventilation, this period may need to be 24–48 h, or even longer, while patients ventilated for less than 12–24 h can often be extubated within 10–15 minutes. During this 'trial of spontaneous respiration' the patient should be closely observed for any signs of respiratory distress.

ADULT RESPIRATORY DISTRESS SYNDROME (ARDS)

DEFINITION AND CAUSES

This syndrome was originally described in 1967 as acute respiratory distress in adults characterized by severe dyspnoea, tachypnoea, cyanosis refractory to oxygen therapy, loss of lung compliance and diffuse alveolar infiltrates seen on the chest x-ray. ARDS can therefore be defined as diffuse pulmonary infiltrates, refractory hypoxaemia and respiratory distress. A PCWP less than 16 mmHg is often included in the definition in an attempt to exclude cardiogenic pulmonary oedema. ARDS can occur as a non-specific reaction of the lungs to a wide variety of insults, including shock (especially septic shock), fat embolism, trauma, burns, pancreatitis, cardiopulmonary bypass, lung contusion, inhalation of smoke or toxic gases, Goodpasture's syndrome, amniotic fluid embolism and aspiration pneumonia. Superadded infection is a common feature of ARDS.

PATHOPHYSIOLOGY

Non-cardiogenic pulmonary oedema

This is the main feature of ARDS and is associated with an increased pulmonary capillary permeability. This can be partly explained by the microcirculatory stasis and disseminated intravascular coagulation which can occur in shock, as well as the effects of activated platelets and blood coagulation products. A number of vasoactive substances (histamine, 5-HT, prostaglandins) are released in shock, and some of these can cause platelet aggregation and increased capillary permeability. However, the loss of pulmonary capillary integrity is currently thought to be largely caused by polymorphonuclear leucocytes which have been stimulated by activated complement. It is possible that the capillary endothelium is then damaged by toxic oxygen radicals produced by these activated cells. For example, the free radical superoxide ($O_2^{\bullet-}$) can participate in a number of chemical reactions, yielding hydrogen peroxide (H_2O_2) and hydroxyl radicals ($OH^{\bullet-}$). These can damage cell membranes and interfere with the function of a number of enzyme systems. This may be valuable when directed against bacteria but detrimental when capillary endothelium is the target.

Pulmonary hypertension

This is a common feature of ARDS. Initially, mechanical obstruction of the pulmonary circulation may occur as a result of vascular compression by interstitial oedema and subsequently oedema of the vessel wall itself. Later, constriction of the pulmonary vasculature may develop in response to increased autonomic nervous activity and circulating substances such as catecholamines, 5-HT, thromboxane, fibrin/fibrinogen degradation products, complement and activated leucocytes. Those vessels supplying alveoli with low oxygen tensions constrict (the 'hypoxic vasoconstrictor response'), diverting pulmonary blood flow to better oxygenated areas of lung, thus limiting the degree of shunt. In some patients with ARDS and pulmonary hypertension, angiography will reveal 'beading' of the arterioles and peripheral 'pruning' of the pulmonary vasculature. This suggests fibrin deposition and is associated with a marked increase in dead space and a poor prognosis, despite attempts to reverse the process using heparin and streptokinase. In this situation, subpleural lung segments are infarcted but continue to be ventilated and are therefore liable to rupture. In others, angiography is normal, pulmonary hypertension is absent, and in these the 'wet lung' usually responds to dehydration and respiratory support.

Hyaline membranes

These are seen microscopically in the lungs of patients with ARDS and consist of necrotic type I pneumocytes and coagulated intra-alveolar proteins derived from the pulmonary exudate.

Fibrosis

Within 7 days of the onset of ARDS, activated fibroblasts are seen in the interstitial spaces. Subsequently, interstitial fibrosis progresses, with loss of elastic tissue and obliteration of the lung vasculature. These changes are probably irreversible, although lung function often returns virtually to normal in patients who recover from ARDS, particularly in the young and non-smokers; residual x-ray changes are usually limited to a few linear scars.

CLINICAL PRESENTATION

The first sign of the development of ARDS is often an unexplained tachypnoea, followed by increasing hypoxaemia. Later, the chest x-ray shows bilateral, diffuse shadowing with an alveolar pattern and air bronchograms which may then progress to the picture of complete 'white-out'.

MANAGEMENT

This is based on treatment of the underlying condition (e.g. eradication of sepsis), and supportive measures such as oxygen, CPAP, and IPPV/IMV with PEEP. Oedema formation should be minimized by controlling left atrial pressure and, if possible, maintaining plasma proteins, particularly albumin, close to the normal range. However, once plasma enters the interstitial space, the transvascular oncotic gradient disappears and the main determinants of interstitial oedema formation become the microvascular hydrostatic pressure and lymphatic drainage. There is therefore some controversy concerning the relative merits of colloids or crystalloids for volume replacement in patients likely to develop ARDS, or in whom the condition is established. Cardiovascular support and the reduction of oxygen requirements are also important.

There is some evidence to suggest that the early administration of high-dose steroids to those at risk may prevent, or limit, the severity of pulmonary damage, but the use of these agents remains controversial.

PROGNOSIS

Despite the treatment outlined, the mortality from established severe ARDS remains high at more than 50% overall. Approximately 40% of uncomplicated cases die, but the mortality rises with increasing age and failure of other organs.

Brain death

Brain death means 'the irreversible loss of the capacity for consciousness combined with the irreversible loss of the capacity to breathe'. Both these are essentially functions of the brain stem. Death, if thought of in this way, can arise either from causes outside the brain (i.e. respiratory and cardiac arrest) or from causes within the head. With the advent of artificial ventilation it became possible to support such a dead patient temporarily, although in all cases cardiovascular failure eventually supervenes and progresses to asystole.

Before considering such a diagnosis it is essential that certain preconditions and exclusions are fulfilled.

Preconditions
- The patient must be in apnoeic coma (i.e. unresponsive and on a ventilator, with no spontaneous respiratory efforts).
- Irremediable structural brain damage due to a disorder which can cause brain stem death must have been diagnosed with certainty (e.g. head injury, intracranial haemorrhage).

Exclusions
- The possibility that unresponsive apnoea is the result of poisons, sedative drugs or neuromuscular blocking agents must be excluded.
- Hypothermia must be excluded as a cause of coma. The central body temperature should be more than 35°C.
- There must be no significant metabolic or endocrine disturbance that could produce or contribute to coma. There should be no profound abnormality of the plasma electrolytes, acid–base balance, or blood glucose levels.

Diagnostic tests for the confirmation of brain death

All brain stem reflexes are absent in brain death.

The following tests should not be performed in the presence of seizures or abnormal postures.

- The pupils should be fixed and unresponsive to bright light. Both direct and consensual light reflexes should be absent. The size of the pupils is irrelevant, although most often they will be dilated.
- Corneal reflexes should be absent.
- Oculocephalic reflexes should be absent, i.e. when the head is rotated from side to side, the eyes move with the head and therefore remain stationary relative to the orbit. In a comatose patient whose brain stem is intact the eyes will rotate relative to the orbit (i.e. doll's eye movements will be present).
- There are no vestibulo-ocular reflexes on caloric testing (see p. 802).
- There should be no motor responses within the cranial nerve territory to painful stimuli applied centrally or peripherally. Spinal reflexes may be present.
- There must be no gag or cough reflex in response to pharyngeal, laryngeal or tracheal stimulation.

- Spontaneous respiration should be absent. The patient should be ventilated with 5% CO_2 in 95% O_2 for 10 min and then disconnected from the ventilator for a further 10 min. Oxygenation is maintained by insufflation with 100% oxygen at high flow rates via a catheter placed in the endotracheal tube. The patient is observed for any signs of spontaneous respiratory efforts. A blood gas sample should be obtained during this period to ensure that the P_aCO_2 is sufficiently high to stimulate spontaneous respiration (>6.7 kPa [50 mm Hg]).

The examination should be performed (and repeated after a few hours) by two doctors of senior status a minimum of 6 h after the onset of coma or, if due to cardiac arrest, at least 24 h after restoration of an adequate circulation.

It is not necessary to perform confirmatory tests such as EEG and carotid angiography, as these may be misleading.

In suitable cases and provided the patient was carrying a donor card and/or the consent of relatives has been obtained, the organs of those in whom brain stem death has been established may be used for transplantation. In all cases the coroner's consent must be obtained.

Results, costs and patient selection for intensive care

For many critically ill patients intensive care is undoubtedly life-saving and resumption of a normal lifestyle is to be expected.

In the most seriously ill patients, however, immediate mortality rates are high, a significant number die soon after discharge from the intensive care unit, and the quality of life for some of those who do survive may be poor. Moreover, intensive care is expensive, particularly for those with the worst prognosis.

Inappropriate use of intensive care facilities has other implications. The patient may experience unnecessary suffering and loss of dignity, while relatives may also have to endure considerable emotional pressures. In some cases treatment may simply prolong the process of dying, or sustain life of dubious quality, and in others the risks of interventions may outweigh the potential benefits.

Rational selection of those patients most likely to benefit from intensive care is therefore clearly desirable, both for a humane approach to the management of the critically ill and to ensure optimal use of relatively scarce resources.

Currently decisions to limit therapy, or not to resuscitate in the event of cardiorespiratory arrest, are made jointly by the medical staff of the unit, the primary physician or surgeon and the nurses, normally in consultation with the patient's family.

Acknowledgement

Figs. 13.1, 13.2, 13.5, 13.6, 13.7, 13.8, 13.9, 13.11, 13.12, 13.13, 13.14 and 13.15 are from Hinds CJ (1987) *Intensive Care: A Concise Textbook*. London: Baillière Tindall. Used with permission.

Further reading

Hinds CJ (1987) *Intensive Care: A Concise Textbook*. London: Baillière Tindall.

Tinker J & Rapin M (eds) (1983) *Care of the Critically Ill Patient*. Berlin: Springer-Verlag.

14

Adverse Drug Reactions and Poisoning

Adverse drug reactions

The size of the problem

Any substance that possesses useful therapeutic effects may also produce unwanted, toxic or adverse effects. The incidence of adverse drug reactions in the population is not really known. A survey of 1160 patients given a variety of drugs showed that the incidence of adverse reactions increased with age from about 3% in patients 10–20 years of age to about 20% in patients 80–89 years of age. It has been estimated that about 0.5% of patients who die in hospital do so as a result of their treatment rather than the condition for which they were admitted.

CLASSIFICATION

Adverse drug reactions can be classified in several ways. They may be divided into reactions due to:
- Overdosage
- Intolerance
- Side-effects
- Secondary effects
- Idiosyncrasy
- Hypersensitivity

Another system of classification divides them into two types:
- Type A—the results of an exaggerated but otherwise normal pharmacological action of a drug

- Type B—totally aberrant effects not expected from the known pharmacological actions of a drug

In this chapter adverse drug reactions are divided into three types (see Table 14.1):
- Dose dependent
- Dose independent
- Pseudoallergic

The mechanisms underlying many drug reactions, however, are unclear and these reactions cannot at present be classified easily, e.g. hepatotoxicity, analgesic nephropathy and practolol fibrosis.

Dose-dependent reactions

These occur in all patients given sufficiently large doses of any drug. The effects produced may be further subdivided into:
- Reactions that are predictable, being exaggerated therapeutic actions, e.g. depression of cardiac contractility by lignocaine or quinidine, or central nervous depression by barbiturates or narcotics
- Reactions that appear to be unrelated to their therapeutic effects, e.g. the ototoxicity produced by streptomycin

Table 14.1 Comparison between dose-dependent, dose-independent and pseudo-allergic reactions.

	Dose-dependent	Dose-independent	Pseudoallergic
All patients	Yes	No	No
All drugs	Yes	No	No
Previous exposure necessary	No	Yes	No
Treatment	Reduce dose	Stop drug	Avoid drug or Reduce dose

The first group, being predictable, can be anticipated and looked for without much difficulty. The second unpredictable group poses serious problems of recognition and quantification, particularly with a new drug.

Factors that influence the dose at which these dose-dependent effects appear are described on p. 652.

Dose-independent reactions

These occur in only a small proportion of patients and tend to be limited to certain well-defined manifestations. The possibility, however, of new syndromes occurring must never be overlooked. These reactions usually occur in patients who have previously been exposed and sensitized to the drug itself, to another drug of the same chemical class, or to one of another class of drugs that shares similar antigenic properties. For example, exposure to one form of penicillin usually produces a state of hypersensitivity to other penicillin derivatives, and, in a small proportion of patients, also to cephalosporin derivatives which share cross-antigenicity with the 6-amino-penicillanic acid nucleus.

Most drugs are of relatively low molecular weight and only become antigenic when they are combined covalently and irreversibly with other substances of high molecular weight, usually proteins. The drug is then said to be a *hapten*. Sometimes it is a metabolite of the drug or an impurity produced during manufacture which acts as the hapten. The most common of these dose-independent reactions are acute hypersensitivity reactions. These are due to the release of histamine and other mediators following the interaction of antigen with antibody (IgE) produced by B lymphocytes and bound to the cell membranes of mast cells or circulating basophils. The released substances cause rashes, oedema and the more serious effects of bronchospasm, peripheral vasodilatation and cardiovascular collapse—the anaphylactic reaction.

Circulating antigen–antibody complexes (immune complexes) cause the serum sickness syndrome. They are deposited in the basement membrane of the renal glomerulus and elsewhere.

Delayed hypersensitivity reactions, such as contact dermatitis, are due to the formation of sensitized T lymphocytes, which activate a cell-mediated immune response.

Other forms of dose-independent reactions include various blood dyscrasias. These may involve the production of antibodies to circulating blood elements, leading to:
- Thrombocytopenic purpura (e.g. with quinine)
- Haemolytic anaemia (e.g. with methyldopa)
- Depression of bone marrow function, either selective (e.g. agranulocytosis) or total (aplastic anaemia). For example, chloramphenicol is a very effective antibiotic, but about one person in every

---

Anaphylaxis

Anaphylaxis usually follows injections or occasionally insect bites.

Clinical features
Bronchospasm
Laryngeal spasm
Breathlessness
Cyanosis
Hypotension
Nausea, vomiting, diarrhoea

Treatment
Lay patient head down
Ensure airway free
Monitor blood pressure

Give:

Adrenaline i.m. 0.5–1.0 mg every 15 min
Intravenous infusion
Oxygen by variable concentration mask
Chlorpheniramine 10–20 mg slow i.v. infusion over 24 h
Hydrocortisone 100 mg i.v. every 4 h
In severe cases, prednisolone 20 mg every 6 h

---

20 000 develops a fatal aplastic anaemia which is unrelated to the dose administered and which cannot at present be predicted by any pre-dose screening test. The exact mechanism of this aplasia is unknown.

Pseudoallergic reactions

In some susceptible patients, substances mimic the allergic reactions described under dose-independent reactions but without the same immunological mechanisms occurring. Unlike allergic reactions they occur on first contact with a drug rather than after previous sensitizing exposure. Susceptibility to such a reaction appears to be determined by genetic and environmental factors. These reactions are produced by compounds that are able to release histamine and other mediators directly from mast cells without involving an antigen–antibody reaction. Examples are:
- The itching, bronchospasm and vasodilatation due to histamine release by morphine
- The flushing, urticaria, angio-oedema, conjunctivitis, rhinitis, bronchial asthma, hypotension and even fatal shock produced by aspirin

It is probable that reactions to many other drugs are also due to this mechanism (see Table 14.2). An interesting example is the anaphylactic response produced by aspirin in one patient with urticaria pigmentosa and generalized mastocytosis.

If use of the particular drug to which the pseudoallergic reaction occurs cannot be avoided, its

Table 14.2 Agents that are believed to be capable of producing pseudoallergic reactions through release of histamine and other mediators.

Aspirin and other non-steroidal anti-inflammatory drugs
Barbiturates
Anaesthetics (intravenous)
Neuromuscular blocking drugs
Morphine
Chlorpropamide/alcohol interaction (p. 751)
Sodium cromoglycate
Polypeptides, gamma globulin
Dextrans and other colloids
Radiographic contrast media
Cremophor (solvent for some intravenous drugs)
Tartrazine

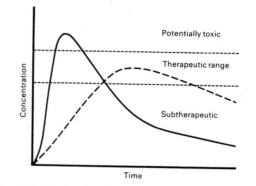

Fig. 14.1 Relationships between drug blood concentration and effect and time after oral administration.

dose should be kept as low as possible, or, in the case of intravenous administration, it should be given by slow infusion rather than rapid injection. Sometimes it is possible to desensitize a patient by starting with a small dose of the drug and gradually increasing it under supervision.

FACTORS INFLUENCING DOSE-DEPENDENT ADVERSE DRUG REACTIONS

Formulation

The active agent represents only a small proportion of the total weight of a tablet or capsule. Similarly, drugs for injection require solubilization or suspension in a fluid vehicle of varying complexity. Other constituents of dosage forms, called *excipients*, are not necessarily inert, and may play an important part in facilitating or hindering the absorption of a drug. The proportion of an administered drug dose that reaches its site of action in the systemic circulation is known as its bioavailability. If the drug is given intravenously its bioavailability is 100%.

The dose-dependent adverse effects of many drugs are related to higher blood levels than those necessary for their therapeutic action (see Fig. 14.1). A formulation that results in such high blood levels may, therefore, produce unacceptable effects. In the case of a poorly soluble drug, its physical form may be important in determining its dissolution rate and, therefore, its rate of absorption. For example, when the particle size of digoxin was reduced by a manufacturer, many patients experienced digitalis toxicity because the rate and extent of absorption was increased. Similarly, the influence of a change of the excipient on a drug's bioavailability was seen in Australia when a manufacturer of phenytoin cap-

sules changed from using the relatively water-insoluble calcium sulphate to the much more soluble lactose. This led to an increase in the bioavailability of phenytoin, which was even more marked because of the 'saturation kinetics' that phenytoin exhibits (see p. 655).

Modification of the physical form of a drug, and changes in other constituents, permits the development of 'controlled release' formulations. These produce sustained levels within the therapeutic range and prevent early peak blood levels which enter the toxic range (see Fig. 14.1). This effect is particularly useful in drugs with a short half-life.

Route of administration

Parenteral administration of a drug may produce higher peak levels than are produced by oral administration, and may therefore produce more marked concentration-related adverse effects. For example, the intravenous administration of many drugs, particularly as bolus injections, may produce unwanted cardiac or central nervous effects. Intrathecal penicillin can produce encephalopathy and convulsions due to the toxic effects of high concentrations on the central nervous system; this route is nowadays seldom used.

Adverse reactions may occur due to accidents during administration; for example, arterial rather than venous injection of thiopentone results in vascular spasm, arterial thrombosis and gangrene.

Pregnancy

Some drugs given in the first three months of pregnancy may cause congenital abnormalities and are said to be teratogenic. The best known example of a teratogenic drug is thalidomide, which resulted in bizarre and therefore easily recognizable abnormalities such as absent or grossly abnormal limbs (amelia, phocomelia). Stilboestrol administration during pregnancy produced adenosis and adenocarcinoma of the vagina in the female offspring when they reached their late teens or early twenties. This was recognized because of the normally relatively low incidence of this carcinoma in this age group. Low-grade teratogens that cause only minor deformities infrequently are likely to be unrecognized or demonstrated only with difficulty. Other drugs that are known or suspected to be teratogenic are given in Table 14.3.

Drugs given after the period of organogenesis may affect the growth or function of normally-formed fetal tissues or organs. The more important of these drugs are given in Table 14.4.

Age

Some drugs produce specific adverse effects at the extremes of life.

Neonates

In the neonatal period, drug-metabolizing enzymes may be deficient for at least a month after birth, particularly in the premature neonate. Neonates have problems in effectively metabolizing vitamin K analogues, sulphonamides, barbiturates, morphine and curare. One of the most dramatic examples is the production of the 'grey baby' syndrome by chloramphenicol in premature infants. This consists of circulatory collapse and muscular hypotonia and is thought to be due to a combination of defective hepatic conjugation of chloramphenicol and accumulation of unconjugated drug because of immature renal excretion.

In addition to hepatic immaturity, newborn infants have a relatively lower glomerular filtration rate and renal plasma flow than adults, which results in reduced excretion of drugs such as aminoglycosides and digoxin.

Table 14.3 Agents known or suspected to be teratogenic in man.

Definite or strongly suspected teratogens
Thalidomide
Anticonvulsants
Antineoplastic drugs
Folic acid antagonists
Alcohol
Warfarin
Lithium
Oestrogens
Stilboestrol
Androgenic steroids
Etretinate
Isotretinoin
Podophyllum resin
Organic mercury
Possible teratogens
Inhalational anaesthetics
Vitamin A
Progestogens
Live vaccines (some)

Table 14.4 Drugs that may have unwanted effects on the fetus during intrauterine life if given to the mother.

Drug	Effect
Antibacterial drugs	
Tetracyclines	Dental discoloration
Aminoglycosides	Eighth nerve damage
Novobiocin	
Sulphonamides	Jaundice, kernicterus
Antithyroid drugs	
Iodides	
Carbimazole	Neonatal hypothyroidism,
Lithium	goitre
Povidone-iodine	
Anticoagulants	Fetal and neonatal
Warfarin	haemorrhage
Hypoglycaemics	Fetal and neonatal
Sulphonylureas	hypoglycaemia
Cardiovascular drugs	Fetal tachycardia, delayed
Beta-agonists	labour
	Fetal and neonatal
Beta-antagonists	bradycardia, impaired
Reserpine	adrenergic responses
Central nervous system drugs	
Narcotics	Central nervous
Alcohol	depression, withdrawal
Barbiturates	syndromes
Benzodiazepines	
Corticosteroids and sex hormones	Fetal and neonatal adrenal suppression, virilization of female fetus
Non-steroidal anti-inflammatory drugs	Premature closure of fetal
Aspirin	ductus arteriosus,
Indomethacin	delayed labour, increased blood loss

The elderly

Elderly patients are more susceptible to most dose-related adverse drug reactions.

Reduced hepatic drug extraction and metabolism occurs with increasing age. This contributes to the increased incidence of adverse effects in older patients following the administration of central depressant drugs such as sedatives, tranquillizers and hypnotics. Age-related changes in the sensitivity of the central nervous system to the effects of these compounds may also be involved.

Glomerular filtration rate falls with age, leading to the accumulation of drugs principally excreted unchanged by the kidney. In view of this, doses of digoxin, lithium and aminoglycosides have to be reduced in elderly patients.

Increasing age is also associated with changes in body composition, as well as with a general tendency to a decrease in body weight. Both of these may influence the distribution and tissue levels of administered drugs.

Differences in enzyme activity

Differences in enzyme activity between individuals may be either inherited or acquired.

Inherited

There are marked differences in the rates of drug metabolism between individuals. Some of these are known to be due to polymorphic genetic control of the metabolic pathways involved (see Table 14.5).

Other examples include the exacerbation of acute intermittent porphyria by barbiturates and the occurrence of a rare familial resistance to coumarin anticoagulants.

Acquired enzyme inhibition

Many adverse drug reactions occur due to the administration of drugs which cause inhibition of enzymes.

Monoamine oxidase. This is a widely distributed enzyme that is responsible for the intracellular degradation of, amongst other monoamines, adrenaline, noradrenaline, dopamine and 5-hydroxy-tryptamine (serotonin). Its inhibition by monoamine oxidase inhibitors (MAOIs) may, therefore, give rise to serious adverse effects from the following agents if taken concurrently (see Fig. 14.2):

- Indirectly acting sympathomimetic amines, such as ephedrine and phenylpropanolamine, whose pressor and cardiac actions are due to the release of noradrenaline from adrenergic nerve terminals and are potentiated by MAO inhibition
- Foods which contain tyramine, such as cheeses, wines, meat and yeast products. Tyramine is an indirectly acting amine with similar actions to phenylpropanolamine.
- Monoamine-reuptake inhibiting (tricyclic) anti-depressants, which can cause serious central nervous stimulation, convulsions and circulatory collapse if given together with an MAOI
- Antihypertensive drugs such as reserpine, guanethidine and bethanidine which release noradrenaline from its neuronal stores and so can produce serious hypertension
- Pethidine, which may produce severe narcotic effects with coma and hyperthermia in patients receiving MAOIs, possibly owing to raised levels of cerebral 5-hydroxytryptamine

Xanthine oxidase. Inhibition of xanthine oxidase by allopurinol can lead to reduced breakdown of

Table 14.5 Adverse drug reactions associated with inherited enzyme deficiencies.

Deficient enzyme	Drugs involved	Adverse effects
Cholinesterase	Succinylcholine	Prolonged neuromuscular blockade, apnoea
N-Acetyltransferase	Isoniazid	Peripheral neuropathy
	Procainamide Phenelzine Hydralazine	Systemic lupus erythematosus
Glucose-6-phosphate dehydrogenase	Primaquine Sulphonamides Nitrofurantoin Quinine Chloramphenicol	Haemolysis
Glutathione peroxidase	Sulphonamides	Haemolysis
Methaemoglobin reductase	Sulphonamides Nitrites	Methaemoglobinaemia
Mixed function oxidase (cytochrome P450)	Debrisoquine	Hypotension
	Phenformin (withdrawn)	Lactic acidosis
	Perhexilene	Peripheral neuropathy, liver damage
	Metoprolol	Bradycardia, marked beta-blockade

Fig. 14.2 Mechanisms by which monoamine oxidase inhibitors and monoamine reuptake inhibitors influence indirectly and directly acting sympathomimetic amines. a=granular stores of catecholamine; b= free cytoplasmic catecholamine; c=catecholamine released into synaptic cleft by nerve impulse or indirectly acting amine such as ephedrine or tyramine; d=exogenously administered directly acting amine such as noradrenaline; e=reuptake of catecholamine into the neurone, terminating its action. 1. Normal synapse; 2. Monoamine oxidase inhibition leads to increased catecholamine release by nerve impulse or sympathomimetic amine; 3. Monoamine reuptake inhibition leads to increased effects of transmitter or administered amine.

purines such as 6-mercaptopurine and azathioprine, with an increased risk of their dose-dependent adverse effects, for example on the bone marrow.

Aldehyde dehydrogenase. This is inhibited by disulfiram, resulting in an accumulation of acetaldehyde after ingestion of alcohol, with the resulting 'antabuse' reaction of flushing, hypotension, headache, sweating, nausea, vomiting and even cardiovascular collapse. This forms the basis of one approach to the management of alcohol dependence (see p. 892). A similar reaction may occur with the antimicrobial drug metronidazole.

Competition by drugs for hepatic drug-metabolizing pathways is not uncommon and is becoming increasingly recognized as a basis for adverse drug interactions. For example, cimetidine increases the anticoagulant effect of warfarin, the sedative effect of diazepam and the beta-adrenoceptor blocking action of propranolol by inhibiting their hepatic metabolism. Sulphonamides decrease phenytoin metabolism so that toxic levels may be reached.

Acquired enzyme induction
The activity of hepatic drug-metabolizing enzymes may be increased by a large number of common substances, including insecticides, pesticides, polycyclic aromatic hydrocarbons, and some drugs such as barbiturates, phenytoin, carbamazepine and rifampicin. Such enzyme induction results in increased drug metabolism and breakdown, reducing the therapeutic activity of certain drugs. Examples include oral anticoagulants, corticosteroids and the contraceptive pill. The importance of enzyme induction lies in the exaggerated effects that can occur if the inducing drug is discontinued and the drug whose metabolism was being induced, e.g. warfarin, continues to be given in an increased dosage.

Protein binding

Many drugs are loosely bound to plasma and tissue proteins. The free unbound fraction is pharmacologically active. This fraction is increased in conditions in which hypoproteinaemia occurs (see Table 14.6). Competition between drugs for common binding sites can lead to a transient increase in free levels of one following its displacement by another, but the clinical importance of this is uncertain because increased clearance of the free fraction occurs, which tends to re-establish the original equilibrium between free and bound drug levels.

Route and kinetics of metabolism

Adverse reactions are particularly likely to occur where the relationship between drug dose and blood level is non-linear, so that relatively small increments in the dose given may lead to unexpectedly large increases in the blood level. Such a relationship is typical of saturation kinetics, in which hepatic metabolizing pathways become saturated or exhausted at a certain dose. Above this dose proportionately more unchanged drug enters the systemic circulation. An important example of this phenomenon is seen with phenytoin (Fig. 14.3).

Some adverse effects are due not to the parent compound but to highly reactive metabolites. For example, when paracetamol is taken in overdose, the capacity of hepatic conjugating mechanisms is exceeded and a hepatotoxic metabolite is formed and accumulates (see p. 665).

Excretion

Many drugs are excreted by the kidney, while others are reabsorbed. Changes in urinary pH affect elimination; for example, the excretion of the acidic drug aspirin is increased, while that of the basic drug mexiletine is reduced, by alkalinization of the urine. This may be important clinically in patients who have a persistently high urine pH from renal disease

Table 14.6 Influence of disease on drug toxicity through changes in pharmacokinetics.

Disease	Mechanism	Drugs involved	Effects
Liver disease; renal disease; cancer	Reduced serum albumin	Acidic drugs, e.g. aspirin	Increased free drug, risk of increased toxicity
Acute and chronic inflammation, myocardial infarction, surgery, trauma, cancer	Increased alpha-1-acid glycoprotein	Basic drugs, e.g. beta-antagonists, anti-arrhythmics	Reduced free drug, possibility of reduced therapeutic and toxic effects
Renal disease; cardiac failure	Reduced renal excretion	Digoxin, aminoglycosides, lithium	Increased therapeutic and toxic effects
Chronic liver disease; cardiac failure	Reduced hepatic uptake and clearance	Centrally acting drugs, steroids, warfarin, propranolol, tolbutamide, theophylline, lignocaine	Increased therapeutic and toxic effects
Cardiac failure	Reduced gastrointestinal perfusion and drug absorption	Digoxin	Possibility of reduced absorption and therapeutic effects, but importance uncertain

or a vegetarian diet. Competition for renal tubular excretion also occurs, e.g. penicillin competes with probenecid.

Fig. 14.3 Saturation kinetics as exhibited by phenytoin. The measurements were obtained from one patient on several maintenance doses of phenytoin and show a curvilinear relationship between dose and serum concentration. Note the relatively small dose range compatible with a therapeutic concentration. Modified from Turner P & Richens A (1981) *Clinical Pharmacology*, 4th edn. Edinburgh: Churchill Livingstone. With permission.

Local factors

The therapeutic action of some drugs is markedly dependent on the local physiological environment at its site of action. A good example is the effect of myocardial potassium concentration on the cardiac actions of digitalis glycosides, hypokalaemia leading to enhancement of their action, with the risk of toxicity. Another example is the influence of changes in sodium and potassium status on the response to lithium.

Drug interactions

Drugs can interact within the body in many ways that may lead to adverse effects. Some important examples are given in Table 14.7.

Patient compliance

Patient compliance is also a factor in adverse reactions. Compliance is influenced by the drug formulation, frequency of dosage, number of drugs prescribed, and by the patient's age and ability to comprehend instructions.

Table 14.7 Some clinically important drug interactions leading to adverse effects.

Drug A *may interact with*	Drug B	Potential results	Mechanism
Reduced hepatic excretion			
Carbamazepine Phenytoin Diazepam Propranolol Theophylline Coumarin anticoagulants	Cimetidine Sodium valproate Chloramphenicol Phenylbutazone Sulphonamides Tolbutamide Indomethacin Clofibrate	Potentiation of drug A	Inhibition of hepatic enzymes by drug B
Reduced renal excretion			
Penicillins Cephalosporins Dapsone	Probenecid	Increased plasma levels of drug A	Reduced tubular secretion of drug A
Mexiletine Amphetamine	Antacids (systemically absorbed)	Increased plasma levels of drug A	Reduced excretion of drug A in alkaline urine
Inhibition of neuronal uptake			
Monoamine reuptake inhibiting anti-depressants, e.g. imipramine, amitriptyline Mazindol	Noradrenaline Adrenaline Phenylephrine	Potentiation of pressor action of drug B	Inhibition by drug A of neuronal uptake of drug B (see Fig. 14.2)
Inhibition of monoamine oxidase			
MAOIs e.g. phenelzine	Amphetamine Ephedrine Phenylpropanolamine Pseudoephedrine Fenfluramine Levodopa Tyramine-containing food and wines	Acute hypertensive crisis	Release by drug B of monoamine stores increased by drug A (see Fig. 14.2)
	Pethidine and other narcotics	Central nervous excitation, coma	Uncertain
Summation of effects			
Barbiturates Benzodiazepines	Alcohol Other CNS depressants	Increased CNS depression	Summation of CNS depression
Monoamine reuptake inhibiting antidepressants, e.g. imipramine, amitriptyline	Anticholinergics Antihistamines Antiparkinsonian drugs	Excessive central and peripheral atropine-like effects	Summation of anti-cholinergic actions
	Monoamine oxidase inhibitors e.g. phenelzine	Central nervous excitation, coma	Increased central monoamine activity
Thiazide and loop diuretics	Corticosteroids Carbenoxolone	Hypokalaemia	Renal potassium loss
Angiotensin-converting enzyme inhibitors, e.g. captopril, enalapril	Potassium-sparing diuretics	Hyperkalaemia	Potassium retention
Anti-arrhythmic drugs	Beta-adrenoceptor blocking drugs, particularly propranolol	Myocardial depression	Summation of myocardial depression

Table 14.7 (*continued*)

Drug A *may interact with*	Drug B	Potential results	Mechanism
Antihypertensive drugs	Vasodilators Alcohol Fenfluramine Levodopa Bromocriptine	Hypotension	Summation of hypotensive effects
Loop diuretics	Aminoglycosides Cephaloridine Cephalothin	Increased nephrotoxicity and ototoxicity	Uncertain
Others			
Digoxin	Thiazide and loop diuretics	Toxicity of drug A	Hypokalaemia
	Quinidine Amiodarone Nifedipine Verapamil	Toxicity of drug A	Clearance of drug A reduced by drug B
Lithium	Haloperidol	Involuntary movements	Uncertain
Competitive neuromuscular blocking drugs, e.g. tubocurarine	Aminoglycosides Propranolol Lithium Quinidine	Potentiation of drug A	Uncertain
Metronidazole Chlorpropamide	Alcohol	Flushing, hypotension	Uncertain
Alcohol	Disulfiram	'Antabuse' reaction: flushing, hypotension, tachycardia, arrhythmias	Inhibition by drug B of metabolism of drug A, producing acetaldehyde accumulation
Azathioprine 6-Mercaptopurine	Allopurinol	Toxicity of drug A	Xanthine oxidase inhibition by drug B

INFLUENCE OF DISEASE ON ADVERSE DRUG REACTIONS

Disease processes may increase the risk and severity of adverse drug reactions in several ways:
- Disease may lead to changes in the pharmacokinetics of a drug. A reduction in protein binding or reduced renal or hepatic clearance will potentiate the effects of certain drugs (Table 14.6).
- Changes in receptor density and function may occur. For example, there is evidence that the enhanced bronchoconstrictor effects of beta-adrenoceptor antagonists in asthmatic patients may be due to a reduction ('down regulation') in beta receptor number produced by long-term treatment with beta-agonists such as salbutamol. The sensitivity of patients with myasthenia gravis to the neuromuscular blocking effects of streptomycin, neomycin or kanamycin may be due to drug-induced changes in cholinergic receptors.
- Some inherited diseases are associated with enhanced drug toxicity (see Table 14.8).

There are also several examples of disease-related enhanced drug toxicity the nature of which is not yet understood (see Table 14.9).

MONITORING ADVERSE DRUG REACTIONS

Clinical trials of new drugs are conveniently classified into:
- Phase 1, in which the drug is given to a small number of normal volunteers in closely controlled and supervised conditions to study its kinetics and pharmacological effects
- Phase 2, in which the drug is given to a relatively small number of patients with the disease for which its use is proposed. The therapeutic efficacy, correct dosage and pharmacokinetics of the drug are determined by comparing the data with those for normal subjects to obtain some evidence of its safety.
- Phase 3, in which the clinical evaluation of the drug is extended to larger numbers of patients (perhaps hundreds). Trials include comparisons with placebos and with established treatments.
- Phase 4 (post-marketing surveillance, PMS), in

Table 14.8 Some examples of enhanced drug toxicity associated with inherited diseases.

Inherited disease	Drug	Reaction
Haemophilia and von Willebrand's disease	Salicylates	Prolongs bleeding time
Hereditary myopathies, myotonia congenita	Halothane Caffeine Succinylcholine Potassium chloride	Malignant hyperthermia (malignant hyperpyrexia)
Osteogenesis imperfecta	Halothane Succinylcholine	Pyrexia
Periodic paralysis	Potassium chloride Insulin Adrenaline Ethanol Liquorice derivatives	Paralysis
Familial dysautonomia	Cholinergic and adrenergic agonists	Denervation supersensitivity

Table 14.9 Some examples of drug toxicity associated with disease states, the nature of which is not yet understood.

Disease	Drug	Reaction
Glandular fever (infectious mononucleosis)	Ampicillin Amoxycillin	Rash
Hypothyroidism Respiratory failure	CNS depressants	Enhanced CNS depression and respiratory failure
Burns Renal failure Peripheral neuropathy	Succinylcholine	Release of potassium-producing cardiac arrhythmias
Rheumatoid arthritis and other connective tissue diseases	Salicylates	Hepatotoxicity (rare)
Cystic fibrosis	Isoprenaline Theophylline	Bronchospasm
Renal failure	Clofibrate (withdrawn)	Severe myopathy
	Benzodiazepines Monoamine reuptake inhibiting antidepressants	Fatal dialysis dementia

which long-term assessment of the safety and efficacy of the drug is made in thousands of patients, following the licensing of the drug for marketing

Experience has shown that careful observation of patients in phase 2 and phase 3 clinical trials is only likely to detect those adverse reactions that occur in 1% or more of patients exposed to a drug. Adverse reactions with an incidence of less than 1% require detection in phase 4 (PMS) studies.

Several countries have developed systems for collecting information about suspected adverse drug reactions. In the UK two systems are of particular interest.

Prescription event monitoring (PEM)

This scheme involves identifying doctors and their patients as the prescriptions for a particular drug pass through the central Prescription Pricing Authority office. Relevant prescriptions are photocopied and the copies sent in confidence to the Drug Surveillance Research Unit in Southampton. Each 'test' drug under investigation is matched with a 'control' drug which is chemically or pharmacologically similar and already marketed for the same indications. Similar numbers of patients receiving each drug are selected and a simple questionnaire is sent to their general medical practitioners, requesting information on age, new diagnoses or events that have come to the doctor's attention, and reasons for any referral to a consultant or admission to hospital. PEM should be able to identify adverse drug reactions that have an incidence of 1 in 3000 or greater.

Yellow card system

This voluntary system has been the most productive to date in the UK for identifying important adverse drug reactions. Yellow reply-paid cards are supplied to doctors and dentists, who are encouraged to use them to report any suspected adverse drug reactions to the government's advisory Committee on Safety of Medicines. Although the rate of reporting is low, this system has drawn attention to the association of oral contraceptives and thromboembolism, hepatitis and methyldopa, jaundice and halothane, and extra-pyramidal effects and metoclopramide. At present, only this system is potentially capable of detecting risk at all levels of incidence.

When suspicion has been aroused through the yellow card system, the existence or otherwise of a true association between a reported event and the implicated drug must be demonstrated epidemiologically by case control or cohort studies, and by clinical pharmacological and toxicological studies of the possible mechanisms involved.

The problems associated with long-term surveillance of many thousands of patients must not be underestimated. Such studies are costly in both time and money, and it is difficult to maintain the integrity of the study cohort, the interest and commitment of the doctors, and the compliance of the patients.

REDUCTION OF ADVERSE DRUG REACTIONS

The incidence of adverse drug reactions can be reduced by:
- The development and marketing of safer drugs by the pharmaceutical industry
- Tighter control by drug-regulatory authorities within government on the licensing, promotion and marketing of drugs

In addition, the doctor must think carefully about every drug he or she prescribes.

The hazards of adverse drug reaction can be substantially reduced by:
- Understanding the mechanisms underlying the reactions
- Excluding a history of adverse reaction
- Individualizing drug dosage

Prescribing manuals and therapeutic textbooks give recommended ranges of drug doses. The choice of dose for an individual patient, however, depends on a large variety of factors, including genetic and environmental factors, most of which are still only poorly understood. The prescribing doctor must, therefore, determine the optimum drug dose for the patient from the advised range given by considering the factors already discussed and on the basis of his or her own experience. In some cases the dose can be decided by monitoring its therapeutic effect; for example, prothrombin time can be measured when using an oral anticoagulant drug, or blood sugar when using insulin or an oral hypoglycaemic drug. In addition, for drugs with a narrow therapeutic ratio (i.e. the ratio of the dose necessary to produce a therapeutic effect to that necessary to produce a toxic effect), or whose kinetics are not linear, titration of the dose to obtain a desirable blood level may be of value. Such control is called 'therapeutic drug monitoring', and is particularly helpful with digoxin, gentamicin, lithium and phenytoin, whose potentially toxic concentrations are relatively close to the therapeutic range (see Table 14.10).

Table 14.10 Drugs for which plasma concentration monitoring may be helpful.

Drug	Therapeutic plasma concentration range	Toxic levels	Optimum time for sampling after dose (h)
Carbamazepine	21–42 µmol·l^{-1}	>42 µmol·l^{-1}	>8
Digoxin	1.3–2.6 nmol·l^{-1}	>2.6 nmol·l^{-1}	>8
Gentamicin	Trough <2 mg·l^{-1} Peak 4–8 mg·l^{-1}	>2 mg·l^{-1} >12 mg·l^{-1}	6–8 1
Lithium	0.6–1.4 mmol·l^{-1}	>1.5 mmol·l^{-1}	>10
Phenytoin	40–80 µmol·l^{-1}	>80 µmol·l^{-1}	>10
Theophylline	55–110 µmol·l^{-1}	>110 µmol·l^{-1}	>4

Maintaining a low threshold of suspicion

Most important of all is that all prescribing doctors should be continually aware of the possibility that any clinical or life event (e.g. an accident) may be associated in some way with a patient's treatment. The lower the threshold of suspicion on the part of the doctor, the lower the risk of serious long-term adverse drug reactions in the patient.

Poisoning

In most hospitals in the Western World the commonest reason for acute admission to a medical ward is poisoning. Such poisoning is usually by self-administration of prescribed or over-the-counter medicines. Occasionally, however, toxic agents are accidentally ingested or inhaled at home or work or are administered with criminal intent.

Types of poisoning

Self-poisoning. This refers to the deliberate ingestion of a drug or some other substance not meant for consumption.

The terms 'parasuicide' and 'attempted suicide' are inappropriate and should not be used; most patients have no wish to kill themselves.

Accidental poisoning. This occurs mostly in children below 5 years of age, but can occur in adults, e.g. from the accidental inhalation of a gas, ingestion of fluid from a wrongly labelled bottle, stings and bites, or eating poisonous food (such as mushrooms).

Non-accidental poisoning. This is the deliberate administration of a poison to a child.

Homicidal poisoning.

Self-poisoning is often a cry for help, in which the patient takes whatever drug is easily available at home. Doctors should therefore always prescribe limited amounts of drugs, and it is advisable to keep only small amounts of tablets, preferably foil-wrapped, in the home.

The majority of cases (80%) of self-poisoning do not require intensive medical management, but all require a sympathetic and caring approach to their problems. Both the patient and the family may require psychiatric help (see p. 884) and the social services should be contacted to help with social and domestic problems.

In England there were 97 000 hospital admissions in 1982 for self-poisoning, the commonest being with psychotropics (29 000), and analgesics and anti-rheumatic drugs (26 000). In the same year in England and Wales there were 2208 deaths from poisoning, of which 237 were due to Distalgesic (paracetamol and dextropropoxyphene), 163 to paracetamol alone and 131 to amitriptyline. This pattern is reflected in many other countries where similar medicines are available.

Information from other continents is difficult to compare, but in Asia and Africa it seems that poisoning is a significant medical problem, with children a particularly vulnerable group. In Cairo, over half of the enquiries at the poisons reference centre involve the poisoning of children.

In countries where barbiturates are available without a prescription, their increased use is reflected in their involvement in self-poisoning.

The number of admissions from self-poisoning is increasing. However, as a result of good supportive care and the reduced availability of coal gas and barbiturates, the mortality of patients is declining and is now well under 1%. Studies of the drugs involved reveal that:

- Acute overdoses usually involve more than one drug.
- Alcohol is the most commonly implicated second 'drug' in mixed self-poisonings; 60% of men and 45% of women consume some alcohol at the same time as the drug.
- There is a poor correlation between the drug history and the toxicological findings. Therefore, patients' statements about the type and amount of drug ingested should not be relied on.
- The use of minor tranquillizers and antidepressants is increasing, but there is a decrease in the number of overdoses with barbiturates.

HISTORY

Eighty per cent of adults are conscious on arrival at hospital and the diagnosis of self-poisoning can usually be made easily from the history. In the unconscious patient a history from friends or relatives is helpful and the diagnosis can often be inferred from tablet bottles or a suicide note brought by the ambulance attendants.

It should be emphasized that in any patient with an altered conscious level, drug overdose must always be considered in the differential diagnosis.

EXAMINATION

On arrival at hospital the patient must be assessed urgently in the Casualty Department. The following should be evaluated:

- Level of consciousness—a useful practical grading is:
  - I Drowsy but responds to commands
  - II Unconscious but responds to mild stimulation

III Unconscious and responds only to maximal painful stimuli
IV Unconscious and no response
● Respiratory effort and cyanosis
● Blood pressure and pulse rate
● Pupil size and reaction to light (NB opiates constrict)
● Evidence of head injury or drug addiction

If the patient is unconscious the following should also be checked:
● Presence or absence of cough and gag reflex
● Temperature—measured with a low-reading rectal thermometer

The physical signs that may aid identification of the agents responsible for poisoning are shown in Fig. 14.4.

PRINCIPLES OF MANAGEMENT

Most patients with self-poisoning require only general care and support of the vital systems. However, for a few drugs additional therapy is required.

Blood and urine samples should always be taken on admission for the determination of drug levels, as these are invaluable for the management of certain poisons and are helpful in legal problems. Drug screens of blood and urine are occasionally indicated in the seriously ill, unconscious patient in whom the cause of coma is unknown.

Routine haematological and biochemical investigations are of value, particularly in the differential diagnosis of coma.

Care of the unconscious patient

In all cases the patient should be nursed in the lateral position, with the lower leg straight and the upper leg flexed; in this position the risk of aspiration is reduced. A clear passage for air should be encouraged by the removal of any obstructing object, vomit or dentures, and by backward elevation of the mandible. Nursing care of the mouth, pressure areas and bladder should be instituted.

Respiratory support

If respiratory depression is minimal, oxygen (approximately 60%) should be administered via a mask. A naso- or oropharyngeal airway should be inserted and constant observation is mandatory to detect any further depression of ventilation.

Loss of the cough or gag reflex is the prime indication for intubation. The gag reflex is assessed by positioning the patient on his side and making him gag using a sucker. In most patients the reflexes are depressed sufficiently to allow intubation without the use of sedatives or relaxants. The complications of endotracheal tubes are discussed on p. 644.

If ventilation remains inadequate, intermittent positive pressure ventilation (IPPV) should be instituted (see p. 642). Blood gas analysis is useful to confirm the need for IPPV. Hypoxaemia is common in the unconscious patient, particularly after the ingestion of opiates and barbiturates, and can easily go undetected without blood gas analysis.

Cardiovascular support

Hypotension is a common feature of drug overdose and is caused by the physiological effects listed in Table 14.11. The classic features of shock—tachy-

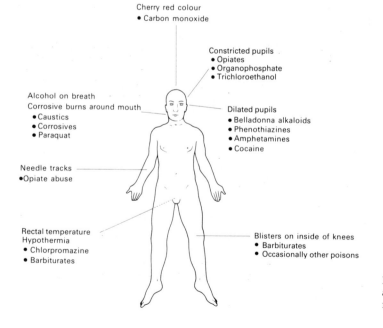

Fig. 14.4 Physical signs which may aid the identification of agents responsible for poisoning.

Table 14.11 Causes of hypotension after drug overdose.

An expanded venous bed due to venous vasodilatation
Hypovolaemia due to inadequate fluid intake in prolonged coma
Institution of IPPV in an already hypovolaemic patient
Myocardial depression due to the direct effect of the drug, exaggerated by hypoxia, acidosis and hypothermia

cardia and pale cold skin—may be present, but vasodilatation may also be seen, e.g. with barbiturate overdose.

In the majority of cases, hypotension is mild and elevation of the feet is the only treatment required. In patients with more severe hypotension, volume expanders such as dextran should be used. In severely hypotensive patients, the measurement of central venous pressure (CVP) is helpful. Urine output (aiming for $0.5\ ml \cdot kg^{-1} \cdot h^{-1}$) is also an important longer-term guide to the adequacy of the circulation, as many vasodilated overdose patients are adequately perfused with a systolic blood pressure of as low as 90–100 mmHg. Some patients may need to be catheterized in order to monitor urine output.

If a patient fails to respond to the above measures, intensive therapy is required (see p. 635).

Arrhythmias are commonly seen with tricyclic antidepressants (see p. 666). Known arrhythmogenic factors such as hypoxia, acidosis and hypokalaemia should be corrected.

Special problems
Hypothermia. Defined as a rectal temperature of below 35°C, this is a common problem, especially in older patients or those poisoned with chlorpromazine or a similar neuroleptic. Hypothyroidism should always be excluded. Hypothermia is compounded by drug-induced vasodilatation and environmental exposure. The patient should be covered with a 'space blanket' and given intravenous and intragastric fluids at normal body temperature. Inspired gases should also be warmed to 37°C.

Rhabdomyolysis. Rhabdomyolysis can occur from pressure necrosis in drug-induced coma or it may complicate heroin abuse without coma. The risk of renal failure from myoglobinaemia is potentiated by dehydration and acidosis.

Convulsions. These may occur in serious tricyclic antidepressant poisoning, and in antihistamine, anticonvulsant or phenothiazine poisoning. Diazepam 10 mg i.v. is the standard treatment for fits of any cause. The patient should also receive a loading dose of phenytoin (1 g administered intravenously over 4 h via a central vein) and a maintenance dose of 100 mg 8-hourly if the fits are not immediately controlled. Persistent fits must be controlled rapidly, as they may otherwise result in severe hypoxia, brain damage and laryngeal trauma.

Stress bleeding. Measures to prevent stress ulceration of the stomach should be started on admission in all patients who are unconscious and require intensive care. Administration of antacid by intragastric tube is usually adequate.

SPECIFIC MANAGEMENT

Many techniques have been developed to decrease drug absorption and increase drug elimination, but most of these manoeuvres are only helpful with a few drugs. These, as well as antidotes to specific drugs, are described below.

Decreasing drug absorption
Vigorous attempts to empty the gastrointestinal tract are indicated when drugs that cause potentially fatal complications other than coma or respiratory depression have been ingested. Examples of such drugs are aspirin, paracetamol, colchicine, organophosphates, iron salts and tricyclic antidepressants. It is important to remember that the risk of aspiration into the lungs associated with the use of gastric lavage may well cause more problems than the effects of the drugs themselves.

Induced emesis. Induced emesis may be useful in small children, as they are more difficult to lavage. It is rarely used in adults, as only small amounts of drug are recovered.

Paediatric ipecacuanha emetic mixture (*not* the undiluted fluid extract) is the emetic of choice. The dose is 10 ml for a child. Other emetics such as apomorphine, saline, copper sulphate and mustard are dangerous and should not be used.

Gastric lavage. This procedure is of most help when performed within 4 h of drug ingestion. It may, however, still be carried out for certain drugs when the time elapsed is between 4 and 12 h (see Table 14.12). Lavage is contraindicated for some poisons, e.g. corrosives, petrol or paraffin.

Absorbants. If administered promptly and in sufficiently large amounts, activated charcoal significantly reduces the gastrointestinal absorption of many drugs. It is an adjunct to emesis or lavage but

Table 14.12 Drugs for which gastric lavage is useful more than 4 h after ingestion.

Salicylates
Basic drugs such as quinidine or tricyclic antidepressants, where gastric emptying is delayed
Paracetamol

Technique of gastric lavage

- The way in which lavage is performed is important.
- The main danger is from pulmonary aspiration, and it is vital that the tracheobronchial tree is protected either by an intact cough reflex or by a cuffed endotracheal tube.
- The patient should be positioned lying on his left side, with his head over the end or side of the bed so that the mouth and throat are at a lower level than the larynx and trachea.
- A wide-bore tube (Jacques' gauge 30) is lubricated with glycerine or Vaseline and passed into the stomach. Aspiration is performed first, and then followed by lavage using 300 ml of water at body temperature for the first washing.
- This process should be repeated at least three or four times, using up to 500 ml of water on each occasion.
- An aliquot of the washing should be saved in case it is needed for drug analysis.

---

does not replace them. It is not often used but occasionally can be useful in severe poisoning with tricyclic antidepressants, theophylline derivatives, phenothiazine and antihistamines.

Increasing drug elimination
Forced alkaline diuresis. This potentially lethal technique is rarely necessary, as few drugs are excreted in their unchanged form. Its benefits have been shown to be outweighed by its serious complications. It is mainly used in salicylate poisoning, which is discussed on p. 665.

Peritoneal dialysis. The use of this technique is limited by its low efficacy but it may be indicated for patients severely poisoned by ethylene glycol.

Haemodialysis. This technique may be useful for patients with severe poisoning by lithium salts or methyl or ethyl alcohols. Rarely, patients with severe salicylate poisoning (blood salicylate level > 900 mg$\cdot$l^{-1} or 6.5 mmol$\cdot$l^{-1}) refractory to forced alkaline diuresis may be helped by haemodialysis.

Haemoperfusion. This is very rarely used. It involves the passage of blood through devices containing absorbent particles, such as activated charcoal or resins, to which drugs are adsorbed. Its use should be considered in patients severely poisoned with certain drugs, e.g. theophylline, and who fail to improve despite the use of adequate supportive measures.

Antagonizing the effects of poisons
These techniques will be considered under the individual drugs. Specific antidotes are available for

a small number of drugs. Antidotes act in a number of ways:

- Interaction with poison to form an inert complex which is then excreted, e.g. desferrioxamine in iron overdose
- Acceleration or detoxification of a poison, e.g. N-acetylcysteine in paracetamol poisoning
- Prevention of the formation of a more toxic compound, e.g. ethanol used as a competitive substrate for the metabolizing enzyme to prevent formation of toxic metabolites in methanol poisoning
- Competition with the poison for essential receptors, e.g. naloxone in opiate poisoning
- Blockade of receptors through which the toxic effects are mediated, e.g. atropine used to block cholinergic receptors in organophosphate poisoning

---

Specific drug problems

ANALGESICS

Analgesic poisoning is common in some areas, accounting for one-third of all cases of self-poisoning admitted to hospital. Salicylate poisoning has decreased over the past decade, while paracetamol poisoning has increased.

Combinations of aspirin or paracetamol and narcotic analgesics such as codeine or dextropropoxyphene are frequently taken. Distalgesic, a combination of paracetamol and dextropropoxyphene can cause severe respiratory distress and is a major cause of death.

Accidental poisoning with analgesics has decreased since the introduction of child-proof bottles.

Salicylates

Salicylates are well absorbed from the stomach and small intestine. They are metabolized to form salicyluric acid and salicyl phenolic glucuronides, a process that is saturated at therapeutic dosage. At high doses renal excretion becomes important. Overdosage stimulates the respiratory centre, directly increasing the depth and rate of respiration and thereby producing a respiratory alkalosis. Compensatory mechanisms include renal excretion of bicarbonate and potassium, which result in a metabolic acidosis. Salicylates also interfere with carbohydrate, fat and protein metabolism, as well as with oxidative phosphorylation. This gives rise to increased lactate, pyruvate and ketone bodies, all of which contribute to the acidosis.

Symptoms and signs of salicylate poisoning include tinnitus, nausea and vomiting, overbreathing, hyperpyrexia, and sweating with a tachycardia. Alternatively, the patient may appear completely well, even with high blood levels of salicylate.

With severe intoxication (salicylate levels 800–1000 mg·l^{-1}; 5.6–7.2 mmol·l^{-1}), confusion, delirium, convulsions and coma result. It should be remembered that consciousness is not impaired unless the blood salicylate level is very high or, more commonly, another drug has been taken.

Cerebral and pulmonary oedema are serious complications, and may be exacerbated by forced diuresis.

TREATMENT

Aspirin delays gastric emptying and gastric lavage should be performed up to 12 h after ingestion in all but the mildest cases.

Intravenous fluids may be necessary to correct dehydration and hypokalaemia. Occasionally intramuscular vitamin K is required to correct hypoprothrombinaemia.

Forced alkaline diuresis is used if the blood level exceeds 500 mg·l^{-1} (3.6 mmol·l^{-1}). Increasing the pH of the urine from 7 to 8 increases the renal excretion of salicyclic acid by about a factor of ten. In the first hour 1500 ml of fluid should be given as 500 ml 5% dextrose, 500 ml 1.4% sodium bicarbonate and then 500 ml 5% dextrose again. Sufficient potassium should be mixed with each 500 ml bag to keep the serum potassium level above 3.5 mmol·l^{-1}. Bolus intravenous injections of frusemide 20 mg may be needed to initiate and maintain a urine flow of above 500 ml·h^{-1}. If less than 200 ml of urine is produced in the first hour, diuresis should be discontinued. The urine pH should be measured regularly—every 15 or 30 min—and kept at between 7.5 and 8.5. The plasma pH should be monitored at least 2-hourly to ensure that it does not rise above 7.6; the plasma electrolytes should also be measured. If facilities are not available for constant observation by medical and nursing staff, forced alkaline diuresis may be more dangerous than the salicylate poisoning itself and should not be used.

Paracetamol (see also p. 247)

Self-poisoning with paracetamol is common and the outcome can often be fatal. Paracetamol is converted to a toxic metabolite, which is normally rapidly conjugated with reduced glutathione. After a large overdose, glutathione is depleted and the reactive intermediate binds covalently to liver cells, causing necrosis. Marked liver necrosis can occur with as little as 10 g (20 tablets), and death with 15 g. The prothrombin time is the best guide to the severity of the damage.

The clinical features in the first 24 h include nausea and vomiting, but consciousness is preserved. Most patients recover within 48 h, but some develop liver failure which becomes apparent in 72–96 h.

TREATMENT

The most reliable way to determine which patients need specific treatment is by reference to a normogram (Fig. 14.5); this relates the measurement of plasma paracetamol to the likely prognosis. Significant liver damage is likely if the paracetamol level 4 h after ingestion exceeds 200 µg·ml^{-1} (1.35 mmol·l^{-1}) and the antidote should be given.

Methionine and N-acetylcysteine are sulphydryl group doners that increase the availability of hepatic glutathione. Treatment with intravenous N-acetylcysteine should be started in all patients whose paracetamol levels are in the toxic range, provided that no more than 10 h have elapsed since ingestion of the overdose. Side-effects of treatment include convulsions and bronchoconstriction. The use of oral sulphydryl donor compounds such as methionine or cysteamine is controversial.

In addition to using specific antidotes, gastric

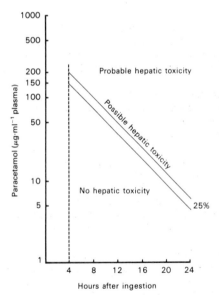

Fig. 14.5 Nomogram for paracetamol. Cautions for use of this chart:
- Serum levels drawn before 4 h may not represent peak levels.
- The graph should be used only in relation to a single acute ingestion.
- The lower solid line 25% below the standard nomogram is included to allow for possible errors in paracetamol plasma assays and estimated time from ingestion of an overdose.

From Duffy JP & Rumack BH (1984) Effects and treatment of acetaminophen overdosage. *Monitor* (Syva International) 1 (2): 5, and Crome P, Volans GN, Vale JA, Widdop B & Goulding R (1976) Oral methionine in the treatment of severe paracetamol (acetaminophen) overdose. *Lancet ii:* 829–830. With permission.

lavage, a 5% dextrose drip, correction of any electrolyte imbalance and, if the prothrombin time is prolonged, the administration of vitamin K may be necessary.

Poisoning with paracetamol and dextropropoxyphene (Distalgesic) is complicated by respiratory depression. Since dextropropoxyphene is an opiate, naloxone should be given intravenously in an initial dose of 0.4–2.0 mg, and repeated at 2–3 min intervals up to a total of 10 mg if necessary.

OTHER DRUGS

Table 14.13 shows some specific features associated with overdose of particular drugs, some of which are discussed in more detail below.

Psychotrophic drugs

Benzodiazepines
These are commonly taken in cases of self-poisoning, accounting for 40% of all drug overdosages in the UK. On their own they are remarkably safe, but they potentiate the CNS-depressant effects of other drugs taken with them, such as barbiturates or ethanol. Benzodiazepines produce drowsiness, ataxia, dysarthria, nystagmus and sometimes coma. Mild hypotension and respiratory depression may occur.

Treatment is, however, usually unnecessary and most patients recover within 24 h. Deaths from benzodiazepines alone are rare.

Antidepressants
Monoamine oxidase inhibitors (MAOIs). Self-poisoning with MAOIs is extremely uncommon. Symptoms do not usually develop for at least 12 h after the overdose, when catecholamine levels in the tissues have risen. The clinical features include central nervous system overactivity, with agitation, hallucinations and restlessness. Facial grimacing and writhing movements of the limbs and trunk may occur. There is usually dilatation of the pupils, tachycardia, a rising blood pressure and profuse sweating, although hypotension may occur. Muscle tone may be exaggerated and convulsions are common. Hyperpyrexia also occurs.

Gastric lavage is performed and supportive measures undertaken. Beta-adrenoceptor blocking drugs are usually given.

Tricyclic antidepressants. Most of the features of self-poisoning with these agents are due to the anticholinergic effects of the drugs. Clinical features include a decrease in the level of consciousness, but deep coma does not usually occur. Convulsions, increased muscle tone, hyperreflexia and extensor plantar responses sometimes occur. The pupils are

Table 14.13 Some specific management techniques that may be required for common overdoses.

Poison	Additional clinical features	Management			
		Gastric lavage	Antiarrhythmics	Anticonvulsants	Antidote
Tricyclic antidepressants	Arrhythmias, hypotension	Yes	Yes	Yes	—
Benzodiazepines		Yes	—	—	—
Opiates		Yes	—	—	Naloxone 0.4–1.2 mg i.v.
Theophylline		Yes	Yes	Yes	Absorbent, e.g. activated charcoal
Phenothiazines	Hypotension, hypothermia, dyskinesia	Yes	—	—	Benztropine 2 mg i.v. for dystonic reactions
Iron	GI symptoms, e.g. vomiting, bloody diarrhoea	—	—	—	Desferrioxamine 5 g orally to bind iron in the gut; 2 g i.m. for absorbed iron, and slow i.v. infusion of 15 mg·kg^{-1}·h^{-1} (maximum 80 mg·kg^{-1} in 24 h)
MAOIs	CNS overactivity	Yes	—	—	Beta-adrenoceptor blocking agent
Phenytoin	Ataxia, nystagmus, dysarthria	Yes	—	—	—

usually fixed and dilated and there may be oph-thalmoplegia and gaze paralysis. Urinary retention may be present. Cardiovascular effects include hypotension and sinus tachycardia. More serious tachyarrhythmias and conduction defects are uncommon and are thought to be due to the quinidine-like action of these drugs. Ventricular dysrhythmias are a cause of death in the first few hours following overdose.

If more than 15 tablets have been taken or if the patient is unconscious, gastric lavage should be per-formed within 4 h of admission to hospital. Cardiac dysrhythmias may need treatment, but often this is not necessary. Anti-arrhythmic therapy is often not effective; correction of any accompanying acidosis and hypoxia is more important.

Most patients recover consciousness within 24 h, while most cardiac abnormalities settle within 12 h.

Newer antidepressants such as mianserin and nomifensine produce only mild clinical effects, with drowsiness, hypotension and sinus tachycardia, which are much less severe than with the tricyclic antidepressants.

Lithium

Self-poisoning with this agent usually occurs in patients on long-term maintenance therapy. It is sometimes accidental or due to:
- Impairment of lithium elimination by the kidney, owing to the administration of a diuretic
- Other factors affecting water and electrolyte balance, such as nausea, vomiting or diarrhoea

Clinical features include nausea, vomiting, diar-rhoea, apathy and decreased consciousness. There may be ataxia with increased muscle tone and rigidity. Electrolyte disturbances, such as hypokalaemia, occur with ECG changes. Acute renal failure is a rare complication. Coma is associated with a bad prognosis.

Serum lithium concentrations correlate poorly with the severity of lithium poisoning, but neverthe-less levels in excess of $1.5 \ mmol \cdot l^{-1}$ are often serious.

Treatment is supportive. Intravenous fluids are necessary to maintain a good urinary output. Forced diuresis should not be used, but haemodialysis may be helpful in severe cases.

Cardiorespiratory drugs

These may be taken deliberately or sometimes accidentally by the elderly, often when one tablet is mistaken for another.

Beta-adrenoceptor blocking drugs

A small overdose of these drugs produces a brady-cardia, but a large overdose can produce convul-sions, coma, severe bradycardia and hypotension. Treatment is supportive. Atropine 0.6–1.2 mg i.v. is given. Glucagon in a bolus dose of 10 mg i.v. fol-lowed by an infusion of $3 \ mg \cdot h^{-1}$ should be used for severe hypotension. This agent activates adenyl cyclase, promoting formation of cAMP, which is a direct beta-stimulant of the heart.

Digoxin

Self-poisoning with this agent is uncommon, but chronic poisoning in patients on digoxin is frequent. Clinical features include nausea, vomiting and cardiac arrhythmias, such as heart block and various tachyarrhythmias, including ventricular tachycardia.

Treatment is supportive. Cardiac abnormalities are treated, and any hypokalaemia should be corrected.

Purified Fab fragments of digoxin antibody are now available for the treatment of digoxin toxicity.

HOUSEHOLD AND DOMESTIC POISONS

Virtually all substances found in the home have been ingested either by adults because of poorly labelled bottles or accidentally by children. Occasionally household agents are deliberately taken. Many kitchen products contain bleaches (sodium hypochlorite or hydrogen peroxide), acids or alkalis and the main problem after poisoning with them is their corrosive action on the gut. There is an immed-iate burning pain in the lips, mouth, throat, retrosternal area and stomach, and ulceration may follow. Vomiting may occur, with blood in severe cases. The major long-term complication is oesopha-geal stricture. Poisoning with sodium hypochlorite should be treated with sufficient water or milk to dilute it. Gastric lavage is contraindicated unless very substantial quantities have been taken. Alkalis should not be neutralized.

Some household products contain solvents, e.g. acetone in nail varnish remover or toluene in paints, which may be sniffed accidentally or intentionally (see p. 672).

Paraquat

Over the last few years, accidental poisoning with paraquat has become less common and deliberate self-poisoning now accounts for most cases. Paraquat is found in commonly used brands of weedkiller as an aqueous 20% solution (Gramoxone) or 2.5% solution (Weedol). A dose of 1.5 g may be fatal. Clinical features include ulcers in the mouth and oesophagus, diarrhoea and vomiting, epistaxis, pulmonary oedema, and later pulmonary fibrosis, respiratory failure and renal failure. Treatment is with gastric lavage with Fuller's earth and purging with magnesium sulphate. Haemodialysis may be useful in removing the paraquat if the plasma level is high.

The outcome can be predicted by relating the plasma paraquat concentration to the number of hours that have elapsed since ingestion. It is doubtful whether any treatment affects the prognosis.

CARBON MONOXIDE

This is a world-wide problem. Domestic gas in the UK (except in Northern Ireland) does not contain carbon monoxide, but the combustion of any fuel gas in the absence of adequate oxygen and ventilation may lead to domestic carbon monoxide poisoning. The other common sources of carbon monoxide are the exhaust fumes of petrol engines and from certain gas appliances which use propane and butane gases.

Carbon monoxide combines readily with haemoglobin to form carboxyhaemoglobin, thus preventing the formation of oxyhaemoglobin. The clinical features of carbon monoxide poisoning include mental impairment, including coma in severe cases. Headache, nausea and vomiting, and the classical pink colour of the skin due to the carboxyhaemoglobin are seen. More severe toxicity produces widespread effects, including myocardial damage and respiratory distress. Treatment consists of removing the patient from the carbon monoxide source, and giving as high a concentration of oxygen as possible together with general supportive therapy.

INSECTICIDES

Carbamates and organophosphate insecticides are used extensively in agriculture. They may be ingested accidentally, inhaled, or absorbed through the skin when protective clothing is not worn. These agents are potent inhibitors of cholinesterase and produce an accumulation of acetylcholine. Carbamate poisoning is generally less severe and of shorter duration.

The clinical features are due to the muscarinic and nicotinic effects of acetylcholine. They include nausea, vomiting, hypersalivation, muscle weakness, bronchospasm, and respiratory failure; convulsions may also occur. The plasma cholinesterase activity will be low.

Treatment involves washing any contaminated skin. Atropine 2 mg i.v. is given repeatedly to obtain full atropinization. Pralidoxime mesylate 1 g i.v., a cholinesterase reactivator, is used in severe cases.

CYANIDE

Ingestion or inhalation of this agent produces rapid onset of dizziness and headache, followed by acute shortness of breath, shock and eventual coma. Cyanosis is not present and the skin colour is red. There may be an odour of bitter almonds. Cyanide inhibits cytochrome oxidase, preventing cellular respiration, which leads to hypoxia, metabolic acidosis and frequently death. Treatment is urgent; 600 mg of dicobalt edetate should be given intravenously over 1 min and 300 mg given a minute later if no recovery occurs. General supportive treatment, including oxygen, should be given.

METHANOL, ETHANOL AND ETHYLENE GLYCOL

These agents are all chiefly metabolized by alcohol dehydrogenase in the liver. In poisoning, there is increased lactate formation, which increases the metabolic acidosis found after methanol (due to formate) or ethylene glycol ingestion (due to glycolate).

Minor poisoning with methanol causes headache, breathlessness and photophobia. In severe poisoning there is papilloedema and eventually optic atrophy and blindness. Poisoning with methanol is treated with gastric lavage and correction of acidosis with bicarbonate infusion. Ethanol infusion and haemodialysis are used to remove methanol in patients who have taken more than 30 g of methanol and who have a blood level of methanol greater than 500 mg·l^{-1} (15.6 mmol·l^{-1}). Intravenous folinic acid may prevent ocular toxicity.

Ethanol poisoning produces severe depression of consciousness and hypoglycaemia, particularly in children. Treatment usually only consists of gastric lavage with an endotracheal tube in position. The use of fructose is no longer advised and peritoneal or haemodialysis is only indicated for very severe cases.

Poisoning with ethylene glycol (antifreeze) causes gastrointestinal upset and neurological involvement, including coma, followed by cardiorespiratory collapse and acute renal failure. Treatment is by gastric lavage and correction of the acidosis with intravenous sodium bicarbonate and of the hypocalcaemia with intravenous calcium solutions. Ethanol is given orally or intravenously in severe cases to inhibit the metabolism of ethylene glycol. Haemodialysis is indicated in patients who have taken more than 50 g of ethylene glycol or who have plasma levels greater than 500 mg·l^{-1} (8.1 mmol·l^{-1}).

HEAVY METALS

Mercury

Chronic mercury poisoning causes tremor (hatters' shakes), excessive salivation, scanning speech, anxiety and depression. In the hatters' trade a rabbit fur was stirred in vats of hot mercuric nitrate to make felt, and inhalation of the vapour led to signs of chronic mercury poisoning.

Acute mercury poisoning is seen after the ingestion of mercuric salts (e.g. mercuric chloride), inhalation of mercuric vapours or the ingestion of mercury oxide in 'button' batteries. It is treated by induced emesis, lavage and injections of dimercaprol or penicillamine.

Lead

Acute lead poisoning is rare. Chronic lead poisoning, however, commonly occurs.

Occupational lead poisoning

This is a notifiable disease in the UK and work with lead is covered by strict regulations. Most lead poisoning occurs in scrap metal or smelting workers. Blood levels in these workers should be lower than 800 $\mu g \cdot l^{-1}$ (4 $mmol \cdot l^{-1}$).

Domestic lead poisoning

This usually occurs in children due to the ingestion of old lead-based paint around the home. Most toys now have lead-free paint. Chronic ingestion of water from lead pipes and acute accidental ingestion of fluid from car batteries are other frequent causes of lead poisoning.

After absorption, lead interferes with haem and globin synthesis (see p. 267). It also binds to bone, and in patients suffering from chronic exposure, small amounts of lead can be found in many tissues.

CLINICAL FEATURES

- Anorexia, nausea and vomiting
- A blue line on the gums
- Constipation and severe abdominal colic
- Dense metaphyseal bands at the growing ends of long bones, particularly the wrist and knee in children (lead lines)
- Anaemia, with erythrocytes showing basophil stippling
- Peripheral nerve lesions giving wrist drop and foot drop, with muscle involvement
- Lead encephalopathy, with eventual seizures and impairment of consciousness

The diagnosis is made on the basis of the clinical features. The blood level of lead is very variable; levels above 800 $\mu g \cdot l^{-1}$ (4 $mmol \cdot l^{-1}$) are toxic.

TREATMENT

It is most important to remove the source of lead intoxication. Sodium calciumedetate (calcium EDTA), D-penicillamine and dimercaprol have all been used for treatment.

Arsenic

Acute poisoning with arsenic causes vomiting, abdominal pain and diarrhoea. It is treated with rehydration and dimercaprol. Chronic poisoning causes excess salivation, weakness, anorexia and polyneuritis. There is a 'raindrop' pigmentation of the skin. Arsenic accumulates in the hair and the nails.

VENOMOUS ANIMALS

Snakes

The adder (*Vipera berus*) is the only poisonous snake native to the UK. However, a number of dangerous snakes are kept as pets, and world-wide venomous snakes still cause significant mortality. There are three types of venomous snake:

- Viperidae, which have long erectile fangs. They are subdivided into two types:
  (a) *Viperidae* (true vipers, e.g. Russell's viper [dabora], European adder), which are found in all parts of the world except America and the Asian Pacific
  (b) *Crotalidae* (pit-vipers, e.g. rattlesnakes, Malayan pit-viper), which are found in Asia and America. They have small heat-sensitive pits between the eyes and the nostrils.
  The venom of both of these classes of snake is vasculotoxic
- Elapidae (cobras, mambas, kraits, coral-snakes), which are found in all parts of the world except Europe. They have short, unmoving fangs and the venom produces neurotoxic features. Venom from the Asian cobra and the African spitting cobra also produces local tissue necrosis
- Hydrophidae (sea-snakes), which are found in Asian Pacific coastal waters. They have short fangs and flattened tails. The venom is myotoxic.

CLINICAL FEATURES

Viperidae

Russell's viper is the most important cause of snakebite mortality in India, Pakistan and Burma. There is local swelling at the site of the bite, which may become massive. Local tissue necrosis may occur, particularly with cobra bites. Evidence of systemic involvement occurs within 30 min, including vomiting, evidence of shock and hypotension; haemorrhage due to incoaguable blood can be fatal.

Elapidae

There is not usually any swelling at the site of the bite. Vomiting and shock occur and are followed by muscle weakness, with paralysis of the respiratory muscles in severe cases. Cardiac muscles can also be involved.

Hydrophidae

Systemic features are muscle involvement, myalgia and myoglobinuria, which can lead to acute renal failure. Cardiac and respiratory paralysis may occur.

MANAGEMENT

A firm pressure bandage should be placed over the bite and the limb immobilized. This greatly delays the spread of the venom. Arterial tourniques should not be used and incision or excision of the bite area should not be performed. The type of snake should be identified if possible.

Often no venom has been injected by the snake bite and antivenoms are not generally indicated unless systemic effects are present. Antivenoms can cause severe allergic reactions and should not be given purely because a bite has occurred. Nevertheless, careful observation for 12–24 h is necessary and antivenom must always be given when indicated, as the mortality of snake bite is 10–15% with certain snakes.

General supportive measures should be given as necessary, as for all poisoning. These include diazepam for anxiety and intravenous fluids with volume expanders for hypotension. Treatment of acute respiratory, cardiac and renal failure is instituted as necessary.

Specific measures, i.e. antivenoms, can rapidly neutralize venom, but only if an amount in excess of the amount of venom is given. Antivenoms cannot reverse the effects of the venom so they must be given early. They do minimize some of the local effects and may prevent necrosis at the site of the bite. Antivenoms should be administered intravenously by slow infusion, the same dose being given to children and adults.

Allergic reactions are frequent, and adrenaline (1 in 1000 solution) should be available. Antivenoms are usually rapidly effective. In severe cases the antivenom infusion should be continued even with allergic reactions, with subcutaneous injections of adrenaline being given as necessary. Large quantities of antivenom may be required.

Local wounds often require little treatment. If necrosis is present, antibiotics should be given together with initially minimal surgical treatment. Skin grafting may be required later. Antitetanus prophylaxis must be given.

Antivenoms must be kept readily available in all snake-infested areas.

Scorpions

Scorpion stings are a serious problem in the tropics and cause 1000 deaths per year in Mexico. The poison glands are situated in the end of the tail.

Severe pain occurs immediately at the site of puncture, followed by swelling. This should be treated by a firm pressure bandage to avoid the spread of the neurotoxic venom. Signs of systemic involvement include vomiting, respiratory depression and haemorrhage. Treatment is supportive. Antivenom is available in certain countries.

Spiders

The black widow spider (*Latrodectus mactans*) is found in North America and the tropics and occasionally in Mediterranean countries. The bite quickly becomes painful and generalized muscle pain, sweating, headache and shock occur. No systemic treatment is required except in cases of severe systemic toxicity, when specific antivenom should be given where this is available.

Loxosceles causes many bites in Central and South America. *L. reclusa*, the brown recluse spider, is also found in the southern USA. Spiders are often found in bedrooms, so that patients are often bitten at night. There is a burning pain at the site of the bite, followed by a necrotic ulcer in some cases. Systemic effects, which include fever, vomiting and haemolysis, are rare. No treatment is indicated except in severe cases, when an antivenom should be given if available.

Phoneutria nigriventer, the banana spider, and *Atrax robustus*, the Sydney funnel-web spider, can both give nasty bites, which are occasionally fatal.

Insects

Insect stings, e.g. from wasps and bees, and bites, e.g. from ants, produce pain and swelling at the puncture site. Death rarely occurs and is usually due to anaphylaxis, which requires urgent treatment (see p. 651).

Marine animals

There are many poisonous fish that can be dangerous. They are usually found in tropical waters, but cases have been described world-wide. Stingrays and scorpion fish are two examples that sting by injecting venom through barbed spines. There is immediate severe local pain and swelling, which may be followed by tissue necrosis. Systemic effects include diarrhoea, vomiting, hypotension and cardiac arrhythmias. Treatment is supportive. Care should always be taken in waters where these fish are known to be present.

Venomous Coelenterata include jellyfish, sea anemones and the Portuguese man-of-war. The tentacles contain toxin which, following a sting, produces painful wheals at the site of contact. These wheals may become necrotic. Rarely there are systemic side-effects, including abdominal pain, diarrhoea and vomiting, hypotension and convulsions. Treatment consists of removing the tentacles, having first applied acetic acid (vinegar) to them. Alcohol compounds should not be used.

Molluscs

Only the octopus and cone-shells are venomous to man. The blue-ringed octopus, which is found in Australia, has toxic saliva, which flows into the wounds from the beak of the octopus and can cause serious systemic effects.

In cone-shells the venom is found in association with their radular teeth. A bite initially produces local numbness, which can then spread over the body and may eventually lead to paralysis.

Seafood poisoning

This can occur with fish and shellfish. In some cases it is attributable to toxins, but most poisonings occur as a result of pathogens such as *Salmonella* or hepatitis A virus. Ichthyosarcotoxic fish contain toxins in their blood, skin and muscle and are the commonest cause of poisoning.

Ciguatera. Poisoning occurs chiefly with the reef-dwelling fish from around the Pacific and Caribbean. The fish contain ciguatoxins from the plankton *Gambier discus*. Most cases of poisoning are due to the red snapper, grouper, barracuda and amberjack fish, but many other species may be responsible. The poisonous fish cannot be distinguished from identical fish that do not contain the poison. The toxin is unaffected by cooking.

Symptoms occur from a few minutes to 30 h after ingestion of the fish. They include numbness and paraesthesia of the lips, abdominal pain, nausea, vomiting and diarrhoea. Visual blurring, photophobia, a metallic taste in the mouth, myalgia and eventual hypotension and shock can also occur.

Treatment is symptomatic, but symptoms can last for up to 2 weeks.

Scrombroid fish. Fish such as tuna, mackerel and skipjack contain a high degree of histidine. This is decarboxylated by bacteria to histamine, and, particularly if the fish are allowed to spoil, large amounts can accumulate in the fish, producing flushing, burning, pruritus, headache, urticaria, nausea, vomiting and bronchospasm 2–3 h after ingestion. Treatment is symptomatic; care should be taken only to eat fresh fish.

Tetrodotoxin-containing puffer-fish are found in both sea- and freshwater areas of Asia, India and the Caribbean. Symptoms which follow ingestion are circumoral paraesthesia, malaise and hypotension, with more severe cases producing ataxia and neuromuscular paralysis. The mortality is 50–60%.

Shellfish. Bivalve molluscs, e.g. mussels, oysters, scallops and clams, can acquire the neurotoxin saxitoxin from the dinoflagellate *Gonoyaulax*. These protozoa colour the sea red and molluscs should never be taken from such areas. Symptoms are similar to those caused by tetrodotoxin, but are usually less severe. Treatment is symptomatic.

PLANTS

Many plants are known to be poisonous, but in practice it is unusual for severe poisoning to occur. Children are the usual victims. Only two people are known to have died from plant poisoning in the UK over the last 15 years. The commonest effects of nettles, poison ivy, etc. are dermatitis followed by vomiting. Poisonous plants commonly ingested include hemlock, labernum, deadly nightshade and green potatoes. Deadly nightshade (*Atropa belladonna*) contains hyoscyamine and hyoscine. When ingested these cause the anticholinergic effects of a dry mouth, nausea and vomiting, eventually leading to blurring of the vision, hallucinations, confusion and hyperpyrexia.

Mushrooms

There are many poisonous mushrooms that can be confused with edible fungi and be eaten by mistake. Nevertheless, apart from transient nausea, vomiting and diarrhoea, which can occur with many species, very severe reactions are rare.

Fatal mushroom poisoning is almost invariably due to *Amanita phalloides* (the death cap mushroom). This fungus contains phallotoxins and amatoxins, both of which interfere with cell metabolism. Toxicity is increased if the mushrooms are eaten raw, as some toxins are inactivated by heat. In general, the sooner the symptoms occur, the less serious the poisoning, depending on the type of mushroom ingested. Within 2 h, nausea, vomiting, diarrhoea and sweating occur. After about 6 h, patients complain of headache and dizziness, and severe vomiting occurs at about 12 h. After 72 h, the more serious complications of hepatocellular and renal failure may occur, which have a high mortality.

The diagnosis is made by obtaining a careful history, with identification of the mushroom if possible. Amatoxins can be measured in the blood by radioimmunoassay.

Treatment should include gastric aspiration and lavage and general support. There is some evidence that haemodialysis may be of some value.

Other mushrooms that are poisonous include:

- *Amanita muscaria* (fly agaric), which contains a little muscarine and other hallucinogenic substances
- *Coprinus atramentarius* (ink cap), which contains a dehydrogenase inhibitor with a disulfiram-like effect, producing flushing, swelling, a rash on the face and hands, and cardiovascular effects, particularly after alcohol
- *Amanita pantherina* (false blusher), which produces similar features to deadly nightshade because of its atropine-like effects

Drug abuse

Solvents

Solvent abuse has become a common problem, particularly in teenagers who inhale volatile organic solvents such as toluene in glues ('glue sniffing'). Many other solvents, such as aerosols (hair lacquer), antifreeze and petrol, can also be misused. Solvents are applied to a piece of cloth or put into a plastic bag and inhaled, often until consciousness is lost. The patient presents either in the acute intoxicated state or as a chronic abuser with excoriation and rashes over the face and a peripheral neuropathy. Death can occur and is probably due to cardiac arrhythmias. Stigmata of solvent abuse include sores or a rash round the nose and mouth and glue on the clothing.

Other drugs

Drug addicts frequently overdose themselves and are commonly admitted to hospital with the signs of opiate injection. Tell-tale injection sites and pinpoint pupils are important clues. Naloxone is given in the same dosage as for Distalgesic overdose (p. 666).

Cannabis

Cannabis is usually smoked and often taken casually. Initially there is euphoria, followed by drowsiness and sleep. Redness of the conjunctivae and pupil dilatation are seen. No specific treatment is required.

Amphetamines

Amphetamines are taken for their stimulatory effect. In overdose there is confusion, delirium, hallucinations and violent behaviour. Cardiac arrhythmias can be a major problem. Treatment is with sedatives, such as diazepam. Forced acid diuresis may be used but is rarely required.

Cocaine

Cocaine can be taken by injection, inhalation or ingestion. It produces excitement, over-alertness, euphoria and restlessness. This is followed by delirium, tremor, convulsions and cardiac arrhythmias, which may cause cardiac failure. Respiratory failure may also occur.

Treatment is symptomatic and supportive. There is no specific antidote.

Poison information services

Information on poisoning can be obtained from the poisons information services at the following numbers:

National Poisons Information Service

Belfast	0232 240503
Cardiff	0222 569200
Dublin	0001 745588
Edinburgh	031 229 2477
	031 229 2441 (Viewdata)
London	01 407 7600 or 01 635 9191

Other centres

Birmingham	021 554 3801
Leeds	0532 430715 or 0532 432799
Newcastle	0632 325131

Laboratory analysis may help in the diagnosis and management of some cases. Information on the available services can be obtained from the National Poisons Information Service in London.

Further reading

Henry J & Volans G (1984) *ABC of Poisoning. Part 1. Drugs.* London: British Medical Association.

Byth PL (1983) General management of drug overdose and poisoning. *Current Therapeutics* 24 July: 99–115.

Crome P (1982) Antidepressant overdosage. *Drugs* **23**: 431–461.

Davies DM (ed.) (1986) *Textbook of Adverse Drug Reactions,* 3rd edn. Oxford: Oxford University Press.

Kallos P & West GB (1983) Pseudo-allergic reactions in man. In Turner P & Shand DG (eds) *Recent Advances in Clinical Pharmacology,* vol. 3, pp 235–252. Edinburgh: Churchill Livingstone.

Prescott LF (1978) Drug toxicity. In Turner P & Shand DG (eds) *Recent Advances in Clinical Pharmacology,* vol. 1, pp 189–209. Edinburgh: Churchill Livingstone.

Turner P, Richens A & Routledge P (1986) *Clinical Pharmacology,* 5th edn. Edinburgh: Churchill Livingstone.

Vale JA & Meredith TJ (1985) *Concise Guide to the Management of Poisoning,* 3rd edn. Edinburgh: Churchill Livingstone.

15

Environmental Disorders

Heat

In health, the core temperature of man is maintained by the thermoregulatory centre in the hypothalamus at a constant 37°C. Heat is produced by cellular metabolism, and is lost through the skin by vasodilatation and sweating and in air expired from the lungs. Sweating occurs when the ambient temperature is greater than 32.5°C and during exercise. The evaporation of sweat is an important mechanism in keeping the skin cool and the body temperature down.

Acclimatization
Acclimatization to a hotter climate takes from 1–2 weeks. There is a gradual increase in sweating, and the sweat has a lower salt content. This process allows increased evaporation.

Heat cramps

These are painful cramps in the muscles (usually of the legs) after exercise. They often occur in fit young people who are well acclimatized when they take vigorous exercise in hot weather. The symptoms are thought to be the result of a low extracellular sodium caused by replenishment of water but not salt during prolonged sweating. The cramps respond to salt and water replacement.

Heat exhaustion

This usually occurs in subjects who are not acclimatized and who undertake heavy exercise. It typically occurs in troops who are suddenly landed in a hot climate without prior acclimatization. Heat exhaustion is caused by water depletion, or salt and water depletion, due to sweating. Water loss can be as high as 5–6 l per day, and up to 20 g of salt can be lost.

Common symptoms are giddiness, generalized fatigue, weakness and syncope. Many patients are not seriously affected, but they may go on to develop hypotension, a rise in body temperature of 38–40°C, and signs of volume depletion. Dehydration and delirium can eventually occur. Sweating usually continues until the late stages. The serum sodium can be high in water depletion, but is normal or low if both water and salt are depleted.

TREATMENT

The patient is removed from the heat and cooled using cold sponging and fans.

Oral rehydration with both salt and water may be all that is required; 25 g of sodium chloride and 5 l of water in the first 24 h is given, with adequate replacements thereafter. In severe heat exhaustion, intravenous fluid is required. Isotonic saline is usually given, depending on the level of sodium in the serum. Careful monitoring is required and any subsequent potassium loss must be corrected.

Heat stroke

Heat stroke is an acute life-threatening situation when the body temperature is above 41°C. The patient suffers from headache, nausea, vomiting and weakness. The skin is hot. Sweating is often absent, but this is not invariable, even in severe heat stroke. Neurological involvement leads to confusion, delirium and eventually coma.

Heat stroke occurs in hot humid climates with little cooling wind, even without exercise. Patients are usually unacclimatized; in some, sweating is limited due to prickly heat (i.e. inflammation of the sweat glands after prolonged exposure to high temperatures). Old age, diabetes and alcohol are all further precipitating factors.

The diagnosis is clinical. The patient must be rapidly removed from the hot area, and then cooled with sponging and ice if available.

Unconscious patients need to be managed in intensive care (see p. 624) and rapid cooling with ice packs started. Fluids may be required, but these must be given with care as hypovolaemia is not present in many patients.

Prompt treatment is essential and can lead to a rapid and complete recovery; any delay may be fatal.

COMPLICATIONS

- Shock
- Cerebral oedema
- Renal and hepatic failure

Treatment of the complications is described in the appropriate chapters.

Malignant hyperpyrexia

This is discussed on p. 866.

Cold

Hypothermia is defined as a fall in the core (i.e. rectal) temperature to below 35°C. It is frequently lethal when the core temperature falls below 32°C.

Frostbite is local cold injury which occurs when tissue freezes.

Hypothermia

Hypothermia occurs in a variety of clinical settings:

- *In the home environment.* Hypothermia may occur in cold climates when there is poor heating, inadequate clothing and poor nutrition. Depressant drugs (e.g. hypnotics), alcohol, hypothyroidism or intercurrent illness may also contribute. Hypothermia is commonly seen in the poor and elderly, the latter having a diminished ability to feel cold and often a decrease in the insulating fat layer. Infants and neonates become hypothermic very rapidly at normal room temperature because of their relatively large surface area and lack of subcutaneous fat.
- *During exposure to extremes of temperature outside.* Hypothermia is a prominent cause of death in climbers, skiers, Arctic and Antarctic travellers and in wartime. Wet, cold conditions and windchill, physical exhaustion and inadequate clothing are common contributory factors.
- *Following immersion in cold water.* Dangerous hypothermia can develop after several hours immersion at temperatures of 15–20°C. Below 12°C the patient's limbs become anaesthetized and paralysed and take a long time to recover after the patient is rescued.

CLINICAL FEATURES

Mild hypothermia (32–35°C) causes shivering and initially a feeling of intense cold. The subject is alert and usually takes appropriate action to rewarm, e.g. huddling, extra clothing or exercise. As the core temperature falls, severe hypothermia (below 32°C) initially causes impairment of judgement (including awareness of the cold) and later leads to altered consciousness and coma. Death follows, usually from ventricular fibrillation.

DIAGNOSIS

If a thermometer is available (which must be low reading), the diagnosis is straightforward. If not, a rapid clinical assessment should be made. The hypothermic patient feels cold to the touch—the abdomen, groin and axillae are cold and clammy. If consciousness is impaired (i.e. the patient is uncooperative, sleepy or in a coma) the core temperature is almost certainly below 32°C; this is a medical emergency.

SEQUELAE

The pulse rate and volume fall, and respiration becomes shallow and slow. Muscle stiffness develops and the tendon reflexes are depressed. The systemic blood pressure falls. As coma ensues, the pupillary and other brainstem reflexes are lost (the pupils are fixed and may be dilated in severe hypothermia).

Metabolic changes are variable, with either metabolic acidosis or alkalosis occurring. Arterial oxygen tension readings may appear normal since they are measured at room temperature, but these measurements are falsely high as the arterial Po_2 falls 7% per °C fall in temperature.

Ventricular dysrhythmias (tachycardia and fibrillation) or asystole are the usual cause of death and may occur during treatment. 'J' waves—rounded waves above the isoelectric line immediately after the QRS complex—are pathognomic of hypothermia. Prolongation of the PR interval, QT interval and QRS complex also occur.

MANAGEMENT

The principles of management of this serious emergency are to rewarm the patient gradually whilst correcting metabolic abnormalities and treating cardiac dysrhythmias. Hypothyroidism must always be looked for (see p. 714).

If the patient is awake, with a temperature above 32°C, rewarming can be achieved by placing the patient in a warm room, using 'space blankets', and giving warm fluids orally. Outdoors, the same result can be achieved by adding extra clothing, huddling with the casualty, and using a warmed sleeping bag.

Rewarming may take several hours. Alcohol should be avoided—it may add to confusion, boost confidence factitiously, cause peripheral vasodilatation (and further heat loss) or precipitate hypoglycaemia.

Severe hypothermia

In severe hypothermia, the patient may appear dead. (Hypothermia should always be excluded before brain death is diagnosed.) Warming should take place gradually, aiming at an increase in temperature of 1°C per hour. The patient should be covered with a 'space blanket' and placed in a warm room. Direct surface heat from an electric blanket is also helpful. Any underlying condition should be treated promptly. Drug overdose should always be excluded.

Warmed intravenous fluids are given slowly and metabolic disturbances corrected. Hypothyroidism, if present, should be treated with triiodothyronine 10 µg i.v. 8-hourly. Various methods of artificial rewarming have been suggested—warm humidified air by inhalation, gastric or peritoneal lavage, or haemodialysis—but in practice these are rarely used. The cardiac rhythm should be monitored and dysrhythmias corrected.

Careful monitoring of all vital functions is required; appropriate treatment and intensive care is given as necessary.

PREVENTION

Prevention of hypothermia is particularly important in the elderly, who should be advised to try and improve general heating and insulation in the house. Heat should be provided in the bedrooms, and the use of safe electric blankets advised. Financial help will be needed by many patients. Constant supervision should be given during cold spells, when warm food and extra blankets must be provided. Patients who have been treated previously for hypothermia are especially at risk.

Frostbite

The formation of ice crystals in the skin and superficial tissues begins when the temperature there falls to −3°C; ambient temperatures generally have to be below −6°C for this to occur.

RECOGNITION

Frostbitten tissue is pale, greyish and initially doughy to the touch. Later it freezes hard, when it looks (and feels) like meat taken from a deep freeze. This condition may occur when working or exercising in low temperatures and typically develops without the patient's knowledge. Hands and feet which have 'lost their feeling' is an important feature when the temperature is below −5°C, as frostbite may then develop insidiously.

MANAGEMENT

The frostbitten patient should, if possible, be transported (or walk, even on frostbitten feet) to a place of safety before treatment commences. Warming using the body heat of a companion or by immersion in water at 39 to 42°C should be continued until obvious thawing occurs. This may be painful. Blisters will form within several days and, depending on the degree of frostbite, a blackened carapace or shell develops as the blisters regress or burst. Dry, nonadherent dressings and strict aseptic precautions are essential. Frostbitten tissues are anaesthetic and are at risk from infection and further trauma. Recovery takes place over many weeks. Surgery may be required, but should be avoided in the early stages, as it is difficult to predict the eventual amount of recovery.

High altitudes

The partial pressure of ambient (and hence alveolar and arterial) oxygen falls in a near-linear relationship to atmospheric pressure (see Fig. 15.1).

Below 3000 m there are few important clinical effects. Commercial aircraft are pressurized to 2750 m and the resulting hypoxia causes breathlessness only in those with severe cardiorespiratory disease. The incidence of thromboembolism is, however, slightly greater than at sea level in sedentary travellers on long flights.

Above 3000–3500 m, hypoxia causes a spectrum of related clinical syndromes which affect visitors to high altitudes, principally climbers, trekkers, skiers and troops (Table 15.1). These conditions, which often coexist, occur largely during the acclimatization process. This may last some weeks, but enables man to live (permanently if necessary) at altitudes up

Fig. 15.1 Diagram to show the decrease in oxygen and barometric pressure with increasing altitude.

Table 15.1 Conditions caused by sustained hypoxia.

Condition	Incidence	Usual altitude
Acute mountain sickness	70%	3500–4000 m
Acute pulmonary oedema	2%	4000 m
Acute cerebral oedema	1%	4500 m
Retinal haemorrhages	50%	5000 m
Deterioration	100%	5600 m
Chronic mountain sickness	Rare	4500 m

to about 5600 m. At greater heights, although man can survive for days or weeks, deterioration due to chronic hypoxia is inevitable.

It has now been demonstrated on several occasions that ascent to the highest of the world's summits is possible without the use of supplementary oxygen. At the summit of Everest the barometric pressure is 34 kPa (253 mmHg). This enables an acclimatized mountaineer to have an alveolar Po_2 of 4.0–4.7 kPa (30–35 mmHg)—near the physiological limits of man.

Acute mountain sickness (AMS)

This term is used to describe the malaise, nausea, headache and lassitude which is common above 3500 m. Following arrival at this altitude there is usually a latent interval of 6–36 h before the onset of symptoms. Treatment is rest, with analgesics being given if necessary; recovery is almost invariable.

Prophylactic treatment with the carbonic anhydrase inhibitor acetazolamide is of value in reducing the symptoms of AMS, since these are partly due to the development of alkalosis.

In a minority of cases, the more serious sequelae of high-altitude pulmonary oedema (HAPO) and high-altitude cerebral oedema (HACO) occur (see below).

High-altitude pulmonary oedema (HAPO)
Predisposing factors include youth, rapidity of ascent, heavy exertion and a previous history of mountain sickness. Breathlessness, with frothy blood-stained sputum indicates established HAPO. Unless treated rapidly this leads to cardiorespiratory failure, collapse and death. Milder forms of HAPO are common, presenting with breathlessness which is not severe; it is important to recognize them.

High-altitude cerebral oedema (HACO)
Cerebral oedema is a poorly understood sequel of hypoxia. It is probably the result of the abrupt increase in cerebral blood flow which occurs even at modest altitudes of 3500–4000 m. Headache is usual, and is accompanied by varying disturbances of cerebral function; drowsiness, ataxia, nystagmus

and papilloedema are common. Coma and death follow if the condition progresses.

Treatment
Any but the milder forms of AMS require urgent treatment. Oxygen should be given if it is available, and descent to a lower altitude should take place as quickly as possible. Dexamethasone or betamethasone are effective treatment in HAPO or HACO. Diuretics are of little value.

Retinal haemorrhages

Small 'flame' haemorrhages in the nerve fibre layer of the retina are common above 5000 m. They are usually symptomless unless they cover the macula, when there is painless loss of central vision. Recovery is usual.

Deterioration

Prolonged residence between 5600 and 7000 m leads to a syndrome of weight loss, anorexia and listlessness after several weeks. Above 7500 m deterioration develops more quickly, although it is possible to survive for a week or more at altitudes over 8000 m.

Chronic mountain sickness

This rare syndrome occurs in long-term residents of high altitudes after several decades. It has been described clearly only in the Andes, but may occur in Tibet and elsewhere in central Asia.

Polycythaemia, drowsiness, cyanosis, finger clubbing, congested cheeks and ear lobes, and right ventricular enlargement occur. The condition is gradually progressive.

By way of contrast, coronary artery disease and hypertension are rare in the native populations of high altitude.

Diving

The increases in ambient pressure to which a diver is exposed at various depths are summarized in Table 15.2.

Table 15.2 Pressure in relation to sea depth.

Sea depth (m)	Absolute pressure (atmospheres)	mmHg
0	1	760
10	2	1520
50	6	4560
90	10	7600

Various methods are used to supply air to the diver. With the simplest, e.g. a snorkel, the limiting factor, which occurs below 0.5 m, is the respiratory effort required to suck air into the lungs. At greater depths this 'forced negative-pressure ventilation' ultimately results in pulmonary capillary damage and haemorrhagic pulmonary oedema. Scuba tanks, the method commonly used for sporting diving down to 50 m, carry compressed air at a pressure balanced with the water pressure.

Divers who work at great depths for commercial purposes or for underwater exploration breathe helium/oxygen or nitrogen/oxygen mixtures delivered by hose from the surface.

A wide variety of complex medical problems may affect divers at all depths. These are summarized below.

PROBLEMS DURING COMPRESSION
(i.e. descent)

Barotitis ('ear squeeze') and barosinusitis ('sinus squeeze')

Barotitis is the term used to describe acute vertigo occurring due to otitis media or the passage of water into the middle ear at depths of from 5 to 20 m. It is prevented by inflating the middle ear (by blowing or swallowing with an open glottis against closed lips and nostrils). Treatment of serious otitis media is with nasal vasoconstrictor drops (phenylephrine). Rupture of the tympanic membrane may occur.

Barosinusitis is the term used to describe the sinus pain and the later damage to the walls of paranasal air sinuses which occurs during compression. It can be prevented by avoiding diving when the respiratory airways are blocked, e.g. due to upper respiratory infection or allergic rhinitis.

Nitrogen narcosis

When compressed air is breathed below 30 m the narcotic effects of nitrogen cause impairment of cerebral function with changes of mood and performance which may be life-treatening. The condition reverses rapidly on ascent.

Nitrogen narcosis is avoided by replacing air with helium/oxygen mixtures, which can enable divers to descend to 700 m.

At these great depths neurological disturbances occur which are believed to be the result of the direct effects of pressure on neurones. Tremor, hemiparesis and psychological changes may occur.

Oxygen narcosis

Pure oxygen cannot be used for diving because oxygen becomes toxic to the lungs when the alveolar oxygen pressure exceeds 1.5 atmospheres absolute (5 m of water) and to the nervous system at around 10 m of water.

In the lungs, linear atelectasis appears and there is endothelial cell damage with exudation and pulmonary oedema. In the nervous system there is initially a feeling of apprehension, nausea and sweating, followed by muscle twitching and generalized convulsions, which may be fatal under water.

PROBLEMS DURING DECOMPRESSION

Decompression sickness ('the bends') occurs on returning to the surface and is caused by the release of inert gases, usually nitrogen or helium, which form bubbles in the tissues as the ambient pressure falls. It only occurs when the diver ascends too rapidly. Decompression tables are available for calculating the time needed to come to the surface safely from any given depth.

Decompression sickness

This can take a mild form (type 1 'bends'), with skin irritation, mottling or limb pain only, or be more serious (type 2 'bends'), in which a variety of neurological features appear. Patients with type 2 'bends' may develop cortical blindness, hemiparesis, sensory disturbances or cord lesions. If nitrogen bubbles occur in the pulmonary vessels, divers experience retrosternal discomfort, dyspnoea and cough ('the chokes'). These symptoms develop within minutes or hours of a dive.

Treatment is with oxygen. In addition, all but the mildest forms of decompression sickness (i.e. skin mottling alone) require recompression, usually in a pressure chamber.

A long-term problem is aseptic necrosis caused by infarction due to nitrogen bubbles lodging in nutrient arteries supplying bone. It is seen in 5% of deep sea divers.

Lung rupture, pneumothorax and surgical emphysema

These emergencies occur principally when divers 'breath-hold' while making emergency ascents after losing their gas supply. Following lung rupture the patient notes severe dyspnoea, cough and haemoptysis. Pneumothorax and emphysema usually respond to 100% oxygen. Air embolism may occur and should be treated with recompression.

Ionizing radiation

Ionizing radiation is either penetrating (x-rays, gamma rays or neutrons) or non-penetrating (alpha or beta particles). Penetrating radiation affects the whole body, while non-penetrating radiation only affects the skin. All radiation effects, however, depend on the type of radiation, the distribution of dose and the dose rate.

Absorption of doses greater than 100 rads of gamma radiation, e.g. following survival from a nuclear explosion or nuclear power plant accident, causes acute radiation syndromes of varying severity. Long-term effects also occur, sometimes decades after exposure, as radiation increases the rate of mutagenesis.

Radiation is measured in joules per kilogram $(J \cdot kg^{-1})$; $1 J \cdot kg^{-1}$ is also known as 1 Gray (1 Gy). This is equivalent to 100 rads. Radioactivity is measured in becquerels (Bq); 1 Bq is equal to the amount of radioactive material in which there is one disintegration per second. 1 curie (Ci) is equal to 3.7×10^{10} Bq.

Mild acute radiation sickness

Nausea, vomiting and malaise follow doses of 75–125 rad (approximately 1 Gy). Lymphopenia occurs within several days, followed 2–3 weeks later by a fall in all white cells and platelets. There is a late risk of leukaemia and solid tumours.

Severe acute radiation sickness

Many systems are affected; the extent of the damage depends on the dose of radiation received. The effects of radiation are summarized in Table 15.3.

Table 15.3 The effects of radiation.

Acute effects
Haemopoietic syndrome
Gastrointestinal syndrome
CNS syndrome
Radiation dermatitis
Delayed effects
Infertility
Teratogenesis
Cataract
Neoplasia
Non-lymphocytic leukaemia
Thyroid
Salivary glands
Skin
Others

Haemopoietic syndrome

Absorption of doses between 200 and 1000 rad (2 to 10 Gy) is followed by early and transient vomiting in some individuals, followed by a period of relative well-being. Lymphocytes are particularly sensitive to radiation damage and severe lymphopenia develops over several days. A decrease in granulocytes and platelets occurs 2–3 weeks later as no new cells are being formed by the damaged marrow. Thrombocytopenia with bleeding develops and frequent, overwhelming infections occur, with a very high mortality.

Gastrointestinal syndrome

Absorption of doses greater than 600 rad (6 Gy) causes vomiting several hours after exposure. This then stops, only to recur some 4 days later accompanied by severe diarrhoea. Due to radiation inhibition of cell division, the villous lining of the intestine becomes denuded. Intractable bloody diarrhoea follows, with dehydration, secondary infection and death.

Radiation dermatitis

Skin erythema, purpura, blistering and secondary infection occur. Total loss of body hair is a bad prognostic sign and usually follows an exposure of at least 500 rad (5 Gy).

CNS syndrome

Exposures above 3000 rad (30 Gy) are followed rapidly by nausea, vomiting, disorientation and coma; death due to severe cerebral oedema follows in 36 h.

Late effects of radiation exposure

The survivors of the nuclear bombing of Hiroshima and Nagasaki have provided information on the long-term effects of radiation. The risk of developing acute granulocytic leukaemia or cancer, particularly of the skin, thyroid and salivary glands, increases.

Infertility, teratogenesis and cataract are also late sequelae of radiation exposure.

TREATMENT

As well as nuclear explosions, people may be exposed to ionizing radiation due to accidents in hospital, in industry or at nuclear power plants (e.g. Chernobyl) and reactors. Acute radiation sickness is a medical emergency. Hospitals should be immediately informed of the type and length of exposure so that suitable arrangements can be made to receive the patient. The initial radiation dose absorbed can be reduced by removing clothing contaminated by radioactive materials.

Treatment of radiation sickness is largely supportive and consists of prevention and treatment of infection, haemorrhage and fluid loss. Storage of the patient's white cells and platelets for future use should be considered, if feasible.

Accidental ingestion or exposure to bone-seeking radioisotopes (e.g. strontium-90 and caesium-137) should be treated with chelating agents (e.g. EDTA) and massive doses of oral calcium. Radioiodine contamination should be treated immediately with potassium iodide 133 mg per day. This will block 90% of radioiodine absorption by the thyroid if given immediately before exposure.

Electric shock

Electric shock may produce clinical effects in three ways:
- *Pain and psychological sequelae.* The common 'electric shock' is usually a painful but harmless stimulus which is an unpleasant and frightening experience. It produces no lasting neurological damage or cutaneous evidence of damage.
- *Disruption of specific biological processes.* Ventricular fibrillation, muscular contraction and spinal cord damage follow a major shock. These are seen typically following a lightning strike.
- *Electrical burns.* These are either superficial burns (e.g. lightning may cause a fern-shaped burn), or necrosis of subcutaneous tissues due to the heat generated by the electricity.

Noise

The intensity of sound is expressed in terms of the square of the sound pressure. The bel is a ratio and is equivalent to a 10-fold increase in sound intensity; a decibel (dB) is one-tenth of a bel. Sound is made up of a number of frequencies ranging from 30 hertz (Hz) to 20 kHz, with most being between 1 and 4 kHz. When measuring sound, these different frequencies must be taken into account. In practice a scale known as A-weighted sound is used; sound levels are reported as dB(A). A hazardous sound source is defined as one with an overall sound pressure greater than 90 dB(A).

Repeated prolonged exposure to loud noise, particularly in the frequency range of 2 to 6 kHz, causes first temporary and later permanent hearing loss due to damage to the organ of Corti, with destruction of hair cells and, eventually, the auditory neurones. This is a common occupational problem, not only in industry and the armed forces, but also in the home (e.g. electric drills and sanders), in sport (e.g. motor racing) and in entertainment (pop stars, their audiences and disc jockeys).

Serious noise-induced hearing loss is almost wholly preventable by personal protection (ear muffs, ear plugs); little treatment can be offered once deafness becomes established.

Drowning and near drowning

This is a common cause of accidental death, accounting for over 100 000 deaths annually world-wide. Approximately 40% of drownings occur in children under 5 years of age. Exhaustion, alcohol, drugs and hypothermia all contribute to the problem.

'Dry' drowning
Ten to twenty per cent of drownings occur without aspiration of water into the lungs. Laryngeal spasm is thought to occur, which leads to asphyxia and cerebral anoxia from airway blockage. This can occur in both salt and fresh water.

'Wet' drowning
Fresh water aspiration. Fresh water is hypotonic to plasma so that after entry into the lungs it is rapidly absorbed into the circulation. This results in hypervolaemia, haemolysis (water enters the red cells) and electrolyte disturbances.

Fresh water aspiration also damages the alveolar membrane, leading eventually to pulmonary oedema and hypoxia. Cerebral anoxia, oedema and coma occur. Cardiac dysrhythmias and arrest occur as a result of the hypoxia.

Sea water aspiration. Sea water contains three to four times the salt concentration of plasma and thus when aspirated into the lungs leads to fluid entering the lungs from the circulation, producing pulmonary oedema and hypoxia. Hypovolaemia and electrolyte changes occur.

Hypoxia eventually leads to neurological and cardiac problems as in fresh water aspiration.

EMERGENCY TREATMENT

It must be remembered that patients can survive up to 45 minutes under water without suffering damage. The exact reasons for this are not clearly understood, but it is probably related to the protective role of the diving reflex. It has been shown experimentally that submersion in water causes a reflex slowing of the pulse and vasoconstriction. In addition, hypothermia decreases oxygen consumption of both the heart and brain.

Patients should be turned to one side and the mouth cleared of any debris. Mouth-to-mouth respiration should be immediately started together with cardiac resuscitation if this is appropriate (see p. 473).

Mouth-to-mouth resuscitation should always be attempted, even in the absence of a pulse and the presence of fixed dilated pupils, as patients can frequently make a dramatic recovery.

All patients should be subsequently admitted to hospital for intensive monitoring. Intensive care therapy may be required, and patients are liable to develop the adult respiratory distress syndrome (ARDS).

PROGNOSIS

The prognosis is good if the patient is fully conscious on admission to hospital but poor if the patient is still in a coma.

Motion sickness

This common problem, particularly in children, is caused by repetitive stimulation of the labyrinth of the ear. It occurs frequently at sea and in cars, but may occur on horseback or on less usual forms of transport such as camels or elephants. Nausea, sweating, dizziness and profuse vomiting occur, accompanied by an irresistible desire to stop moving.

Prophylactic antihistamines or vestibular sedatives (hyoscine or cinnarizine) are of some value.

Further reading

Auerbach PS & Geehr EC (1983) *Management of Wilderness and Environmental Emergencies*. London: Macmillan.

Nelson RN, Rund DA & Keller MD (1985) *Environmental Emergencies*. Philadelphia: W.B. Saunders.

16

Endocrinology

Introduction

Hormones

Hormones are chemical messengers that are produced by a variety of specialized secretory cells. They may be transported in the blood to a distant site of action (the classical endocrine effect) or may act directly upon nearby cells (paracrine activity). In addition, in the hypothalamus and elsewhere in the brain there are many cells that secrete hormones, some of which have true endocrine or paracrine activity while others behave more like neurotransmitters.

Synthesis, storage and release of hormones
Under either neural or endocrine stimulation, the cell increases production of its specific hormone product. This signal is often in the form of a precursor molecule which may itself be biologically inactive. The hormone is often further processed intracellularly before being packaged into granules, which are then transported to the basement membrane and released.

Plasma transport
Most hormones are secreted into the systemic circulation, but in the hypothalamus they are released into the pituitary portal system. Much higher concentrations of the releasing factors thus reach the pituitary than occur in the systemic circulation.

Many hormones are bound to proteins within the circulation. Only the free (unbound) hormone is available to the tissues and thus biologically active. The binding to proteins serves to buffer against very rapid changes in plasma levels of the hormone. The levels of binding proteins are frequently altered in disease states and this is important in interpreting many tests of endocrine function, which often measure total rather than free hormone levels. Binding proteins frequently comprise both specific, high-affinity proteins of limited capacity, such as thyroxine-binding globulin (TBG), and other less specific low-affinity ones, such as prealbumin and albumin (Table 16.1).

Action
Hormones may act at the cell surface and/or within the cell. Many protein hormones in particular bind to specific cell surface receptors where they trigger internal messengers ('second messengers', for example working via cyclic AMP or calcium), which leads either to rapid alterations in membrane ion transport or to slower responses such as DNA, RNA and protein synthesis. Other hormones, especially steroids, enter most cells of the body where they act on intracellular receptors.

Some characteristics of these hormone systems are shown in Table 16.2.

Table 16.1 Plasma hormones with important binding proteins.

Hormone	Binding protein(s)
Thyroxine (T$_4$)	Thyroxine-binding globulin (TBG) Thyroxine-binding prealbumin (TBPA) Albumin
Triiodothyronine (T$_3$) (less bound than T$_4$)	Thyroxine-binding globulin (TBG) Albumin
Cortisol	Cortisol binding globulin (CBG)
Testosterone Oestradiol	Sex hormone binding globulin (SHBG)

Table 16.2 Characteristics of different hormone systems.

	Peptides and catecholamines	Steroids and thyroid hormones
Protein binding:	No	Yes
Changes in plasma concentrations:	Rapid changes	Slow fluctuations
Half-life:	Short (seconds to minutes)	Long (minutes to days)
Type of receptors:	Cell membrane	Intracellular
Mechanism:	Activate pre-formed enzymes	Stimulate protein synthesis
Speed of effect:	Rapid (seconds to minutes)	Slow (hours to days)

The sensitivity and/or number of receptors to a hormone is often decreased after prolonged exposure to a high hormone concentration ('down-regulation'). The reverse is also true when stimulation is absent or minimal, the receptors showing increased numbers or sensitivity.

Control and feedback

Most hormone systems are controlled by some form of feedback. An example is the hypothalamic–pituitary–thyroid axis (Fig. 16.1):

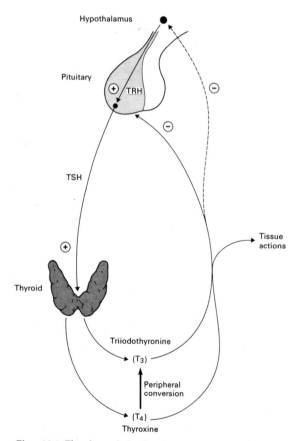

Fig. 16.1 The hypothalamic–pituitary–thyroid feedback system. The dotted line indicates *probable* negative feedback at hypothalamic level.

- Thyrotrophin-releasing hormone (TRH) is secreted in the hypothalamus and travels via the portal system to the pituitary, where it stimulates the thyrotrophs to produce thyroid-stimulating hormone (TSH).
- TSH is secreted into the systemic circulation, where it stimulates increased thyroidal iodine uptake, and increased thyroxine (T_4) and triiodothyronine (T_3) synthesis and release.
- Serum levels of T_4 and T_3 are thus increased by TSH; in addition the conversion of T_4 to T_3 (the more active hormone) in peripheral tissues is stimulated.
- T_4 and T_3 then enter cells, where they bind to nuclear receptors and promote increased metabolic and cellular activity.
- Blood levels of T_3 and T_4 are sensed by receptors in the pituitary and possibly the hypothalamus. If they rise above the normal range, the production of TRH and TSH is suppressed, leading to less T_4 and T_3 secretion.
- Peripheral T_3 and T_4 levels thus fall to normal.
- If, however, T_3 and T_4 levels are low (e.g. post-thyroidectomy) increased amounts of TRH, and thus TSH, are secreted, stimulating the remaining thyroid to produce more T_3 and T_4. Blood levels of T_4 and T_3 may be restored to normal, although this will be at the expense of an increased TSH drive, reflected by a high TSH level.

This is known as a negative feedback system, a term which refers to the effect of T_4 and T_3 on the pituitary and hypothalamus. There are also positive feedback systems, classically seen in the regulation of the normal menstrual cycle (see pp. 695–697).

Pattern of secretion

Hormone secretion may be continuous or intermittent. The former is shown by the thyroid hormones, where T_4 has a half-life of 7–10 days and T_3 of about 1 day. Levels over the day, month and year show very little variation. In contrast, secretion of the gonadotrophins, luteinizing hormone (LH) and follicle-stimulating hormone (FSH) is normally pulsatile, with one pulse being released every 2 h or so. Continuous infusion of LH to produce a steady equivalent level does not produce the same result (e.g. ovulation in the female) as the intermittent pulsatility, and may indeed produce down-regulation and amenorrhoea.

Biological rhythms. The most important are the circadian rhythm and the menstrual cycle.

The circadian rhythm involves changes over the 24 h of the day/night cycle. A good example is glucocorticoid activity. Fig. 16.2 shows plasma cortisol levels measured over 24 h—levels are highest in the early morning and lowest overnight. Additionally, cortisol release is pulsatile, corresponding to the pulses of pituitary adrenocorticotrophic hormone. Thus 'normal' cortisol levels (stippled areas in Fig. 16.2) vary during the day and great variations can be seen in samples taken only 30 min apart.

The menstrual cycle (see pp. 695–697) is the best example of a longer (28-day) biological rhythm.

Other regulatory factors
The following factors also play a part in regulating the secretion of some hormones:
- *Stress.* Though difficult to define, stress can produce rapid increases in adrenocorticotrophic hormone (ACTH) and cortisol, growth hormone, prolactin, adrenaline and noradrenaline.
- *Sleep.* Secretion of growth hormone and prolactin is increased during sleep.

Testing endocrine function

Blood levels
Assays for all the important hormones are now available. Obviously the time, day and conditions when the sample is taken may make great differences to the hormone levels. The correct method and timing of samples will depend upon the characteristics of the endocrine system involved.

Basal levels are especially useful for hormone systems with long half-lives, e.g. T_4 and T_3. These vary little in the short term and random samples are therefore satisfactory. Basal samples may also be satisfactory for other hormones if interpreted with respect to normal ranges for the time of day or month, the diet and the posture concerned. Examples are follicle-stimulating hormone, oestrogen and progesterone, and aldosterone. All relevant details must be recorded at the time of sampling.

Stress-related hormones (e.g. catecholamines, prolactin, growth hormone and cortisol) may require samples to be taken via an indwelling needle some time after venepuncture to avoid high levels being produced artefactually.

Levels in urine
Collections of urine taken over 24 h have the advantage of providing an 'integrated mean' of a day's secretion, but are often incomplete or wrongly timed.

Levels in saliva
Saliva is sometimes used for steroid estimations, especially in children.

Stimulation and suppression tests
These are valuable in instances of hormone deficiency or excess, respectively.

Stimulation tests. Where the secretory capacity of a gland is damaged, maximal stimulation by the trophic hormone will give a diminished output. Thus in the ACTH stimulation test for adrenal reserve (Fig. 16.3a), a patient with primary hypoadrenalism (Addison's disease) will demonstrate an impaired response to ACTH.

Suppression tests. A patient with a hormone-producing tumour usually fails to show normal negative feedback. A patient with Cushing's disease (excess pituitary ACTH) will thus fail to suppress ACTH and cortisol production when given a dose of synthetic steroid, as would normal subjects (see Fig. 16.3b).

All these tests must be performed exactly as laid down, as slight variations in technique will produce variations in results. Details and the results of common tests are given in the Appendices on p. 959.

Measurement of hormone concentrations
Circulating levels of most hormones are very low (10^{-6} to 10^{-12} mol$\cdot$l^{-1}) and cannot be measured by simple chemical techniques. The most widely used method is radioimmunoassay, which is illustrated in Fig. 16.4.

Radioimmunoassay has limitations; in particular the immunological activity of a hormone, as used in developing the antibody, may not necessarily correspond to its biological activity. Nevertheless, reliable radioimmunoassays for most hormones are available, many at local hospitals and others at

Fig. 16.2 Plasma cortisol levels during a 24-h period. Note both the pulsatility and the shifting baseline.

Fig. 16.3 (a) Short ACTH stimulation test showing a normal response in a healthy subject (A) and a decreased response in a patient with Addison's disease (B). (b) Dexamethasone suppression tests in a normal subject (A) and a patient with Cushing's disease (B), showing inadequate suppression.

national level (in the UK at the Supraregional Assay Service).

Recent advances such as labelling of the antibody, enzyme-linked immunoadsorbent assays (ELISA) or using the biological activity of the hormone to produce colour reactions in tissue slices are becoming more widely used.

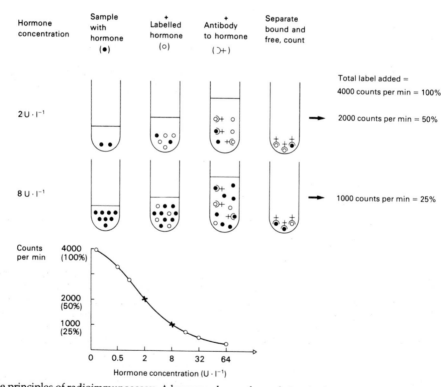

Fig. 16.4 The principles of radioimmunoassay. A known volume of sample is mixed with a known amount of radioactively labelled hormone. To this is added a known amount of specific antibody to the hormone. The antibody will attach to labelled and unlabelled hormone in proportion to their relative concentrations. Antibody-bound hormone and remaining free hormone can be separated and the bound or free radiolabelled part can be counted. In the instance shown, bound label is counted—the amount will vary depending on the hormone concentration in the sample.

A set of 'standards' of known hormone level is included with the unknown samples; all are treated in exactly the same way. From the standards a 'standard curve' is produced, showing the variation in counts per minute, or percentage total binding, with increasing concentrations of hormone. The 'unknown' samples will produce a number of counts; by reading off the graph the concentration of hormone originally present in the sample can be determined.

An introduction to endocrine disease

Most endocrine disease is extremely simple to understand—there is either too much of a hormone or too little! The underlying pathology (such as a tumour) may also cause local symptoms.

EPIDEMIOLOGY

The commonest endocrine conditions are:
- Diabetes (see Chapter 17)
- Thyroid disorders, affecting four to eight new patients per general practitioner per year
- Children with short stature or delayed puberty
- Subfertility, affecting 5–10% of all couples trying to conceive; among these endocrine causes are common
- Disorders of menstruation and excessive hair growth in young women
- Primary hyperparathyroidism, affecting about 0.1% of the population
- Osteoporosis

While other endocrine conditions are uncommon, they often affect young people and are usually curable or completely controllable with appropriate therapy.

Hormones are also widely used therapeutically:
- Oral contraceptives are the contraceptive choice of about 50% of women aged 18–35.
- Corticosteroid therapy is widely used for non-endocrine disease such as asthma.

SYMPTOMS

Common presenting symptoms are shown in Table 16.3. This table demonstrates the many effects that hormonal abnormality can produce.

Hormones produce widespread effects upon the body, and focal symptoms are less common than with other types of disease. Many endocrine symptoms are diffuse and vague, and the differential diagnosis is often wide.

In addition, there are close physiological, and sometimes anatomical, relationships between different glands. Thus excessive growth *may* be caused by excess pituitary growth hormone production, *possibly* from a pituitary tumour, which *might* affect control of gonadal, breast, thyroid and adrenal function. If the tumour is large it *could* cause visual field defects and even affect the hypothalamus, *perhaps* producing diabetes insipidus. These possible connections and implications need to be recognized. Other examples are shown in Fig. 16.5.

HISTORY AND EXAMINATION

Specific dates of onset of symptoms, how they were noticed and how they have progressed is vital. Not

Table 16.3 Common presenting complaints in endocrine disease.

Body size and shape
Short stature
Tall stature
Excessive weight or weight gain
Loss of weight

'Metabolic' effects
Tiredness
Weakness
Increased appetite
Decreased appetite
Polydipsia/thirst
Polyuria/nocturia
Tremor
Palpitation
Anxiety

Local effects
Swelling in the neck
Carpal tunnel syndrome
Bone or muscle pain
Protrusion of eyes
Visual loss (acuity and/or fields)
Headache

Reproduction/sex
Loss or absence of libido
Impotence
Oligomenorrhoea/amenorrhoea
Subfertility
Galactorrhoea
Gynaecomastia
Delayed puberty
Precocious puberty

Skin
Hirsuties
Hair thinning
Pigmentation
Dry skin
Excess sweating

all questions are necessary or relevant for all patients—the skill is to ask the right ones!

Examination too must be selective and thoughtful, though general observation is vital. Conditions such as acromegaly and Cushing's syndrome are usually immediately apparent to the alert. However, 'lateral thinking' is often needed (Fig. 16.5).

Physical signs are listed under the relevant diseases, and Table 16.4 describes the details to be elicited from the past, family and social histories. It must always be remembered that endocrine problems can be iatrogenic (Table 16.5).

Specific points about endocrine disease

As with other systems, endocrine disease may be congenital or acquired and may be caused by a

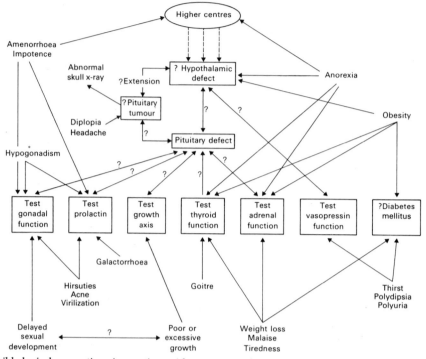

Fig. 16.5 Possible logical connections in a patient with common endocrine presenting symptoms. Not all possibilities are indicated.

Table 16.4 Endocrine disease—past, family and social histories.

Past history
Necessary details may include:
Previous pregnancies (ease of conception, postpartum haemorrhage)
Relevant surgery (e.g. thyroidectomy, orchidopexy)
Radiation (e.g. to neck, gonads, thyroid)
Drug exposure (e.g. chemotherapy, sex hormones, oral contraceptives)
In childhood, developmental milestones

Family history
Family history of:
Autoimmune disease
Endocrine disease
Essential hypertension

Family details of:
Height
Weight
Body habitus
Hair growth
Age of sexual development

Social history
Detailed records of alcohol intake (e.g. subfertility, obesity)
Drug abuse (e.g. cannabis and subfertility)
Full details of occupation, access to drugs, chemicals, etc.
Diet, e.g. salt, liquorice, iodine

variety of pathologies. However, several forms of illness are commoner than in other systems.

Autoimmune disease
Organ-specific autoimmune disease has now been shown for every major endocrine organ (Table 16.6). Such diseases are characterized by the presence of specific antibodies in the serum, often present years before clinical symptoms are evident. The conditions are usually commoner in women and have a strong genetic component, often with an identical twin concordance rate of up to 50% and with marked HLA associations.

Endocrine tumours
Hormone-secreting tumours occur in all endocrine organs, most commonly in the pituitary, thyroid and parathyroid. Fortunately they are more commonly benign than malignant. While often considered to be 'autonomous', many do show evidence of feedback occurring at a higher than normal 'set-point'.

Enzymatic defects
The biosynthesis of most hormones involves many stages. Deficient or abnormal enzymes involved in this pathway can lead to absent or reduced production of the terminal hormone. In general, severe deficiencies present early in life with obvious signs, whereas partial deficiencies present later with mild signs or are only evident when the pathway is put

Table 16.5 Drugs and endocrine disease.

Drug*	Effect
Drugs inducing endocrine disease	
Chlorpromazine Metoclopramide Oestrogens	Increase prolactin, causing galactorrhoea
Iodine Amiodarone	Hyperthyroidism
Lithium Amiodarone	Hypothyroidism
Chlorpropamide	Inappropriate ADH secretion
Drugs simulating endocrine disease	
Sympathomimetics Amphetamines	Mimic thyrotoxicosis or phaeochromocytoma
Liquorice	Mineralocorticoid activity; can simulate aldosteronism
Purgatives Diuretics	Hypokalaemia Secondary aldosteronism
Exogenous hormones Use, abuse or misuse, by patient or doctor, of the following:	
Steroids	Cushing's syndrome Diabetes
Thyroxine	Thyrotoxicosis factitia
Vitamin D preparations Milk and alkali preparations	Hypercalcaemia
Insulin	Hypoglycaemia

* Drugs causing gynaecomastia are listed in Table 16.18.

Table 16.6 Types of autoimmune disease.

Organ	Antibody	Clinical syndrome
Stimulating Thyroid	Thyroid stimulating immunoglobulin (TSI, TSAb) Thyroid growth immunoglobulin	Graves' disease, neonatal thyrotoxicosis Goitre
Destructive Thyroid	Thyroid microsomal antibody Thyroglobulin	Primary hypothyroidism (myxoedema)
Adrenal	Adrenal cortex	Primary hypoadrenalism (Addison's disease)
Pancreas	Islet cell	Type I (insulin-dependent) diabetes
Stomach	Gastric parietal cell Intrinsic factor	Pernicious anaemia
Skin	Melanocyte	Vitiligo
Ovary	Ovary	Primary ovarian failure
Testis	Testis	Primary testicular failure
Parathyroid	Parathyroid chief cell	Primary hypoparathyroidism
Pituitary	Pituitary-specific cells	Selective hypopituitarism, e.g. GH deficiency, hyperprolactinaemia

NB Other related diseases include myasthenia gravis and autoimmune liver disease.

under stress. An example of an endocrine condition due to an enzyme defect is congenital adrenal hyperplasia (see p. 729).

Receptor abnormalities

There are rare conditions where hormone secretion and control are normal but the cellular receptors are defective. Thus if androgen receptors are defective, normal levels of androgen will not produce masculinization (e.g. as in testicular feminization, see p. 708).

Central control of endocrine function

Anatomy

Many of the peripheral hormone systems are controlled by the hypothalamus and pituitary. The hypothalamus is sited at the base of the brain around the third ventricle and above the pituitary stalk, which leads down to the pituitary itself.

Fig. 16.6 shows the important anatomical relationships of the hypothalamus and pituitary. The optic chiasm is just above the pituitary fossa; any expanding lesion from the pituitary or hypothalamus can produce visual field defects by exerting pressure on the chiasm. The pituitary is itself encased in a bony box; any lateral, anterior or posterior expansion of the pituitary must therefore cause bony erosion. Upward expansion of the gland through the diaphragma sellae is termed suprasellar extension. The normal fossa is of very variable size but a true lateral x-ray should show a well-defined outline with a single floor.

Embryologically, the anterior pituitary is formed from Rathke's pouch; this meets an outpouching of the third ventricular floor, which becomes the posterior pituitary.

Physiology

The hypothalamus contains many vital control centres for such functions as appetite, thirst, thermal regulation and sleep/waking. It acts as an integrator of many neural and endocrine inputs, which control the release of releasing factors. Among other important influences it has control over are the circadian rhythm, menstrual cyclicity, stress, exercise and mood. From the hypothalamus a portal venous system runs down the stalk to the pituitary, through which releasing factors are transported.

The release of most anterior pituitary hormones is controlled in a similar way. Peptide releasing factors (Table 16.7) are produced in the hypothalamus, travel down the portal system and stimulate specific cells within the pituitary. These cells then produce increased amounts of the trophic hormones, which stimulate the peripheral glands. This pattern is illustrated in Fig. 16.7. The major exception is prolactin secretion, which is predominantly under inhibitory control by dopamine from the hypothalamus.

In contrast the posterior pituitary acts merely as a storage organ. Antidiuretic hormone (ADH, vasopressin) and oxytocin, both nonapeptides, are synthesized in the supraoptic and paraventricular nuclei in the anterior hypothalamus. They are then transported along a single axon and stored in the posterior pituitary. This means that damage to the stalk or pituitary does not prevent synthesis and release of vasopressin and oxytocin. ADH is discussed in more detail on pp. 730–732; oxytocin produces milk ejection and uterine myometrial contraction.

Elucidation of the structures of the hypothalamic hormones, mainly by molecular biological techniques, has allowed their synthesis and the production of agonist and antagonist analogues. Thus gonadotrophin-releasing hormone (LHRH), corticotrophin-releasing hormone (CRH), growth hormone releasing hormone (GHRH), vasopressin and their analogues are increasingly used both in testing function and therapeutically.

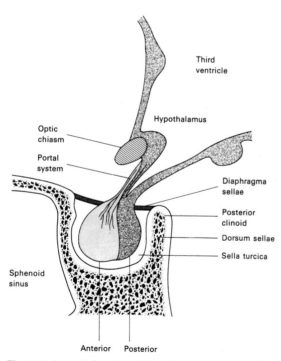

Fig. 16.6 A sagittal section of the pituitary fossa, showing the important anatomical relationships.

Table 16.7 Nomenclature and biochemistry of hypothalamic, pituitary and peripheral hormones.

Hypothalamic hormones	Pituitary hormones	Peripheral hormones
Gonadotrophin-releasing hormone (LHRH, GnRH) *Structure*: Decapeptide	Luteinizing hormone (LH) Follicle-stimulating hormone (FSH) *Structure*: Two-chain (α, β) peptides MW 32 000	Oestrogens/androgens *Structure*: Steroids
Prolactin inhibiting factor (PIF) *Structure*: Dopamine	Prolactin (PRL) *Structure*: Single peptide chain MW 23 000	—
Growth homone-releasing factor (GRF) *Structure*: 40 amino acids Somatostatin (GHRIH) *Structure*: Cyclic peptide, 14 amino acids	Growth hormone (GH) *Structure*: Single chain peptide MW 23 000	Somatomedin C and others *Structure*: Small peptides MW 5000–9000
Thyrotropin-releasing hormone (TRH) *Structure*: Tripeptide	Thyroid-stimulating hormone (TSH) *Stucture*: Two-chain (α, β) peptide MW 28 000	Thyroxine, triiodothyronine (T₄, T₃) *Structure*: Thyronines
Corticotrophin-releasing factor (CRF) *Structure*: 41 amino acids	Adrenocorticotrophic hormone (ACTH) *Structure*: Single chain peptide, 39 amino acids MW 4500	Cortisol *Structure*: Steroid
Vasopressin, anti-diurectic hormone (ADH) *Structure*: Nonapeptide	—	—
Oxytocin *Structure*: Nonapeptide	—	—

NB The alpha chains of LH, FSH and TSH are identical.

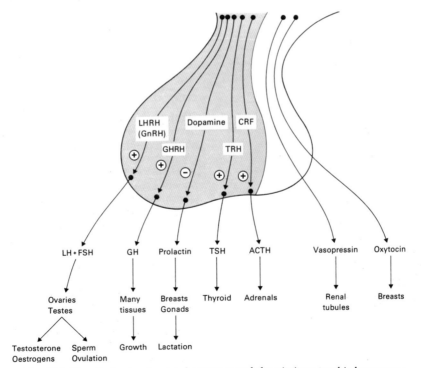

Fig. 16.7 Hypothalamic releasing hormones and the pituitary trophic hormones.

Endorphins and the ACTH families of peptides
Recently discovered hypothalamic hormones include the endorphins (*endogenous morphine*), some of which are derived from part of the ACTH precursor molecule (Fig. 16.8). This scheme demonstrates some of the complex processing of pituitary peptides including the role of a 'prohormone', from which the major hormone, ACTH, is split. The endorphins have opioid activity and are thought to be mediators of stress-induced analgesia.

They have also been found within the gut but their physiological role is still uncertain.

Presentations of hypothalamic and pituitary disease

Overproduction of hypothalamic–pituitary hormone. There are three major types:
- Growth hormone (GH) excess leading to acromegaly or gigantism
- Prolactin excess (prolactinoma or hyperprolactinaemia)
- Cushing's disease (excess adrenocorticotrophic hormone secretion)

Tumours producing luteinizing hormone (LH), follicle-stimulating hormone (FSH) or thyroxine-stimulating hormone (TSH) are very rare. Some 'non-functioning' tumours may produce the alpha subunit of LH, FSH and TSH alone (see Table 16.7).

Underproduction of hormone. This may be due to disease at the level of either the hypothalamus or the pituitary.

Local effects. Pituitary and hypothalamic lesions, hormonally active or not, can cause symptoms by infiltration of or pressure on:

- The visual pathways, resulting in field defects and visual loss
- The cavernous sinus, resulting in lesions of the third, fourth and sixth cranial nerves
- Bony structures surrounding the fossa, resulting in headache
- The hypothalamic centres, resulting in altered appetite, obesity, thirst, somnolence/wakefulness or precocious puberty

HYPOPITUITARISM

PATHOPHYSIOLOGY

Deficiency of hypothalamic releasing hormones or of pituitary trophic hormones may be either selective or multiple. There are, for example, rare congenital isolated deficiencies of LH/FSH and ACTH. Multiple deficiencies usually result from tumour growth or other destructive lesions. With the latter, there is generally a progressive loss of anterior pituitary function in the order shown from left to right in Fig. 16.7: GH and the gonadotrophins are usually affected first, hyperprolactinaemia occurs relatively early because of the loss of tonic inhibitory control by dopamine, TSH is usually next, and ACTH last. Panhypopituitarism refers to deficiency of all anterior pituitary hormones and is most commonly caused by pituitary tumours.

ADH and oxytocin secretion will only be significantly affected if the hypothalamus is involved.

CAUSES

Disorders causing hypopituitarism are listed in Table 16.8.

CLINICAL FEATURES

Symptoms and signs depend upon the extent of hypothalamic and/or pituitary deficiencies. Loss of libido, amenorrhoea and impotence are symptoms of gonadotrophin deficiency with signs of reduced secondary sexual characteristics, while hyperprolactinaemia may cause galactorrhoea. GH deficiency is clinically 'silent' except in children. Secondary thyroid and adrenal failure lead to tiredness, slowness of thought and action, and mild hypotension. Panhypopituitarism may give the classical picture of pallor with hairlessness ('alabaster skin').

Particular syndromes related to hypopituitarism include:
- *Kallman's syndrome* (isolated gonadotrophin deficiency). This leads to primary hypogonadism. It is often familial and associated with anosmia and colour blindness.
- *Sheehan's syndrome.* This situation, now rare, is pituitary infarction following postpartum haemorrhage.

Fig. 16.8 Processing of the ACTH precursor molecule (proopiocortin) illustrating some of the products. MSH= melanocyte-stimulating hormone; LPH=lipotrophin.

Table 16.8 Causes of hypopituitarism.

Congenital
Isolated deficiency of pituitary hormones (e.g. Kallmann's syndrome)

Infective
Basal meningitis (e.g. tuberculosis)
Encephalitis
Syphilis

Vascular
Pituitary apoplexy
Sheehan's syndrome (postpartum necrosis)
Carotid artery aneurysms

Immunological
Pituitary antibodies

Neoplastic
Pituitary or hypothalamic tumours
Craniopharyngioma
Meningiomas
Gliomas
Pinealoma
Secondary deposits, especially breast

Traumatic
Skull fracture
Surgery, especially transfrontal

Infiltrations
Sarcoidosis
Histiocytosis X
Haemochromatosis

Others
Radiation damage
Fibrosis
Chemotherapy

'Functional'
Anorexia nervosa
Starvation
Emotional deprivation

- *Pituitary apoplexy*. A pituitary tumour may infarct or haemorrhage into itself. This may produce severe headache, sometimes followed by acute life-threatening hypopituitarism.
- *The empty sella syndrome*. This is sometimes due to a defect in the diaphragma and extension of the subarachnoid space or it may follow spontaneous infarction of a tumour. All or most of the sella turcica does not contain pituitary tissue, but despite this pituitary function may be normal.

INVESTIGATION

Each axis of the hypothalamic–pituitary system may require separate investigation. The presence of normal gonadal function (ovulatory menstruation or normal libido/erections) renders multiple defects of anterior pituitary function unlikely. Tests range from the simple basal levels, e.g. T_4 for the thyroid axis, to stimulatory tests for the pituitary and tests of feedback for the hypothalamus (Table 16.9).

TREATMENT

Steroid and thyroid hormones are essential for life. Both may be given as oral replacement drugs, aiming to restore the patient to clinical and biochemical normality (Table 16.10). Growth hormone therapy may be given if necessary in the growing child, and sex hormone production may be restored with testosterone and oestrogens for symptomatic control. If necessary, human chorionic gonadotrophin (HCG) (mainly LH) and Pergonal or Metrodin (mainly FSH) can be given if fertility is desired; pulsatile luteinizing hormone releasing hormone (LHRH) therapy may shortly supplant this.

Table 16.9 Tests for hypothalamic–pituitary (HP) function.

Axis	Tests for end-organ product	Feedback hormone	Tests for pituitary reserve	Tests for hypothalamic feedback
Anterior pituitary				
HP–ovarian	Oestradiol levels Progesterone levels Ultrasound (pelvic)	LH FSH	LHRH test	Clomiphene test
HP–testicular	Testosterone levels Sperm count	LH FSH	LHRH test	Clomiphene test
Growth	GH/somatomedin C levels	SmC	GRF test	Insulin tolerance test
Breast	Prolactin levels		—	—
Thyroid	T_4/T_3 levels	TSH	TRH test	—
Adrenal	Cortisol levels	ACTH	CRF test	Insulin tolerance test
Posterior pituitary				
Thirst	Plasma and urine osmolalities	Vasopressin response to small amounts of hypertonic saline (300 mmol·l^{-1})		

SmC = somatomedin C.

Table 16.10 Replacement therapy for hypopituitarism.

Axis	Usual replacement	Additional therapy
Gonadal	Males: testosterone 500 mg every 3–4 weeks Females: cyclical oestrogen/progestogen	HCG plus FSH (Pergonal) to produce testicular development, spermatogenesis or ovulation; used for infertility (Pulsatile LHRH used in both sexes)
Breast (prolactin)	Bromocriptine 3–15 mg daily as replacement inhibition	—
Growth	None needed in adult	For growth, GH injections or ? GRF analogues
Thyroid	Thyroxine 0.1–0.2 mg daily	—
Adrenal	Hydrocortisone 15–40 mg daily Prednisolone 5–10 mg daily (Normally no need for mineralocorticoid replacement)	ACTH (tetracosactrin) to prevent or reverse adrenal suppression
Thirst	Desmopressin 10–20 μg once or twice daily	Carbamazepine, thiazides or chlorpropamide sometimes useful in mild diabetes insipidus

HCG = Human chorionic gonadotrophin (mainly LH); GRF = growth hormone releasing factor.

Two warnings are necessary:
- Thyroid replacement should not commence until normal glucocorticoid function has been demonstrated or replacement steroid therapy initiated, otherwise acute adrenal failure may be precipitated.
- Glucocorticoid deficiency may mask impaired urine concentrating ability, diabetes insipidus only becoming apparent *after* steroid replacement.

PITUITARY TUMOURS

Tumours are amongst the commonest causes of hypopituitarism. Investigation of a possible tumour involves three lines of questioning:

1 *Is there a hormonal excess?*
The clinical features of acromegaly and Cushing's disease or hyperprolactinaemia are usually, but not always, obvious. Hyperprolactinaemia may be clinically 'silent'.

2 *Are any hormones deficient?*
Clinical examination may give clues; thus short stature in a child with a pituitary tumour is likely to be due to GH deficiency. A slow, lethargic adult with pale skin is likely to be TSH and/or ACTH deficient. Milder deficiencies may not be obvious, and require specific testing (Table 16.9).

3 *Is there a tumour?* How big is it and what anatomical effects is it exerting?
Investigations include:
- Lateral skull x-rays. These may show enlargement of the fossa. However, this is a common incidental finding and requires further investigation (Fig. 16.9).
- Visual fields. These should be plotted formally; common defects are upper temporal quadran-

Fig. 16.9 Lateral skull x-ray showing double floor and enlargement of the pituitary fossa in a patient with acromegaly.

tanopias and bitemporal hemianopias (see p. 793).
- High-resolution CT scanning with reconstruction. This is the investigation of choice (Fig. 16.10).

The common types of pituitary tumour (see Table 16.11) are:
- Prolactinomas (histologically chromophobe adenomas)
- Non-functioning tumours, usually chromophobe adenomas
- Acidophil adenomas, causing acromegaly
- Basophil adenomas or hyperplasia, causing Cushing's disease or Nelson's syndrome.

Fig. 16.10 CT scan (sagittal reconstruction) showing a pituitary tumour with suprasellar extension.

The differential diagnosis includes craniopharyngioma. This is a usually cystic hypothalamic tumour arising from Rathke's pouch and often mimicking an intrinsic pituitary lesion. Though it can present at any age, it is the commonest tumour in children and is often calcified. Less common are meningiomas, gliomas, pinealomas and carotid artery aneurysms masquerading as tumours.

TREATMENT

Therapy has three aims:

1 *Reduction of excessive hormone secretion.* This may be ultimately achieved by eradication of the tumour, but medical control is often possible in the short-term and, occasionally, as long-term therapy:
- Prolactinomas usually respond to bromocriptine, a dopamine agonist, which often also produces significant tumour shrinkage as well as control of the galactorrhoea (see p. 705).
- Acromegaly also responds with some lowering of GH levels on bromocriptine, though the response is often incomplete and tumour shrinkage less likely (see p. 712).

- ACTH secretion cannot usually be controlled medically, but the peripheral effects of cortisol can be ameliorated by the 11β-hydroxylase blocker, metyrapone (see p. 728).

2 *Replacement of deficient hormone production* (see Table 16.10).

3 *Removal/control of the tumour* (see Table 16.12).
- Surgical removal is ideal and can be performed transsphenoidally or by the open transfrontal route. The former is suitable when the tumour is small, confined within or a little above the fossa and when there is no major suprasellar extension. The transfrontal route is used for significant suprasellar extensions or when there is a hypothalamic tumour. When surgical removal is incomplete, radiotherapy should be given to prevent recurrence. Immunostaining of the removed material may allow confirmation of the tumour cell type and its hormonal activity.
- Radiotherapy can be given as conventional external therapy, using a three-beam technique (40–45 Gy, i.e. 4000–4500 rad, not exceeding 180 rad per fraction). An alternative is the transsphenoidal implantation of radioactive yttrium needles, which provide high-level local radioactivity at the tumour site. This requires great expertise and has best been used for Cushing's disease. Radiotherapy cannot be given when a tumour extends much above the sella as there is a danger of visual pathway and hypothalamic damage.
- Medical means may shrink or control a tumour, especially if it is considered inoperable, and is sometimes used for long-term therapy (especially for prolactinomas). Bromocriptine, mentioned above, is often used to obtain shrinkage of a large tumour before deciding on the possibility of sub-

Table 16.11 Clinical and cellular characteristics of pituitary tumours.

Tumour/condition	Usual size	Commonest clinical presentation
Prolactinoma	Most <10 mm (microprolactinoma)	Galactorrhoea, amenorrhoea, hypogonadism, impotence
	Some >10 mm (macroprolactinoma)	As above, plus headaches, visual field defects, hypopituitarism
Acromegaly	Medium–large (90%+ of skull x-rays abnormal)	Change in appearance, visual field defects, chance observation, hypopituitarism
Cushing's disease	Most small, or hyperplasia rather than tumour	Central obesity, chance observation (local symptoms rare)
Nelson's syndrome	Often large	Post-adrenalectomy, pigmentation, sometimes local symptoms
Non-functional tumours	Often large	Headaches, visual field defects, hypopituitarism (small ones often found incidentally at post mortem)
Craniopharyngiomas	Often very large and cystic (skull x-ray abnormal in 50%+, calcification common)	Headaches, visual field defects, growth failure (50% below age 20, about 15% arise within sella)

Table 16.12 Comparisons of primary treatment for pituitary tumours.

	Advantages	Disadvantages
Surgical		
Transsphenoidal adenomectomy or hypophysectomy	Relatively minor procedure	Limited value if significant suprasellar extension Needs considerable expertise
Transfrontal	Good access to suprasellar region	Major procedure Danger of frontal lobe damage High chance of subsequent hypopituitarism
Radiotherapy		
External (40–50 Gy)	Non-invasive Prevents recurrence	Slow action May not be effective
Yttrium implantation	High local dose	Later hypopituitarism Great expertise needed
Medical		
Bromocriptine (for prolactinomas and acromegaly)	Non-invasive Reversible	Not curative Significant side-effects in minority Expensive

sequent transsphenoidal surgery or radiotherapy.

- With small tumours producing no pressure symptoms and without endocrine deficit, observation alone may be indicated.

WEIGHT, EXERCISE AND STRESS

The importance of these factors in hypothalamic–pituitary function has only recently been realized. Anorexia nervosa, the 'slimming disease' commonly affecting young females, is associated with major functional hypopituitarism (see p. 896). Anorexia nervosa often presents as amenorrhoea, without which the diagnosis is extremely unlikely. Anorexia nervosa is an extreme example, but more marginal degrees of underweight are a cause of anovulation, secondary amenorrhoea and oligomenorrhoea.

Similar effects are seen in female athletes undergoing heavy training; menstrual irregularity may occur but invariably reverts to normal when training stops.

Stress, though difficult to define, also affects endocrine function, especially menstruation. Emotional deprivation in childhood is an important cause of growth retardation and may be mediated by reduced GH secretion.

Reproduction and sex

Embryology

Until 8 weeks the sexes share a common development, with a primitive genital tract including the wolffian and müllerian ducts. There are additionally a primitive perineum and primitive gonads. In the presence of a Y chromosome the potential testes develop while the ovaries regress. In the absence of a Y chromosome, the potential ovaries develop and related ducts form a uterus and the upper vagina. Production of certain factors from the early 'testes' in the male produces atrophy of the müllerian duct, while the wolffian duct differentiates into an epididymus, vas deferens, seminal vesicle and prostate. Androgens induce transformation of the perineum to include a penis, penile urethra and scrotum containing the testes, which descend in response to androgenic stimulation. At birth testicular volume is 0.5–1 ml.

Definitions

Relevant terminology is shown in Table 16.13.

Physiology

The male
An outline of the hypothalamic–pituitary–testicular axis is shown in Fig. 16.11:

- Pulses of LHRH (GnRH) are released from the hypothalamus and stimulate LH and FSH release from the pituitary.
- LH stimulates testosterone production from the Leydig cells of the testis.
- Testosterone acts systemically to produce male secondary sexual characteristics, anabolism and the maintenance of libido. It also acts locally within the testis to aid spermatogenesis.
- FSH stimulates the Sertoli cells in the seminiferous tubules to produce mature sperm.
- Testosterone feeds back on the hypothalamus/ pituitary to inhibit LHRH secretion.

Table 16.13 Definitions in reproductive medicine.

Menarche	Age at first period
Primary amenorrhoea	Failure to begin spontaneous menstruation by age 16
Secondary amenorrhoea	Absence of menstruation for 3 months in a woman who has previously had cycles
Oligomenorrhoea	Irregular long cycles; often used for any length of cycle above 32 days
Dyspareunia	Pain or discomfort in the female during intercourse
Libido	Sexual interest or desire; often difficult to assess and is greatly affected by stress, tiredness and psychological factors
Impotence	Inability of the male to achieve or sustain an erection adequate for satisfactory intercourse
Azoospermia	Absence of sperm in the ejaculate
Oligospermia	Reduced numbers of sperm in the ejaculate; normal values are disputed

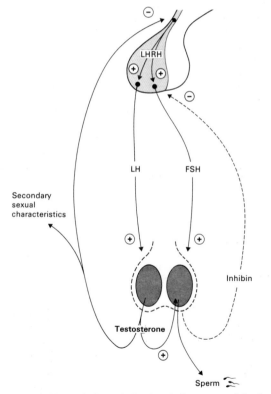

Fig. 16.11 The male hypothalamic–pituitary–gonadal axis.

● 'Inhibin', as yet uncharacterized, appears to feedback to decrease FSH secretion.

The secondary sexual characteristics of the male for which testosterone is necessary are the growth of

pubic, axillary and facial hair, enlargement of the external genitalia, deepening of the voice, sebum secretion and frontal balding.

The female
The female situation is more complex (Figs. 16.12 and 16.13):
● In the adult female higher brain centres impose a menstrual cycle of 28 days upon the activity of hypothalamic LHRH.
● Pulses of LHRH stimulate release of pituitary LH and FSH.
● LH stimulates ovarian oestrogen production.
● FSH stimulates the follicles, normally producing one dominant follicle which enlarges during the early (follicular) stage of the cycle.
● Oestrogens show a double feedback action on the pituitary, initially inhibiting gonadotrophin secretion (negative feedback) but later high level exposure results in increased LHRH secretion and increased LH sensitivity to LHRH (positive feedback). This leads to the mid-cycle LH surge, which induces ovulation (Fig. 16.13).
● The follicle then differentiates into a corpus luteum, which secretes both progesterone and oestradiol during the second half of the cycle (luteal phase).
● This causes uterine endometrial proliferation in preparation for possible implantation. If implantation does not occur, the corpus luteum regresses, progesterone secretion falls and the endometrium is shed.
● If pregnancy does occur, the placenta will, by then, be making sufficient oestrogens and progesterone to support itself.

Oestrogens also induce secondary sexual character-

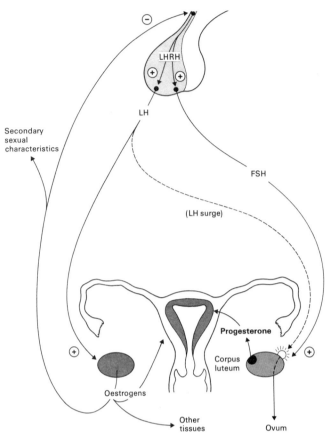

Fig. 16.12 The female hypothalmic–pituitary–gonadal axis.

istics, especially the development of the breasts and nipples, vaginal and vulval growth and pubic hair development. They also induce growth and maturation of the uterus and fallopian tubes.

Puberty

The mechanisms initiating puberty are poorly understood. LH and FSH are both low in the prepubertal child. FSH begins to rise first, initially in nocturnal pulses. This is followed by a rise in LH, with a subsequent increase in testosterone/oestrogen levels.

In boys, pubertal changes begin between 10 and 14 years and are complete between 15 and 17 years. The genitalia develop, the testes enlarge and the area of pubic hair increases. Peak height velocity is reached betweeen age 12 and 17 years. Full spermatogenesis occurs comparatively late.

In girls, events start a year earlier. Breast bud enlargement begins at age 9–13 and continues to 12–18 years. Pubic hair growth commences at ages 9–14 and is completed at 12–16½ years. Menarche occurs relatively late (age 11–15) but peak height velocity is reached much earlier than in boys (age 10–13½ years).

Precocious puberty

Development of menarche (girls) or secondary sexual characteristics (boys) before age 9 is premature, and may take the following forms:

● Idiopathic precocity (common in girls). This is a diagnosis of exclusion, with no apparent cause for premature entry into puberty and an early growth spurt. Treatment is with cyproterone acetate, an anti-androgen with progestational activity, but LHRH analogues causing suppression of sex hormone production are likely to supercede this.
● Cerebral precocity. Many causes of hypothalamic disease, especially tumours, may present in this way. In boys this must be rigorously excluded.
● Albright's syndrome. This usually occurs in girls and presents with precocity and polyostotic fibrous dysplasia.

Premature thelarche is early breast development alone; it is usually transient and occurs between ages 2 and 4 years. Premature adrenarche is early development of pubic hair without other significant changes.

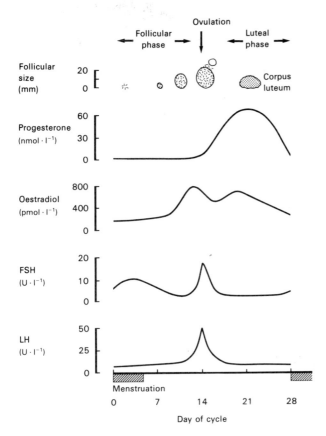

Fig. 16.13 Hormonal and follicular changes during the normal menstrual cycle.

Delayed puberty

Over 95% of children show signs of pubertal development by age 14 years. In its absence, investigation should begin by age 15. Causes of hypogonadism (see below) are clearly relevant but most cases are simply due to idiopathic delay.

In constitutional delay, pubertal development, bone age and stature should be in parallel. In boys, a testicular volume greater than 5 ml indicates the onset of puberty. A rising serum testosterone level is an earlier clue. In girls the breast bud is the first sign. Ultrasound allows assessment of ovarian and uterine development.

Basal LH/FSH levels may identify the site of a defect, and LHRH tests can indicate the stage of early puberty.

If puberty appears to be occurring, continued observation is all that is required.

The menopause

The menopause or cessation of periods occurs about age 50 years. During the late 40s, FSH and LH concentrations begin to rise, probably as follicle supply diminishes. Oestrogen levels fall and the cycle becomes disrupted. Most women notice irregular scanty periods coming on over a variable period,

though, in some, sudden amenorrhoea or menorrhagia occur. Eventually the menopausal pattern of low oestradiol levels with grossly elevated LH and FSH (usually >50 and >25 $u \cdot l^{-1}$ respectively) is established.

Features of oestrogen deficiency include hot flushes, which occur in most women and can be disabling, vaginal dryness and atrophy of the breasts. Patients become very liable to osteoporosis (see p. 735) and the premenopausal protection from ischaemic heart disease disappears.

There may also be vaguer symptoms of loss of libido, loss of self-esteem, non-specific aches and pains, irritability, loss of concentration and weight gain. The oestrogen-deficient symptoms respond well to oestrogen replacement, but the vaguer symptoms respond less well. The oestrogen should be given cyclically with a progestogen to prevent endometrial carcinoma due to unopposed oestrogen action. The usual hazards of oestrogens apply (see below); many physicians only use treatment for the period when symptoms are particularly disabling.

Premature menopause

The commonest cause of early menopause in the 20s and 30s is ovarian failure, which is apparently autoimmune in nature.

The ageing male

In the male there is no sudden 'change of life'. However, there is a progressive loss of sexual function, with a reduction in morning erections and frequency of intercourse. The age of onset varies widely, but overall testicular volume diminishes and gonadotrophin levels gradually rise.

Physiology of prolactin secretion

The hypothalamic–pituitary control of prolactin secretion is illustrated in Fig. 16.14. It is under tonic dopamine inhibition; other factors known to increase prolactin secretion (e.g. thyrotrophin-releasing hormone) are probably of little importance.

Prolactin stimulates milk secretion but also reduces gonadal activity. It decreases LHRH pulsatility at the hypothalamic level and, to a lesser extent, blocks the action of LH on the ovary or testis, producing hypogonadism. These actions may be clinically important.

Fig. 16.14 The control of prolactin secretion.

DISORDERS OF SEX AND REPRODUCTION

CLINICAL FEATURES

A detailed history and examination of all systems is required.

Sexual and menstrual disorders

History
Libido
Potency
Frequency of intercourse
Menstruation—relation of symptoms to cycle
Breasts (? galactorrhoea)
Hirsuties

Physical signs
Evidence of systemic disease
Secondary sexual characteristics
Genital size (testes, ovaries, uterus)
Cliteromegaly
Breast development, gynaecomastia
Galactorrhoea
Extent/distribution of hair

INVESTIGATION

The patient is his or her own best assay for gonadal endocrine function. A man having regular satisfactory intercourse or a woman with regular ovulatory periods is most unlikely to have significant *endocrine* disease.

When symptoms are present, much can be deduced by basal measurements of the gonadotrophins, oestrogen or testosterone, and prolactin:

- A low serum testosterone or oestradiol level with high gonadotrophins implies primary gonadal disease.
- In contrast, low levels of LH/FSH and testosterone or oestradiol imply hypothalamic and/or pituitary disease.
- Confirmation of normal female reproductive endocrinology requires the demonstration of ovulation; this is achieved by measurement of luteal phase serum progesterone and by ovarian ultrasound.
- Demonstration of normal male function requires healthy sperm showing good motility and few abnormal forms as well as adequate numbers.
- Hyperprolactinaemia can be confirmed or excluded by direct measurement. Levels may increase with stress; ideally a cannula should be inserted and samples taken through it 30 min later.
- The clomiphene test examines hypothalamic negative feedback. Clomiphene is a competitive oestrogen antagonist which binds to, but does not activate, oestrogen receptors, thus inducing a rise in gonadotrophin secretion in the normal subject.

More detailed tests are indicated in Table 16.14.

Table 16.14 Tests of gonadal function.

	Uses/comments
Male Basal testosterone	Normal levels exclude hypogonadism
Sperm count	Normal count excludes any deficiency Motility and abnormal sperms should be noted
Female Basal oestradiol	Normal levels exclude hypogonadism
Luteal phase progesterone (days 18–24)	If >30 mmol·l^{-1}, suggests ovulation
Ultrasound of ovaries	To confirm ovulation

Both sexes
Basal LH/FSH
	Demonstrates state of feedback system for
	  hormone production (LH) and germ cell
	  production (FSH)

LHRH test	Shows adequacy (or otherwise) of LH and FSH stores in pituitary

HCG test (testosterone or
  oestradiol measured)
	Response shows potential of ovary or
	  testis; failure demonstrates primary
	  gonadal problem

Clomiphene test (LH and FSH measured)	Tests negative feedback system
Post-coital test	Demonstrates state of sperm and sperm– mucus interaction

DISORDERS IN THE MALE

Hypogonadism

CLINICAL FEATURES

Male hypogonadism may be a presenting complaint or an incidental finding, e.g. during investigation for infertility. Except with infertility, the complaints are usually of androgen deficiency (see Table 16.15) rather than deficiency of sperm production. Sperm only makes up a very small proportion of seminal fluid volume.

CAUSES

Causes of male hypogonadism are shown in Table 16.16.

INVESTIGATION

Testicular disease may be initially apparent, but basal levels of testosterone, LH and FSH should be measured. These measurements will allow the distinction between primary gonadal (testicular) failure and hypothalamic–pituitary disease to be made. Closer examination or biopsy of the testes may then be necessary.

Skull radiology, pituitary CT scan, prolactin levels and other pituitary function tests may be needed. Semen analysis, chromosomal analysis and bone age estimation may be required.

TREATMENT.

The cause can rarely be reversed. Replacement therapy should therefore be commenced (Table 16.17). Primary gonadal failure should be treated with androgens. Patients with hypothalamic–pituitary disease may be given LH and FSH or pulsatile LHRH if fertility is required; otherwise they should receive androgen replacement.

Particular causes of hypogonadism include:
- *Cryptorchidism.* By the age of 5 years both testes should be in the scrotum. After that age the germinal epithelium is increasingly at risk, and lack of descent by puberty is associated with infertility. Surgical exploration and orchidopexy are usually undertaken, but a short trial of HCG occasionally induces descent. Intra-abdominal testes have an increased risk of developing malignancy; if presentation is after puberty orchidectomy is advised.
- *Klinefelter's syndrome* (see p. 104). This chromosomal disorder (47XXY) affects both the

Table 16.15 Effects of androgens and consequences of androgen deficiency in the male.

Physiological effect	Consequences of deficiency
General	
Maintenance of libido	Loss of libido
Deepening of voice	High-pitched voice*
Frontotemporal balding	Smooth skin
Facial, axillary and limb hair	Decreased hair
Pubic hair	
Maintenance of male pattern	Thinning and loss of pubic hair
Testes and scrotum	
Maintenance of testicular size/ consistency	Small soft testes
Rugosity of scrotum	Poorly developed penis/scrotum
Maintenance of erectile/ejaculatory function	Loss of erections/ejaculation
Stimulation of spermatogenesis	Subfertility
Skeletal	
Epiphyseal fusion	Eunuchoidism*
Maintenance of muscle bulk	Decreased muscle bulk and power

* If pre-pubertal.

Table 16.16 Causes of male hypogonadism.

Reduced gonadotrophins (hypothalamic–pituitary disease)
   Hypopituitarism
   Selective gonadotrophic deficiency (Kallmann's syndrome)

Hyperprolactinaemia

Primary gonadal disease (congenital)
   Anorchia/Leydig cell agenesis
   Chromosome abnormality (e.g. Klinefelter's syndrome)
   Enzyme defects
   5α-Reductase deficiency

Primary gonadal disease (acquired)
   Testicular torsion
   Castration
   Local testicular disease
   Chemotherapy/radiation toxicity
   Renal failure
   Cirrhosis/alcohol
   Sickle cell disease

Androgen receptor deficiency

Leydig cells and the seminiferous tubules. Patients usually present with poor sexual development, small or undescended testes, gynaecomastia or infertility. They are sometimes mentally retarded. Clinical examination shows small but firm testes, often gynaecomastia and usually signs of androgen deficiency. Confirmation is by chromosomal analysis. Treatment is androgen replacement therapy, though, if the patient is mentally subnormal, this should be used carefully. No treatment is possible for the infertility.

- *Isolated deficiency of LHRH or LH/FSH (Kallman's syndrome)*. Also known as hypogonadotrophic hypogonadism, this is often associated with decreased sense of smell and sometimes with bony, renal and cerebral abnormalities (e.g. colour blindness). Management is that of secondary hypogonadism; fertility is possible.
- *Oligospermia or azoospermia*. These abnormalities may be secondary to androgen deficiency, and corrected by replacement but, more often, they result from primary testicular disease which is rarely treatable. Azoospermia with low FSH levels suggests a vas deferens block.

Lack of libido and impotence

Many patients with impotence have no definable organic cause. A careful history of physical disease, related symptoms, stress and psychological factors, together with drug use must be taken. The presence of nocturnal emissions and frequent, satisfactory morning erections largely excludes endocrine disease as a cause.

True erectile difficulty may be psychological, neurogenic, vascular, endocrinological or related to drugs. Vascular disease may be more common than realized, and is often associated with vascular problems elsewhere. The endocrine causes are those of hypogonadism (see above) and can be excluded by normal testosterone, gonadotrophin and prolactin levels. Autonomic neuropathy, most commonly

Table 16.17 Androgen replacement therapy.

Preparation	Dose	Remarks
Testosterone mixed esters	250–500 mg i.m. every 3–6 weeks	Injection can be painful Usual maintenance therapy
Testosterone propionate	50–100 mg i.m. every 1–2 weeks	Frequent injections needed as half-life is short Good initial therapy
Testosterone undecanoate	80–240 mg daily, orally in divided doses	Variable dose, irregular absorption Very expensive

NB Mesterolone and methyltestosterone are no longer advised; they are weakly active and can cause cholestasis.

from diabetes mellitus, is the commonest identifiable cause on examination. Many drugs can be responsible—cannabis, diuretics, bethanidine/guanethidine, methyldopa, beta-blockers and alcohol all produce impotence. Apart from cessation of the offending drug, there is no treatment other than mechanical devices and penile implants.

If no organic disease is found the problem is probably psychosexual; this is discussed on p. 898.

Gynaecomastia

Gynaecomastia is development of breast tissue in the male. Causes are shown in Table 16.18.

Pubertal gynaecomastia occurs in perhaps 50% of normal boys, often asymmetrically. It usually resolves spontaneously within 6–18 months, but if it persists surgical removal may be required, as fibrous

Table 16.18 Causes of gynaecomastia.

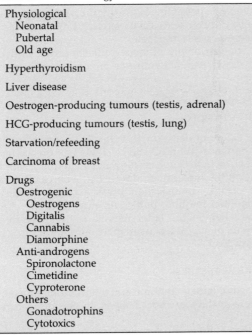

Physiological
  Neonatal
  Pubertal
  Old age

Hyperthyroidism

Liver disease

Oestrogen-producing tumours (testis, adrenal)

HCG-producing tumours (testis, lung)

Starvation/refeeding

Carcinoma of breast

Drugs
  Oestrogenic
    Oestrogens
    Digitalis
    Cannabis
    Diamorphine
  Anti-androgens
    Spironolactone
    Cimetidine
    Cyproterone
  Others
    Gonadotrophins
    Cytotoxics

tissue will have been laid down. The cause is thought to be relative oestrogen excess.

In the older male gynaecomastia requires a full assessment to exclude potentially serious underlying disease. Drug effects are common, but once these have been excluded, most cases have no definable cause.

DISORDERS IN THE FEMALE

Hypogonadism

Impaired ovarian function, whether primary or secondary, will lead both to oestrogen deficiency and abnormalities of the menstrual cycle. The menstrual cycle is very sensitive to disruption, cycles becoming anovulatory and irregular before disappearing altogether. Symptoms will depend on the age at which the failure develops: before puberty, primary amenorrhoea, possibly with delayed puberty, will occur, whereas after puberty secondary amenorrhoea and possibly hypogonadism will result.

Oestrogen deficiency
The physiological effects of oestrogens and symptoms/signs of deficiency are shown in Table 16.19.

Amenorrhoea

Absence of periods or markedly irregular, infrequent periods (oligomenorrhoea) is a common presentation, often the earliest, of female gonadal disease.

Important factors in clinical assessment of such patients are shown in Table 16.20. Causes include:
- Pregnancy. This must *always* be considered.
- Genital tract abnormalities such as imperforate hymen, especially in primary amenorrhoea
- Weight-related amenorrhoea. A minimum body weight is necessary for regular menstruation. This condition is common and may be seen at weights within the 'normal' range. Many of these subjects may have additional minor endocrine disease (e.g. polycystic disease) but restoration of body weight to above the 50th centile is often

Table 16.19 Effects of oestrogens and consequences of oestrogen deficiency.

Physiological effect	Consequence of deficiency
Breast Development of connective and duct tissue Nipple enlargement and areolar pigmentation	} Small, atrophic breasts
Pubic hair Maintenance of female pattern	Thinning and loss of pubic hair
Vulva and vagina Vulval growth Vaginal glandular and epithelial proliferation Vaginal lubrication	Atrophic vulva Atrophic vagina Dry vagina and dyspareunia
Uterus and tubes Myometrial and tubal hypertrophy Endometrial proliferation	} Small, atrophic uterus and tubes
Skeletal Epiphyseal fusion Maintenance of bone mass	Eunuchoidism* Osteoporosis

* If pre-pubertal.

Table 16.20 Clinical assessment of amenorrhoea.

History
? Pregnant
Age of onset
Age of menarche, if any
Sudden or gradual onset
General health
Weight, absolute and changes
Stress (job, lifestyle, exams, relationships)
Excessive exercise
Drugs
Hirsuties, acne, virilization
Headaches/visual symptoms
Sense of smell
Past history of pregnancies
Past history of gynaecological surgery

Examination
General health
Body shape and skeletal abnormalities
Weight and height
Hirsuties and acne
Evidence of virilization
Maturity of secondary sexual characteristics
Galactorrhoea
Normality of vagina, cervix and uterus

helpful. Similar problems occur with intensive physical training (see p. 694).

- Hypothalamic amenorrhoea. Some dispute the existence of this condition, linking all cases to low weight or increased stress. A few patients, however, do appear to have defective cycling mechanisms without apparent explanation.
- Severe illness, even in the absence of weight loss
- After stopping the contraceptive pill

INVESTIGATION

Basal levels of FSH, LH and prolactin allow initial distinction between primary gonadal and hypothalamic–pituitary causes (Table 16.21). When oligomenorrhoea is present, FSH/LH samples should be taken in the follicular phase. Secondary investigations are shown in Table 16.21.

TREATMENT

The cause of amenorrhoea should be treated wherever possible (e.g. hypothyroidism, low weight, stress or excessive exercise). Primary ovarian disease is rarely treatable.

The treatment of hyperprolactinaemia and of polycystic ovarian syndrome are discussed below.

Hirsuties (see p. 947)

PATHOPHYSIOLOGY

The extent of hair growth varies between individuals, families and races. Soft vellous hair on the face and elsewhere is not sex hormone dependent, nor is hair on the forearm and lower leg, whereas that on the beard, moustache, breast, chest, axillary, abdominal midline, pubic and thigh areas is. Any excess hair in the latter regions is thus usually a marker of increased ovarian or adrenal androgen production.

CLINICAL FEATURES

The complaint is common and often accompanied by severe anxiety and social stress. Important features are:

- Age and speed of onset. Rapid progression and

Table 16.21 Differential diagnosis and investigation of amenorrhoea.

Diagnosis	Biochemical markers	Secondary tests
Ovarian failure		
Ovarian dysgenesis*	High FSH	Repeat FSH
Premature ovarian failure*	High LH	Karyotype (see p. 104)
Steroid biosynthetic defect*		Laparoscopy/biopsy of ovary
(Ovariectomy)		Serum oestradiol
(Chemotherapy)		HCG stimulation
Partial ovarian failure		
Resistant ovary syndrome	High LH	Serum oestradiol
Polycystic ovarian syndrome*		Serum testosterone, androgens, SHBG
		Ultrasound of ovary
		Serum prolactin
		Laparoscopy and biopsy of ovary
Gonadotrophin failure		
Hypothalamic–pituitary disease*	Low LH	X-ray pituitary fossa
Kallmann's syndrome*	Low FSH	Serum oestradiol
Anorexia*		LHRH test
Weight loss*		Clomiphene test
General illness*		Serum thyroxine
Hypothyroidism*		Serum prolactin
Hyperprolactinaemia		
Prolactinoma*		Repeat prolactin (if >2000 mU·l^{-1} then
Idiopathic hyperprolactinaemia	High prolactin	tumour probable)
Hypothyroidism*		Pituitary fossa x-ray
Polycystic ovarian disease*		CT scan of pituitary fossa
Drugs		Serum thyroxine
Others (Cycle defect? Other endocrine disease?)		
Hypothalamic cause*		Serum thyroxine
Weight gain/loss*	Normal LH	Serum testosterone, SHBG
Mild polycystic disease	Normal FSH	Laparoscopy and biopsy of ovary
Cushing's syndrome	Normal prolactin	
Thyrotoxicosis		
Post-pill amenorrhoea		
Androgen excess		
Gonadal tumour	High androgen	Androgen measurement
Uterine/vaginal abnormality		
Imperforate hymen*		Examination under anaesthesia plus
Absent uterus*		endometrial biopsy
Lack of endometrium		Progestogen challenge

* These conditions may present as primary amenorrhoea.

prepubertal or late onset suggest a more serious cause.
- Accompanying virilization (cliteromegaly, frontal balding, male phenotype). This implies considerable androgen excess.
- The disruption of menstruation. Considerable disruption implies a more serious cause.

CAUSES

A summary of causes is given in Table 16.22.

INVESTIGATION

These are shown in Table 16.22.

TREATMENT

The underlying cause should be removed when possible (e.g. drugs, adrenal or ovarian tumours). Other therapy is local or systemic.

Local therapy
Plucking, bleaching, depilatory cream or wax and

Table 16.22 Conditions causing hirsuties.

Condition	Clinical presentation	Menstruation	Investigations (results)
Hirsuties without virilization			
Familial/racial	Family history often present Long history, beginning after menarche	Normal	Normal
Idiopathic	Long history, beginning after menarche	Normal	Normal
Polycystic ovarian syndrome (mild)	Long history, beginning after menarche Sometimes acne or greasy skin	Normal to chaotic	Androgens ($\uparrow$) SHBG ($\downarrow$) LH ($\uparrow$) Ultrasound of ovary
Late-onset congenital adrenal hyperplasia	Often before menarche Often short stature Sometimes acne or greasy skin	Variable	17-Hydroxyprogesterone ($\uparrow$)
Hirsuties with virilization			
Polycystic ovarian syndrome (severe)	Long history, beginning after menarche	Chaotic or amenorrhoea	Androgens ($\uparrow$) SHBG ($\downarrow$) LH ($\uparrow$) Ultrasound
Ovarian neoplasms	Short history, any adult age	Usually amenorrhoea	Ultrasound of ovary Laparoscopy and biopsy of ovary
Congenital adrenal hyperplasia	Infancy or childhood	—	17-Hydroxyprogesterone ($\uparrow$) Pregnanetriol ($\uparrow$) ACTH ($\uparrow$)
Adrenal tumours	Any age	Usually amenorrhoea	CT scan of adrenal

Drugs causing hirsuties include androgens, phenytoin, diazoxide, minoxidil, cyclosporin and some progestogens.

shaving may all help. Electrolysis is slow and expensive.

Systemic therapy

Oestrogens (e.g. oral contraceptives) reduce free androgens by increasing sex hormone-binding globulin (SHBG) levels when these are low (e.g. in the polycystic ovarian syndrome).

Cyproterone acetate (50–200 mg daily) is an anti-androgen, but is also teratogenic and a weak gluco-corticoid and progestogen. Given continuously it produces amenorrhoea, so it is normally only given for the first 14–21 days of each cycle.

Other agents of doubtful efficacy include spironolactone, bromocriptine and cimetidine. Prednisolone may rarely improve hirsuties associated with polycystic ovarian syndrome.

Polycystic ovarian syndrome

PATHOPHYSIOLOGY

This very common condition, originally known in its severe form as the Stein–Leventhal syndrome, is characterized by multiple ovarian cysts and by excess androgen production from the ovaries and adrenals, though whether the basic defect is ovarian, adrenal or pituitary remains unknown.

CLINICAL FEATURES

Polycystic ovarian syndrome is a common cause of amenorrhoea/oligomenorrhoea, hirsuties or acne, usually beginning shortly after menarche. It is sometimes associated with obesity. Mild virilization occurs in severe cases.

INVESTIGATION

The levels of free androgens are increased, though the total testosterone may be normal. SHBG levels are low.

The LH to FSH ratio is raised ($>2:1$), but the FSH is normal or low. Mild hyperprolactinaemia is common.

Ovarian ultrasound scanning is useful to confirm polycystic changes.

TREATMENT

This depends upon whether the aim is to produce fertility, regularize periods or reduce hirsuties:

- Prednisolone (2.5 mg in the morning, 5 mg at night) is given to reverse the circadian rhythm and thereby suppress the adrenal androgens. Regular ovulatory cycles often ensue, but hirsuties is little affected.

- Oestrogens/oral contraceptives may be used for hirsuties (see above).
- Clomiphene 50–200 mg daily may be given from days 2–6 of the menstrual cycle (or tamoxifen 10–40 mg daily) plus HCG 5000 units i.m. on day 12 or 13 in order to produce fertility. This can cause ovarian hyperstimulation and requires careful monitoring.
- Rarely, wedge resection of the ovary may be performed to produce fertility.

HYPERPROLACTINAEMIA

Increased prolactin levels (>360 mu·l^{-1}) may be physiological, pathological or secondary to drug therapy (Table 16.23). Not all patients with galactorrhoea have hyperprolactinaemia, but the other causes are poorly understood ('normoprolactinaemic galactorrhoea').

CLINICAL FEATURES

Hyperprolactinaemia per se usually presents with:
- Galactorrhoea, spontaneous or expressible (60% of cases)
- Oligo- or amenorrhoea
- Decreased libido in both sexes
- Decreased potency
- Subfertility
- Symptoms or signs of oestrogen or androgen deficiency. In the long-term, osteoporosis may result.
- Delayed or arrested puberty in the peri-pubertal patient

Additionally there may be headaches and/or visual field defects if a pituitary tumour is present (more common in men).

INVESTIGATION

If physiological and drug causes of galactorrhoea have been excluded:
- At least three prolactin levels should be measured. Mean levels >2000 mu·l^{-1} suggest a prolactinoma.
- A good quality skull x-ray should be obtained.
- The visual fields should be checked.
- Anterior pituitary function should be assessed if there is any clinical evidence of hypopituitarism or radiological evidence of tumour.
- A CT scan of the pituitary is necessary if there is an obvious tumour, and desirable if not.

Macroprolactinoma refers to tumours of >10 mm diameter, microprolactinoma to smaller ones. The size of the prolactinoma may affect the choice of treatment.

TREATMENT

Hyperprolactinaemia should be reduced with bromocriptine, a dopamine agonist. Initial doses should be small (e.g. 1 mg) and taken *with* food, the first dose being taken at night. The dose should be gradually increased, usually to 2.5 mg three times daily, depending on clinical response and prolactin levels. Maintenance doses are 2–15 mg daily in divided doses. Side-effects include nausea and vomiting, dizziness and syncope, constipation and cold peripheries.

If a tumour is present this is likely to shrink with bromocriptine. Definitive therapy is controversial, and will depend upon the size of the tumour, the patient's wish for fertility and local facilities:
- Transsphenoidal surgery often restores normoprolactinaemia but there is a considerable late recurrence rate.
- Radiotherapy is only slowly effective and can sometimes eventually cause hypopituitarism.
- Small tumours and asymptomatic patients may only need observation.
- Rarely, tumours enlarge during pregnancy, producing headaches and visual defects. Bromocriptine should be given.

Table 16.23 Causes of hyperprolactinaemia.

Physiological
Sleep (REM phase)
Pregnancy
Suckling
Nipple stimulation
Stress
Coitus

Pathological
Production by tumours
    Prolactinomas
    Occurs in some acromegalics
Interference with stalk
    Any hypothalamic/pituitary tumour
Idiopathic hyperprolactinaemia
Polycystic ovarian syndrome
Primary hypothyroidism
Chest wall injury
Renal failure
Liver failure

Drug-induced
Dopamine antagonists
    (e.g. metoclopramide)
Phenothiazines
Oestrogens
Opiates
Cimetidine
Methyldopa
Reserpine

ORAL CONTRACEPTION

The combined oestrogen–progestogen pill is widely used for contraception and has a low failure rate (<1 per 100 women-years). Pills in current use usually contain 20–30 µg of oestrogen, usually in the form of ethinyl oestradiol, together with a variable amount of one of several progestogens. The mechanism of action is two-fold:

- Suppression by oestrogen of gonadotrophins, thus preventing follicular development, ovulation and luteinization
- Progestogen effects on cervical mucus, making it hostile to sperm

Side-effects of these preparations are shown in Table 16.24. Most of the serious side-effects are rare. While some effects require immediate cessation of the pill,

Table 16.24 Adverse effects and drug interactions of oral contraceptives (mixed oestrogen/progesterone combinations).

General
Weight gain
Loss of libido
Pigmentation (chloasma)
Breast tenderness
Increased growth rate of some malignancies
Cardiovascular
Increased blood pressure*
Deep vein thrombosis*
Myocardial infarction
Stroke
Gastrointestinal
Nausea and vomiting
Abnormal liver function*
Gallbladder disease
Hepatic tumours
Nervous system
Headache
Migraine*
Depression*
Gynaecological
Amenorrhoea
'Spotting'
Cervical erosion
Haematological
Increased clotting tendency
Endocrine/metabolic
Impaired glucose tolerance
Worsened lipid profile
Drug interactions (*reduced contraceptive effect*)
Antibiotics
Barbiturates
Phenytoin
Carbamazepine
Rifampicin

* Common reasons for *stopping* oral contraceptives.

the importance of other milder side-effects must be judged against the hazards of pregnancy occurring with inadequate contraception, especially if other effective contraceptive methods are not practicable or acceptable. It is, however, clear that the hazards of the combined pill are much greater in women over 35, especially in smokers and those with other risk factors for cardiovascular disease (e.g. hypertension, hyperlipidaemias).

SUBFERTILITY

This term, which is kinder than infertility, is defined as the inability of a couple to conceive after one year of unprotected intercourse.

Investigation requires the combined skills of a gynaecologist and an endocrinologist. Both partners must be considered and every aspect of the whole train of events critically examined.

CAUSES (Fig. 16.15)

- About 30% of cases have an identifiable male factor.
- Female tubal problems account for perhaps 20% of cases; a similar proportion have ovulatory disorders.
- Cervical mucus, inadequate intercourse and vaginal factors are uncommon (5%).
- There is no apparent explanation in 15% of cases ('idiopathic' subfertility).
- A significant proportion of cases have both male and female problems.

CLINICAL ASSESSMENT

Both partners should be seen and the following factors checked:
- *The man:* previous testicular damage (e.g. orchitis), urethral symptoms and venereal problems, local surgery and use of alcohol and drugs
- *The woman:* previous pelvic infection, regularity of periods, previous surgery, alcohol intake and smoking
- *Together:* frequency and adequacy of intercourse, use of lubricants

Examination should include an assessment of secondary sexual characteristics, body habitus and general health. In men, size and consistency of the testes are important, plus exclusion of a varicocele. In women, vaginal examination allows a check on the uterus and ovaries.

INVESTIGATION

Appropriate tests for particular defects are shown in Fig. 16.15.

Fig. 16.15 The major factors involved in subfertility and their investigation. SCMC=sperm–cervical mucus contact test.

TREATMENT

Any defect(s) found should be treated if possible. In vitro fertilization (IVF) is becoming widely used, especially for instances of tubal blockage and oligospermia.

DISORDERS OF SEXUAL DIFFERENTIATION

An individual's sex can be defined in several ways:
- *Chromosomal sex*—the normal female is 46XX, the normal male 46XY. The Y chromosome confers male sex; if it is not present, development follows female lines.
- *Gonadal sex*—obviously determined predominantly by chromosomal sex but requires normal embryological development
- *Phenotypic sex*—the normal physical appearance and characteristics of male and female body shape. This in turn is a manifestation of gonadal sex and subsequent sex hormone production.
- *Social sex (gender)*—heavily dependent on phenotypic sex and normally assigned on appearance of the external genitalia at birth
- *Sexual orientation*—heterosexual, homosexual (male/male or female/female) or ambisexual (both sexes)

Disorders of sexual differentiation are rare but may involve abnormalities of chromosomal, gonadal, endocrine and phenotypic development (Table 16.25, see p. 708).

The growth axis

Physiology and control of growth hormone
(Fig. 16.6)

Growth hormone (GH) is the pituitary factor responsible for the stimulation of body growth in man. Its secretion is stimulated by growth hormone releasing hormone (GHRH), which is released into the portal system from the hypothalamus; it is also under inhibitory control by growth hormone release inhibiting hormone (GHRIH; somatostatin). GH stimulates the hepatic production of the intermediates, somatomedins, which actually stimulate growth. The metabolic actions of the system are:
- Increasing collagen and protein synthesis
- Promoting retention of calcium, phosphorus and nitrogen, necessary substrates for anabolism
- Opposing the action of insulin

GH release is intermittent and mainly nocturnal, especially during sleep. The frequency and size of GH pulses increase during the growth spurt of adolescence and decline thereafter. Acute stress and

Table 16.25 Disorders of sexual differentiation.

Condition	Chromosomes	Gonads	Phenotype	Remarks
Turner's syndrome	45XO	Streak	Female	Often morphological features (short stature, web neck)
Gonadal dysgenesis	46XY	Streak or minimal testes*	Immature female	
Congenital adrenal hyperplasia	46XX	Ovary	Female with variable virilization	Obvious androgen excess
Virilizing tumour	46XX	Ovary	Female with variable virilization	Obvious androgen excess
True hermaphroditism	46XX/XY or mosaic	Testis and ovary	Male or ambiguous	
Klinefelter's syndrome	47XXY	Small testes	Male, often with gynaecomastia	Many are hypogonadal
Testicular feminization	46XY	Testes*	Ambiguous or infantile female	Androgen receptor defective
Testicular synthetic defects	46XY	Testes*	Cryptorchid, ambiguous	
5α-Reductase deficiency	46XY	Testes	Cryptorchid, ambiguous	Impaired conversion of testosterone to dihydroxytestosterone
Anorchia	46XY	Absent	Immature female	

* Gonadectomy advised because of high risk of malignancy.

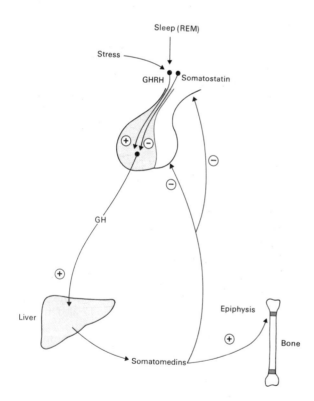

Fig. 16.16 The control of growth hormone and somatomedin secretion.

exercise both stimulate GH release while, in the normal subject, hyperglycaemia suppresses it.

Normal growth

Factors other than GH that are involved in growth in the human are:

- *Genetic*. Children of two short parents will probably be short.
- *Nutritional*. Adequate nutrients must be available; impaired growth can result from inadequate dietary intake or small bowel disease (e.g. coeliac disease).
- *General health*. Any serious systemic disease in

childhood is likely to reduce growth (e.g. renal failure).

- *Emotional deprivation and psychological factors.* These can impair growth by complex, poorly understood mechanisms.

Assessment of growth

Charts showing the range of height and weight with age for normal British children are available (Fig. 16.17).

More important is the height velocity, which requires at least two serial measurements. This is a measure of current growth rate, while attained height is largely dependent upon previous growth. Height must be measured very carefully, ideally at the same time of day on the same instrument.

The future height of a child can be predicted approximately from the parental heights:

- For a boy, 5 in (13 cm) is *added* to his *mother's* height and the mean parental height then calculated.
- For a girl, 5 in (13 cm) is *subtracted* from the *father's* height before taking the mean.

Thus, for a boy with a father of height 5 ft 10 in and

Fig. 16.17 A height chart for boys. Child A illustrates the course of a child with hypopituitarism, initially treated with cortisol and thyroxine, but showing growth only after growth hormone treatment. Child B shows the course of a child with constitutional growth delay without treatment. The open circles show the data corrected for bone age. Based on a Tanner–Whitehouse chart, reference 1A, reproduced by permission of Castlemead Publications.

mother of 5 ft 1 in, the corrected heights are 5 ft 10 in and 5 ft 6 in, and his predicted height is 5 ft 8 in. A daughter of the same parents would be expected to be 5 ft 3 in (the mean of 5 ft 5 in and 5 ft 1 in).

GROWTH FAILURE (SHORT STATURE)

When a child or his parents complain of short stature, particular attention should focus on:

- Possible systemic disorders, especially small bowel disease
- Evidence of skeletal or other congenital abnormalities
- Endocrine status, particularly primary hypo-thyroidism
- Dietary intake and use of drugs, especially steroids for asthma
- Emotional, psychological, family and school problems

School, clinic and home records of height and weight should be obtained whenever possible, to allow growth velocity calculation. If unavailable, such data must be obtained prospectively.

The clinical features of the commoner causes of growth failure are given in Table 16.26.

A child with normal growth velocity is unlikely to have significant endocrine disease.

However, low growth velocity without apparent systemic cause requires further investigation. Sudden cessation of growth suggests major physical disease; if no gastrointestinal, respiratory, renal or skeletal abnormality is apparent then a cerebral tumour or hypothyroidism are the likeliest causes. Slow-growing children require a full endocrine assessment.

Problems of growth and development

History
Rate of growth (home/school records, e.g. heights on kitchen door)
Change in appearance (old photos)
Change in shoe/glove/hat size
Age of appearance of pubic hair, breasts, menarche

Physical signs
Evidence of systemic disease
Body size, relative weight, proportions
 (span versus height)
Skin thickness, interdental separation
Facial features
Spade hands/feet
Grading of secondary sexual characteristics

INVESTIGATION

Having excluded systemic disease, the following should be undertaken:

- *Thyroid function tests*—serum T$_4$ and TSH

Table 16.26 Clinical features of common causes of short stature.

	Family history	Growth pattern	Clinical features	Time of puberty	Bone age	Remarks
Constitutional delay	Often present	Rather slow from birth	Immature but appropriate	Late but spontaneous	Moderate delay but maturing	Often difficult to differentiate from GH deficiency; growth velocity measurement vital
Familial short stature	Positive	Slow from birth	Normal	Normal	Normal	Need heights of all family members
GH deficiency	Rare	Slow	Immature, often overweight	Delayed	Moderate to marked delay; not progressing	Early investigation and treatment vital; increased suspicion if child is plump
Primary hypothyroidism	Rare	Slow	Immature	Delayed	Markedly delayed	Measure T_4 and TSH in all cases of short stature; clear clinical signs often not present
Small bowel disease	Sometimes	Slow	Immature, usually thin	Delayed	Delayed	Diarrhoea plus macrocytosis/anaemia; occasionally no gastrointestinal symptoms

- *GH status*. Basal levels are of little value. The GH response to Bovril, exercise, clonidine, arginine and insulin are all used; a normal peak response is >20 mu·l^{-1}.
- *Assessment of bone age*. Left hand and wrist x-rays allow an assessment of bone age; x-rays of the knee show the state of epiphysial closure.

TREATMENT

Systemic illness should be treated.

Primary hypothyroidism is treated with replacement thyroxine 0.05–0.2 mg daily. GH deficiency was treated with human GH, but this has been withdrawn, as cases of Creutzfeldt–Jakob disease (see p. 839) due to viral contamination have been reported. It has been superseded by biosynthetic GH, and growth hormone releasing hormone (GHRH) analogues are also being evaluated.

GROWTH HORMONE EXCESS—GIGANTISM AND ACROMEGALY

Growth hormone stimulates skeletal and soft tissue growth. GH excess therefore produces gigantism in children (if acquired before epiphysial fusion) and acromegaly in adults.

The commonest causes of tall stature are hereditary (two tall parents) and idiopathic (constitutional). It can occasionally be due to thyrotoxicosis. GH excess is a rare cause and is usually clinically apparent.

Acromegaly

CLINICAL FEATURES

The symptoms and signs of acromegaly are shown in Fig. 16.18. One-third of patients present with changes in appearance and one-quarter with visual field defects or headaches; in the remainder the diagnosis is made by an alert observer when the patient is seen for another problem, e.g. diabetes or hypertension.

INVESTIGATION

- GH is usually undetectable in adults, except during stress or as occasional spikes. Undetectable GH levels on present assays thus exclude the diagnosis, but a detectable random level does not confirm it.
- The glucose tolerance test is diagnostic. Acromegalics fail to suppress GH measured during this test to below 1 mu·l^{-1}, and about 25% of acromegalics have abnormal glucose tolerance.

Symptoms of acromegaly

Change in appearance
Increased size of hands/feet
Headaches
Visual deterioration
Tiredness
Weight gain
Amenorrhoea/oligomenorrhoea
Galactorrhoea
Impotence or poor libido
Deep voice
Goitre
Breathlessness
Galactorrhoea
Excessive sweating
Pain/tingling in hands
Polyuria/polydipsia
Muscular weakness
Joint pains

Old photographs are frequently useful.
Symptoms of hypopituitarism may be present as well.

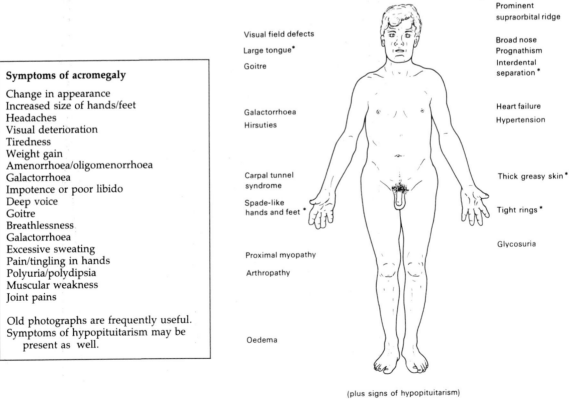

(plus signs of hypopituitarism)

Fig. 16.18 The signs of acromegaly.
*indicates signs of greater discriminant value.

- Lateral skull x-rays are abnormal in 90% as the tumours are relatively large.
- Visual field defects are common (see p. 793).
- High-resolution CT scans are virtually never normal.
- Partial or complete anterior hypopituitarism is common.
- Hyperprolactinaemia occurs in 30% of patients.

MANAGEMENT

Untreated acromegaly results in markedly reduced survival, with most deaths caused by heart failure, coronary artery disease and hypertension-related conditions. Treatment is therefore indicated in all except the elderly or those with minimal abnormalities. The general advantages and disadvantages of surgery, radiotherapy and medical treatment are discussed on p. 694.

Which treatment should be performed is controversial and complete cure is often slow, if possible at all. The choice lies between:

- Transsphenoidal surgery, with subsequent radiotherapy if excision is incomplete
- Transfrontal surgery for big tumours causing pressure effects, usually with postoperative radiotherapy
- External radiotherapy (takes 3–10 years) plus bromocriptine
- Bromocriptine alone, which is usually reserved for the elderly and frail. It is also given to shrink tumours prior to definitive therapy or to control symptoms and persisting GH secretion. The maintenance dose is 10–60 mg daily, but should start slowly.

Hypopituitarism should be corrected (see p. 691). Concurrent diabetes and/or hypertension should be treated conventionally; both usually improve with treatment of the acromegaly.

The thyroid axis

The metabolic rate of many tissues is controlled by the thyroid hormones, and overactivity and underactivity of the gland are common clinical problems.

Anatomy

The thyroid gland consists of two lateral lobes connected by an isthmus. It is closely attached to the thyroid cartilages and to the upper end of the trachea, and thus moves on swallowing. It is often palpable in normal women.

Embryologically it originates from the base of the tongue and descends to the middle of the neck. Remnants of thyroid tissue can sometimes be found at the base of the tongue (lingual thyroid) and along the line of descent. The gland has a rich blood supply from the superior and inferior thyroid arteries.

The thyroid consists of follicles lined by cuboidal epithelioid cells. Inside the follicles is the colloid, which is an iodinated glycoprotein, thyroglobulin, synthesized by the follicular cells. Each follicle is surrounded by a basement membrane, between which are parafollicular cells containing calcitonin-secreting C cells.

Biochemistry

The thyroid hormones, thyroxine (T_4) and triiodothyronine (T_3) are synthesized within the gland (Fig. 16.19).

More T_4 than T_3 is produced, but T_4 is converted in some peripheral tissues (liver, kidney and muscle) to the more active T_3 by 5'-monodeiodination; alternatively 3'-monodeiodination yields the inactive reverse T_3 (rT_3).

In plasma, 99% of all T_4 and T_3 is bound to hormone-binding proteins (thyroxine-binding globulin, TBG; thyroid-binding prealbumin, TBPA; and albumin—see p. 681). Only free hormone is available to the tissues, where T_3 binds to specific nuclear receptors within the cell.

Physiology of the hypothalamic–pituitary–thyroid axis (see Fig. 16.1)

- Thyrotrophin-releasing hormone (TRH) is released in the hypothalamus and stimulates release of thyroid-stimulating hormone (TSH) from the pituitary.
- TSH stimulates the TSH receptor in the thyroid to increase synthesis of both T_4 and T_3 and also to release stored hormone, producing increased plasma levels of T_4 and T_3.
- T_4 and T_3 feed back on the pituitary, and perhaps the hypothalamus, to reduce TSH secretion.

Thyroid function tests

Radioimmunoassays for total T_4, free T_4, total T_3, free T_3 and TSH are widely available. There are only minor circadian rhythms and measurements may therefore be made at any time.

Particular uses of the tests are summarized in Table 16.27. Tests include:

- *Thyroid hormone uptake tests*. There are many forms of this measurement of free protein binding sites, which is used to calculate the 'free thyroxine index' (FTI). TBG is sometimes measured directly.
- *TSH measurement*. Immunoassays for TSH were too insensitive to differentiate between normal and low levels. New immunoradiometric assays

Fig. 16.19 The synthesis and metabolism of the thyroid hormones. The shaded areas denote the side chain shown for tyrosine.

Table 16.27 Advantages and limitations of usual thyroid function tests.

Test	Most useful in	Not useful or possibly misleading in
Total thyroxine (T_4)	Hypothyroidism* Thyrotoxicosis*	Pregnancy Oestrogen therapy Oral contraceptive use 'Sick euthyroid syndrome' Drug therapy, e.g. NSAIDS Neonates
Total triiodothyronine (T_3)	Thyrotoxicosis*	Hypothyroidism
TSH (conventional immunoassay)	Primary hypothyroidism* Neonatal screening*	Thyrotoxicosis
TSH (immunoradiometric assay)	Thyrotoxicosis* Primary hypothyroidism* Neonatal screening* Hypothalamic–pituitary disease	
TRH test	Doubtful function (pregnancy, drugs)	Thyroid eye disease Non-toxic adenoma Hypothalamic–pituitary disease

* Tests of first choice in this situation.

(IRMA) are more sensitive and can distinguish between normal and low levels. They are reducing the need for TRH tests. The TSH IRMA is now probably the most useful single test of thyroid function; it can accurately detect both primary hypothyroidism and hyperthyroidism.

- *TRH test.* Hypothyroid patients show a high basal TSH level with an excessive rise in response to TRH, whereas hyperthyroid subjects show suppression with a minimal increment of TSH (Fig. 16.20). Flat responses are also seen with solitary autonomous nodules, Graves' eye disease and excessive thyroxine replacement.

Problems in interpretation of thyroid function tests
There are three major areas of difficulty, mainly related to alterations in TBG levels or binding (Table 16.28).

Serious acute or chronic illness. Thyroid function is affected in several ways;
- Reduced concentration and affinity of binding proteins
- Decreased peripheral conversion of T_4 to T_3 with more rT_3 being produced
- Reduced hypothalamic–pituitary TSH production

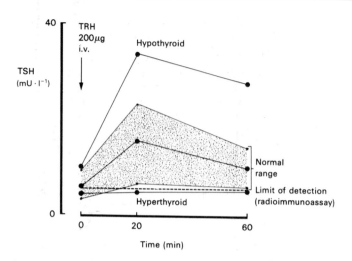

Fig. 16.20 Normal and abnormal responses to the TRH test using a conventional TSH radioimmunoassay.

Systemically ill patients can therefore have apparently low total and free T_4 and T_3 levels with a normal basal TSH (the 'sick euthyroid' syndrome). Levels are usually only mildly below normal and the tests should be repeated after resolution of the underlying illness.

Pregnancy and oral contraceptives. These lead to greatly increased TBG, and thus to high or high-normal total T_4 and high thyroid hormone uptake test (THUT) levels. The normal physiological changes during pregnancy are not well understood.

Drugs. Many drugs affect thyroid function tests by interfering with protein binding. The commonest are listed in Table 16.28. Basal TSH levels, and TRH tests if needed, should be performed if clinical doubt persists.

Table 16.28 Factors affecting thyroxine binding globulin (TBG) levels.

Increased TBG
Hereditary
Pregnancy
Oestrogen therapy
Oral contraceptive use
Hypothyroidism
Phenothiazines
Acute viral hepatitis
Decreased TBG
Hereditary
Androgens
Corticosteroid excess
Thyrotoxicosis
Nephrotic syndrome
Major illness
Malnutrition
Chronic liver disease
Drugs causing altered binding
Non-steroidal anti-inflammatory drugs
Phenytoin

Thyroid autoimmunity

Antibodies to the thyroid are common and may be either destructive or stimulating; both occasionally coexist in the same patient.

Destructive antibodies may be directed against the microsomes or against thyroglobulin. They may be detected by haemagglutination techniques. They are found in up to 20% of the population, especially older women, but only 10–20% of these develop overt hypothyroidism.

A heterogeneous group of stimulatory antibodies, termed thyroid-stimulating immunoglobulin or antibody (TSI or TSAb), also exist. These may stimulate the TSH receptor, producing Graves' disease, and/or increased cell division and goitre formation.

Long-acting thyroid stimulator (LATS) and LATS-protector (LATS-P) have also been described but bear little correlation to clinical thyroid disease.

HYPOTHYROIDISM

Underactivity of the thyroid may be *primary*, from disease of the thyroid, or *secondary* to hypothalamic–pituitary disease (reduced TSH) (Table 16.29).

Causes of primary hypothyroidism
Atrophic (autoimmune) hypothyroidism. This is the commonest cause of hypothyroidism and is associated with microsomal autoantibodies leading to lymphoid infiltration of the gland and eventual atrophy and fibrosis. It is six times more common in females and the incidence increases with age. This condition is associated with other autoimmune diseases such as pernicious anaemia.

Hashimoto's thyroiditis. This form of autoimmune thyroiditis, again commoner in women and commonest in late middle-age, produces atrophic

Table 16.29 Causes of hypothyroidism.

Primary
Congenital
  Agenesis
  Ectopic thyroid remnants

Defects of hormone synthesis
  Iodine deficiency
  Dyshormonogenesis
  Antithyroid drugs

Autoimmune
  Atrophic thyroiditis
  Hashimoto's thyroiditis

Infective
  Post subacute thyroiditis

Post-surgery

Post-irradiation
  ^{131}I therapy
  External neck irradiation

Infiltration
  Tumour

Peripheral resistance to thyroid hormone

Secondary
Hypopituitarism
Isolated TSH deficiency

changes with regeneration, leading to goitre formation. The thyroid is usually firm and rubbery, but may range from soft to hard. Thyroid microsomal antibodies are again present, often in very high titres. Patients may be hypothyroid or euthyroid.

Thyroxine therapy may shrink the goitre even when the patient is not hypothyroid, though this may take a long time.

Iodine deficiency. In mountainous areas (in the Alps, the Himalayas, South America, central Africa) dietary iodine deficiency still exists and goitre, occasionally massive, is common. It was formerly seen in the UK as 'Derbyshire neck'. Patients may be euthyroid or hypothyroid, depending on the severity of iodine deficiency.

Dyshormonogenesis. This rare condition is due to genetic defects in the synthesis of thyroid hormones. Patients develop hypothyroidism with a goitre. One particular form is associated with deafness (Pendred's syndrome).

CLINICAL FEATURES OF HYPOTHYROIDISM (Fig. 16.21)

Hypothyroidism may produce symptoms throughout the body. The classical picture of the slow, dry-haired, thick-skinned, deep-voiced patient with weight gain, cold intolerance, bradycardia and constipation makes the diagnosis easy; the term 'myxoedema' refers to the accumulation of mucopolysac-

Symptoms of primary hypothyroidism

Tiredness/malaise
Weight gain
Anorexia
Cold intolerance
Poor memory
Change in appearance
Depression
Psychosis
Coma
Deafness
Poor libido
Goitre
Puffy eyes
Dry, brittle, unmanageable hair
Dry, coarse skin
Arthralgia
Myalgia
Constipation
Menorrhagia or oligomenorrhoea

A history from a relative is often revealing.
Symptoms of other autoimmune disease may be present.

Mental slowness*
Psychosis/dementia
Large tongue
'Peaches and cream complexion'
Ataxia
Dry thin hair*

Hypertension

Hypothermia
Heart failure
Bradycardia*
Pericardial effusion*

Carpal tunnel syndrome

Myotonia

Muscular hypertrophy*

Oedema

Poverty of movement
Loss of eyebrows
Deafness
Periorbital oedema
Deep voice
(Goitre)

Anaemia

Dry skin
Mild obesity

Cold peripheries

Proximal myopathy

Slow-relaxing reflexes

Fig. 16.21 The signs of hypothyroidism.
*indicates signs of greater discriminant value.

charide in subcutaneous tissues. Milder symptoms are, however, more common.

Special difficulties in diagnosis may arise:

- Children with hypothyroidism may not show classical features but often have a slow growth velocity, poor school performance and, sometimes, arrest of pubertal development.
- Young women with hypothyroidism may not show obvious signs. Hypothyroidism must be considered in all patients with oligomenorrhoea/amenorrhoea, menorrhagia, infertility or hyperprolactinaemia.
- Among the elderly many of the clinical features are difficult to differentiate from normal ageing.

INVESTIGATION OF PRIMARY HYPOTHYROIDISM
(Table 16.27)

The total or free T_4 level is the test of choice. If low, then the basal TSH level should be measured—a high TSH level confirms primary hypothyroidism. A low TSH level should be followed by a TRH test and consideration of secondary hypothyroidism.

Thyroid and other organ-specific antibodies may be present. Other abnormalities include:

- Anaemia. This is usually normochromic and normocytic in type, but it may be macrocytic (occasionally due to associated pernicious anaemia) or microcytic (in women, due to menorrhagia).
- Hyponatraemia due to an increase in antidiuretic hormone (ADH) and impaired free water clearance
- Increased aspartate aminotransferase levels

TREATMENT OF PRIMARY OR SECONDARY HYPOTHYROIDISM

Replacement therapy with thyroxine (T_4) is given for life. The starting dose will depend upon the age and fitness of the patient, especially the cardiac performance. In the young and fit 0.1 mg is suitable, while 0.05 mg is more appropriate for the old or frail; both are given as a single daily dose. T_3 administration offers no significant advantage over T_4.

Patients with ischaemic heart disease require more gradual therapy, especially if the hypothyroidism is severe and long-standing. Most physicians would begin with 0.025 mg daily and perform serial ECGs, increasing the dose at 2–6-week intervals if angina does not occur or worsen and the ECG does not deteriorate. Some, however, would use T_3, beginning with 2.5–5 µg every 8 h, and doubling the dose every 48 h up to 10 µg three times daily. If progress is satisfactory T_4 (0.1 mg daily) is then started.

Adequacy of replacement should be assessed clinically and by thyroid function tests (T_4, T_3 and TSH) after at least 6 weeks on a steady dose. If the

serum T_4 remains low and the TSH levels are high, the dose should be increased to 0.15 mg daily and the tests repeated 6 weeks later. This stepwise progression, to 0.2 and (rarely) 0.3 mg daily, should be continued until the TSH is just suppressed into the normal range. TSH cannot be used in this way in secondary hypothyroidism. The normal maintenance dose is 0.1–0.2 mg daily; excessive replacement is probably dangerous.

Clinical improvement may not begin for 2 weeks and full resolution of symptoms may take 6 months. The importance of lifelong therapy should be emphasized. The possibility of other autoimmune endocrine disease developing, especially Addison's disease, should be considered.

Myxoedema coma

Severe hypothyroidism, especially in the elderly, may present with confusion or even coma. Hypothermia is often present and the patient may have severe cardiac failure, hypoventilation, hypoglycaemia and hyponatraemia.

The mortality is at least 50% and patients require full intensive care. Optimal treatment is controversial, most physicians advising T_3 orally or intravenously in doses from 2.5 µg every 8 h. A single large dose (e.g. 300 µg) should not be used as it can be dangerous.

Additional measures should include:

- Oxygen (ventilation if necessary)
- Monitoring of cardiac output
- Gradual rewarming (see p. 674)
- Hydrocortisone 100 mg i.v. 8-hourly
- Dextrose infusion to prevent associated hypoglycaemia

Myxoedema madness

Depression is common in hypothyroidism, but occasionally, with severe hypothyroidism in the elderly, the patient may become frankly demented or psychotic. This may occur shortly after starting thyroxine replacement.

Screening for hypothyroidism

The incidence of congenital hypothyroidism is approximately 1 in 3500 births. Untreated, severe hypothyroidism leads to permanent neurological and intellectual damage ('cretinism'). Routine screening of the newborn using a blood-spot, as in the Guthrie test, to detect a high TSH level as an indicator of primary hypothyroidism is efficient; cretinism is prevented if thyroxine is started within the first months of life.

Screening of elderly patients is controversial, but there is little doubt that the prevalence of unsuspected hypothyroidism in the over 65s is 1–3%.

GOITRE

Goitre (thyroid enlargement) is more common in women than in men, and may be either physiological or pathological.

CLINICAL FEATURES

Most commonly a goitre is noticed as a cosmetic defect by the patient or by friends and relatives. The majority are painless, but pain or discomfort can occur in acute varieties. It can produce dysphagia and difficulty in breathing, implying oesophageal or tracheal compression. Clinical examination should record the size, shape, consistency and mobility of the gland, as well as whether its lower margin can be demarcated (thus implying the absence of retrosternal extension). A bruit may be present. Associated lymph nodes should be sought and the tracheal position determined if possible. Examination should never omit an assessment of the patient's clinical thyroid status.

Specific enquiry should be made about any medication, especially iodine-containing preparations.

ASSESSMENT

Two questions must be answered about any goitre: its pathological nature, and the patient's thyroid status.

The nature can often be judged clinically. Goitres are usually separable into diffuse and nodular types. Causes of goitre are shown in Table 16.30. Particular points of note are:

● Puberty produces a diffuse increase in the size of the thyroid.
● In Graves' disease (autoimmune hyperthyroidism), the gland is again diffusely enlarged, often somewhat firm, and frequently associated with a bruit.
● Tenderness in a diffuse swelling is suggestive of a viral thyroiditis (de Quervain's thyroiditis). This is usually associated with a systemic viral illness and may produce transient clinical hyperthyroidism with an increase in serum T_4.
● Pain in a goitre may be caused by thyroiditis, bleeding into a cyst or (rarely) a thyroid tumour.
● In simple goitre no clear cause is found for enlargement of the thyroid, which is usually smooth and soft. It may be associated with growth-stimulating antibodies.
● Nodular goitres may have multiple or solitary nodules. Commonest is the multinodular goitre, especially in older patients. The patient is usually euthyroid, but may be hyperthyroid. Multinodular goitre is the commonest cause of tracheal and/or oesophageal compression and may cause laryngeal nerve palsy. It may also extend retrosternally.
● Solitary nodules present a difficult problem. A

Table 16.30 Causes of goitre.

Physiological
  Puberty
  Pregnancy

Autoimmune
  Graves' disease
  Hashimoto's disease

Thyroiditis
  Acute (de Quervain's thyroiditis)
  Chronic fibrotic (Reidel's thyroiditis)

Iodine deficiency (endemic goitre)

Dyshormonogenesis

Goitrogens (e.g. sulphonylureas)

Multinodular goitre

Diffuse goitre
  Colloid
  Simple

Cysts

Tumours
  Adenomas
  Carcinoma
  Lymphoma

Miscellaneous
  Sarcoidosis
  Tuberculosis

history of pain, rapid enlargement or associated lymph nodes in such a situation suggests the possibility of thyroid carcinoma. The majority of such nodules are, however, cystic or benign and indeed may simply be the largest solitary nodule of a multinodular goitre. Risk factors for malignancy include previous irradiation, long-standing iodine deficiency and occasional familial cases. Solitary toxic nodules are quite uncommon.
● Fibrotic goitre (Reidel's thyroiditis) is a rare condition, usually producing a 'woody' gland. It is associated with other mid-line fibrosis and is often difficult to distinguish from carcinoma, being irregular and hard.
● Excessive doses of carbimazole or propylthiouracil will induce goitre.
● Iodine deficiency and dyshormonogenesis can also cause goitre (see above).

INVESTIGATION

The clinical findings will dictate which tests are performed initially. Investigations include:
● *Thyroid function tests*—T_4 plus TSH or T_4 plus T_3 (Table 16.27).
● *Chest and thoracic x-rays*—to detect tracheal compression and large retrosternal extensions
● *Thyroid scan (iodine or technetium)*. This demonstrates active thyroid tissue and is most

useful for showing single toxic nodules (with suppression of the remaining gland uptake) and multinodular goitres. 'Cold' areas (without uptake) are likely to be cysts, fibrotic areas or tumours. The chance of a 'cold nodule' being malignant is about 10%. Iodine scans are useful in demonstrating retrosternal extension, ectopic thyroid tissue and biologically active thyroid carcinoma.

- *Ultrasound scan.* This technique, with improving resolution, can distinguish cystic from solid thyroid nodules; completely cystic lesions are very rarely malignant.
- *Fine needle biopsy.* With fine needles and expert cytology this technique is of increasing value. Local complications are rare. The theoretically high risk of missing small areas of malignant change in cold nodules has not proved to be so.

TREATMENT

During puberty and pregnancy, a goitre associated with euthyroidism rarely requires intervention; the patient should be reassured that spontaneous resolution is likely.

In other situations, the patient should be rendered euthyroid.

Indications for intervention are:

- *The possibility of malignancy.* A history of rapid growth, pain, cervical lymphadenopathy or previous irradiation to the neck warrant surgical exploration. Until recently removal of all 'cold nodules' was advised because of the 10% risk of carcinoma, but needle biopsy and cytology render this unnecessary.
- *Pressure symptoms.* Pressure on the trachea or, more rarely, the oesophagus also warrants surgery. A retrosternal goitre should be considered.
- *Cosmetic reasons.* A large goitre often causes considerable anxiety to the patient even if it is functionally and anatomically benign.

THYROID CARCINOMA

The different types of thyroid malignancy, their characteristics and treatment are listed in Table

16.31. The tumour is relatively uncommon, being responsible for 400 deaths annually in the UK.

Particular points are:

- In papillary and follicular carcinomas:
  (a) Iodine is taken up, which can be shown by scanning.
  (b) After total thyroidectomy, a therapeutic radioiodine dose will be taken up by remaining thyroid tissue or metastatic lesions.
  (c) Replacement thyroxine will be needed after surgery and should suppress TSH to prevent stimulation of any residual differentiated carcinoma.
  (d) Lungs and bone are the commonest sites of metastasis. Local invasion is often a problem.
- Anaplastic carcinomas and lymphoma do not respond to radioactive iodine.
- Medullary carcinoma, often associated with multiple endocrine neoplasia (see p. 742), is usually treated by total thyroidectomy. The patient's family should be screened for this and other endocrine neoplastic conditions.
- After total thyroidectomy, estimation of thyroglobulin, a marker released by thyroid tissue, may be useful in detecting recurrence.

HYPERTHYROIDISM

Hyperthyroidism is common, affecting about 2–5% of all females at some time. Nearly all cases are caused by intrinsic thyroid disease; a pituitary cause is extremely rare (see Table 16.32).

Graves' disease

Graves' disease is the commonest cause of hyperthyroidism. It is an autoimmune process where serum IgG antibodies behave like TSH, binding to the thyroid TSH receptor and producing stimulation of thyroid hormone production. The antibodies, known as thyroid-stimulating immunoglobulins or antibodies (TSI or TSAb), can be measured in serum.

Associated with the thyroid disease in many cases are eye changes (see below) and other signs such as pretibial myxoedema. Graves' disease is also associated with other autoimmune disorders such as pernicious anaemia and myasthenia gravis (see p. 269 and p. 864).

Table 16.31 Types of thyroid malignancy.

Cell type	Frequency	Behaviour	Spread	Prognosis
Papillary	70%	Occurs in young people, slow-growing	Local, sometimes lung/bone secondaries	Good, especially in young
Follicular	20%	Commoner in females	Metastases to lung/bone	Good if resected
Anaplastic	<5%	Aggressive	Locally invasive	Very poor
Lymphoma	<2%	Variable		Sometimes responsive to radiotherapy
Medullary cell	5%	Often familial	Local and metastases	Poor

Table 16.32 Causes of hyperthyroidism.

Graves' disease
Solitary toxic nodule (adenoma)
Toxic multinodular goitre

Acute thyroiditis
  Viral
  Autoimmune
  Post-irradiation

Thyrotoxicosis factitia (secret T$_4$ consumption)
Exogenous iodine
Metastatic differentiated thyroid carcinoma
TSH-secreting tumours (e.g. pituitary)
HCG-producing tumours
Hyperfunctioning ovarian teratoma (struma ovarii)

The natural history is one of fluctuation, many patients showing a pattern of alternating relapse and remission; perhaps only 40% of subjects have just one episode.

Toxic solitary nodule
This is the cause of about 5% of cases of hyperthyroidism.

Toxic multinodular goitre
This commonly occurs in older women.

CLINICAL FEATURES

The symptoms of hyperthyroidism affect many systems; the symptoms and relevant signs are shown in Fig. 16.22.

Symptomatology and signs vary with age and with the underlying aetiology. Important points are as follows:
- The eye signs, pretibial myxoedema and thyroid acropachy only occur in Graves' disease. Pretibial myxoedema is an infiltration of mucopolysaccharides in the subcutaneous tissues of the shin and only occurs with eye disease (see below). It appears as a pink to purplish-brown, raised, well-demarcated area. Thyroid acropachy is very rare and consists of clubbing, swollen fingers and periosteal new bone formation.
- In the elderly a frequent presentation is with atrial fibrillation, other tachycardias and/or heart failure, often with few other signs. Thyroid function tests are mandatory in any patient with unexplained atrial fibrillation.
- Children frequently present with excessive height or an excessive growth rate, or with behavioural problems such as hyperactivity. They may also show weight gain rather than loss.

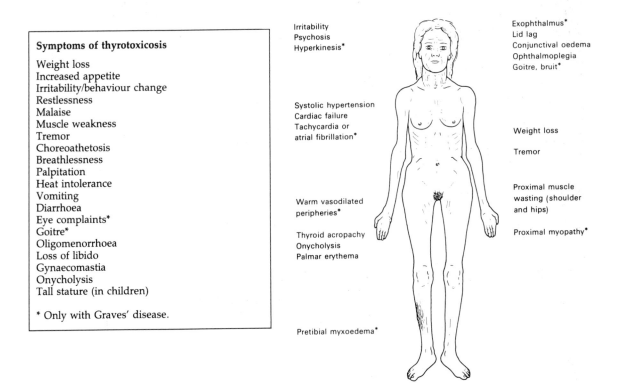

Symptoms of thyrotoxicosis
Weight loss
Increased appetite
Irritability/behaviour change
Restlessness
Malaise
Muscle weakness
Tremor
Choreoathetosis
Breathlessness
Palpitation
Heat intolerance
Vomiting
Diarrhoea
Eye complaints*
Goitre*
Oligomenorrhoea
Loss of libido
Gynaecomastia
Onycholysis
Tall stature (in children)
* Only with Graves' disease.

Irritability
Psychosis
Hyperkinesis*

Exophthalmus*
Lid lag
Conjunctival oedema
Ophthalmoplegia
Goitre, bruit*

Systolic hypertension
Cardiac failure
Tachycardia or
atrial fibrillation*

Weight loss

Tremor

Warm vasodilated
peripheries*

Proximal muscle
wasting (shoulder
and hips)

Thyroid acropachy
Onycholysis
Palmar erythema

Proximal myopathy*

Pretibial myxoedema*

Fig. 16.22 The signs of hyperthyroidism.
*indicates signs of greater discriminant value.

● Some elderly patients present with a clinical picture more like hypothyroidism—so-called 'apathetic thyrotoxicosis'.

DIFFERENTIAL DIAGNOSIS

Thyrotoxicosis is often clinically obvious, but treatment should *never* be instituted without biochemical confirmation.

Differentiation of the mild case from anxiety states may be difficult; useful positive clinical markers are eye signs, proximal myopathy and wasting, and the hyperdynamic circulation with warm peripheries seen in thyrotoxicosis compared with the clammy hands of anxiety.

INVESTIGATION

The total or free T_3 is more often raised than T_4. TSI estimation should be performed if available.

If doubt persists (e.g. the 'pill', drug effects, TBG abnormalities; see Table 16.27), a basal TSH (IRMA) is valuable. If then real doubt remains, the TRH test is still helpful. A normal TSH rise excludes the diagnosis; a flat response is characteristic but not diagnostic.

TREATMENT

Three possibilities are available: antithyroid drugs, surgery and radioiodine. Practices and beliefs differ widely within and between countries, and also depend on patient preference and local expertise. Some general guidelines are:
● Large goitres, and single or multiple nodular goitres are unlikely to remit after a course of antithyroid drugs.
● In the UK radioiodine is rarely given to those under age 40.

Antithyroid drugs
Carbimazole and propylthiouracil are most often used. They inhibit the formation of thyroid hormones and also have other minor actions (Table 16.33).

Initial doses and side-effects are detailed in Table 16.33. Though thyroid hormone synthesis is reduced very quickly, the long half-life of T_4 (7 days) means that clinical benefit is not apparent for 10–20 days.

As many of the manifestations of hyperthyroidism are mediated via the sympathetic system, beta-blockers are used to provide rapid partial symptomatic control; they also decrease peripheral conversion of T_4 to T_3. Drugs preferred are those without intrinsic sympathomimetic activity (Table 16.33). They should not be used alone for hyperthyroidism except when the condition is self-limiting, e.g. in subacute viral thyroiditis.

Subsequent management is as follows:
● The situation is reviewed after 4–6 weeks, and the dose of carbimazole reduced depending on the patient's clinical state and T_4/T_3 levels.
● When the patient is euthyroid, beta-blockers should be stopped.
● If the hyperthyroidism is controlled after 2–3 months, the dose of carbimazole can be reduced and can be given once daily.
● The dose is gradually reduced to 5 mg daily over 12–18 months if the thyrotoxicosis remains controlled.
● When the patient is euthyroid on 5 mg of carbimazole daily, drug treatment can be discontinued.
● About 50% of patients will relapse, mostly within the next 2 years. Long-term antithyroid therapy is sometimes required.
● Propylthiouracil is used in similar fashion but doses required are 10-fold higher (50–600 mg daily).

Toxicity (Table 16.33). The major side-effect of antithyroid drugs is agranulocytosis, which occurs in approximately 1 in 1000 patients within 3 months of treatment. Patients should be warned to seek

Table 16.33 Drugs used in the treatment of thyrotoxicosis.

Drug	Usual starting dose	Side-effects	Remarks
Anti-thyroid drugs			
Carbimazole	10–20 mg 8-hourly	Rash, nausea, vomiting, arthralgia, agranulocytosis (0.1%), jaundice	Active metabolite is methimazole Mild immunosuppressive activity
Propylthiouracil	100–200 mg 8-hourly	Rash, nausea, vomiting, agranulocytosis	Also blocks conversion of T_4 to T_3
Beta-blockers for symptomatic control			
Propranolol	40–80 mg 6- to 8-hourly	Avoid in asthma; use with care in heart failure Usual beta-blocker side-effects	Use beta-blocking agents *without* intrinsic sympathomimetic activity
Nadolol	40–240 mg daily		May need higher doses in hyperthyroidism as metabolism is increased

immediate medical attention if they develop unexplained fever or sore throat. If toxicity occurs with carbimazole, propylthiouracil may be used and vice versa; side-effects rarely occur with both drugs.

Subtotal thyroidectomy

Thyroidectomy should only be performed in patients who have previously been rendered euthyroid. Conventional practice is to stop the antithyroid drug 10–14 days before the operation and to give potassium iodide (60 mg three times daily) to reduce the vascularity of the gland.

Particular indications for surgery are:
- A large goitre
- Peristent drug side-effects
- Poor compliance with drug therapy
- Recurrent hyperthyroidism after drugs
- Patient choice

The operation should be performed by an experienced surgeon so as to reduce the chance of complications. These include:
- Early postoperative bleeding, causing tracheal compression and asphyxia. This is a rare emergency requiring immediate removal of all clips or sutures to allow escape of the blood or haematoma.
- Laryngeal nerve palsy (1% of cases). Vocal cord movement should be checked preoperatively. Mild hoarseness is a more common complication.
- Transient hypocalcaemia (up to 10% of cases); permanent hypoparathyroidism occurs in less than 1%
- Recurrent hyperthyroidism (less than 5% of cases)
- Hypothyroidism. About 10% of patients are hypothyroid within 1 year and this percentage increases with time. It is more likely to occur if microsomal antibodies are found.

Radioactive iodine

Iodine-131, in an empirical dose (usually 18–40 × 10^{10} Bq), accumulates in the thyroid and destroys the gland by local irradiation. Early discomfort in the neck and immediate worsening of hyperthyroidism are sometimes seen. If the latter occurs, the patient should not receive carbimazole for 2–3 days after radioiodine administration as it will prevent uptake of the radioiodine by the gland. They should receive propranolol (Table 16.33), until carbimazole can be restarted.

Apart from the immediate problems above, a major complication of radioactive iodine therapy is the progressive incidence of subsequent hypothyroidism, affecting the majority of subjects over the following 20 years. Though 75% of patients are rendered euthyroid in the short term, a small proportion remain hyperthyroid.

Special situations in hyperthyroidism

Thyroid crisis

This rare condition is a rapid deterioration of thyrotoxicosis, with hyperpyrexia, severe tachycardia and extreme restlessness; the mortality is 10%. It is usually precipitated by stress, infection, surgery in an unprepared patient, or radioiodine therapy. With careful management it should no longer occur.

Treatment is urgent. Propranolol in full doses is started immediately, together with potassium iodide, antithyroid drugs, corticosteroids (which suppress many of the manifestations of hyperthyroidism) and full supportive measures.

Hyperthyroidism in pregnancy and neonatal life

Maternal hyperthyroidism during pregnancy is uncommon and is usually mild. The diagnosis can be difficult to make because of misleading thyroid function tests (see above); a TRH test should be performed if necessary. The pathogenesis is almost always Graves' disease. In this condition TSI crosses the placenta to stimulate the fetal thyroid. Carbimazole also crosses the placenta, but thyroxine does so poorly. The smallest dose of carbimazole necessary is used and the fetus must be monitored (see below). The paediatrician should be informed and the infant checked immediately after birth. Overtreatment with carbimazole can cause fetal goitre.

If necessary (due to poor patient compliance or drug side-effects) partial thyroidectomy can be performed, preferably in the second trimester. Radioactive iodine is absolutely contraindicated.

The fetus and maternal Graves' disease

Any mother with a history of Graves' disease may have circulating TSI. Even if she has been treated (e.g. by surgery), the immunoglobulin may still be present. It stimulates the fetal thyroid, and the fetus can thus become hyperthyroid while the mother remains euthyroid.

Any such patient should therefore be monitored during pregnancy. Fetal heart rate provides a direct biological assay of thyroid status, and monitoring should be performed at least monthly. Rates above 160 beats per minute are strongly suggestive of fetal hyperthyroidism, and maternal treatment with carbimazole and/or propranolol may be used. To prevent the mother becoming hypothyroid, thyroxine may be given as this does not easily cross the placenta. Sympathomimetics, used to prevent premature labour, are contraindicated as they may provoke fatal tachycardias in the fetus.

Thyrotoxicosis may also develop in the neonatal period as TSI has a half-life of approximately 3 weeks. Manifestations in the newborn include irritability, failure to thrive and persisting weight loss, diarrhoea and eye signs. Thyroid function tests are difficult to interpret as neonatal normal ranges vary with age.

Untreated neonatal thyrotoxicosis is thought to be a cause of hyperactivity in later childhood.

Thyroid eye disease

This is also known as dysthyroid eye disease or ophthalmic Graves' disease.

PATHOPHYSIOLOGY

Recent evidence suggests that the exophthalmos of Graves' disease is due to specific antibodies which cause retro-orbital inflammation and subsequent oedema. Histology of this shows the classical lymphocytic infiltration of autoimmune disease. It is not due to TSH, LATS or LATS-P. While often associated with Graves' hyperthyroidism, it need not be so and patients may be hyperthyroid, euthyroid or hypothyroid.

CLINICAL FEATURES

The clinical appearances are characteristic (Fig. 16.23). Proptosis and limitation of eye movements (ophthalmoplegia) are direct effects of the inflammation, while conjunctival oedema, lid lag and corneal scarring are secondary to the proptosis and lack of eye cover.

Eye manifestations often do not parallel the clinical course of Graves' disease.

Eye complaints

History
Difficulty in reading/distant vision
Double vision
Grittiness
Protrusion

Physical signs
Acuity
Eye movements
Conjunctivitis/chemosis
Lid lag/lid retraction
Exophthalmos

INVESTIGATION

Few investigations are necessary if the appearances are characteristic and bilateral. If they are markedly different in the two eyes, other retro-orbital space-occupying lesions should be considered.

The total T_4, T_3 and TSH should be measured.

CT scanning of the orbits will exclude other causes and show the enlarged muscles and oedema. The exophthalmos should be measured to allow progress to be monitored.

TREATMENT

If abnormal, the thyroid function should be normalized. Direct treatment may be either local or systemic, depending upon severity:
- Methylcellulose eye drops are given to aid lubrication.
- Lateral tarsorrhaphy aids closure of the eye lids.
- If more severe, systemic steroids (prednisolone 30–120 mg daily) may reduce inflammation.
- Irradiation of the orbits is also used in very severe instances.
- Surgical decompression of the orbit(s) is occasionally needed.
- Corrective eye muscle surgery may improve diplopia due to ocular palsies.

The glucocorticoid axis

Anatomy and function

The human adrenal comprises an outer cortex with three zones (zona reticularis, fasciculata and glomerulosa) producing steroids, and an inner medulla, which synthesizes, stores and secretes catecholamines (see p. 741). The adrenal steroids are grouped into three classes based on their predominant physiological effects:
- *Glucocorticoids*. These are named after their effects

Symptoms		Signs
Protruding eyes		Lid lag
Grittiness		Lid retraction
Weeping eyes		Exophthalmos
Double vision		Ocular palsies
Visual impairment		Conjunctival oedema
		Chemosis
		Incomplete cover
		Corneal ulceration

Fig. 16.23 The signs of thyroid eye disease.

Table 16.34 The actions of glucocorticoids.

Increased or stimulated
Gluconeogenesis
Glycogen deposition
Protein catabolism
Fat deposition
Sodium retention
Potassium loss
Free water clearance
Uric acid secretion
Circulating neutrophils

Decreased or inhibited
Protein synthesis
Host response to infection
Lymphocyte transformation
Delayed hypersensitivity
Circulating lymphocytes
Circulating eosinophils

Table 16.35 Glucocorticoid and mineralocorticoid potency of equal amounts of common steroids.

Steroid	Glucocorticoid effect*	Mineralocorticoid effect*
Cortisol (hydrocortisone)	1	1
Prednisolone	4	0.7
Dexamethasone	40	2
Aldosterone	0.1	400
Fludrocortisone	10	400

* Cortisol is arbitrarily defined as 1.

on carbohydrate metabolism; their major actions are listed in Table 16.34.

● *Mineralocorticoids.* The predominant effect of mineralocorticoids is on the extracellular balance of sodium and potassium in the distal tubule of the kidney. Aldosterone is the predominant mineralocorticoid in man; corticosterone makes a small contribution. The weak mineralocorticoid activity of cortisol is also important as it is present in considerable excess. Aldosterone is produced solely in the zona glomerulosa.

● *Androgens.* Though secreted in considerable quantities, most have only relatively weak androgenic activity.

The relative potency of common steroids is shown in Table 16.35.

Biochemistry

All steroids have a single basic skeleton (Fig. 16.24a)

and the chemical differences between them are slight. The major biosynthetic pathways are shown in Fig. 16.24b.

Physiology

Glucocorticoid production by the adrenal is under hypothalamic/pituitary control (Fig. 16.25). Corticotrophin-releasing factor (CRF) is secreted in the hypothalamus in response to circadian rhythm, stress and other stimuli. It travels down the portal system to stimulate adrenocorticotrophic hormone (ACTH) release from the anterior pituitary. Circulating ACTH stimulates cortisol production in the adrenal. The cortisol secreted (or any other synthetic corticosteroid) feeds back on the hypothalamus and pituitary to inhibit further CRF/ACTH release. The set point of this system clearly varies through the day according to the circadian rhythm, and is usually overridden by severe stress.

Following adrenalectomy or Addison's disease cortisol secretion will be absent or reduced; ACTH levels will therefore rise.

Mineralocorticoid secretion is mainly controlled by the renin–angiotensin system (see p. 739).

Fig. 16.24 (a) The steroid molecule. (b) The major steroid biosynthetic pathways.

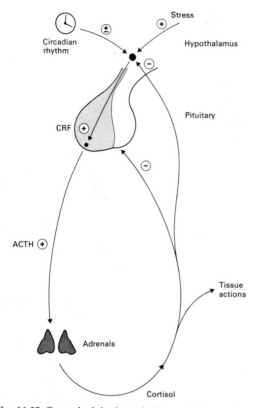

Fig. 16.25 Control of the hypothalamic–pituitary–adrenal axis. CRF=corticotrophin releasing factor.

Investigation of glucocorticoid abnormalities

Basal levels
ACTH and cortisol are released episodically; the following precautions are therefore necessary when taking a blood sample:

- The sampling time should be accurately recorded.
- Stress should be minimized.
- Sampling should be delayed for 48 h after admission if Cushing's syndrome is suspected.
- Appropriate normal ranges (for the time of day) should be used.

Suppression and stimulation tests are used in instances of excess and deficient cortisol production, respectively.

Dexamethasone suppression tests
Administration of synthetic glucocorticoid to a normal subject produces prompt feedback suppression of CRF and ACTH levels and thus suppression of endogenous cortisol secretion (prednisolone and dexamethasone are not measured by cortisol assays). Three forms of the test are used in the diagnosis and differential diagnosis of Cushing's syndrome (see Table 16.36).

ACTH stimulation tests
Synthetic ACTH (tetracosactrin, which consists of the first 24 amino acids of human ACTH) is given to stimulate adrenal cortisol production (see p. 723). Details are given in Table 16.36.

ADDISON'S DISEASE—PRIMARY HYPOADRENALISM

PATHOPHYSIOLOGY AND CAUSES

In this rare condition there is destruction of the entire adrenal cortex. Glucocorticoid, mineralocorticoid and sex steroid production are all reduced. This differs from hypothalamic–pituitary disease, where mineralocorticoid secretion remains largely intact, being predominantly stimulated by angiotensin II.

Table 16.36 Details of dexamethasone suppression and ACTH tests.

Test	Protocol	Measure	Criteria for suppression	Use
Dexamethasone				
Overnight	Take 1–2 mg on going to bed on day −1	Plasma cortisol at 0900 h on day 0	Plasma cortisol <180 nmol·l^{-1}	Outpatient screening test
'Low-dose'	0.5 mg 6-hourly × 8 doses from 0900 h on day 0	Plasma cortisol at 0900 h on days 0 and +2	Plasma cortisol <180 nmol·l^{-1} on second sample	For diagnosis of Cushing's syndrome May not suppress in obesity and depression
'High-dose'	2 mg 6-hourly × 8 doses from 0900 h on day 0	Plasma cortisol at 0900 h on days 0 and +2 (24 h urinary steroids on days −1 and +2)	Plasma cortisol on day +2 $<50\%$ of that on day 0	Differential diagnosis of Cushing's syndrome; pituitary-dependent disease suppresses in about 90%
ACTH				
Short	Tetracosactrin 0.25 mg i.m. at time 0	Plasma cortisol at time 0, +30 and +60 min	Cortisol at +30 min >690 nmol·l^{-1} Rise >330 nmol·l^{-1}	To exclude primary adrenal failure
Long	Depot tetracosactrin 1 mg i.m. at time 0	Plasma cortisol at time 0, +1, +2, +3, +4, +5, +8 and +24 h	Maximum >1000 nmol·l^{-1}	To demonstrate/exclude adrenal suppression

Table 16.37 Causes of primary hypoadrenalism.

Autoimmune disease
Tuberculosis
Surgical removal

Haemorrhage/infarction
   Meningococcal septicaemia
   Venography

Infiltration
   Malignant destruction
   Amyloid

Schilder's disease (adrenal leukodystrophy)

Also, hypothalamic–pituitary disease does not affect sex steroid production by the adrenals as this is largely independent of pituitary action.

Reduced cortisol levels lead, through feedback, to increased ACTH production, which is responsible for the hyperpigmentation.

Primary hypoadrenalism shows a marked female preponderance and is now most often caused by autoimmune disease, but in the past tuberculosis was an important cause (see Table 16.37).

CLINICAL FEATURES

The clinical features of Addison's disease are shown in Fig. 16.26. The symptomatology is often vague —weakness, tiredness, weight loss and anorexia predominate. Important features are as follows:

Symptoms of primary hypoadrenalism
Weight loss
Anorexia
Malaise
Weakness
Fever
Depression
Impotence/amenorrhoea
Nausea/vomiting
Diarrhoea
Confusion
Syncope from postural hypotension
Abdominal pain
Constipation
Myalgia
Joint or back pain
Features of other autoimmune disease (e.g. vitiligo)   are quite common.

- Pigmentation (dull slaty grey-brown) is the predominant sign. It occurs in the mouth (opposite the molars), on the hands and on all flexural regions. It is particularly significant if it occurs in a recent scar.
- Postural hypotension due to hypovolaemia and sodium loss is usually present, even if the supine blood pressure is normal.

INVESTIGATION

Once Addison's disease is suspected, investigation is urgent. If the patient is seriously ill or hypotensive, hydrocortisone 100 mg should be given intramuscularly; ideally a blood sample is taken before the hydrocortisone is given for the measurement of plasma cortisol. Full investigation should be delayed until emergency treatment has improved the patient's condition. Tests are as follows:

- Single cortisol measurements are of virtually no value, unless the level is very low (<180 $nmol \cdot l^{-1}$).
- The short ACTH stimulation test should be performed (see Table 16.36), when an absent or impaired cortisol response is seen. This can be confirmed if necessary by a long ACTH stimulation test to exclude adrenal suppression by steroids.
- A plasma ACTH level should be measured at 0900 h; a high level (>80 $ng \cdot l^{-1}$) with low or low-normal cortisol confirms primary hypoadrenalism.

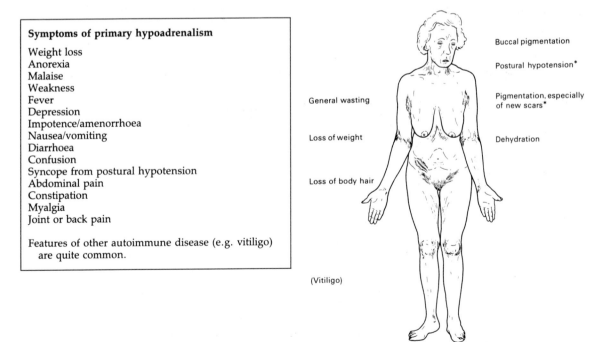

Fig. 16.26 The signs of primary hypoadrenalism (Addison's disease).
*indicates signs of greater discriminant value.

- Electrolyte and urea concentrations are measured. These classically show hyponatraemia, hyperkalaemia and a high urea level, but can be normal.
- Serum aldosterone is reduced, with high plasma renin activity.
- Blood glucose may be low, with symptomatic hypoglycaemia.
- Adrenal antibodies are present in many cases of autoimmune adrenalitis.
- Chest and abdominal x-rays may show evidence of tuberculosis and/or calcified adrenals.
- Hypercalcaemia and anaemia (after rehydration) are sometimes seen.

TREATMENT

Long-term treatment is with replacement glucocorticoid and mineralocorticoid; dosage details are shown in Table 16.38.

Tuberculosis must be treated if present or suspected (see p. 602).

Adequacy of the glucocorticoid dose is judged by:
- Clinical well-being and restoration of normal weight
- Cortisol levels during the day while on replacement hydrocortisone (this cannot be used for synthetic steroids)

Fludrocortisone replacement is assessed by:
- Blood pressure response to posture—it should not fall
- Suppression of plasma renin activity to normal

Patient advice
All patients requiring replacement steroids should:
- Carry a steroid card
- Wear a Medic-Alert bracelet; this gives details of their condition so that emergency replacement therapy can be given if they are found unconscious.
- Keep an ampoule of hydrocortisone and a syringe at home in case oral therapy is impossible

Table 16.38 Average replacement steroid dosages for adults with primary hypoadrenalism.

Drug	Dose
Glucocorticoid	
Cortisol	30 mg daily—20 mg on waking, 10 mg at 1800 h
or Prednisolone	7.5 mg daily—5 mg on waking, 2.5 mg at 1800 h
or Dexamethasone	0.75 mg daily—0.5 mg on waking, 0.25 mg at 1800 h
Mineralocorticoid	
Fludrocortisone	0.05—0.4 mg daily

Acute hypoadrenalism
The major deficiencies are of salt, steroid and glucose.
- Assuming normal cardiovascular function, 1 l of normal saline should be given over 30–60 min with 100 mg of intravenous hydrocortisone.
- Dextrose should be infused if hypoglycaemia is present.
- Subsequent saline requirements may be for several litres within 24 h (assessing with CVP line if necessary) plus hydrocortisone 100 mg i.m. 6-hourly until the patient is clinically stable.
- Oral replacement medication is then started, initially hydrocortisone 20 mg 8-hourly or equivalent, reducing the amount over a few days.
- Fludrocortisone is unnecessary acutely as the high cortisol doses provide sufficient mineralocorticoid activity—it should be introduced later.

SECONDARY HYPOADRENALISM

This may arise from hypothalamic–pituitary disease or from long-term steroid therapy leading to hypothalamic–pituitary–adrenal suppression.

Most patients with the former have panhypopituitarism (see p. 691) and need thyroxine replacement as well as cortisol; in this case hydrocortisone *must* be started before thyroxine.

The commonest cause of secondary hypoadrenalism is long-term corticosteroid medication for non-endocrine disease. The hypothalamic–pituitary axis and the adrenal may both be suppressed and the patient may have vague symptoms of feeling unwell. The long ACTH stimulation test should demonstrate a delayed cortisol response.

CUSHING'S SYNDROME

Cushing's syndrome (named after Harvey Cushing, a Boston neurosurgeon) is the term used to describe the clinical state of increased free circulating glucocorticoid. It occurs most often following the therapeutic administration of synthetic steroids (see below); all the spontaneous forms of the syndrome are rare.

PATHOPHYSIOLOGY AND CAUSES

The causes of Cushing's syndrome are usually subdivided into two groups (Table 16.39):
- Increased circulating ACTH from the pituitary, ectopic tumour or medical administration, with consequential glucocorticoid excess
- A primary excess of endogenous or exogenous glucocorticoid hormone alone, with subsequent (physiological) suppression of ACTH

Table 16.39 Causes of Cushing's syndrome.

ACTH-dependent disease
Pituitary-dependent (Cushing's disease)
Ectopic ACTH-producing tumours
ACTH administration

Non-ACTH-dependent causes
Adrenal adenomas
Adrenal carcinomas
Glucocorticoid administration

Others
Alcohol-induced pseudo-Cushing's syndrome

CLINICAL FEATURES

The predominant clinical features of Cushing's syndrome are those of glucocorticoid excess and are illustrated in Fig. 16.27. Particular points include the following:

- Pigmentation only occurs with ACTH-dependent causes.
- A Cushingoid appearance can be caused by excess alcohol consumption (pseudo-Cushing's syndrome); the pathophysiology is poorly understood, but cortisol levels are raised.
- Impaired glucose tolerance or frank diabetes are common, especially in the ectopic ACTH syndrome.
- Hypokalaemia due to the mineralocorticoid activity of cortisol is common with ectopic ACTH secretion.

INVESTIGATION

There are two phases to the investigation:
- Confirmation of the presence or absence of Cushing's syndrome
- Differential diagnosis of its cause

Confirmation of Cushing's syndrome
Confirmation rests on demonstrating inappropriate cortisol secretion which is not suppressed by exogenous glucocorticoid; difficulties occur with obesity and depression, when cortisol dynamics are often abnormal. Random cortisol measurements are of no value.

Outpatient screening methods include:
- Urinary free cortisol measurements. Repeatedly normal 24-h values (corrected for body mass) render the diagnosis most unlikely.
- The overnight dexamethasone suppression test (Table 16.36). Normal suppression reliably excludes the diagnosis, but failure to suppress is not diagnostic.

Inpatient tests include:
- Circadian rhythm. After 48 h in hospital, cortisol samples are taken at 0900 h and 2400 h (without warning the patient). Normal subjects show a pronounced circadian variation (Fig. 16.2, see p. 683); those with Cushing's syndrome have high evening cortisol levels, though the 0900 h value may be normal.

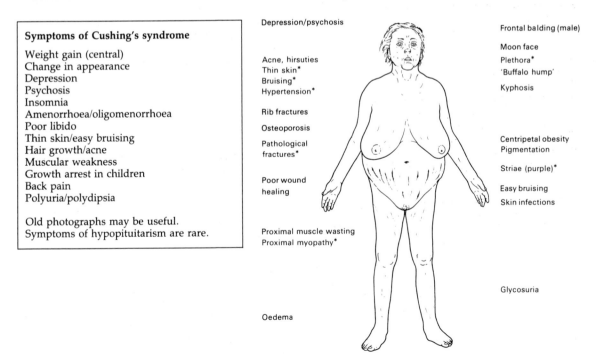

Symptoms of Cushing's syndrome

Weight gain (central)
Change in appearance
Depression
Psychosis
Insomnia
Amenorrhoea/oligomenorrhoea
Poor libido
Thin skin/easy bruising
Hair growth/acne
Muscular weakness
Growth arrest in children
Back pain
Polyuria/polydipsia

Old photographs may be useful.
Symptoms of hypopituitarism are rare.

Depression/psychosis

Acne, hirsuties
Thin skin*
Bruising*
Hypertension*

Rib fractures

Osteoporosis

Pathological
fractures*

Poor wound
healing

Proximal muscle wasting
Proximal myopathy*

Oedema

Frontal balding (male)

Moon face
Plethora*
'Buffalo hump'

Kyphosis

Centripetal obesity
Pigmentation

Striae (purple)*

Easy bruising

Skin infections

Glycosuria

Fig. 16.27 The signs of Cushing's syndrome.
*indicates the signs of most value in discriminating Cushing's syndrome from simple obesity and hirsuties.

- Low-dose dexamethasone test (Table 16.36). Patients with Cushing's syndrome fail to suppress plasma or urinary cortisol levels.
- Insulin tolerance test. This is useful in depression or obesity, when abnormal circadian and suppression responses are seen. The normal rise of cortisol with hypoglycaemia does not occur in patients with Cushing's syndrome.

Differential diagnosis of the cause
The cause of Cushing's syndrome can be extremely difficult to establish. The classical ectopic ACTH syndrome is distinguished by a short history, pigmentation and weight loss, unprovoked hypokalaemia, clinical or chemical diabetes, and plasma ACTH levels above 200 ng·l^{-1}.

Severe hirsuties/virilization suggests an adrenal tumour.

Biochemical and radiological procedures for diagnosis include:

- Plasma potassium measurement. All diuretics must be stopped. Hypokalaemia is common with ectopic ACTH secretion.
- Adrenal CT scan. Adrenal adenomas and carcinomas causing Cushing's syndrome are relatively large and always detectable by CT scanning. Carcinomas are distinguished by their large size, irregular outline and signs of infiltration or metastases.
- High dose dexamethasone test (Table 16.36). Failure of urinary or plasma cortisol suppression suggests an ectopic source of ACTH or an adrenal tumour. The metyrapone test has been shown to be of little value.
- Plasma ACTH levels. Low or undetectable ACTH levels <10 ng·l^{-1}) on two or more occasions are a reliable indicator of non-ACTH dependent disease.
- Pituitary CT scan. This is of less value than the adrenal CT scan; only a minority of tumours of significant size are detected with confidence.
- Skull x-ray. This is also of little value as 80% of patients with a pituitary tumour have a normal x-ray.
- Chest x-ray. This is mandatory to demonstrate a carcinoma of the bronchus or a bronchial carcinoid. Lesions may be very small; if ectopic ACTH is suspected, whole lung and mediastinal CT scans should be performed.

Further investigation may involve selective catheterization of the jugular veins and the inferior petrosal sinus for pituitary lesions, or throughout the body in a search for ectopic sources. Bronchoscopy, cytology and regional arteriograms are sometimes necessary.

TREATMENT

Untreated Cushing's syndrome has a very bad prognosis, with death occurring from hypertension, myocardial infarction, infection and heart failure. Whatever the underlying cause, cortisol hypersecretion should be controlled prior to surgery or radiotherapy. Considerable morbidity and mortality is otherwise associated with operating on unprepared patients. The usual drug used is metyrapone, an 11β-hydroxylase blocker, which is given in doses of 0.75–4.0 g daily in three to four divided doses. Plasma cortisol should be monitored, aiming to reduce the mean level during the day to 300–400 nmol·l^{-1} (equivalent to normal production rates). Other, less satisfactory drugs include aminoglutethimide and trilostane.

Choice of treatment depends upon the cause.

Cushing's disease (pituitary-dependent hyperadrenalism)
Treatment options are surgery, radiotherapy and medical control; the choice between them remains controversial.

Transsphenoidal removal of the tumour is probably the treatment of choice. Selective surgery nearly always leaves the patient ACTH-deficient immediately postoperatively and this is considered a good prognostic sign. Transfrontal surgery is rarely necessary because most tumours are small, though they may occasionally be locally invasive.

Yttrium implantation of radioactive needles in the fossa produces good results but it is not generally available.

External irradiation alone is slow, only effective in 20–50%, and of little value except in those unfit for, or unwilling to have, surgery. Medical therapy to reduce ACTH (e.g. bromocriptine, cyproheptadine) is rarely effective.

Other causes
Adenomas should be resected after preparation with metyrapone. Contralateral adrenal suppression may last for years.

Carcinomas are highly aggressive and the prognosis is poor. In general, if there are not widespread metastases, the tumour bulk should be reduced surgically and the adrenolytic drug mitotane (*o,p'*DDD) given; its side-effects (nausea/vomiting, ataxia) are often a problem.

Ectopic tumour sources should be removed if possible. Otherwise chemotherapy/radiotherapy should be used, depending on the tumour. Control of Cushing's syndrome with metyrapone is beneficial.

If the source is not clear, cortisol hypersecretion should be controlled with medical therapy until a diagnosis can be made.

Nelson's syndrome

This is a syndrome of increased pigmentation associated with an enlarging pituitary tumour occurring after bilateral adrenalectomy. The tumour may be locally invasive, but most physicians believe it can be prevented by radiotherapy at the time of adrenalectomy.

CONGENITAL ADRENAL HYPERPLASIA (CAH)

PATHOPHYSIOLOGY

This condition results from a deficiency of an enzyme in the steroid synthetic pathways, most commonly 21-hydroxylase. As a result, cortisol secretion is reduced and feedback leads to increased ACTH secretion to maintain adequate cortisol; this in turn leads to diversion of the steroid precursors into the androgenic steroid pathways (Fig. 16.28). Thus 17-hydroxyprogesterone, androstenedione and testosterone levels are increased, leading to virilization. Rarely aldosterone synthesis is impaired, with resultant salt wasting.

CLINICAL FEATURES

If severe, CAH presents at birth with sexual ambiguity or adrenal failure. In the female, clitoral hypertrophy, urogenital abnormalities and labioscrotal fusion are common, but the syndrome may be unrecognized in the male. Precocious puberty with hirsutism is a later presentation, while some milder cases only present in adult life, usually accompanied by primary amenorrhoea. Hirsutism developing before menarche is suggestive of CAH.

INVESTIGATION

- 17-Hydroxyprogesterone levels are increased (Fig. 16.28).

- Urinary pregnanetriol excretion is increased.
- Basal ACTH levels are raised.

TREATMENT

Replacement of glucocorticoid activity, and mineralocorticoid activity if deficient, is as for primary hypoadrenalism (see above). Correct dosage is often difficult to establish in the child, but should ensure normal 17-hydroxyprogesterone and ACTH levels while allowing normal growth; excessive replacement leads to stunting of growth.

USES AND PROBLEMS OF THERAPEUTIC STEROID THERAPY

Apart from their use as therapeutic replacement, synthetic glucocorticoids are widely used for many non-endocrine conditions (Table 16.40).

Short-term use (e.g. for acute asthma) carries little risk of significant side-effects except for the simultaneous suppression of immune responses.

Long-term therapy with synthetic or natural steroids will, in most respects, mimic endogenous Cushing's syndrome. Exceptions are the relative absence of hirsutism, acne and severe sodium retention, as the synthetic steroids have low androgenic and mineralocorticoid activity. Excessive doses of steroids may also be absorbed from skin when strong

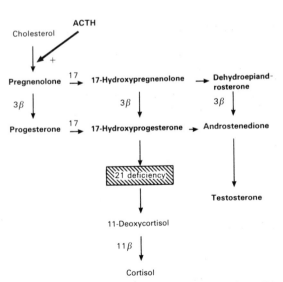

Fig. 16.28 Effects of congenital adrenal hyperplasia (21-hydroxylase deficiency) on steroid biosynthesis. Precursors and products present in excess appear in bold type. Those present in normal or reduced quantities appear in light type.

Table 16.40 Common therapeutic uses of glucocorticoids.

Respiratory disease
Asthma
Chronic bronchitis and emphysema
Sarcoidosis
Hay fever (usually topical)
Cardiac disease
Post-myocardial infarction syndrome
Renal disease
Some nephrotic syndromes
Gastrointestinal disease
Ulcerative colitis
Crohn's disease
Chronic active hepatitis
Rheumatological disease
Systemic lupus erythematosus
Polymyalgia rheumatica
Neurological disease
Cerebral oedema
Skin disease
Tumours
Hodgkin's lymphoma
Other lymphomas
Transplantation
Immunosuppression

dermatological preparations are used, but inhaled steroids very rarely cause Cushing's syndrome, though they may cause adrenal suppression.

The major hazards are detailed in Table 16.41; in

Table 16.41 Adverse effects of corticosteroid therapy.

PHYSIOLOGICAL
Adrenal and/or pituitary suppression
PATHOLOGICAL
Cardiovascular Increased blood pressure
Gastrointestinal Peptic ulceration exacerbation (possible) Pancreatitis
Renal Polyuria Nocturia
Central nervous Depression Euphoria Psychosis Insomnia
Endocrine Weight gain Glycosuria/hyperglycaemia/diabetes Impaired growth Amenorrhoea
Bone and muscle Osteoporosis Proximal myopathy and wasting Aseptic necrosis Pathological fractures
Skin Thinning Easy bruising
Eyes Cataracts
Infections (increased susceptibility) (signs and fever are frequently masked) Septicaemia TB Skin, e.g. fungi

the long-term many are of such severity that the clinical need for high-dose steroids should be continually and critically assessed.

Supervision of steroid therapy

All patients receiving steroids should carry a steroid card and should know that:
- Long-term steroid therapy must never be stopped suddenly. Doses should be reduced very gradually, the dose being given entirely in the morning.
- Doses need increasing in times of serious intercurrent illness (defined as presence of a fever), accident and stress. Double doses should be taken during these times.
- Other physicians, anaesthetists and dentists *must* be told they are on steroid therapy.

Steroids and surgery

Any patient who is receiving steroids, or who has recently received them and whose adrenal glands may still be suppressed, requires careful control of steroid medication around the time of surgery. For all operations hydrocortisone 100 mg i.m. is given preoperatively. This is followed by a suitable dose intramuscularly every 6 h for 24–72 h depending on the degree of surgery performed (see Table 16.42).

The thirst axis

Thirst and water regulation is largely controlled by antidiuretic hormone (ADH, vasopressin). This is synthesized in the hypothalamus and migrates in neurosecretory granules along axonal pathways to the posterior pituitary.

Changes in plasma osmolality are sensed by osmoreceptors in the anterior hypothalamus. Vasopressin secretion is suppressed at levels below 280 mosmol·kg^{-1}, thus allowing maximal water diuresis. Above this level, plasma vasopressin

Table 16.42 Steroid cover for operative procedures.

Procedure	Premedication	Per- and postoperative	Resumption of normal maintenance dosage
Simple procedures, e.g. gastroscopy, simple dental extractions	Hydrocortisone 100 mg i.m.	—	Immediately if no complications
Minor surgery, e.g. varicose veins, hernias	Hydrocortisone 100 mg i.m.	Hydrocortisone 100 mg i.m. every 6 h for 24 h	After 24 h if no complications
Major surgery, e.g. hip replacement, vascular surgery	Hydrocortisone 100 mg i.m.	Hydrocortisone 100 mg i.m. every 6 h for 72 h	After 72 h if normal progress and no complications; perhaps double normal dose for next 2–3 days
GI tract surgery or major thoracic surgery (not eating or ventilated)	Hydrocortisone 100 mg i.m.	Hydrocortisone 100 mg i.m. every 6 h for 72 h or longer if still unwell	When patient eating normally again; until then higher doses (50 mg 6-hourly) may be needed

Table 16.43 Factors affecting vasopressin release.

Increased by:
Increased osmolality
Hypovolaemia
Hypotension
Nausea
Hypothyroidism
Angiotensin II
Adrenaline
Cortisol
Nicotine
Antidepressants
Decreased by:
Decreased osmolality
Hypervolaemia
Hypertension
Ethanol
Alpha-adrenergic stimulation

increases in direct proportion to plasma osmolality. At the upper limit of normal (295 mosmol·kg^{-1}), maximum antidiuresis is achieved and thirst is experienced at about 298 mosmol·kg^{-1}.

Other factors affecting vasopressin release are shown in Table 16.43.

At normal concentrations the kidney is the predominant site of action. Via a cyclic AMP mechanism, it allows the collecting tubule to become permeable to water, thus permitting reabsorption of hypotonic luminal fluid. At high concentrations vasopressin also causes vasoconstriction.

Disorders of vasopressin secretion or activity include:

● Inappropriate excess of the hormone (syndrome of inappropriate antidiuretic hormone; SIADH)
● Deficiency as a result of hypothalamic disease (diabetes insipidus)
● 'Nephrogenic diabetes insipidus'—a condition where the renal tubules are insensitive to vasopressin due to a receptor abnormality

Syndrome of inappropriate antidiuretic hormone (SIADH)

CLINICAL FEATURES

The presentation is usually vague, with confusion, nausea, irritability and, later, fits and coma. There is no oedema. Mild symptoms usually occur with plasma sodium levels of below 125 mmol·1^{-1} and serious manifestations are likely below 115 mmol·1^{-1}.

BIOCHEMISTRY

Usual features are:
● Dilutional hyponatraemia due to excessive water retention
● Low plasma osmolality with higher 'inappropriate' urine osmolality
● Continued urinary sodium excretion
● Absence of hypertension or hypokalaemia
● Normal renal and adrenal function

CAUSES

The causes of SIADH are listed in Table 16.44.

DIFFERENTIAL DIAGNOSIS

The differential diagnosis of hyponatraemia is listed on p. 436.

TREATMENT

The underlying cause should be corrected where possible. For symptomatic relief the fluid intake should be restricted to 500–1000 ml daily. The plasma osmolality, sodium and body weight are measured frequently.

● If water restriction is poorly tolerated or ineffective, demeclocycline 600–1200 mg daily may be given; this inhibits the action of vasopressin on the kidney, causing a reversible form of diabetes insipidus. It may, however, cause photosensitive rashes.
● When the hyponatraemia is very severe, hypertonic saline 300 mmol·1^{-1} slowly i.v. and frusemide may be used. These should be used with extreme caution (see p. 437).

Table 16.44 Causes of the syndrome of inappropriate ADH (SIADH).

Tumours
Small cell carcinoma of lung
Prostate
Thymus
Pancreas
Lymphomas
Pulmonary lesions
Pneumonia
Tuberculosis
Lung abscess
CNS causes
Meningitis
Tumours
Head injury
Subdural
Cerebral abscess
SLE vasculitis
Metabolic causes
Alcohol withdrawal
Porphyria
Drugs
Chlorpropamide
Carbamazepine
Cyclophosphamide
Vincristine

Table 16.45 Causes of diabetes insipidus.

Cranial diabetes insipidus
Congenital

Idiopathic

Tumours
  Craniopharyngioma
  Pituitary with suprasellar extension
  Hypothalamic tumour, e.g. glioma
  Metastases, especially breast
  Lymphoma/leukaemia

Infections
  Tuberculosis
  Meningitis
  Cerebral abscess

Infiltrations
  Sarcoidosis
  Histiocytosis X

Post-surgical
  Transfrontal
  Transsphenoidal

Post-radiotherapy

Vascular
  Haemorrhage/thrombosis
  Sheehan's syndrome

Nephrogenic diabetes insipidus
Idiopathic

Renal tubular acidosis

Hypokalaemia

Hypercalcaemia

Drugs, e.g.
  Lithium
  Demethylchlortetracycline (demeclocycline)
  Glibenclamide

Diabetes insipidus (DI)

CLINICAL FEATURES

A deficiency of vasopressin leads to polyuria, nocturia and compensatory polydipsia. Urine output may reach as much as 10–15 l daily, leading to dehydration, which may be very severe if the thirst mechanisms are impaired or the patients are denied fluid.

Causes of DI are listed in Table 16.45. The commonest cause is following hypothalamic–pituitary surgery; the DI is usually transient, frequently remitting afer a few days or weeks. Primary overdrinking (polydipsia) is a common differential diagnosis.

DI may be masked by simultaneous cortisol deficiency—cortisol replacement allows a water diuresis and DI then becomes apparent.

DIDMOAD syndrome (Wolfran syndrome) is a rare recessive condition comprising diabetes insipidus, diabetes mellitus, optic atrophy and deafness.

BIOCHEMISTRY

Features include:
- High or high-normal plasma osmolality with low urine osmolality (in primary polydipsia the plasma osmolality tends to be low)
- Resultant high or high-normal plasma sodium
- Failure of urinary concentration with fluid deprivation
- Restoration of urinary concentration with vasopressin or an analogue

The latter points may be studied with a formal water deprivation test. In normal subjects plasma osmolality remains normal while urine osmolality rises above 700 mosmol·kg^{-1}; in DI, plasma osmolality rises while the urine remains dilute, only concentrating *after* exogenous vasopressin is given.

TREATMENT

Synthetic vasopressin (desmopressin; DDAVP) is now the treatment of choice. It is given intranasally, 10–20 µg once or twice daily, or intramuscularly 2–4 µg. The response is variable and must be monitored carefully, with measurement of the osmolality.

Alternative agents in mild disease, probably working by sensitizing the tubules to endogenous vasopressin, include thiazide diuretics, carbamazepine 200–400 mg daily and chlorpropamide 200–350 mg daily; the latter may cause hypoglycaemia.

Nephrogenic diabetes insipidus

The renal tubules are resistant to normal or high levels of plasma vasopressin. It may be inherited as a sex-linked recessive trait or can be acquired as a result of renal disease, drug ingestion, hypercalcaemia or hypokalaemia. Wherever possible the cause should be reversed.

Skeletal endocrinology

Bone forms 25% of the normal adult's weight; its major mineral constituents are calcium, phosphate and, to a much lesser extent, magnesium. In the adult there is a continuous process of bone remodelling and resorption. While exchange of calcium between bone and plasma is only 10–15 mmol daily, over a year 20% of total bone calcium is exchanged.

Physiology, structure and function of bone

Bone is a collagen-based matrix with mineral laid down upon it. Its structural strength depends upon both components; uncalcified bone is soft (e.g. in osteomalacia), while defective collagen leads to brittle bones (e.g. in osteogenesis imperfecta).

Bone deposition is carried out by osteoblasts, while resorption depends on osteoclasts. The local factors controlling the relative activity of these processes is poorly understood, but is certainly dependent on hormonal factors. Procollagen is synthesized in osteoblasts and modified to yield collagen, which is a semi-rigid rod-like molecule with the general formula of 333 × (glycine–proline–amino acid), which polymerizes in a staggered linear fashion and is joined by cross-linkages. After formation, calcium hydroxyapatite crystallization occurs between and around the collagen fibrils.

Osteoclasts are stimulated by parathormone (PTH), appear on the surface of bone and cause bone resorption.

Bone metabolism and mineralization is thus dependent on:
- Collagen synthesis
- Absorption and availability of calcium, affected by vitamin D
- Bone resorption and deposition, largely under hormonal control

Calcium absorption and distribution

Normal adult Western calcium consumption is approximately 20–25 mmol (800–1000 mg) daily, though intake is much lower in some less affluent countries. Calcium deficiency does not appear to be a significant cause of bone disease, probably because calcium absorption increases in states of dietary calcium deficiency. Absorption is occasionally reduced by generalized malabsorption.

Calcium fluxes between gut, plasma, bone and kidney are shown in Fig. 16.29. The circulating pool of calcium is tiny compared with the bony reservoir, and small compared with the daily fluxes.

Vitamin D metabolism (see Chapter 3)

Vitamin D metabolism is illustrated in Fig. 3.4 (see p. 135). The predominant active metabolite is 1,25-dihydroxycholecalciferol.

Cholecalciferol (vitamin D_3) from the diet and a precursor synthesized in the skin from cholesterol under ultraviolet light stimulation (usually sunlight) are hydroxylated within the liver to form the principal circulating metabolite, 25-hydroxycholecalciferol. This is further hydroxylated within the kidney to either 1,25-dihydroxycholecalciferol, the active metabolite, or to a similar but physiologically inactive product 24,25-dihydroxycholecalciferol. The relative amount of 1,25-dihydroxycholecalciferol produced compared with 24,25-dihydroxycholecalciferol increases with low plasma calcium, partially under PTH control.

Regulation of plasma calcium

PTH is secreted by the four parathyroid glands. Levels of PTH rise as the plasma calcium falls. The actions of PTH are several, all serving to raise the plasma calcium. It results in:
- Increased tubular reabsorption of calcium
- Increased excretion of phosphate

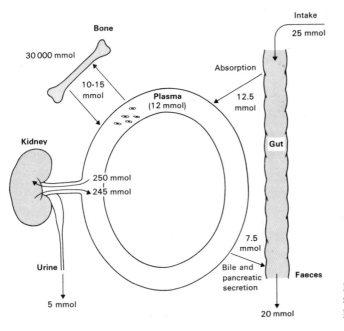

Fig. 16.29 Calcium exchange in the normal human. The fluxes shown are per day.

- Increased osteoclastic resorption of bone
- Increased absorption of calcium
- Increased synthesis of 1,25-dihydroxychole-calciferol

The effects are mediated at membrane receptors on the target cells, with resultant increased adenyl cyclase activity.

Other calcium regulatory factors
Calcitonin. This hormone is produced by thyroid C-cells. Its physiological importance in man as a hypocalcaemic hormone remains uncertain. Plasma levels of calcitonin rise with increasing plasma calcium, and it is known to inhibit osteoclastic bone resorption and increase renal excretion of calcium and phosphate. However, total thyroidectomy (absent calcitonin) and medullary carcinoma (excess calcitonin) have few skeletal effects. It is used in the treatment of Paget's disease (see p. 367) and in the emergency treatment of hypercalcaemia.

Glucocorticoids. Steroids have complex actions on bone, essentially leading to excessive bone resorption and osteoporosis.

Sex hormones. Androgens and/or oestrogens have several effects on the skeleton:
- In puberty they induce the growth spurt and subsequent epiphysial closure.
- Both influence skeletal calcium content, especially oestrogen; deficiency post-menopausally leads to progressive bone loss.

Growth hormone. Acting via the somatomedins (see p. 708) growth hormone stimulates the growth of cartilage.

Thyroid hormones. Excess T_4 and T_3 cause increased bone turnover, while hypothyroidism leads to growth delay.

The role of magnesium

Total body magnesium is about 25 g. Plasma magnesium ranges between 0.7–1.0 mmol·l^{-1}, and generally follows plasma calcium levels. Magnesium deficiency occurs, especially in malabsorption; the level should be measured when there are signs or symptoms of hypocalcaemia that are unresponsive to conventional correction.

The role of phosphate

Phosphate forms an essential part of most biochemical systems from nucleic acids downwards. About 80% of all body phosphorus is within bone, plasma phosphate normally ranging from 0.80–1.40 mmol·l^{-1}. Phosphate reabsorption from the kidney is decreased by PTH, thus hyperparathyroidism is associated with low plasma phosphate levels. High levels are found in hypoparathyroidism and in renal failure, when normal reabsorption does not occur.

Measurement of plasma calcium and phosphate

The total plasma calcium is normally 2.2–2.6 mmol·l^{-1}. Usually only 40% of the total plasma calcium is ionized and physiologically relevant; the remainder is protein-bound or complexed and thus is unavailable to the tissues. Ionizable calcium is difficult to measure but very dependent upon protein, in particular albumin, concentration. An approximate correction for plasma calcium is to add or subtract 0.02 mmol·l^{-1} for every gram per litre by which the simultaneous albumin concentration lies below or above a standard figure (normally 40 or 47 g·l^{-1}). Thus a total calcium of 2.22 mmol·l^{-1} with an albumin of 35 g·l^{-1} will become 2.32 mmol·l^{-1} (corrected to 40 g·l^{-1}). The normal range will obviously vary depending on whether the correction is made to 40 or 47 g·l^{-1}.

For critical measurement, samples should be taken in the fasting state without use of a cuff (as this would affect albumin concentration).

PTH assays are available in special centres; interpretation requires simultaneous plasma calcium and phosphate measurements.

METABOLIC BONE DISEASE

Osteomalacia

PATHOPHYSIOLOGY

Osteomalacia results from inadequate mineralization of the osteoid framework, leading to soft bones. It is thus usually caused by a defect in vitamin D availability or metabolism. The effect on bone is shown in Fig. 16.30. Rickets is the term for childhood osteomalacia with resultant bony deformities.

CAUSES

- Deficiency of vitamin D—dietary plus inadequate sunlight exposure, often occurring in Asian immigrant females in the UK
- Malabsorption—patients after gastric surgery, those with coeliac disease and those with deficient bile salt production
- Renal disease, leading to inadequate conversion of 25-hydroxycholecalciferol to 1,25-dihydroxy-cholecalciferol (see p. 419)

Less common causes are hepatic failure (reduced 25-hydroxycholecalciferol) and phenytoin or barbiturate therapy (affects vitamin D metabolism). Vitamin D-resistant rickets (familial hypophosphataemia) is an X-linked disorder with hypophosphataemia, phosphaturia and rickets.

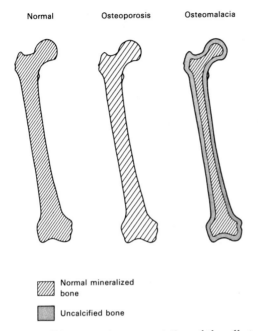

Normal   Osteoporosis   Osteomalacia

Normal mineralized bone

Uncalcified bone

Fig. 16.30 Diagrammatic representation of the effects of osteoporosis and osteomalacia on the density and calcification of bone.

CLINICAL FEATURES

Childhood rickets usually presents with bony deformity or failure of adequate growth. In the adult, osteomalacia may produce bone and muscle pain and tenderness, often due to subclinical fractures. There is often a marked proximal myopathy.

INVESTIGATION

The only certain diagnosis is made by bone biopsy, with demonstration of increased unmineralized bone; undecalcified bone must be used for examination. The following findings are characteristic:
- Low or low-normal plasma calcium
- Low serum phosphate
- Increased alkaline phosphatase
- X-rays showing a defective mineralization, especially in the pelvis, long bones and ribs, often with Looser's zones (linear areas of low density)

TREATMENT

Vitamin D replacement is given, usually as calciferol 500–5000 units daily or the newer active metabolite, 1α-hydroxycholecalciferol 1–3 μg daily. Plasma calcium *must* be checked regularly. Higher doses are needed where renal disease or resistance to vitamin D is present.

Osteoporosis

PATHOPHYSIOLOGY

Osteoporosis is reduced bone mass per unit bone volume (Fig. 16.30). This leads to reduced strength and increased risk of fracture, often with even minor trauma. Measurement of bone mass by densitometry and similar techniques is difficult and not generally available, and plain radiography gives only very crude clues to the presence of osteoporosis.

The following factors are relevant:
- Bone mass decreases with increasing age.
- Osteoporosis is commonest in post-menopausal women, as oestrogens prevent bone resorption. This group has a high prevalence of osteoporosis and fractures, most commonly Colles' fractures and fractures of the femoral neck or vertebrae.
- Inadequate dietary calcium intake is thought to be important, with the average adult intake of 500–700 mg (12.5–17.5 mmol) daily being only half that required to maintain balance.
- Physical activity, especially during growth, may promote increased bone mass. Excessive exercise in women, however, may produce hypogonadism (see p. 702).

Other factors causing osteoporosis are listed in Table 16.46.

CLINICAL FEATURES

The commonest presentation is of acute bone pain secondary to a suspected or actual fracture.

INVESTIGATION

- Plain radiology is of limited value—the reduction in density must be extreme before it can be detec-

Table 16.46 Causes of osteoporosis.

Old age
Post-menopausal

Endocrine causes
    Cushing's syndrome
    Diabetes mellitus
    Thyrotoxicosis
    Hypogonadism
    Acromegaly

Rheumatoid arthritis (localized only)
Immobilization   Long-term bed rest
Weightlessness
Chronic renal failure

Drugs
    Glucocorticoids
    Heparin ⎫
    Diuretics ⎬ long-term

ted with certainty. Crush fractures and complete vertebral collapse are common. There tends to be vertebral biconcavity.

- Fresh fractures may be highlighted by bone scanning using technetium-99m.
- Plasma calcium, phosphate and alkaline phosphatase are all normal, except following a recent fracture when the latter may be raised. The disorder is one of bone mass not of calcium metabolism per se.
- Secondary deposits or multiple myeloma may need to be excluded.
- The possibilities of thyrotoxicosis, Cushing's syndrome and diabetes mellitus may require investigation.
- Histological examination by transiliac biopsy is sometimes used to confirm the diagnosis. Coincident osteomalacia is sometimes present.
- Bone mass measurement is not widely available and CT scanning little used.

TREATMENT

Treatment of the established disease is unsatisfactory as bone mass has already been lost. Prophylaxis for high-risk individuals is therefore preferable.

Fractures should be treated by conventional orthopaedic means. Fresh fractures of the spine require short-term bed rest with adequate analgesia and, if necessary, muscle relaxants.

Treatment of the underlying osteoporosis is the same as that for prophylaxis, though coincident osteomalacia should be treated as above.

PROPHYLAXIS

This area is controversial and the scientific evidence conflicting. The following measures have been suggested but, apart from the first, are not widely accepted:

- Oestrogen therapy is of proven value but, in view of potential side-effects (thrombosis, endometrial carcinoma), is only normally given to those with premature menopause or ovariectomy, those with high-risk factors, e.g. those who are nulliparous, have hypogonadism or who have a family history of osteoporosis.
- Dietary calcium may be increased to >1.5 g daily, especially in postmenopausal women.
- Moderate exercises against gravity, e.g. walking, running and competitive sports, may also retard bone loss. This is often painful or impossible in those with established disease.

Fluoride, calcitonin and diphosphonates are being investigated but their use cannot be advised at present.

HYPOCALCAEMIA

PATHOPHYSIOLOGY

Hypocalcaemia may be due to deficiencies of calcium homeostatic mechanisms or secondary to high phosphate levels (Table 16.47). Hypoparathyroidism is uncommon.

CAUSES

- Renal failure. This is the commonest cause of hypocalcaemia.
- Postoperative. Transient hypocalcaemia may follow thyroid, parathyroid or other neck operations, but may become permanent.
- Idiopathic hypoparathyroidism. This is one of the rarer autoimmune disorders. Vitiligo, cutaneous moniliasis and other autoimmune disease are often seen.
- DiGeorge's syndrome. This is a familial condition associated with intellectual impairment, cataracts, calcified basal ganglia and occasionally with organ-specific autoimmune disease.
- Pseudohypoparathyroidism. This is a syndrome of end-organ resistance to PTH. It is associated with short stature, short metacarpals and intellectual impairment. Pseudo-pseudohypoparathyroidism is the situation of the phenotypic defects without the calcium abnormalities.

CLINICAL FEATURES

The symptoms are those of neuromuscular irritability and neuropsychiatric manifestations. Parasthesiae, circumoral numbness, cramps, anxiety and

Table 16.47 Causes of hypocalcaemia.

Increased phosphate
Chronic renal failure
Phosphate therapy
Drugs
Calcitonin
Diphosphonates
Miscellaneous
Acute pancreatitis
Citrated blood in massive transfusion
Hypoparathyroidism
Congenital deficiency (DiGeorge's syndrome)
Idiopathic hypoparathyroidism (autoimmune)
After neck operations
Severe hypomagnesaemia
Resistance to PTH
Pseudohypoparathyroidism
Vitamin D
Deficiency
Resistance to vitamin D

tetany are followed by convulsions, laryngeal stridor, dystonia and psychosis.

Two important signs of hypocalcaemia are Chvostek's sign, where gentle tapping over the facial nerve causes twitching of the facial muscles, and Trousseau's sign, where inflation of a sphygmomanometer cuff above diastolic blood pressure for 3 min induces tetanic spasm of the fingers and wrist. Severe hypocalcaemia may cause papilloedema and a prolonged QT interval on the ECG.

INVESTIGATION

The clinical picture is usually diagnostic and is confirmed by a low serum calcium. The following may be helpful in finding the cause:
- High phosphate levels
- Absent or low PTH levels
- Parathyroid antibodies (not widely available)
- Vitamin D metabolites
- X-rays of metacarpals showing short fourth metacarpal (occurs in pseudohypoparathyroidism)

TREATMENT

Urgency of treatment depends upon the severity of symptoms and the degree of hypocalcaemia. If severe (e.g. tetany) intravenous calcium (10 ml initially, then 10–40 ml of 10% calcium gluconate in a litre of saline over 4–8 h) is given. Oral calcium supplements (4–20 mmol [2–10g] daily) are rarely sufficient alone.

1-Hydroxylated derivatives of vitamin D are now preferred for treatment because of their shorter half-life. Usual daily maintenance doses are 1–3 μg for 1α-hydroxycholecalciferol and 1,25-dihydroxycholecalciferol and 0.25–2 mg for dihydrotachysterol. During treatment, the plasma calcium *must* be monitored frequently to prevent hypercalcaemia.

HYPERCALCAEMIA

Hypercalcaemia is much commoner than hypocalcaemia, and is increasingly detected incidentally with multichannel chemical analysers. Mild, asymptomatic hypercalcaemia occurs in approximately 0.1% of the population and is usually due to primary hyperparathyroidism.

True hypercalcaemia should be confirmed on a carefully collected specimen (see above).

PATHOPHYSIOLOGY AND CAUSES

Major causes of hypercalcaemia are listed in Table 16.48; primary hyperparathyroidism and malignant disease are the commonest.

Hyperparathyroidism can be primary, secondary or tertiary:
- Primary hyperparathyroidism is caused by single

Table 16.48 Causes of hypercalcaemia.

Excess PTH
Primary hyperparathyroidism
Tertiary hyperparathyroidism
Ectopic PTH secretion (very rare)

Excess action of vitamin D
Iatrogenic or self-administered excess
Sarcoidosis

Excess calcium intake
'Milk alkali' syndrome

Drugs
Thiazides

Malignant disease
Secondary deposits
Production of osteoclastic factors
Myeloma

Other endocrine disease
Thyrotoxicosis
Addison's disease

Miscellaneous
Long-term immobility
Familial hypocalcuric hypercalcaemia

(80+% of cases) or multiple (5%) parathyroid adenomas or by hyperplasia (10%). Parathyroid carcinoma is rare (2%).
- Secondary hyperparathyroidism is physiological compensatory hypertophy of all four parathyroid glands due to hypocalcaemia (e.g. in renal failure or vitamin D deficiency). PTH levels are raised but calcium levels are low or normal; PTH levels fall to normal after correction of the cause of hypocalcaemia.
- Tertiary hyperparathyroidism is the development of apparently autonomous parathyroid hyperplasia after long-standing secondary hyperparathyroidism, most often in renal failure on dialysis. Plasma calcium and PTH are both raised, the latter often grossly so. Parathyroidectomy is necessary at this stage.

CLINICAL FEATURES

The symptoms and signs of hypercalcaemia are:
- General—malaise, depression, hypertension
- Renal—renal colic from stones, polyuria/nocturia, haematuria
- Bones—bone pain
- Abdominal—abdominal pain, sometimes peptic ulceration

Particular points of note are:
- Malignant disease is usually advanced by the time hypercalcaemia occurs as a result of lytic bony metastases. The common tumours are bronchus, breast, myeloma, oesophagus, thyroid, prostate, lymphoma and renal cell carcinoma. Ectopic PTH secretion is very rare.

- Severe hypercalcaemia (>3 mmol·l^{-1}) is usually associated with malignant disease, hyperparathyroidism, renal dialysis or vitamin D therapy.
- Corneal calcification is a marker of long-standing hypercalcaemia.
- In primary hyperparathyroidism only 5–10% have definite bony lesions and 20–40% renal involvement.

INVESTIGATION AND DIFFERENTIAL DIAGNOSIS

- Several fasting calcium and phosphate samples should be taken. Hypophosphataemia is common in primary hyperparathyroidism.
- PTH levels should be measured. Detectable levels during hypercalcaemia are inappropriate and imply hyperparathyroidism.
- Abdominal x-rays may show renal calculi or nephrocalcinosis. Renal function must be measured.
- High-definition hand x-rays may show subperiosteal erosions in the middle or terminal phalanges.
- Protein electrophoresis is performed to detect myeloma, serum thyroxine to detect thyrotoxicosis, biopsy of the appropriate tissue to detect, for example, sarcoidosis or malignant tissue.
- A hydrocortisone suppression test is performed. Plasma calcium in hyperparathyroidism is resistant to suppression by steroids (10 days of hydrocortisone 40 mg three times daily); this also occurs with some malignancies. In sarcoidosis, vitamin D-mediated hypercalcaemia and most malignancies, suppression to normal or near-normal levels is seen.
- PTH reduces the renal tubular reabsorption of bicarbonate, thereby slighty reducing the plasma level. As a consequence plasma chloride is elevated in primary hyperparathyroidism.

If primary hyperparathyroidism is confirmed, the following may be helpful in localization, though adenomas are usually small:

- A barium swallow—may show indentation of the oesophagus by an adenoma
- Ultrasound
- CT scan, though very high resolution is needed
- Radioisotope 'subtraction' scans—a picture of the parathyroid tissue is derived from the difference in uptake between thallium-201 (taken up by thyroid and parathyroid) and technetium-99m (taken up by thyroid only)
- Venous catheterization for local PTH levels—usually reserved for previous operative failures

TREATMENT

Primary hyperparathyroidism

Indications for surgery in hyperparathyroidism remain controversial. All agree that, with renal disease or bone involvement, surgery is indicated, there being no long-term medical treatment. The situation when the plasma calcium is mildly raised (2.65–2.9 mmol·l^{-1}) is disputed; most physicians feel that probable symptoms of hypercalcaemia, which may be mild and non-specific, should lead to parathyroidectomy. Those who are asymptomatic should receive careful follow-up; development of renal, bone or other symptoms then warrants surgery.

Parathyroid surgery should only be performed by experienced surgeons. Ninety per cent of these patients have adenomas rather than hyperplasia, but the minute glands may be very difficult to define. It is also difficult to distinguish between an adenoma and a normal parathyroid.

If initial exploration is unsuccessful, venous catheterization for PTH levels may be helpful; a few parathyroid glands lie in ectopic sites elsewhere in the neck and upper mediastinum.

The main danger postoperatively is hypocalcaemia (see above):

- Chvostek's and Trousseau's signs should be sought.
- Daily plasma calcium measurements are needed for 2–5 days.
- Mild transient hypoparathyroidism often occurs for 1 or 2 weeks, possibly due to suppression of the other parathyroids. Depending on severity, oral or intravenous calcium should be given temporarily.
- A few patients develop long-standing surgical hypoparathyroidism.

Secondary hyperparathyroidism

Treatment of other causes depends upon the primary pathology, though steroids are often useful.

Acute hypercalcaemia

This is an emergency leading to nausea and vomiting, nocturia and polyuria, drowsiness and altered consciousness. The serum calcium is greater than 3 mmol·l^{-1}.

While investigation of the cause is underway, immediate treatment is mandatory:

- Adequate rehydration (3–4 l daily of saline for 2–3 days) is given.
- Prednisolone 30–60 mg daily is effective in some states, especially myeloma, sarcoidosis and vitamin D excess.

If the levels of calcium are very high (e.g. 3.2–3.5 mmol·l^{-1}), the following hypocalcaemic agents may be used:

- Calcitonin 200 units 6 hourly i.v. has an acute but very short-lived hypocalcaemic action.
- Mithramycin 25 µg·kg^{-1} over 4–6 h is often effective for 48 h.
- Intravenous diphosphonates (e.g. amino-

propylidene diphosphonate) lower the plasma calcium but their place is as yet undefined.

- Oral phosphate (sodium cellulose phosphate 5 g three times daily) produces diarrhoea and is of dubious value in lowering calcium; intravenous phosphate rapidly lowers calcium levels but is dangerous.

Once the calcium is reduced to levels where the patient is no longer acutely ill, routine investigation can proceed.

Endocrinology of blood pressure control

The control of blood pressure (BP) is complex and involves neural, cardiac, hormonal and many other mechanisms.

BP is dependent upon cardiac output and peripheral resistance. Although cardiac output can be increased in endocrine disease (e.g. thyrotoxicosis), the main role of hormonal mechanisms is control of peripheral resistance and of circulating blood volume.

When to investigate for secondary hypertension?

Endocrine causes account for less than 5% of all hypertension (Table 16.49). Therefore not all

Table 16.49 Endocrine causes of hypertension.

Excessive renin, and thus angiotensin II, production Renal artery stenosis Other local renal disease Renin-secreting tumours
Excessive production of catecholamines Phaeochromocytoma
Excessive GH production Acromegaly
Excessive aldosterone production Adrenal adenoma (Conn's syndrome) Idiopathic adrenal hyperplasia Dexamethasone-suppressible hyperaldosteronism

Excessive production of other mineralocorticoids
Cushing's syndrome (massive excess of cortisol, a
  weak mineralocorticoid)
Congenital adrenal hyperplasia (in some cases)
Tumours producing other mineralocorticoids, e.g.
  corticosterone

Exogenous 'mineralocorticoids' Liquorice ingestion Abuse of mineralocorticoid preparations

hypertensives should be fully investigated endocrinologically. The highest chances of endocrine causes are in:

- Subjects under 35 years old, especially those without a family history of hypertension
- Those with accelerated (malignant) hypertension
- Those with hypertension resistant to conventional triple therapy
- Those with indications of renal disease (e.g. proteinuria, unequal renal sizes)
- Those with unprovoked hypokalaemia
- Those with unusual symptoms (e.g. sweating attacks, weakness)

The renin–angiotensin–aldosterone axis

The renin–angiotensin–aldosterone system is illustrated in Fig. 16.31. Angiotensinogen, an alpha-2-globulin of hepatic origin, circulates in the plasma. The enzyme renin is secreted by the kidney in response to decreased renal perfusion pressure or flow; it cleaves the decapeptide angiotensin I from angiotensinogen. Angiotensin I is inactive, but is further cleaved by converting enzyme (present in lung and vascular endothelium) into the active peptide, angiotensin II, which has two major actions:

- It causes powerful vasoconstriction (within seconds)
- It causes stimulation of the adrenal zona glomerulosa to increase aldosterone production. Aldosterone then causes sodium retention and urinary potassium loss (hours to days).

The vasoconstrictor action of angiotensin II is short-term, while the sodium retention induced by aldosterone increases total body sodium and the BP in the long term.

As the BP increases and sodium is retained, the stimuli to renin secretion are reduced (by negative feedback). Dietary sodium excess will tend to suppress renin secretion, whereas sodium deprivation or urinary sodium loss will increase it.

RENIN (AND ANGIOTENSIN)-DEPENDENT HYPERTENSION

Many forms of unilateral and bilateral renal disease are associated with hypertension. The classic example is renal artery stenosis; the major hypertensive effects of this and other situations such as renin-secreting tumours are directly or indirectly due to angiotensin II.

Renal artery stenosis

This is discussed on p. 398.

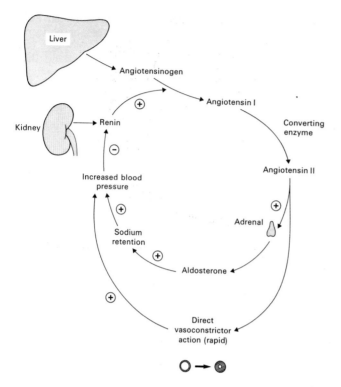

Fig. 16.31 The renin–angiotensin–aldosterone system.

DISORDERS OF ALDOSTERONE

Primary hyperaldosteronism

PATHOPHYSIOLOGY

This rare condition (<1% of all cases of hypertension) is caused by excess aldosterone production, leading to sodium retention, hypertension, potassium loss and thus hypokalaemia.

CAUSES (Table 16.49)

Adrenal adenomas (Conn's syndrome) account for 60% of cases, and 30% are due to bilateral adrenal hyperplasia, which may be secondary to an excess of a pituitary aldosterone-stimulating factor.

CLINICAL FEATURES

The usual presentation is hypertension and hypokalaemia (<3.5 mmol·l^{-1}), though 20% of patients have potassium levels of 3.5–4.2 mmol·l^{-1}. The few symptoms are non-specific; muscle weakness, nocturia and tetany are rarely seen. The hypertension may be severe and associated with renal and retinal damage.

Adenomas, often very small, are commoner in young females, while bilateral hyperplasia rarely occurs before age 40 and is commoner in males.

INVESTIGATION

The characteristic features are:
- Hypokalaemia. A high-salt diet should be given for several days before the blood sample is taken and plasma samples must be separated quickly. Diuretics must be stopped 3 weeks before investigation; bethanidine may be used for temporary control.
- Increased urinary potassium loss. Levels >30 mmol·day^{-1} during hypokalaemia are inappropriate.
- Elevated plasma aldosterone levels which are not suppressed with saline infusion (300 mmol over 4 h) or fludrocortisone administration
- Suppressed plasma renin activity. Beta-blockers and other drugs can also interfere with renin activity.

Once a diagnosis of hyperaldosteronism is established, differentiation of adenoma from hyperplasia involves adrenal CT scanning (not infallible as tumours are small), adrenal scintillation scanning and venous catheterization.

TREATMENT

An adenoma should be surgically removed; the BP falls in 70% of cases. Those with hyperplasia should be treated with the aldosterone antagonist spironolactone 100–400 mg daily; side-effects include nausea, rashes and gynaecomastia. Amiloride 10–40 mg daily is an alternative.

Secondary hyperaldosteronism

This situation arises when there is excess renin and hence excess angiotensin II causing stimulation of the zona glomerulosa. Common causes are accelerated hypertension and renal artery stenosis, when the patient will be hypertensive. Causes associated with normotension include congestive cardiac failure and cirrhosis, where excess aldosterone production contributes to sodium retention.

Spironolactone is of value in both situations. Converting enzyme inhibitors, e.g. captopril or enalapril, may be used in heart failure.

Hypoaldosteronism

Except as part of primary hypoadrenalism (Addison's disease, see p. 724), this is very uncommon.

Atrial natriuretic factor/peptide

This recently discovered peptide is secreted from the atrium and produces marked effects on the kidney, increasing sodium and water excretion and glomerular filtration rate and lowering the BP, plasma renin activity and plasma aldosterone. Active analogues are being investigated.

THE ADRENAL MEDULLA

The major catecholamines, noradrenaline and adrenaline, are produced in the adrenal medulla (Fig. 16.32). While noradrenaline and adrenaline undoubtedly produce hypertension when infused, they probably play little part in BP regulation in normal man.

Phaeochromocytoma

Phaeochromocytomas, tumours of the sympathetic nervous system, are very rare (less than 1 in 1000 cases of hypertension). Ninety per cent arise in the adrenal, 25% are multiple and 10% are malignant. Some are associated with multiple endocrine neoplasia syndromes (see p. 742).

CLINICAL FEATURES

The clinical features are those of catecholamine excess (see Table 16.50) and are frequently intermittent.

Table 16.50 Symptoms and signs of phaeochromocytoma.

Symptoms
Anxiety or panic attacks
Palpitations
Tremor
Sweating
Headache
Flushing
Nausea and/or vomiting
Weight loss
Constipation or diarrhoea
Raynaud's phenomenon
Chest pain
Polyuria/nocturia

Signs
Hypertension—intermittent or constant
Tachycardia plus arrhythmias
Bradycardia
Orthostatic hypotension
Pallor or flushing
Glycosuria
Fever
(Signs of hypertensive damage)

Fig. 16.32 The synthesis and metabolism of catecholamines.

INVESTIGATION

The possibility of phaeochromocytoma needs to be frequently considered in those with hypertension. Specific tests are as follows:

● Measurement of urinary metabolites (vanillyl-mandelic acid and metanephrines; see Fig. 16.32) is a useful screening test. Normal levels on three 24 h collections virtually exclude the diagnosis. Many drugs and dietary vanilla interfere with these tests.
● If high levels of vanillylmandelic acid are found, plasma catecholamines may be estimated.
● CT scans, initially of the abdomen, are usually helpful as the tumours are often large.
● A recent development is scanning with ^{131}I-metaiodobenzylguanidine, which produces specific uptake in sites of sympathetic activity.

TREATMENT

Tumours should be removed if this is possible. Medical pre- and perioperative treatment is vital and includes complete alpha- and beta-receptor blockade with phenoxybenzamine (20–40 mg daily initially) *then* propranolol (120–240 mg daily) plus transfusion of whole blood to re-expand the contracted plasma volume. Surgery in the unprepared patient is fraught with dangers of both hyper- and hypotension; sodium nitroprusside should be available in case sudden severe hypertension develops.

When operation is not possible, combined alpha- and beta-receptor blockade can be used long-term.

Other endocrinological disorders

Diseases of many glands

Multiple gland failure
This is caused by autoimmune disease (see Table 16.6, p. 687).

Multiple tumours
There are two rare groups of endocrine adenomas (MEA) affecting multiple glands; the conditions are frequently familial. Details of the clinical syndromes are given in Table 16.51.

Ectopic hormone secretion

Ectopic hormone secretion from a non-endocrine cell is most usually seen in tumours that have some degree of embryological resemblance to specialist endocrine cells. The clinical effects will be those of the hormone produced, with or without manifestations of systemic malignancy.

The commonest situations seen are:

● Hypercalcaemia of malignant disease. This is often associated with squamous cell tumours of lung and breast with bone metastases. It is sometimes mediated by various factors (rarely PTH).
● Syndrome of inappropriate ADH secretion (see p. 731). Again this is commonest from a primary tumour of the lung.
● The ectopic ACTH syndrome (see p. 728). Small-cell carcinoma of the lung, carcinoid tumours and medullary thyroid carcinomas are the commonest causes.
● Production of insulin-like activity, which may produce hypoglycaemia (see p. 768).

Table 16.51 Multiple endocrine neoplasia (MEN) syndromes.

Organ involved	Frequency of involvement	Commonest tumours and/or manifestations
Type 1		
Parathyroid	90%	Parathyroid adenomas/hyperplasia
Pituitary	70%	Prolactinoma, acromegaly
Pancreas	50%	Zollinger–Ellison syndrome, insulinoma
Adrenal	40%	Non-functional adenoma
Thyroid	20%	Multiple or single adenoma
Type 2 (sometimes split into 2A and 2B)		
Adrenal	Most	Phaeochromocytoma, 70% bilateral
Thyroid	Most	Medullary carcinoma (calcitonin production)
Parathyroid	60%	Parathyroid hyperplasia

Cushing's syndrome and diarrhoea (2A), neuromas and marfanoid facies (2B) may also occur.

Further reading

Beardwell C & Robertson GL (eds) (1981) *The Pituitary*. London: Butterworths.

Besser GM & Cudworth AG (eds) (1986) *A Colour Atlas of Endocrinology*. London: Gower Medical.

Clinics in Endocrinology and Metabolism—a series of reviews of specific topics published by WB Saunders, London.

DeGroot LJ, Reed Larsen P, Refetoff S & Stanbury JB (1984) *The Thyroid and its Disorders*, 5th edn. New York: Wiley.

Greenspan FS & Forsham PH (eds.) (1986). *Basic and Clinical Endocrinology*, 2nd edn. Los Altos: Lange Medical Publishers.

Hall R, Anderson, J, Smart GA & Besser GM (eds) (1987) *Fundamentals of Clinical Endocrinology*, 4th edn. London: Pitman Medical.

Martin CR (1985) *Endocrine Physiology*. Oxford: Oxford University Press.

Wilson JD & Foster DW (eds) (1985) *Williams' Textbook of Endocrinology*, 7th edn. Philadelphia: WB Saunders.

Diabetes and other Disorders of Metabolism

Diabetes mellitus

Introduction

Diabetes means excessive urination. Earlier generations of physicians, obliged to taste the urine, distinguished the honey flavour of diabetes mellitus from the tasteless urine of diabetes insipidus. Diabetes mellitus is a group of metabolic disorders characterized by chronic hyperglycaemia. The metabolic disturbance involves the metabolism of fat and protein as well as that of carbohydrates, reflecting a state of insulin deprivation. This in turn may be due to deficient insulin secretion, to factors opposing the tissue effects of insulin, or to both. Untreated diabetes results in characteristic clinical symptoms; these vary in intensity, and may culminate in the hyperglycaemic emergencies of diabetic ketoacidosis or non-ketotic hyperosmolar coma. Diabetes is usually irreversible, and while it allows the patient to have a reasonably normal lifestyle, its late complications result in a considerably reduced life expectancy. These complications include accelerated arterial disease and a characteristic microangiopathy. Macrovascular disease leads to an increased prevalence of coronary artery disease and peripheral vascular disease, while microvascular damage contributes to diabetic retinopathy and diabetic nephropathy.

Diabetes is common, affecting some 30 million people world-wide. Its causes are incompletely understood, but it is clear that the disease is often multifactorial and that both genetic and environmental factors are involved. Primary diabetes mellitus has two main forms: insulin-dependent (IDDM) and non-insulin-dependent (NIDDM), which are also referred to as type I and type II diabetes.

Insulin secretion

Insulin is the key hormone involved in the storage and controlled release within the body of the chemical energy available from food. It is synthesized in the beta cells of the pancreatic islets in the form of pro-insulin, which is stored in secretory granules close to the cell membrane. A biochemically inert peptide fragment known as connecting (C) peptide breaks off from pro-insulin (Fig. 17.1) in the secretory

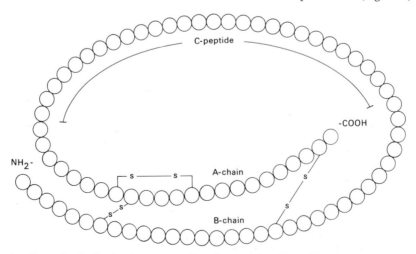

Fig. 17.1 The pro-insulin molecule. During the process of insulin secretion, C-peptide (connecting-peptide) breaks off and insulin is released as two peptide chains linked by disulphide bridges.

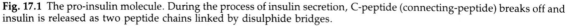

process, so that equimolar quantities of insulin and C-peptide are released into the circulation. Insulin enters the portal circulation, and is carried to the liver, its prime target organ. About 50% of secreted insulin is extracted and degraded in the liver; the residue is broken down by the kidney. C-peptide is only partially extracted by the liver (and hence provides a useful index of the rate of insulin secretion), but is mainly degraded by the kidney.

An outline of glucose metabolism
Blood glucose levels are closely regulated in health and rarely stray outside the range of 3.5–8.0 mmol·l^{-1}, despite the varying demands of food, fasting and exercise. The principal organ of glucose homeostasis is the liver, which absorbs and stores glucose (as glycogen) in the post-absorptive state and releases it into the circulation between meals to match the rate of glucose utilization by peripheral tissues.

Glucose production. About 200 g of glucose is produced and utilized each day. More than 90% is derived from the liver, three-quarters from glycogen and one-quarter from gluconeogenesis. The remaining 5–10% derives from renal gluconeogenesis.

Glucose utilization. The brain is the major consumer of glucose. Its requirement is 1 mg·kg^{-1} body weight per minute, or 100 g daily in a 70 kg man. Glucose uptake by the brain is obligatory and is not dependent on insulin, and the glucose used is oxidized to carbon dioxide and water.

Other tissues such as muscle and fat are facultative glucose consumers. The effect of insulin peaks associated with meals is to lower the threshold for glucose entry into cells; at other times energy requirements are largely met by fatty acid oxidation. Glucose taken up by muscle is stored as glycogen or broken down to lactate, which re-enters the circulation and becomes an important substrate for hepatic gluconeogenesis. Glucose is used by fat tissue as a source of energy and as a substrate for triglyceride synthesis; lipolysis releases fatty acids from triglyceride together with glycerol, another substrate for hepatic gluconeogenesis.

Hormonal regulation. Insulin is the major regulator of intermediary metabolism, although its actions are modified in important respects by other hormones. Dose–response curves for the production and utilization of glucose are shown in Fig. 17.2.

At low insulin levels, glucose production is maximal and utilization is minimal; at high levels the situation is reversed. At intermediate plasma insulin levels of 40–50 mU·l^{-1}, glucose production is largely suppressed but utilization remains low. This observation forms the theoretical basis for the low dose insulin regimen used to treat diabetic ketoacidosis (see below).

Fig. 17.2 The effect of different insulin levels upon glucose production and glucose utilization. Hepatic glucose production rises as insulin levels fall. Conversely, peripheral uptake of glucose is promoted at high insulin levels.

The effect of counter-regulatory hormones (glucagon, adrenaline, cortisol and growth hormone) is to shift the dose–response curves to the right, resulting in greater production of glucose and less utilization for a given level of insulin.

The opposing actions of insulin and two of its antagonists are summarized in Table 17.1.

Table 17.1 Opposing actions of insulin and two of its antagonists—glucagon and adrenaline.

Insulin	Action	Glucagon and adrenaline
	Glucose production:	
↓	Glycogenolysis	↑
↓	Gluconeogenesis	↑
	Glucose utilization by:	
↑	fat and muscle	↓
↓	Lipolysis	↑
↓	Ketogenesis	↑

TYPES OF DIABETES

Diabetes may be primary or secondary (see Table 17.2). Although both IDDM (type I diabetes) and NIDDM (type II diabetes) represent two distinct diseases from the epidemiological point of view, clinical distinction may sometimes be difficult. The two disease processes could, in clinical terms, be visualized as opposite ends of a continuous spectrum (Table 17.3).

Insulin-dependent diabetes mellitus (IDDM; type I diabetes)

EPIDEMIOLOGY

Approximately one person in 400 in the UK is treated with insulin, but some of these would be considered

Table 17.2 Causes of secondary diabetes.

Liver disease
Cirrhosis

Pancreatic disease
Chronic pancreatitis
Tropical diabetes
Pancreatectomy
Haemochromatosis

Endocrine disease
Cushing's syndrome
Acromegaly
Thyrotoxicosis
Phaeochromocytoma

Drug-induced disease
Thiazide diuretics
Steroid therapy

Insulin-receptor abnormalities
Congenital lipodystrophy
Acanthosis nigricans

Genetic syndromes, e.g.
Glycogen storage disease

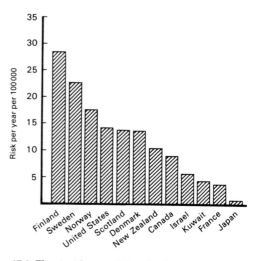

Fig. 17.3 The incidence of insulin-dependent diabetes mellitus (type I diabetes) in different countries.

to have NIDDM by the criteria shown in Table 17.3. IDDM is most common in populations of European extraction, and within Europe there is a marked increase in incidence as one moves north from the Mediterranean—the highest incidence occurs in northern Scandinavia. The frequency of IDDM in various countries is shown in Fig. 17.3.

The incidence in childhood is maximal at 11–12 years of age. Presentation is more common in the spring and autumn than in the summer, and it has been suggested that this might be related to the greater prevalence of viral infections at these times.

AETIOLOGY

Genetic susceptibility
IDDM is not genetically predestined, but an

Table 17.3 The spectrum of diabetes: a comparison of insulin-dependent diabetes mellitus (IDDM) and non-insulin-dependent diabetes mellitus (NIDDM).

	IDDM (type I)	NIDDM (type II)

Epidemiology:	Patients are:
	  Younger
	  Usually lean
	  European extraction
	    (Most commonly)
		Patients are:
		  Older
		  Often overweight
		  All racial groups
		    (Increasing incidence
		      in affluent immigrants)

	Seasonal incidence	
	? Viral aetiology	
Heredity:	HLA-DR3 or DR4 in 95%	No HLA links

	30–50% concordance in
	  identical twins
		90% concordance in
		  identical twins

Pathogenesis:	Autoimmunity Islet cell antibody Insulitis	No evidence
Clinical:	Insulin deficiency	Partial insulin deficiency, insulin resistance
	May develop ketoacidosis	May develop non-ketotic hyperosmolar state
	Always need insulin	Sometimes need insulin

DR3 ⟨ B8 — CW7 — A1
        B18 — CW5

DR4 ⟨ B15 — CW3 — A2
        B40 — CW3

Fig. 17.4 HLA axes of susceptibility for diabetes.

increased susceptibility to the disease may be inherited.

Identical twins. The identical twin of a patient with IDDM has a 30–50% chance of developing the disease. This implies that non-genetic factors must also be involved.

HLA system. Ninety five per cent of IDDM patients carry HLA-DR3, HLA-DR4 or both. Other reported HLA associations in the A and B regions are secondary to linkage disequilibrium (Fig. 17.4).

DR3 and DR4 are common antigens present in 50–60% of the UK population. The relative risk conferred by DR3 is estimated at 7, that of DR4 at 9, and that of both DR3 and DR4 at 14 times normal. Since this risk is additive, a model based on two susceptibility genes (one associated with DR3 and one with DR4) has been proposed.

In contrast, individuals with HLA-DR2 have a considerably reduced risk (0.12 times normal) of developing diabetes. The reasons for this protective effect are unclear.

The insulin gene. Associations between IDDM and other chromosomes (apart from chromosome 6) have been described. A polymorphous DNA region close to the insulin gene on chromosome 11 (Fig. 17.5) has been studied, and short, intermediate and long insertions (see p. 98) have been reported. Homozygosity of the short (class I) allele is found in some 80% of patients with IDDM as against 40% of controls.

Fig. 17.5 Map of the banding pattern of one chromatid of chromosome 11, showing the position of the insulin gene (INS). Apo AI/CIII=apolipoproteins; CAT=catalase; c-ras^H=c-Harvey *ras* oncogene; LDHA=lactate dehydrogenase; NAG=*N*-acetylglucosamine. From Galton DJ (1985) *Molecular Genetics of Common Metabolic Disease.* London: Edward Arnold. With permission.

Immunological aspects
Several pieces of evidence suggest that autoimmune processes are involved in the pathogenesis of IDDM.

Association with other autoimmune disease. Autoimmune thyroid disease, Addison's disease and pernicious anaemia are more common in patients and their relatives.

Immunogenetic associations. The association between DR3, DR4 and diabetes, and the protective effect of DR2 might represent idiosyncracies in the immune process which result in increased (or reduced) susceptibility.

The insulitis process. Autopsies of patients who died soon after diagnosis are characterized by infiltration of the pancreatic islets by mononuclear cells. A similar pattern occurs in other autoimmune diseases, e.g. thyroiditis.

Immune abnormalities at diagnosis. About 70% of newly presenting patients have islet cell antibodies. These react with human islets and can be detected by immunofluorescence. They usually become undetectable within a few years of diagnosis. In such patients increased numbers of activated T lymphocytes are also present in the circulation at diagnosis.

Environmental factors
A viral aetiology has been suspected for many years. This is based on the seasonal incidence of the condition, anecdotal associations, and analysis of viral antibody titres at diagnosis. IgM antibodies to coxsackie B4 have been reported in 20–30% of new cases. However, in view of the long prodromal period (see below), it seems likely that viruses precipitate rather than initiate the onset of diabetes.

The diabetes prodrome
Prospective study of first degree relatives of children with diabetes has revealed that islet cell antibodies may appear in the circulation months or even years before diagnosis. Insulin antibodies have also been reported in this period, and abnormalities of insulin secretion in response to intravenous glucose may develop.

The sequence of events leading to diagnosis may be as shown in Fig. 17.6. Better understanding of this sequence may in time permit strategies of prevention to be tested.

Non-insulin-dependent diabetes mellitus (NIDDM; type II diabetes)

EPIDEMIOLOGY

Unlike IDDM this is relatively common in all populations enjoying an affluent lifestyle. Large differences in prevalence have been reported. The disease may

Genetic predisposition

↓

Initiating event (? environmental)

↓

Immune activation

↓

Progressive beta cell loss

↓

Abnormalities of insulin secretion

↓

? Second trigger ? viral

↓

Clinical onset

↓

'Remission' (partial recovery of beta cell function)

↓

Loss of insulin secretion

Fig. 17.6 The possible sequence of events leading to the development of IDDM.

be present in a subclinical form for years before diagnosis, and the incidence increases markedly with age and degree of obesity. The onset may be accelerated by the stress of pregnancy, drug treatment or intercurrent illness. Estimates of prevalence using the WHO criteria would suggest an overall prevalence of around 2% in the UK; the rate is about five-fold higher in Asian immigrants.

The rates shown in Table 17.4 have been reported in various populations.

Epidemiological surveys have shown that indolent well-fed populations are 2–20 times as likely to develop NIDDM as lean populations of the same race.

AETIOLOGY

Genetics
Identical twins of a patient with NIDDM have an almost 100% chance of developing diabetes. Patients

Table 17.4 Frequency of non-insulin-dependent diabetes mellitus in various populations (WHO criteria).

Group	Age (years)	Rate (%)
USA	20–74	6.9
USA—Mexican immigrants	25–65	17.0
USA—Pima Indians	25+	25.5
Malta	15+	7.7
Indonesia	15+	1.7
New Guinea (highlands)	20+	0.0

are significantly more likely to have a first degree relative with NIDDM than control populations. Certain families exist in which diabetes appears to travel as an autosomal dominant characteristic, but study has been limited by the lack of a useful genetic marker for the condition.

Immunology
There is no evidence of immune involvement in its pathogenesis.

Insulin secretion and action
Patients with NIDDM, unlike those with IDDM, are seen to still have about 50% of their beta cell mass at autopsy.

Abnormalities of insulin secretion develop early in the course of the disease. Normal subjects have a biphasic insulin response to intravenous glucose. In NIDDM the first-phase insulin response to intravenous glucose is lost, and insulin secretion in response to oral glucose is delayed and exaggerated. The majority of patients manifest reduced insulin secretion relative to the prevailing glucose concentration, and progressive beta cell loss occurs in many patients, although not to the extent seen in IDDM. It is not known whether this is due to 'exhaustion' of surviving beta cells or to some independent process of damage.

Insulin resistance is also present. Obesity is present in 80% of such patients, but resistance may also be marked in lean patients. The nature and cause of this resistance remain uncertain.

Impaired glucose tolerance

If an oral glucose tolerance test is administered at random to a large population, 1–2% will be found to have unsuspected diabetes. A much larger group—5% or more (depending on the age, race and nutritional state of the population)—fall into an intermediate category now referred to as impaired glucose tolerance (IGT). The criteria for this category are given below. Follow-up of patients in this case shows that some (2–4% yearly) go on to develop diabetes, but that the abnormality does not progress in the majority. This group is certainly heterogeneous, e.g. some are obese, some have liver disease, and others are on medication that impairs glucose tolerance; individuals in this category are at increased risk of arterial disease but do not develop the specific microvascular complications of diabetes.

Tropical diabetes

A distinct variety of diabetes has recently been described. This is found only in Third World countries on or near the equator. The following features have been described:
● Onset is before the age of 30.
● There is a history of severe malnutrition.
● There is insulin dependence, sometimes with severe but fluctuating insulin resistance.

The oral glucose tolerance test

After an overnight fast, 75 g of glucose are taken in 250–350 ml of water. Blood samples are taken in the fasting state and 2 h after the glucose has been given.

A specific enzymatic glucose assay must be used. Plasma glucose levels are 10% higher than whole blood.

Diabetes
This is present when the fasting *blood* glucose is over 6.7 mmol·l^{-1} and/or when the 2-h value is over 10 mmol·l^{-1}. Corresponding values for *plasma* glucose are 7.8 mmol·l^{-1} and 11.1 mmol·l^{-1}.

Impaired glucose tolerance
This is present when the fasting blood glucose is below 6.7 mmol·l^{-1} and when the 2-h value is between 6.7 and 10 mmol·l^{-1}. Corresponding values for *plasma* glucose are 7.8 and 11.1 mmol·l^{-1}. Impaired glucose tolerance can only be diagnosed using the oral glucose tolerance test.

Intermediate sampling times (e.g. 30 min and 60 min) are not needed for the diagnosis of diabetes by WHO criteria. However, simultaneous blood and urine glucose measurements can be used to define a low renal threshold for glucose.

Diabetes can usually be diagnosed on the basis of fasting or random blood glucose measurements (see text). *The glucose tolerance test should be reserved for borderline cases only.*

- Ketoacidosis does not develop when insulin is withdrawn.

There are two main variants:
- *Fibrocalculous pancreatic diabetes*. This is associated with exocrine pancreatic deficiency, pancreatic fibrosis (often leading to calcification) and the presence of stones in the pancreatic duct. There may be a history of recurrent abdominal pain, and in 75% of cases there is evidence of pancreatic calcification on plain abdominal x-ray. Most populations in which this condition arises are subject to malnutrition and have a diet based on cassava. Cyanates are present in the cassava root and may be a factor in the pancreatic damage.
- *Protein-deficient pancreatic diabetes*. This form appears to be a direct consequence of malnutrition. The main differences from the fibrocalculous variant are that exocrine pancreatic function is unimpaired and there is no evidence of pancreatic fibrosis or calcification. Abdominal pain is not a feature.

In both forms of tropical diabetes insulin secretion is preserved, although impaired; this is the likely explanation for the observed resistance to ketosis.

CLINICAL PRESENTATION OF DIABETES

Acute presentation
Young people often present with a brief, 2- to 4-week history and report the classic triad of symptoms:
- *Polyuria*, due to the osmotic diuresis that results when blood glucose levels exceed the renal threshold
- *Thirst*, due to the resulting loss of fluid and electrolytes
- *Weight loss*, due to fluid depletion and the accelerated breakdown of fat and muscle secondary to insulin deficiency

Ketoacidosis may be the presenting feature if these early symptoms are not recognized and treated.

Subacute presentation
The clinical onset may be over several months, particularly in older patients. Thirst, polyuria and weight loss are usual features, but medical attention is sought for such symptoms as lack of energy, visual blurring due to refractive errors, or pruritus vulvae or balanitis due to *Candida* infection.

Complications
Complications may be the presenting feature. These include:
- Staphylococcal skin infections
- Retinopathy noted during a visit to the optician
- Peripheral neuropathy causing paraesthesia in the feet
- Impotence
- Arterial disease, resulting in myocardial infarction or peripheral gangrene

Asymptomatic diabetes
Glycosuria or a raised blood glucose may be detected on routine examination (e.g. for insurance purposes) in individuals who deny any symptoms of ill health.

Physical examination

This is often unrewarding, but evidence of weight loss and dehydration may be present, and the breath may smell of ketones. Older patients may present with established complications, and the presence of the characteristic retinopathy is diagnostic of diabetes.

INVESTIGATION OF DIABETES

The diagnosis is usually simple. Blood glucose levels are so closely controlled by the body that even small deviations become important:
- In *symptomatic* patients, a single elevated blood glucose, measured by a reliable method, indicates diabetes.

- In *asymptomatic* or *mildly symptomatic* patients, the diagnosis is made on:
  - (a) One, preferably two, fasting venous *blood* glucose levels above 6.7 mmol·l^{-1} (120 mg·dl^{-1}); the equivalent venous *plasma* level is 7.8 mmol·l^{-1} (140 mg·dl^{-1})
  - (b) One, preferably two, random values above 10 mmol·l^{-1} (180 mg·dl^{-1}) in venous whole blood or 11.1 mmol·l^{-1} (200 mg·dl^{-1}) in venous plasma
- A glucose tolerance test (GTT) is *unnecessary* when the criteria above are satisfied, and should be reserved for true borderline cases.
- Glycosuria is measured using sensitive glucose-specific dip-stick methods. Glycosuria is not diagnostic of diabetes but indicates the need for further investigation. About 1% of the population have renal glycosuria. This is an inherited low renal threshold for glucose, transmitted either as a mendelian dominant or recessive trait.

Other investigations

No further tests are needed to diagnose diabetes. Other routine investigations include screening the urine for proteinuria, a full blood count, urea and electrolytes, and a fasting blood sample for cholesterol and triglycerides. The latter test is useful to exclude an associated hyperlipidaemia but should only be performed after blood glucose levels have been brought under control.

It is important to remember that diabetes may be *secondary* to other conditions (see Table 17.2), may be *precipitated* by underlying illness, and be *associated* with autoimmune disease or hyperlipidaemia.

TREATMENT OF DIABETES

Guidelines to therapy

All patients with diabetes require diet therapy. Good glycaemic control is unlikely to be achieved with insulin or oral therapy when diet is neglected, especially when the patient is also overweight.

Insulin is always indicated in a patient who has been in ketoacidosis, and is usually indicated in patients who present under the age of 40. Insulin is also indicated in older patients following primary or secondary failure of oral therapy (see below). Tablets should be avoided in younger patients and are contraindicated in pregnancy.

In older patients the approach to therapy is empirical. Diet alone should be tried in the first instance, and dietary knowledge and compliance should always be reassessed with care before proceeding to the next step. This is of particular importance in the obese patient who fails to lose weight.

When diet fails to achieve satisfactory control, thin patients are usually treated with a sulphonylurea drug, and obese patients with a biguanide. Primary failure of treatment occurs when these agents (alone or in combination) never achieve the desired level of control. Other patients may show a good initial response followed by progressive loss of control over the succeeding months or years; this is referred to as secondary failure of treatment.

Since this approach is largely empirical, it is not surprising that practice differs from one country to another. For example metformin (the only biguanide in common use) is very widely employed in France, tends to be used less in the UK, and is not licensed in the USA. Criteria of control also vary, so that what is classed as primary failure at one centre may be seen as a success in another. The most widespread error in management is procrastination; the patient whose control is inadequate on tablets should start insulin without undue delay.

Diet

The diet for a diabetic patient is no different from the diet considered healthy for the population as a whole.

Carbohydrate

This should consist of unrefined carbohydrate rather than simple sugars such as sucrose. Carbohydrate is absorbed relatively slowly from fibre-rich foods, preventing the rapid swings in circulating glucose seen when refined sugars are ingested. For example, the glucose peak seen after eating an apple is much flatter than that seen after drinking the same amount of carbohydrate as apple juice.

The total amount of carbohydrate in the diet should provide 50–55% of the total calories.

Fat

The traditional diabetic diet was low in carbohydrates and therefore high in fat (Table 17.5). Not only was this high fat content inappropriate for patients already predisposed to arterial disease, but glucose tolerance actually deteriorates rather than improves on a low carbohydrate diet.

Table 17.5 Comparison of the composition of the traditional and modern diabetic diet.

	Percentage of calories	
	Traditional diet	Modern diet
Protein	12	15
Fat	66	35
Carbohydrate	22	50

Calories

These should be tailored to the needs of the patient:
- The overweight diabetic patient is started on a

reducing diet of approximately 1000–1600 kcal per day (4000–6000 kJ).

- The lean patient is put on an isocaloric diet.
- Patients who are underweight because of untreated diabetes require energy supplementation.

Prescribing a diet

Most people find it extremely difficult to modify their eating habits, and repeated advice and encouragement is needed if this is to be achieved. A diet history is taken, and the diet prescribed should involve the least possible interference with the lifestyle of the patient. It is important to stress that patients on insulin or oral agents should eat the same amount at the same time each day. Patients on insulin require snacks between meals and at bedtime to buffer the effect of injected insulin. Alcohol is not forbidden but its calorific content should be taken into account. Patients on insulin should be warned to avoid alcoholic binges since these may precipitate severe hypoglycaemia.

The role of patient education

The care of diabetes is based on self-management by the patient, who is helped and advised by those with specialized knowledge. The quest for improved glycaemic control has made it clear that whatever the technical expertise applied, the outcome depends on willing cooperation by the patient. This in turn depends on an understanding of the risks of diabetes and the potential benefits of glycaemic control and other measures such as maintaining a lean weight, stopping smoking and taking care of the feet.

If accurate information is not supplied, misinformation from friends and other patients will take its place. For this reason many patients have exaggerated fears of, for example, blindness (about 1 patient in 10 is blind after 30 years of diabetes), death during hypoglycaemia (extremely rare), or the risk of passing diabetes on to their children (2–5% of offspring develop IDDM).

Organized training programmes involving nurse specialists, dietitians and chiropodists as well as physicians are now a recognized part of good modern diabetes care.

Tablet treatment (see Table 17.6)

Sulphonylureas

These have two main actions:

- They increase basal and stimulated insulin secretion.
- They reduce peripheral resistance to insulin action.

The effects upon insulin secretion are most marked in the early stages of treatment, but the peripheral effects are more important for maintenance therapy. The sulphonylureas should be avoided in young ketotic patients, who require early insulin therapy, and are contraindicated in pregnancy. Insulin should be substituted during major surgery or severe intercurrent illness.

These drugs have similar actions and potency. All should be used with care in patients with liver disease, and only tolbutamide or glibornuride should be given to patients with renal impairment. Tolbutamide is the safest drug in the very elderly because of its short duration of action. Chlorpropamide is still widely used but has the disadvantages of a long duration of action and a wider range of side-effects.

Drug interactions (see p. 658). All sulphonylureas bind to circulating albumin and may be displaced by other drugs such as sulphonamides which compete for their binding sites. Their clinical effect may be reduced by thiazide diuretics or steroid therapy.

Side-effects. Hypoglycaemia is the most common side-effect and may be severe and prolonged. Skin rashes and other sensitivity reactions may occur.

Chlorpropamide use is often associated with a facial flush when alcohol is taken. It may also cause a cholestatic jaundice and (at high doses) a dilutional hyponatraemia.

Table 17.6 Drugs used in non-insulin-dependent diabetes mellitus.

	Duration of action	Excretion	Dose per 24 h
Sulphonylureas			
Tolbutamide	6–8 h	Hepatic	1–2 g
Chlorpropamide	36–48 h	Hepatic and renal	100–500 mg
Glibenclamide	12–20 h	Hepatic and renal	2.5–20 mg
Glibornuride	16 h	Hepatic	12.5–75 mg
Gliclazide	10–12 h	Hepatic and renal	40–320 mg
Biguanides			
Metformin	12–20 h	Unchanged in urine	1–2 g in 2–3 doses

Biguanides

Metformin acts by reducing glucose absorption from the gut and by increasing insulin sensitivity. Unlike the sulphonylureas it does not induce hypoglycaemia in normal volunteers. It is usually reserved for patients in middle or old age, particularly for the overweight. It may be given in combination with sulphonylureas when a single agent has proved to be ineffective.

Its side-effects include anorexia, epigastric discomfort and diarrhoea. Lactic acidosis has occurred in patients with severe hepatic or renal disease, and metformin is contraindicated when these are present.

Insulin treatment

Injections

Most people have a fear of injecting themselves, and insulin therapy should begin with a lesson in injection technique. A disposable 10–16 mm needle (depending on adiposity) should be used to its full depth at 90° to the skin. The thighs and abdomen are the most convenient areas, and the injection site used should be changed regularly to prevent areas of lipohypertrophy. The rate of insulin absorption depends on local subcutaneous blood flow, and is accelerated by exercise, local massage or a warm environment. Absorption is more rapid from the arm than from the abdomen, and is slowest from the thigh. All these factors can influence the shape of the insulin profile.

All patients need careful training for a life with insulin, but routine hospital admission is unnecessary where facilities for community support exist.

Choice of insulin

Species. Insulin is found in every creature with a backbone, and the central part of the molecule is constant. (For example, fish insulin produces hypoglycaemia in man.) Differences in the amino acid sequence alter the antigenicity of the molecule. Beef insulin has three amino acids that are different from human insulin, and pork insulin has only one; the latter is therefore less antigenic.

Human insulin is produced by:

- Chemical substitution of an amino acid in position 30 of the beta-chain of pork insulin
- DNA coding of *Escherichia coli* to produce alpha- and beta-chains, combining the chains in vitro (bio-engineering)

All forms of injected insulin, even human, may result in antibody formation, but insulin antibodies usually have little clinical importance. Human insulin is likely to replace the other varieties in the course of time.

Purity. Earlier preparations of insulin contained glucagon and other impurities. Modern insulins are now of high purity, having only a single sharp peak on electrophoresis.

Formulation (see Table 17.7). There are two main types of insulin:
- Insulin prepared in a clear solution (soluble or crystalline). These insulins are short-acting and are the only insulins to be used in emergencies such as ketoacidosis or for surgical operations.
- Insulins pre-mixed with retarding agents (either protamine or zinc) which precipitate crystals of varying size according to the conditions employed. These insulins are intermediate or long-acting.

All insulins are available in solutions containing 40, 80 and 100 units per millilitre, but in the UK the standard insulin available is 100 units per millilitre.

Clinical use

In normal subjects a sharp rise in insulin occurs after meals; this is superimposed on a constant background of insulin secretion (Fig. 17.7). Insulin therapy attempts to reproduce this pattern. In order to achieve this, an intermediate-acting insulin is given to control the afternoon and night blood sugar level, and short-acting insulins are given morning and evening to match mealtimes (Fig. 17.8a).

Ideal control is often hard to achieve for the following reasons:
- The insulin is given into the systemic circulation rather than the portal circulation.

Table 17.7 Some insulin preparations.

| | Action | Source | | |
		Beef	Pork	Human
Soluble	Short	Neusulin Velosulin	Actrapid Humulin S	Human Actrapid
Isophane (protamine)	Intermediate	Neuphane	Protaphane Insulatard	Humulin I
Lente (zinc)	Long	Neulente Ultratard	Monotard MC	Human Monotard Human Ultratard Humulin Zn

Fig. 17.7 Non-diabetic glucose and insulin profiles.

- Subcutaneous soluble insulin takes 60–90 min to achieve peak plasma levels—the onset and off-set of action are too slow.
- The absorption of subcutaneous insulin into the circulation is variable; the longer-acting the preparation, the more erratic the absorption.
- Basal insulin levels are constant in the normal state, but injected insulin invariably peaks and declines, with resulting swings in metabolic control.

Individuals vary and therapy must be tailored accordingly. One approach to therapy is outlined here:

- Young patients are started on two injections daily of an intermediate insulin. Some recovery of endogenous insulin secretion may occur over the first few months ('the honeymoon period') and the insulin dose may need to be reduced. Requirements rise thereafter and soluble insulin is added to the regimen. As a rule of thumb, two-thirds of the daily dose is given in the morning, and two-thirds of each injection is given as intermediate insulin.
- Older patients may sometimes manage adequately on a single daily injection.

If glycaemic control is inadequate with the standard approach, the alternatives are multiple insulin injections or continuous subcutaneous insulin infusion (CSII). Both methods require a planned approach to life, with special attention to diet and exercise and frequent blood glucose testing.

Multiple injections. The introduction of 'pen injection' devices has made this approach more acceptable to patients. Three variants are shown diagramatically in Fig. 17.8b–d.

Infusion devices. CSII is delivered by a small pump strapped around the waist which infuses a constant trickle of insulin under the skin. Mealtime doses are

delivered when the patient touches a button on the side of the pump.

This approach has the advantage of smoothing blood glucose levels to prevent swings to hyper- and hypoglycaemia, and is particularly useful in the overnight period. It also has the advantage of flexibility concerning mealtimes, which is of great value to patients in busy jobs who cannot always live by the clock. Disadvantages include the nuisance of being attached to a gadget, skin infections, and the risk of ketoacidosis if the flow of insulin is broken (since these patients have no protective reservoir of depot insulin). Infusion pumps should only be used by specialized centres able to offer a round-the-clock service to their patients.

Social implications
Patients starting on insulin need to inform the driving licence authorities and their insurance companies. They are also wise to inform their employers. Certain types of work are unsuitable for insulin-treated patients, including driving a heavy goods vehicle, working at heights, or working close to dangerous machinery in motion. Certain professions such as the police and the armed forces are barred to all diabetic patients, but there are few other limitations, although a considerable amount of ill-informed prejudice still exists.

Complications
At the injection site. Shallow injections result in intradermal insulin delivery and scarring. Injection site abscesses occur but are rare.

Local allergic responses sometimes occur early in therapy but usually resolve spontaneously. Generalized allergic responses are exceptionally rare.

Lipodystrophies which may occur include lipoatrophy, a local allergic response now virtually abolished by the use of highly purified insulins, and lipohypertrophy, occurring as a result of over-use of a single injection site with any type of insulin.

Insulin resistance. The most common cause of mild insulin resistance is obesity. Occasional unstable patients require massive insulin doses, often with a fluctuating requirement. Subcutaneous degradation of injected insulin is one of several postulated causes. Insulin resistance associated with antibodies directed against the insulin receptor has been reported in patients with acanthosis nigricans.

Weight gain. Patients with NIDDM who are non-compliant with their diet and predisposed to weight gain may show progressive weight gain on treatment, especially if the insulin dose is increased inappropriately.

Hypoglycaemia. This is the most common complication of insulin therapy and is a major cause of anxiety

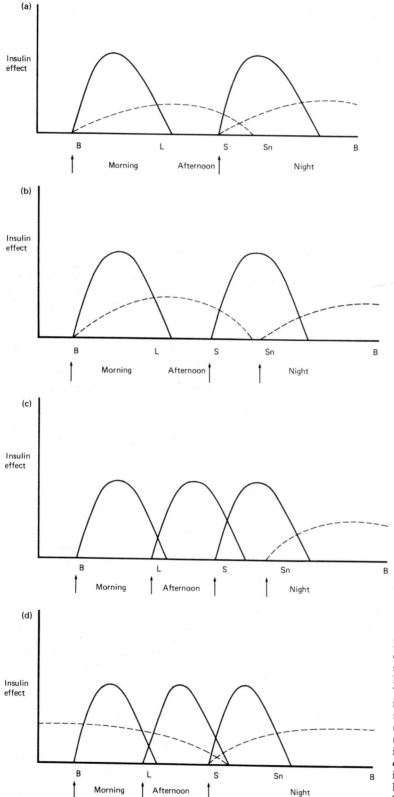

Fig. 17.8 Insulin regimens. Profiles of soluble insulin are shown as solid lines and intermediate or long-acting insulin as broken lines. The arrows indicate when the injections are given. (a) Twice daily soluble and intermediate. (b) Splitting the evening injection. (c) Thrice daily soluble with intermediate overnight. (d) Thrice daily soluble with long-acting insulin given before supper. B=breakfast; L=lunch; S=supper; Sn=snack (bedtime).

for patients and relatives. Symptoms typically develop over a few minutes, and most patients experience adrenergic features of sweating, tremor and a pounding heart beat. Physical signs include pallor and a cold sweat. A minority of long-standing patients report loss of these warning symptoms and may in consequence drift into severe hypoglycaemia. Such patients appear pale, drowsy or detached, signs which their relatives quickly learn to recognize. Behaviour is clumsy or inappropriate, and some become irritable or even aggressive. Others slip rapidly into hypoglycaemic coma.

Occasionally, patients develop convulsions during hypoglycaemic coma, especially at night. It is important not to confuse this with idiopathic epilepsy, especially since patients with frequent hypoglycaemia often have abnormalities on the EEG. Another presentation is with hemiparesis or hemiplegia, which resolves within a few minutes when glucose is administered.

Hypoglycaemia is a common problem. Virtually all patients experience intermittent symptoms, and one in three is likely to go into coma at some stage of therapy. A minority suffer attacks that are so frequent and severe as to be virtually disabling.

Hypoglycaemia results from an imbalance between injected insulin and a patient's normal diet, activity and basal insulin requirement. The times of greatest risk are before meals and during the night. Irregular eating habits, unusual exertion and alcohol excess may precipitate episodes; others appear to be due simply to variation in insulin absorption.

A further problem is that diabetic patients have an impaired ability to counter-regulate glucose levels after hypoglycaemia. The glucagon response is invariably deficient, even though the alpha cells are preserved and respond normally to other stimuli. The adrenaline response may also fail in patients with a long duration of diabetes.

Nocturnal hypoglycaemia is commonly caused by attempts to compensate for the slight increase in insulin requirements from 4 a.m. (the 'dawn phenomenon') (Fig. 17.9). Attempts to improve fasting blood glucose levels by raising the insulin dose can cause hypoglycaemia earlier in the night. It was widely believed that this hypoglycaemia caused a rebound hyperglycaemia (the 'Somogyi effect') due to an unbalanced counter-regulatory response, but in practice fasting hyperglycaemia is usually due to insulin deficiency.

The diagnosis of hypoglycaemia is simple and can usually be made on clinical grounds. Patients should carry a card or wear a bracelet or necklace identifying themselves as diabetic, and these should be looked for in unconscious patients. If real doubt exists, it will do no harm to administer glucose whilst a laboratory blood glucose result is awaited.

Any form of rapidly assimilated carbohydrate will relieve the early symptoms, and patients should always carry sugar or sweets. Drowsy patients will

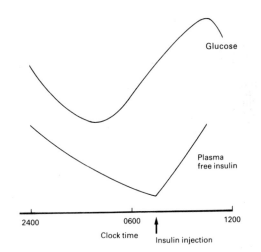

Fig. 17.9 Injected insulin 'fades' overnight, whereas insulin requirements increase after about 4 a.m. (the 'dawn phenomenon'). As a result, nadir glucose values occur around 3 a.m. and the risk of hypoglycaemia is greatest at this time. Conversely, glucose levels rise sharply before breakfast and peak 1–2 h after this meal.

often be able to take carbohydrate in liquid form, e.g. Lucozade. Unconscious patients should be given intravenous glucose (50 ml of 50% dextrose solution) or intramuscular glucagon (1 mg). Glucagon acts by mobilizing hepatic glycogen, and works almost as rapidly as glucose. It is simple to administer and can be given at home by relatives. Glucose reserves should be replenished with oral glucose once the patient revives.

Measuring control

The 'artificial pancreas' is a system of blood glucose control that works by continuous blood glucose analysis. This is fed into a computer which delivers an appropriate amount of insulin into the circulation. Patients on insulin need to devise their own simplified form of this feedback loop.

Urine tests
Urine tests are simple to perform, and it can usually be assumed that a patient with consistently negative tests and no symptoms of hypoglycaemia is well controlled. Even so, the correlation between urine tests and simultaneous blood glucose is poor. This is because:

- Changes in urine glucose lag behind changes in blood glucose.
- The mean renal threshold is around 10 mmol·l^{-1} but the range is wide (7–13 mmol·l^{-1}). The threshold also rises with age.
- Urine tests can give no guidance concerning blood glucose levels below the renal threshold.

Dip-stick tests based on specific enzymatic reactions

for glucose have now superseded the older tablet method for testing the urine.

Urinary ketones may also be measured by a dip-stick test. This is rarely helpful in routine outpatient management, but can be useful in special situations such as intercurrent infections. Heavy ketonuria can inhibit some dip-stick tests for glucose, and a combined stick (measuring both glucose and ketones) may be of value.

Blood glucose levels

Blood glucose levels provide the best assessment of day-to-day control. A fasting glucose level is a useful guide to therapy in NIDDM since it correlates well with other measures of control, but this is not the case in IDDM.

A random blood glucose test (e.g. in the clinic) is of limited value, but patients may easily be taught to provide their own profiles by testing fingerprick blood samples with reagent strips and reading these with the aid of a visual scale or reflectance meter. It has been amply demonstrated that most patients are willing and able to provide reasonably accurate results provided they have been properly taught how to do so.

Blood is taken from the side of a finger pulp (*not* from the tip, which is densely innervated) using a special lancet such as a Monolet, which can be fitted to a spring-loaded device. The standard flat steel lancets provided in many hospitals are unsuitable for this technique. Patients are asked to take regular profiles (e.g. four daily samples on 2 days each week) and to note these in a diary or record book. They are encouraged to adjust their insulin dose as appropriate and should ideally be able to obtain advice over the telephone when needed.

Glycosylated haemoglobin (HbA$_{1c}$)

Glycosylation of haemoglobin occurs as a two-step reaction resulting in the formation of a covalent bond between the glucose molecule and the terminal valine of the beta chain of the haemoglobin molecule. The rate at which this reaction occurs is related to the prevailing glucose concentration. Glycosylated haemoglobin can be distinguished by techniques such as electrophoresis, and is expressed as a percentage of the normal haemoglobin. The usefulness of this test is that it condenses all the changes in blood glucose levels over several weeks into a single value which is related to the mean blood glucose over the same period. The figure will, however, be misleading if the lifespan of the red cell is reduced. HbA$_{1c}$ provides a rapid assessment of the level of glycaemic control in a given patient, but blood glucose testing is needed before the clinician can know what to do about it.

Does good glycaemic control matter?

The answer to this question involves a number of separate issues.

1 Is poor control associated with an increased risk of diabetic complications?

Retrospective studies have repeatedly shown that those with the worst control have the highest rate of complications.

2 Is this increased risk reversible?

There are many difficulties in answering this question:
● The gestation of diabetic complications is lengthy, often 10–20 years.
● Control was difficult to quantify before HbA$_{1c}$ tests were introduced.
● Good control is difficult to achieve, so comparisons have usually been between 'poor and worse' control rather than between 'good and bad'.
● Some patients are easier to bring into good control than others, so the groups selected as 'well' or 'poorly' controlled in previous studies were not strictly comparable.

Prospective randomized studies are therefore needed. Studies in experimental animals strongly suggest that improved control is protective. Studies in man are now under way but face considerable technical problems.

3 Can established complications be halted or reversed by intensive insulin therapy?

Insulin infusion devices have made near-normal blood glucose control possible for closely supervised groups of patients. Studies in patients with established retinopathy or nephropathy have shown that early retinopathy benefits from 2–3 years of intensive therapy, but that patients with more advanced retinal changes or proteinuria do not. Retinopathy may show a transient deterioration in the most strictly controlled group. These observations suggest that microvascular lesions may be self-perpetuating once a threshold level of damage has been reached.

4 Is large vessel disease influenced by control?

Patients with impaired glucose tolerance have an increased rate of large vessel disease but rarely develop microvascular lesions. This might be because large arteries are more sensitive to elevated glucose levels, but it has also been suggested that hyperinsulinaemia (present in many patients with NIDDM and a common consequence of insulin treatment) is a cause of accelerated atherogenesis. At present there is little evidence that good glycaemic control protects against arterial disease.

DIABETIC METABOLIC EMERGENCIES

The main terms used are defined in Table 17.8.

Table 17.8 Terms used in diabetes.

Ketonuria	Detectable ketone levels in the urine; it should be appreciated that ketonuria occurs in fasting non-diabetics and may be found in relatively well-controlled patients with IDDM
Ketosis	Elevated plasma ketone levels in the absence of acidosis
Diabetic ketoacidosis	A metabolic emergency in which hyperglycaemia is associated with a metabolic acidosis due to greatly raised (>5 mmol·l^{-1}) ketone levels
Non-ketotic hyperosmolar coma	A metabolic emergency in which uncontrolled hyperglycaemia induces a hyperosmolar state in the absence of significant ketosis
Lactic acidosis	A metabolic emergency in which elevated lactate levels induce a metabolic acidosis; in diabetic patients this is rare and associated with biguanide therapy

Diabetic ketoacidosis

CAUSES

Diabetic ketoacidosis is the hallmark of IDDM. Its main causes can be grouped as follows:
- Previously undiagnosed diabetes
- Interruption of insulin therapy
- The stress of intercurrent illness

It is important to note that the majority of cases reaching hospital could have been *prevented* by earlier diagnosis, better communication between patient and doctor, and better patient education.

The most common error of management is for a patient to reduce or omit insulin because he feels unable to eat due to nausea or vomiting. This is a factor in at least 25% of all hospital admissions. Insulin should never be stopped.

PATHOGENESIS

Ketoacidosis is a state of uncontrolled catabolism associated with insulin deficiency. Insulin deficiency is a necessary precondition since only a modest elevation in insulin levels is sufficient to inhibit hepatic ketogenesis. Even so, stable patients do not readily develop ketoacidosis when insulin is withdrawn. Other factors include counter-regulatory hormone excess and fluid depletion. The combination of insulin deficiency with excess of its hormonal antagonists leads to the parallel processes shown in Fig. 17.10.

In the absence of insulin, hepatic glucose production accelerates and peripheral uptake by tissues such as muscle is reduced. Rising glucose levels lead to an osmotic diuresis, loss of fluid and electrolytes, and dehydration. Plasma osmolality rises and renal perfusion falls.

In parallel, rapid lipolysis occurs, leading to elevated circulating free fatty acid levels. The free fatty acids are broken down to fatty acyl-CoA within the liver cells, and this in turn is converted to acetoacetate (ketone bodies) within the mitochondria (Fig. 17.11).

Accumulation of ketone bodies produces a

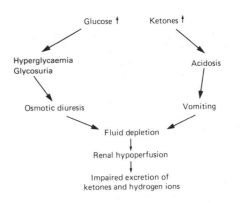

Fig. 17.10 Dehydration occurs during ketoacidosis as a consequence of two parallel processes. Hyperglycaemia results in osmotic diuresis, and hyperketonaemia results in acidosis and vomiting. Renal hypoperfusion then occurs and a vicious circle is established as the kidney becomes less able to compensate for the acidosis.

metabolic acidosis. This is typically associated with nausea and vomiting, leading to further loss of fluid and electrolytes. The excess ketones are excreted in the urine but also appear in the breath, producing a distinctive smell similar to that of acetone. Respiratory compensation for the acidosis leads to hyperventilation, graphically described as 'air hunger'. Progressive dehydration impairs renal excretion of hydrogen ions and ketones, aggravating the acidosis. As the pH falls below 7.0 ($[H^+] > 100$ nmol·l^{-1}), pH-dependent enzyme systems in many cells function less effectively. Untreated, severe ketoacidosis is invariably fatal.

CLINICAL FEATURES

The features of ketoacidosis are those of uncontrolled diabetes with acidosis, and include prostration, hyperventilation (Kussmaul respiration), nausea, vomiting and, occasionally, abdominal pain. The latter is sometimes so severe as to cause confusion with a surgical acute abdomen.

Some patients are mentally alert at presentation, but confusion and stupor are common. About 5%

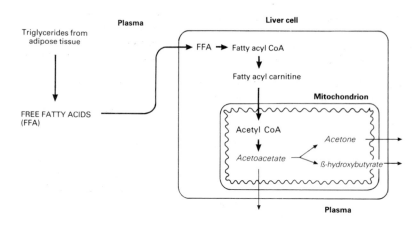

Fig. 17.11 Ketogenesis. During insulin deficiency lipolysis accelerates and FFA taken up by liver cells form the substrate for ketone formation (acetoacetate, acetone and β-hydroxybutyrate) within the mitochondrion.

present in coma. Evidence of marked dehydration is present and the eyeball is lax to pressure in severe cases. Hyperventilation is present but becomes less marked in very severe acidosis due to respiratory depression. The smell of ketones on the breath allows an instant diagnosis to be made by those able to detect the odour. The skin is dry and the body temperature is often subnormal, even in the presence of infection; in such cases, pyrexia manifests in the course of treatment.

DIAGNOSIS

This is confirmed by demonstrating hyperglycaemia with ketonaemia or heavy ketonuria, and acidosis. No time should be lost and treatment is started as soon as the first blood sample has been taken.

Hyperglycaemia is demonstrated by Stix testing, while a blood sample is sent to the laboratory for confirmation. Ketonaemia is confirmed by centrifuging a blood sample and testing the plasma with Ketostix or Acetest tablets. An arterial blood sample is taken for blood gas analysis.

Further investigations are detailed below.

MANAGEMENT

The principles of management are as follows:
- *Replace the fluid losses.*
- *Replace the electrolyte losses.* Potassium levels need to be monitored with great care to avoid the cardiac complications of hypo- or hyperkalaemia.
- *Restore the acid–base balance.* A patient with healthy kidneys will rapidly compensate for the metabolic acidosis once the circulating volume is restored. Bicarbonate is seldom necessary, although it is usual for this to be given at a pH below 7.0 ([H$^+$] > 100 nmol·l^{-1}).
- *Replace the deficient insulin.* Traditionally therapy was given as a bolus with half the dose injected into a vein and half into muscle. Modern treatment is with a low dose regimen, given as an intravenous infusion or as hourly intramuscular injections. The subcutaneous route is avoided because subcutaneous blood flow is reduced in shocked patients. The low dose regimen lowers blood glucose by suppressing hepatic glucose production, whereas the high dose regimen also promotes rapid entry of glucose and potassium into muscle cells. As might be expected, the high dose regimen can lead to severe hypoglycaemia or hypokalaemia, complications largely avoided by the low dose approach.
- *Replace the energy losses.* Dextrose can be given with insulin cover once blood glucose levels are brought under control.
- *Seek the underlying cause.* Physical examination may reveal a source of infection, e.g. a perianal abscess. Two common markers of infection are misleading: fever is unusual even when infection is present and polymorpholeucocytosis is present even in the absence of infection. Relevant investigations include a chest x-ray, urine and blood cultures, and an ECG (to exclude myocardial infarction). If infection is suspected, broad-spectrum antibiotics are started once the appropriate cultures have been taken.

Problems of management
- *Hypotension.* This may lead to renal shutdown. Plasma expanders (or whole blood) are therefore given if the systolic blood pressure is below 80 mmHg. A central venous pressure line is useful in this situation. A bladder catheter is inserted if no urine is produced within 4 h, but routine catheterization is unnecessary.
- *Coma.* The usual principles apply (see p. 789). It is essential to pass a nasogastric tube to prevent the rare but often fatal complication of acute gastric dilatation.
- *Cerebral oedema.* This rare but feared complication has mostly been reported in children or young adults. The mortality is high.
- *Hypothermia.* Severe hypothermia with a core temperature below 33°C may occur and may be

overlooked unless a rectal temperature is taken with a low-reading thermometer.

- *Late complications.* These include stasis pneumonia and deep vein thrombosis, and occur especially in the comatose or elderly patient.
- *Complications of therapy.* These include hypoglycaemia and hypokalaemia. Over-enthusiastic fluid replacement may precipitate pulmonary oedema in older patients. Hyperchloraemic acidosis, usually mild, may develop in the course of fluid therapy. The nature of a persistent acidosis may be overlooked if the plasma chloride level has not been estimated.

Subsequent management
Intravenous fluids are stopped once the metabolic condition is under control and the patient is able to take the necessary fluids by mouth. Insulin is given as three or four soluble subcutaneous doses per day until a maintenance regimen can be restarted. Sliding scale regimens are often unnecessary and may even delay the establishment of stable blood glucose levels.

The treatment of diabetic ketoacidosis is incomplete without a careful enquiry into the causes of the episode and advice as to how to avoid its recurrence.

Non-ketotic hyperosmolar coma

This condition, in which severe hyperglycaemia develops without significant ketosis, is the metabolic emergency characteristic of uncontrolled NIDDM. Patients present in middle or later life, often with previously undiagnosed diabetes. Common precipitating factors include consumption of glucose-rich fluids (e.g. Lucozade), concurrent medication

---

Guidelines for the diagnosis and management of diabetic ketoacidosis

Diagnosis
Hyperglycaemia—measure blood glucose
Ketonaemia—test plasma with Ketostix/Acetest
Acidosis—measure blood gases

Investigations
Blood glucose
Urea and electrolytes
Osmolality
Full blood count
Blood gases
Blood and urine culture
Chest x-ray
ECG

Management
Insulin: i.v. 6 units stat, then 6 units hourly by infusion
OR
i.m. 20 units stat, then 6 units hourly by i.m. injection

Fluid replacement: Normal saline (0.9%—150 mmol each of Na^+ and Cl^- per litre) 4 l in 4 h, then 1 l 4-hourly
Add KCl 20 mmol to each litre

IF:
- Blood pressure below 80 systolic, give 2 units whole blood or plasma
- pH below 7.0 ([H^+] >100 $nmol \cdot l^{-1}$), give sodium bicarbonate 1·4% (167 mmol each of Na^+ and HCO_3^- per litre) 500 ml over 1 h. Add KCl 20 mmol; rate should not exceed 20 $mmol \cdot l^{-1}$ over 1 h.
- Plasma Na^+ over 150 $mmol \cdot l^{-1}$, give 1 l of $\frac{1}{2}$ normal (0.45%) saline

Special measures:
- Broad spectrum antibiotics if infection is likely
- Bladder catheter if no urine is passed after 4 h
- Nasogastric tube if in coma
- CVP line in elderly or shocked patients

Subsequent management:
- Monitor glucose hourly $\left.\right\}$ for 8 h
  Monitor electrolytes 2-hourly
- Adjust K^+ replacement according to results. (Use ECG monitor as additional check.)
- When blood glucose falls to 10–12 $mmol \cdot l^{-1}$, change infusion fluid to 10% dextrose plus 20 mmol KCl, 500 ml 4-hourly. Continue insulin 3 units hourly by infusion or 6 units 2-hourly by i.m. injection.

Electrolyte changes in diabetic ketoacidosis and non-ketotic hyperosmolar coma

Examples with sample values:

	Severe ketoacidosis	Non-ketotic hyperosmolar coma
Na^+ (mmol·l^{-1})	140	155
K^+ (mmol·l^{-1})	5	5
Cl^- (mmol·l^{-1})	100	110
HCO_3^- (mmol·l^{-1})	5	30
Urea (mmol·l^{-1})	8	15
Glucose (mmol·l^{-1})	30	50
Arterial pH	7.0	7.35

The *osmolality* can be measured directly, or can be calculated approximately from the formula:

$$Osmolality = 2(Na^+ + K^+) + glucose + urea$$

The normal range is 285–300 mmol·l^{-1}.

For example, in the example of severe ketoacidosis given above:

$$Osmolality = 2(140 + 5) + 30 + 8 = 328 \text{ mmol·l}^{-1}$$

and in the example of non-ketotic hyperosmolar coma:

$$Osmolality = 2(155 + 5) + 50 + 15 = 385 \text{ mmol·l}^{-1}$$

The *anion gap* is calculated as $(Na^+ + K^+) - (Cl^- + HCO_3^-)$ (see p. 443). The normal anion gap is less than 17. In the example of ketoacidosis the anion gap is 40, and in the example of non-ketotic hyperosmolar coma the anion gap is 20.

---

such as thiazide diuretics or steroids, and intercurrent illness.

Non-ketotic coma and ketoacidosis represent two ends of a spectrum rather than two distinct disorders. The biochemical differences may partly be explained as follows:

- The extreme dehydration characteristic of non-ketotic coma may be related to age. Old people experience thirst less acutely, and more readily become dehydrated. In addition, the mild renal impairment associated with age results in increased urinary losses of fluid and electrolytes.
- The degree of insulin deficiency is less severe in non-ketotic coma. Endogenous insulin levels are sufficient to inhibit hepatic ketogenesis, whereas glucose production is unrestrained.

CLINICAL PRESENTATION

The characteristic clinical features are dehydration and stupor or coma. Impairment of consciousness is directly related to the degree of hyperosmolality. Evidence of underlying illness such as pneumonia or pyelonephritis may be present, and the hyperosmolar state may predispose to stroke, myocardial infarction or arterial insufficiency in the lower limbs.

INVESTIGATION AND TREATMENT

These are according to the guidelines for ketoacidosis, but care must be taken with the amount of fluid and insulin given. Plasma osmolality is monitored and half-normal saline (i.e. 0.45%) is used for initial rehydration in severe cases. Normal saline (0.9%) remains the standard fluid for rehydration.

PROGNOSIS

The reported mortality is around 30–50%, mainly because of the advanced age of the patients and the frequency of intercurrent illness. Unlike ketoacidosis, non-ketotic coma is not an absolute indication for subsequent insulin therapy, and survivors may do well on diet and oral agents.

Lactic acidosis

Lactic acidosis may occur in diabetic patients on biguanide therapy. Phenformin, the agent responsible in the great majority of reported cases, has now been withdrawn. The risk in patients taking metformin is extremely low provided that the therapeutic dose is not exceeded and the drug is withheld in patients with advanced hepatic or renal dysfunction.

Patients present with a severe metabolic acidosis, usually without significant hyperglycaemia or ketosis, and treatment is by rehydration and infusion of bicarbonate. The mortality is in excess of 50%.

COMPLICATIONS OF DIABETES

When insulin was introduced it was assumed that it would provide complete and adequate replacement therapy, just as thyroxine does in hypothyroidism.

Time proved that insulin-treated patients still have a considerably reduced life expectancy. Those diagnosed before the age of 20 have only a 50–60% chance of living past the age of 45, although there are recent indications of improved survival. The excess deaths are mainly due to diabetic nephropathy, but there is also a considerable excess cardiovascular mortality. Heart disease, peripheral vascular disease and stroke are the major causes of death in patients over the age of 50.

Large vessel disease
Diabetes is a risk factor in the development of atherosclerosis. This risk is related to that of the background population. For example, Japanese diabetics are much less likely to develop athero-sclerosis than patients in Europe but are much more likely to develop it than non-diabetic Japanese. The excess risk to diabetics compared with the general population increases as one moves down the body:
● Stroke is twice as likely.
● Myocardial infarction is three to five times as likely.
● Women with diabetes lose their pre-menopausal protection from coronary artery disease.
● Amputation of a foot for gangrene is 50 times as likely.

Diabetes is additive with other risk factors for large vessel disease. In other words, the diabetic who smokes or is obese, hypertensive or hyperlipidaemic adds the risks conferred by these conditions to that of diabetes itself.

Microvascular complications
In contrast to macrovascular disease, which is prevalent in Western populations as a whole, microvascular disease is specific to diabetes. Small blood vessels throughout the body are affected, but the disease process is of particular danger in three sites:
● The retina
● The renal glomerulus
● The nerve sheath

Diabetic retinopathy, nephropathy and neuropathy tend to manifest 10–20 years after diagnosis in young patients. They present earlier in older patients, probably because these have had unrecognized diabetes for months or even years prior to diagnosis.

Diabetic eye disease

Diabetes can affect the eyes in a number of ways. The most common and characteristic form of involvement is diabetic retinopathy. About one in three young patients is likely to develop visual problems, and 10% are blind after 30 years of diabetes; diabetes is the commonest cause of blindness in the population as a whole up to the age of 60.

Other forms of eye disease may also occur:
● The lens may be affected by reversible osmotic changes in patients with acute hyperglycaemia, causing blurred vision, or by cataracts.
● Rubeosis iridis (new vessel formation in the iris) may develop as a late complication of diabetic retinopathy and can cause glaucoma.
● External ocular palsies, especially of the sixth nerve, can occur.

The natural history of retinopathy (Fig. 17.12)
Diabetes causes increased thickness of the basement membrane and increased permeability of the retinal capillaries. Aneurysmal dilatation may occur in some vessels while others become occluded. These changes are first detectable by fluorescein angiography, a technique in which a fluorescent dye is injected into an arm vein and photographed in transit through the retinal vessels.

Background retinopathy. The first abnormality visible through the ophthalmoscope is the appearance of dot 'haemorrhages', which are actually due to capillary microaneurysms. Leakage of blood into the deeper layers of the retina produces the characteristic 'blot' haemorrhage, while exudates of fluid rich in lipids and protein give rise to hard exudates. These have a bright yellow-white colour and a sharply defined margin.

These changes rarely develop in young patients with a duration of diabetes under 10 years, but by 20 years virtually all eyes will show changes on fluorescein angiography, and most will at least manifest the occasional dot haemorrhage on careful ophthalmoscopy. In contrast, retinopathy may be present at diagnosis or shortly thereafter in older patients, suggesting that presentation may have been preceded by a long period of undiagnosed diabetes.

Background retinopathy does not in itself con-

Fig. 17.12 Almost all patients show some evidence of retinopathy within 20 years of diagnosis; angiography and retinal photography are more sensitive than ophthalmoscopy.

stitute a threat to vision, but may progress to two other distinct forms of retinopathy: maculopathy or proliferative retinopathy.

Diabetic maculopathy. This may lead to blindness in the absence of proliferation in the older patient with NIDDM. It is characterized by strings of hard exudates arranged in horseshoe or circular fashion around the central and lateral part of the macula. These may cause loss of visual acuity by occluding the central part of the retina. Oedema and ischaemia of the macula may also occur. Maculopathy can usually be diagnosed by measurement of visual acuity and use of the ophthalmoscope, but more elaborate techniques are needed to diagnose macular oedema and ischaemia.

Proliferative retinopathy. This dangerous form of retinopathy appears to develop on a basis of retinal ischaemia. The earliest sign is the appearance of 'cotton-wool spots', representing patches of retinal oedema. Unlike hard exudates they may also occur in severe hypertensive retinopathy. The term 'soft exudate' is often used synonymously, but is best avoided. Cotton-wool spots are greyish-white, have indistinct margins and a dull matt surface, unlike the glossy appearance of hard exudates. Venous beading and/or venous loops are other recognized pre-proliferative changes.

Hypoxia is thought to be the signal for formation of new vessels. These lie superficially or grow forward into the vitreous, resembling fronds of seaweed. They branch repeatedly, are fragile, bleed easily (because they lack the normal support-ive tissue) and may give rise to a fibrous tissue reaction.

Haemorrhages can be pre-retinal or into the vitreous. A vitreous haemorrhage presents as a loss of vision in one eye, sometimes noticed on waking, or as a floating shadow affecting the field of vision. Ophthalmoscopy gives the appearance of a feature-less, grey haze. Partial recovery of vision is the rule, as the blood is reabsorbed, but repeated bleeds may occur.

Loss of vision may also result from fibrous pro-liferation associated with new vessel formation. This may give rise to traction bands which contract in the course of time, producing retinal detachment.

Cataracts

Senile cataracts develop some 10–15 years earlier in diabetic patients than in the remainder of the population.

Juvenile or 'snowflake' cataracts are much less common. These are diffuse, rapidly progressive cataracts associated with very poorly controlled diabetes. They should be distinguished from temporary lens changes which occasionally appear during hyperosmolar coma and resolve when the coma is brought under control.

Examination of the eye

Careful systematic examination of the eye is essen-tial. Visual fields, acuity and eye movements are tested, and the pupils are dilated with a quick-acting mydriatic such as tropicamide 0.5%. Dilating drugs should not be used in patients with a history of glaucoma or cataract surgery, except with the advice of an ophthalmologist.

The examination begins at arm's length. At this distance, cataracts are silhouetted against the red reflex of the retina. The ophthalmoscope is advanced until the retina is in focus. The examination begins at the optic disc, moves through each quadrant in turn, and ends with the macula (since this is least comfort-able for the patient). The ophthalmoscope is then adjusted to the +10 dioptre lens for examination of the cornea, anterior chamber and lens. The location of abnormalities should always be sketched in the notes for future reference.

Management of diabetic eye disease

There is no specific medical treatment for back-ground retinopathy, but patients are advised not to smoke and hypertension should be treated. Rapid progression may occur in pregnant patients and in those with nephropathy, and these groups need frequent monitoring. All patients with retinopathy should be examined regularly in the clinic and, if possible, also supervised by an ophthalmologist. Referral to an ophthalmologist is particularly import-ant in the following circumstances:
- Deteriorating visual acuity
- Extensive hard exudates
- Pre-proliferative changes (cotton-wool spots or venous beading)
- New vessel formation

The ophthalmologist may perform fluorescein angio-graphy to define the extent of the problem. Maculopathy and proliferative retinopathy are treat-able by retinal photocoagulation with lasers; in the latter condition early effective therapy reduces the risk of visual loss by about 50%. Pituitary ablation was used, but now most physicians advise photocoagulation.

The diabetic kidney

The kidney may be damaged by diabetes in three main ways:
- Glomerular damage
- Ischaemia due to hypertrophy of afferent and efferent arterioles
- Ascending infection

Diabetic glomerulosclerosis

Clinical nephropathy secondary to glomerular disease usually manifests 15–25 years after diagnosis and affects 30–40% of patients diagnosed under the age of 30. It is the leading cause of premature death in

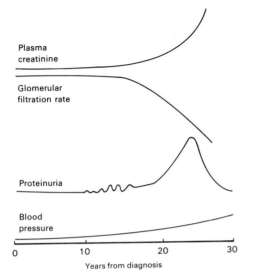

Fig. 17.13 Schematic representation of the natural history of nephropathy. The typical onset is 15 years after diagnosis. Intermittent proteinuria leads to persistent proteinuria. In time, the plasma creatinine rises as the glomerular filtration rate falls.

young diabetic patients. Older patients may also develop nephropathy, but the proportion affected is much smaller.

The earliest functional abnormality in the diabetic kidney is renal hypertrophy associated with a raised glomerular filtration rate; this appears soon after diagnosis and is related to poor glycaemic control.

The initial structural lesion in the glomerulus is thickening of the basement membrane. Associated changes may result in disruption of the protein cross-linkages which make the membrane an effective filter. In consequence, a progressive leak of protein into the urine occurs. The earliest evidence of this is 'microalbuminuria' (i.e. amounts of urinary albumin so small as to be detectable only by special techniques), which in turn progresses to frank proteinuria. Light microscopic changes of glomerulosclerosis become manifest; both diffuse and nodular glomerulosclerosis can occur. The latter is sometimes known as the Kimmelstiel–Wilson lesion. At a later stage still, the glomerulus is replaced by hyaline material. The clinical stages that parallel this process are shown in Fig. 17.13. Microalbuminuria is followed by intermittent Albustix-positive proteinuria, and then persistent proteinuria. At this stage the plasma creatinine is normal, but the average patient is only some 8–10 years from terminal renal failure. The proteinuria may become so heavy as to induce a transient nephrotic syndrome, with the associated features of peripheral oedema and hypoalbuminaemia. Patients will typically show a normochromic, normocytic anaemia and a raised ESR. Hypertension is a common development and may itself damage the kidney still further. A rise in

plasma creatinine is a late feature which progresses inevitably to renal failure, although the rate of progression may vary widely between individuals.

The natural history of this process is shown in Fig. 17.13. A curious feature is that almost all patients with long-established diabetes have abnormalities on renal biopsy, but only a proportion develop the features of a progressive renal disease.

Ischaemic lesions
Arteriolar lesions, with hypertrophy and hyalinization of the vessels, affect both afferent and efferent arterioles. The appearances are similar to those of hypertensive disease, but are not necessarily related to the blood pressure in patients with diabetes.

Infective lesions
Urinary tract infections are more common in women but not men with diabetes. Ascending infection may occur because of bladder stasis due to autonomic neuropathy, and infections more easily become established in damaged renal tissue. Autopsy material frequently reveals interstitial changes suggestive of infection, but ischaemia may produce similar changes and the true frequency of pyelonephritis in diabetes remains uncertain.

Untreated infections in diabetics can result in renal papillary necrosis, in which renal papillae are shed in the urine, but this complication is rare.

Diagnosis and management of diabetic nephropathy
The earliest clinical feature is proteinuria. Unfortunately, this is a sign of established and progressive disease. Poor glycaemic control is undoubtedly a risk factor in the development of nephropathy, but the established disease does not respond to improved control. For this reason it is now common for patients to be screened for microalbuminuria and there are indications that the process may still be reversible at this early stage. In patients with diabetes, proteinuria usually, but not invariably, implies diabetic nephropathy. It is important to consider and exclude other possible causes of renal disease. Clinical suspicion may be provoked by an atypical history, the absence of diabetic retinopathy (usually but not invariably present with diabetic nephropathy) and the presence of haematuria. Renal biopsy should be considered in such cases, but in practice is rarely necessary or helpful. The risk of intravenous urography is increased in diabetes, especially if patients are allowed to become dehydrated prior to the procedure, and a renal ultrasound is preferable. Other investigations include repeated microscopy and culture of the urine, 24-h urine collections to quantify protein loss and to measure creatinine clearance, and regular measurement of the plasma creatinine level.

Management of diabetic nephropathy is similar to that of other causes of renal failure, with the following provisos:

- Oral hypoglycaemic agents partially excreted via the kidney (e.g. chlorpropamide) must be avoided.
- Insulin sensitivity increases and drastic reductions in dosage may be needed.
- Meticulous control of hypertension may help to postpone renal failure.
- Diabetic retinopathy tends to progress rapidly and frequent ophthalmic supervision is essential.

Management of end-stage disease is complicated by the fact that patients often have other complications of diabetes such as blindness, autonomic neuropathy or peripheral vascular disease. Vascular shunts tend to calcify rapidly, hence chronic ambulatory peritoneal dialysis may be preferable to haemodialysis, and the failure rate of renal grafts is somewhat higher than in non-diabetic patients. A recent trend is to perform a segmental pancreatic graft at the same time as a renal graft. Although pancreatic grafts have a limited viability, due to progressive fibrosis within the graft, they may give the patient a year or so of freedom from insulin injections.

Recent evidence suggests that diabetic nephropathy is becoming less common as diabetes care improves.

Diabetic neuropathy

Diabetes can damage peripheral nervous tissue in a number of ways. The vascular hypothesis postulates occlusion of the vasa nervorum as the prime cause. This seems likely in isolated mononeuropathies, but the diffuse symmetrical nature of the common forms of neuropathy implies a metabolic cause. Since hyperglycaemia leads to increased formation of sorbitol and fructose in Schwann cells, accumulation of these sugars may disrupt function and structure.

The earliest functional change in diabetic nerves is delayed nerve conduction velocity; the earliest histological change is segmental demyelination, due to damage to Schwann cells. In the early stages axons are preserved, implying prospects of recovery, but at a later stage irreversible axonal degeneration develops.

The following varieties of neuropathy may occur (Fig. 17.14):
- Symmetrical sensory polyneuropathy (distal)
- Mononeuropathy and multiple mononeuropathy:
  - (a) Cranial nerve lesions
  - (b) Isolated peripheral nerve lesions
  - (c) Diabetic amyotrophy
- Autonomic neuropathy

Symmetrical sensory polyneuropathy
This is often unrecognized by the patient in its early stages. Early clinical signs are loss of vibration sense, pain sensation (deep before superficial) and

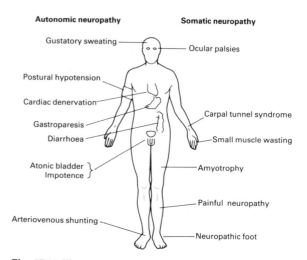

Fig. 17.14 The neuropathic man.

temperature sensation in the feet. At later stages patients may complain of a feeling of 'walking on cotton wool' and can lose their balance when washing the face or walking in the dark due to impaired proprioception. Involvement of the hands leads to the familiar 'stocking and glove' distribution. Complications include unrecognized trauma, beginning as blistering due to an ill-fitting shoe or a hot water bottle, and leading to ulceration.

A diffuse, painful neuropathy is a rare but unpleasant complication. The patient describes burning or crawling pains in the feet, shins and anterior thighs. These symptoms are typically worse at night, and pressure from the bedclothes may be intolerable. Acute painful neuropathy is an occasional presenting feature, which usually responds to improved glycaemic control. A more chronic form, developing later in the course of the disease, is sometimes resistant to almost all forms of therapy. Neurological assessment is difficult because of the hyperaesthesia experienced by the patient, but muscle wasting is not a feature and objective signs can be minimal.

Involvement of motor nerves to the small muscles of the feet gives rise to interosseous wasting. Unbalanced traction by the long flexor muscles leads to a characteristic shape of the foot, with a high arch and clawing of the toes, which in turn leads to abnormal distribution of pressure on walking, resulting in callus formation under the first metatarsal head or on the tips of the toes and perforating neuropathic ulceration.

Neuropathic arthropathy (Charcot's joints) may sometimes develop in the ankle. The hands show small muscle wasting as well as sensory changes, but it is important to differentiate these signs and symptoms from those of the carpal tunnel syndrome, which occurs with increased frequency in diabetes and may be amenable to surgery.

Mononeuropathy and multiple mononeuropathy
Cranial nerve lesions. Isolated or multiple palsies of nerves to the external eye muscles, especially the third and sixth nerves, are more common in diabetes. A characteristic feature of diabetic third nerve lesions is that pupillary reflexes are retained owing to sparing of pupillomotor fibres. Full recovery is the rule.

Isolated peripheral nerve lesions. Manifestations may be sensory, motor, or mixed, and multiple nerves may be involved ('mononeuritis multiplex'). The onset is usually abrupt and sometimes painful; recovery is typically slow and incomplete. Lesions are more likely to occur at common sites for external pressure palsies or nerve entrapment, e.g. the median nerve in the carpal tunnel.

Diabetic amyotrophy. This condition is usually seen in older men with diabetes. Presentation is with painful wasting, usually asymmetrical, of the quadriceps muscles. Features include extreme wasting with loss of the knee jerks, and extreme tenderness of the affected area. An extensor plantar response sometimes develops and CSF protein content is elevated. Diabetic amyotrophy is usually associated with periods of poor glycaemic control and may be present at diagnosis; unlike other forms of diabetic neuropathy, amyotrophy often resolves in time with careful control of the blood glucose.

Autonomic neuropathy
Patients with evidence of somatic neuropathy will also have damage of the sympathetic and parasympathetic nervous systems. In the early stages these autonomic lesions are asymptomatic and can only be detected with special tests, but they may later give rise to disabling symptoms.

The cardiovascular system. Vagal neuropathy results in tachycardia at rest and loss of sinus arrhythmia. At a later stage the heart may become denervated (resembling a transplanted heart). Cardiovascular reflexes such as the Valsalva manoeuvre are impaired.

Postural hypotension occurs due to loss of sympathetic tone to peripheral arterioles. A warm foot with a bounding pulse is sometimes seen in peripheral neuropathy as a result of this peripheral vasodilatation.

Gastrointestinal tract. Vagal damage can lead to gastroparesis, often asymptomatic, but sometimes leading to intractable vomiting. Diarrhoea often occurs at night accompanied by urgency and incontinence. Diarrhoea and steatorrhoea may occur due to bacterial overgrowth and treatment is with antibiotics.

Bladder involvement. Loss of tone, incomplete emptying, and stasis (predisposing to infection) can occur, and may ultimately result in an atonic, painless, distended bladder.

Impotence. This is common. The first manifestation is incomplete erection which may in time progress to total impotence; retrograde ejaculation also occurs. However, impotence in diabetes is not always due to autonomic neuropathy. Other causes include anxiety, depression, alcohol excess, drugs, primary or secondary gonadal failure and (rarely) disease of the iliac vessels. Treatment is difficult and depends largely on sympathetic counselling of both partners.

The diabetic foot

Many amputations in diabetes could be delayed or prevented by more effective patient education and medical supervision. Ischaemia, infection and neuropathy combine to produce tissue necrosis. Although these factors may coexist, it is important to distinguish between the ischaemic and the neuropathic foot (Table 17.9).

Management of the diabetic foot
Many diabetic foot problems are avoidable, so patients need to learn the principles of foot care and should be advised concerning appropriate footwear and the risks of smoking. Older patients should visit a chiropodist regularly and should not cut their own toe-nails.

Once tissue damage has occurred in the form of ulceration or gangrene, the aim is preservation of viable tissue. The two main threats are:
- *Infection.* This rapidly takes hold in a diabetic foot, and early effective antibiotic treatment is essential. Collections of pus are drained and excision of infected bone is needed if osteomyelitis develops. Regular x-rays of the foot are needed to check on progress.
- *Ischaemia.* The blood flow to the feet is assessed clinically or with the Doppler ultrasound stethoscope. Femoral arteriography may be performed, since localized areas of occlusion may be amenable to bypass surgery.

Table 17.9 Distinguishing features between ischaemia and neuropathy in the diabetic foot.

	Ischaemia	Neuropathy
Symptoms:	Claudication Rest pain	Usually painless Sometimes painful neuropathy
Inspection:	Dependent rubor Trophic changes	High arch Clawing of toes No trophic changes
Palpation:	Cold Pulseless	Warm Bounding pulses
Ulceration:	Painful Heels and toes	Painless Plantar

Foot problems are the major cause of hospital bed occupancy by diabetic patients. Good liaison between surgeon and physician is essential if this period in hospital is to be used efficiently. When irreversible arterial insufficiency is present, it is often quicker and kinder to opt for an early major amputation rather than subject the patient to a debilitating sequence of conservative procedures.

Infections

There is no evidence that diabetic patients with good glycaemic control are more prone to infection than normal subjects. However, poorly controlled diabetes entails increased susceptibility to the following infections:

- *Skin:*
  (a) Staphylococcal infections (boils, abscesses, carbuncles)
  (b) Mucocutaneous candidiasis
- *Urinary tract:*
  (a) Urinary tract infections (in women)
  (b) Pyelonephritis
  (c) Perinephric abscess
  (d) Genital infections (Bartholin's abscess)
- *Lungs:*
  (a) Staphylococcal and pneumococcal pneumonia
  (b) Gram-negative pneumonia
  (c) Tuberculosis

One reason why poor control lends to infection is that chemotaxis and phagocytosis by polymorphonuclear leucocytes is impaired at high blood glucose levels.

Conversely, infections may lead to loss of glycaemic control, and are a common cause of ketoacidosis. Insulin-treated patients need to increase their dose by up to 25% in the face of infection, and non-insulin-treated patients may need insulin cover while the infection lasts. Patients should be told never to omit their insulin dose, even if they are nauseated and unable to eat; instead they should seek urgent medical advice.

Skin and joints (see p. 934 and p. 355)

Joint contractures in the hands are a common consequence of childhood diabetes. The sign may be demonstrated by asking the patient to join his hands as if in prayer; the metacarpophalangeal and interphalangeal joints cannot be apposed. Thickened, waxy skin can be noted on the backs of the fingers. These features may be due to glycosylation of collagen and are not progressive.

Osteopenia in the extremities is also described in IDDM but rarely leads to clinical consequences.

SPECIAL SITUATIONS

Surgery

Smooth control of diabetes minimizes the risk of infection and balances the catabolic response to anaesthesia and surgery. The procedure for insulin-treated patients is simple:

- Soluble insulin only is given for 2–3 days before surgery.
- Whenever possible, diabetic patients should be first on the morning theatre list.
- An infusion of glucose, insulin and potassium is given during surgery. The insulin can be injected into the glucose solution or administered by syringe pump. A standard combination is 16 units of soluble insulin with 10 mmol KCl in 500 ml of 10% dextrose, infused at $100 \text{ ml} \cdot \text{h}^{-1}$.
- Postoperatively, the infusion is maintained until the patient is able to eat. Glucose levels are checked 2- to 4-hourly and potassium levels are monitored.

The same approach is used in the emergency situation, with the exception that an insulin infusion or subcutaneous injections of 4–6 units of soluble insulin hourly may be needed to bring the blood glucose under control prior to surgery.

Non-insulin-treated patients should stop medication 2 days before the operation. Patients with mild hyperglycaemia (fasting blood glucose below 8 $\text{mmol} \cdot \text{l}^{-1}$) can be treated as non-diabetic. Those with higher levels are treated with soluble insulin prior to surgery, and with glucose, insulin and potassium during and after the procedure, as for insulin-treated patients.

Pregnancy and diabetes

Modern management has transformed the outcome of pregnancy in women with diabetes. Thirty years ago one pregnancy in three ended with the death of the fetus or neonate. Today, the results in specialized centres approach those of non-diabetic pregnancy. This improvement is due to meticulous glycaemic control and careful medical and obstetric management.

Glycaemic control in pregnancy
The patient should perform daily home blood glucose profiles; the renal threshold falls in pregnancy and urine tests are therefore of little or no value. Insulin requirements rise, and intensified insulin regimens may become necessary. The aim is to maintain blood glucose and HbA_{1c} levels within the normal range.

When the pregnancy is planned, good control is sought prior to conception.

General management

The patient is seen at intervals of 2 weeks or less at a clinic managed jointly by obstetrician and physician. Routine admission at 32 weeks is no longer necessary, and, circumstances permitting, the aim should be outpatient management with a spontaneous vaginal delivery at term.

Obstetric problems associated with diabetes

Poorly controlled diabetes is associated with macrosomia, hydramnios, pre-eclampsia and intrauterine death. Ketoacidosis in pregnancy carries a 50% fetal mortality, but maternal hypoglycaemia is relatively well tolerated.

Neonatal problems

Maternal diabetes, especially when poorly controlled, is associated with fetal macrosomia. The infant of a diabetic mother is more susceptible to hyaline membrane disease than non-diabetic infants of similar maturity. In addition, neonatal hypoglycaemia may occur. The mechanism is as follows: maternal glucose crosses the placenta, but insulin does not; the fetal islets hypersecrete to combat maternal hyperglycaemia, and a rebound to hypoglycaemic levels occurs when the umbilicus is severed.

These complications are due to hyperglycaemia in the third trimester. Poor glycaemic control in the first trimester carries an increased risk of congenital malformations, particularly of the cardiovascular and central nervous systems. For this reason, women with diabetes should be advised to achieve optimum glycaemic control before conception.

Genetic aspects

The child of an insulin-dependent diabetic patient has an increased chance of developing IDDM. This risk, curiously, is greater with a diabetic father (between 1 in 20 and 1 in 40) than with a diabetic mother (1 in 40–80). The overall risk for a second sibling is 1 in 20, rising to 1 in 8 for an HLA-identical sibling.

Gestational diabetes

This term refers to diabetes that develops in the course of pregnancy and remits following delivery.

The diabetes is typically asymptomatic and is demonstrated biochemically on the basis of random testing or an oral glucose tolerance test. Since the renal threshold for glucose falls during normal pregnancy and glucose tolerance deteriorates, the condition may easily be misdiagnosed. Current practice in many centres is to screen for this condition using glucose levels in blood samples taken at antenatal clinics. A value above 6.4 mmol·l^{-1} within 2 h of a meal, or above 5.8 mmol·l^{-1} thereafter, represents a deviation above the ninety-ninth percentile and indicates the need for an oral glucose tolerance test.

Treatment is with diet in the first instance, but most patients require insulin cover during the pregnancy. Oral agents are avoided because of the potential risk to the fetus.

Gestational diabetes has been associated with a higher frequency of obstetric problems, fetal macrosomia and neonatal hypoglycaemia. It is likely to recur in subsequent pregnancies, and non-insulin-dependent diabetes may develop later in life.

Not all diabetes presenting in pregnancy is gestational. True IDDM may develop, and swift diagnosis is essential to prevent the development of ketoacidosis. Hospital admission is required if the patient is symptomatic, or has ketonuria or a markedly elevated blood glucose level.

Brittle diabetes

There is no precise definition for this term, which is used to describe patients with recurrent ketoacidosis and/or recurrent hypoglycaemic coma. Of these, the largest group is made up of those who experience recurrent severe hypoglycaemia.

Recurrent severe hypoglycaemia

This affects 1–3% of insulin-dependent patients. Most are adults who have had diabetes for more than 10 years. By this stage endogenous insulin secretion is negligible in the great majority of patients. Pancreatic alpha cells are still present in undiminished numbers, but the glucagon response to hypoglycaemia is virtually absent. Long-term patients are thus subject to fluctuating hyperinsulinaemia due to erratic absorption of insulin from injection sites, and lack a major component of the hormonal defence against hypoglycaemia. In this situation adrenaline secretion becomes vital, but this too may become impaired in the course of diabetes. Loss of adrenaline secretion has been attributed to autonomic neuropathy, but this is unlikely to be the sole cause; central failure of sympathetic–medullary activation (as brain cells adapt to recurrent hypoglycaemia) may be responsible.

The following factors may also predispose to recurrent hypoglycaemia:

- *An unrecognized low renal threshold for glucose.* Attempts to render the urine sugar free will inevitably produce hypoglycaemia.
- *Excessive insulin doses.* A common error is to increase the *dose* when a patient needs more frequent injections to overcome a problem of *timing*.
- *Endocrine causes.* These include pituitary insufficiency, adrenal insufficiency and premenstrual insulin sensitivity.
- *Alimentary causes.* These include exocrine pancreatic failure and diabetic gastroparesis.
- *Renal failure.* This is associated with falling insulin requirements and unstable control.

- *Patient causes.* The patient may be unintelligent, feckless or may manipulate his therapy.

Recurrent ketoacidosis

This usually occurs in adolescents or young adults, and the most severe form is more common in girls. Although metabolic decompensation may develop very rapidly, it is often impossible to pin-point an underlying abnormality. Many theories exist concerning the causes of this condition, but all agree that it is heterogeneous. The following categories have been suggested:

- *Iatrogenic.* Inappropriate insulin combinations may be a cause of swinging glycaemic control. For example, a once-daily regimen may cause hypoglycaemia during the afternoon or evening and pre-breakfast hyperglycaemia due to insulin deficiency.
- *Intercurrent illness.* Unsuspected infections, including urinary tract infections and tuberculosis, may be present. Thyrotoxicosis can also manifest as unstable glycaemic control.
- *Psychosocial causes.* These certainly form the largest category. It has been suggested that neuroendocrine mechanisms such as catecholamine secretion might mediate the metabolic disturbance. Other patients undoubtedly manipulate their illness, whether consciously or unconsciously.
- *Unknown aetiology.* The most 'brittle' patients of all are usually female, aged 15–25 and often overweight, and typically suffer from amenorrhoea. The insulin requirement is variable but is often high. Sophisticated 'cheating' has been detected in some of these patients, but this should never be assumed without convincing proof.

Hypoglycaemia

Hypoglycaemia develops when hepatic glucose output falls below the rate of glucose uptake by peripheral tissues. Hepatic glucose output may be reduced by:

- The inhibition of hepatic glycogenolysis and gluconeogenesis by insulin
- The depletion of hepatic glycogen reserves by malnutrition, fasting, exercise or advanced liver disease
- Impaired gluconeogenesis (e.g. following alcohol ingestion)

In the first of these categories, insulin levels are raised and the liver contains adequate glycogen stores, and the hypoglycaemia can be reversed by injection of glucagon. In the other two situations, insulin levels are low and glucagon is ineffective.

Peripheral glucose uptake is accelerated by high insulin levels and by exercise, but these conditions are normally balanced by increased glucose output. Insulin or sulphonylurea therapy for diabetes accounts for the vast majority of cases of severe hypoglycaemia encountered in a casualty department.

The commonest symptoms and signs of hypoglycaemia are neurological. The brain consumes about 50% of the total glucose produced by the liver. This high energy requirement is needed to generate ATP used to maintain the potential difference across axonal membranes.

Insulinomas

Insulinomas are pancreatic islet cell tumours which secrete insulin. Most are sporadic but some patients have multiple tumours arising from neural crest tissue (multiple endocrine adenomatosis). Some 95% of these tumours are benign. The classic presentation is with fasting hypoglycaemia, but early symptoms may also develop in the late morning or afternoon. Recurrent hypoglycaemia is often present for months or years before the diagnosis is made, and the symptoms may be atypical or even bizarre; the presenting features in one series are given in Table 17.10. Common misdiagnoses include psychiatric disorders, epilepsy and cerebrovascular disease.

Table 17.10 Presenting features of insulinoma.

Diplopia
Sweating, palpitations, weakness
Confusion or abnormal behaviour
Loss of consciousness
Grand mal seizures

DIAGNOSIS

Whipple's triad remains the basis of clinical diagnosis. This is satisfied when:

- Symptoms are associated with fasting or exercise
- Hypoglycaemia is confirmed during these episodes
- Glucose relieves the symptoms

A fourth criterion—demonstration of inappropriately high insulin levels during hypoglycaemia—may usefully be added to these.

In practice, the diagnosis is confirmed by the demonstration of hypoglycaemia in association with inappropriate and excessive insulin secretion. Hypoglycaemia is demonstrated by:

- Measurement of overnight fasting (16 h) glucose and insulin levels on three occasions. About 90%

of patients with insulinomas will have low glucose and non-suppressed (normal or elevated) insulin levels.
- Performing a prolonged supervised fast. Whipple's triad can be demonstrated in about 95% of patients in the course of a 48-h fast.

Autonomous insulin secretion is demonstrated by lack of the normal feedback suppression during hypoglycaemia. This may be shown by:
- Measuring insulin, C-peptide or pro-insulin levels during a spontaneous episode of hypoglycaemia
- Inducing hypoglycaemia. Since pharmaceutical insulin does not contain C-peptide, an insulin tolerance test is performed and C-peptide is assayed as an index of endogenous insulin secretion. An alternative is to infuse fish insulin, which does not interfere with the assay for human insulin, and to measure circulating insulin levels. These tests are potentially hazardous, and should be resorted to only when real doubt exists concerning the diagnosis.

Many patients also have an abnormal (diabetic) glucose tolerance test, but this has no diagnostic value.

TREATMENT

The most effective therapy is surgical excision of the tumour. It is usual to perform pancreatic angiography preoperatively in an attempt to localize the tumour, but the majority of insulinomas can be palpated by a skilled surgeon. Localization is also possible using a rapid insulin assay on blood sampled at different levels from the pancreatic vein.

Medical treatment with diazoxide is useful when the insulinoma is malignant, in patients in whom a tumour cannot be located, and in elderly patients with mild symptoms.

Hypoglycaemia with other tumours

Hypoglycaemia may develop in the course of advanced cachectic disease, and has been described in association with many tumour types. Certain massive tumours, especially sarcomas, are associated with hypoglycaemia, possibly because the tumour is consuming large amounts of glucose. Other tumour types appear to secrete substances with insulin-like action, but true ectopic insulin secretion is extremely rare.

Post-prandial hypoglycaemia

If frequent *venous* blood glucose samples are taken following a prolonged glucose tolerance test, about one in four subjects will have at least one value below 3 mmol·l^{-1}. The arteriovenous glucose difference is quite marked during this phase, so that very few are truly hypoglycaemic in terms of arterial (or capillary) blood glucose content. Failure to appreciate this simple fact led some authorities to believe that post-prandial (or reactive) hypoglycaemia was a potential 'organic' explanation for a variety of complaints that might otherwise have been considered psychosomatic. An epidemic of 'non-hypoglycaemia' followed, particularly in the USA. Later work showed a poor correlation between symptoms and biochemical hypoglycaemia. Even so, a number of otherwise normal people occasionally become pale, weak and sweaty at times when meals are due, and report benefit from advice to take regular snacks between meals.

True post-prandial hypoglycaemia may develop in the presence of alcohol, which 'primes' the beta cells to produce an exaggerated insulin response to carbohydrate. The person who substitutes gin and tonic for lunch is particularly at risk. Post-prandial hypoglycaemia sometimes occurs after gastric surgery, due to rapid gastric emptying and mismatching of food and insulin. This is referred to as 'dumping' but it is rarely a clinical problem (see p. 167).

Hepatic and renal causes of hypoglycaemia

The liver can maintain a normal glucose output despite extensive damage, and hepatic hypoglycaemia is uncommon. It is particularly a problem with fulminant hepatic failure following poisoning with, for example, paracetamol.

The kidney has a subsidiary role in glucose production (via gluconeogenesis in the renal cortex), and hypoglycaemia is sometimes a problem in terminal renal failure.

Endocrine causes of hypoglycaemia

Endocrine disorders resulting in deficiencies of hormones antagonistic to insulin are rare but well-recognized causes of hypoglycaemia. These include hypopituitarism, isolated ACTH deficiency and Addison's disease.

Drug-induced hypoglycaemia

Many drugs have been reported to produce isolated cases of hypoglycaemia, but usually only when other predisposing factors are present. The following are among the more important:
- *Sulphonylureas* may be used in the treatment of diabetes or may be taken by non-diabetics in suicide attempts.
- *Quinine* may produce severe hypoglycaemia in the course of treatment for falciparum malaria.
- *Salicylates* may cause hypoglycaemia following accidental ingestion by children, but this complication is very rare in adults.
- *Propranolol* has been reported to induce hypogly-

caemia in the presence of strenuous exercise or starvation.

Alcohol-induced hypoglycaemia

Alcohol-induced hypoglycaemia was first described in poorly-nourished chronic alcoholics but may also present in binge drinkers and in children who have taken relatively small amounts of alcohol. Alcohol inhibits gluconeogenesis and is most likely to induce hypoglycaemia when taken by fasting or malnourished individuals or children, who have no hepatic glycogen reserve. The clinical presentation is with coma and hypothermia.

Factitious hypoglycaemia

This is a relatively common variant of self-induced disease. Hypoglycaemia is produced by surreptitious self-administration of insulin or sulphonylureas. Many patients in this category have been extensively investigated for an insulinoma. Measurement of C-peptide levels during hypoglycaemia should identify patients who are injecting insulin; sulphonylureas may be picked up by chromatography of plasma or urine.

Lipid disorders

Cholesterol and triglyceride are insoluble and are transported between the intestine, liver and periphery in the form of soluble complexes known as lipoproteins. These circulate as spherical particles with an envelope of phospholipid and apoproteins and a non-polar lipid core. They can be divided by density, configuration and electrophoretic mobility into four major classes: chylomicrons, very low density lipoproteins (VLDLs), low density lipoproteins (LDLs) and high density lipoproteins (HDLs) (Table 17.11).

Chylomicrons are large particles composed mainly of triglyceride. They are synthesized in the walls of the small intestine and provide the main form of transport for dietary fat. Their presence gives post-prandial plasma a lactescent appearance which normally clears within a few hours.

VLDLs are relatively large particles with a high proportion of triglyceride. These are produced in the liver and represent endogenous triglyceride synthesis. Chylomicrons and VLDLs are catabolized by lipoprotein lipase in peripheral tissues and by hepatic lipase. Partial breakdown and exchange of apoproteins gives rise to smaller, denser particles with a high cholesterol content.

LDLs are the major cholesterol-carrying lipoproteins in normal plasma and are mostly derived from partial catabolism of VLDLs. Peripheral uptake is mainly in the liver by a receptor-dependent mechanism; the LDLs are then internalized and metabolized to release free cholesterol.

HDLs are produced in the liver and intestine and contain 20–30% of circulating cholesterol. This heterogeneous group of particles may be involved in reverse cholesterol transport (i.e. from the periphery back to the liver). If so, this might explain their apparent protective role in atherosclerosis.

The enzyme lipoprotein lipase is situated in the capillary endothelium of skeletal muscle and adipose tissue. It is activated by apoprotein C-II (apo C-II) on the surface of chylomicrons and VLDLs, and hydrolyses the triglyceride content of these particles to free fatty acids.

Apoproteins
The apoprotein genes are encoded on chromosome 11 (see Fig. 17.5) and at least eight different apolipoproteins have been found so far.

Apoproteins were originally thought only to have a structural role in lipoproteins and to contribute to the solubility of the lipid complex. They are now known to also be involved in binding the particles to cell surface receptors and in activating enzymes important for their metabolism. Examples of apoproteins performing these functions are given below:
- Cofactors for enzymes involved in lipoprotein metabolism:
  (a) Apo A-I (cofactor for lecithin cholesterol acyltransferase)
  (b) Apo C-II (cofactor for lipoprotein lipase)
  (c) Apo A-II (cofactor for hepatic lipase)
- Ligands for binding lipoprotein particles to specific cell surface receptors:
  (a) Apo B-100 (LDL pathway)
  (b) Apo E (chylomicron remnant pathway)
- Structural proteins in lipoprotein particles:

Table 17.11 Composition of major lipoprotein classes.

	Protein	Triglyceride	Cholesterol	Phospholipid	Major apoproteins
Chylomicrons	2%	85%	4%	9%	B, CI, CII, CIII
VLDL	10%	50%	15%	18%	B, CI, CII, CIII, E
LDL	23%	10%	45%	20%	B
HDL	55%	4%	17%	24%	A–I, A–II

(a) Apo B-100 (VLDLs and LDLs)
(b) Apo B-48 (chylomicrons)
(c) Apo A-I (HDLs)

Lipids, lipoproteins and atherosclerosis
There is a well-established association between atherosclerosis and plasma cholesterol, but even stronger associations appear when the cholesterol-carrying LDL and HDL lipoprotein fractions are considered. LDL-cholesterol levels are predictive of coronary heart disease, but an inverse relationship is seen with HDL-cholesterol, so that high levels appear to be protective.

Cholesterol deposited in atheromatous lesions is derived from LDL and enters the lesion at a rate dependent upon the plasma concentrations. The protective role of HDL may be in mediating hepatic cholesterol excretion by reverse transport of cholesterol from the periphery.

The atherogenicity of triglyceride-rich lipoproteins is less clear, but there are strong epidemiological associations with ischaemic heart disease and peripheral vascular disease.

The hyperlipidaemias

CLINICAL FEATURES

Features associated with hyperlipidaemia include:
- Xanthelasmas (cholesterol deposits on the eyelid)
- Premature arcus in the cornea
- Xanthomas (cholesterol deposits in the skin)
- Rarely, lipaemia retinalis (turbid blood in the retinal vessels)

Evidence of possible underlying disorders such as hypothyroidism should be sought.

INVESTIGATION

Initial investigation involves measurement of the fasting cholesterol and triglyceride levels. The patient follows his normal diet for the preceding 2 weeks, and drugs that may affect lipid metabolism are withdrawn. The result may be influenced by acute illness, but the test may be performed soon after myocardial infarction and any high levels followed up.

Values should be assessed according to the age of the patient. Results over the ninety-fifth percentile should be investigated further, including measurement of HDL-cholesterol and lipoprotein electrophoresis.

Examination of stored serum provides useful information: a diffuse milky appearance usually means raised VLDL, whereas a creamy upper layer with clear plasma beneath indicates chylomicronaemia. Family members should be investigated when a primary hyperlipidaemia is suspected.

CLASSIFICATION

The classification of the hyperlipidaemias (Table 17.12) is complex and many find it confusing. This is because the standard Fredrickson/WHO classification is based on patterns found during laboratory analysis rather than on disease entities. These patterns may result from a variety of disease processes and sometimes overlap.

Rapid progress is taking place in analysis of the underlying genetic and molecular disorders. In general, the hyperlipidaemias constitute a group of rare but relatively well-defined single-gene disorders and a larger group, presumably polygenic, in which genetic and environmental factors overlap.

Secondary causes of raised lipid levels (Table 17.13) must be excluded before a primary disorder can be diagnosed.

Type I hyperlipidaemia
This rare condition is characterized by the presence of chylomicrons in fasting plasma. The primary form is transmitted as an autosomal recessive trait. Patients are unable to metabolize chylomicrons due to deficiency of extrahepatic lipoprotein lipase or its cofactor apoprotein C-II.

Patients present in childhood with hepatosplenomegaly, eruptive xanthomas and lipaemia retinalis; some experience recurrent pancreatitis. Despite the raised triglyceride levels there is little evidence of premature vascular disease. Treatment is with a low fat diet.

Table 17.12 Classification of hyperlipidaemia.

	Plasma cholesterol	Plasma triglyceride	Lipoprotein abnormality
Type I	+	+++	Chylomicrons
Type IIa	+++	−	LDL
Type IIb	++	++	LDL, VLDL
Type III	++	++	IDL
Type IV	+	++	VLDL
Type V	+	+++	Chylomicrons, VLDL

Table 17.13 Secondary causes of raised cholesterol and triglyceride.

Raised cholesterol
Diet
Hypothyroidism
Liver disease
Nephrotic syndrome
Porphyria
Raised triglyceride
Obesity
Poorly controlled diabetes
Alcohol excess
High carbohydrate diet
Renal failure
Oestrogen therapy

Type IIa hyperlipidaemia

This is characterized by hypercholesterolaemia with normal triglycerides and clear plasma. LDL levels are raised but VLDL levels are normal. The best-known genetic cause is familial hypercholesterolaemia, which is an autosomal dominant trait. Heterozygotes make up 1 in 500 of the population; homozygotes are correspondingly very rare. The metabolic defect is related to binding and internalization of LDL to its receptor.

Heterozygotes often develop coronary artery disease between the third and fifth decade of life and account for 5% of survivors of myocardial infarction under the age of 60. Premature arcus and xanthomas may be present, and cholesterol levels are markedly elevated. Homozygotes have grossly elevated cholesterol (usually >16 mmol·l^{-1}) and marked xanthomatosis, and develop coronary artery disease whilst in their teens.

Treatment is with a low cholesterol diet, cholestyramine and nicotinic acid (Table 17.14), and can be very effective if this regimen is followed conscientiously.

Type IIb hyperlipidaemia

In this condition both LDL and VLDL levels are raised. Most patients have familial combined hyperlipidaemia—an autosomal dominant trait with a variable expression—which may give rise to type IIa (raised LDL), type IV (raised VLDL) or type IIb hyperlipidaemia (raised LDL and VLDL) within members of the same family. Patients are at risk from premature coronary artery disease, and 15% of survivors of myocardial infarction under the age of 60 have been reported to suffer from this disorder.

Type III hyperlipidaemia

This is characterized by raised cholesterol and triglyceride levels due to a particle of intermediate density between VLDL and LDL known as intermediate-density lipoprotein (IDL). The metabolic defect is a failure of chylomicron remnant removal. The disease develops in adult life, and is often associated with obesity, glucose intolerance and hyperuricaemia. Palmar xanthomas may be present and are diagnostic. The risk of coronary artery and peripheral vascular disease is increased. Most patients are homozygous for a variant form of apoprotein E known as apoprotein E-2.

Treatment is by weight reduction and reduced dietary cholesterol and fat. Nicotinic acid may also be necessary.

Type IV hyperlipidaemia

This is relatively common, is associated with diabetes, and may be exacerbated by a number of environmental factors including diet, alcohol and medication such as thiazide diuretics and oral contraceptives.

Some patients have familial combined hyperlipidaemia (see above); the other major primary cause is familial hypertriglyceridaemia. This is an autosomal dominant disorder associated with raised VLDL, normal LDL and reduced HDL. Both overproduction and underutilization of VLDL contribute to the high plasma levels.

Treatment is with weight reduction, a low fat diet, careful control of diabetes when present, and alcohol avoidance.

Type V hyperlipidaemia

Chylomicronaemia is present as in type I, but in addition the underlying plasma is turbid due to elevated VLDL levels. The condition is usually seen in adults who are also obese, diabetic and hyperuricaemic. Pancreatitis and arthritis may develop, and eruptive xanthomas can appear. Lipoprotein lipase and apoprotein C-II are normal, but a rare variant—apoprotein E-4—is often present.

Table 17.14 Lipid-lowering agents used in hyperlipidaemia.

	Usual dose	Indications	Side-effects	Contraindications and precautions
Nicotinic acid (niacin)	1 g × 3 daily (max. 6 g daily)	Types II, III, IV and V	Flushing; irritation of skin and eyes	Contraindicated in liver disease, peptic ulceration and pregnancy
Clofibrate (withdrawn)	1 g × 2 daily	Types III and IV	Abdominal discomfort; cholesterol cholelithiasis; myositis (rare)	Avoid in liver and kidney disease and pregnancy; potentiates action of warfarin
Bezafibrate	200 mg × 3 daily			
Cholestyramine	8 g × 3 daily (max. 32 g daily)	Type II	Flatulence; bowel disturbance	Reduces absorption of some drugs (e.g. digoxin, warfarin); avoid in pregnancy

Treatment is by a low fat diet, weight reduction, avoidance of alcohol, and careful control of diabetes when present. Some patients benefit from treatment with nicotinic acid.

MANAGEMENT OF HYPERLIPIDAEMIAS

General principles are:
- The maintenance of a lean body weight
- A low fat diet
- The avoidance of alcohol
- The avoidance of oestrogens and thiazides
- The avoidance of smoking
- The treatment of diabetes and hypertension when present

Lipid-lowering agents (see Table 17.14)

These may be effective in one of three ways:
- Reduced synthesis of VLDLs and LDLs (e.g. nicotinic acid)
- Enhanced VLDL clearance (e.g. bezafibrate)
- Enhanced LDL catabolism (e.g. cholestyramine, which is a non-absorbable anion exchange resin which binds bile acids in the gut lumen, thus reducing the enterohepatic circulation and enhancing cholesterol conversion to bile acids)

The actions and indications for the use of these agents are given in Table 17.14. All three agents have been shown to reduce the incidence of coronary artery disease in prospective studies, but clofibrate increased the frequency of gallbladder disease and there was an associated increased mortality from non-cardiovascular causes. As a consequence, bezafibrate is now used. Cholestyramine has been shown to markedly reduce the incidence and progression of coronary disease in a large cohort of American men with raised cholesterol levels.

Hypolipidaemia

Low lipid levels can be found in severe protein–energy malnutrition. They are also seen occasionally with severe malabsorption and in intestinal lymphangiectasia.

Abetalipoproteinaemia

This is described on p. 184.

Familial alpha-lipoprotein deficiency (Tangier disease)

One of the two HDL apoproteins, apo A-I, is deficient in homozygotes with this very rare disease so that there is little HDL in plasma. Tangier disease is inherited as an autosomal recessive. The serum cholesterol is low but serum triglycerides are normal or high. Cholesterol accumulates in reticulo-endothelial tissue, although the mechanism is uncertain, producing enlarged and orange-coloured tonsils and hepatosplenomegaly. There are also corneal opacities and a polyneuropathy.

Inborn errors of carbohydrate metabolism

Glycogen storage disease

All mammalian cells can manufacture glycogen, but the main sites of its production are the liver and muscle. Glycogen is a high molecular weight glucose polymer. In glycogen storage disease, there is either an abnormality in the molecular structure or an increase in glycogen concentration due to a specific enzyme defect. All these conditions are autosomal recessive in inheritance and present in infancy, except for McArdle's disease, which presents in adults.

Table 17.15 shows the classification and clinical features of these diseases.

Galactosaemia

Galactose is normally converted to glucose. However, a deficiency of the enzyme galactose-1-phosphate uridyl transferase results in accumulation of galactose-1-phosphate in the blood. This deficiency, inherited as an autosomal recessive, results in hypoglycaemia and acidosis in the neonate. Progressive hepatosplenomegaly, cataracts, renal tubular defects and mental retardation occur.

Treatment is with a galactose-free diet which, if started early, results in normal development. Untreated patients die within a few days. Prenatal diagnosis and diagnosis of the carrier state are possible by measurement of the level of galactose-1-phosphate in the blood.

Galactokinase deficiency also results in galactosaemia and early cataract formation.

Defects of fructose metabolism

Absorbed fructose is chiefly metabolized in the liver to lactic acid or glucose. Three defects of metabolism occur; all are inherited as autosomal recessive traits:
- *Fructosuria* is due to fructokinase deficiency. It is a benign condition.
- *Fructose intolerance* is due to fructose-1-phosphate aldolase deficiency. Fructose-1-phosphate accumulates after fructose ingestion, resulting in symptoms of hypoglycaemia. Hepatomegaly and renal tubular defects occur but are reversible on a fructose-free diet. Intelligence is normal.
- *Fructose-1,6-diphosphate deficiency* leads to a failure of gluconeogenesis, and hepatomegaly.

Table 17.15 Glycogen storage diseases.

Type	Affected tissue	Enzyme defect	Clinical features	Tissue needed for diagnosis*	Outcome
I (Von Gierke)	Liver, intestine, kidney	Glucose-6-phosphatase	Hepatomegaly, hypoglycaemia, stunted growth, obesity, hypotonia	Liver	If patients survive initial hypoglycaemia, prognosis is good; hyperuricaemia is a late complication
II (Pompé)	Liver, muscle, heart	Lysosomal α-glucosidase	Heart failure, cardiomyopathy	Leucocytes, liver, muscle	Death in first 6 months; juvenile and adult variants seen
III (Forbes)	Liver, muscle (abnormal glycogen structure)	Amylo-1, 6-glucosidase	Like type I	Leucocytes, liver, muscle	Good prognosis
IV (Anderson)	Liver (abnormal glycogen structure)	1, 4-α-glucan branching enzyme	Failure to thrive, hepatomegaly, cirrhosis and its complications	Leucocytes, liver, muscle	Death in first 3 years
V (McArdle)	Muscle only	Phosphorylase	Muscle cramps and myoglobinuria after exercise (in adults)	Muscle	Normal life span; exercise must be avoided

* Tissue obtained is used for the biochemical assay of the enzyme.

Pentosuria

Pentosuria is due to L-xylulose reductase deficiency. It has no clinical significance.

Inborn errors of amino acid metabolism

Inborn errors of amino acid metabolism are chiefly inherited as autosomal recessive conditions. The major ones are shown in Table 17.16.

AMINO ACID TRANSPORT DEFECTS

Amino acids are filtered by the glomerulus but 95% of the filtered load is reabsorbed in the proximal convoluted tubule by an active transport mechanism.

Aminoaciduria results from:
- Abnormally high amino acid plasma levels (e.g. phenylketonuria)
- Any inherited disorder that damages the tubules secondarily (e.g. galactosaemia)
- Tubular reabsorptive defects, either generalized (e.g. Fanconi syndrome) or specific (e.g. cystinuria)

Amino acid transport defects can be congenital or acquired.

Generalized aminoacidurias

Fanconi syndrome
This occurs in a juvenile form (De Toni–Fanconi–Debré syndrome) or in adult life. There is defective tubular reabsorption of:
- Most amino acids
- Glucose
- Phosphate, resulting in hypophosphataemic rickets
- Bicarbonate, with failure to transport hydrogen ions, causing renal tubular acidosis which then produces a hyperchloraemic acidosis

Other abnormalities include:
- Hypouricaemia
- Potassium depletion, primary or secondary to the acidosis
- Polyuria
- Increased excretion of immunoglobulins and other low molecular weight proteins

Various combinations of the above abnormalities have been described.

The juvenile form begins at the age of 6–9 months, with failure to thrive, vomiting and thirst. There is also acidosis, dehydration and vitamin D resistant rickets.

In the adult the disease is similar to the juvenile form, but osteomalacia is a major feature.

Table 17.16 Inborn errors of amino acid metabolism.

Disease	Enzyme defect	Incidence	Biochemical and clinical features	Treatment	Prognosis
Albinism	Tyrosinase	1 in 13 000	Amelanosis—whitish hair, pink-white skin, grey/blue eyes; Nystagmus, photophobia, strabismus	Symptomatic	—
Alkaptonuria	Homogentisic acid oxidase	1 in 100 000	Homogentisic acid polymerizes to produce a black-brown product which is deposited in cartilage and other tissue (ochronosis); Urine darkens on standing; Sweat stains clothing; Arthritis	None	Good
Homocystinuria Type I	Cystathionine synthetase		Homocystine is excreted in urine; Mental handicap; Marfan-like syndrome; Thrombotic episodes	—	—
Type II	Methylene tetrahydrofolate reductase		Survivors have mental retardation	—	Mainly die as neonates
Phenylketonuria	Phenylalanine-4-hydroxylase	1 in 20 000	Brain damage with mental retardation and epilepsy; Phenylpyruvate and its derivatives excreted in urine	Diet low in phenylalanine in first few months of life prevents damage	—
Histidinaemia	Histidine deaminase	Very rare	Mental retardation	—	—
'Maple syrup' disease	Branched-chain ketoacid decarboxylase	Very rare	Failure to thrive; Fits, neonatal acidosis and severe cerebral degeneration; Valine, isoleucine, leucine and their derivatives are excreted in urine; A milder form is seen	—	Early death
Oxalosis (hyperoxaluria)	Glyoxylic acid dehydrogenase	Very rare	Nephrocalcinosis, renal stones, renal failure due to deposition of calcium oxalate	—	Death occurs in first two decades

There are many other enzyme defects producing, for example, alaninaemia, ammonaemia, argininaemia, citrullinaemia, isovaleric acidaemia, lysinaemia, ornithinaemia or tyrosinaemia.

Treatment is with large doses of vitamin D (e.g. 1–2 µg of 1-alpha-hydroxycholecalciferol with regular blood calcium monitoring).

Lowe's syndrome (oculocerebrorenal dystrophy)
In this syndrome there is generalized aminoaciduria combined with mental retardation, hypotonia, congenital cataracts and an abnormal skull shape.

Specific aminoacidurias

Cystinuria
There is defective tubular reabsorption and jejunal absorption of cystine and the dibasic amino acids lysine, ornithine and arginine. Inheritance is either completely or incompletely recessive, so that heterozygotes who have increased excretion of lysine and cystine only can occur. Cystine absorption from the jejunum is impaired but, nevertheless, cystine in peptide form can be absorbed. Cystinuria leads to urinary stones and is responsible for approximately 1–2% of all urinary calculi. The disease often starts in childhood although most cases present in adult life.

Treatment is with a high fluid intake in order to keep the urinary cystine concentration low. Patients are encouraged to drink up to 3 l over 24 h and to drink even at night. Penicillamine should be used for patients who cannot keep the cystine concentration of their urine low.

The condition cystinosis (see p. 777) must not be confused with cystinuria.

Hartnup's disease
There is defective tubular reabsorption and jejunal absorption of most neutral amino acids but not their peptides. The resulting tryptophan malabsorption produces nicotinamide deficiency (see p. 138). Patients can be asymptomatic but others develop evidence of pellagra, with cerebellar ataxia, psychiatric disorders and skin lesions. Treatment is with nicotinamide and often brings about considerable improvement.

Tryptophan malabsorption syndrome (blue diaper syndrome)
This is due to an isolated transport defect for tryptophan; the tryptophan excreted oxidizes to a blue colour on the baby's diaper.

Familial iminoglycinuria
This occurs when there is defective tubular reabsorption of glycine, proline and hydroxyproline. It seems to have few clinical effects.

Methionine malabsorption syndrome
This is due to failure to absorb and excrete methionine, and results in diarrhoea, vomiting and mental retardation. Patients characteristically have an oasthouse smell.

Mucopolysaccharide disorders

Mucopolysaccharide disorders are inherited clinical syndromes due to the failure of the normal breakdown of complex carbohydrates. Partially degraded glycosaminoglycans accumulate in the skeleton, connective tissues and central nervous system.

Hurler's syndrome

This is inherited as a recessive disorder. Affected infants deteriorate after the first few months of life, both mentally and physically. Patients are short and have a characteristic facial appearance (gargoylism) with a flattened nose bridge and an open mouth with a large tongue. Death occurs in late childhood, usually from pneumonia.

Hunter's syndrome

This is similar to Hurler's syndrome but it is inherited in an X-linked recessive manner.

Morquio syndrome

In this syndrome the child becomes progressively more deformed and dwarfed. Intelligence is normal.

Lysosomal storage diseases (sphingolipidoses)

Lysosomal storage diseases are due to inborn errors of metabolism which are inherited in a sex-linked recessive manner.

Sphingolipids are degraded by a series of lysosomal enzymes, and accumulate, when there is a deficiency of these enzymes.

Gaucher's disease
In Gaucher's disease there is an accumulation of glucocerebroside in the reticuloendothelial system, particularly the liver, bone marrow and spleen. There are three clinical types, the commonest presenting in adult life with an insidious onset of hepatosplenomegaly. There is a high incidence in Ashkenazi Jews (1 in 3000 births), and patients have a characteristic pigmentation on exposed parts, particularly the forehead and hands. Typical Gaucher cells are found in the bone marrow, which are glucocerebroside-containing reticuloendothelial histiocytes. Patients develop anaemia, evidence of hypersplenism and pathological fractures due to bone involvement. Nevertheless, many have a normal lifespan.

Acute Gaucher's disease presents in infancy or childhood with rapid onset of hepatosplenomegaly with neurological involvement due to Gaucher cells in the brain. The outlook is poor.

Niemann–Pick disease

This is due to the accumulation of sphingomyelin in reticuloendothelial macrophages in many organs, particularly the liver, spleen, bone marrow and lymph nodes. The disease usually presents within the first 6 months of life with mental retardation and hepatosplenomegaly. Typical foam cells are found in the marrow, lymph nodes, liver and spleen.

Tay–Sachs disease (familial amaurotic idiocy)

In this condition there is accumulation of GM2 gangliosides in the central nervous system and peripheral nerves. It is particularly common in Ashkenazi Jews. There is a progressive degeneration of all cerebral function, with fits, epilepsy, dementia and blindness and death usually before 2 years of age. The macula has a characteristic cherry spot appearance.

Fabry's disease

This is due to a deficiency of alpha-galactosidase, causing an accumulation of alpha-galactosyl-lactosyl-ceramide in various tissues including the liver, kidney, blood vessels and the ganglion cells of the nervous system. The patients present with peripheral nerve involvement, but eventually most patients develop renal problems in adult life.

DIAGNOSIS

Many of the sphingolipidoses can be diagnosed by demonstrating the enzyme deficiency in the appropriate tissue.

Prenatal diagnosis is becoming possible in a number of the conditions by obtaining specimens of amniotic cells (see p. 105). Carrier states can also be identified, so that sensible genetic counselling can be given.

Cystinosis

In cystinosis, cystine accumulates in the reticuloendothelial cells. It is inherited in an autosomal recessive manner. The exact defect is unknown but it is thought to be a defect of cystine transport across the lysosomal membrane. Three forms are recognized: the infantile form is usually fatal in the first year owing to renal failure; the intermediate form presents in early/young adult life with fever and renal problems; and the adult form is benign. The generalized aminoaciduria seen in these patients often causes confusion with the Fanconi syndrome. Corneal deposits of cystine are seen.

The porphyrias

This heterogeneous group of rare inborn errors of metabolism is caused by abnormalities of enzymes involved in the biosynthesis of haem resulting in overproduction of the intermediate compounds called porphyrins (Fig. 17.15).

Structurally, porphyrins consist of four pyrrole rings. These pyrrole rings are formed from the precursors glycine and succinyl-CoA, which are converted to δ-aminolaevulinic acid (δ-ALA) in a reaction catalysed by the enzyme δ-ALA synthetase. Two molecules of δ-ALA condense to form a pyrrole ring.

Porphyrins can be divided into uro-, copro- or protoporphyrins depending on the structure of the side-chain. They are termed type I if the structure is symmetrical and type III if it is asymmetrical. Both uro- and coproporphyrins can be excreted in the urine.

The sequence of enzymatic changes in the production of haem is shown in Fig. 17.15. The chief rate-limiting step is the enzyme δ-ALA synthetase, as an increase in this enzyme results in an overproduction of porphyrins. Haem provides a negative feedback mechanism on this enzyme.

In porphyria the excess production of porphyrins occurs either in the liver (hepatic porphyrias) or in the bone marrow (erythropoietic porphyria), but porphyrias can also be classified in terms of clinical presentation as acute or non-acute. Acute porphyrias usually produce neuropsychiatric problems and are associated with excess production and urinary excretion of δ-ALA and porphobilinogen; these metabolites are not increased in non-acute porphyrias. The second control mechanism is therefore uroporphyrinogen-I–synthetase (see Fig. 17.15); this is depressed or normal in the acute porphyrias and raised in non-acute cases.

A classification of porphyrias is given in Table 17.17.

Acute intermittent porphyria

This is an autosomal dominant disorder. Presentation is in early adult life, usually around the age of 30, and women are affected more than men. It may be precipitated by alcohol and drugs such as barbiturates and oral contraceptives, but a wide range of lipid-soluble drugs have also been incriminated. The abnormality lies at the level of porphobilinogen synthetase in the haem biosynthetic pathway (see Fig. 17.15).

Fig. 17.15 Porphyrin metabolism. The numbers indicate the blocks occurring in various forms of porphyria. 1=acute intermittent porphyria; 2=congenital (erythropoietic) porphyria; 3=porphyria cutanea tarda; 4=hereditary coproporphyria; 5=variegate porphyria; 6=erythropoietic protoporphyria.

Table 17.17 The classification of porphyrias.

	Hepatic	Erythropoietic
Acute:	Acute intermittent porphyria Variegate porphyria Hereditary coproporphyria	
Non-acute:	Porphyria cutanea tarda	Congenital porphyria Erythropoietic protoporphyria

Presentation is with:
- Abdominal pain, vomiting and constipation (90%)
- Peripheral polyneuropathy (sensory and motor) (70%)
- Hypertension and tachycardia (70%)
- Neuropsychiatric disorders (such as depression, anxiety, and frank psychosis) (50%)

The diagnosis should be considered whenever there is a combination of these cardinal features or:
- A family history of porphyria
- The urine turns red-brown or red on standing. A classic bedside test for excess porphobilinogen may be performed by adding one volume of urine to one volume of Ehrlich's aldehyde, which produces a pink colour. If excess porphobilinogen is present the pink colour persists when two volumes of chloroform are added.
- Normal blood count; occasional neutrophil leucocytosis
- Abnormal liver function tests—elevated bilirubin and transaminases
- Blood urea often raised

MANAGEMENT

Management of the acute episodes is largely supportive. A high carbohydrate intake is maintained (this has an indirect effect on porphyrin overproduction), and a narcotic may be given for pain. Intravenous haematin infusion also appears to be of benefit.

Management in the remission period is by avoidance of possible precipitating factors.

Other acute porphyrias

Variegate porphyria

This combines many of the features of acute intermittent porphyria with those of a cutaneous porphyria. A bullous eruption develops on exposure to sunlight owing to the activation of porphyrias deposited in the skin. There is an increased production of protoporphyrinogens owing to an abnormality of protoporphyrinogen oxidase in the haem biosynthetic pathway (see Fig. 17.15).

Hereditary coproporphyria

This is extremely rare and broadly similar in presentation to variegate porphyria. The distinction is based on biochemical analysis.

Porphyria cutanea tarda (cutaneous hepatic porphyria) (see p. 936)

This condition, which has a genetic predisposition, presents with a bullous eruption on exposure to sunlight; the eruption heals with scarring. Alcohol is the most common precipitating agent. There is an abnormality in hepatic uroporphyrinogen decarboxylase. Evidence of biochemical or clinical liver disease may also be present. Polychlorinated hydrocarbons have been implicated and porphyria cutanea tarda has been seen in association with benign or malignant tumours of the liver.

The diagnosis depends on demonstration of increased levels of urinary uroporphyrin. Histology of the skin shows subepidermal blisters with perivascular deposition of PAS-staining material. The serum iron and transferrin saturation are often raised. The liver biopsy shows mild iron overload as well as features of alcoholic liver disease.

Remission can be induced by venesection; this should be repeated if the urinary uroporphyrin rises in the remission phase. Chloroquine may also have a useful role in promoting urinary excretion of uroporphyrins.

Erythropoietic porphyrias

Congenital porphyria

This is extremely rare and is transmitted as an autosomal recessive trait. Its victims show extreme sensitivity to sunlight and develop disfiguring scars. Dystrophy of the nails, blindness due to lenticular scarring, and brownish discoloration of the teeth also occur.

Erythropoietic protoporphyria

This is commoner than congenital porphyria and is inherited as an autosomal dominant trait. It presents with irritation and burning pain in the skin on exposure to sunlight. Hepatic involvement may also occur. Diagnosis is made by fluorescence of the peripheral red blood cells and by increased protoporphyrin in the red cells and stools. Oral β-carotene provides effective protection against solar sensitivity; the reason for this is not known.

Further reading

Bliss M (1983) *The Discovery of Insulin*. Edinburgh: Paul Harris.

Bloom A & Ireland J (1980) *A Colour Atlas of Diabetes*. London: Wolfe Medical.

Galton DJ (1985) *Molecular Genetics of Common Metabolic Disease*. London: Edward Arnold.

Havel JR (ed.) (1982) *Lipid Disorders*. Medical Clinics of North America, vol. 66, No. 2. Philadelphia: WB Saunders.

Keen H & Jarrett J (eds) (1982) *Complications of Diabetes*, 2nd edn. London: Edward Arnold.

McColl KEL, Moore MR & Goldberg A (1982) Porphyrin metabolism—the porphyrias. In Hardisty RN & Weatherall DJ (eds) *Blood and its Disorders*. 2nd edn. Oxford: Blackwell Scientific.

Stanbury JB, Wyngaarden JB, Fredrickson DS, Goldstein JL & Brown MS (eds) (1982) *The Metabolic Basis of Inherited Disease*, 5th edn. New York: McGraw-Hill.

World Health Organization (1985) *Diabetes Mellitus. Report of a WHO study group*. WHO Technical Report series 727, Geneva.

18

Neurology and Muscle Disease

Introduction

THE EPIDEMIOLOGY OF NEUROLOGICAL DISEASE

The spectrum of diseases seen in neurological practice over the last four decades has been dramatically changed by advances in treatment. Some previously common fatal diseases of the nervous system are now rarities. Examples of some of these advances are given in Table 18.1. Nevertheless, in many conditions therapeutic neurology still remains in its infancy and often no curative treatment is available.

Table 18.1 Some advances in treatment in neurological disease.

Condition	Advance in treatment
Neurosyphilis	Penicillin (1940s) Neurosyphilis now rare
Poliomyelitis	Immunization (1950s) Polio now exceptional in Britain
Subacute combined degeneration of cord	Fatal prior to B_{12} therapy
Myasthenia gravis	Advances in receptor chemistry and neuro-immunology (1970s)
Intracranial aneurysms and pituitary tumours	Advances in neurosurgery and anaesthesia

The neurological diseases seen commonly in the UK and some of the important rarer conditions are summarized in Table 18.2.

Despite the serious nature of many of the diseases, the majority of patients attending neurologists do not have sinister conditions. Tension headaches, migraine, dizziness and malaise are common presenting symptoms and frequently cause anxiety. 'Neurological' symptoms may be the presenting features of common psychological illnesses (e.g. depression or anxiety) which require sympathy, interpretation and treatment.

Prevalence rates often differ widely from annual incidence rates; these will be mentioned under the individual diseases.

Neurology in developing countries. In developing countries low standards of nutrition and hygiene with widespread economic under-privilege contribute to the different patterns of disease which are seen. Common neurological conditions of the Indian subcontinent, south-east Asia, and Africa include:

- Leprosy
- Tuberculosis (meningitis, tuberculoma)
- Meningococcal meningitis
- Tetanus
- Rabies
- Cerebral malaria
- Multiple vitamin deficiencies
- Cysticercosis

Of these, only TB and meningococcal infection are seen commonly in Europe.

Table 18.2 Neurological diseases: annual incidence rates per 100 000 population in the UK.

Disorder	Rate
Herpes zoster	400
Back pain and sciatica	300
Stroke	150
Epilepsy and single seizures	50
Dementia	50
Polyneuropathy	40
Transient ischaemic attacks	30
Bell's palsy	25
Parkinson's disease	20
Alcoholism (neurological complications)	20
Meningitis	15
Encephalitis	15
Subarachnoid haemorrhage	15
Metastatic brain tumour	15
Benign brain tumour	10
Primary malignant brain tumour	5
Metastatic cord tumour	5
Trigeminal neuralgia	4
Multiple sclerosis	3
Motor neurone disease	2
All primary muscle disease	1.5
Intracranial abscess	1
Benign spinal cord tumour	1
Huntington's disease	0.4
Myasthenia gravis	0.4

SOME COMMON NEUROLOGICAL SYMPTOMS

Headache

Headache at some time is an almost universal experience. It varies from an infrequent and trivial nuisance to a symptom of serious intracranial disease. The diagnosis is usually made by taking a careful history in which the patient should be questioned about the onset, duration, site and characteristics of the headache.

Mechanism of headache
The brain itself is almost devoid of pain receptors and thus, a priori, it is unusual for intracranial masses to cause headache.

Pain receptors are found in the vessels at the base of the brain (both arterial and venous) and in the meninges. These receptors are also present in extracranial vessels, the muscles of the scalp, neck and face, the paranasal sinuses, the eyes and the teeth.

Pain is caused by stimulation of pain receptors and/or the liberation of local chemicals such as histamine and 5-hydroxytryptamine.

Pressure headaches
Intracranial mass lesions displace the meninges and the basal vessels. When these structures are physically moved by changes in cerebrospinal fluid pressure (e.g. coughing), pain is exacerbated. Cerebral oedema, which accumulates around mass lesions, causes further shift. Headache is typically worse after lying down for some hours, i.e. on waking in the morning.

Any headache, however mild, which is present on waking and which is made worse by coughing, straining or sneezing may well be due to displacement or dilatation of the intracranial vessels and *may* be due to a mass lesion. These are often called 'the headaches of raised intracranial pressure'. They may be accompanied by vomiting.

Single episodes of severe headache
When patients complain only of a single episode of severe headache, the following should be considered:
● Migraine
● Subarachnoid haemorrhage
● Meningitis and encephalitis
● Sinusitis
● Hangover
● Migrainous neuralgia
● Tension headache
● Hydrocephalus (rare)

Particular attention should be paid to the presence of neck stiffness, rashes, vomiting and fever, which suggest meningeal irritation.

Recurrent severe headache
Most conditions that cause single episodes of headache can recur. However, migraine and tension headaches (see p. 845) are the commonest causes of recurrent pain.

Intermittent hydrocephalus due to an intraventricular tumour is a rare cause of recurrent prostrating headaches and weakness of the legs.

Headache of subacute onset
The onset and progression of a headache over days or weeks with or without the features of 'pressure headaches' should always raise the suspicion of an intracranial mass lesion or serious intracranial disease.

Encephalitis (see p. 837) and viral meningitis (see p. 836) should also be considered. Giant cell arteritis (see p. 847) should also be considered, particularly in the elderly.

Post-traumatic headaches frequently last several weeks. A subdural haematoma (see p. 822) should be considered when the nature of these headaches is suggestive of a mass lesion.

Chronic headaches

Almost all recurring headaches with a history going back for several years or more are due to muscle tension and/or migraine (see p. 845).

Dizziness and vertigo

'Dizziness' is a word patients use for a wide variety of complaints ranging from a vague feeling of unsteadiness to severe, acute vertigo. It is also frequently used to describe the light-headedness that is felt in anxiety and 'panic attacks', during palpitations, and in syncope or chronic ill health. Therefore, the *site* of this symptom must be determined, i.e. whether it is perceived in the limbs, the chest or the head.

Vertigo (an illusion of movement) is a more definite symptom. It is usually a sensation of rotation in which the patient feels that he or his surroundings are spinning or moving. Vertigo indicates disease of the labyrinth, vestibular pathways or their central connections.

Blackouts

Like dizziness, 'blackouts' is a vague, descriptive term implying either altered consciousness, visual disturbance or falling. Epilepsy, syncope, hypoglycaemia and other conditions must be considered (see p. 826).

Difficulty in walking

This is a common complaint in neurological disease; the main causes are given in Table 18.3. Arthritis and muscle pain also alter the gait, making it stiff and slow.

Spasticity

Spasticity (see p. 806) with or without pyramidal weakness causes stiffness and jerkiness of gait which is maintained on a narrow base. The toes catch level ground, causing wearing down and scuffing of the toes of the shoes. The pace shortens. Clonus may be noticed as involuntary extensor jerking of the legs.

Table 18.3 Common neurological causes of difficulty in walking.

Spasticity
Parkinson's disease
Cerebellar ataxia
Sensory loss (joint position)
Distal weakness
Proximal weakness
Apraxia of gait

When the problem is predominantly unilateral and weakness is marked (in a hemiparesis), the weaker leg drags stiffly and is circumducted around obstacles.

Parkinson's disease (see p. 828)

Here there is rigidity in both the extensors and the flexors of the limbs. Power remains normal. The gait slows; the pace shortens to a shuffle. The base remains narrow and falls occur. A stoop is apparent and swinging of the arms is diminished. The gait is 'festinant', i.e. hurried, as small rapid steps are taken. There is particular difficulty in initiating movement, in turning quickly and in stopping. Sometimes when the patient stops or is halted, a few rapid, small and unsteady backward steps are taken; this is known as retropulsion.

Cerebellar ataxia

In disease of the lateral lobes of the cerebellum the stance becomes broad-based, unstable and tremulous. The gait tends to veer towards the side of the more affected cerebellar lobe (see p. 808).

In disease of the cerebellar vermis (a midline structure), the trunk becomes unsteady and there is a tendency to fall backwards (truncal ataxia).

Sensory ataxia

The ataxia of peripheral sensory lesions (e.g. polyneuropathy, p. 857) is due to diminution of the sense of proprioception (joint position). The patient cannot perceive accurately the position of the legs. The gait becomes broad-based and high-stepping or 'stamping'.

The ataxia is made worse by removal of additional sensory input, e.g. in the dark or when the eyes are closed. This is the basis of a positive Romberg's test, which was first described in the sensory ataxia of tabes dorsalis (see p. 838).

Weakness of the lower limbs

With distal weakness the affected leg is lifted over obstacles. If the dorsiflexors of the foot are weak, such as in a common peroneal nerve palsy (see p. 857), the foot, having been lifted, returns to the ground with a visible and audible 'slap'.

Weakness of proximal lower limb muscles leads to difficulty in rising from the sitting position. Once upright the patient walks with a waddling gait, the pelvis being ill-supported by each lower limb as it carries the full weight of the body.

Apraxia of gait

In frontal lobe disease (e.g. tumours, hydrocephalus, infarction) the central organization of walking is disturbed. The patient is able to move the legs normally while sitting or lying but cannot walk in an organized way. This is known as 'apraxia of gait'—a failure of the skilled movement of walking.

NEUROLOGICAL EXAMINATION

There are two fundamental questions to be answered in any neurological problem:
1 What is the site or sites of lesions?
2 What is the likely pathology?

A full history, including past illnesses, family and social history, should first be obtained. The following headings summarize the essential elements of the clinical examination:
- State of consciousness
- Appearance, attitude, involuntary movements
- Orientation in time and place
- Recall of recent and distant events
- Level of intellect—a rough guide
- Language and speech disorders
- Cerebral dominance
- Disorders of higher function (e.g. apraxia)
- Mental state (see p. 869)
- The skull—shape, circumference, presence of bruits
- The neck—stiffness, palpation and auscultation of carotid arteries
- The cranial nerves
- The motor system
  - (a) Upper limbs:
    Wasting and fasciculation
    Posture of the outstretched arms—drift, rebound, tremor
    Tone—if increased, is it spasticity or 'extra-pyramidal' rigidity?
    Power—weakness may be graded roughly into 'slight', 'moderate' or 'severe' or, where appropriate, into grades devised by the Medical Research Council (Table 18.4)
    Tendon reflexes: + or ++ = normal; +++ = increased; 0 = absent with reinforcement
  - (b) Thorax and abdomen:
    Respiration
    Abdominal reflexes and muscles
  - (c) The lower limbs:
    Wasting and fasciculation
    Tone, power and tendon reflexes
    Plantar responses
    Gait
    Romberg's test

- The sensory system. Firstly, the patient is asked whether or not the feeling in the limbs, face and trunk is entirely normal.
  - (a) Posterior columns:
    Light touch
    Vibration (using a 128 Hz tuning fork)
    Joint position
    Two-point discrimination (normal: 0.5 cm on fingertips, 2 cm on soles) is sometimes valuable
  - (b) Spinothalamic tracts:
    Pain (pin prick)—use a clean pin
    Temperature
    A chart of areas of abnormal sensation is a valuable record.
- Co-ordination and fine movements

Short neurological examination

A detailed neurological examination is time-consuming and is not necessary in all patients, particularly those without symptoms suggestive of neurological disease. A short examination should however be carried out routinely and will detect the majority of defects.

Short neurological examination

Look at the patient
- General demeanour
- Speech
- Gait
- Arm swinging

Examine head
- Fundi
- Pupils
- Eye movements
- Facial movements
- Tongue

Examine upper limbs
- Posture of outstretched arms
- Wasting, fasciculation
- Co-ordination
- Reflexes

Examine lower limbs
- Power (hip flexion, ankle dorsiflexion)
- Reflexes
- Plantar responses

Assess sensation
- Ask the patient

INVESTIGATION

The history and examination remain the most important single 'test' in neurology, but specialist investigations such as computed tomography have

Table 18.4 Medical Research Council grades of muscle weakness.

Grade	Definition
0	No contraction
1	Flicker of contraction
2	Active movement with gravity eliminated
3	Active movement against gravity
4	Active movement against gravity and resistance
5	Normal power

revolutionized the management of patients during the last decade and have reduced the number of invasive tests performed.

Preliminary investigation

Examples of helpful routine investigation are given in Table 18.5.

Table 18.5 Preliminary investigations in neurological disease, with examples.

Test	Yield
Urinalysis	Glycosuria (polyneuropathy), ketones (coma), Bence Jones proteins (cord compression)
Blood picture	Macrocytosis (B_{12} deficiency), high ESR (giant cell arteritis)
Serum electrolytes	Hyponatraemia, hypokalaemia (weakness)
Blood glucose	Hypoglycaemia (coma), diabetes mellitus (coma)
Serum calcium	Hypocalcaemia, tetany
Chest x-ray	Bronchial carcinoma, spinal or rib lesions, thymoma

Specialized tests

Skull x-rays
Plain x-rays should not be done unnecessarily: they should only be performed if a fracture or intracranial pathology is suspected. The following lesions may be seen:
- Fractures and lesions of the vault (e.g. osteolytic lesions)
- Enlargement or destruction of the sella turcica (e.g. intrasellar tumour, raised intracranial pressure)
- Intracranial calcification (e.g. tuberculoma, oligodendroglioma, wall of an aneurysm, cysticercosis)
- Pineal calcification (to show midline shift)

Spinal x-rays
These show fractures and degenerative, destructive and congenital lesions.

Computed tomography (CT)
Method. This technique uses a collimated x-ray beam moving synchronously with detectors across a slice of brain between 2 mm and 13 mm thick. The transmitted x-irradiation from an 'element' of that slice (<1 mm^2) is processed by computer and a numerical value (the Hounsfield number) assigned to its density (air $= -1000$ units; water $= 0$; bone $= +1000$ units).

The difference in x-ray attenuation between bone, brain and CSF makes it possible to distinguish normal and infarcted tissue, tumour, extravasated blood and oedema. Examples of normal CT scans are shown in Fig. 18.1.

The image can be enhanced with intravenous contrast media to show areas of increased blood supply and oedema more clearly. Additional information about the subarachnoid space and the cerebral ventricles is obtained by scanning after the intrathecal injection of water-soluble contrast media (e.g. metrizamide) or air. In general, lesions of the order of 1 cm in diameter can be visualized on CT scans.

The method is safe (apart from occasional systemic reactions to contrast); the irradiation involved is comparable to a skull x-ray.

Uses. CT scanning is used for the diagnosis of:
- Cerebral tumours
- Intracerebral haemorrhage and infarction
- Subdural and extradural haematoma
- Subarachnoid haemorrhage
- Lateral shift of midline structures and displacement of the ventricular system
- Cerebral atrophy
- Pituitary lesions
- Spinal lesions

The CT scan can also be used to show a brain is anatomically normal with a high degree of accuracy.

Limitations. These are:
- Lesions under 1 cm in diameter may be missed.
- Lesions with attenuation close to that of bone may be missed if they are near the skull.
- Lesions with attenuation similar to that of brain may be difficult to diagnose (e.g. 'isodense' subdural haematoma).
- The results are poor when the patient does not cooperate; a general anaesthetic may occasionally be necessary.

Magnetic resonance imaging (MRI) (nuclear magnetic resonance scanning)
This technique makes use of the properties of protons aligned in a strong magnetic field. The protons are bombarded with radio-frequency waves at right angles to generate images. The equipment is expensive and restricted to specialized units.

The particular value of MRI scanning is its ability to distinguish between white matter and grey matter (Fig. 18.2). Brain tumours, syringomyelia, the lesions of multiple sclerosis and lesions in the posterior fossa and at the foramen magnum are demonstrated well.

Cerebral angiography
This shows the cerebral arterial and venous systems. Contrast is injected intra-arterially. It has been largely superseded by CT scanning for the investigation of cerebral tumours.

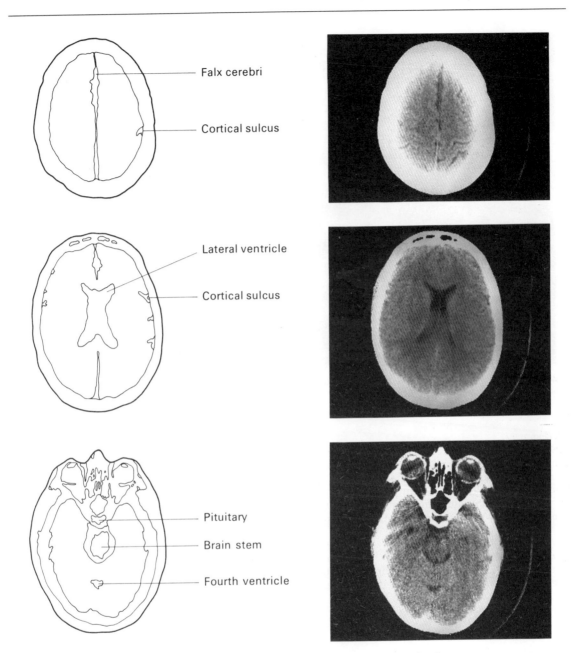

Fig. 18.1 Normal CT head scans: transverse sections at three levels.

Angiography is useful for the demonstration of aneurysms, arteriovenous malformations and venous occlusion. Films of the aortic arch and the carotid and vertebral arteries demonstrate occlusion, stenoses and atheromatous plaques. Spinal angiography is used to investigate arteriovenous malformations of the cord.

Angiography is invasive and requires a general anaesthetic; it should rarely be performed outside a specialist centre. It carries a mortality of around 1% and a 1% risk of stroke.

Digital vascular imaging (DVI) using computerized subtraction has recently been developed. Contrast is injected intravenously and no anaesthetic is necessary. The technique is of great value in the diagnosis of extracranial arterial disease. Intracranial vessels are less well seen.

Lumbar air encephalography
This once common neurological investigation is now rarely performed.

Fig. 18.2 MRI scan showing lesions of multiple sclerosis. Courtesy of MRI Ltd, London.

Myelography
A water-soluble radiopaque dye is injected into the lumbar (or rarely cisternal) subarachnoid space. This is used in the diagnosis of tumours of the spinal cord and other causes of cord compression.

Radiculography is an examination confined to the lumbar region to show compression of nerve roots.

Isotope brain and bone scanning
Labelled technetium in the form of $^{99}Tc^m$-pertechnate is injected intravenously and can be detected in the following vascular abnormalities in the head:
● Vascular tumours
● Arteriovenous malformations
● Cerebral infarcts
● Subdural haematoma

The method is safe, non-invasive and cheap, but is insensitive compared with CT scanning.

Isotope bone scanning is useful for detecting vertebral lesions (e.g. metastases).

Electroencephalography
Electroencephalograms (EEGs) are recorded from scalp electrodes on 16 channels simultaneously for 10–30 minutes. Their main value since the introduction of CT scans is in the diagnosis of epilepsy and diffuse brain diseases.

Epilepsy (see p. 822). It should be remembered that patients with epilepsy may have a normal EEG between fits.

Diffuse brain disorders. Slow-wave EEG abnormalities are seen in encephalitis, dementia and metabolic states (e.g. hypoglycaemia and hepatic coma).

Brain death (see p. 648). The EEG is isoelectric (i.e. flat). An EEG is no longer necessary to confirm the diagnosis of brain death in the UK.

Electromyography and nerve conduction studies
Electromyography. A concentric needle electrode is inserted into voluntary muscle. The recording is viewed on an oscilloscope and amplified through a speaker. The following can be demonstrated:
● Normal interference pattern
● Denervation
● Myopathic, myotonic or myasthenic changes (see p. 862)

Peripheral nerve conduction. Three measurements are of principal value in the diagnosis of neuropathies and nerve entrapment:
● Mean conduction velocity (motor and sensory) (see Fig. 18.3)
● Distal motor latency
● Sensory action potentials

Cerebral-evoked potentials
Visual-evoked potentials record the time taken for the response to a retinal stimulus to travel to the occipital cortex. Their value is chiefly in documenting previous retrobulbar neuritis (see p. 835), which causes a permanent delay in the latency despite clinical recovery of vision.

Similar techniques exist for the measurement of auditory and somatosensory potentials (from an arm or leg), though in general these techniques are less highly developed than those for detecting the visual-evoked response.

Examination of the CSF
With newer techniques lumbar puncture (LP) and examination of the CSF is carried out less frequently than in former years.

Indications for lumbar puncture. These now include:
● The diagnosis of meningitis and encephalitis
● The diagnosis of neurosyphilis and multiple sclerosis
● The intrathecal introduction of contrast media and drugs
● The diagnosis of suspected subarachnoid haemorrhage (sometimes)
● To remove CSF therapeutically (e.g. in benign intracranial hypertension) (rare)
● The diagnosis of miscellaneous conditions (e.g. certain polyneuropathies, sarcoidosis, intrathecal neoplastic involvement)

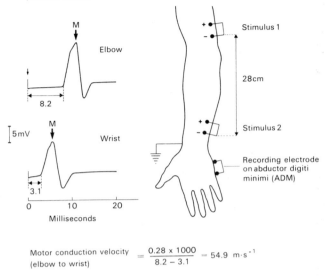

Motor conduction velocity (elbow to wrist) $= \dfrac{0.28 \times 1000}{8.2 - 3.1} = 54.9 \text{ m·s}^{-1}$

Fig. 18.3 Measurement of motor conduction velocity of the ulnar nerve. A recording electrode on abductor digiti minimi records the muscle action potential from the ulnar nerve at the elbow (stimulus 1) and at the wrist (stimulus 2). From these values the motor conduction velocity can be calculated.

Lumbar puncture

Lumbar puncture should not be performed in the presence of raised intracranial pressure or when an intracranial mass lesion is a possibility.

Technique
- The patient is placed on the edge of the bed in the left lateral position with the knees and chin as close together as possible.
- The third and fourth lumbar spines are marked. The fourth lumbar spine usually lies on a line joining the iliac crests.
- Using sterile precautions, 2% lignocaine is injected into the dermis by raising a bleb in either the third or fourth lumbar interspace.
- The special lumbar puncture needle is pushed through the skin in the midline. It is pressed steadily forwards and slightly towards the head.
- When the needle is felt to penetrate the dura mater, the stylet is withdrawn and a few drops of CSF are allowed to escape.
- The CSF pressure can now be measured by connecting a manometer to the needle. The patient's head must be on the same level as the sacrum. Normal CSF pressure is 60–150 mmH$_2$O. It rises and falls with respiration and the heart beat.
- Specimens of CSF are collected in three sterilized test tubes and sent to the laboratory. An additional sample in which the sugar level can be measured, together with a simultaneous blood sample for blood sugar measurement, should be taken when relevant (e.g. in meningitis).
- The patient should lie flat for about 8 h after the procedure to reduce the headache which may follow a lumbar puncture.

Contraindications for lumbar puncture. These are:
- Suspicion of a mass lesion of the brain or spinal cord. 'Coning' sometimes occurs if a mass is present and the pressure below it is relieved by LP.
- Any cause of raised intracranial pressure
- Local infection near the site of puncture
- Congenital lesions in the lumbosacral region (e.g. meningomyelocele)
- Platelet count below $40 \times 10^9 \cdot l^{-1}$ and other clotting abnormalities

These contraindications are relative, i.e. there are rare circumstances when LP should be performed in spite of the contraindications.

The composition of the normal CSF is shown in Table 18.6. Changes of diagnostic importance are mentioned under the sections on individual diseases.

Table 18.6 The normal CSF.

Appearance	Crystal clear Colourless
Pressure	5–15 cm of CSF with patient recumbent
Cell count	<5 per mm^3 No polymorphs Mononuclear cells only
Protein	0.2–0.4 g·l^{-1}
IgG	<15% of total CSF protein
Oligoclonal bands	Absent

Biopsy
Muscle. Biopsy is useful in the diagnosis of inflammatory and dystrophic disorders of muscle (see p. 862).

Peripheral nerve. Sural nerve biopsy is carried out to aid diagnosis in certain polyneuropathies (see p. 857), but it seldom helps with therapy.

Brain. Brain biopsy (e.g. of a non-dominant frontal lobe) is undertaken to diagnose inflammatory and degenerative brain diseases. It is rarely performed. Suspected herpes simplex encephalitis is a potential indication.

Psychometric assessment
Formal psychometric testing is used to assess intellectual function. Preservation of the verbal IQ (a measure of past attainments) in the presence of deterioration of the performance IQ (a measure of present abilities) is a useful indicator of dementia. Low subtests scores (e.g. for block design, speech or constructional skills) indicate impaired function of specific regions of the brain. The main limitation of these techniques is that depression and lack of concentration can also impair scores.

Miscellaneous tests
Certain specialized tests are employed in the diagnosis of individual (and often rare) neurological diseases. Examples are:
- Serum enzymes liberated from muscle—greatly raised in many primary muscle diseases (see p. 862). Creatine phosphokinase is the enzyme usually assayed in most laboratories.
- Serum copper and caeruloplasmin in Wilson's disease
- Antibodies to acetylcholine receptor protein in myasthenia gravis

Unconsciousness and coma

The central reticular formation which extends from the brain stem to the thalamus controls the state of consciousness. This complex process involves interactions between the reticular formation, the cortex and brain stem, and all sensory pathways.

Disturbed consciousness

Definitions
- *Consciousness* means awareness of oneself and the surroundings in a state of wakefulness.
- *Clouding of consciousness* is reduced wakefulness or awareness.
- *Sleep* (see p. 791) is a state of mental and physical inactivity from which the subject can be roused.
- *Stupor* is an abnormal, sleepy state from which the patient can be aroused by stimuli which may need to be repeated or vigorous.
- *Confusion* is the state of altered consciousness in which patients are bewildered and misinterpret the world around them.
- *Delirium* is a state of high arousal (seen typically in delirium tremens, see p. 893) in which there is confusion and often visual hallucinations.
- *Coma* is a state of unrousable unresponsiveness. A useful grading system for coma is shown in Table 18.7. An alternative grading system is given on p. 661.

Table 18.7 Glasgow 'coma' scale.

	Score
Eye opening (E)	
Spontaneous	4
To speech	3
To pain	2
Nil	1
Best motor response (M)	
Obeys	6
Localizes	5
Withdraws	4
Abnormal flexion	3
Extensor response	2
Nil	1
Verbal response (V)	
Orientated	5
Confused conversation	4
Inappropriate words	3
Incomprehensible sounds	2
Nil	1

Coma score = E+M+V (minimum = 3; maximum = 15)

Causes of coma

Altered consciousness is produced by three types of process affecting the brain stem, reticular formation and the cerebral cortex.
- *Diffuse cortical dysfunction.* Generalized metabolic (e.g. uraemia) or toxic (e.g. septicaemia) disorders can depress brain function.
- *Direct effect on the brain stem.* Lesions of the brain stem itself damage the reticular activating system.
- *Indirect effect on the brain stem.* Mass lesions above the tentorium cerebelli compress or damage the ascending reticular activating system in the brain stem.

It is important to understand that single focal brain lesions of the cerebral hemispheres do not produce coma unless they compress the brain stem. Oedema frequently surrounds hemisphere lesions, contributing greatly to their effects.

The 'locked-in syndrome' is a state of unresponsiveness but wakefulness due to massive brain stem

Table 18.8 Principal causes of coma and stupor.

Diffuse brain dysfunction
Drug overdose, alcohol
CO poisoning, anaesthetic gases
Hypoglycaemia, hyperglycaemia
Hypoxic/ischaemic brain injury
Hypertensive encephalopathy
Renal failure
Hepatic failure
Respiratory failure with CO_2 retention
Hypercalcaemia, hypocalcaemia
Hypoadrenalism, hypopituitarism and hypothyroidism
Hyponatraemia, hypernatraemia
Metabolic acidosis
Hypothermia, hyperpyrexia
Trauma—following closed head injury
Epilepsy—following a generalized seizure
Encephalitis, cerebral malaria
Subarachnoid haemorrhage
Porphyria

Direct effect on brain stem
Brain stem haemorrhage or infarction
Brain stem neoplasm
Brain stem demyelination
Wernicke–Korsakoff syndrome
Trauma

Indirect effect on brain stem
Hemisphere tumour, infarction, abscess, haematoma, encephalitis or trauma
Cerebellar lesions

infarction. The patient is unable to communicate or move but has a functioning cortex.

Unresponsiveness of psychological origin may cause difficulty in the differential diagnosis of apparent coma.

The principal causes of coma and stupor are shown in Table 18.8. A common cause of coma is self-poisoning (see p. 661).

THE UNCONSCIOUS PATIENT

Immediate assessment

Immediate assessment, which takes only seconds, is essential (Table 18.9).

Table 18.9 Immediate assessment of coma patients (see also p. 661).

Examine	Action
Airway	Clear, and intubate if necessary
Pulse (? absent) Pupils (? fixed, dilated)	Perform cardiopulmonary resuscitation if appropriate
For presence of trauma	If head injury present, anticipate deterioration

A history should then be obtained from accompanying relatives, friends, ambulance drivers or the police. Many patients with diabetes mellitus, epilepsy, hypoadrenalism and those who take corticosteroids wear or carry identifying discs or cards; these should be looked for.

Further examination

- The depth of coma should be recorded (Table 18.7).
- A full general and neurological examination should then be carried out.

GENERAL EXAMINATION

Temperature
This is raised in infection and hyperpyrexia and low in hypothermia.

Skin
The following should be noted:
- Colour (cyanosis, jaundice, purpura, rashes, pigmentation)
- Texture (coarse and dry in hypothyroidism)
- Presence of injection sites (diabetics, drug addicts)

Breath
Alcohol or ketones may be smelt on the patient's breath. Foetor may suggest hepatic failure or uraemia.

Respiration
Depressed but regular respiration occurs in most states of stupor and coma. The presence of particular types of respiration may point to the diagnosis:
- *Cheyne–Stokes respiration (periodic respiration)* is alternating hyperpnoea and apnoea. In neurological disease it implies bilateral cerebral dysfunction, usually deep in the hemispheres or in the upper brain stem, and may be a sign of incipient 'coning'. It may occur in metabolic comas, particularly if there is CO_2 retention from pulmonary disease.
- *Kussmaul (acidotic) respiration* is deep-sighing hyperventilation which occurs principally in diabetic ketoacidosis and uraemia.
- *Central neurogenic (pontine) hyperventilation* describes the sustained, rapid, deep breathing seen in patients with pontine lesions.
- *Ataxic respiration* is the shallow, halting respiration which occurs when the medullary respiratory centre is damaged. It is frequently a preterminal event.
- *Vomiting, hiccup and excessive yawning* may indicate a lesion in the lower brain stem in a stuporose patient.

NEUROLOGICAL EXAMINATION

Head and neck
The patient should be examined for evidence of trauma and neck stiffness.

Pupils
The size of the pupils and their reaction to light should be recorded. The following patterns may be seen:
- Dilatation of one pupil which becomes fixed to light indicates herniation of the uncus of the temporal lobe ('coning') and compression of the third nerve. This is a potential neurosurgical emergency.
- 'Pinpoint' light-fixed pupils occur with pontine lesions (e.g. a pontine haemorrhage) which interrupt the sympathetic pathways.
- Mid-position or slightly dilated pupils (4–6 mm) fixed to light and sometimes irregular are seen when damage to the midbrain interrupts the pupillary light reflex.
- Horner's syndrome (ipsilateral pupillary constriction and ptosis, see p. 796) occurs with lesions of the hypothalamus and also in 'coning'.
- Fixed, dilated pupils are a cardinal sign of brain death. They also occur in deep coma, particularly coma due to barbiturate intoxication or hypothermia.

Pupillary changes due to drugs are described on p. 662.

NB   No mydriatic drugs should be given to the unconscious patient.

Fundi
Any papilloedema should be recorded.

Ocular movements
In most cases of coma the eyes are slightly divergent. Slow, roving eye movements, usually horizontal, are seen in light coma.

The doll's head reflex and caloric reflex. Passive head rotation causes conjugate ocular deviation in the direction opposite to the induced head movement (doll's head reflex). This reflex is lost in very deep coma and is absent in brain stem lesions. It is absent in brain death.

Conjugate ocular deviation is seen when ice-cold water is run into the external auditory meatus; this is known as the caloric or vestibulo-ocular reflex and indicates that the brain stem is intact. In coma, this test is used mainly in the diagnosis of brain death (see p. 648).

Abnormalities of conjugate gaze (see p. 796). Sustained conjugate lateral gaze occurs towards the side of a destructive hemisphere lesion ('the eyes look *towards the normal limbs'*) because of damage to supranuclear pathways. In a pontine brain stem lesion, sustained conjugate lateral gaze occurs away from the side of the lesion, '*towards the paralysed limbs'*.

Rarely, an irritative lesion in the frontal region (e.g. an epileptic focus) may drive the eyes away from the hemisphere lesion, i.e. conjugate deviation may occur away from the side of the lesion.

Skew deviation (where one eye is deviated upwards and the other down) is a rare sign. It indicates a brain stem lesion.

Spontaneous eye movements. Spontaneous eye movements (other than roving eye movements) are distinctly unusual in coma of any cause.

The sudden, brisk, downward-'diving' eye movement seen in pontine (or cerebellar) haemorrhage is known as ocular 'bobbing'.

Motor responses
Impairment of consciousness makes it difficult to recognize focal neurological signs. The following should be looked for:
- The response to visual threat in a stuporose patient—this may show a hemianopia
- Tone—the only evidence of a hemiparesis may be abnormal flaccidity on the affected side
- The response to painful stimuli—this may be asymmetrical
- The facial appearance—drooping of one side of the face, unilateral dribbling, or blowing in and out of the paralysed cheek may occur
- Asymmetry of the tendon reflexes
- Asymmetry of the plantar responses. However, both are frequently extensor in coma of any cause.
- Asymmetry of decerebrate and decorticate posturing

INVESTIGATION

In many instances the cause of coma will be evident from the history and examination (e.g. head injury, cerebral haemorrhage, self-poisoning), and appropriate investigations should be carried out.

If the cause is still unclear, further investigations will be necessary.

Blood and urine
- Drugs screen, e.g. salicylates, diazepam (see p. 662)
- Routine biochemistry, e.g. urea, electrolytes, glucose, calcium, liver function
- Metabolic and endocrine studies, e.g. thyroid function tests, serum cortisol
- Blood cultures

Rare conditions such as cerebral malaria or porphyria should also be considered.

CT head scan
This may indicate an otherwise unsuspected mass lesion or intracranial haemorrhage.

CSF examination

Lumbar puncture should only be performed in coma after careful assessment of the case. It is contraindicated if an intracranial mass lesion is a possibility. A CT scan is often necessary to exclude this. CSF examination is likely to alter therapy only if undiagnosed meningo-encephalitis is present.

Management

The unconscious patient needs careful nursing with 2-hourly turns and frequent nursing observations to detect any change in vital functions or deterioration of conscious level.

Longer-term management requirements are:
- *Skin*—turning, skin care, avoidance of pressure sores, removal of rings
- *Oral hygiene*—mouthwashes, suction
- *Eye care*—taping of lids, prevention of corneal damage
- *Fluids*—prevention of dehydration (intragastric or i.v. fluids)
- *Calories*—liquid diet through a fine intragastric tube, 3000 kcal (1255 kJ) daily
- *Sphincters*—catheterization only if necessary (Paul's tubing if possible); avoidance of constipation (evacuate rectum manually if necessary)

Brain death

This is described on p. 648.

Sleep

Sleep is required on a regular basis. The reason for this is unclear; it is postulated that the laying down of memory is one important component. Complex pathways between the cortex and reticular formation are involved in the production and maintenance of sleep. During a normal night's sleep there are periods of deep sleep associated with rapid eye movement (REM). Dreaming occurs during REM sleep.

In *insomnia* sleep is fitful. Less time than usual is spent in REM sleep.

In *sleep apnoea* the normal short periods of apnoea seen during REM sleep are prolonged. This occurs with brain stem lesions and with upper airways obstruction, when it is accompanied by snoring. This is particularly important in patients with chronic obstructive airways disease who may become severely hypoxic (see p. 583).

Narcolepsy is irresistible episodes of sleep at inappropriate times (see p. 827).

The cerebral cortex

Lesions of the cerebral cortex cause symptoms by three processes:
- Destruction or impairment of function of cortical neurones and surrounding structures
- Irritation of neurones, causing partial seizures which may become generalized
- Displacement of the intracranial contents.

Cerebral localization

Cerebral dominance

The concept of cerebral dominance arose with the observation that right-handed patients with speech disorders had destructive lesions within the left hemisphere.

We now understand that the overall function of the left fronto-temporo-parietal region is communication. Destructive lesions at different sites within this region cause disorders of:
- Language (known as aphasia)
- Writing (known as agraphia)
- Reading (known as alexia)
- Calculation (known as acalculia)

Disorders in right-handed patients with *right* hemisphere lesions are more difficult to define, but consist of abnormalities of spatial perception and apraxia, i.e. loss of the ability to perform *patterns* of movement, though the patient understands their purpose and has neither loss of sensation nor weakness. Such patients tend to lose their way in familiar surroundings. They may fail to put on clothing correctly ('dressing apraxia') or to recognize once familiar faces.

Gerstmann's syndrome

This rare syndrome consists of an inability to name parts of the body, agraphia, acalculia and right–left disorientation. It is usually bilateral and is due to damage to the left hemisphere involving the supramarginal gyrus. It seldom occurs alone.

Table 18.10 summarizes the principal disorders seen with a local destructive lesion of the cortex.

Irritative lesions

The site of a lesion may also be suggested by specific irritative effects on the cortex and the surrounding structures. Table 18.11 summarizes these effects.

Speech, aphasia and dysarthria

Speech is communication by language. Aphasia (or dysphasia) is a loss or defect in language and is

Table 18.10 Principal disorders seen with a destructive lesion of the cortex in a right-handed individual.

Site of lesion	Disorder
Either frontal region	Intellectual impairment Personality change Urinary incontinence Mono- or hemiparesis
Left frontal region	Broca's aphasia
Left temporoparietal region	Acalculia Alexia Agraphia Wernicke's aphasia Right–left disorientation Homonymous field defects
Right temporal region	Confusional states Failure to recognize faces Homonymous field defects
Right parietal region	Dressing apraxia Failure to recognize faces Neglect of left limbs
Either parietal region	Contralateral sensory loss or neglect Constructional apraxia* Agraphaesthesia† Failure to recognize surroundings Limb apraxia Homonymous field defects
Occipital lobes and occipitoparietal region	Visual field defects Visuospatial defects Disturbances of visual recognition

* Inability to draw or construct shapes and patterns.
† Inability to recognize shapes drawn on the palm.

Table 18.11 Effects of an irritative lesion of the cortex.

Site of lesion	Effects
Frontal region	Partial seizures – focal motor seizures of contralateral limbs Conjugate deviation of head and eyes away from the lesion
Temporal region	Formed visual hallucinations Complex partial seizures Memory disturbances (e.g. déjà vu)
Parietal region	Partial seizures – focal sensory seizures of contralateral limbs Crude visual hallucinations, (e.g. shapes in one part of the field)
Occipital region	Visual disturbances (e.g. flashes)

caused by left fronto-temporo-parietal lesions.

Dysarthria, i.e. disordered articulation, should be distinguished from aphasia. Any lesion that produces paralysis, slowing or incoordination of the muscles of articulation or local discomfort will cause dysarthria. Examples are upper and lower motor lesions of the lower cranial nerves, cerebellar lesions, Parkinson's disease and local lesions of the mouth, larynx, pharynx, tongue and teeth. Many aphasic patients are also somewhat dysarthric.

Broca's aphasia (expressive aphasia, anterior aphasia)
This is due to a lesion in the left frontal lobe which causes reduced fluency of speech with comprehension remaining relatively preserved.

The patient is nearly mute and makes great efforts to initiate speech. Language is reduced to a few disjointed words and there is failure to construct sentences.

Patients who recover from this form of aphasia say that they knew what they wanted to say but 'could not get the words out'.

Wernicke's aphasia (receptive aphasia, posterior aphasia)
This is due to a left temporo-parietal lesion. Language is fluent but the words themselves are incorrect. This varies from the insertion of a few incorrect or non-existent words into fluent speech (when it may be difficult to recognize the aphasia) to a profuse outpouring of wholly non-existent words. This may be so bizarre that it can be confused with psychotic behaviour.

Patients who have recovered from Wernicke's aphasia say that when aphasic they found the speech of others like a wholly unintelligible foreign language, and though they knew they were speaking, could neither stop themselves nor understand what they were saying.

Nominal aphasia (anomic aphasia or amnestic aphasia)
This term is used to describe difficulty in naming familiar objects. When it occurs in a severe and isolated form, it is caused by a left posterior temporal/inferior parietal lesion. Naming difficulty is, however, an early sign in many types of aphasia.

Global aphasia (central aphasia)
This is a combination of the expressive disturbance characteristic of Broca's aphasia and the loss of comprehension of Wernicke's aphasia. It is due to widespread damage to the areas concerned with speech and is the commonest form of aphasia after a severe left hemisphere infarct. Writing and reading are also affected.

Memory and its disorders

These are described in Chapter 19.

The cranial nerves

THE OLFACTORY NERVE (FIRST CRANIAL NERVE)

This sensory nerve arises from olfactory (smell) receptors in the nasal mucosa. Branches pierce the cribriform plate and synapse in the olfactory bulb. The olfactory tract then passes to the olfactory cortex in the anteromedial surface of the temporal lobe.

Loss of the sense of smell (anosmia) occurs with head injury and tumours of the olfactory groove (e.g. meningioma).

The sense of smell is often lost, sometimes permanently, after upper respiratory viral infections. It is diminished in nasal obstruction.

THE OPTIC NERVE (SECOND CRANIAL NERVE) AND THE VISUAL SYSTEM

The optic nerve carries axons from the ganglion cells of the retina to the lateral geniculate bodies. The visual pathway is shown in Fig. 18.4. It should be noted that the lens causes the image on the retina to

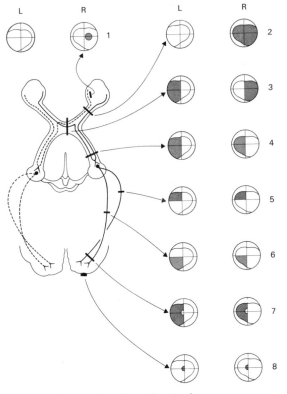

Fig. 18.4 The visual pathway (see text).

be inverted. Thus an object in the lower part of the visual field is projected to the upper retina and an object in the temporal half of the visual field is projected to the nasal half of the retina.

At the optic chiasm, fibres travelling in the nasal portions of the optic nerves cross to the opposite sides, where they join uncrossed temporal fibres from the lateral portion of each optic nerve. One optic tract thus carries fibres from the temporal side of the ipsilateral retina and the nasal side of the contralateral retina.

From the lateral geniculate body, fibres pass in the optic radiation to the visual cortex of the occipital lobe.

The visual field projected to each optic tract, radiation and cortex is called 'homonymous', to indicate the different (i.e. bilateral) origins of each pathway. (A homonym is the same word used to denote different things.)

Field defects are 'hemianopic' when half the field is affected, and 'quadrantanopic' when a quadrant is affected. 'Congruous' denotes symmetry and 'incongruous' lack of symmetry.

Visual acuity

This should be tested with a Snellen test chart and corrected for refractive errors with lenses or a pinhole. The corrected visual acuity should be recorded. The normal acuity should be 6/6 to 6/9 in both eyes.

Visual field defects

These should be charted by confrontation with white- and red-headed pins and, if abnormal or in doubt, recorded in detail with a Goldman (or similar) screen. The common defects are shown in Fig. 18.4.

Retinal and local eye lesions (Fig. 18.4, site 1)
Lesions of the retina produce peripheral visual loss (i.e. tunnel vision) or scotomata (small areas of visual loss). Common causes are diabetic retinal vascular disease, glaucoma and retinitis pigmentosa.

Local lesions of the eye (e.g. cataract) can also cause visual loss.

Optic nerve lesions (Fig. 18.4, site 2)
Unilateral visual loss, commencing as a central or paracentral scotoma, is characteristic of optic nerve lesions. Complete lesions of the optic nerve produce total unilateral visual loss with loss of pupillary light reflex (direct and consensual) when the blind eye is illuminated.

The causes of optic nerve lesions are given in Table 18.12. The principal pathological appearances of the optic disc are:
● Disc swelling (papilloedema)
● Pallor (optic atrophy)

Papilloedema (Table 18.13). This means swelling of the

Table 18.12 Principal causes of an optic nerve lesion.

Optic and retrobulbar neuritis
Optic nerve compression (e.g. tumour or aneurysm)
Toxic optic neuropathy (e.g. tobacco, ethambutol, methyl alcohol, quinine)
Syphilis
Ischaemic optic neuropathy (e.g. in giant cell arteritis)
Papilloedema of any cause
Hereditary optic neuropathies
Severe anaemia
Vitamin B_{12} deficiency (see p. 859)
Trauma
Infective—spread of paranasal sinus infection or orbital cellulitis

Table 18.13 Causes of papilloedema.

Intracranial mass lesions
Encephalitis
Subarachnoid haemorrhage
Benign intracranial hypertension
Metabolic causes, e.g. CO_2 retention, chronic anoxia, hypocalcaemia
Accelerated hypertension
Optic neuritis
Disc infiltration, e.g. leukaemia
Ischaemic optic neuropathy
Retinal venous obstruction (thrombosis, orbital lesions)

papilla—the optic disc. The earliest ophthalmoscopic signs are redness of the disc followed by blurring and heaping up of its margins (the nasal margin first). There is loss of the normal, visible, spontaneous pulsation of the retinal veins. The physiological cup becomes obliterated and the disc engorged, with dilatation of its vessels and the retinal veins. Small haemorrhages surround the disc.

True disc oedema should be distinguished from various conditions which simulate it. Marked hypermetropic (long-sighted) refractive errors make the disc appear pink, distant and ill-defined. Opaque (myelinated) nerve fibres near the disc and hyaline bodies (drusen) can be mistaken for disc swelling.

In difficult cases fluorescein angiography is diagnostic. In papilloedema, fluorescein injected intravenously leaks from the disc capillaries and may be seen and photographed.

Early papilloedema from causes other than optic neuritis (see below) often produces few visual symptoms, the patient's complaints being those of the underlying disease.

As disc oedema develops there is enlargement of the blind spot and blurring of the vision. As the disc becomes engorged its arterial blood flow is reduced and in severe papilloedema, infarction of the nerve occurs, often suddenly, with resulting blindness.

Optic neuritis. Optic neuritis is swelling of the optic disc due to primary inflammation of the optic nerve. The commonest cause is demyelination (e.g. multiple sclerosis). Disc swelling due to optic neuritis is distinguished from other causes of disc oedema by the occurrence of early and severe visual loss.

The term retrobulbar neuritis implies that the inflammatory process is 'behind the bulb' (i.e. the eye), so that no abnormality may be seen with the ophthalmoscope in spite of visual impairment.

Optic atrophy. Disc pallor (optic atrophy) may follow a variety of pathological processes, including infarction of the nerve, optic neuritis, optic nerve compression, syphilis, B_{12} deficiency and toxins (e.g. quinine and methyl alcohol).

Optic atrophy is described as consecutive or secondary when it follows papilloedema. The degree of visual loss depends upon the underlying pathology.

Defects of the optic chiasm (Fig. 18.4, site 3)
Bitemporal hemianopic defects occur when a lesion compresses the central part of the chiasm. Common causes are:
- Pituitary neoplasm
- Craniopharyngioma
- Aneurysm
- Secondary neoplasm

Defects of the optic tract and optic radiation (Fig. 18.4, sites 4, 5 and 6)
Homonymous hemianopia or quadrantanopia are the typical field defects caused by unilateral compression or infarction of these structures. Optic tract lesions are rare.

Temporal lobe lesions (due to tumour or infarction) cause upper quadrantanopic defects; parietal lobe lesions cause lower quadrantanopic defects.

Defects of the occipital cortex (Fig. 18.4, sites 7 and 8)
Homonymous hemianopic defects are caused by unilateral posterior cerebral artery infarction. The macular region (at the occipital pole) is spared because it has a separate blood supply from the middle cerebral artery.

Damage to one occipital pole causes a small, congruous, scotomatous, homonymous hemianopia.

Widespread bilateral occipital lobe damage by tumour, trauma or infarction causes the syndrome of 'cortical blindness' (Anton's syndrome). The patient is blind but characteristically lacks insight into the degree of visual loss and may deny it. The pupillary responses are normal. (See also p. 817.)

The pupils

Sympathetic impulses from fibres in the nasociliary nerve act on the dilator muscle of the pupil (dilator pupillae) and cause the pupil to dilate.

Sympathetic fibres to the eye (and face) originate in the hypothalamus, pass uncrossed through the midbrain and lateral medulla and emerge from the spinal cord at T1 (close to the lung apex). Postganglionic fibres begin in the superior cervical ganglion. These pass to the pupil in the nasociliary nerve from a plexus surrounding the internal carotid artery. Those fibres to the face (sweating and pilo-erection) form a plexus surrounding the external carotid artery. This arrangement is of clinical importance in Horner's syndrome (see p. 796).

Parasympathetic impulses, which pass from the ciliary ganglion in the short ciliary nerves to the sphincter muscle of the pupil (sphincter pupillae), cause the pupil to constrict.

An outline of the arrangement of parasympathetic fibres to the pupils and the mechanism of the light reflex are shown in Fig. 18.5.

The light reflex. Afferent fibres in each optic nerve (some crossing in the chiasm, see Fig. 18.5) pass to both lateral geniculate bodies and relay to the Edinger–Westphal nuclei.

Efferent (parasympathetic) fibres from each Edinger–Westphal nucleus pass via the third nerve to the ciliary ganglion and thence to the pupil.

Light constricts the pupil of the eye being tested (direct reflex) and the contralateral pupil (consensual reflex).

The convergence reflex. Fixation on a near object requires convergence of the ocular axes and is accompanied by pupillary constriction.

The afferent fibres in each optic nerve which pass through both lateral geniculate bodies also relay to the convergence centre. This centre receives 1a spindle afferent fibres from the extra-ocular muscles —principally the medial recti, which are innervated by the third nerve. The efferent route is from the convergence centre to the Edinger–Westphal nucleus, ciliary ganglion and pupils.

Clinical abnormalities of the pupils
Degenerative changes in old age. The pupil tends to become small (3–3.5 mm) in old age (senile miosis) and may be irregular. A bright light is necessary to demonstrate constriction. The convergence reflex is sluggish. A slight difference between the size of the pupils is common (physiological anisocoria), but the

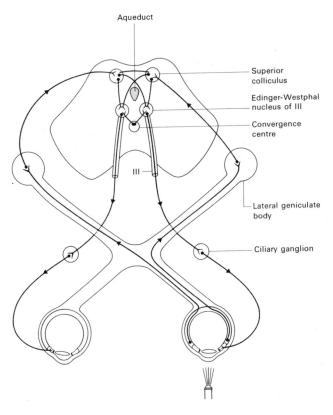

Aqueduct

Superior colliculus

Edinger-Westphal nucleus of III

Convergence centre

III

Lateral geniculate body

Ciliary ganglion

Fig. 18.5 The pupils: afferent and parasympathetic efferent pathways (see text).

changes may cause confusion with the Argyll Robertson pupil.

The Argyll Robertson pupil. This is a small irregular (3 mm or less) pupil which is fixed to light but constricts on convergence. The lesion is believed to be in the area surrounding the aqueduct.

The Argyll Robertson pupil is (almost) diagnostic of neurosyphilis. Similar changes are occasionally seen in diabetes mellitus.

The myotonic pupil (Holmes–Adie pupil). This is a dilated pupil seen most commonly in young women. It is usually unilateral. There is no reaction (or a very slow reaction) to a bright light, and slow and incomplete constriction to convergence. The condition is due to denervation in the ciliary ganglion.

The myotonic pupil is of no pathological significance, but is often associated with diminished or absent tendon reflexes.

Horner's syndrome. This syndrome is due to interruption of sympathetic fibres to one eye. It presents as unilateral pupillary constriction with slight ptosis and enophthalmos. The conjunctival vessels may be injected. There is loss of sweating of the same side of the face or body; the extent depends upon the level of the lesion. The syndrome indicates a lesion of the sympathetic pathway on the same side. Causes of Horner's syndrome are given in Table 18.14.

The level of the lesion is indicated by the distribution of the loss of sweating:
- Central lesions affect sweating over the entire half of the head, arm and upper trunk.

Table 18.14 Causes of Horner's syndrome.

Hemisphere and brain stem lesions
Massive cerebral infarction
Pontine glioma
Lateral medullary syndrome
'Coning' of the temporal lobe
Cervical cord lesions
Syringomyelia
Cord tumours
T1 root lesions
Bronchial neoplasm (apical)
Apical TB
Cervical rib
Brachial plexus trauma
Sympathetic chain in the neck
Following thyroid/laryngeal surgery
Carotid artery occlusion
Neoplastic infiltration
Cervical sympathectomy
Miscellaneous
Congenital
Migrainous neuralgia (usually transient)

- Lesions of the neck proximal to the superior cervical ganglion cause diminished sweating on the face.
- Lesions distal to the superior cervical ganglion do not affect sweating at all.

Pharmacological tests are helpful in indicating the level of the lesion. For example, a lesion distal to the superior cervical ganglion causes denervation hypersensitivity of the pupil which dilates when 1:1000 adrenaline is instilled. This dose has little effect on the normal pupil.

Other abnormalities of the pupils seen in coma are discussed on p. 790.

THE OCULAR MOVEMENTS

The control of ocular movement can be divided into:
- The central upper motor neurone mechanisms which effect the normal yoked parallel movements of the eyes (conjugate gaze)
- The oculomotor, abducens and trochlear nerves and the muscles they supply

Conjugate gaze
Fast voluntary and reflex eye movements originate in each frontal lobe. Fibres pass in the anterior limb of the internal capsule and cross in the pons to end in the parapontine reticular formation (PPRF; Fig. 18.6a); the PPRF was previously known as the centre for lateral gaze.

The PPRF is close to each sixth nerve nucleus. It also receives fibres from:
- The ipsilateral occipital cortex. These pathways are concerned with movements to track or pursue objects within the visual fields.
- Both vestibular nuclei. These pathways are concerned with the relationship between eye movements and the position of the head and neck (doll's head reflexes, see p. 790).

The PPRF coordinates lateral eye movements through the medial longitudinal fasciculus (MLF) (Fig. 18.6b). Fibres from the PPRF pass to both the ipsilateral sixth nerve nucleus and, having crossed the midline, the opposite third nerve nucleus via the MLF. Each sixth nerve nucleus (supplying the lateral rectus) and the opposite third nerve nucleus (supplying the medial rectus and others) are thus linked. The eyes move with parallel axes and at the same velocity.

Abnormalities of conjugate lateral gaze

It is important to understand that a destructive lesion of one side of the brain still allows the eyes to be driven laterally by the intact opposite pathway.

A destructive frontal lobe lesion (e.g. an infarct)

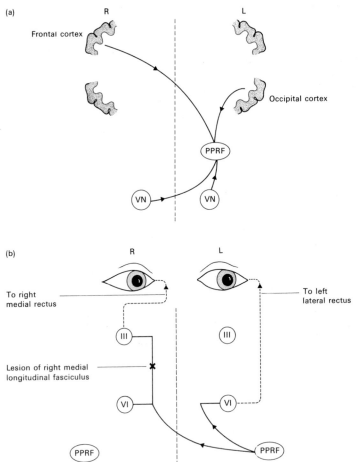

Fig. 18.6 (a) Conjugate lateral gaze: principal input *to* parapontine reticular formation (PPRF). VN = vestibular nucleus. (b) Conjugate lateral gaze: principal output *from* PPRF (see text for explanation). From Bannister R (1985) *Brain's Clinical Neurology*, 6th edn. Oxford: Oxford University Press.

causes failure of conjugate lateral gaze to the side opposite to the lesion (Fig. 18.6a). In an acute lesion the eyes are often deviated past the midline to the side of the lesion and therefore look *towards the normal limbs*. There is usually a contralateral hemiparesis.

An irritative frontal lobe lesion (e.g. an epileptic focus), by stimulating the opposite PPRF, drives the eyes away from the side of the lesion.

A unilateral destructive brain stem lesion involving the PPRF causes failure of horizontal conjugate gaze towards the side of the lesion. There is usually a hemiparesis and the eyes are deviated *towards the paralysed limbs*.

Doll's head reflexes and skew deviation
These may occur in coma (see p. 790).

Internuclear ophthalmoplegia
Internuclear ophthalmoplegia (INO) is one of the commoner complex brain stem signs which involve the oculomotor system. It is due to a lesion within the MLF.

It is a common sign in multiple sclerosis (MS). When present bilaterally it is almost pathognomonic of MS. Unilateral lesions are also caused by small brain stem infarcts. In a right INO there is a lesion of the right MLF (see Fig. 18.6b). On attempted left lateral gaze the right eye fails to adduct. The left eye develops coarse nystagmus in abduction.

The side of the lesion is on the side of impaired adduction, not on the side of the nystagmus.

Abnormalities of vertical gaze

A failure of up gaze is caused by an upper brain stem lesion, such as a supratentorial mass pressing from above, or a tumour of the brain stem (e.g. a pinealoma). When the pupillary convergence reflex fails, this combination is called Parinaud's syndrome.

Defective up gaze also occurs in certain degenerative disorders (e.g. progressive supranuclear palsy, see p. 830).

Impairment of up gaze also occurs as part of normal ageing.

Weakness of the extraocular muscles (diplopia)

Diplopia (double vision) implies that there is weakness of one or more of the extraocular muscles.

The cause is usually a lesion of the third, fourth or sixth cranial nerves (or a combination of these) or their nuclei, or disease of the neuromuscular junction (myasthenia gravis) or the ocular muscles.

Squint (strabismus)

This is the appearance of the eyes when the visual axes fail to meet at the fixation point.

Paralytic squint. Paralytic or 'incomitant' squint occurs when there is an acquired defect of the movement of an eye. There is a squint (and hence diplopia) maximal in the direction of action of the weak muscle.

Non-paralytic squint. Non-paralytic or 'concomitant' squint describes a squint beginning in childhood in which the angle between the visual axes does *not* vary when the eyes are moved, i.e. the squint remains the same in all directions of gaze. Diplopia is almost never a symptom. The deviating eye (the one that does not fixate) usually has defective vision; this is called amblyopia ex anopsia.

Non-paralytic squint may be latent, i.e. only visible at certain times, such as when the patient is tired.

The *cover test* is used to assess squint and to recognize latent squint. The patient is asked to fix on an object. The eye which is apparently fixing the object centrally is covered. If the uncovered eye makes any movement to take up fixation, then a squint must have been present. The test is repeated with the opposite eye—the fixing eye will not move when the other squinting eye is covered or uncovered.

The oculomotor nerve (third cranial nerve)

The nucleus of the third nerve lies ventral to the aqueduct in the midbrain. Efferent fibres to four external ocular muscles (the superior, inferior and medial recti, and the inferior oblique), the levator palpebrae superioris and the sphincter pupillae (parasympathetic) enter the orbit through the superior orbital fissure.

The common causes of an oculomotor nerve lesion are given in Table 18.15. Signs of such a lesion are:
- Unilateral complete ptosis
- The eye facing 'down and out'
- Fixed and dilated pupil

'Sparing of the pupil' means that the parasympathetic fibres which run in a discrete bundle on the superior surface of the nerve are undamaged by the lesion and the pupil reacts normally.

Table 18.15 Common causes of an oculomotor nerve lesion.

Aneurysm of the posterior communicating artery
'Coning' of the temporal lobe

Infarction of the nerve
    In diabetes mellitus
    Atheroma

Midbrain infarction
Midbrain tumour

In diabetes, infarction of the nerve usually spares the pupil.

In a third nerve palsy the eye can still abduct (sixth nerve) and 'intort' (fourth nerve). When a patient with a right third nerve lesion attempts to converge and look downwards, the conjunctival vessels of the right eye can be seen to twist clockwise; this is 'intortion' and indicates that the trochlear nerve is intact.

The trochlear nerve (fourth cranial nerve)

The trochlear nerve supplies the superior oblique muscle.

An isolated fourth nerve lesion is a rarity. The head is tilted away from the side of the lesion. The patient complains of diplopia when attempting to look down and away from the affected side.

The abducens nerve (sixth cranial nerve)

The abducens nerve supplies the lateral rectus muscle.

In a sixth nerve lesion there is a convergent squint with diplopia maximal on looking to the side of the lesion. The eye cannot be abducted beyond the midline.

There are many causes of a sixth nerve lesion. The nerve may be damaged in the brain stem as in multiple sclerosis, due to raised intracranial pressure, when it is compressed against the tip of the petrous temporal bone, or by infiltration by tumours, particularly nasopharyngeal carcinoma. An isolated sixth nerve palsy may occur in diabetes mellitus.

THE TRIGEMINAL NERVE (FIFTH CRANIAL NERVE)

The trigeminal nerve is mainly sensory but contains some motor fibres.

Sensory fibres (see Figs 18.7 and 18.11) from the three divisions—ophthalmic (V_1), maxillary (V_2) and mandibular (V_3)—pass to the trigeminal ganglion at the apex of the petrous temporal bone. From here central fibres enter the brain stem. Ascending fibres

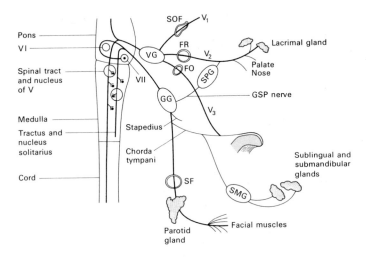

Fig. 18.7 Fifth and seventh cranial nerves and their relationships.
SOF = superior orbital fissure;
FR = foramen rotundum;
FO = foramen ovale;
SF = stylomastoid foramen;
SPG = sphenopalatine ganglion;
GG = geniculate ganglion;
VG = gasserian ganglion;
SMG = submandibular ganglion;
GSP = greater superficial petrosal.

transmitting the sensation of light touch enter the nucleus in the pons. Descending fibres carrying pain and temperature sensation form the spinal tract of the fifth nerve and end in the spinal nucleus in the medulla and upper cervical cord.

Motor fibres arise in the upper pons and join the mandibular branch to supply the muscles of mastication.

Signs of a trigeminal nerve lesion
Diminution of the corneal reflex is often the first sign of a fifth nerve lesion.

A complete fifth nerve lesion causes unilateral sensory loss on the face, tongue and buccal mucosa. The jaw deviates to the side of the lesion when the mouth is opened.

Central (brain stem) lesions of the lower trigeminal nuclei (e.g. in syringobulbia, see p. 850) produce a characteristic circumoral sensory loss.

When the spinal tract (or spinal nucleus) alone is involved, the sensory loss is restricted to pain and temperature sensation, i.e. 'dissociated' (see p. 812).

Causes of trigeminal nerve lesions
Brain stem. Lesions at this site involve the nuclei and central connections, and include:
● Brain stem glioma
● Multiple sclerosis
● Infarction
● Syringobulbia

Cerebello-pontine angle. Here the nerve is compressed by:
● Acoustic neuromas
● Meningiomas
● Secondary neoplasms

Apex of the petrous temporal bone. Infection from chronic middle ear disease involves the nerve at this

site. The combination of this and a sixth nerve lesion is called Gradenigo's syndrome.

Cavernous sinus. Here the trigeminal ganglion is compressed by:
● Aneurysm
● Extension of a pituitary neoplasm
● Cavernous sinus thrombosis
● Secondary neoplasm

The trigeminal ganglion is infected in ophthalmic herpes zoster (see p. 838), the commonest lesion of the ganglion.

Peripheral branches of the trigeminal nerve. These are affected by neoplastic infiltration of the skull base.

Trigeminal neuralgia

Trigeminal neuralgia ('tic douloureux') is a condition of unknown cause, seen most commonly in old age. It is almost always unilateral.

SYMPTOMS

Severe paroxysms of knife-life or electric-shock-like pain, lasting seconds, occur within the distribution of the fifth nerve. The pain tends to commence in the mandibular division (V_3) and spread to the maxillary (V_2) and (rarely) to the ophthalmic division (V_1). It occurs many times a day.

Each paroxysm is stereotyped, brought on by stimulation of a specific 'trigger zone' in the face. Washing, shaving, a cold wind or eating are examples of the trivial stimuli that may provoke the pain. The face may be screwed up in agony (hence 'tic'—an involuntary movement).

The pain characteristically does not occur at night. Spontaneous remissions last for months or years before recurrence.

SIGNS

There are no signs of trigeminal nerve dysfunction. The corneal reflex is preserved. Diagnosis is on clinical grounds alone.

TREATMENT

The anticonvulsant carbamazepine 600–1200 mg daily suppresses attacks in the majority of patients. It does not, however, prevent the tendency of the neuralgia to recur. Phenytoin and clonazepam are less effective.

If drug therapy fails, alcohol injection into the trigeminal ganglion or peripheral branches of the nerve can be carried out. Other surgical procedures (radio-frequency extirpation of the ganglion, nerve decompression or sectioning of the sensory root) are useful in difficult cases.

'Secondary' trigeminal neuralgia

Trigeminal neuralgia also occurs in multiple sclerosis (see p. 833), with lesions of the cerebello-pontine angle (see below), with tumours of the fifth nerve (e.g. neuroma) or when the nerve is compressed by an aneurysm. These lesions are usually accompanied by physical signs (e.g. a depressed corneal reflex).

Idiopathic trigeminal neuropathy

A chronic and isolated fifth nerve lesion may sometimes develop without any apparent cause. When sensory loss is severe, trophic changes (facial scarring and corneal ulceration) occur.

Post-herpetic neuralgia (see p. 838)

This may occur in the distribution of a division of the trigeminal nerve.

THE FACIAL NERVE (SEVENTH CRANIAL NERVE)

This nerve is largely motor in function, supplying the muscles of facial expression. The nerve carries sensory taste fibres from the anterior two-thirds of the tongue. The complex arrangement of the nerves to the face, their nuclei and connections is shown in Fig. 18.7.

The facial nerve arises from the seventh nerve nucleus in the pons and leaves the skull through the stylomastoid foramen.

Part of each facial nucleus supplying the upper face (principally the frontalis muscle) receives some supranuclear fibres from each hemisphere.

Signs of facial weakness
Lower motor neurone (LMN) lesions. A unilateral LMN lesion causes weakness of *all* the muscles of facial expression on the same side. The face, especially the angle of the mouth, falls, and dribbling occurs from the corner of the mouth. There is weakness of eye closure since the upper facial musles are weak. Corneal ulceration may occur if the cornea is exposed during sleep. The platysma muscle is also weak.

Upper motor neurone (UMN) lesions. UMN lesions cause weakness of the lower part of the face on the side opposite the lesion. The frontalis muscle is spared: the normal furrowing of the brow is preserved and eye closure and blinking are not affected.

In UMN lesions there is relative preservation of spontaneous 'emotional' movement (e.g. smiling) compared with voluntary movement.

Causes of facial weakness
The commonest cause of facial weakness is a supranuclear lesion, e.g. cerebral infarction, leading to UMN weakness.

Lesions at four other levels may be recognized by the associated signs.

Pons. The sixth nerve nucleus is encircled by the seventh nerve fibres and is therefore often involved in pontine lesions of the seventh nerve, causing a lateral rectus palsy.

If there is accompanying damage to the neighbouring PPRF (see p. 796) and corticospinal tract, there is the combination of:
● LMN facial weakness
● Failure of conjugate lateral gaze (towards the lesion)
● Contralateral hemiparesis

Causes include pontine tumours (e.g. glioma), demyelination and vascular lesions.

The facial nucleus is affected in poliomyelitis (see p. 54) and in motor neurone disease (see p. 851); the latter usually causes bilateral weakness.

Cerebellopontine angle. The fifth, sixth and eighth nerves are affected with the seventh nerve in lesions in the cerebellopontine angle. Causes are acoustic neuroma and meningioma.

Within the petrous temporal bone. The geniculate ganglion (a sensory ganglion for taste) lies at the genu of the facial nerve (see Fig. 18.7). Fibres join the facial nerve in the chorda tympani and carry taste from the anterior two-thirds of the tongue. The (motor) nerve to the stapedius muscle leaves the facial nerve distal to the genu.

Lesions within the petrous temporal bone cause:
● Loss of taste on the anterior two-thirds of the tongue
● Hyperacusis (an unpleasantly loud distortion of hearing) due to paralysis of the stapedius muscle

Causes include:
- Bell's palsy
- Trauma
- Infection of the middle ear
- Herpes zoster (Ramsay Hunt syndrome)
- Tumours (e.g. glomus tumour)

Within the face. Branches of the facial nerve pierce the parotid gland and supply the muscles of facial expression. The nerve can be damaged here by parotid gland tumours, mumps (epidemic parotitis) and sarcoidosis (see p. 603).

The nerve is also affected in polyneuritis (e.g. Guillain–Barré syndrome, see p. 857).

Weakness of the muscles of the face also occurs in primary muscle disease and disease of the neuromuscular junction. Weakness is usually bilateral. Causes include:
- Dystrophia myotonica
- Facio-scapulo-humeral dystrophy
- Myasthenia gravis

Bell's palsy

This is a common, acute, isolated facial nerve palsy believed to be due to a viral infection which causes swelling of the nerve within the petrous temporal bone.

SYMPTOMS

The patient notices marked unilateral facial weakness, often on waking. There is pain behind the ear. Hyperacusis and distortion of taste may occur.

SIGNS

There is a complete LMN facial weakness, sometimes with loss of taste on the anterior two-thirds of the tongue. The diagnosis is made on clinical grounds. *No* other cranial nerves are involved.

MANAGEMENT AND COURSE

Some improvement usually occurs towards the end of the second week. Thereafter, continuing recovery occurs, but this may take 12 months to become complete. About 15% of patients are left with a severe, unsightly, residual weakness.

Electrophysiological tests are of some help in predicting the outcome. After the third week the absence of an evoked potential from muscle (the nerve is stimulated over the parotid gland) indicates that recovery is unlikely.

Steroids (e.g. prednisolone 60 mg daily, reducing to 0 over 10 days) or ACTH reduce the proportion of patients left with a severe deficit, provided the drugs are given at the onset.

A tarsorrhaphy (suturing of the upper to the lower lid) may be necessary if there is prolonged corneal exposure.

Cosmetic surgery and/or re-innervation (e.g. anastomosis of the lingual nerve to the facial nerve) are sometimes indicated after a year has elapsed from the initial attack if there is severe residual paralysis.

The condition occasionally recurs and is very rarely bilateral.

Ramsay Hunt syndrome

This is herpes zoster (shingles) of the geniculate ganglion.

There is a facial palsy (identical to Bell's palsy) with herpetic vesicles in the external auditory meatus (which receives a sensory twig from the facial nerve) and sometimes in the soft palate. Deafness may occur.

Treatment for shingles should be given (see p. 925).

Hemifacial spasm

This is an irregular clonic spasm of the facial muscles, usually occurring in middle-aged women. It varies in severity from a mild inconvenience to a severe and disabling condition when it affects all the facial muscles of one side.

The causes are:
- Idiopathic
- Acoustic neuroma
- Paget's disease of the skull
- Following Bell's palsy
- Pressure from aberrant vessels in the cerebello-pontine angle

SIGNS

There are clonic spasms of the facial muscles on one side. A mild LMN facial weakness is common.

MANAGEMENT

Mild cases require no treatment. In severe cases various destructive or decompressive procedures on the facial nerve in the cerebello-pontine angle are helpful. Drugs are of no value.

Myokymia

Facial myokymia is a rare, continuous, fine, sinuous movement of the lower face which is seen in brain stem lesions (e.g. multiple sclerosis).

The term myokymia is also used to describe the innocent twitching around the eye which commonly occurs in fatigue.

THE VESTIBULOCOCHLEAR NERVE (EIGHTH CRANIAL NERVE)

This nerve has two parts—cochlear and vestibular.

Cochlear nerve

Auditory fibres from the spiral organ (of Corti) in the cochlea pass to the cochlear nuclei in the pons. Fibres from these nuclei cross the midline and pass upwards through the medial lemnisci to the medial geniculate bodies and the temporal gyri.

The symptoms of a cochlear nerve lesion are deafness and tinnitus. The signs are of hearing loss, with bone conduction decreased as well as air conduction. This is called sensorineural or perceptive deafness.

Vestibular nerve

Vestibular fibres from the three semi-circular canals, the saccule and the utricle pass to the vestibular nuclei in the pons. Vestibular nerve fibres also pass directly to the cerebellum.

The vestibular nuclei are connected to the spinal cord, the cerebellum, the nuclei of the ocular muscles and the parapontine reticular formation (PPRF), the spinal muscles and the temporal lobe.

The maintenance of balance and posture depends in part upon impulses passing between the neck and spinal muscles and the vestibular system.

The main symptom of a vestibular lesion is vertigo. Vomiting frequently accompanies acute vertigo of any cause. Nystagmus is the principal physical sign, often with loss of balance.

Vertigo

Vertigo (see p. 782) indicates a disturbance of vestibular, brain stem or, rarely, cortical function. The principal causes are given in Table 18.16.

Deafness and tinnitus accompanying vertigo

Table 18.16 Principal causes of vertigo.

Ménière's disease
Drugs (e.g. streptomycin, anticonvulsant intoxication)
Toxins (e.g. ethyl alcohol)
'Vestibular neuronitis'
Multiple sclerosis
Migraine
Acute cerebellar lesions
Cerebellopontine angle lesions
Partial seizures (temporal lobe focus)
Brain stem ischaemia or infarction
Benign positional vertigo

indicate that its origin is from the ear or the eighth cranial nerve.

Nystagmus

Nystagmus is a rhythmic oscillation of the eyes. It is a sign of disease of either the ocular or the vestibular system and its connections. Nystagmus is described as either 'pendular' or 'jerk'.

For true nystagmus to be present it must be sustained and demonstrable within binocular gaze.

Pendular nystagmus. Pendular movement means movements to and fro which are similar both in velocity and amplitude. Pendular nystagmus is always binocular, horizontal and present in all directions of gaze.

It is seen when there is poor visual fixation (e.g. long-standing, severe visual impairment) or as a congenital lesion, when it is sometimes associated with head-nodding. It does not occur in 'neurological' diseases.

Jerk nystagmus. Jerk nystagmus (the usual nystagmus of neurological disease) has a fast and a slow component to the rhythmic movement. It is seen in vestibular, brain stem, cerebellar and (very rarely) cortical lesions.

The direction of the nystagmus is named after the *fast* component, which can be thought of as a reflex attempt to correct the slower component.

Considerable difficulties exist when attempts are made to use the direction of jerk nystagmus alone as a localizing sign, although it is both a common and valuable indication of abnormality. The following statements help in the interpretation of jerk nystagmus.

In peripheral lesions:
- The nystagmus is horizontal or rotary, and is directed away from the affected labyrinth. Vertical nystagmus is not seen in peripheral lesions.
- In benign positional vertigo there is nystagmus after a delay of several seconds on testing. When the test is repeated, nystagmus is not elicited.

In central lesions:
- Nystagmus is vertical, horizontal, obliquely beating, down beating or different in type in the two eyes.
- On positional testing the nystagmus is immediate and does not fatigue.
- Nystagmus in a unilateral cerebellar lesion is towards the side of the lesion. It is greater in amplitude and slower in rate when the eyes are deviated towards the side of the lesion.

Investigation of vestibulocochlear nerve lesions

Audiometry is of value in distinguishing sensorineural deafness from conductive deafness.

Caloric tests are used to assess function of the

labyrinth. These record the evoked nystagmus when, first cold, then warm, water is run into the external meatus. Decreased or absent nystagmus indicates ipsilateral labyrinth, eighth nerve or brain stem involvement. In the normal caloric test:

- *Cold* water in the *left* ear causes nystagmus to the *right*
- *Warm* water in the *left* ear causes nystagmus to the *left*.

The right ear would give opposite responses.

Auditory-evoked potentials record the response from a repetitive 'click' stimulus. The level of the lesion may be detected by abnormalities in the response.

Causes of lesions of the vestibulocochlear nerve and its central connections

Lesions at five levels can be recognized by the associated signs.

Cortex. Vertigo sometimes occurs as an aura in a partial seizure of temporal lobe origin.
Deafness is very rare.

Pons. Vertigo is common with demyelinating or vascular lesions of the brain stem which involve the vestibular nuclei and their connections. A sixth or seventh nerve lesion, internuclear ophthalmoplegia or contralateral hemiparesis help localization. Nystagmus is frequently present.
Deafness is very rare.

Cerebellopontine angle and cerebellum. Perceptive deafness occurs. Sixth, seventh and fifth nerve lesions develop, followed by cerebellar signs (ipsilateral) and later 'pyramidal' signs (contralateral). Nystagmus is usually present; it may be to either side and/or vertical.
Causes include acoustic neuroma, meningioma and secondary neoplasm.

Petrous temporal bone. A seventh nerve lesion may be present. Causes include trauma, middle ear infection and Paget's disease of bone.

End organ disease. The main causes are:
- Ménière's disease
- Drugs (e.g. streptomycin)
- Noise
- Infection (middle ear)
- Intrauterine rubella
- Congenital syphilis
- Mumps
- 'Vestibular neuronitis'

Ménière's disease

This condition is characterized by recurrent attacks of the three symptoms—vertigo, tinnitus and deafness. It is associated with a dilatation of the endolymph system of unknown cause.

SYMPTOMS

The sudden, unprovoked attacks of vertigo with vomiting and loss of balance last from minutes to hours. Tinnitus and deafness accompany an attack but may be overshadowed by the degree of vertigo. The attacks are recurrent over months or years. Ultimately deafness develops and the vertigo ceases.

SIGNS

Nystagmus often accompanies an attack. Sensorineural deafness may be found.

MANAGEMENT

Medical treatment with vestibular sedatives (e.g. cinnarizine or prochlorperazine) is unsatisfactory. Each attack is, however, self-limiting. Betahistine 8 mg three times daily is sometimes helpful.
Recurrent severe attacks may require surgery, (e.g. ultrasound destruction of the labyrinth or vestibular nerve section).

Vestibular neuronitis

This common syndrome describes an acute attack of severe vertigo with nystagmus, often with vomiting, but without loss of hearing. It is believed to follow or accompany viral infections which affect the labyrinth.
The disturbance lasts for several days or weeks but is self-limiting and rarely recurs. Treatment is with vestibular sedatives. The condition is sometimes followed by benign positional vertigo. Very similar symptoms may be caused by demyelination or vascular lesions within the brain stem.

Benign positional vertigo

Positional vertigo is vertigo precipitated by movement, usually into a particular position. It may occur when turning in bed or on sitting up. The vertigo is transient, lasting seconds or minutes.
Vertigo can be produced by moving the patient's head suddenly. There is a latent interval of a few seconds, followed by nystagmus.
The syndrome of benign positional vertigo sometimes follows 'vestibular neuronitis', head injury or ear infection. It usually lasts for some months. There are no sequelae, although the condition sometimes recurs. Treatment is with vestibular sedatives.
Positional nystagmus (and vertigo) without a latent interval and which does not fatigue is

occasionally seen with neoplasms of the posterior fossa.

THE GLOSSOPHARYNGEAL AND VAGUS NERVES (NINTH AND TENTH CRANIAL NERVES)

The glossopharyngeal nerve

This mixed nerve arises in the medulla and leaves the skull through the jugular foramen with the vagus and accessory nerves.

Its sensory fibres supply all sensation to the tonsillar fossa and pharynx (the afferent pathway of the gag reflex), and taste to the posterior third of the tongue.

Motor fibres supply the stylopharyngeus muscle, autonomic fibres supply the parotid gland, and a sensory branch supplies the carotid sinus.

Isolated lesions are most unusual since lesions at the jugular foramen also affect the vagus and sometimes the accessory nerves.

Glossopharyngeal neuralgia

This is a rare, severe, paroxysmal neuralgia. Pain involves the pharynx and is triggered by swallowing.

The vagus nerve

This mixed nerve supplies the striated muscle of the pharynx (efferent pathway of the gag reflex), the larynx (including the vocal cords via the recurrent laryngeal nerves) and the upper oesophagus.

There are some sensory fibres from the larynx.

Parasympathetic fibres supply the heart and abdominal viscera.

Ninth and tenth nerve lesions

Unilateral lesions of the ninth nerve cause diminished sensation on one side of the pharynx. Unilateral tenth nerve lesions cause unilateral failure of voluntary and reflex elevation of the soft palate, which is drawn to the side opposite the lesion. Individual lesions of these nerves are unusual.

Bilateral combined lesions of the ninth and tenth nerves cause weakness of elevation of the palate, depression of palatal sensation and loss of the gag reflex. The cough is depressed and the vocal cords paralysed. The patient complains of difficulty in swallowing, choking (particularly with fluids) and hoarseness.

The causes of ninth and tenth nerve lesions are given in Table 18.17.

Lesions of the recurrent laryngeal nerves

Unilateral paralysis of this important branch of each vagus causes hoarseness (dysphonia) and depres-

Table 18.17 Principal causes of lesions of the ninth, tenth and eleventh cranial nerves.

Site	Pathology
Brain stem	Infarction
	Syringobulbia
	Motor neurone disease (motor fibres)
	Poliomyelitis (motor fibres)
Jugular foramen	Tumours
	Carcinoma of nasopharynx
	Glomus tumour
	Internal jugular vein thrombosis
Neck and nasopharynx	Tumours
	Carcinoma of nasopharynx
	Metastases
	Polyneuropathy

sion of the forceful, explosive part of the cough reflex. Bilateral lesions are a serious emergency and cause respiratory obstruction.

The left recurrent laryngeal nerve (which loops beneath the aorta) is more commonly affected than the right.

Causes of recurrent laryngeal nerve lesions include:

- Mediastinal tumours
- Aneurysm of the aorta
- Trauma or surgery to the neck

THE ACCESSORY NERVE (ELEVENTH CRANIAL NERVE)

This motor nerve to the trapezius and sternomastoid muscles arises in the medulla and leaves the skull through the jugular foramen with the ninth and tenth nerves.

Lesions of the eleventh nerve cause weakness of the sternomastoid (neck turning) and the trapezius (shoulder shrugging). The principal causes are shown in Table 18.17.

THE HYPOGLOSSAL NERVE (TWELFTH CRANIAL NERVE)

The motor nerve to the tongue arises in the medulla and leaves the skull through the anterior condylar foramen.

Twelfth nerve lesions

Lower motor neurone lesions of the twelfth nerve lead to unilateral weakness, wasting and fasciculation of the tongue. When protruded the tongue deviates towards the weaker side.

Some causes of a hypoglossal nerve (or nucleus) lesion are:

- *In the brain stem:*
  Motor neurone disease
  Syringobulbia
  Poliomyelitis
- *At the skull base:*
  Trauma
  Tumours
     Nasopharyngeal carcinoma
     Glomus tumour
- *In the neck:*
  Trauma
  Tumours

Bilateral supranuclear (upper motor neurone) lesions cause the tongue movements to be slow; in addition the tongue cannot be protruded very far. There is no fasciculation.

BULBAR AND PSEUDOBULBAR PALSY

A *bulbar palsy* is weakness of lower motor neurone type of the muscles supplied by the lower cranial nerves whose nuclei lie in the medulla (the 'bulb'). The weakness is caused by lesions of the lower cranial nerve nuclei, the (ninth to twelfth) cranial nerves themselves or by neuromuscular diseases.

    The symptoms, signs and causes of a bulbar palsy are mentioned under the sections on the ninth to twelfth cranial nerves. Isolated lesions of these nerves are rare.

    In *pseudobulbar* palsy, bilateral supranuclear (upper motor neurone) lesions of the lower cranial nerves cause weakness and poverty of movement of the tongue and the pharyngeal musculature. Signs of

a pseudobulbar palsy are a stiff, slow, spastic tongue (which is not wasted) and dysarthria with a 'gravelly' voice which is slow and sounds 'dry'. The gag reflex and palatal reflex are preserved. The jaw jerk is exaggerated. Emotional lability often accompanies pseudobulbar palsy. The principal causes are:

- Motor neurone disease (see p. 851), in which there are often both upper and lower motor neurone lesions
- Multiple sclerosis, in which it occurs mainly as a late (preterminal) event
- Cerebrovascular disease, in which it may occur with multi-infarct dementia

Severe difficulty with swallowing, dysarthria and a slow-moving tongue also occur in the late stages of Parkinson's disease and this should be distinguished from both pseudobulbar and bulbar palsy.

The motor system

THE CORTICOSPINAL TRACTS

The corticospinal tracts originate from the neurones of the fifth layer of the cortex and terminate on the motor nuclei of the cranial nerves and anterior horn cells of the spinal cord. The pathways of importance (see Fig. 18.8) in clinical diagnosis decussate in the medulla and pass to contralateral halves of the cord as the crossed lateral corticospinal tracts. This is the

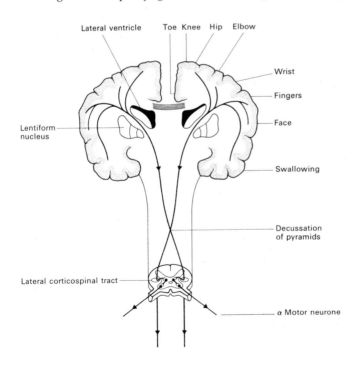

Fig. 18.8 The crossed corticospinal ('pyramidal') tracts.

'pyramidal' system, disease of which causes upper motor neurone (UMN) lesions.

A small proportion of the corticospinal outflow remains uncrossed (the anterior corticospinal tracts).

Characteristics of UMN lesions (Table 18.18)

Table 18.18 Signs of an upper motor neurone lesion.

Weakness with a characteristic distribution
Increase in tone of the spastic type
Exaggerated tendon reflexes
An extensor plantar response
Loss of abdominal reflexes
No muscle wasting
Normal electrical excitability of muscle

Weakness
A UMN ('pyramidal') lesion above the decussation causes weakness of the contralateral limbs, i.e. a hemiparesis. In an acute, severe lesion such as an infarct of the internal capsule, this weakness will be dense, but in partial lesions there is a characteristic *pattern* of weakness in the limbs: in the upper limb the flexors are stronger than the extensors, and in the lower limb the extensors are stronger than the flexors. In the upper limb the weaker movements are thus shoulder abduction and elbow extension; in the forearm and hand, the wrist and finger extensors and abductors are weaker than their antagonists. In the lower limb the weaker movements are flexion and abduction of the hip, flexion of the knee, and dorsiflexion and eversion of the ankle.

When the UMN lesion is below the decussation, the hemiparesis is on the same side as the lesion.

Increase in tone (spasticity)
An acute lesion of one pyramidal tract causes a flaccid paralysis (and areflexia). An increase in tone follows within several days due to loss of the inhibitory effect of the corticospinal pathway and an increase in spinal reflex activity. This increase in tone affects all muscle groups on the affected side but is most easily detected in the stronger muscles. It is of 'clasp knife' type, changing suddenly from increased to decreased resistance. The tendon reflexes are exaggerated on passive movement and clonus can commonly be demonstrated.

Changes in superficial reflexes
The plantar response becomes extensor. In a severe lesion (e.g. an infarct of the internal capsule causing hemiplegia) this response can be elicited from a wide area of the affected limb. As recovery occurs the area which is sensitive becomes smaller until only the posterior third of the lateral aspect of the sole is receptive. The stimulus may have to be unpleasant

(an orange stick is the correct instrument to use). For the response to be certainly extensor the dorsiflexion of the great toe should be accompanied by fanning of the toes.

The abdominal (and cremasteric reflexes) are abolished on the affected side. When the UMN lesion is above the fifth nerve motor nuclei the jaw jerk becomes exaggerated and pouting and facial reflexes appear.

The signs of a pyramidal lesion may be minimal. Weakness, spasticity or changes in superficial reflexes may predominate and the absence of one group of signs does not exclude a UMN lesion.

Clinical patterns of upper motor neurone disorders

Two main patterns of clinical features occur in UMN (pyramidal) disorders: hemiparesis and paraparesis.

Hemiparesis means weakness of the limbs of one side; paraparesis means weakness of both lower limbs.

The terms hemiplegia and paraplegia strictly indicate total paralysis, but the terms are often used to describe severe weakness.

Hemiparesis
The level of a unilateral lesion of the corticospinal tracts may be determined by the accompanying features.

Motor cortex. Weakness localized to a contralateral limb (monoplegia) or part of a limb is characteristic of an isolated lesion of the motor cortex. There may be a defect in higher cortical function (e.g. aphasia). Focal epilepsy may occur.

Internal capsule. Since the corticospinal fibres are tightly packed in the internal capsule, occupying about 1 cm^2, a small lesion causes a large deficit.

An infarct of a small branch of the middle cerebral artery (see p. 817) causes a sudden, dense, contralateral hemiplegia which includes the face.

Pons. A pontine lesion is rarely confined to the corticospinal tract alone. Adjacent structures such as cranial nerve nuclei (e.g. of the sixth or seventh nerve) are involved, causing ipsilateral cranial nerve lesions with contralateral hemiparesis.

Spinal cord. A lesion of one lateral corticospinal tract in the cord causes an ipsilateral UMN lesion and is indicated by a reflex level in the upper limbs (e.g. absent biceps jerk) or the presence of a Brown-Séquard syndrome (see p. 812).

Paraparesis. Paraparesis (or tetraparesis, when the four limbs are involved) indicates bilateral damage to the corticospinal tracts. This is due either to spinal cord compression (see p. 812) or to other diseases

Table 18.19 Causes of a spastic paraparesis.

Spinal cord compression (see Table 18.47)
Multiple sclerosis, myelitis
Motor neurone disease
Subacute combined degeneration of the cord
Syringomyelia
Syphilis
Familial or sporadic paraparesis
Vascular disease of the cord

Parasagittal cortical lesions
  Meningioma
  Venous sinus thrombosis

Hydrocephalus
Multiple cerebral infarction
Non-metastatic manifestation of malignancy

that cause bilateral UMN lesions as part of their clinical picture (see Table 18.19). Exceptionally bilateral weakness is caused by two separate lesions, one in each motor cortex.

THE EXTRAPYRAMIDAL SYSTEM AND THE CONTROL OF MOVEMENT

The extrapyramidal system is a general term for the basal ganglia and the cerebellum. In disorders of this system, the commonest of which is Parkinson's disease, there is a combination of:
● Reduction in movement, i.e. bradykinesia (slow movement) or akinesia (no movement)
● Involuntary movements (tremor, chorea, dystonia or athetosis)
● Rigidity

Anatomy and physiology

Structure
The corpus striatum, consisting of the caudate nucleus, globus pallidus and putamen (the latter two forming the lentiform nucleus) lies close to the substantia nigra, thalami and subthalamic nuclei. There are interconnections between these structures and the cerebral cortex, the cerebellum and the reticular formation, the cranial nerve nuclei (particularly the vestibular nerve) and the spinal cord (Fig. 18.9).

The overall function of this complex system is the initiation and modulation of movement. The system modulates cortical motor activity by a series of hypothetical servo loops.

It is now clear that the clinical picture of many basal ganglia disorders is the result of biochemical changes in neurotransmitters rather than discrete anatomical lesions. In Parkinson's disease there is:

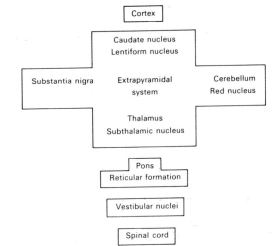

Fig. 18.9 The relationship of the extrapyramidal system to related structures.

● Reduction (to 10% of normal) of dopamine in the putamen and substantia nigra.
● Reduction of noradrenaline and 5-hydroxytryptamine (to 40% of normal) in the putamen.
● Reduction in substantia nigra and cerebral cortex of glutamic acid decarboxylase (GAD), the enzyme responsible for synthesizing gamma-aminobutyric acid (GABA).

Cholinergic activity is relatively well preserved in Parkinson's disease.

Changes in the balance between neurotransmitters are associated with characteristic clinical patterns. For example:
● In Parkinson's disease an increase in dopamine activity (due to levodopa therapy) relieves rigidity. In excess (in both normal people and those with Parkinson's disease), levodopa therapy causes chorea.
● In Huntington's disease (chorea) there is a marked reduction in acetylcholine and GABA activity in the striatum. Dopamine activity is normal.
● In normal people an increase in acetylcholine activity or a decrease in dopamine activity causes rigidity and bradykinesia (parkinsonism). For example, reserpine (which depletes neurones of dopamine) and phenothiazines or butyrophenones (which block dopaminergic neurones) cause or exacerbate parkinsonism.

Extrapyramidal disorders can be divided into the akinetic-rigid syndromes (see p. 827), in which poverty of movement predominates, and the dyskinesias, in which there are a variety of involuntary movements.

CEREBELLUM

The cerebellum receives afferent fibres from:
- Proprioceptive organs in joints and muscles
- The vestibular nuclei
- The basal ganglia
- The corticospinal system

Efferent fibres pass from the cerebellum to:
- Each red nucleus
- The vestibular nuclei
- The basal ganglia
- The anterior horn cells

Each lateral lobe of the cerebellum coordinates movement of the ipsilateral limb. The vermis (a midline structure) is concerned with maintenance of axial (midline) posture and balance.

Cerebellar lesions

Expanding mass lesions within the cerebellum produce hydrocephalus, causing severe headaches, vomiting and papilloedema. 'Coning' of the cerebellar tonsils through the foramen magnum and respiratory arrest occur, often within hours. Very rarely 'tonic seizures' of the limbs occur with cerebellar masses.

Lateral cerebellar lobes
A lesion within one cerebellar lobe (e.g. a tumour or infarction) causes disruption of the normal sequence of movements (dyssynergia) on the side of the lesion.

Posture and gait. The outstretched arm is held still in the early stages of a cerebellar lesion but there is rebound overshoot when the limb is pressed downwards by the examiner and released. As the lesion progresses, coarse tremor develops. Gait is ataxic with a broad base; the patient falters towards the side of the lesion.

Tremor and ataxia. Movement is imprecise in direction, in force and in distance (dysmetria).
Rapid alternating movements (tapping, clapping or rotary movements of the hand) are clumsy and disorganized (dysdiadochokinesis).
'Intention tremor' (action tremor) is produced when the 'finger–nose–finger' and 'heel–shin' tests are performed.

Nystagmus (see p. 802). Coarse horizontal nystagmus appears with cerebellar lobar lesions. Its direction is towards the side of the lesion and it is most marked on looking towards this side. Postural nystagmus sometimes occurs.

Dysarthria. Speech is affected (usually with bilateral lesions). A halting, jerking dysarthria results—the 'scanning speech' of cerebellar lesions.

Other signs. Titubation—rhythmic tremor of the head in either to and fro ('yes–yes') movements or rotary ('no–no') movements—also occurs, mainly when cerebellar connections are involved (e.g. in essential tremor or demyelination).
Hypotonia and depression of reflexes are also sometimes seen with cerebellar disease but are usually of little value as localizing signs. 'Pendular', i.e. slow, reflexes also occur.

Midline cerebellar lesions
Lesions of the cerebellar vermis have a dramatic effect on the equilibrium of the trunk and axial musculature. Truncal ataxia causes difficulty in

Table 18.20 Principal causes of cerebellar syndromes.

Cause	Comments

Primary or secondary neoplasm, e.g.
    Haemangioblastoma
    Medulloblastoma
    Secondary neoplasm
    Compression by acoustic
    neuroma
	Unilateral involvement

Cerebellar haemorrhage	Unilateral involvement
Cerebellar infarction	Unilateral involvement
Cerebellar abscess	Unilateral involvement

Development lesions, e.g.
    Arnold–Chiari malformation
    Basilar invagination
	Unilateral and bilateral involvement

Multiple sclerosis	Unilateral or bilateral involvement
Hydrocephalus	
Paget's disease of the skull	Basilar invagination

'Toxic' cerebellar syndromes
    Anticonvulsant drugs
    Alcohol
    Carbon monoxide poisoning
    Lead poisoning	

Inherited cerebellar disease, e.g.
    Friedreich's ataxia
    Ataxia telangiectasia
    Essential tremor	

Post-infective cerebellar syndrome of childhood	Transient ataxia occurring after exanthemata or infectious mononucleosis
Hypothyroidism	
Non-metastatic manifestation of malignancy	
Cerebral oedema of chronic hypoxia	

standing and sitting unsupported, with a rolling, broad, ataxic gait.

Lesions of the flocculonodular region cause vertigo, vomiting and ataxia of gait if they extend to the roof of the fourth ventricle.

Table 18.20 summarizes the main causes of cerebellar disease.

TREMOR

Tremor is an oscillation, regular and sinusoidal, of a part of the body. Different varieties are outlined below.

Postural tremor
Everyone has a physiological tremor of the outstretched hands at 8–12 Hz. This is increased with anxiety, hyperthyroidism and certain drugs (lithium, sodium valproate and sympathomimetics) or in mercury poisoning. A coarse, postural tremor is seen in chronic alcoholism and in benign essential tremor (usually at 5–8 Hz). Postural tremor does not worsen on movement.

Intention tremor
Tremor which is exacerbated by action, with past-pointing and accompanying slowness and incoordination of rapid alternating movement (dysdiadochokinesis), occurs in cerebellar lobe disease and with lesions of cerebellar connections. Titubation (tremor of the head) and nystagmus may be present.

Rest tremor
This occurs primarily in Parkinson's disease and is sometimes described as 'pill-rolling' between the thumb and index finger. It is present at rest, is between 4–7 Hz, and is not made worse by action.

Other tremors
Tremor is seen following lesions of the red nucleus (e.g. infarction, demyelination) and rarely with frontal lobe lesions.

LOWER MOTOR NEURONES

The lower motor neurone (LMN) is the motor pathway from the anterior horn cell (or cranial nerve nucleus) via a peripheral nerve to the motor end plate.

The motor unit consists of a single anterior horn cell, the single fast-conducting alpha motor nerve fibre which leaves the spinal cord via the anterior root, and the group of muscle fibres (100–2000) being supplied via the mixed peripheral nerve. The anterior horn cell is activated by the impulses from:
- The corticospinal tracts

- The extrapyramidal system (basal ganglia and cerebellum)
- Afferent fibres from the posterior roots

Signs of an LMN lesion

Voluntary muscle depends upon the motor unit for all movement and also for its metabolic integrity. Signs follow rapidly if the LMN is interrupted at any point in its course (Table 18.21). Wasting appears within three weeks of the development of an LMN lesion. Fasciculation (fine twitching of muscle) also occurs at this time and is due to sprouting of surviving axons re-innervating muscle cells that have lost their nerve supply.

Table 18.21 Signs of a lower motor neurone lesion.

Weakness of muscle or muscles supplied
Wasting
Hypotonia
Reflex loss confined to the reflex arc affected
Fasciculation
Fibrillation potentials (detected electromyographically, see p. 862)
Contractures of muscle
'Trophic' changes in skin and nails

Causes of an LMN lesion

Examples of LMN lesions at various levels are:
- Anterior horn cell—poliomyelitis, motor neurone disease
- Spinal root—cervical and lumbar root lesions, neuralgic amyotrophy
- Peripheral (or cranial) nerve—nerve trauma or compression, polyneuropathy

THE SPINAL REFLEX ARC

The components of the spinal reflex arc are illustrated in Fig. 18.10. The stretch reflex is the physiological basis for the tendon reflexes. For example, in the knee jerk, a tap on the patellar tendon activates stretch receptors in the quadriceps. Impulses in first-order sensory neurones pass directly to lower motor neurones (L3 and L4) which activate the quadriceps, causing a contraction.

Loss of a tendon reflex is caused by a lesion anywhere along the spinal reflex path. The reflex lost indicates the level of the lesion (Table 18.22).

Reinforcement
Distraction of the patient's attention, clenching the teeth or pulling of the interlocked fingers increases the activity of the stretch reflex. Such 'reinforcement'

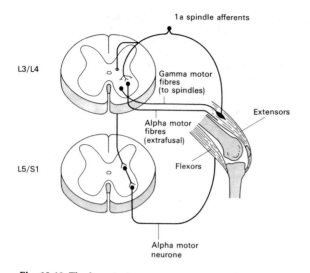

Fig. 18.10 The knee jerk: an example of a spinal reflex arc.

Table 18.22 Spinal levels of tendon reflexes.

Spinal level	Reflex
C5–6	Brachioradialis
C5–6	Biceps
C7	Triceps
L3–4	Knee
S1	Ankle

manoeuvres should be carried out before a reflex is recorded as absent.

The sensory system

Peripheral nerves and spinal roots

Peripheral nerves carry all modalities of sensation from either free or specialized nerve endings to the dorsal root ganglia and thus to the cord.

The sensory distribution of the spinal roots (dermatomes) is shown in Fig. 18.11.

The spinal cord (Fig. 18.12)

Posterior columns
For clinical purposes the sensory modalities of vibration sense, joint position, light touch and two-point discrimination travel uncrossed in the posterior columns to the gracile and cuneate nuclei in the medulla. Axons from second-order neurones cross the midline in the brain stem to form the medial lemniscus and pass to the thalamus.

Spinothalamic tracts
Fibres carrying pain and temperature sensation synapse in the dorsal horn of the cord, cross the cord and pass as the spinothalamic tracts to the thalamus and reticular formation.

The sensory cortex

The projection of fibres from the thalamus to the sensory cortex of the parietal region is shown in Fig. 18.12. Connections also exist between the thalamus and the motor cortex.

LESIONS OF THE SENSORY PATHWAYS

Paraesthesiae, numbness and pain are the principal symptoms of lesions of the sensory pathways below the level of the thalamus. The quality and distribution of the symptoms may suggest the site of the lesion.

Peripheral nerve lesions

The symptoms are felt in the distribution of the affected peripheral nerve (see p. 855).

Fig. 18.11 The dermatomes. The inset shows the distribution of the sensory loss in lesions of the peripheral branches of the fifth cranial nerve.

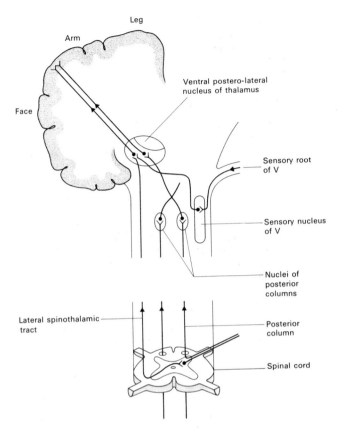

Fig. 18.12 The principal sensory pathways. The posterior columns remain uncrossed until the medulla. The spinothalamic tracts cross close to their entry into the spinal cord.

Section of a nerve is followed by complete sensory loss. Nerve entrapment (see p. 856) causes numbness, pain and tingling. Tapping the site of compression sometimes causes a sharp, electric-shock-like pain in the distribution of the nerve (Tinel's sign). All peripheral nerve lesions can cause neuralgia—a local pain of great severity. Examples are:

- Trigeminal neuralgia
- Migrainous neuralgia
- Post-herpetic neuralgia
- Causalgia

Spinal root lesions

Root pain
The pain of spinal root compression is felt around the affected root. The pain is referred to the myotome supplied by the root, and causes a tingling discomfort in the dermatome. The pain is made worse by manoeuvres that either stretch the nerve root (as in straight leg raising) or which increase the pressure in the spinal subarachnoid space (as in coughing and straining).

Examples of compressive root lesions are cervical or lumbar disc protrusions (see p. 860).

Dorsal root lesions
Section of a dorsal root causes loss of all modalities of sensation in the appropriate dermatome. However, the overlap with adjacent dermatomes may make it difficult to detect anaesthesia.

Lightning pain. Tabes dorsalis (now a rarity) is a form of neurosyphilis which causes a low-grade inflammation of the dorsal roots, posterior columns and root entry zone of the cord. Its presentation includes irregular, sharp, momentary stab-like pains which involve one or two spots, typically in a calf, thigh or ankle.

Spinal cord lesions

Posterior column lesions
Posterior column lesions cause:
- Tingling of a limb
- Electric-shock-like sensations
- Clumsiness
- Numbness
- Band-like sensations

These symptoms are often felt vaguely without a clear sensory level on the side of the lesion.

Position sense, vibration sense, light touch and

two-point discrimination are lost below the level of the lesion. Loss of position sense produces sensory ataxia (see p. 782).

L'Hermitte's sign

This is an electric-shock-like sensation radiating down the trunk and limbs which is produced by neck flexion. It indicates a cervical cord lesion. L'Hermitte's sign is common in acute exacerbations of multiple sclerosis (see p. 833). It also occurs in cervical spondylotic myelopathy (see p. 860) and subacute combined degeneration of the cord (see p. 859).

Spinothalamic tract lesions

Pure spinothalamic lesions cause isolated contralateral loss of pain and temperature sensation below the level of the lesion. This is called 'dissociated sensory loss'.

The spinal level is modified by the lamination of fibres within the spinothalamic tracts. Fibres from the lower spinal roots lie superficially and are therefore damaged first by compressive lesions from outside the cord. As an external compressive lesion (e.g. a midthoracic spinal meningioma; see Fig. 18.13) enlarges, the spinal sensory level ascends as deeper fibres become involved. Conversely, a central lesion

of the cord (e.g. a syrinx, see p. 850) affects the deeper fibres first.

Symptoms of spinothalamic tract lesions are the absence of pain (resulting in painless burns and minor injuries) or the loss of temperature sensation. Perforating ulcers and neuropathic joints may follow.

Spinal cord compression

This important syndrome causes a progressive spastic paraparesis (or tetraparesis) with sensory loss below the level of the lesion. Sphincter disturbance is common.

Root pain is frequent but not invariable. It is felt characteristically at the site of compression. It radiates in a band around the chest with thoracic cord lesions (e.g. meningioma) and is made worse by coughing, straining and jarring as the meningeal sheath of the root is stretched.

Involvement of one spinothalamic tract (contralateral loss of pain and temperature) together with one corticospinal tract (ipsilateral 'pyramidal' signs) is known as the 'Brown-Séquard syndrome' of hemisection of the cord.

Paraparesis and spinal cord disease are discussed on pp. 806 and 848.

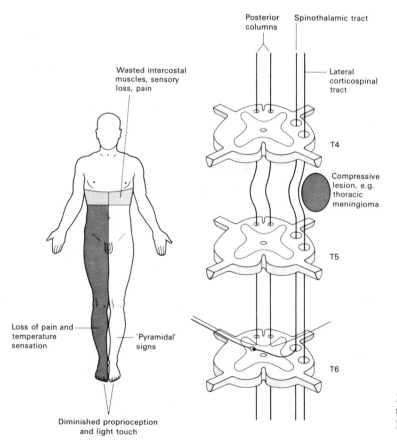

Fig. 18.13 The clinical features of spinal cord compression and their production.

Pontine lesions

Pontine lesions lie above the decussation of the posterior columns. Since the medial lemniscus and spinothalamic tracts are close together, there is loss of all forms of sensation on the side opposite the lesion. The upper cranial nerve nuclei are often also involved.

Thalamic lesions

Thalamic lesions may produce loss of sensation to all modalities of sensation on the opposite side of the body; this is an unusual clinical picture.

Spontaneous pain may also occur. Thalamic pain, sometimes called the 'thalamic syndrome', is usually caused by a small thalamic infarct. The patient develops a hemiparesis which recovers partially. There remains a constant deep-seated pain which affects the paretic limbs. It is often very severe. Movement does not change the pain, which continues night and day. Extreme anguish is usual and the secondary depression that follows may lead to suicide.

Cortical lesions

Pain is not a feature of destructive cortical lesions.

Irritative phenomena (e.g. partial seizures) in the parietal cortex cause tingling sensations in the affected part.

Sensory loss, neglect of one side and subtle disorders of sensation may occur with lesions of the parietal cortex.

PAIN AND DISTURBANCE OF SENSATION

Pain fibres

Primary afferent axons (2–5 μm, A-delta, thinly myelinated fibres and smaller, unmyelinated C fibres) pass in the peripheral nerves to the dorsal horn of the spinal cord. Some axons synapse in the substantia gelatinosa of the dorsal horn.

The gate theory of pain
This suggests that pain sensation is altered by other afferent impulses (e.g. touch, pressure, vibration) which enter the spinal cord and have a 'gating' or inhibitory effect on impulse transmission. Thus, pain sensation may be modulated by other sensory modalities.

Local heat and transcutaneous electrical stimulation are sometimes useful in the management of chronic pain.

Opioid peptides
Naturally occurring opioid peptides act as neurotransmitters and are widely distributed within

Table 18.23 Opioid peptides.

Peptide	Receptor
Enkephalins	Delta receptors
Dynorphins	Kappa receptors
Endorphins	Mu receptors

the central nervous system. They are found mainly within the substantia gelatinosa of the dorsal horn, in the periaqueductal grey matter and in the midline raphe nuclei of the brain stem. Three classes of peptide and receptor have now been recognized (Table 18.23). β-Endorphin is the most potent known endorphin and has a powerful analgesic action. Morphine and other opiates also act at the mu receptor.

Psychological aspects of pain

Pain is difficult to quantify and its interpretation depends not only on the patient's description but also on the experience, personality and mood of the doctor. Depression is an almost invariable companion of chronic pain.

Control of the bladder and sexual function

Afferent fibres (T12–S4) record changes in pressure within the bladder and tactile sensation in the genitalia.

The efferent pathways are shown in Table 18.24.

Table 18.24 Efferent nerve supply of the bladder and genitalia.

Type of nerve supply	Source	Structure/function supplied
Parasympathetic	S2–S4	Detrusor muscle contraction Genitalia (penile erection, engorgement of clitoris)
Somatic	Pudendal nerves	External sphincter
Sympathetic	T12–L2	Trigone Ejaculation, orgasm

Disorders of micturition

Bilateral upper motor neurone lesions cause frequency of micturition and incontinence. The bladder is small and unusually sensitive to small changes in intravesical pressure.

Lower motor neurone lesions (which must be

bilateral to cause urinary symptoms) cause a flaccid, atonic bladder, which overflows without warning.

Frontal lobe lesions (e.g. dementia, hydrocephalus) cause a disturbance of awareness of micturition, resulting in incontinence.

Impotence

Failure of erection of the penis (or clitoris) and ejaculation is caused by bilateral upper or lower motor lesions. Depression is also a common cause of impotence.

Cerebrovascular disease

Disease of the vessels of the brain includes the following conditions:
- Thromboembolic infarction
- Primary intracranial haemorrhage
- Subarachnoid haemorrhage
- Subdural and extradural haemorrhage and haematoma
- Cortical venous and dural venous sinus thrombosis

During the last 30 years clinical and pathological studies have demonstrated that arterial thromboembolism is the commonest cause of 'stroke'.

Strokes cause about 10 deaths per 100 000 population per annum in those aged 40 years, rising to 1000 deaths per 100 000 in those aged 75.

Definitions
Stroke. This is a focal neurological deficit due to a vascular lesion. It is usually of rapid onset and, by definition, lasts longer than 24 h if the patient survives. A hemiplegia due to middle cerebral arterial thromboembolism is a common example.

A stroke is said to be 'completed' when the deficit has reached its maximum, usually within 6 h of onset. It is 'in-evolution' when it is becoming worse, usually within 24 h of onset.

These definitions, although valuable, are arbitrary. The clinical picture of 'stroke' may also be caused by tumour, abscess, subdural haematoma or, rarely, by demyelination.

Transient ischaemic attack (TIA). This is a focal deficit lasting less than 24 h. There is complete recovery. The attack is usually of sudden onset. TIAs have a tendency to recur.

Pathophysiology
Difficulties occur in the diagnosis of cerebrovascular disease because similar clinical events can be caused by different pathological processes.

Completed stroke. A completed stroke is caused by:
- Embolism from a distant site and subsequent infarction
- Thrombosis of a cerebral vessel and infarction
- Haemorrhage into the brain

TIAs. TIAs are caused either by the passage of microemboli or, less commonly, by a fall in cerebral perfusion (e.g. due to a cardiac dysrhythmia, postural hypotension or decreased flow through atheromatous vertebral arteries, which are sometimes associated with cervical spondylosis). Small areas of infarction or even haemorrhages may also present with features identical to an embolic TIA.

The underlying risk factors and predisposing pathology are shown in Table 18.25.

Thromboembolism from vascular disease outside the brain is the cause of about 70% of strokes and 90% of TIAs.

The principal sources of emboli are atheromatous plaques within the great vessels, the carotid and vertebral systems, or the heart (from mitral or aortic valves, or from mural thrombi forming on diseased heart muscle).

Table 18.25 Risk factors and predisposing causes in cerebrovascular disease.

Risk factors
Hypertension
Diabetes mellitus
Obesity
Family history
Smoking
Hyperlipidaemia
Oral contraceptives
Alcohol
Predisposing causes
Extracranial atheroma
Intracranial atheroma
Heart disease
Low cerebral perfusion
Berry aneurysms
Arteriovenous malformation
Miscellaneous:
Hyperviscosity
Arteritis
Trauma
Congenital lesions
Metabolic diseases
Bleeding disorders

Vascular anatomy
An understanding of normal arterial anatomy and the likely sites of atheromatous plaques and stenotic lesions is important.

The circle of Willis (Fig. 18.14) is supplied by the two internal carotid arteries and by the basilar artery, which is formed by the union of the two vertebral arteries. Proximal to the circle, atheromatous

Other important arteries

Principal arteries

Fig. 18.14 The arteries supplying
the brain.

- Anterior
communicating
- Medial striate
- Superior
cerebellar
- Pontine
- Labyrinthine
- Anterior inferior
cerebellar
- Posterior inferior
cerebellar

Circle
of
Willis

- Anterior cerebral
- Middle cerebral
- Posterior
communicating
- Internal carotid
- Posterior cerebral
- Basilar
- Vertebral
- Anterior spinal

plaques and stenoses are common at the following
sites (see Fig. 18.16, p. 817):
- The origin of the common carotid arteries
- The origin of the internal carotid arteries
- Within the carotid syphon (in the cavernous
  sinus)
- Within the subclavian vessels

The distribution of the anterior, middle and posterior
cerebral arteries, which supply the cerebrum, is
shown in Fig. 18.15.

Autoregulation. The smooth muscle of small intracerebral arteries responds directly to changes in
pressure gradient across the vessel wall. In the nor-

(a)

Anterior cerebral artery

(b)

Frontal pole

Occipital pole

Posterior cerebral
artery

Speech area   Middle cerebral artery

Fig. 18.15 The distribution of the
three major cerebral arteries.
(a) Medial view. (b) Lateral view.

mal situation, constant cerebral blood flow (CBF) can be maintained with systolic blood pressures between 80 and 170 mmHg (i.e. the CBF is independent of perfusion pressure).

In disease states CBF autoregulation may fail. The contributory causes are:
- Severe hypotension (systolic BP <75 mmHg)
- Severe hypertension (systolic BP >180 mmHg)
- Increase in blood viscosity (polycythaemia, hyperviscosity syndromes)
- Raised intracranial pressure
- Changes in arterial Po_2 and Pco_2

Transient ischaemic attacks (TIAs)

Symptoms. TIAs cause sudden loss of function in one region of the brain. Symptoms usually reach their peak in seconds and last for minutes or hours (but by definition <24h).

The general site of the cerebral lesion is often suggested by the clinical pattern of the attack.

Signs. The diagnosis of a TIA is often based upon a description of it as a past event. During an attack the loss of function can be demonstrated. Consciousness is usually preserved.

There may be clinical evidence of a source of embolus, such as:
- Valvular heart disease or endocarditis
- Recent myocardial infarction
- Atrial fibrillation (or other dysrhythmia)
- Carotid artery stenosis (arterial bruit)
- Difference between right and left brachial blood pressure (subclavian stenosis)

There may be other clinical evidence of associated disease, such as:
- Atheroma
- Hypertension
- Postural hypotension
- Bradycardia or low cardiac output
- Diabetes mellitus
- Arteritis (rare)
- Polycythaemia (rare)

Specific types of TIA
The clinical features of many of the forms of TIA are given in Table 18.26. Hemiparesis, vertigo or aphasia are the commonest complaints.

Some specific examples of the manifestations of TIAs are given below.

Amaurosis fugax. This is the sudden loss of vision in one eye due to the passage of emboli through the retinal arteries. The emboli are sometimes visible through an ophthalmoscope. Amaurosis fugax is suggestive of a TIA in the anterior circulation and is often the first clinical evidence of carotid stenosis. It may also herald a hemiparesis.

Table 18.26 Features of transient ischaemic attacks.

Anterior circulation (carotid system)	Posterior circulation (vertebrobasilar system)
Amaurosis fugax	Diplopia, vertigo, vomiting
Aphasia	Choking and dysarthria
Hemiparesis	Ataxia
Hemisensory loss	Hemisensory loss
Hemianopic visual loss	Hemianopic visual loss
	Transient global amnesia
	Tetraparesis
	Drop attacks
	Loss of consciousness (rare)

Drop attacks. These sudden episodes of weakness of the lower limbs with falls, but without loss of consciousness, occur most commonly in middle-aged and elderly females. They are believed to be due to transient ischaemia in the brain stem due to microemboli or, less commonly, decreased perfusion in the vertebrobasilar system.

Transient global amnesia. Episodes of amnesia with confusion lasting for several hours are caused by ischaemia in the posterior circulation.

Differential diagnosis
TIAs must be distinguished (usually on wholly clinical grounds) from other causes of transient loss of function.

Focal epilepsy is usually accompanied by 'irritative phenomena' (e.g. jerking of the limbs) and characteristically there is a 'march' of events, with some progression. In a TIA the maximum deficit is usually apparent immediately.

Migraine, with a focal prodrome, sometimes causes diagnostic confusion. Headache is distinctly unusual in a TIA and there are usually no visual disturbances suggestive of migraine.

Prognosis
A TIA is an important prognostic event. Studies have shown that 5 years after the TIA:
- One out of six patients will have suffered a stroke
- One out of four patients will have died (usually from heart disease or stroke)

A TIA in the anterior circulation is generally of more serious prognostic significance than a TIA in the posterior circulation.

CEREBRAL INFARCTION

Cerebral infarction from thromboembolism usually produces a stroke, but small infarcts may present as TIAs or may even be symptomless. The clinical picture is very variable and depends on the site and extent of the infarct. It is no longer usual to attempt to subdivide the site into the precise distribution of a single branch vessel. Nevertheless, the site of cerebral infarction may be inferred from the pattern of the physical signs (e.g. cortex, internal capsule, brain stem).

SYMPTOMS AND SIGNS

The commonest stroke is the hemiplegia caused by infarction of the internal capsule following thromboembolism of a branch of the middle cerebral artery. A similar picture is caused by internal carotid occlusion (Fig. 18.16).

The signs are those of an acute upper motor neurone lesion of one side, including the face. Aphasia is usual when the dominant hemisphere is affected. The limbs are at first flaccid and areflexic. Headache is unusual and consciousness is not lost.

After a variable period the reflexes recover and become exaggerated, and an extensor plantar response appears. Weakness is maximal at first, and recovers gradually over the course of days, weeks or months.

Brain stem infarction
Infarction in the brain stem causes complex patterns of dysfunction depending on the site of the lesion and its relationship to the cranial nerve nuclei, long tracts and brain stem connections (see Table 18.27):

Table 18.27 Features of brain stem infarction.

Clinical feature	Structure involved
Hemiparesis or tetraparesis	Corticospinal tracts
Sensory loss	Medial lemniscus and spinothalamic tracts
Diplopia	Oculomotor system
Facial numbness	Fifth nerve nuclei
Facial weakness (LMN)	Seventh nerve nucleus
Nystagmus	Vestibular connections
Dysphagia, dysarthria	Ninth and tenth nerve nuclei
Dysarthria, ataxia, hiccups, vomiting	Brain stem and cerebellar connections
Horner's syndrome	Sympathetic fibres
Altered consciousness	Reticular formation

- *The lateral medullary syndrome*, formerly called posterior inferior cerebellar artery (PICA) thrombosis, or Wallenberg's syndrome, is the most widely recognized syndrome of brain stem infarction. It is caused by PICA or vertebral artery thromboembolism (Fig. 18.17). There is sudden vertigo, vomiting and ipsilateral ataxia, with contralateral loss of pain and temperature sensation (see Table 18.28).
- *Coma* may be caused by bilateral brain stem infarction which damages the reticular formation.
- *The 'locked-in' syndrome* is caused by upper brain stem infarction; despite being conscious the patient can neither speak, swallow nor move the limbs.
- *Pseudobulbar palsy* (see p. 805) may be caused by brain stem infarct.

Other types of infarction
Lacunar infarction. Lacunae are small (<1.5 cm) areas of infarction seen at post mortem in patients with hypertension. They may be symptomless but can cause stroke of a mild degree. Pure motor stroke, pure sensory stroke, sudden unilateral ataxia and sudden dysarthria with a clumsy hand are typically caused by single lacunar infarcts.

Multi-infarct dementia. Multiple lacunes or larger infarcts cause the picture of generalized intellectual loss which is sometimes seen in patients with cerebrovascular disease. The condition tends to occur with a stepwise progression with each subsequent infarct. The final picture is of dementia, pseudobulbar palsy and a shuffling gait with small steps. There may be confusion clinically with Parkinson's disease, and this syndrome has been termed 'atherosclerotic parkinsonism' in the past.

Hemianopic visual loss or cortical blindness (Anton's

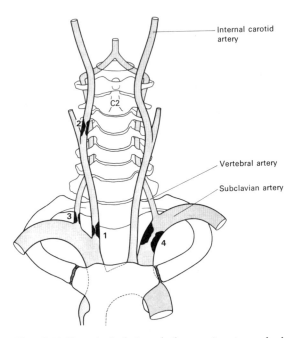

Fig. 18.16 The principal sites of atheroma in extracerebral vessels. 1 = common carotid artery; 2 = internal carotid artery; 3 = vertebral artery; 4 = subclavian artery.

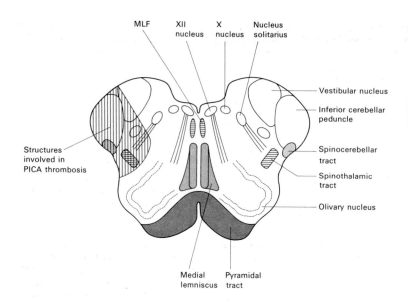

MLF   XII   X   Nucleus
       nucleus nucleus   solitarius

Vestibular nucleus

Inferior cerebellar
peduncle

Structures
involved in
PICA thrombosis

Spinocerebellar
tract

Spinothalamic
tract

Olivary nucleus

Medial   Pyramidal
lemniscus tract

Fig. 18.17 A cross-section of medulla showing posterior inferior cerebellar artery (PICA) thrombosis. MLF = medial longitudinal fasciculus. Modified from Ross Russell RW & Wiles CM (1986) *Neurology* (Integrated Clinical Science Series). London: Heinemann.

Table 18.28 Features of the lateral medullary syndrome.

Ipsilateral
Trigeminal sensory loss
Sixth nerve palsy
Nystagmus
Ataxia
Horner's syndrome
Ninth and tenth nerve lesions
Contralateral
Spinothalamic sensory loss in limbs
Hemiparesis (mild and unusual)

syndrome, see p. 794). This may follow infarction of the posterior cerebral arteries.

Weber's syndrome. This consists of an ipsilateral third nerve paralysis with a contralateral hemiplegia due to a lesion in one half of the midbrain. Paralysis of upward gaze, due to a lesion localized in the region of the red nucleus, may also occur.

Watershed infarction. This describes the multiple cortical infarcts that occur during prolonged episodes of very low cerebral perfusion (e.g. following massive myocardial infarction or hypotensive therapy). The border zones between the areas supplied by the anterior, middle and posterior cerebral arteries are damaged. A syndrome of cortical visual loss, and memory and intellectual impairment is typical.

IMMEDIATE MANAGEMENT

The initial decision of whether to admit a stroke patient to hospital depends upon the clinical state and facilities available at home. It is often the practical difficulties of caring for the disabled for what may be a prolonged period that determine these immediate decisions. If possible, a TIA or a mild stroke can be managed at home and specialist advice sought when necessary.

The management of the unconscious patient is described on p. 789.

EXAMINATION

In the examination, particular care should be taken to find a possible source of embolus (e.g. carotid bruit, atrial fibrillation, valve lesion or evidence of endocarditis) and to determine whether hypertension or postural hypotension is or has been present. There may be evidence of other emboli or a history of previous TIAs.

The brachial blood pressure should be measured in each arm; a difference of more than 20 mmHg is suggestive of stenosis of a subclavian artery.

INVESTIGATION

The investigations listed in Table 18.29 should be carried out in all cases.

Table 18.29 Preliminary investigation in stroke.

Test	Yield
Urinalysis, blood sugar	Diabetes mellitus
Haemoglobin	Polycythaemia
White cell count	Infection
ESR	Inflammation
Serology for syphilis	Possible neurosyphilis
Chest x-ray	Neoplasms
ECG	Recent infarct, dysrhythmia

Blood cultures should be taken if there is any possibility of endocarditis.

Special investigations

Lumbar puncture is no longer a routine investigation in stroke. It is indicated only in special circumstances (e.g. when syphilitic serology in blood is positive).

Investigation such as CT scanning and angiography are expensive and the information gained rarely changes the management in the elderly patients in whom stroke and TIAs are most common. These studies are not often indicated in patients over 65 years unless there is doubt about the aetiology of the stroke.

All young stroke and TIA patients (<60 years) should be considered for both CT scanning and angiography. A specialist opinion may be necessary to decide the timing and indications.

CT scanning. CT scanning will usually demonstrate the site of a lesion and distinguish between haemorrhage and infarction. It will also rule out (or show unexpected) mass lesions such as subdural haematoma, tumour or abscess.

Angiography. Carotid arteriography is valuable in anterior circulation TIAs to diagnose surgically accessible arterial stenoses (mainly internal carotid stenosis) (see Fig. 18.18). It may also show inaccessible lesions within the cranium. There is a high probability of finding a carotid stenosis when there is a loud localized carotid bruit in the neck.

The majority of normotensive young patients (below 60 years of age) with TIA or stroke in the anterior circulation who recover well should be considered for angiography. In more elderly patients the risks of the procedure and the relatively poor results of vascular surgery in preventing further stroke usually make further investigation unwise.

Vertebral and arch angiography are now rarely performed following posterior circulation TIAs and strokes unless there is a clinical suggestion of subclavian artery disease.

Fig. 18.18 Carotid arteriogram showing a tight stenosis of internal carotid artery (arrow).

Digital vascular imaging can be used to demonstrate disease of the extracranial vessels and is an alternative to percutaneous arteriography.

TREATMENT

Surgical approaches

Internal carotid endarterectomy. This is considered in patients who are shown to have an internal carotid artery stenosis that narrows the arterial lumen by more than 70%. The results of surgery are still being evaluated, but early results are not encouraging. The procedure has a mortality of under 3%.

Extracranial–intracranial bypass. Anastomosis of the superficial temporal artery (external carotid) through a burr-hole to a cortical branch of the middle cerebral artery (internal carotid) is considered when there is internal carotid occlusion. The indications for the procedure are still being assessed, but a recent trial suggests little benefit.

Medical therapy

All risk factors (see Table 18.25) should be treated if possible.

Hypertension. The control of high blood pressure is the single most important factor in the prevention of stroke. The incidence of stroke is falling in countries where active treatment of hypertension is undertaken.

Other measures. Anticoagulants are indicated when there is atrial fibrillation or other paroxysmal dysrhythmias, uninfected cardiac valve lesions or cardiomyopathy. Anticoagulants are sometimes used in 'stroke-in-evolution'. They are potentially dangerous in the 2 weeks following cerebral infarction because of the risk of provoking cerebral haemorrhage.

Polycythaemia should be treated (see p. 289).

Aspirin and dipyridamole (see p. 297) may offer some protection against further episodes of TIA or cerebral infarction. The evidence supporting their use remains controversial.

Baclofen (a GABA antagonist) is sometimes helpful in the management of severe spasticity following stroke.

PROGNOSIS

Approximately one-third of hospitalized patients will die in the first month following infarction and one-half by 6 months. A poor outcome is likely when there is coma, a defect in conjugate gaze and a severe hemiplegia. Recurrent strokes are common (10% in the first year) and in addition many patients die of a myocardial infarction. Overall only 50% of initial survivors are alive after 3 years.

Gradual improvement usually follows stroke, although the patient may be left with a severe residual deficit. Of those who survive a stroke, about one-third return to independent mobility and one-third have severe disability requiring permanent institutional care.

Global aphasia may begin to recover noticeably during the first week, when there is often return of some spontaneous speech. The outlook is variable but many stroke patients who recover are left with word-finding difficulties.

REHABILITATION

Physiotherapy and speech therapy
Skilled physiotherapy is of particular value in the first few months following the stroke. It is helpful in relieving spasticity, preventing contractures and teaching stroke patients to use walking aids. The effect of physiotherapy on the longer-term outcome is debatable.

Speech therapy is frequently recommended in aphasia. Its value is difficult to assess. It is probable that the spontaneous return of speech is hastened as much by normal conversation with a relative as by skilled manoeuvres on the part of a therapist.

Both physiotherapy and speech therapy have an undoubted psychological role. Stroke is frequently a devastating event and, particularly when it occurs during working life, radically alters the pattern of the patient's remaining years. Many patients become unemployable and cannot lead independent lives. The financial consequences to the sufferer are usually considerable. The loss of self-esteem makes secondary depression common. *Any* attempts to speed improvement are thus greatly welcomed by these patients.

Following recovery from stroke, various aids and modifications may be necessary at home, such as:
- Stair rails
- Portable lavatories
- Bath rails
- Hoists
- Sliding boards
- Wheelchairs
- Tripods
- Modification of doorways and sleeping arrangements
- Stair lifts
- Kitchen modifications

A visit to the patient's home with the occupational therapist and family doctor to discuss these problems is valuable.

PRIMARY INTRACRANIAL HAEMORRHAGE

Intracerebral haemorrhage

AETIOLOGY

Rupture of small arteries affected by 'lipohyaline degeneration' is the principal cause of primary intracerebral haemorrhage. This occurs typically in patients with hypertension and occurs at well-defined sites—basal ganglia, pons, cerebellum and subcortical white matter. Saccular ('berry') aneurysms and arteriovenous malformations also bleed into the brain (see p. 821).

RECOGNITION

There is no entirely reliable way of distinguishing between haemorrhage and infarction, as both produce a stroke. Cerebral haemorrhage, however, tends to be accompanied by a severe headache and to be followed by coma. Meningism occurs when blood leaks into the ventricular or subarachnoid CSF, and is usually accompanied by altered consciousness.

MANAGEMENT

The management of cerebral haemorrhage is as for cerebral infarction, although the immediate prognosis is not as good. Only when an intracerebral haematoma behaves as an expanding mass lesion, causing deepening coma and coning, should surgical removal be considered.

Cerebellar haemorrhage

It is important to recognize cerebellar haemorrhage because it causes an acute hydrocephalus. There is headache and rapid reduction of consciousness with signs of brain stem origin (e.g. nystagmus, ocular palsies). The gaze deviates to the side of the lesion. Emergency surgery may be necessary to remove a cerebellar haematoma.

SUBARACHNOID HAEMORRHAGE

The term subarachnoid haemorrhage (SAH) describes spontaneous rather than traumatic arterial bleeding into the subarachnoid space.

INCIDENCE

SAH accounts for 10% of cerebrovascular disease and has an annual incidence of 15 per 100 000.

CAUSES

The causes of SAH are shown in Table 18.30.

It is unusual to find any contributing disease,

Table 18.30 Causes of subarachnoid haemorrhage.

Saccular ('berry') aneurysms	70%
Arterio-venous malformation	10%
No lesion found	20%

Rare causes
Bleeding disorders
Mycotic aneurysms (endocarditis, see p. 526)
Acute bacterial meningitis
Brain tumours
Arteritis (e.g. systemic lupus erythematosus)
Spinal SAH from a spinal arteriovenous malformation

though coarctation of the aorta, the Ehlers–Danlos syndrome, Marfan's syndrome and other inherited disorders of collagen may be associated with SAH.

Saccular ('berry') aneurysms (Fig. 18.19)
Saccular aneurysms form on the circle of Willis and its adjacent branches. The common sites of aneurysms are:

- Junction of the posterior communicating and the internal carotid artery—posterior communicating artery aneurysm
- Junction of the anterior communicating artery and the anterior cerebral artery—anterior communicating artery aneurysm
- Branching point of the middle cerebral artery—middle cerebral artery aneurysm

Fig. 18.19 Carotid arteriogram showing a large aneurysm of the anterior communicating artery (bottom arrow). The top arrow indicates the anterior cerebral arteries.

Other sites are on the basilar artery, the posterior inferior cerebellar artery, the intracavernous internal carotid artery and the ophthalmic artery. Saccular aneurysms are an incidental finding in 1% of autopsies and may be multiple.

Aneurysms cause symptoms either by spontaneous rupture (when there is usually no preceding history) or by pressure effects on surrounding structures, e.g. a posterior communicating aneurysm may cause a painful third nerve palsy (see p. 798).

Arteriovenous malformation
These are lesions of developmental origin, usually within the hemisphere. They may cause epilepsy, which is often focal. Once they have ruptured to cause a SAH, there is a tendency to rebleed at a rate of 10% per year.

CLINICAL FEATURES

The onset is sudden with a devastating occipital headache. This is usually followed by vomiting and often by loss of consciousness. The patient remains comatose or drowsy for several hours to several days.

On examination there is neck stiffness and a positive Kernig's sign. Papilloedema is sometimes present, and may be accompanied by retinal haemorrhages and subhyaloid haemorrhage (massive retinal haemorrhage tracking beneath the hyaloid membrane).

INVESTIGATION

CT scanning shows subarachnoid or intraventricular blood. Lumbar puncture is no longer carried out routinely.

Carotid and vertebral angiography is usually performed in all patients who are potentially fit for surgery (i.e. those who are young—below 55–60 years—and not in coma) to establish the site of the bleeding.

DIFFERENTIAL DIAGNOSIS

SAH must be differentiated from acute meningitis and severe migraine. It is sometimes difficult to distinguish between SAH and primary intracerebral haemorrhage.

MANAGEMENT

Some 10% of cases of SAH are either dead or moribund before they reach hospital and 30% die during the first episode. Of the remainder, a further 20% will die in the early weeks in hospital from further bleeding.

Patients who are comatose or who have severe neurological deficits have a poor prognosis. In others, where angiography can demonstrate aneurysms, a direct neurosurgical approach and clipping of the neck of the aneurysm is possible.

The immediate treatment of patients with SAH is bed rest and supportive measures. Hypertension should be controlled. Dexamethasone and anti-fibrinolytic agents are often prescribed, but their place in therapy is dubious.

It is usual to refer all cases to a specialist centre for a decision about angiography and possible surgery.

SUBDURAL AND EXTRADURAL HAEMORRHAGE AND HAEMATOMA

These conditions are of great neurosurgical import-ance as both may cause death unless treated promptly.

Chronic subdural haematoma (SDH) (see Fig. 18.21b, p. 841)
This occurs when blood accumulates in the subdural space following rupture of a vein. It is almost always due to head injury, which may be minor, but the latent interval between injury and symptoms may be weeks or months. Chronic SDH is common in the elderly and the alcoholic.

Headache, drowsiness and confusion are com-mon, and the symptoms often fluctuate. Focal defi-cits such as hemiparesis or sensory loss may develop and epilepsy may occur. Stupor and coma gradually ensue.

Extradural haemorrhage (see Fig. 18.21a, p. 841)
This follows a tear of a branch of a middle meningeal artery, usually underlying a linear skull fracture. Blood accumulates in the extradural space. The most characteristic picture is of a head injury with a brief duration of unconsciousness followed by the so-called 'lucid interval' of recovery. The patient then develops a progressive hemiparesis and stupor, and rapidly occurring transtentorial 'coning', with first an ipsilateral dilated pupil followed by fixed dilated pupils, tetraplegia and death.

An acute subdural haemorrhage presents in a similar way.

MANAGEMENT

The diagnosis of extradural or subdural haemor-rhage or haematoma is confirmed by CT scan and/or arteriography.

Surgical drainage is carried out through burr-holes. If performed early the outlook is excellent. When far from specialist help (e.g. in war time or at sea), drainage should be carried out when the diagnosis is suspected on clinical grounds alone; this procedure has frequently been life-saving.

In the elderly some SDHs resolve spontaneously and can be monitored with serial CT scans.

CORTICAL VENOUS AND DURAL VENOUS SINUS THROMBOSIS

These are unusual complications of skull and paranasal (air) sinus infection, dehydration or severe intercurrent illness. They are also associated with pregnancy and the contraceptive pill.

Cortical venous thrombosis
The venous infarct caused by the thrombosis leads to focal signs (e.g. hemiparesis) and epilepsy. There is often a fever.

Dural venous sinus thromboses
Cavernous sinus thrombosis. This causes ocular pain, proptosis and chemosis. An external and internal ophthalmoplegia with papilloedema develop.

Lateral and sagittal sinus thrombosis. This causes symptoms of raised intracranial pressure (including headache), papilloedema and often epilepsy.

MANAGEMENT

Treatment and investigation is directed at the under-lying cause of the thrombosis. Anticonvulsants are used in epilepsy and antibiotics in infection. Anti-coagulants are rarely indicated.

Epilepsy and other causes of recurrent loss of consciousness

EPILEPSY

An epileptic seizure is a convulsion or transient abnormal feeling experienced by the subject due to a paroxysmal discharge of cerebral neurones. Epi-lepsy, by definition, is the continuing tendency to have such seizures, even if a long interval separates attacks.

INCIDENCE

Epilepsy is a common condition. Some 3% of the population have two or more seizures during their lives. In Britain approximately 65 people suffer from their first seizure each day. Around a quarter of a million people in Britain take anticonvulsants. In Asia the prevalence is similar to Western nations; the condition is, however, over twice as common in Africa.

PATHOPHYSIOLOGY

The spread of electrical activity between cortical neurones is normally restricted. Synchronous discharge of neurones in normal brain takes place in small groups only; these limited discharges are responsible for the normal rhythms of the electro-encephalogram (EEG).

During a seizure, large groups of neurones are activated repetitively and 'hypersynchronously'. There is a failure of inhibitory synaptic contact between neurones. This causes high voltage spike-and-wave activity on the EEG.

Epileptic activity confined to one area of the cortex is associated with specific symptoms and signs (partial seizures). This activity may remain focal or may spread to cause paroxysmal activity in both hemispheres and a generalized convulsion. This is called secondary generalization of a partial seizure.

Generalized seizure activity without a focal onset arises from the cortex when the overall excitability is increased.

Seizure threshold

Each individual has a threshold for seizure activity. Experimentally some chemicals (e.g. pen-tylenetetrazol) induce seizures in all those who inhale them. Individuals who are more likely than others in the population to have seizures in response to various stimuli are said to have a 'low seizure threshold', although this is a concept, not an actual measurement.

CLASSIFICATION

Epilepsy can be divided according to the clinical type of seizure rather than the possible cause (see Table 18.31); this replaces older classifications.

Generalized seizures

Tonic–clonic seizures (grand mal seizures, generalized convulsions). Following a vague warning, the body enters a rigid tonic phase which lasts for up to a minute. The subject may utter a cry and fall, sometimes injuring himself. The tongue may be bitten and there may be incontinence of urine or faeces.

This is followed by a convulsion (the clonic phase) in which the muscles jerk rhythmically. This lasts a few seconds to a few minutes. Seizures are usually self-limiting, leaving the patient drowsy or in coma for several hours.

Tonic–clonic seizures may be a variety of generalized epilepsy or may follow a partial seizure.

Typical absences (petit mal). This type of generalized epilepsy is almost invariably a disorder of childhood, and by definition an attack is accompanied by 3 Hz spike-and-wave in the EEG. The child ceases activity, stares and pales slightly. The eyelids may twitch. The attack lasts for a few seconds only. A few jerks may occur.

After an attack the child carries on as if nothing

Table 18.31 Classification of epilepsy.

Generalized seizures
Absence seizures*
Typical absences with 3 Hz spike-and-wave
discharge (petit mal)
Atypical absences with other EEG changes
Myoclonic seizures
Tonic–clonic seizures (grand mal, major convulsions)*
Tonic seizures
Akinetic seizures
Partial seizures
These start by activation of a group of neurones in one part of one hemisphere. They are also called focal seizures.
Simple partial seizures (no impairment of consciousness)*
Complex partial seizures (with impairment of consciousness)*
Partial seizures evolving to tonic–clonic seizures*
Apparent generalized tonic–clonic seizures, with EEG but not clinical evidence of focal onset*

* Common varieties of epilepsy.

had happened. Typical absence attacks are never due to identifiable focal lesions. Children with typical absence attacks may in adult life develop generalized seizures.

The term *petit mal* should not be used to describe the absence attacks of partial seizures.

Partial seizures (focal seizures)

The hallmark of a partial seizure is a discharge from a focal group of neurones. The seizure frequently has clinical features which provide evidence of its site of origin.

When these features precede a grand mal fit, the warning they give to the patient or relatives is called the 'aura' and the seizure is said to become secondarily generalized.

Jacksonian (motor) seizures. These seizures originate in the motor cortex. Jerking movements typically begin at the angle of the mouth or in the thumb and index finger, spreading to involve the limbs on the side opposite the epileptic focus. Conjugate gaze (see p. 796) may deviate away from a frontal lobe focus (an 'adversive seizure').

Paralysis of the affected limbs may follow for several hours (Todd's paralysis).

Temporal lobe seizures. These are associated with strange disturbances of smell, or feelings of unreality ('jamais vu') or undue familiarity ('déjà vu') with the surroundings. Visual hallucinations (visions or faces) may be seen. Absence attacks or vertigo may occur.

Many other types of partial seizure are known, e.g. autonomic disturbances with pilo-erection or flushing, sensory disturbances (parietal cortex), crude visual shapes (occipital cortex) or strange sounds (auditory cortex).

AETIOLOGICAL AND PRECIPITATING FACTORS
(Table 18.32)

A cause for epilepsy is found in under one-quarter of patients. A number of secondary factors may trigger seizures in those with a low seizure threshold.

Family history. About 30% of patients with epilepsy have a history of seizures in first degree relatives. Usually the mode of inheritance is vague; a low seizure threshold appears to run in some families. Generalized typical absence seizures (petit mal) are sometimes inherited as an autosomal dominant trait with variable penetrance.

Trauma and surgery. Perinatal trauma (causing cerebral contusion and haemorrhage) and fetal anoxia are common causes of seizures in childhood. Hypoxic damage to the medial temporal lobes (medial temporal sclerosis) is an important cause.

Head injury is sometimes followed by epilepsy within the first week ('early' epilepsy) or many months or years later ('late' epilepsy). To cause epilepsy the injury must almost always be sufficient to cause coma. The presence of early epilepsy, a depressed skull fracture, cerebral contusion, a dural tear or intracranial haematoma increases the incidence of late post-traumatic epilepsy.

Surgery to the cerebral hemispheres is followed by epilepsy in 20–30% of cases.

Pyrexia. High fevers in children under 5 years are sometimes associated with generalized seizures ('febrile convulsions'). In the majority there is no tendency for the seizures to recur in adult life.

Intracranial mass lesions. All mass lesions affecting the cerebral cortex may cause epilepsy—either partial or secondarily generalized seizures. If the onset of seizures is in adult life, the chance of an unsuspected mass lesion being present is around 3%. Raised intracranial pressure from other causes (e.g. hydrocephalus) may cause seizures.

Cerebral infarction. Seizures may follow cerebral infarction, especially in the elderly.

Drugs, alcohol and drug withdrawal. Phenothiazines, monoamine oxidase inhibitors, tricyclic antidepressants, amphetamines, lignocaine and nalidixic acid may occasionally provoke fits either in overdose or in therapeutic doses in individuals with a low seizure threshold.

Alcoholism is a common cause of seizures. They occur either with chronic alcohol excess or during a period of abstention. Alcohol-induced hypoglycaemia can also provoke attacks.

Withdrawal of anticonvulsant drugs (especially phenobarbitone) and withdrawal of benzodiazepines may provoke seizures.

Encephalitis and other inflammatory conditions of the brain. Seizures are frequently the presenting feature of encephalitis, cerebral abscess, cortical venous thrombosis and neurosyphilis.

Metabolic abnormalities. Seizures may occur with the following metabolic abnormalities:
- Hypocalcaemia
- Hypoglycaemia
- Hyponatraemia
- Acute hypoxia
- Porphyria
- Uraemia
- Hepatic failure

Degenerative brain disorders. Seizures occur in Alzheimer's disease and in many rarer degenerative diseases. Epilepsy is three times more common in patients with multiple sclerosis than in the general population.

Photosensitive and other types of reflex epilepsy. Seizures are sometimes precipitated by flashing lights or a flickering television screen. This photosensitivity can be seen on the occipital recording of the EEG. Very rarely other stimuli provoke attacks.

INVESTIGATION

The diagnosis should be made on the clinical description. The electroencephalogram (EEG) is the single most useful investigation in the study of a seizure, though it has distinct limitations.

The electroencephalogram in epilepsy
- During a seizure the EEG is almost invariably

Table 18.32 Aetiological and precipitating factors in epilepsy.

Family history
Trauma and surgery
Pyrexia
Intracranial mass lesions
Cerebral infarction
Drugs, alcohol and drug withdrawal
Encephalitis
Metabolic abnormalities
Degenerative brain disorders
Photosensitivity and auditory stimuli

abnormal because epileptic activity reaches the surface of the brain.

- EEG evidence of seizure activity is shown typically by a cortical spike focus (e.g. in a temporal lobe) or by generalized spike-and-wave activity.
- In petit mal 3 Hz spike-and-wave activity is seen. It is always present during an attack and is frequently seen in the inter-ictal intervals (i.e. between attacks).
- A normal EEG between attacks does not exclude epilepsy. Many people suffering from epilepsy have normal inter-ictal EEG activity. In addition, an abnormal inter-ictal EEG does not prove that an attack was epileptic.
- The EEG unfortunately does not indicate the effect of anticonvulsant drugs or determine the prognosis in epilepsy.
- EEG telemetry, with tape or disk recordings for hours or days, has greatly added to the value of this investigation in the study of attacks of disturbed consciousness whose nature is uncertain.

Other investigations

Routine investigations (blood picture, serum biochemistry, chest x-ray) may indicate an underlying metabolic or structural cause. Such tests are normal in idiopathic epilepsy.

CT scanning is always indicated in adults who have seizures of recent onset with physical signs, but in general the diagnostic yield of scanning after single or recurrent seizures is low.

TREATMENT

Emergency measures

The emergency treatment of a seizure is simply to ensure that the patient harms himself as little as possible and that the airway is patent in a prolonged seizure and in post-ictal coma. Wooden mouth gags, tongue forceps and physical restraint frequently cause injury rather than prevent it.

If there is any suspicion of hypoglycaemia, blood should be taken for the measurement of glucose, and intravenous glucose given.

Long-term anticonvulsant drugs

Anticonvulsant drugs are indicated in recurrent seizures. Phenytoin, carbamazepine and sodium valproate are the commonest drugs prescribed. Phenobarbitone, primidone and the benzodiazepine clonazepam are also used. There are differences in opinion about the most appropriate drugs for each particular variety of seizure; one suggested scheme is given in Table 18.33.

Phenytoin has the advantage of being cheap and effective. Its therapeutic level in serum is well defined, and the serum level of phenytoin should be monitored in the majority of patients (Table 18.34). The therapeutic serum levels of other anticonvul-

Table 18.33 Suggested scheme for the use of anticonvulsant drugs.

Type of seizure	Drug
Generalized tonic–clonic seizures	Phenytoin
Generalized absence (petit mal) seizures	Sodium valproate
Partial seizures	Carbamazepine Sodium valproate

Table 18.34 Therapeutic levels of anticonvulsant drugs.

Drug	Adult daily dose	Therapeutic level
Phenytoin	300 mg	40–80 μmol·l^{-1}
Carbamazepine	200 mg ×3	20–50 μmol·l^{-1}
Sodium valproate	200 mg ×3	200–700 μmol·l^{-1}*

* Poorly defined.

sants are less clearly defined and routine estimations are not usually performed.

It is preferable to try to use one drug alone in the treatment of epilepsy, although a second (or third) drug may be needed in resistant cases.

Unwanted effects. Intoxication with all anticonvulsants causes a syndrome of ataxia, nystagmus and dysarthria.

Chronic administration of phenytoin can cause:
- Gum hypertrophy
- Hypertrichosis
- Osteomalacia
- Folate deficiency
- Polyneuropathy
- Encephalopathy

The more common idiosyncratic (non-dose-related) side-effects are summarized in Table 18.35.

Status epilepticus

This is when seizures follow each other without recovery of consciousness. It is a medical emergency. When grand mal seizures follow one another there is

Table 18.35 Idiosyncratic unwanted effects of anticonvulsant drugs.

Drug	Side-effects
Phenytoin	Rashes Blood dyscrasias Lymphadenopathy Systemic lupus erythematosus
Carbamazepine	Rashes Blood dyscrasias
Sodium valproate	Anorexia Hair loss Liver damage

a serious risk of death from cardiorespiratory failure. Immediate treatment with diazepam 10 mg i.v. followed by an intravenous infusion of 200 mg·l^{-1} over 24 h is essential. Chlormethiazole 0.8% should be given by intravenous infusion if status epilepticus continues or returns. Ventilatory support must be available.

'Status' can also occur in absence seizures and in focal epilepsy ('epilepsy partialis continua').

Neurosurgical treatment

Several surgical approaches have been used in epilepsy. The most important is amputation of the anterior temporal lobe (usually of the non-dominant side) in those with partial seizures or partial seizures that are secondarily generalized. Indications include poor control on drug therapy and a clearly defined focus of abnormal electrical activity.

The social consequences of epilepsy

The great majority of patients with epilepsy can be managed by a general practitioner or as an out-patient, and have infrequent seizures that alter relatively little the pattern of their lives. In a small minority who have exceedingly frequent seizures, treatment in hospital or residential care is necessary.

There remains, however, a considerable social stigma attached to the diagnosis, an important fact to be considered when the nature of attacks of disturbed consciousness is uncertain. Employers are reluctant to take on patients with seizures.

Present trends are to encourage both adults and children with epilepsy to lead lives as unrestricted as possible, though with simple, sensible provisos such as avoiding swimming alone and dangerous sports such as rock-climbing or solo canoeing. It is also wise to advise on simple domestic matters, e.g. that the bathroom door should remain unlocked.

Driving and epilepsy

Those who have suffered from seizures are unable to hold a driving licence in Britain unless they satisfy the following criteria:
- They shall have been free from *any* form of epileptic attack whilst awake for a period of 2 years prior to the issue of a licence.
- In the cases of attacks whilst asleep, the attacks must have occurred only whilst asleep for a period of at least 3 years prior to the issue of a licence.

The rules for those holding public service vehicle licences and heavy goods vehicle licences are stricter: any attack after the age of 3 automatically bars an applicant from holding such a licence indefinitely.

It is the duty of a doctor to inform patients of these regulations.

OTHER CAUSES OF RECURRENT ATTACKS OF DISTURBED CONSCIOUSNESS (Table 18.36)

Episodes of transient loss or disturbance of consciousness are common clinical problems. It is usually possible to distinguish between a 'fit' (a seizure), a 'faint' (syncope) and other types of attack from the history given by the patient and the account of an eye witness.

Table 18.36 Causes of recurrent attacks of disturbed consciousness.

Epilepsy
Syncope
Micturition syncope
Cough syncope
Breath holding (children)
Postural hypotension
Carotid sinus syncope
Transient cerebral ischaemia
Cardiac dysrhythmias
Effort syncope
Narcolepsy and cataplexy
Night terrors in children
Psychogenic attacks
Panic attacks
Hyperventilation
Hypoglycaemia
Hypocalcaemia
Vertigo

Syncope ('fainting') and related disorders

Sudden reflex bradycardia and peripheral and splanchnic vasodilatation leading to loss of consciousness occurs commonly in response to prolonged standing, fear, venesection or pain. It almost never occurs in the recumbent posture. The subject falls to the ground and is unconscious for less than 2 min. Recovery is rapid. A few jerking movements are uncommon, but do occur. Incontinence of urine is exceptional.

Other forms

Syncope may occur after micturition in men (particularly at night), when the venous return to the heart is obstructed by breath-holding and severe coughing.

The syndrome of carotid sinus syncope is believed to be due to excessive sensitivity of the sinus to external pressure. It may occur in elderly patients who, on touching the neck, lose consciousness.

Postural hypotension occurs in patients with impaired autonomic reflexes, e.g. in the elderly, in autonomic neuropathy, or with ganglion–blocking drugs used in hypertension, phenothiazines, levodopa or tricyclic antidepressants.

Transient cerebral ischaemia, usually due to thromboembolism in the posterior cerebral circulation, may cause episodes of loss of consciousness or 'drop attacks' (see p. 816).

Cardiac dysrhythmias (cardiac syncope, Stokes–Adams attacks—see p. 482) are important causes of recurrent episodes of loss of consciousness, particularly in the elderly. There is sometimes a preceding warning of palpitation (either fast or slow). The loss of consciousness is sudden and accompanied by pallor. Exceptionally, there are convulsive movements ('anoxic convulsions'). Flushing may occur when the patient recovers. The usual cardiac dysrhythmias to cause loss of consciousness are paroxysmal bradycardias (e.g. in complete heart block) or tachycardias (e.g. ventricular tachycardias, ventricular fibrillation). Supraventricular tachycardias are unusual causes of loss of consciousness.

Effort syncope (syncope on exertion) is of cardiac origin (e.g. aortic stenosis, hypertrophic obstructive cardiomyopathy).

INVESTIGATION

Syncope and related conditions where cerebral blood flow is impaired can usually be distinguished from epilepsy on the clinical history alone.

Cardiac monitoring may sometimes be necessary to detect a dysrhythmia.

MANAGEMENT

The immediate management of syncope, or impending syncope, is to lay the patient down, to elevate the lower limbs and record the pulse. In the rare circumstances where cerebral blood flow cannot be restored, e.g. in a dentist's chair, syncope may be followed by cerebral infarction.

Narcolepsy and cataplexy

Narcoleptic attacks are periods of irresistible sleep. They may occur when there is little distraction, after meals, while travelling in a vehicle, or without obvious cause. Genetically, narcolepsy is strongly associated with HLA-DR2.

Cataplexy is a sudden loss of tone in the lower limbs with preservation of consciousness. Attacks are set off by sudden surprise or emotion.

The two conditions are related and may be accompanied by hypnagogic hallucinations (terrifying hallucinations on falling asleep), hypnapompic hallucinations (on waking) and sleep paralysis (a frightening inability to move whilst drowsy). The EEG is normal in these attacks.

Treatment is with methyl phenidate, other amphetamine-like drugs, or small doses of tricyclic antidepressants.

Panic attacks, night terrors and psychogenic attacks

Panic attacks are usually associated with an autonomic disturbance, e.g. tachycardia, sweating and pilo-erection. Consciousness is usually preserved, Hyperventilation (see below) is common.

Night terrors are sudden episodes seen in children who awake as if from a dream in a state of terror.

Psychogenic attacks cause considerable difficulty in diagnosis. Attacks resembling grand mal fits may occur but more usually there are bizarre and irregular limb movements.

Hypoglycaemia

Hypoglycaemia causes attacks in which the patient either feels unwell or may lose consciousness, sometimes with a convulsion. There is often some warning, with hunger, shaking and sweating.

Hypoglycaemic attacks unrelated to diabetes are rare. Most patients who feel unwell after fasting or in the early morning have no serious organic disease.

Hypocalcaemia and hyperventilation

A grand mal fit may accompany hypocalcaemia (see p. 736).

The alkalosis accompanying hyperventilation leads to a feeling of lightheadedness which may be accompanied by circumoral and peripheral tingling and tetany (e.g. carpopedal spasm) (see p. 886).

Vertigo

Acute episodes of vertigo (see p. 782) sometimes cause loss of consciousness for a few seconds.

Choking

Sudden prostration sometimes follows choking, particularly when a large bolus of meat obstructs the larynx. The patient goes blue, is speechless and may die in the attack if the obstruction is not relieved.

Treatment involves immediately grasping the patient around the abdomen and squeezing hard in an effort to eject the food (see p. 576).

Parkinson's disease and other movement disorders

Disorders of movement can be classified broadly into akinetic-rigid syndromes, where there is loss of movement with increase in muscle tone, and dyskinesias, where there are added movements outside voluntary control. Both are due to disorders of the extrapyramidal system.

Parkinson's disease is much the commonest of these conditions. A classification of movement disorders is given in Table 18.37.

Table 18.37 A classification of movement disorders.

Akinetic-rigid syndromes
Parkinson's disease
Drug-induced parkinsonism, e.g. phenothiazines
MPTP-induced parkinsonism
Post-encephalitic parkinsonism
'Parkinsonism plus'
Childhood akinetic-rigid syndromes
Dyskinesias
Essential tremor
Chorea
Hemiballismus
Myoclonus
Tick or 'habit spasms'
Torsion dystonias

AKINETIC-RIGID SYNDROMES

Parkinson's disease

In 1817, James Parkinson, a physician in Hoxton, London, described the clinical appearance of patients with the 'shaking palsy'. The disease is common and world-wide, with prevalence increasing sharply with age to about 1 in 200 in those over 70 years. The condition is clinically distinct from other 'parkinsonian' syndromes.

There are few clues as to its cause:
- Patients who develop the disease have smoked less and die less frequently from lung cancer than the normal population.
- Minute doses of a pyridine compound (see p. 830) cause a severe parkinsonian syndrome. The significance of this to idiopathic Parkinson's disease is not clear.
- The condition is not inherited.
- Survivors of encephalitis lethargica, which is presumed to be a viral disease, develop parkinsonism. However, it is not thought that the idiopathic disease is related to this or to another infective agent.

PATHOLOGY

In the pars compacta of the substantia nigra there is progressive cell degeneration and the appearance of eosinophilic inclusion bodies (Lewy bodies). Degeneration also occurs in other brain stem nuclei. Biochemically there is loss of dopamine (and melanin) in the striatum which correlates well with the areas of cell loss and also with the degree of

akinesia. The underlying cause of these biochemical changes remains obscure.

CLINICAL FEATURES

There is a combination of tremor, rigidity and akinesia, together with important changes in posture.

Symptoms
The commonest symptoms are tremor and slowness of movement. Patients also complain that the limbs feel stiff and ache and that fine movements are difficult. The slowness of movement causes the characteristic symptoms of difficulty in rising from a chair or getting in or out of bed. Writing becomes small (micrographia) and spidery, with a tendency to tail off at the end of a line. Other evidence of the disease often comes from relatives who have noted slowness and an impassive facial expression.

Signs
Tremor. This is a characteristic 4–7 Hz rest tremor which is usually decreased by action and increased by emotion. 'Pill-rolling' movements of the fingers and thumbs may be seen. The shaking is sometimes unilateral or more prominent on one side.

Rigidity. Stiffness of the limbs develops which can be felt throughout the range of movement and equally in opposing groups of muscles (in contrast to the selective increase in tone found in spasticity). This 'lead-pipe' rigidity is often more marked on one side and is present in the neck and axial muscles (where it is difficult to examine).

The rigidity is usually more easily felt when a joint is moved slowly and gently. Simultaneous active movement of the opposite limb increases the tone of the side under examination. When combined with tremor, the smooth plasticity of the increase in tone is broken up into a jerky resistance to passive movement, a phenomenon known as 'cogwheeling'.

Akinesia. The poverty and slowing of movement (bradykinesia) is an additional handicap, distinct from rigidity. There is difficulty in initiating movement. Rapid finger movements (such as piano-playing movements) become indistinct, slow and tremulous. The immobility of the face gives a mask-like facies with the appearance of depression. The frequency of spontaneous blinking is reduced, causing a 'serpentine stare'.

Postural changes. A stoop is characteristic and the gait is shuffling, festinant and with poor arm swinging. The posture is sometimes, perhaps unfairly, called 'simian' to describe the forward flexion, immobility of the arms and lack of facial expression. The patient sits with the trunk bent forward and motionless, without gesture or animation, but the limbs are tremulous. Balance is impaired, but despite this the gait remains on a narrow base. Falls are common as the usual corrective righting reflexes fail, the sufferer falling stiffly 'like a telegraph pole'.

Speech. Speech is altered to a monotonous slurring dysarthria, due to the combination of akinesia, tremor and rigidity. Dribbling is frequent, and dysphagia occurs as the disease progresses.

Other findings. Constipation is usual and urinary difficulties are common, especially in men. The skin is greasy and sweating is excessive.

Power remains normal until advanced akinesia makes its assessment difficult. There is no sensory loss, although patients often complain of discomfort in the limbs. The reflexes are normal (though they may be asymmetrical, following an asymmetrical increase in tone). The plantar responses are flexor.

Cognitive function is preserved, at least in the early stages. In the late stages dementia sometimes occurs.

Natural history

Parkinson's disease progresses over a period of years, beginning as a mild inconvenience but slowly overtaking the patient. Remissions are unknown except for rare and remarkable short-lived periods of release. These tend to occur at times of great emotion, fear or excitement, when the sufferer is released for seconds or minutes and able to move quickly.

The rate of progression is very variable, with a benign form running over several decades. Usually the course is over 10–15 years, with death resulting from bronchopneumonia.

DIFFERENTIAL DIAGNOSIS

There is no laboratory test for the disease. The diagnosis is made on clinical grounds alone. The condition must be distinguished from other akinetic-rigid syndromes. Hypothyroidism and depression also cause slowing of movement.

Certain diffuse or multifocal brain diseases cause some features of 'parkinsonism' (i.e. the slowing, rigidity and tremor). Alzheimer's disease, multi-infarct dementia, and the sequelae of repeated head injury (e.g. in boxers) or hypoxia are the commoner examples.

TREATMENT

Older treatments with anticholinergic drugs altered the disease little, and frequently caused mental confusion. Benzhexol is still used in mild cases and as an adjunct to other therapy. Amantadine, originally introduced as an antiviral agent, is also sometimes effective.

Levodopa

The introduction of levodopa in the late 1960s was a revolutionary therapeutic approach, apparently replacing the lost neurotransmitter dopamine. Today levodopa is usually combined with a peripheral decarboxylase inhibitor—benserazide (as Madopar) or carbidopa (as Sinemet). This combined therapy reduces the peripheral side-effects, principally nausea, of levodopa and its metabolites.

Treatment is commenced gradually (Madopar 125 mg or Sinemet '110' one tablet three times daily) and increased until either an adequate improvement has taken place or side-effects limit further increase in dose.

The great majority of patients with Parkinson's disease (but not other parkinsonian syndromes) improve initially with levodopa. The response in severe, previously untreated disease may be dramatic.

Unwanted effects of levodopa therapy. Nausea and vomiting within an hour of treatment are the commonest symptoms of the dose being too large. Confusion and visual hallucinations also occur. Chorea occurs in acute overdose.

As there are considerable problems with long-term treatment, levodopa therapy should not be started until necessary. Sometimes the drug appears to become ineffective, even with increasing doses. The disease progresses and the patient suffers from severe episodes of 'freezing' and falls. Fluctuation in the response to levodopa may also occur. The duration of action of the drug contracts, and the patient begins to suffer from a 'chronic levodopa syndrome', fluctuating between dopa-induced dyskinesias (chorea and dystonic movements) and severe and sometimes sudden immobility (on–off syndrome).

These are major and often insoluble problems in management. Approaches to treatment of the complications include the following:

- The interval between levodopa doses can be shortened and the individual doses reduced.
- Selegiline—a type B monoamine oxidase inhibitor—inhibits the catabolism of dopamine in the brain. This sometimes has the effect of smoothing out the response to levodopa.
- 'Drug holidays'—periods of drug withdrawal—are sometimes helpful. They require close supervision since severe rigidity and akinesia follow the withdrawal of levodopa.

Alternative drugs to levodopa are directly acting dopaminergic agonists such as bromocriptine, which is similar in efficacy to levodopa although much more costly.

Psychiatric aspects

Depression is common in Parkinson's disease as the symptoms become worse and unresponsive to treatment. It is particularly difficult to treat as type A monoamine oxidase inhibitor antidepressants (e.g. phenelzine) are absolutely contraindicated with levodopa, and tricyclic antidepressants (e.g. amitriptyline) have extrapyramidal side-effects.

All anti-parkinsonian drugs, particularly in high doses, may cause confusion with visual hallucinations, which may exacerbate an associated dementia.

Neurosurgery

Stereotactic placement of small lesions in the ventrolateral nucleus of the thalamus was commonly used in the two decades preceding the development of levodopa. The procedure was effective in reducing tremor, but poor for relieving akinesia; it is now rarely performed.

Physiotherapy and physical aids

Skilled and determined physiotherapy can improve the gait and help the patient to overcome particular problems.

Sensible guidance should be given about:

- Clothing—avoiding zips, fiddly buttons and lace-up shoes
- Cutlery—using built-up handles
- Chairs—high, upright chairs are easier to rise from than a deep, comfortable armchair
- Rails—should be fitted near the lavatory and bath
- Shoes—should be easy to put on and have smooth soles
- Flooring—patients' feet sometimes 'stick' to carpets and rugs and they prefer to walk on vinyl or linoleum
- Walking aids—often a hindrance in the early stages, but later a frame or a tripod may be helpful

Drug-induced movement disorders

Parkinsonism

Reserpine, phenothiazines and butyrophenones induce a parkinsonian syndrome, with slowness and rigidity but usually little tremor. Methyldopa and tricyclic antidepressants also cause some slowing of movement. These syndromes tend not to progress. They respond poorly to levodopa. They disappear when the drug is stopped.

MPTP-induced parkinsonism. MPTP (1-methyl-4-phenyl-1,2,3,6-tetrahydropyridine) is an impurity produced inadvertently when opiate analgesics are synthesized illicitly. A few cases of a severe and largely irreversible parkinsonian syndrome have followed ingestion of minute quantities of MPTP. The relevance of this to idiopathic Parkinson's disease is not clear.

Other movement disorders due to neuroleptic drugs

Neuroleptic drugs (i.e. phenothiazines and butyrophenones) also produce other varieties of movement disorder.

Akathisia. This is a restless, repetitive and irresistible need to move.

Acute dystonic reactions. These sometimes follow, unpredictably, single doses of these drugs, even those used as antiemetics or vestibular sedatives, (such as prochlorperazine and metoclopramide). Spasmodic torticollis, trismus and oculogyric crises (i.e. episodes of sustained upward gaze) may occur. These acute dystonias respond promptly to the intravenous injection of an anticholinergic drug (e.g. benztropine 1–2 mg).

Chronic tardive dyskinesias. These disabling disorders consist of mouthing and smacking of the lips, grimaces and contortion of the face and neck. They tend to occur some 6 months after commencing neuroleptic therapy and may be made temporarily worse when the offending drug is stopped. Only about half of the cases eventually recover.

Post-encephalitic parkinsonism

An epidemic of an encephalitic illness (encephalitis lethargica) occurred in 1918–1930 which left in its wake a severe extrapyramidal syndrome of parkinsonism with added dystonic movement disorders. Many of the survivors were permanently disabled. No recent cases of the disease have been recorded in the UK; a recent epidemic may have occurred in Bulgaria.

'Parkinsonism plus'

This describes rare disorders in which there is parkinsonism and evidence of a separate pathology.

Progressive supranuclear palsy is the commonest disorder and consists of axial rigidity, dementia and signs of parkinsonism together with a striking inability to move the eyes vertically or laterally.

Other examples of 'parkinsonism plus' are the rare multiple system atrophies, e.g. olivo-ponto-cerebellar degeneration and primary autonomic failure (Shy–Drager syndrome).

Akinetic-rigid syndromes in children

A group of extremely rare disorders may cause an akinetic-rigid syndrome in those under 20 years of age. The most important are Wilson's disease and athetoid cerebral palsy.

Wilson's disease

This is a rare and treatable disorder of copper metabolism which is inherited as an autosomal recessive disease. There is deposition of copper in the brain (particularly in the basal ganglia), in the cornea and in the liver (see p. 240). It is most important that all young patients with cirrhosis are screened for this condition as the neurological damage is irreversible unless early treatment is instituted.

Children with the disease have an akinetic-rigid syndrome and/or dyskinesias followed by progressive intellectual impairment.

The condition may be recognized by the Kayser–Fleischer ring—a deposit of brownish-green pigment around the margin of the cornea in Descemet's membrane. In the early stages it can only be seen with a slit lamp.

Treatment is with penicillamine. Provided this is started early enough, the disease does not progress and may improve.

Athetoid cerebral palsy

Writhing movements of the limbs, sometimes with an increase in tone, are seen in cerebral palsy following kernicterus. This is now much less common following the prophylactic treatment of rhesus haemolytic disease.

DYSKINESIAS

Benign essential tremor

This common condition, often inherited as an autosomal dominant trait, causes tremor at 5–8 Hz which is usually worse in the upper limbs. The head and trunk may be involved. Pathologically there is patchy neuronal loss in the cerebellum and cerebellar connections. Tremor is seen when the hands adopt a posture, such as holding a glass or a spoon. Oscillations are not usually present at rest nor do they worsen on movement.

Essential tremor may be seen at any age but occurs most frequently in the elderly. It is slowly progressive but rarely produces a severe disability. Writing is shaky and untidy but there is no micrographia. Anxiety exacerbates the tremor, sometimes dramatically.

Treatment is often unnecessary. Many of those affected are reassured to find they do not have Parkinson's disease, with which the condition is often confused.

Small doses of alcohol and beta-adrenergic blockers such as propranolol often reduce the tremor. The anticonvulsant primidone also helps some patients. Sympathomimetics (e.g. salbutamol) make the tremor worse.

Chorea

Chorea consists of jerky, quasi-purposive and sometimes explosive movements, following each other but flitting from one part of the body to another. The causes of chorea are listed in Table 18.38; the commoner conditions are outlined below.

Huntington's disease

Relentlessly progressive chorea and dementia in

Table 18.38 Causes of chorea.

Huntington's disease
Sydenham's chorea
Benign hereditary chorea
Abetalipoproteinaemia (see p. 184) and chorea
Chorea associated with:
Drugs—phenytoin, levodopa, alcohol
Thyrotoxicosis
Systemic lupus erythematosus
Polycythaemia vera
Encephalitis lethargica
Stroke
Trauma (subdural haematoma)
Tumour

middle life are the hallmarks of this inherited disease which was first described in 1872 by George Huntington shortly after he qualified in medicine.

The prevalence of the disease is about 1 in 20000. It occurs world-wide. Inheritance is as an autosomal dominant trait with full penetrance; the children of an affected parent have a 50% chance of inheriting the disease as it rarely, if ever, jumps a generation. The family history of the disease in previous generations is often concealed, either by design or default. Recent advances in gene mapping and linkage association suggest a gene defect, possibly at the G8 locus of chromosome 4.

Pathology. There is cerebral atrophy with marked loss of small neurones in the caudate nucleus and putamen. Important changes in neurotransmitters occur:

● There is reduction in the enzymes synthesizing acetylcholine and GABA in the striatum.
● There is depletion of GABA, angiotensin-converting enzyme and met-enkephalin in the substantia nigra.
● Somatostatin levels are high in the corpus striatum.

These changes may be secondary to the cell damage. In contrast to Parkinson's disease, dopamine and tyrosine hydroxylase activity are normal.

Management and course. There is steady progression, of both the dementia and chorea. No treatment arrests the disease, although phenothiazines may reduce the chorea by causing drug-induced parkinsonism. Tetrabenazine 25 g three times daily is also used to control the chorea. Death usually occurs between 10 and 20 years after the onset.

There are at present no predictive tests for Huntington's chorea and some families choose to be sterilized in an effort to eradicate the gene. The discovery of a DNA marker makes prenatal diagnosis possible, but the exact inheritance is still being evaluated. Thus great caution must be taken in advising families as there are great legal and social implications of preclinical diagnosis.

Sydenham's chorea (St Vitus' dance)

Thomas Sydenham described this transient chorea of adolescence and childhood in 1686. Less than half of the cases follow within 3 months of rheumatic fever (see p. 512). It may recur, or appear, in adult life during pregnancy (chorea gravidarum) or in those taking oral contraceptives. In each case there is a diffuse encephalitis.

The onset of the chorea is usually gradual. Irritability, insolence and inattentiveness herald the onset of fidgety movements which are sometimes predominantly unilateral. A minority of patients are confused. Although rheumatic heart disease is sometimes found, the child usually does not have a fever or other features of rheumatic fever. The ASO titre and ESR are rarely raised.

Recovery occurs spontaneously within weeks or months.

Hemiballismus

Hemiballismus (also called hemiballism) describes violent swinging movements of one side of the body caused usually by infarction or haemorrhage in the ipsilateral subthalamic nucleus.

Myoclonus

Myoclonus is the sudden, involuntary jerking of a single muscle or a group of muscles. It occurs in a wide range of disorders and is sometimes provoked by a sudden stimulus such as a loud noise.

Benign essential myoclonus

Nocturnal myoclonus, i.e. sudden jerking of a limb or the body on falling asleep, is extremely common and not pathological.

'Paramyoclonus multiplex' is widespread, random muscle jerking usually occurring in adolescence. Fits do not occur.

Myoclonic epilepsy

Muscle jerking is a feature of many different forms of epilepsy.

Progressive myoclonic epilepsies

These very rare conditions include various familial and metabolic disorders where myoclonus accompanies a progressive encephalopathy.

An example is Lafora body disease, a syndrome of myoclonus, epilepsy and dementia, with mucopolysaccharide inclusion bodies in neurones, liver cells and intestinal mucosa.

Static myoclonic encephalopathies

Myoclonus may follow a severe brain insult such as severe cerebral anoxia following cardiac arrest.

Tics

Repetitive twitching movements of the face, neck or hand are part of our normal motor gestures. Patients or their relatives seek advice about them when they become too frequent or irritating. Simple transient tics, e.g. sniffing or a particular facial grimace, are common in childhood, but may persist into adult life.

The rare Gilles de la Tourette syndrome is the occurrence of multiple tics accompanied by sudden explosive barking and grunting with the utterance of sexually related obscenities. The condition develops in childhood or adolescence, in either sex, and is usually lifelong. This is thought to be due to an organic disorder of the basal ganglia. Treatment with haloperidol is sometimes helpful.

Torsion dystonias

Dystonia implies a movement caused by a prolonged muscular contraction when a part of the body is thrown into spasm. A classification of the dystonias is given in Table 18.39.

Table 18.39 A classification of dystonias.

Generalized dystonia
Idiopathic dystonia musculorum deformans
Drug-induced dystonia (e.g. metoclopramide)
Symptomatic dystonia (e.g. after encephalitis lethargica or in Wilson's disease)
Paroxysmal dystonia (very rare, familial, with marked fluctuation)
Focal dystonia
Spasmodic torticollis
Writer's cramp
Oromandibular dystonia
Blepharospasm
Hemiplegic dystonia (e.g. following stroke)

Dystonia musculorum deformans

This rare disease is frequently inherited (there are various modes of transmission) and commences in childhood as dystonic spasms of the limbs which affect gait and posture. It is gradually progressive, spreading to all parts of the body over one or two decades. Intellect is not impaired. Spontaneous remissions occasionally occur.

Spasmodic torticollis

Dystonic spasms gradually develop around the neck, usually in the third to fifth decade. They cause the head to turn (torticollis) or to be drawn backwards (retrocollis) or forwards.

Minor dystonic movements can also affect the trunk or limbs. A curious feature is that some patients have a 'trigger area', often on the jaw. Gentle pressure at this site relieves the involuntary movement.

Various psychiatric explanations have been

advanced for this and other movement disorders, but it is now felt that they are organic conditions. Torticollis may remit but many cases remain for life.

Writer's cramp

This is a specific inability to perform a previously highly developed skilled movement, especially writing, due to a curious dystonic posturing. It occurs particularly in those who spend many hours each day writing, and is thus seen less frequently now than in former years. Other skilled functions of the hand are normal and there are no other neurological signs. Prolonged rest sometimes seems to help the condition but it may become a major disability.

Blepharospasm and oromandibular dystonia

These related conditions consist of spasms of forced blinking or involuntary movement of the mouth and tongue, e.g. lip-smacking and protrusion of the tongue and jaw. Speech may be affected.

TREATMENT

All dystonic movement disorders are particularly difficult to treat. Butyrophenones (e.g. haloperidol) are sometimes helpful. Blepharospasm can be helped by minute injections of botulinum toxin into the orbicularis oculi muscle.

Multiple sclerosis

Multiple sclerosis (MS) is a common disease of unknown cause in which there are multiple areas of demyelination within the brain and spinal cord. These are 'disseminated in time and place' (hence the old name 'disseminated sclerosis'). An acquired defect in the oligodendroglial cells which produce myelin may be responsible.

The commonest age of onset is between 20 and 35 years. In the UK MS causes disability of varying degree in over 50 000 people.

PREVALENCE

The disease occurs world-wide, but the prevalence varies widely, being directly proportional to the distance from the equator. At 50–65° N (roughly Land's End to Iceland) the prevalence is 60–100 per 100 000 people; at latitudes less than 30° N the prevalence is less than 10 per 100 000; and at the equator it is a rarity. In the southern hemisphere the variation is similar.

AETIOLOGY

The cause of the disease is unknown.

Familial incidence and HLA linkage

First degree relatives of a patient have an increased chance of developing MS, although there is no clearcut pattern of inheritance.

In caucasians in northern Europe and the USA, there is a positive association between MS and antigens HLA-A3, B7 and DR2.

Infection

Although efforts to transmit MS experimentally have been uniformly unsuccessful, there is an abnormal immune response in MS patients, with an increase in the titres of serum and CSF antibodies to many common viruses, particularly measles.

Certain epidemic transmissable zoonoses, such as scrapie, a demyelinating disease in sheep, are pathologically similar to MS.

Diet

It has been suggested that MS is related to the consumption of large quantities of animal fats. Surveys in Norway have shown that MS is distinctly uncommon in coastal fishing communities compared with agricultural areas. However, the role of diet is particularly difficult to evaluate.

PATHOLOGY

The essential features are plaques of demyelination, initially 2–10 mm in size (see Fig. 18.20). These lesions are perivenular and have a predelection for the following sites within the brain and spinal cord:
- Optic nerves
- Brain stem and its cerebellar connections
- Cervical cord
- Periventricular region

Plaques very rarely occur in the neighbourhood of anterior horn cells, and never occur in the myelin sheaths of peripheral nerves.

Fig. 18.20 Multiple sclerosis. Cross-section of the spinal cord showing demyelination (arrows) in the posterior column and lateral corticospinal tracts. Courtesy of Professor W.I. Macdonald.

CLINICAL FEATURES

Common presentations of MS are described below.

Optic neuropathy (ON)

Symptoms. The patient complains of blurring of vision in one eye. Mild ocular pain is usual. The symptoms progress, usually over days, to produce severe visual loss. Recovery occurs, typically within a month. Bilateral ON sometimes occurs.

Signs. The signs of ON depend upon the site of the plaque. When the lesion is in the optic nerve head there is disc swelling (optic neuritis). If the lesion is several millimetres proximal to the disc there are often no ophthalmoscopic features ('the doctor sees nothing and the patient sees nothing'); this is known as retrobulbar neuritis.

Optic neuritis is easily distinguished from papilloedema of other cause by the presence of early visual loss.

A relative afferent pupillary defect is often present in the early stages. This persists after recovery.

Sequelae. There are usually no residual symptoms, but small scotomata and defects in colour vision can be demonstrated. Following the attack, disc pallor appears (optic atrophy), first in the temporal region and then spreading to affect the whole disc.

Brain stem demyelination

An acute episode affecting the brain stem causes diplopia, vertigo, facial numbness or dysphagia. 'Pyramidal' signs in the limbs occur when the corticospinal tracts are involved.

A typical picture is sudden diplopia and vertigo with nystagmus, but without tinnitus or deafness. This lasts for some weeks before recovery. Diplopia may be caused by many different lesions—a sixth nerve lesion and an internuclear ophthalmoplegia are two examples.

Cord lesion

A spastic paraparesis is caused by demyelination in the cord. There is difficulty in walking and sensory disturbance. Urinary symptoms are common.

No single group of signs is diagnostic of MS. Despite this the disease is often recognizable on clinical grounds. There are two patterns of MS:
- Relapsing and remitting, with lesions occurring in different parts of the CNS at different times so that no single lesion can account for the different signs
- Chronic progressive

The distinction between the two is often difficult.

In the initial episode it may be impossible to decide, even with specialized tests, whether or not a lesion is due to demyelination. The appearance of subsequent lesions confirms the diagnosis. Remissions may last for many years; their length is unpredictable.

The later stages of the disease are characterized by progressive disability with a spastic tetraparesis, ataxia, brain stem signs, pseudobulbar palsy and incontinence of urine. Dementia is common. Death follows from uraemia and/or bronchopneumonia.

DIFFERENTIAL DIAGNOSIS

Few other neurological diseases of young people follow a similar relapsing and remitting course. Thromboembolism causes symptoms which are characteristically more sudden in onset. Other degenerative conditions such as Friedreich's ataxia are gradually progessive, without remissions.

Initially individual plaques (e.g. in the optic nerve, brain stem or cord) may cause diagnostic difficulty; they must be distinguished from compressive, inflammatory, mass or other lesions.

CNS sarcoidosis and systemic lupus erythematosus are very rare but may mimic the relapsing pattern of MS.

INVESTIGATION

There is no single diagnostic test for MS. Examination of the peripheral blood and urine is unhelpful and there are no features on plain x-rays.

Examination of the CSF has long been used to support the diagnosis. Table 18.40 summarizes the investigations that are usually performed. The appearance and pressure of the fluid and the level of

Table 18.40 The CSF in multiple sclerosis (MS).

Constituent	Normal	MS	Comments
Cell count	<5 per mm^3	5–60 per mm^3	Rarely up to 100 per mm^3, typically mononuclear cells
Total protein	0.2–0.4 g·l^{-1}	0.4–1.0 g·l^{-1}	Normal in 40% of cases
IgG	<15% of total protein	>15% of total protein	Normal in 60% of cases
Oligoclonal IgG	Negative	Positive	Bands present in 80% of cases

The Pandy test and Lange colloidal gold curve are obsolete.

glucose are normal, and serological tests for syphilis are negative. The presence of oligoclonal bands of IgG indicate the production of immunoglobulin (to unknown antigens) within the central nervous system.

Electrophysiological tests

Delay in the visual-evoked response (VER) follows optic neuropathy. As some attacks are subclinical, a delayed VER may provide evidence of a second lesion within the central nervous system in, for example, an undiagnosed cord lesion.

Brain stem and somatosensory-evoked potentials are also sometimes measured.

Peripheral nerve studies are normal. EEG recordings are unhelpful.

CT and MRI scanning

Plaques of demyelination are sometimes seen as low attenuation lesions on CT scans, although this is unusual. With chronic disease cerebral atrophy is seen.

MRI scanning identifies plaques readily in this disease and may be valuable in cases where there is doubt about the diagnosis (see Fig. 18.2).

MANAGEMENT AND PROGNOSIS

Once diagnosed, practical decisions need to be taken about employment, home and plans for the future in the face of a potentially disabling disease. It is now usual practice to inform patients of the diagnosis.

There is no method of predicting the course of MS but there is wide variation in its severity. Many MS patients live self-sufficient, productive lives while others are gravely disabled.

Wise counsel and honesty, tempered with reassurance of the benign course of many cases of MS, is important.

MANAGEMENT

Many forms of therapy have been suggested for MS, including cryotherapy, pyrotherapy, vaccines, purified protein derivative (PPD), transfer factor, electrical stimulation, gluten-free diets, sunflower seed oil, arsenicals and hyperbaric oxygen. None of these has been shown to benefit patients.

Short courses of ACTH and corticosteroids are used widely in exacerbations and do sometimes appear to reduce temporarily the effect of a relapse. They do not influence the outlook in the long term. Immunosuppressants (azathioprine, cyclophosphamide) are also used, but there is no agreement about their value.

In any chronic neurological disease, treatment of intercurrent infections is important. Urinary infection frequently exacerbates the symptoms.

Muscle relaxants (e.g. baclofen, benzodiazepines and dantrolene) reduce the pain and discomfort of spasticity, particularly when there are flexor spasms of the lower limbs.

Other measures

There is much that should be done for a patient with any chronic neurological disease. Practical advice at work, on walking aids, wheelchairs, car conversions, alterations to houses and gardens can be given. Support in a wide range of areas from fear and reactive depression to the sexual difficulties of the disabled is also helpful.

Infective and inflammatory disease

MENINGITIS

Meningitis (inflammation of the meninges) may be caused by:

- Bacteria
- Viruses
- Fungi
- Other organisms
- Neoplastic cells
- Drugs and contrast media
- Blood (following subarachnoid haemorrhage)

The term is usually restricted to inflammation due to infective agents (see Table 18.41). Microorganisms reach the meninges either by direct extension from the ears, nasopharynx, a cranial injury or congenital meningeal defect, or by spread via the bloodstream.

Table 18.41 Infective causes of meningitis in the UK.

BACTERIA
Neisseria meningitidis*
Haemophilus influenzae*
Streptococcus pneumoniae*
Mycobacterium tuberculosis
Treponema pallidum
VIRUSES
Echo
Coxsackie
Epstein–Barr virus
Mumps
(Polio)
FUNGI
Cryptococcus neoformans
(*Coccidioides immitis, Histoplasma capsulatum, Blastomyces dermatitidis* in USA)

* These organisms account for 70% of acute bacterial meningitis outside the neonatal period. A wide variety of bacteria are responsible for the remaining 30% of cases.

PATHOLOGY

In acute bacterial meningitis the pia-arachnoid is congested with polymorphs. A layer of pus forms which may organize to form adhesions, causing cranial nerve palsies and hydrocephalus. In tuberculous infection the brain is covered in a viscous grey-green exudate; numerous tubercles are found on the meninges. Cerebral oedema is common in bacterial meningitis.

In viral meningitis there is a predominantly lymphocytic inflammatory reaction in the CSF without the formation of pus or adhesions. There is no cerebral oedema unless viral encephalitis develops.

CLINICAL FEATURES (Table 18.42)

Meningitic syndrome
There is intense malaise, fever, rigors, severe headache, photophobia and vomiting. The patient is irritable and often prefers to lie still.

Neck stiffness and a positive Kernig's sign appear within a few hours. In milder cases (and many viral meningitides) there are few other signs, but it is most unreliable to rely on the clinical impression alone when assessing the severity of the infection.

In uncomplicated meningitis, consciousness is not impaired, although the patient may be delirious with a high fever. The appearance of drowsiness, lateralizing signs and cranial nerve lesions including papilloedema indicate a complication such as a venous sinus thrombosis (see p. 822), severe cerebral oedema or hydrocephalus, or an alternative diagnosis such as a cerebral abscess (see p. 840) or encephalitis (see p. 837).

Specific varieties of meningitis
Particular attention should be paid to rashes and associated clinical features (see Table 18.42), and a search should be made for infected foci.

Table 18.42 Clinical clues in meningitis.

Clinical feature	Probable cause
Petechial rash	Meningococcal infection
Skull fracture Ear disease Congenital CNS lesion	Pneumococcal infection
Previous antibiotics	Partially treated bacterial infection
Rash or pleurodynia	Enterovirus infection
International travel	Poliomyelitis (Malaria)
Occupational history (working with infected water), prostration, myalgia, conjunctivitis and jaundice	Leptospirosis

Acute bacterial meningitis. The onset is sudden, with rigors and a high fever. A petechial rash, often sparse, is strong evidence of meningococcal meningitis. Septicaemia may present with acute septicaemic shock.

Viral meningitis. This is almost always a benign, self-limiting condition lasting 4–10 days. Headache may follow for some weeks but there are no serious sequelae.

Tuberculous meningitis. TB causes a chronic meningitis commencing with vague headache, lassitude, anorexia and vomiting. Meningitic signs may appear only after some weeks. Drowsiness, focal signs and seizures may occur. A similar picture occurs in cryptococcal meningitis.

Malignant meningitis. Malignant cells sometimes cause a subacute or chronic meningitic process. Meningitis, cranial nerve palsies, paraparesis and root lesions are seen, often in complex patterns. The CSF shows increased cells and protein and often a low glucose. Treatment is with intrathecal methotrexate. The prognosis is poor.

DIFFERENTIAL DIAGNOSIS

Acute meningitis may resemble subarachnoid haemorrhage, severe migraine and other causes of a sudden severe headache. Meningitis should be considered in all patients who have headache and fever.

MANAGEMENT

Meningitis is an emergency which has a high mortality even in countries with highly developed systems of health care. Although viral meningitis is a self-limiting condition, untreated bacterial meningitis is lethal; in most series the death rate is around 15%. An accurate diagnosis is vital.

If there is no suggestion of an intracranial mass lesion (when CT scanning should be performed), immediate lumbar puncture should be carried out. Typical changes in the CSF are shown in Table 18.43. Blood should be drawn for culture and glucose as well as for routine tests. Chest and skull films should be taken if possible.

Gram-staining of the CSF demonstrates organisms (e.g. gram-positive intracellular diplococci—pneumococcus; gram-negative cocci—meningococcus). Ziehl Neelsen stain demonstrates acid-fast bacilli (TB), though these organisms are rarely numerous. Indian ink stains fungi.

Many serological tests are now available for CSF. Syphilitic serology should always be carried out.

The clinical picture and CSF examination should allow at least a presumptive diagnosis of the cause of the meningitis to be made.

Table 18.43 Typical changes in the CSF in meningitis.

	Normal	Viral	Pyogenic	TB
Appearance	Crystal clear	Clear/turbid	Turbid/purulent	Turbid/viscous
Mononuclear cells	<5 per mm^3	10–100 per mm^3	<50 per mm^3	100–300 per mm^3
Polymorph cells	Nil	Nil*	200–3000 per mm^3	0–200 per mm^3
Protein	0.2–0.4 g·l^{-1}	0.4–0.8 g·l^{-1}	0.5–2.0 g·l^{-1}	0.5–3.0 g·l^{-1}
Glucose	>½ of blood glucose	>½ of blood glucose	<⅓ of normal blood glucose	<⅓ of normal blood glucose

* Some polymorph cells may be seen in the early stages of viral meningitis.

Treatment of bacterial meningitis

It is often possible to distinguish between viral, pyogenic, tuberculous and other organisms from the clinical setting and immediate examination of the CSF. If bacterial meningitis is suspected, high doses of antibiotics are imperative. There should be close liaison with a microbiologist.

In an undiagnosed pyogenic infection in an adult, intravenous benzylpenicillin 2 g 2-hourly and intravenous chloramphenicol 75 mg·kg^{-1} is given. If the diagnosis of pneumococcal or meningococcal infection has been made, penicillin alone may be used. Chloramphenicol alone may be used in *Haemophilus* infections.

Tuberculous meningitis is treated for at least 12 months with antituberculous drugs; rifampicin, isoniazid and pyrazinamide is the usual combination (see p. 602).

It is no longer usual to use intrathecal antibiotics.

Local infection (e.g. an infected paranasal sinus) should also be treated, surgically if necessary.

Differential diagnosis of CSF pleocytosis

Difficulties occur in meningitis when a raised, often mixed (lymphocyte and polymorph) picture is found but no infecting organism. This is sometimes called 'aseptic meningitis'. The conditions listed in Table 18.44 should be considered.

Table 18.44 Causes of CSF pleocytosis.

Partially treated bacterial meningitis
Viral meningitis
TB or fungi
Neoplastic meningitis
Parameningeal foci (e.g. paranasal sinus)
Syphilis
Intracranial abscess
Cerebral venous or arterial infarction
Encephalitis
Rare causes (e.g. cerebral malaria, sarcoidosis, Behçet's syndrome)

ENCEPHALITIS

Encephalitis is inflammation within the brain. It is caused by a wide variety of viruses and may also occur in bacterial and other infections.

Acute viral encephalitis

In many cases viral aetiology is presumed but not confirmed serologically or by culture. The usual organisms cultured from cases of viral encephalitis in adults in Britain are echo, coxsackie, mumps and herpes simplex viruses.

Adenovirus, varicella zoster, influenza, measles and other viruses are rarer causes.

CLINICAL FEATURES

Many of these infections cause a mild self-limiting illness with headache and drowsiness. In a minority there is a more serious illness accompanied by focal signs, seizures and coma. Herpes simplex virus (herpesvirus hominis type 1) accounts for many of these severe infections in Britain and has a mortality of around 25%. In the Far East the Japanese B arbovirus is a more usual, and epidemic, cause of severe encephalitis, with a high mortality.

DIFFERENTIAL DIAGNOSIS

This includes:
- Bacterial meningitis complicated by cerebral oedema and/or cerebral venous thrombosis
- Cerebral abscess
- Acute disseminated encephalomyelitis
- Toxic confusional states in febrile illnesses and in septicaemia

INVESTIGATION

Investigation in severe cases includes CT scanning (which characteristically shows areas of oedema), EEG (which shows slow wave changes) and viral studies of blood and CSF.

Brain biopsy is seldom performed in the UK.

TREATMENT

Suspected herpes simplex encephalitis is treated with intravenous acyclovir, the active form of which inhibits DNA synthesis. Phosphorylation of this drug is dependent upon the presence of viral thymidine kinase; thus the drug is specific for certain viral infections. If the patient is in coma the outlook is poor whether or not drugs are given.

Supportive measures are required for comatose patients. Seizures are treated with anticonvulsants. Prophylactic immunization is possible against Japanese B encephalitis.

Acute disseminated encephalomyelitis (ADE)

This follows many common viral infections (e.g. measles, varicella zoster, mumps and rubella) and immunization against rabies, smallpox, influenza or pertussis. The clinical syndrome is often similar to acute viral encephalitis, with added focal brain stem and/or spinal cord lesions due to demyelination, but in which viral particles are not usually present. The prognosis is variable. Mild cases recover completely, but in severe cases (those in coma) mortality is around 25% and the survivors often have permanent brain damage. Treatment is supportive, with steroids and/or anticonvulsants when necessary.

VIRAL MYELITIS

Myelitis means inflammation of the spinal cord causing paraparesis or tetraparesis. It occurs with varicella zoster or as part of a post-infective encephalomyelitis. Poliomyelitis is a specific enterovirus infection of anterior horn cells (see p. 54).

Transverse myelitis is described on p. 849.

HERPES ZOSTER (SHINGLES)

This is a recrudescence of infection with varicella zoster virus within the dorsal root ganglia (or certain cranial nerves), the original infection having been acquired in an attack of chickenpox many years previously.

CLINICAL FEATURES

The skin changes are described on p. 925.

In the cranial nerves, herpes zoster has a predeliction for the fifth and seventh nerve. 'Ophthalmic herpes' is infection of the first division of the fifth nerve, and may lead to corneal scarring and secondary panophthalmitis. 'Geniculate herpes' (the Ramsay-Hunt syndrome, see p. 801) leads to facial palsy accompanied by vesicles on the pinna, external auditory meatus and fauces.

The local complications of shingles are secondary bacterial infection, very rarely purpura and necrosis in the affected segment ('purpura fulminans'), generalized herpes zoster, and post-herpetic neuralgia.

A myelitis, meningoencephalitis or motor radiculopathy may be caused by varicella zoster.

Post-herpetic neuralgia

Post-herpetic neuralgia is pain in the zone of the previous eruption; it occurs in some 10% of patients. It is a burning, continuous pain responding poorly to all analgesics. Depression is almost universal. Treatment is unsatisfactory but there is a trend towards gradual recovery over 2 years.

NEUROSYPHILIS

Syphilis is described on p. 42.

Before penicillin therapy, some 10% of patients infected at sexual contact by the spirochaete *Treponema pallidum* developed tertiary neurological disease, often 10–25 years after the primary infection. A wide variety of syndromes were described, all of which are now clinical rarities. Neurosyphilis does, however, still occur, particularly in those who may have had many sexual partners.

For practical purposes, negative serological tests for syphilis in blood exclude the disease.

The main tertiary syphilitic syndromes are described below.

Asymptomatic neurosyphilis

This is the term used to describe positive CSF serology without signs.

Meningovascular syphilis

This presents as:

- A subacute meningitis often with cranial nerve palsies and papilloedema
- A focal form in which a gumma, an expanding intracranial mass, causes epilepsy, raised pressure and focal deficits, e.g. hemiplegia
- A paraparesis caused by a spinal meningovasculitis

Tabes dorsalis

This is a complex syndrome in which demyelination occurs in the dorsal roots. Many of the features are due to 'de-afferentation'. The elements of the syndrome are:

- Lightning pains (see p. 811)
- Ataxia, loss of reflexes, widespread sensory loss and some muscle wasting
- Neuropathic joints (Charcot's joints)
- Argyll Robertson pupils
- Ptosis and optic atrophy

General paralysis of the insane (GPI)

The grandiose title indicates that this is a syndrome of madness and weakness. The dementia is often similar to that associated with Alzheimer's disease (see p. 852). Progressive dementia, brisk reflexes, extensor plantar reflexes and tremor occur. Death follows within 3 years of the onset.

Argyll Robertson pupils are usually present. Seizures may occur.

Other forms

Mixtures of the syndromes described above occur.

In congenital neurosyphilis (acquired in utero) there are features of both tabes dorsalis and GPI in childhood; this is known as taboparesis.

In secondary syphilis a self-limiting meningeal reaction occurs which may be symptomless or may cause a subacute meningitis.

TREATMENT

Benzylpenicillin 1 g daily by injection for 10 days in primary infection eliminates future tertiary syphilis. Established neurological disease can be arrested but not usually reversed with penicillin. Allergic reactions (Jarisch–Herxheimer reactions) may occur; high-dose steroid cover is usually given with penicillin to reduce their severity.

OTHER INFECTIONS

The central nervous system is involved in many infective diseases.

Rabies (see p. 61)

This is transmitted to man via penetrating wounds. The rabies virus multiplies in the wound and migrates via the peripheral nerves and dorsal root ganglia to the central nervous system. A fatal encephalitis follows in which, at autopsy, characteristic neuronal inclusion bodies (Negri bodies) are observed.

Tetanus (see p. 24)

This may follow even a trivial wound. There is liberation of a powerful toxin which travels within motor nerves to reach the central nervous system where it binds irreversibly with certain sialic acid-containing gangliosides. The toxin blocks inhibition of spinal reflexes, resulting in spasms.

Botulism (see p. 25)

The paralytic symptoms of botulism are caused by a presynaptic block in neuromuscular transmission.

Lyme disease (see p. 48)

This produces a chronic radiculopathy. A paraparesis can occur.

Leprosy (see p. 38)

In tuberculoid leprosy a mononeuritis multiplex is seen. The infected nerves become large and palpable as hard cords. The peripheral nerves are also affected in lepromatous leprosy.

Poliomyelitis (see p. 54)

In this condition there is invasion of the anterior horn cells by the pathogenic virus. Many infections are subclinical, but in a minority there is serious paralytic disease involving the respiratory muscles and sometimes giving a bulbar palsy.

Acquired immunodeficiency syndrome (AIDS) (see p. 63)

Opportunistic brain infection may occur in AIDS (e.g. toxoplasmosis, fungal infections, cerebral abscess with mixed organisms). Dementia, cerebellar signs and polyneuropathy are also seen.

Other examples of infections involving the central nervous system are summarized in Table 18.45.

MISCELLANEOUS INFLAMMATORY CONDITIONS

Progressive rubella encephalitis

Some 10 years after the primary infection there is rarely a progressive syndrome of mental impairment, fits, optic atrophy, cerebellar and pyramidal signs. There is evidence of local antibody production against rubella viral antigen within the CNS.

Subacute sclerosing pan-encephalitis (SSPE)

The persistence of measles antigen in the CNS is believed to be the cause of this rare late sequel to measles infection. Progressive mental deterioration, fits, myoclonus and pyramidal signs occur, usually in a child. Diagnosis is confirmed by demonstrating a high titre of measles antibody in the blood and CSF.

Creutzfeldt–Jakob disease (CJD)

This is a slowly progressive dementia characterized pathologically by 'spongiform encephalopathy'. It occurs world-wide and is transmitted by an agent resistant to many of the usual sterilization processes. The name given to such agents is 'slow viruses'. Infection has been transmitted from post-mortem and surgical specimens and corneal grafts, and to the recipients of human growth hormone (which was obtained from human pituitary glands removed at autopsy).

The condition has a long incubation period, sometimes up to several years. Death is almost invariable within 2 years from the onset of symptoms.

Kuru

This is a dementia and cerebellar ataxia occurring in

Table 18.45 Miscellaneous CNS infections.

Organism	Disease	CNS manifestation
Rickettsia	Typhus Scrub typhus Rocky mountain spotted fever	Meningo-encephalitis
Plasmodium falciparum	Malaria	Meningo-encephalitis
Toxoplasma gondii	Toxoplasmosis	Meningo-encephalitis (e.g. in AIDS)
Naegleria fowleri (a freshwater amoeba)		Meningo-encephalitis
Entamoeba histolytica	Amoebiasis	Brain abscess
Trypanosoma rhodesiense *Trypanosoma gambiense*	Trypanosomiasis	Encephalitis
Echinococcus granulosus	Hydatid disease	Intracranial cysts
Taenia solium	Cysticercosis	Multiple intracranial cysts
Schistosoma mansoni	Schistosomiasis	Encephalopathy Cord lesions
Strongyloides stercoralis	Strongyloidiasis	Meningo-encephalitis

the highlands of New Guinea. It is believed to have been spread by ritual cannibalism. Spongiform change occurs in the brain (very similar to Creutzfeldt–Jakob disease). This obscure condition is also believed to be transmitted by a slow virus.

Progressive multifocal leuco-encephalopathy
This is an opportunistic infection with the papovaviruses JC and SV-40 (and others) in patients who are immunosuppressed. Multifocal demyelinating hemisphere lesions develop which contain virus particles. Death is usual after several years.

Reye's syndrome (see also p. 246)
This is a severe encephalitic illness, usually of children, accompanied by fatty infiltration of the liver and hypoglycaemia. A viral cause has been postulated, but other factors, including aspirin therapy, have also been implicated.

Mollaret's meningitis
This term is used to describe recurrent episodes of 'aseptic meningitis' over many years. A viral cause is postulated. Some of these patients are helped by treatment with the mitotic poison colchicine.

Vogt–Koyanagi–Harada syndrome
This is a recurrent inflammatory disease of cells of neural crest origin, causing uveitis, meningo-encephalitis, vitiligo, deafness and alopecia.

Epidemic neuromyasthenia
Headache, fever, lassitude, torpor, myalgia and depression sometimes follow epidemic viral infections. Some patients develop transient ocular palsies. Vacuolar changes in peripheral lymphocytes have sometimes been noted.

Sarcoidosis (see p. 603)
This condition may cause a chronic meningo-encephalitis with sarcoid lesions within the brain and spinal cord, a peripheral neuropathy, cranial nerve palsies (particularly bilateral seventh nerve palsies) or, rarely, a myopathy.

Behçet's syndrome
The three principal features are recurrent oral and genital ulceration, inflammatory ocular disease and neurological syndromes. Brain stem and cord lesions, aseptic meningitis, encephalitis and cerebral venous thrombosis also occur.

ABSCESSES

Brain abscess (see Fig. 18.21c)

A focal area of infection within the cerebrum or cerebellum may present as an expanding mass lesion (see p. 843). The usual organisms are streptococci (aerobic, anaerobic and microaerophilic species), *Bacteroides* spp., staphylococci and enterobacteria. Mixed infections are common. Fungi can also cause brain abscesses. A parameningeal (e.g. ear, nose, paranasal sinus, skull fracture) or distant (e.g. lung, heart, abdomen) focus of infection may be present. Frequently no cause is found.

Tuberculoma
Tubercle bacilli cause chronic caseating intracranial granulomas—tuberculomas—which are the commonest single intracranial masses in areas such as India where TB is common. Tuberculomas either present as mass lesions or occur in the course of tuberculous meningitis. They may also be symptom-

less and appear on skull x-rays as areas of intracranial calcification.

CLINICAL FEATURES

Headache, focal signs (e.g. hemiparesis, aphasia, hemianopia), epilepsy and raised intracranial pressure occur. Fever, leucocytosis and a raised ESR are usual in cerebral abscess but are not always present. The presentation may thus be remarkably similar to many cerebral neoplasms. The symptoms may be indolent, developing over weeks, particularly in the cerebral hemispheres. Cerebellar abscesses develop more acutely.

MANAGEMENT

Urgent CT scanning is essential. The search for a focus of infection should include a detailed examination of the skull, ears and paranasal sinuses.

Lumbar puncture is contraindicated in suspected brain abscess.

Treatment should be carried out with liaison between neurosurgeon and microbiologist. Surgical decompression may be necessary if antibiotics are unsuccessful. Despite treatment the mortality of abscess remains high, at around 25%, and epilepsy is common in survivors.

Spinal epidural abscess

Staphylococcus aureus is the usual organism responsible. It reaches the spine via the bloodstream, e.g. from a boil. There is fever and usually back pain followed by paraparesis or root lesions. Emergency myelography, decompression and antibiotics are indicated.

Subdural empyema

This is usually secondary to local infection. The features are similar to those of a cerebral abscess.

Intracranial epidural abscess

Rarely, a collection of pus tracks along the intracranial epidural space, causing sequential cranial nerve lesions, typically without evidence of raised pressure. There is usually evidence of local infection.

Fig. 18.21 CT scan appearances of various conditions. (a) Extradural haemorrhage. (b) Subdural haemorrhage. (c) Abscess. (d) Meningioma. (e) Secondary neoplasm. (f) Acoustic neuroma.

Intracranial tumours

Primary intracranial tumours account for approximately 10% of all neoplasms. The commoner varieties of tumours are outlined in Table 18.46; around one-quarter are metastases (Fig. 18.21e).

Table 18.46 Relative frequency of common intracranial tumours on the basis of clinical presentation.

Tumour	Relative frequency
Primary malignant (glioma) Astrocytoma Oligodendroglioma	40%
Benign Meningioma Neurofibroma	30%
Metastases Bronchus Breast Stomach Prostate Thyroid Kidney	25%

Differences between overall annual incidence rates (Table 18.2) and presentation as clinical problems (Table 18.46) are accounted for by the fact that small meningiomas and cerebral metastases may be found unexpectedly at post-mortem.

Gliomas

These are malignant, intrinsic tumours which originate in neuroglia, usually within the cerebral hemispheres. Their cause is unknown. They are occasionally associated with neurofibromatosis.

Primary intracranial malignant tumours virtually never metastasize outside the CNS and spread only by direct extension.

Astrocytomas. These tumours arise from astrocytes. They are classified into grades I–IV, depending on malignancy. Grade I astrocytomas grow slowly over many years while grade IV tumours cause death within several months.

Cystic astrocytomas occur in childhood, usually within the cerebellum. They are relatively benign.

Oligodendrogliomas. These arise from oligodendroglia and grow slowly, usually over several decades. Calcification is common.

Meningiomas (Fig. 18.21d)

These benign tumours arise from the arachnoid membrane and may grow to a large size, usually over years. When close to the skull they erode bone. They often occur along the intracranial venous sinuses. They are rare below the tentorium.

Neurofibromas

These arise from Schwann cells and occur principally in the cerebellopontine angle where they arise from the eighth nerve sheath (see p. 800).

Other less common neoplasms include:
- Cerebellar haemangioblastoma
- Ependymoma of the fourth ventricle
- Colloid cyst of the third ventricle
- Pinealoma
- Chordoma of the skull base
- Glomus tumour—a vascular neoplasm of the jugular bulb
- Medulloblastoma—a cerebellar tumour of childhood
- Craniopharyngioma (see p. 693)

Pituitary tumours

These are discussed on p. 692.

CLINICAL FEATURES

Mass lesions within the cranium produce symptoms and signs in three co-existing ways:
- By the direct effects of the mass on surrounding structures which are either destroyed or suffer impairment of function from infiltration, pressure or cerebral oedema
- By the effects of raised intracranial pressure and the shift of intracranial contents
- By provoking either generalized or partial seizures

Although neoplasms, either secondary or primary, are the commonest lesions to cause these effects, cerebral abscess, tuberculoma, subdural haematoma and intracranial haematoma may also produce symptoms and signs that may be clinically indistinguishable.

Direct effects of mass lesions

These will depend upon the site of the mass and its speed of growth. The hallmark of a mass lesion is a *progressive* deterioration of function (see p. 843).

Three examples of possible effects are given below:
- A left frontal meningioma (see Fig. 18.21d) will cause a vague disturbance of personality, apathy and impairment of intellectual function over

several months. If the frontal speech area becomes affected, an expressive aphasia will develop. If the corticospinal pathways become involved, a right hemiparesis will follow.

- A right parietal glioma involving the fibres of the optic radiation will cause a left homonymous field defect. Cortical sensory loss and a left hemiparesis may follow. Partial seizures causing episodes of numbness of the left limbs may develop.
- A left eighth nerve sheath neurofibroma (an 'acoustic neuroma') (see Fig. 18.21f) growing in the cerebellopontine angle will cause progressive perceptive deafness (VIII), vertigo (VIII), numbness of the left side of the face (V) and facial weakness (VII), followed by cerebellar ataxia as the cerebellar connections are compressed.

The direct effects are commonly those which first bring the patient to seek medical attention. The rate of progression will vary greatly from a few days or weeks to several years in the case of a slowly enlarging mass. Since cerebral oedema surrounds many mass lesions it is often difficult on clinical grounds to distinguish its effect from that of the mass itself.

Raised intracranial pressure
The triad of headache, vomiting and papilloedema is an important, though relatively unusual, presentation of a mass lesion. It usually implies that obstruction to CSF pathways has occurred. Typically this picture is produced early by masses within the posterior fossa and as a later event with lesions above the tentorium.

Shift of the intracranial contents produces symptoms and signs which co-exist with the direct effects of an expanding mass:

- Distortion of the upper brain stem, as midline structures are displaced either caudally or laterally by a hemisphere mass (see Fig. 18.21), leads to impairment of consciousness (drowsiness progressing to stupor and coma).
- Compression of the medulla by herniation of the cerebellar tonsils caudally through the foramen magnum (an example of 'coning') causes impairment of consciousness, respiratory depression, bradycardia, decerebrate posturing and death.
- False localizing signs ('false' only because they are not related directly to the site of the mass) appear.

The following are common examples of false localizing signs:

- A sixth nerve lesion, first on the side of a mass and later bilaterally, is caused as the nerve is compressed during its long intracranial course.
- A third nerve lesion develops as the uncus of the temporal lobe herniates caudally, compressing the third nerve against the petroclinoid ligament and stretching it by downward displacement of

the posterior communicating artery. The first sign of this is dilatation of the pupil as the parasympathetic fibres in the nerve are compressed.

- Hemiparesis on the *same* side (i.e. 'the one you don't expect') as a hemisphere tumour is caused by compression of the brain stem (the contralateral cerebral peduncle) on the free edge of the tentorium.

These false localizing signs are of vital importance in clinical neurology as their development indicates that a shift of the brain is taking place. Urgent surgical intervention may be necessary.

Seizures
Partial seizures, simple or complex, which may evolve to generalized tonic–clonic seizures are characteristic features of many hemisphere masses, whether malignant or benign. The site of origin of a partial seizure is frequently of localizing value (see p. 823). Generalized tonic–clonic seizures with EEG (but not clinical) evidence of a focal onset also occur.

INVESTIGATION

CT scan is now the investigation of choice when the diagnosis is suspected.

CT Scan
It is important to emphasize that CT indicates only the site of a mass and not its nature. Cerebral abscess, cerebral infarction, benign and malignant tumour may all appear similar.

Technetium brain scan
This is sometimes useful to confirm the site of a lesion shown on CT, but the test discriminates poorly and misses many tumours. *Very* occasionally this test shows a lesion that has been missed by CT.

MRI scan
MRI scans will almost certainly be more discriminating than other non-invasive tests, although it is unlikely that it will be available on a large scale in the near future.

EEG
The EEG may show electrical abnormalities in the region of a mass, but is rarely of major value in management. The main exception is with cerebral abscess, where the EEG shows characteristic marked slow wave changes.

Skull films
Plain x-rays of the skull are discussed on p. 784. In pituitary and parasellar lesions they do give important information about changes in the dorsum sellae and clinoid processes. In hemisphere lesions, plain

films are frequently abnormal, but the test has little value as a screening process.

'Routine' tests

Since the proportion of cerebral tumours that prove to be metastases is high, 'routine' tests such as a chest x-ray are of great importance.

Specialized neuroradiology

Angiography, ventriculography and other contrast studies may rarely be necessary to define the site or the blood supply of a mass.

Lumbar puncture

Lumbar puncture is contraindicated when the differential diagnosis includes any mass lesion.

Examination of CSF rarely yields diagnostically useful information in this situation, and the procedure may be followed by immediate herniation of the cerebellar tonsils. If there are pressing reasons for the procedure it should be carried out after careful assessment of the consequences and a CT scan has been performed.

TREATMENT

Surgical exploration and either biopsy or removal of the mass is usually carried out to ascertain its nature. Some benign tumours can be removed in their entirety.

In addition, radiotherapy is usually recommended for gliomas and for radio-sensitive metastases. Chemotherapy is of little value in the majority of primary brain tumours.

Cerebral oedema surrounding a tumour is rapidly reduced by corticosteroids; dexamethasone and betamethasone are used by injection in an emergency. Intravenous mannitol may also be used as an osmotic diuretic.

Epilepsy is treated with anticonvulsants.

With all malignant brain tumours the overall outlook is poor, with less than 50% survival at 1 year. Meningiomas are, however, often removed in their entirety and thus cured.

Hydrocephalus

In hydrocephalus there is an excessive amount of CSF within the cranium. Although this also occurs in cerebral atrophy, in practice the term hydrocephalus is used to describe different syndromes in which there is, or has been obstruction to CSF outflow with consequent high pressure and dilatation of the cerebral ventricles. Exceptionally an increase in CSF production occurs.

Fig. 18.22 Hydrocephalus. Stenosis of the aqueduct of Sylvius causing gross ventricular dilatation.

Infantile hydrocephalus

Enlargement of the head in infancy is diagnosed in about 1 in 2000 live births. There are several causes:

- *The Arnold–Chiari malformation.* There is elongation of the medulla and abnormal cerebellar tissue (the tonsils) in the cervical canal. Associated spina bifida is common. Syringomyelia may develop.
- *The Dandy-Walker syndrome.* There is cerebellar hypoplasia and obstruction to the outflow foramina of the fourth ventricle.
- *Stenosis of the aqueduct of Sylvius* (Fig. 18.22). This may be either congenital or acquired following neonatal meningitis or haemorrhage.

Hydrocephalus in adult life

Infantile hydrocephalus not infrequently becomes symptomatic only in adult life. The features are of headache, vomiting, papilloedema, ataxia and bilateral pyramidal signs.

Hydrocephalus in adults also occurs with:

- *Tumours of the posterior fossa and brain stem.* These obstruct the aqueduct or fourth ventricular outflow.
- *Subarachnoid haemorrhage, head injury or meningitis (particularly tuberculous).* The hydrocephalus is often a transient phenomenon.
- *Tumours of the third ventricle.* A colloid cyst of the third ventricle causes enlargement of the lateral ventricles, headache and papilloedema.
- *Normal pressure hydrocephalus.* In this syndrome

enlarged cerebral ventricles occur without cortical atrophy. It presents with dementia, urinary incontinence and apraxia, usually in the elderly. The CSF pressure is characteristically normal. It is currently thought that this syndrome suggests that it is the late result of previous episodes of high pressure, though usually of unknown cause.
- *Papilloma of the choroid plexus.* This is an extremely rare neoplasm which secretes CSF.

Ventriculoatrial or ventriculoperitoneal shunting may be necessary when hydrocephalus is diagnosed.

Benign intracranial hypertension (pseudotumour cerebri)

This important syndrome consists of marked papilloedema without other signs in patients who are subsequently shown to have neither a mass lesion nor an increase in ventricular size. It occurs mainly in obese young women with vague menstrual irregularities. Steroid therapy is sometimes thought to be a cause and many other drugs have been occasionally implicated. Other causes of papilloedema should be excluded.

The condition is benign only in that it is not fatal. Infarction of the optic nerve sometimes occurs (with consequent blindness) when the papilloedema is severe and longstanding. Surgical decompression or shunting may be necessary. Thiazide diuretics appear to reduce the intracranial pressure in this condition. Weight reduction is important.

Headache, migraine and facial pain

Tension headache

The vast majority of chronic and recurrent headaches are due to tension in the scalp muscles. There are no features of raised intracranial pressure. 'Tight band' sensations, pressure behind the eyes, and throbbing and bursting sensations are common.

There may be obvious precipitating factors such as worry, noise, concentrated visual effort or fumes. Depression is also a frequent underlying cause. Tension headaches are often attributed to cervical spondylosis, refractive errors or high blood pressure; the evidence for this is poor. Similar headaches also follow head injuries, which may be minor.

There are no abnormal physical signs other than tenderness and tension in the nuchal and scalp muscles.

MANAGEMENT

This involves:
- Firm reassurance
- Avoiding the causes
- Analgesics
- Physical treatments—massage, relaxation
- Antidepressants—when indicated

Investigation may be needed to confirm the benign nature of the problem.

Migraine

Migraine means recurrent headaches associated with visual and gastrointestinal disturbance; despite the origin of the word, it does not invariably mean unilateral headache.

INCIDENCE

About 10% of any population sampled admit to these symptoms.

MECHANISMS

The cause of migraine is unknown. The headache, often throbbing, is believed to be due to vasodilatation or oedema of blood vessels, with stimulation of nerve endings near affected extracranial and meningeal arteries. The release of vasoactive substances is thought to play a role; for example, the serum level of 5-hydroxytryptamine rises at the onset of the prodromal symptoms and falls during the headache.

Cerebral symptoms and signs (e.g. tingling of limbs, aphasia, weakness) are caused by ischaemia and/or depression of cortical function.

Definite precipitating factors are unusual. Some patients complain of symptoms at times of relaxation (e.g. weekend migraine). Others find that chocolate (high in phenylethylamine) and cheese (high in tyramine) precipitate attacks. Migraine is common around puberty, at the menopause and premenstrually, and sometimes increases in severity or frequency with the contraceptive pill or the development of hypertension.

There is no reason to suppose that migraine is associated with any major intracranial lesion. However, since migraine is such a common symptom complex, an intracranial mass lesion and migraine sometimes both occur in the same patient by coincidence.

Rarely, migraine follows head injuries.

CLINICAL PATTERNS

There are several types of migraine, the attacks varying from intermittent headaches indistinguishable from tension headaches to discrete episodes which mimic thromboembolic cerebral ischaemia. The distinction between the variants is somewhat artificial.

The attack may be divided into:
- Prodromal symptoms
- Headache and associated symptoms

Prior to the attack some patients experience a feeling of well-being.

Classical migraine

Prodromal symptoms are usually visual and are related to ischaemia in the distribution of the intracranial arteries. There are unilateral patchy scotomata (when the retinal vessels are involved), unilateral blindness (involvement of the ophthalmic artery) and sometimes hemianopic field loss (involvement of the posterior cerebral artery). Teichopsia (flashes) and fortification spectra (jagged lines resembling battlements) are common.

Transient aphasia sometimes occurs, together with tingling, numbness or vague weakness of one side. The patient feels nauseated.

The prodrome lasts for 15 minutes to 1 h or more. Headache follows. This is occasionally hemicranial ('splitting the head'), but often begins locally and becomes generalized. Nausea increases and vomiting follows. The patient is irritable and prefers to lie in a darkened room. The superficial temporal artery (either or both) is engorged and pulsating.

After several hours the attack ceases. There is sometimes a diuresis towards the end of an attack. Sleep often follows.

Common migraine

This is the usual variety of migraine. Prodromal visual symptoms are vague. There is recurrent headache accompanied by nausea and malaise. Distinction from tension headache may be impossible.

Basilar migraine

The prodromal symptoms are due to ischaemia in the posterior cerebral circulation. Circumoral tingling, numbness of the tongue, vertigo, diplopia, transient blindness, syncope, dysarthria and ataxia occur.

Hemiplegic migraine

This is a rarity in which classical migraine is accompanied by hemiparesis. Recovery occurs within 24 h. Exceptionally cerebral infarction follows.

Ophthalmoplegic migraine

This is a third (or exceptionally a sixth) nerve palsy occurring in a migraine attack. The condition is rare and is difficult to distinguish from other causes of a third nerve palsy (see p. 798) without investigation.

Facioplegic migraine

This rarity is a seventh nerve palsy occurring during a migraine attack.

DIFFERENTIAL DIAGNOSIS

The sudden onset of headache may be similar to meningitis or subarachnoid haemorrhage.

The hemiplegic, visual and hemisensory symptoms must be distinguished from thromboembolic TIAs (see p. 816). In TIAs the maximum deficit is present immediately and headache is unusual.

Unilateral tingling or numbness should be distinguished from sensory epilepsy (partial seizures). In the latter a distinct 'march' of symptoms is usual.

MANAGEMENT

General measures
These include:
- Reassurance and relief of anxiety
- Avoidance of precipitating dietary factors (rarely helpful)
- In those on oral contraceptives, a change in brand or stopping the drug may help. Severe hemiplegic symptoms are an indication for stopping these drugs.

During the attack
Paracetamol or other simple analgesics should be given, with antiemetics (e.g. metoclopramide) if necessary.

Ergotamine tartrate (1–2 mg orally or rectally, 360 μg by aerosol or 0.25–0.5 mg by injection) is sometimes, though not often, helpful if given early in attack. Ergotamine should not be used in patients with a history of vascular disease.

Prophylaxis
It is particularly difficult to discern the true (as opposed to placebo) effects of prophylactic drugs in migraine. When drugs are necessary, the following are used:
- Pizotifen (a 5-HT antagonist) 0.5 mg at night for several days, increasing to 1.5 mg at night. Common side-effects are slight weight gain and drowsiness.
- Propranolol 10 mg three times daily, increasing to 40–80 mg three times daily.
- Clonidine 0.025 mg three times daily, increasing to 0.075 mg three times daily.
- Methysergide (a 5-HT antagonist) 2–6 mg daily. An occasional side-effect is retroperitoneal fibrosis which precludes its use for longer than 6 months.

Facial pain

The face is richly supplied with pain-sensitive structures—the teeth, gums, sinuses, temporomandibular joints, jaw and eyes—disease of which causes facial pain. Facial pain is also caused by some specific neurological conditions; these are mentioned below.

Trigeminal neuralgia
This is described on p. 799.

Trigeminal nerve lesions
These are described on p. 799.

Post-herpetic neuralgia
This is described on p. 838.

Migrainous neuralgia
This condition causes recurrent bouts of excruciating pain which wake the patient at night and are centred around one eye. It affects adults in the third and fourth decades and is more common in men. Alcohol sometimes precipitates an attack.

The pain lasts for several hours. Vomiting occurs. The face and nostril feel congested. A transient ipsilateral Horner's syndrome is common during the attack.

Despite the pain there are no serious sequelae. Treatment of the attack with analgesics is unhelpful. Prophylactic drugs as for migraine are used.

Atypical facial pain
Facial pain for which no cause can be found is seen in the elderly, mainly in women. It is believed to be a somatic equivalent of depression. Tricyclic anti-depressants are sometimes helpful.

Other causes
Facial pain occurs in unusual variants of migraine and in giant cell arteritis (see below).

Giant cell arteritis (cranial arteritis, temporal arteritis)

This important syndrome is a granulomatous arteritis of unknown aetiology occurring chiefly over the age of 60 and affecting in particular the extra-cranial arteries (see p. 396). Other forms of arteritis, e.g. systemic lupus erythematosus (see p. 340) and polyarteritis nodosa (see p. 345), can present with similar features but with a more generalized arteritis affecting intracranial arteries and vasa nervorum of the cranial nerves.

CLINICAL FEATURES

Headache
Headache is almost invariable. It is felt over the inflamed superficial, temporal or occipital arteries. Touching the skin over the inflamed vessel (e.g. combing the hair) causes pain. The arterial pulsation is soon lost and the artery becomes hard, tortuous and thickened. The skin over the vessels may be red. Rarely, gangrenous patches in the scalp appear.

Facial pain
Pain in the face, jaw and mouth occurs and is caused by inflammation of the facial, maxillary and lingual branches of the external carotid artery. Pain is characteristically worse on eating (jaw claudication). Opening the mouth and protruding the tongue is difficult. A painful, ischaemic tongue occasionally occurs.

Visual problems
Visual loss due to inflammation and occlusion of the ciliary and/or central retinal artery occurs in 25% of untreated cases. The patient complains of sudden uniocular visual loss, either partial or complete, which is painless. Amaurosis fugax (see p. 816) may precede total visual loss, which is usually permanent.

When the ciliary vessels are affected the optic disc becomes swollen and pale (see p. 794). The retinal branch vessels are usually normal. If the central retinal artery is occluded, there is sudden unilateral blindness, pallor of the disc and retinal ischaemia.

Systemic features
Generalized limb pains, proximal limb girdle pain and tenderness, without joint effusion (polymyalgia rheumatica, see p. 346), occur in half the cases. Weight loss, sweating and malaise also occur.

Rare complications
Brain stem ischaemia, cortical blindness, ischaemic neuropathy of peripheral nerves, cranial nerve lesions, and involvement of the aorta, coronary, renal and mesenteric arteries are sometimes seen.

INVESTIGATION

The ESR is greatly elevated, 60–100 mm·h^{-1} being common. Plasma alpha-2-globulins are raised, and the albumin is occasionally reduced. Normochromic, normocytic anaemia occurs.

The diagnosis is usually confirmed by biopsy of a superficial temporal artery. A 1 cm (or greater) segment should be excised because the characteristic granulomatous changes within the walls (lymphocytes, plasma cells, multinucleate giant cells, destruction of the internal elastic lamina) may be patchy.

TREATMENT

The diagnosis should be established without delay because of the risk of blindness. High doses of steroids (prednisolone initially 100 mg daily) should be started and the dose reduced as the ESR falls. A characteristic of the condition is that the headache subsides within hours of the first large dose of steroid.

It is usually possible to stop steroid treatment after some months to several years.

Head injury

Over 100 000 patients with head injury are admitted to hospital in Britain annually. Around 400 of these patients have disturbance of consciousness for longer than 1 month. Road traffic accidents and alcoholism are the principal aetiological factors in this major cause of death and morbidity.

Clinical sequelae

Skull fracture

Linear skull fracture of the vault or base is an indication of the severity of injury, but is not necessarily associated with any neurological sequelae. Healing takes place and surgical intervention is usually unnecessary.

Depressed skull fracture of the vault is followed by a high incidence of post-traumatic epilepsy (see p. 824). Surgical elevation and débridement are usually necessary.

The principal local complications of skull fracture are:

- Rupture of a meningeal artery, causing an extradural haematoma (see p. 822)
- Damage to dural veins, causing a subdural haematoma (see p. 822)
- Dural tears, causing CSF rhinorrhoea and otorrhoea with the risk of meningitis

Brain damage

Concussion (commotio cerebri). This is transient loss of consciousness following head injury. Commonly there are no focal signs and patients usually recover.

The pathology is poorly defined. Massive sudden increase in intracranial pressure at impact, with direct injury to neurones, is thought to be responsible for the signs and symptoms.

There is no absolute distinction between concussion and contusion (see below).

Cerebral contusion (contusio cerebri). Cerebral contusion and oedema with secondary brain stem compression usually, but by no means always, causes prolonged unconsciousness and focal signs. Traumatic subarachnoid haemorrhage is a common accompaniment.

Course

There is a tendency for uncomplicated head injury to improve. The duration of loss of consciousness and post-traumatic amnesia (PTA), i.e. until continuous memory returns to normal, is an index of severity. Injuries with PTA lasting for more than 24 h are regarded as 'severe'.

Patients with uncomplicated head injury require supportive therapy (see p. 791). Patients who are deteriorating on a coma scale (see p. 788) may require urgent neurosurgical intervention and drainage of intracranial haematomas or decompression.

Late sequelae

These are common causes of morbidity and have important medicolegal consequences. They include the following:

- Many patients with severe head injuries have prolonged and incomplete recoveries, and are left with impairment of higher cerebral function, hemiparesis and other deficits.
- Post-traumatic epilepsy may occur (see p. 824).
- 'Chronic traumatic encephalopathy' follows repeated (and often minor) injuries. It presents as dementia with extrapyramidal and pyramidal signs, and is seen mainly in professional boxers.
- The 'post-traumatic syndrome' describes the vague complaints of headache, dizziness and malaise which follow even minor head injuries. Depression is prominent. Symptoms may be prolonged.
- 'Benign positional vertigo' (see p. 803) is a transient sequel of head injury.

Diseases of the spinal cord

The cord extends from C1 (its junction with the medulla) to the vertebral body of L1 (the conus medullaris).

Its blood supply is via the anterior spinal artery and a plexus on the posterior cord. This network is supplied by the vertebral arteries, the thyrocervical trunk and several branches from the lumbar and intercostal vessels.

Spinal cord compression

The clinical features are discussed on p. 812.

Acute cord compression is unmistakable. There is sudden paralysis and sensory loss below the level of the lesion.

Chronic compression of the cord causes progressive difficulty in walking (see p. 782) over weeks, months or years. Spastic paraparesis with sensory loss is found. Sphincter disturbance is common.

It is frequently difficult to distinguish chronic cord compression from other causes of paraparesis and tetraparesis on clinical grounds alone (Tables 18.19 and 18.47).

Spinal cord neoplasms (Table 18.48)

Extramedullary tumours (extradural and intradural) cause cord compression gradually over weeks to

Table 18.47 Causes of spinal cord compression.

Spinal cord neoplasms (see Table 18.48)

Disc and vertebral lesions
    Trauma
    Chronic degenerative

Inflammatory
    Epidural abscess
    Tuberculosis
    Granuloma

Vertebral neoplasms
    Metastases
    Myeloma

Epidural haemorrhage

Rarities
    Paget's disease
    Epithelial, endothelial and parasitic cysts
    Aneurysmal bone cyst
    Vertebral angioma
    Haematomyelia, arachnoiditis
    Osteoporosis

Table 18.48 Principal spinal cord neoplasms.

Extradural
Metastases:
    Bronchus
    Breast
    Prostate
    Lymphoma
    Thyroid
    Melanoma

Extramedullary
Meningioma
Neurofibroma
Ependymoma
Arteriovenous malformation

Intramedullary
Glioma
Ependymoma
Haemangioblastoma
Lipoma
Arteriovenous malformation
Teratoma

months, with local or referred root pain and a sensory level (see p. 812).

Intramedullary tumours (e.g. glioma) typically have a very slowly progressive course over several years. Sensory disturbances similar to syringomyelia (see p. 850) may appear.

Disc and vertebral lesions
Central cervical disc protrusion and lumbar disc protrusion are considered on pp. 860 and 361, respectively.

Epidural abscess
This is described on p. 841.

Epidural haemorrhage
This is a rare complication of anticoagulant therapy and bleeding disorders. A rapidly progressive cord lesion is found.

Tuberculosis
Spinal TB is a frequent cause of cord compression in countries where TB is common (e.g. India, Pakistan, Bangladesh and Africa). There is destruction of vertebral bodies and disc spaces, with spread of infection along the extradural space. Cord compression and paraparesis follows (Pott's paraplegia).

MANAGEMENT

Early recognition of the syndrome is vital. Surgical exploration is frequently necessary and, if this is not performed sufficiently early, irreversible paraplegia may follow.

Plain spinal films show degenerative bone disease and destruction of vertebrae by infection or neoplasm. Routine tests may indicate a primary neoplasm or infection.

Myelography is necessary. It should, if possible, be done promptly in a centre equipped to carry out neurosurgical exploration. The signs of cord compression may increase after lumbar puncture.

The results following the early removal of benign tumours are excellent.

Transverse myelitis

This broad term is used to describe acute inflammation of the cord and paraplegia occurring with viral infection, MS and other inflammatory and vascular disorders (e.g. syphilis, radiation myelopathy, anterior spinal artery occlusion). Myelography is usually required to exclude a compressive lesion.

Anterior spinal artery occlusion

Cord infarction, causing an acute paraparesis or tetraparesis (or -plegia) may occur in any thrombotic or embolic vascular disease (e.g. endocarditis, shock, atheroma, diabetes mellitus, syphilis, polyarteritis nodosa). It sometimes occurs during surgery to the posterior mediastinum, and follows dissection of the aorta. It occasionally occurs as an isolated event.

Radiation myelopathy

A mild paraparesis and sensory loss sometimes develops within several weeks to 1 year of radiotherapy if the cord has been damaged.

Metabolic and toxic cord disease

Subacute combined degeneration of the cord due to vitamin B_{12} deficiency (see pp. 269 and 859) is the most important example of metabolic cord disease.

Cord lesions may also be seen in severe malnutrition, when they are probably due to multiple B vitamin deficiencies.

Lathyrism

This is an endemic, spastic paraparesis of central India caused by the toxin B-(N)-oxalylaminoalanine. It occurs when excessive quantities of a drought-resistant pulse, *Lathyrus sativus*, are consumed.

Syringomyelia and syringobulbia

Fluid-filled cavities within the spinal cord (myelia) and brain stem (bulbia) are the essential features of these conditions.

AETIOLOGY

A history of birth injury is frequent and bony anomalies at the foramen magnum, spina bifida (see p. 853), Arnold–Chiari malformation (see p. 844) or hydrocephalus (see p. 844) are often seen.

It is believed that in the presence of an anatomical abnormality at the foramen magnum, the normal pulsatile CSF pressure waves are transmitted to the delicate tissues of the cervical cord and brain stem, with secondary cavity formation. The cavity, or syrinx, is in continuity with the central canal of the cord.

PATHOLOGICAL ANATOMY

The expanding cavity gradually destroys:
- The second order spinothalamic neurones in the cervical cord
- The anterior horn cells
- The lateral corticospinal tracts

The vestibular system, trigeminal nuclei, sympathetic system and twelfth nerve nuclei may also be affected.

CLINICAL FEATURES

Patients usually present in the third to fourth decade.

Pain in the upper limbs is common. This may be exacerbated by exertion or coughing. Spinothalamic sensory loss in the upper limbs leads to painless burns. Difficulty in walking may occur.

The signs of a cavity in the cervical region are:
- Areas of dissociated sensory loss. These may extend in a bizarre distribution over the trunk and upper limbs.
- Loss of upper limb reflexes
- Wasting of the small muscles of the hand
- Spastic paraparesis. This may initially be mild and symptomless.

Neuropathic joints, trophic skin changes and ulcers may occur.

When the cavity extends through the foramen magnum (syringobulbia) into the brain stem, there is atrophy and fasciculation of the tongue, nystagmus, Horner's syndrome, hearing loss and impairment of facial sensation.

MANAGEMENT AND COURSE

The condition is intermittently progressive over several decades.

Investigation shows widening of the cervical canal on plain films, and frequently ventricular enlargement on CT scan. An MRI scan demonstrates the intrinsic cavity. Myelography (which is sometimes followed by deterioration) shows widening of the cord and herniation of the cerebellar tonsils through the foramen magnum.

There is no curative treatment. Decompression of the foramen magnum sometimes reduces the rate of deterioration.

Paraplegia

The patient who becomes paraplegic from any cause demands skilled and prolonged nursing care. Particular problems are discussed below.

Bladder. Intermittent (or continuous) catheterization is usually necessary initially. A reflexly emptying bladder develops in permanent paraplegia, avoiding the need for catheterization and some of the risks of urinary stasis, infection, and renal and bladder calculi.

Bowel. Constipation and faecal impaction must be avoided. Manual evacuation is necessary following acute paraplegia, but reflex emptying later develops.

Skin care. The risk of pressure sores is great. Meticulous attention must be paid to cleanliness and to turning the patient every 2 h. The sacrum, iliac crests, greater trochanters, heels and malleoli should be inspected frequently. Ripple mattresses and water beds are useful.

If pressure sores develop, plastic surgical repair should be considered.

The lower limbs. Passive physiotherapy is helpful in avoiding contractures. Severe spasticity (with spasms either in flexion or extension), may be helped by dantrolene sodium, baclofen or diazepam.

General considerations

The general health and morale of the patient should be considered carefully and regularly. Any intercurrent infection (urinary or respiratory) is potentially hazardous and should be recognized and treated early, as chronic renal failure is the single most common cause of death in paraplegia.

Rehabilitation

Many patients with traumatic paraplegia or tetraplegia return to partial self-sufficiency and a wheelchair existence. They have demanding practical, psychological and social needs, but with guidance and help can often return to an active role in society.

Other causes of cord lesions

These are:
● Multiple sclerosis (see p. 833)
● Motor neurone disease (see p. 851)
● Familial or sporadic paraparesis
● Non-metastatic manifestation of malignancy (see p. 861)
● Neurosyphilis (see p. 838)
● Rarities, e.g. sarcoidosis (see p. 603), Behçet's syndrome (see p. 356)

Degenerative diseases

Motor neurone disease (MND)

In this disease there is progressive degeneration of motor neurones in the spinal cord, in the somatic motor nuclei of the cranial nerves and within the cortex. The condition is sporadic and of entirely unknown cause. The prevalence is about 6 in 100 000, with an equal sex incidence. The onset is in middle life. The sensory system is not involved.

CLINICAL FEATURES

There are three patterns of clinical presentation:
● Progressive muscular atrophy
● Amyotrophic lateral sclerosis
● Progressive bulbar palsy

Although useful as a means of understanding the disease, these are not distinct aetiological or pathological variants; the three merge later in the course of the condition.

Progressive muscular atrophy

Wasting often begins in the small muscles of one hand and spreads inexorably throughout the arm. Although it may begin unilaterally, wasting soon follows on the opposite side.

Fasciculation is common. It is due to the spontaneous firing of abnormally large motor units formed by the branching fibres of surviving axons which are striving to innervate muscle fibres that have lost their nerve supply. Cramps may occur but pain does not.

The physical signs are of wasting and weakness, with fasciculation which is often widespread. Tendon reflexes are lost when the reflex arc is interrupted (by anterior horn cell loss), but are often preserved or exaggerated because of the loss of motor neurones in the corticospinal tracts.

Amyotrophic lateral sclerosis (ALS)

'Lateral sclerosis' means disease of the lateral corticospinal tracts (i.e. a spastic paralysis). 'Amyotrophy' means atrophy of muscle (which would be unusual in most other forms of spastic tetra- or paraparesis). The clinical picture is thus of a progressive spastic tetra- or paraparesis with added *lower* motor neurone signs and fasciculation. 'ALS' is the term usually given to MND in the USA.

Progressive bulbar palsy

Here the brunt of the onset of the disease falls upon the lower cranial nerve nuclei and their supranuclear connections. Dysarthria, dysphagia, nasal regurgitation of fluids and choking are common symptoms. For reasons unknown, this form of the disease is more common in women than in men. The characteristic features are of a mixture of upper and lower motor neurone signs in the lower cranial nerves, e.g. a wasted fibrillating tongue with a spastic weak palate.

COURSE

Remission is unknown. The disease progresses, spreading gradually, and causes death, often from bronchopneumonia. Survival for more than 3 years is most unusual although there are rare 'benign' forms of the condition where survival is prolonged.

The ocular movements are not affected. There are never cerebellar or extrapyramidal signs. Awareness is preserved and dementia is unusual. Sphincter disturbance occurs late, if at all.

MANAGEMENT

There are no specific diagnostic tests and the diagnosis can often be made on clinical grounds alone. Cervical radiculopathy and myelopathy and the rare (almost extinct) syphilitic cervical pachymeningitis may sometimes cause diagnostic difficulty. Bulbar myasthenia gravis may sometimes appear similar in the early stages.

Denervation may be confirmed by electromyogram studies, which characteristically show chronic partial denervation with preserved motor conduction velocity. The CSF is usually normal (the protein may be slightly raised).

No treatment has been shown to influence the course of this disease and management of these often knowledgeable patients is difficult.

Spinal muscular atrophies

These are a group of rare genetically determined disorders of the motor neurone which give rise to slowly progressive, usually symmetrical, muscle wasting and weakness. An acute infantile type

(Werdnig–Hoffmann disease), a chronic childhood type (Kugelberg–Welander disease) and adult forms are recognized. Clinically these conditions may be confused with muscular dystrophies (see p. 865), hereditary neuropathies or motor neurone disease.

DEMENTIA (see p. 876)

The principal causes of progressive generalized failure of higher cerebral functions are shown in Table 18.49.

Alzheimer's disease

This term is now used for both senile and presenile dementia. It is characterized pathologically by severe cortical neuronal loss, and the presence of amyloid bodies of some 50 μm in diameter known as argyrophil plaques. 'Neurofibrillary tangles' occur in degenerating neurones. Neither are specific for the disease.

The cause of this condition is unknown.

CLINICAL FEATURES

The condition is seldom seen below the age of 50. A familial tendency is unusual. Memory failure, progressive intellectual decline and apathy, and on occasion, features of focal cortical disturbance such as aphasia occur. Severe depression may be present in the early stages. The disease is gradually progressive. 'Pyramidal' signs (e.g. extensor plantar reflexes) are sometimes found together with a stoop and expressionless face suggestive of Parkinson's disease. Epilepsy may occur.

INVESTIGATION

There are no characteristic changes in the peripheral blood, in the CSF or on EEG. Cortical atrophy is seen on a CT scan. Psychometric testing may be valuable in the early stages of the condition.

The purpose of investigation in dementia is to establish the diagnosis and to distinguish those causes for which some treatment may be available (Table 18.49).

TREATMENT

No treatment exists for Alzheimer's disease. Patients can remain at home if family support is adequate, but hospital care often becomes necessary. The few treatable causes of dementia (e.g. hypothyroidism) require urgent therapy.

Pick's disease

Pick's disease is dementia in which the cortical atrophy is initially restricted to the frontotemporal region. The cause is unknown.

Congenital and inherited diseases

Cerebral palsy

This term describes disorders apparent at birth or in childhood due to brain damage in the neonatal period leading to non-progressive deficits.

Mental retardation, varying from severe intellectual impairment to mild learning disorders, is common in all forms of cerebral palsy, but severe physical disability is not necessarily associated with a severe defect in higher cerebral function.

CAUSES

The precise cause of brain damage in an individual child may be difficult to determine. The following may be responsible:
● Hypoxia in utero and/or during parturition
● Trauma, during parturition or in the neonatal period
● Prolonged convulsions or coma (e.g. febrile convulsions, hypoglycaemia) in infancy
● Kernicterus
● Cerebral haemorrhage and infarction

CLINICAL FEATURES

Failure to achieve normal developmental milestones is often the earliest feature. More specific motor syndromes become apparent later in childhood or, rarely, in adult life.

Spastic diplegia
This is spasticity (predominantly of the lower limbs) with 'scissoring' of the gait.

Athetoid cerebral palsy
This is described on p. 830.

Infantile hemiparesis
Hemiparesis may be noted at birth or during childhood. Hemiatrophy of the limbs (and atrophy of the contralateral hemisphere) is usual. Seizures are common.

Congenital ataxia
This is incoordination and hypotonia of the trunk and limbs.

Dysraphism

Failure of normal fusion of the fetal neural tube leads to this group of congenital anomalies.

Anencephaly
Anencephaly is absence of the brain and cranial vault, and is incompatible with life.

Table 18.49 Principal causes of dementia in adults and the features on which the diagnosis is made or excluded.

Condition	Diagnostic features
Alzheimer's disease	Clinical history, CT scan
Hypothyroidism	Serum T4 and TSH levels
Subacute combined degeneration of cord	Serum B_{12} assay
Pellagra	Dietary history
Hypoparathyroidism	Serum calcium level
Multiple cerebral infarction	CT scan
Alcohol/Wernicke–Korsakoff syndrome	Clinical history
Intracranial mass, hydrocephalus (including subdural haematoma)	Clinical features, CT scan
Chronic traumatic encephalopathy	Clinical history, CT scan
Huntington's disease	Family history, chorea
Multiple sclerosis	Clinical features, evoked potentials, examination of CSF
Spongiform encephalopathy	EEG, ?cerebral biopsy
Progressive supranuclear palsy	Clinical features
General paralysis of the insane	Syphilitic serology
Poisoning by: Drugs (chronic barbiturate intoxication) Carbon monoxide Heavy metals (organic mercurials, manganese)	Drug levels and clinical history
Following prolonged anoxia or hypoglycaemia	Clinical history
Chronic hepatic encephalopathy	Clinical features, liver function tests
AIDS encephalopathy	HIV antibodies
Uraemia, dialysis	Blood urea level
Rare metabolic disorders, e.g. Wilson's disease	Serum copper level, caeruloplasmin level

NB Depression may produce a clinical picture that is indistinguishable from dementia (see p. 870).

Meningoencephalocele
This is an extrusion of brain and meninges through a midline skull defect which varies from a minor protrusion to a massive defect.

Spina bifida
In spina bifida there is failure of fusion of the neural tube, usually in the lumbosacral region. Several varieties occur.

Spina bifida occulta. This is failure of fusion of the vertebral arch only. There are rarely neurological abnormalities and a bony anomaly is seen on x-ray. It occurs in 3% of the population. A dimple or a tuft of hair may overlie the lesion.

Meningomyelocele and myelocele with spina bifida. Meningomyeloceles consist of elements of the cord and lumbosacral roots contained within a meningeal sac which herniates through a defect in the vertebrae. In severe cases the lower limbs and sphincters are paralysed. The defect is visible at birth.

Meningocele is a meningeal defect alone.

Hydrocephalus is commonly associated with these abnormalities. Meningitis may follow if a sinus connects the spinal canal with the overlying skin.

Basilar impression of the skull (platybasia)

This is usually a congenital anomaly in which there is

invagination of the foramen magnum and skull base upwards. The lower cranial nerves, medulla, upper cervical cord and roots are affected. It is often complicated by the Arnold–Chiari malformation in which aberrant cerebellar tissue extends through the foramen magnum.

The condition also occurs in Paget's disease and rarely in osteomalacia.

NEURO-ECTODERMAL SYNDROMES

These are disorders in which organs derived from ectoderm show a tendency to form tumours and hamartomas, with lesions in the skin, eye and nervous system.

Neurofibromatosis (von Recklinghausen's disease)

This is characterized by multiple skin neurofibromas and pigmentation. The neurofibromas arise from the neurilemmal sheath. One new case occurs in every 3000 live births. The mode of inheritance is autosomal dominant.

CLINICAL FEATURES (see p. 944)

Skin tumours
Subcutaneous, soft, sometimes pedunculated, tumours appear. They may be multiple.

Skin pigmentation
Multiple café-au-lait patches—pale brown macules 1–20 cm in diameter—are found. These are common in the normal population, but more than five patches is abnormal.

Neural tumours
Many neural tumours occur more frequently in von Recklinghausen's disease than in the general population, including:
- Cutaneous neurofibroma
- Eighth nerve sheath neurofibroma
- Spinal cord and nerve root neurofibroma
- Meningioma
- Glioma (including optic nerve glioma)
- Plexiform neuroma (massive cutaneous overgrowth)

Rarely, the benign tumours undergo sarcomatous change.

Associated abnormalities
These include:
- Scoliosis
- Orbital haemangioma
- Local gigantism of a limb
- Phaeochromocytoma and ganglioneuroma
- Renal artery stenosis
- Pulmonary fibrosis

- Obstructive cardiomyopathy
- Fibrous dysplasia of bone

TREATMENT

Surgery may be necessary for cosmetic reasons. Tumours causing pressure within the nervous system require excision.

Tuberose sclerosis (epiloia)

This is a rare autosomal dominant condition whose principal features are adenoma sebaceum, epilepsy and mental retardation (often severe).

Adenoma sebaceum
These are reddish nodules (angiofibromas) which develop on the cheeks in childhood.

Other lesions
Other lesions include shagreen patches, amelanotic naevi, retinal phakomas (glial masses), renal tumours, glial overgrowth in brain and gliomas. Cardiac rhabdomyomas, hamartomas of lung and kidney, and polycystic kidneys may also occur.

Sturge–Weber syndrome (encephalofacial angiomatosis)

There is an extensive port-wine naevus on one side of the face (usually in the distribution of a division of the fifth nerve) and a leptomeningeal angioma, usually parieto-occipital.

Epilepsy is common. Familial occurrence is exceptional.

Von Hippel–Lindau syndrome (retinocerebellar angiomatosis)

This is the occurrence in families (dominant inheritance with variable penetrance) of retinal and cerebellar haemangioblastomas or, less commonly, haemgioblastomas of the cord and cerebrum. Renal, adrenal and pancreatic cysts (and haemangioblastomas) may also be found. Polycythaemia sometimes occurs.

There are numerous other disorders related to these conditions, for example ataxia telangiectasia (see p. 117) and Osler–Weber–Rendu syndrome (see p. 169).

SPINOCEREBELLAR DEGENERATIONS

The classification of these inherited disorders is complex. Three conditions will be mentioned here.

Friedreich's ataxia

This is a progressive degeneration of dorsal root ganglia, spinocerebellar tracts, corticospinal tracts and Purkinje cells of the cerebellum. Difficulty in walking occurs around the age of 12 and is progressive. The clinical findings are:

- Ataxia of gait and trunk
- Nystagmus (in 25%)
- Dysarthria
- Absent joint position and vibration sense in lower limbs
- Absent reflexes in lower limbs
- Optic atrophy (in 30%)
- Pes cavus
- Cardiomyopathy with T-wave inversion and left ventricular hypertrophy

Death is usual before the age of 40.

Hereditary spastic paraparesis

Isolated progressive paraparesis runs in some families. The inheritance is variable. Additional features including cerebellar signs, pes cavus, wasted hands and optic atrophy are sometimes seen. The conditions are usually mild and progress slowly over many years.

Ataxia telangiectasia (see p. 117)

This is a rare, autosomal recessive condition which produces a progressive ataxic syndrome in childhood and early adult life.

There is striking telangiectasia of the conjunctiva, nose, ears and skin creases. There are also defects in cell-mediated immunity and antibody production. A defect in DNA repair has been demonstrated. Death is usual by the third decade, either from infection or from the development of lymphoreticular malignancy.

PERONEAL MUSCULAR ATROPHY AND OTHER INHERITED NEUROPATHIES

These disorders are classified within a large, rare and complex group—hereditary motor and sensory neuropathies (HMSN).

Peroneal muscular atrophy

Peroneal muscular atrophy (Charcot–Marie–Tooth disease) is a common clinical syndrome in which there is distal limb wasting and weakness that slowly progresses over many years, mostly in the legs, with variable loss of sensation and reflexes. In advanced cases the distal wasting below the knees is so marked that the legs resemble 'inverted champagne bottles'.

Mild cases have only pes cavus and clawing of the toes and may pass unnoticed.

Three forms are recognized:
- HMSN type I—a demyelinating neuropathy
- HMSN type II—an axonal neuropathy
- Distal spinal muscular atrophy

Both autosomal dominant and recessive inheritance is seen in different families. In HMSN type I with dominant inheritance (the commonest form) linkage has been demonstrated for the locus in the long arm of chromosome 1.

Optic atrophy, deafness, retinitis pigmentosa and spastic paraparesis are sometimes seen in variants of these conditions.

HMSN type III

This was formerly known as 'the hypertrophic neuropathy of Déjérine–Sottas'. It is an autosomal recessive demyelinating sensory neuropathy of childhood leading to severe incapacity during adolescence. It is notable because the CSF protein may be greatly elevated to 10 g·l^{-1} or more, and the CSF pathways are obstructed by greatly hypertrophied nerve roots.

Diseases of the peripheral nerves

The different nerve fibre types within a peripheral nerve are shown in Table 18.50. All are myelinated except the C fibres, which carry impulses from painful stimuli.

Two pathological processes affect peripheral nerves—axonal (or wallerian) degeneration and demyelination. Neuropathies are classified according to which process predominates.

Axonal degeneration
Axonal degeneration occurs after a nerve has been

Table 18.50 Fibre types in peripheral nerves.

Type	Fibre diameter (μm)	Conduction velocity (m·s⁻¹)	Function
A	10–18	90	Primary spindle afferents Alpha motor neurones
A	6–12	50	Touch and pressure afferents
A	4–8	30	Gamma afferents
B	2–6	10	Autonomic preganglionic
C	0.2–0.3	2	Pain and temperature afferents Autonomic postganglionic

sectioned or its axon severely damaged. Within 7–10 days the axon and the myelin sheath distal to the injury degenerate and are inexcitable electrically. When a motor nerve is damaged there is atrophy of the muscle fibres in the motor units it supplies. Denervation may be detected by recording fibrillation potentials on EMG.

Regeneration occurs by axonal growth down the nerve sheath and axonal sprouting from the stump. Growth takes place at a rate of up to 1 mm per day. In a chronic neuropathic process (e.g. motor neurone disease or polyneuropathy), sprouts from the terminal axons of *normal* motor axons reinnervate the denervated muscle fibres; giant polyphasic units are then seen on EMG.

Demyelination

Here damage to the myelin sheath (the axon is initially preserved) causes conduction block or marked slowing of conduction; this can be used to distinguish demyelination from axonal degeneration. Local demyelination is caused by pressure (compression and entrapment neuropathies) or by inflammation (e.g. Guillain–Barré syndrome).

Definitions

Neuropathy means a pathological process affecting a peripheral nerve or nerves.

Mononeuropathy is a process affecting a single nerve, and multiple mononeuropathy (or mononeuritis multiplex) is a process affecting several or multiple nerves.

Polyneuropathy is a diffuse, symmetrical disease process, usually progressing proximally. It is either acute, subacute or chronic. Its course may be progressive, relapsing or towards recovery. Polyneuropathy may be motor, sensory, sensorimotor (mixed) or autonomic.

Radiculopathy means a disease process affecting the nerve roots.

MONONEUROPATHIES

Peripheral nerve compression and entrapment (Table 18.51)

Damage to a nerve by compression is either acute (e.g. due to a tourniquet or other sustained pressure) or chronic (entrapment neuropathy). In both, demyelination predominates, but some axonal degeneration occurs.

Acute compression usually occurs to nerves which are exposed anatomically (e.g. the common peroneal nerve at the head of the fibula).

Entrapment occurs where a nerve passes through relatively tight anatomical passages (e.g. the carpal tunnel).

These conditions are diagnosed largely from the clinical features. Diagnosis is confirmed by nerve conduction studies and EMG. The commoner conditions are mentioned below.

Table 18.51 Nerve compression and entrapment.

Nerve	Site of entrapment or compression
Median	Carpal tunnel
Ulnar	Cubital tunnel
Radial	Spiral groove of humerus
Posterior interosseous	Supinator muscle
Lateral cutaneous of thigh ('meralgia paraesthetica')	Inguinal ligament
Common peroneal	Neck of fibula
Posterior tibial	Flexor retinaculum (tarsal tunnel)

Median nerve compression at the wrist (carpal tunnel syndrome)

This common syndrome is sometimes seen in:

- Hypothyroidism
- Diabetes mellitus
- Pregnancy
- Rheumatoid arthritis
- Acromegaly

It is usually idiopathic. It causes nocturnal tingling and pain in the hand (and sometimes forearm) followed by weakness of the thenar muscles. Wasting of abductor pollicis brevis develops, with sensory loss on the palm and radial three-and-a-half fingers. Tinel's sign may be positive, i.e. tapping on the carpal tunnel will reproduce the pain.

Treatment with a splint at night or a local steroid injection in the wrist gives temporary relief. When the condition occurs in pregnancy (due to fluid retention) it is often self-limiting. Surgical decompression of the carpal tunnel is often necessary in other cases.

Ulnar nerve compression

This typically occurs at the elbow, where the nerve is compressed in the cubital tunnel. It follows fracture of the ulna or prolonged or recurrent pressure on the nerve at this site.

Wasting of the ulnar innervated muscles develops (hypothenar muscles and interossei) together with sensory loss in the ulnar one-and-a-half fingers.

Decompression and transposition of the nerve at the elbow may be necessary.

The deep (solely motor) branch of the ulnar nerve may be damaged in the palm by recurrent pressure from tools (e.g. screwdrivers), crutches or cycle handlebars.

Radial nerve compression

The radial nerve is compressed acutely against the humerus, e.g. when the arm is draped over a hard chair for several hours ('Saturday night palsy'). Wrist drop and weakness of finger extension and of the brachioradialis muscle follow. Recovery is usual within 1–3 months.

Meralgia paraesthetica

Burning, tingling and numbness on the anterolateral aspect of the thigh is caused by entrapment of the lateral cutaneous nerve of the thigh beneath the inguinal ligament.

Division of the inguinal ligament is not usually effective in relieving the symptoms. Many of the patients are obese; weight reduction helps.

Common peroneal nerve palsy

When the common peroneal nerve is compressed against the head of the fibula (due to prolonged squatting, plaster casts, prolonged bed rest or coma) there is foot drop and weakness of eversion. A patch of numbness on the anterolateral border of the shin or dorsum of the foot may be found. Recovery is usual (but not invariable) within several months.

Multiple mononeuropathy (mononeuritis multiplex)

Multiple mononeuropathy occurs in:
- Diabetes mellitus
- Leprosy
- Connective tissue disease (polyarteritis nodosa, SLE, giant cell arteritis)
- Sarcoidosis
- Malignancy
- Amyloidosis
- Neurofibromatosis

With the exception of diabetes (and leprosy in Asia and Africa), these are all rare causes of neuropathy.

POLYNEUROPATHIES

Although many toxins and disease processes are known to be associated with polyneuropathy (see below), the cause of the majority of cases remains undetermined. The commonest presentation is a chronic or subacute sensorimotor neuropathy. A

Table 18.52 Classification of polyneuropathy.

Idiopathic chronic sensorimotor neuropathy
Post-infective neuropathy (Guillain–Barré syndrome)
Drugs/toxic, metabolic and vitamin deficiency
  neuropathies
Neoplastic neuropathies
Neuropathies in connective tissue diseases
Autonomic neuropathies
Hereditary sensorimotor neuropathies

classification of polyneuropathy is given in Table 18.52.

Idiopathic chronic sensorimotor neuropathy

The patient complains of a progressive symmetrical numbness and tingling in the hands and feet, which spreads proximally in a 'glove and stocking' distribution. There is distal weakness, which also ascends. Rarely the cranial nerves may be affected. Tendon reflexes involving affected nerves are lost. The symptoms may progress over many months, remain static or remit at any stage. Autonomic features are sometimes seen.

Investigation (nerve conduction studies, EMG) of the neuropathy shows axonal degeneration, demyelination, or features of both of these processes. Some cases of demyelinating (not axonal) chronic sensorimotor neuropathy respond to steroid therapy.

Post-infective polyneuropathy (Guillain–Barré syndrome)

CLINICAL FEATURES

This demyelinating neuropathy, which has an auto-allergic basis, follows 1–3 weeks after a viral infection that is often trivial in nature. The patient complains of weakness of distal limb muscles or distal numbness. This ascends over several days or weeks. In mild cases there is little disability, but in some 20% of cases the respiratory and facial muscles are affected and the patient may become paralysed.

Weakness, areflexia and sensory loss are found.

Autonomic features (see below) are sometimes seen. There is a rare proximal form of the condition which initially affects the ocular muscles and in which ataxia is found (Miller Fisher syndrome).

DIAGNOSIS

This is established on clinical grounds and is confirmed by nerve conduction studies which show the slowing of conduction or conduction block seen in demyelinating neuropathies. The CSF contains a normal cell count and sugar level, but the protein is frequently raised to $1–3 \text{ g·l}^{-1}$.

The differential diagnosis includes other paralytic illnesses such as poliomyelitis, botulism or primary muscle disease.

TREATMENT AND COURSE

Treatment is essentially supportive, with particular attention to compensating for weakness of the respiratory and bulbar muscles and to pressure areas. Ventilation may be necessary.

Corticosteroids used to be recommended in the Guillain–Barré syndrome but are not of value.

Plasmapheresis is sometimes used to remove possible antibodies.

Recovery, though gradual over many months, is almost invariable and complete.

Diphtheria

Demyelinating neuropathy is sometimes caused by the exotoxin of *Corynebacterium diphtheriae*. Palatal weakness followed by pupillary paralysis and a sensorimotor neuropathy occur several weeks after faucial infection. The condition is now rare in countries where immunization against diphtheria is practised.

Metabolic, toxic and vitamin deficiency neuropathies

The commoner of these neuropathies are shown in Table 18.53. All are due to impairment of normal metabolism of the axon, myelin or both.

Table 18.53 Toxic, metabolic and vitamin deficiency neuropathies.

Metabolic
Diabetes mellitus
Uraemia
Hepatic disease
Thyroid disease
Porphyria
Amyloid disease
Malignancy
Refsum's disease
Toxic
Drugs
Alcohol
Industrial toxins
Vitamin deficiency
B_1 (thiamine)
B_6 (pyridoxine)
Nicotinic acid
B_{12}

METABOLIC NEUROPATHIES

Diabetes mellitus
Several varieties of neuropathy occur in diabetes mellitus:
- Symmetrical sensory polyneuropathy
- Mononeuropathy and multiple mononeuropathy
  (a) Cranial nerve lesions
  (b) Isolated peripheral nerve lesions, e.g. median
  (c) Diabetic amyotrophy
- Autonomic neuropathy

These are discussed in more detail on p. 764.

Uraemia
Progressive sensorimotor neuropathy occurs in chronic uraemia (see p. 419). The response to dialysis is variable, but the neuropathy usually improves after renal transplantation.

Thyroid disease
A mild chronic sensorimotor neuropathy is sometimes seen in both hyper- and hypothyroidism.

Porphyria
Acute intermittent porphyria is a rare metabolic disorder (see p. 777) in which there are episodes of a severe, mainly proximal, neuropathy, sometimes associated with abdominal pain, confusion and, later, coma. Alcohol and barbiturates may precipitate attacks.

Amyloidosis
This is described on p. 323.

Refsum's disease
This is a rare condition inherited as an autosomal recessive trait. There is a sensorimotor polyneuropathy with ataxia, retinal damage and deafness. It is due to a defect in the metabolism of phytanic acid.

TOXIC NEUROPATHIES

Alcohol
A polyneuropathy, mainly in the lower limbs, occurs in chronic alcoholics. Calf pain is common. The response to abstention is variable.

Drugs
Many drugs have been reported to be associated with polyneuropathy. The more important ones are shown in Table 18.54.

Table 18.54 Drug-associated neuropathies.

Drug	Neuropathy	Mode/site of action
Phenytoin Chloramphenicol Procarbazine	Sensory	Axon
Isoniazid	Sensory	Pyridoxine metabolism
Dapsone Gold Amphotericin	Motor	Axon
Nitrofurantoin Vincristine Chlorambucil Disulfiram Cisplatin	Sensorimotor	Axon
Perhexiline (not available in UK)	Sensorimotor	Myelin

Industrial toxins
A wide variety of industrial toxins have been shown to cause polyneuropathy:

● Lead poisoning causes a motor neuropathy.
● Acrylamide (plastics industry), trichloroethylene (a solvent), hexane and other fat-soluble hydrocarbons (e.g. those inhaled in glue-sniffing, p. 672) cause a progressive polyneuropathy.
● Arsenic and thallium cause a polyneuropathy.

VITAMIN DEFICIENCY NEUROPATHIES

Vitamin deficiencies are an important cause of neuropathy because they are potentially reversible if treated early (and progressive if not). They occur in malnutrition, when they are commonly multiple.

Thiamine (vitamin B₁)
Deficiency causes the clinical syndrome of beri-beri (see p. 136). The principal features are polyneuropathy, Wernicke's encephalopathy, an amnesic syndrome (Wernicke–Korsakoff psychosis) and cardiac failure. Alcoholism is the commonest cause in Western countries. Other neurological consequences of alcohol are summarized in Table 18.55.

Wernicke–Korsakoff syndrome. This important syndrome is an acute or gradual encephalopathy associated with alcoholism and other causes of thiamine deficiency. The typical triad comprises ocular signs, ataxia and a confusional state, but the condition occurs in partial forms. It is due to ischaemic damage

Table 18.55 Effects of alcohol on the nervous system (see also Table 3.16 and p. 147).

Acute intoxication
Disturbance of balance, gait and speech
Coma
Head injury and its sequelae
Alcohol withdrawal
'Morning shakes'
Tremor of arms and legs
Delirium tremens
Thiamine deficiency
Polyneuropathy
Wernicke–Korsakoff syndrome
Epilepsy
Acute intoxication
Alcohol withdrawal
Hypoglycaemia
Cerebellar degeneration
Cerebral infarction
Cerebral atrophy
Dementia
Central pontine myelinolysis
Marchiafava–Bignami syndrome (primary degeneration of the corpus callosum) (rare)

to the brain stem and its connections. Clinical features include:

● *Ocular signs.* Horizontal nystagmus, bilateral lateral rectus palsies, conjugate gaze palsies, fixed pupils and, rarely, papilloedema are found.
● *Ataxia.* There is a broad-based gait, cerebellar signs in the limbs and vestibular paralysis (absent response to caloric stimulation).
● *Confusion.* Apathy, decreased awareness or restlessness, amnesia, stupor and coma occur.

Hypothermia and hypotension due to hypothalamic damage are rare findings.

The condition is underdiagnosed in alcoholics. Erythrocyte transketolase activity is reduced but is of limited practical value in making the diagnosis.

Thiamine (i.m. or i.v.) should be given immediately if the diagnosis is in question. It is harmless; the condition is not. Untreated Wernicke–Korsakoff syndrome commonly leads to a severe irreversible amnesic syndrome and residual brain stem signs.

Pyridoxine (vitamin B₆)
Deficiency causes a mainly sensory neuropathy. It may be precipitated during isoniazid therapy for TB in those who acetylate the drug slowly.

Vitamin B₁₂
Deficiency causes disease of the brain, spinal cord and peripheral nerves.

Subacute combined degeneration of the cord. This important syndrome of the spinal cord is a sequel of Addisonian pernicious anaemia and rarely other causes of vitamin B₁₂ deficiency (see p. 269). It is frequently associated with a peripheral neuropathy.

The patient complains initially of numbness and tingling of the extremities. The signs are of distal sensory loss (particularly posterior column) with absent ankle jerks (due to the neuropathy) combined with evidence of cord disease (exaggerated knee jerk reflexes, extensor plantar responses). Optic atrophy may occur. In the later stages sphincter disturbance, weakness and dementia are seen.

Macrocytosis and megaloblastic changes in the bone marrow are invariable in subacute combined degeneration of the cord. The cause of the B₁₂ deficiency should be established (see p. 270). Treatment with parenteral B₁₂ reverses the peripheral nerve damage but has little effect on the CNS signs.

Before the advent of B₁₂ therapy, the condition was progressive and fatal.

Neoplastic neuropathy

Polyneuropathy is sometimes seen as a non-metastatic manifestation of malignancy (see p. 861).

In myeloma and other dysproteinaemic states, polyneuropathy occurs, due to impaired perfusion of nerve trunks or to demyelination associated with allergic reactions within peripheral nerves.

Neuropathies associated with connective tissue diseases

Sensorimotor neuropathy occurs in systemic lupus erythematosus, polyarteritis nodosa, rheumatoid disease and giant cell arteritis due to micro-infarction of peripheral nerves. A multiple mononeuropathy may also occur (see above).

Autonomic neuropathy

Autonomic dysfunction causes postural hypotension, retention of urine, impotence, diarrhoea (or occasionally constipation), diminished sweating, impaired pupillary responses and cardiac dysrhythmia.

Many varieties of neuropathy affect autonomic function to a mild, and often subclinical, degree. Occasionally, when there is damage to small myelinated and non-myelinated B and C fibres, the clinical features of the autonomic neuropathy predominate. This situation may occur in diabetes mellitus, in amyloidosis and in the Guillain–Barré syndrome.

Hereditary sensorimotor neuropathies

These are described on p. 855.

PLEXUS LESIONS AND RADICULOPATHY

The common conditions that cause nerve root or lumbar or brachial plexus lesions are summarized in Table 18.56.

Table 18.56 Principal causes of plexus and nerve root lesions.

Plexus
Trauma
Malignant infiltration
Cervical rib
Neuralgic amyotrophy
Nerve root
Trauma
Herpes zoster
Meningeal inflammation (e.g. syphilis)
Tumours (neurofibroma, metastases)
Cervical and lumbar spondylosis

Cervical rib (thoracic outlet syndrome)

A fibrous band or cervical rib extending from the tip of the transverse process of C7 to the first rib stretches the lower roots of the brachial plexus (C8 and T1). There is pain along the ulnar border of the forearm, and sensory loss in the distribution of T1 with wasting of the thenar muscles, principally the abductor pollicis brevis muscle. Horner's syndrome may occur. The rib or band can be excised.

In other patients the rib or band causes sub-clavian artery or venous occlusion. The neurological and vascular problems rarely occur together.

Neuralgic amyotrophy

This is a condition in which severe pain in the muscles of the shoulder is followed by wasting, usually of the infraspinatus, supraspinatus, deltoid and serratus anterior muscles. The cause is unknown, but since the condition follows viral infection or immunization in some cases, an allergic basis is postulated.

Recovery of the wasted muscles occurs over some months.

Malignant infiltration

Metastatic disease of nerve roots of the brachial or lumbosacral plexus causes a painful radiculopathy.

A common example is an apical bronchial neoplasm (Pancoast's tumour) which causes a T1 lesion and involves the sympathetic outflow. There is wasting of the small muscles of the hand, pain and sensory loss in areas supplied by T1, and ipsilateral Horner's syndrome. This condition also occasionally occurs in apical TB.

Cervical and lumbar spondylosis (see Table 8.20)

Spondylosis describes the degenerative changes within vertebrae and intervertebral discs which occur during ageing or secondary to trauma or rheumatoid disease. The changes are common in the lower cervical and lower lumbar region.

Several, often related, factors are important in producing signs and symptoms, including:
● Osteophytes—local overgrowth of bone
● Congenital narrowing of the spinal canal
● Disc degeneration with posterior or lateral disc protrusion
● Ischaemic changes in the cord and nerve roots

The commoner clinical syndromes will be described.

Lateral cervical disc protrusion (Fig. 18.23)
The patient complains of pain in the upper limb. A C7 protusion is the commonest lesion. There is root pain (see p. 811) which radiates into the affected myotome (scapula, triceps and forearm extensors in a C7 lesion) and a sensory disturbance (tingling, numbness) in the affected dermatome. There is weakness and, later, wasting of muscles innervated by the affected root (triceps and finger extensors in a C7 lesion) and reflexes using this root will be lost (the triceps jerk in a C7 lesion).

Fig. 18.23 Cervical spondylosis. Central (a) and lateral (b) disc protrusion.

Although the initial pain is often severe, most cases recover with rest and analgesics. It is usual to immobilize the neck in a collar. Plain x-rays of the cervical spine (oblique views) show encroachment into the exit foraminae by osteophytes. In cases where recovery is delayed, root compression may be demonstrated at myelography and surgical root decompression performed.

Central cervical disc protrusion (cervical myelopathy)
Posterior disc protrusion (Fig. 18.23), which is common at C4/5, C5/6 and C6/7 levels, causes spinal cord compression (see p. 812). Congenital narrowing of the canal, osteophytic bars and ischaemia are contributory factors.

The patient complains of difficulty in walking. Frequently there are no symptoms in the neck. A spastic paraparesis (or tetraparesis) is found, with variable sensory loss. A reflex level in the upper limbs and evidence of lateral disc protrusion may coexist.

Plain films may show narrowing of the sagittal diameter of the spinal canal and osteophytes, but the changes correlate poorly with signs and symptoms. Myelography is necessary to demonstrate the level and extent of cord compression.

Cervical laminectomy or anterior fusion of the vertebral bodies with removal of the disc may be necessary when the cord compression is severe or progressive. The results of surgery are often disappointing. Recovery of the 'pyramidal' symptoms is unusual, although progression may be halted.

A collar should be fitted. Manipulation of the neck shoud be avoided.

Thoracic disc protrusion
Central protrusion of a thoracic disc is a rare cause of paraparesis.

Lateral lumbar disc protrusion
The L5 and S1 roots are commonly compressed by lateral prolapse of the L4/5 and L5/S1 discs respectively. There is low back pain and 'sciatica' (pain radiating down the buttock and lower limb). The onset may be acute and follow lifting a heavy weight, or may be subacute and apparently unrelated to exercise.

Straight leg raising is limited. There may be loss of reflexes (ankle jerk in an S1 root lesion or knee jerk in an L4/5 lesion) and weakness of plantar flexion (S1) or extension of the great toe (L5). Sensory loss may be found in the affected dermatome.

Plain films of the lumbar spine show narrowing of the disc space, osteophytes or a narrow canal. Unsuspected malignancy or infection may be demonstrated.

Most cases resolve with rest and analgesics. In the minority, myelography is necessary and laminectomy is indicated when a root lesion is shown.

Central lumbar disc protrusion
A central disc protrusion causes a lesion of the cauda equina, with back pain, weakness of the lower limbs, sacral numbness, retention of urine, impotence and areflexia. Many nerve roots are involved.

The onset is either acute (a cause of an acute flaccid paraparesis) or chronic, when intermittent claudication occurs.

Neoplasms in the lumbosacral region cause a similar picture.

The condition should be suspected if a patient with back pain develops retention of urine. Urgent myelography and decompression is indicated.

Spinal stenosis
Narrowing of the lumbar spinal canal produces back pain (see p. 363). Congenital narrowing of the cervical canal predisposes to cervical myelopathy from minor disc protrusion.

Non-metastatic manifestations of malignancy

Almost any neurological syndrome may occur as a non-metastatic response to malignancy. Clinical pictures include:
- Sensorimotor neuropathy
- Cerebellar syndrome
- Dementia and encephalopathy
- Myasthenic–myopathic syndrome (Eaton–Lambert syndrome)
- Progressive multifocal leucoencephalopathy
- Mononeuritis multiplex
- Cranial polyneuropathy
- Motor neurone disease variants
- Spastic paraparesis

The cause of most of these remains obscure. The clinical importance is that the neurological syndrome sometimes precedes clinical recognition of the neoplasm, which is often an oat cell carcinoma of the bronchus or a lymphoreticular tumour. The neurological signs may recede if the tumour is resected or treated.

Diseases of voluntary muscle

Weakness is the predominant feature of a myopathy. Its distribution and pattern is of diagnostic importance. A classification of muscle disease is given in Table 18.57. Only the more common conditions are mentioned below.

Table 18.57 Classification of muscle disease.

ACQUIRED MYOPATHIES
Inflammatory myopathy
Polymyositis
Alone
With skin lesions (dermatomyositis)
With collagen disease
With malignancy
Viral, bacterial and parasitic infection
Sarcoidosis
Metabolic and endocrine myopathy, due to:
Corticosteroids/Cushing's syndrome
Thyroid disease
Calcium metabolism disorders
Hypokalaemia
Ethanol
Drugs
Myasthenic disorders
Myasthenia gravis
Myasthenic–myopathic (Eaton–Lambert) syndrome
GENETICALLY DETERMINED MYOPATHIES
Muscular dystrophies
Duchenne muscular dystrophy
Facio-scapulo-humeral dystrophy
Limb girdle dystrophy
Myotonias
Dystrophia myotonica
Myotonia congenita
Periodic paralyses
Hypokalaemic
Hyperkalaemic
Normokalaemic
Specific metabolic myopathies, e.g.
Myophosphorylase deficiency
Other defects of glycogen, fatty acid and
mitochondrial metabolism
Malignant hyperpyrexia

PATHOPHYSIOLOGY

Muscle fibres are affected by:
- Acute inflammation and fibre necrosis (e.g. polymyositis)
- Chronic degeneration of muscle fibres (e.g. Duchenne muscular dystrophy)
- Regeneration and fibre hypertrophy
- Complex immune and metabolic disorders. For example:
  - (a) In myasthenia gravis, there is a reduction in the number of available acetylcholine receptors at the neuromuscular junction due to antibodies to the receptor protein.
  - (b) In myotonias, defective chloride ion membrane conductance is associated with delayed muscle relaxation.
  - (c) Enzyme defects in the glycolytic pathway (e.g. myophosphorylase deficiency) result in impaired force generation.

INVESTIGATION

Diagnosis is possible on clinical grounds alone in some myopathies. The distribution of weakness and the consistency of the muscles should be noted.

Serum muscle enzymes
Serum creatine phosphokinase (and aldolase) is greatly elevated in many dystrophies (e.g. Duchenne muscular dystrophy) and in inflammatory disorders of muscle (e.g. polymyositis). These enzymes are normal in myasthenia, and are usually normal in myotonias and chronic partial denervation.

Electromyography
When a muscle is weak the normal interference pattern is reduced. An EMG is useful to distinguish between primary muscle disease and denervation. The principal abnormalities are:
- *Myopathy.* Short duration 'spiky' polyphasic muscle action potentials are seen. Spontaneous fibrillation is occasionally recorded.
- *Denervation.* Fibrillation potentials of about 1 ms in duration and 50–200 µV in amplitude are seen.

Other changes. Myotonic discharges (in myotonias) consist of high-frequency activity which varies repeatedly to cause a sound likened to a propeller-driven dive-bomber on the loudspeaker.

In myasthenia gravis a characteristic decrement in the evoked muscle action potential follows stimulation of the motor nerve. The reverse is seen in the rare myasthenic–myopathic syndrome (Eaton–Lambert syndrome) which may accompany carcinoma of the bronchus.

Muscle biopsy
Information about muscle fibre types (type 1 = slow; Type 2 = fast), denervation, inflammation,

dystrophic changes and muscle histochemistry is obtained by muscle biopsy. Electron microscopy is sometimes necessary.

In chronic partial denervation, 'fibre type grouping', i.e. groups of atrophic fibres of the same fibre type, is seen. Hypertrophic fibres also occur. In acute denervation, small angulated fibres are seen scattered randomly between normal fibres. In dystrophies and myositis, the muscle fibres are diffusely abnormal, the nuclei become central, and invasion by inflammatory cells and/or necrosis occurs.

Considerable experience is required to assess these changes accurately.

INFLAMMATORY MYOPATHIES

Polymyositis

This group of disorders is characterized by non-suppurative inflammation of skeletal muscle. The muscles are weak and usually painful. In many cases there are skin changes (dermatomyositis, see p. 344) or other connective tissue diseases (see p. 339).

CLINICAL FEATURES

'Polymyositis alone' is a rare disease, most common in the fourth and fifth decades. Symptoms are of difficulty in rising from a chair, climbing stairs or lifting. Weakness is typically proximal. The weak muscles ache and are sometimes tender and indurated.

As the disease progresses there may be widespread weakness and wasting, with dysphagia, respiratory muscle weakness and cardiac involvement.

INVESTIGATION

Preliminary investigations show a raised ESR and a mild normochromic normocytic anaemia. Antinuclear factor is sometimes positive. The serum creatine phosphokinase is usually (but not always) elevated.

The EMG shows myopathic changes. Occasionally fibrillation potentials occur and may cause diagnostic difficulty.

Muscle biopsy shows inflammatory changes with infiltration of the muscle by mononuclear cells.

DIFFERENTIAL DIAGNOSIS

Muscular dystrophies rarely progress as rapidly as polymyositis and there is no muscle pain. Pseudohypertrophy does not occur in polymyositis and there is no family history.

Motor neurone disease is always eventually accompanied by upper motor neurone signs, and prominent fasciculation is common.

TREATMENT

Corticosteroids and/or azathioprine or cyclophosphamide reduce the symptoms in about 75% of cases. Only rarely does the disease progress to cause grave disability or death from respiratory failure or cardiac involvement.

Other inflammatory myopathies

Muscle pain and weakness occur in trichinosis due to the ingestion of pork infected with *Trichinella spiralis* (discovered by Sir James Paget when a medical student).

Acute myositis also occurs with coxsackievirus infections (see p. 55).

Tropical pyomyositis of central Africa is suppurative inflammation of muscle caused by staphylococci and other organisms.

An inflammatory myopathy may occur in sarcoidosis.

METABOLIC AND ENDOCRINE MYOPATHIES

Corticosteroids and Cushing's syndrome
Proximal muscle weakness occurs with prolonged high dose steroid therapy (particularly with 9-α-fluorinated steroids such as dexamethasone and triamcinolone) and in Cushing's syndrome. Selective type 2 fibre atrophy is seen on muscle biopsy.

Thyroid disease
Several muscle diseases may occur:
● Thyrotoxicosis is sometimes accompanied by a severe proximal myopathy.
● In ophthalmic Graves' disease there is swelling and lymphocytic infiltration of the extraocular muscles (see p. 722).
● Hypothyroidism is sometimes associated with muscle pain and stiffness, resembling myotonia. A true proximal myopathy also occurs.
● There is also an association between thyrotoxicosis and myasthenia gravis, and between thyrotoxicosis and hypokalaemic periodic paralysis. Both associations are seen most frequently in south-east Asia.

Disorders of calcium metabolism
Proximal myopathy may occur in osteomalacia of any cause (see p. 735). Vitamin D therapy is sometimes curative.

Hypokalaemia
Acute hypokalaemia (e.g. in diuretic therapy) causes a severe flaccid paralysis (periodic paralysis, see p. 866) which is reversed by correcting the electrolyte disturbance.

Chronic mild hypokalaemia (also commonly

caused by diuretics) gives rise to a mild, mainly proximal, weakness.

Alcohol

Severe myopathy with muscle pain, necrosis and myoglobinuria occurs in acute alcoholic excess. (A similar syndrome occurs in diamorphine and amphetamine addicts.) A subacute proximal myopathy occurs in chronic alcoholism.

Drugs

Many drug-induced muscle disorders have been described (see Table 18.58). Most respond to drug withdrawal.

Table 18.58 Drug-induced muscle disorders.

Disorder	Drugs responsible
Subacute proximal myopathy	Diamorphine
	Clofibrate
	Chloroquine
	Lithium
	Quinine
Myasthenic syndromes	D-Penicillamine
	Lithium
	Propranolol
Malignant hyperpyrexia (see p. 866)	Psychotropic drugs
	General anaesthetics

MYASTHENIC DISORDERS

These are disorders characterized by abnormal fatiguability, i.e. weakness after exercise.

Myasthenia gravis

This is characterized by weakness and fatiguability of proximal limb, ocular and bulbar muscles. The heart is not affected.

The cause is unknown. IgG antibodies to acetylcholine receptor protein are found and cause reduction in the available functional receptors at the nicotinic neuromuscular junction.

Thymic hyperplasia is found in 70% of myasthenic patients below the age of 40. In 10% of patients, a thymic tumour is found, the incidence increasing with age; antibodies to striated muscle can be demonstrated in these patients.

There is an association between myasthenia gravis and thyroid disease, rheumatoid disease, pernicious anaemia and systemic lupus erythematosus. Myasthenia gravis is sometimes caused by D-penicillamine treatment in rheumatoid disease.

The prevalence is about 4 in 100 000. It is twice as common in women as in men, with a peak incidence around the age of 30 years.

CLINICAL FEATURES

Fatiguability is the single most important feature. The proximal limb muscles, the extraocular muscles, and the muscles of mastication, speech, and facial expression are those commonly affected in the early stages. Respiratory difficulties may occur.

Complex extraocular palsies, ptosis and a typical fluctuating proximal weakness are found. The reflexes are initially preserved, but may be fatiguable. Muscle wasting is sometimes seen late in the disease.

INVESTIGATION

The clinical picture of fluctuating weakness may be diagnostic but many cases are initially diagnosed as 'hysterical'.

Tensilon (edrophonium) test

Edrophonium (an anticholinesterase) 10 mg i.v. is injected as a bolus after a test dose of 1–2 mg. Improvement in weakness occurs within seconds and lasts for 2–3 minutes when the test is positive. To be certain it is wise to have an observer present and to perform a control test using an injection of saline.

Occasionally the test itself causes bronchial obstruction, and syncope. It should not therefore be carried out where there is no apparatus for resuscitation.

Acetylcholine receptor antibodies

These are present in 90% of cases of generalized myasthenia gravis. The antibodies are found in no other condition.

Nerve stimulation

There is a characteristic decrement in the evoked muscle action potential following stimulation of the motor nerve.

Other tests

Preliminary tests may show a mediastinal mass on chest x-ray. Tomography and mediastinal CT scanning are sometimes indicated.

Routine peripheral blood studies are normal (the ESR is not raised). Autoantibodies to striated muscle, intrinsic factor or thyroid may be found. Rheumatoid factor and antinuclear antibody tests may be positive.

Muscle biopsy is of limited value.

COURSE AND MANAGEMENT

The severity of myasthenia gravis fluctuates but most cases have a protracted course. It is important to recognize respiratory impairment, dysphagia and nasal regurgitation; emergency-assisted ventilation may be required (myasthenic crisis).

Exacerbations are usually unpredictable but may

be brought on by infections and by aminoglycosides or other drugs. Enemas (magnesium sulphate) may provoke severe weakness.

Oral anticholinesterases
Pyridostigmine (60 mg tablet) is the most widely used drug. Its duration of action is 3–4 h. The dose (usually 4 to 16 tablets daily) is determined by the patient's response.

Overdose of anticholinesterase causes severe weakness (cholinergic crisis).

Colic and diarrhoea sometimes occur with anticholinesterases and it is often necessary to give oral atropine 0.5 mg with each dose.

Although anticholinesterases are of value in treating the weakness, they do not alter the natural history of the disease.

Thymectomy
Thymectomy offers long-term benefit. It improves the prognosis, particularly in patients below 40 years and in those who have had the disease for less than 10 years.

Eighty per cent of non-thymoma cases remit. Only 10% of cases with thymoma remit, although surgery is still indicated to remove a potentially malignant tumour.

Immunosuppressant drugs
Corticosteroids are used when there is an incomplete response to anticholinesterases. There is improvement in 70% of cases, although this may be preceded by an initial relapse.

Azathioprine (and sometimes plasmapheresis to remove antibodies) is combined with prednisolone in steroid-resistant cases.

Myasthenic–myopathic syndrome (Eaton–Lambert syndrome)

This is a rare non-metastatic manifestation of oat cell carcinoma of the bronchus. There is defective acetylcholine release at the neuromuscular junction. Proximal muscle weakness, sometimes involving the ocular and bulbar muscles, is found, with absent knee jerks. Weakness tends to improve after muscular contraction (unlike in myasthenia gravis).

Other myasthenic syndromes

Other rare myasthenic syndromes occur (such as congenital myasthenia).

MUSCULAR DYSTROPHIES

These are progressive, genetically determined disorders of skeletal and sometimes cardiac muscle.

Duchenne muscular dystrophy (DMD)

This is inherited as an X-linked recessive disorder, but one-third of cases arise by spontaneous mutation. Recently the DMD locus has been localized to the Xp21 region of the X chromosome. DMD affects male children, is usually obvious by the fourth year, and causes death by the age of 20.

CLINICAL FEATURES

The child has difficulty in running and in rising to an erect position, when he has to 'climb his legs with his arms' (Gower's sign).

There is initially a proximal limb weakness with pseudohypertrophy of the calves. The myocardium is affected. The boy becomes severely disabled by 10 years.

INVESTIGATION

The diagnosis is often obvious.

The creatine phosphokinase is grossly elevated (100–200 times the normal level). Muscle biopsy shows characteristic variation in fibre size, fibre necrosis, regeneration and replacement by fat. The EMG shows a myopathic pattern.

MANAGEMENT

There is no curative treatment. Passive physiotherapy helps to prevent contractures in the later stages of the disease.

Carrier detection
A female with an affected brother has a 50% chance of carrying the gene. In carrier females, 70% have a raised creatine phosphokinase level and the remainder usually have EMG abnormalities or changes on biopsy. Accurate carrier and prenatal diagnosis can be made using cDNA probes which are co-inherited with the DMD locus.

Genetic advice explaining the inheritance of the condition and counselling about abortion should be given. Determination of the fetal sex by amniocentesis and selective abortion of a male fetus is sometimes carried out. Many proven carrier females choose not to have offspring.

Limb girdle and facio-scapulo-humeral dystrophy

These milder dystrophies are summarized in Table 18.59.

There are many other varieties of muscular dystrophy.

Table 18.59 Limb girdle and facio-scapulo-humeral dystrophies.

	Limb girdle	Facio-scapulo-humeral
Inheritance:	Autosomal recessive	Autosomal dominant
Onset:	10–20 years	10–40 years
Muscles affected:	Shoulder and pelvic girdle	Face, shoulder and pelvic girdle
Progress:	Severe disability within 20–25 years	Normal life expectancy, slow progression
Pseudohypertrophy:	Rare	Very rare
Serum creatine phosphokinase:	Raised (slightly)	Raised (slightly) or normal

MYOTONIAS

These conditions are characterized by myotonia, i.e. continued muscle contraction after the cessation of voluntary effort. The EMG is characteristic (see p. 862). The myotonias are important because patients tolerate general anaesthetics poorly. The commonest two of these rare conditions are mentioned below.

Dystrophia myotonica
This autosomal dominant condition causes progressive distal muscle weakness, with ptosis, weakness and thinning of the face and sternomastoids. Myotonia is usually present. The muscle disease is part of a larger syndrome comprising:
- Cataracts
- Frontal baldness
- Intellectual impairment (mild)
- Cardiomyopathy and conduction defects
- Small pituitary fossa and hypogonadism
- Glucose intolerance
- Low serum IgG

The onset of obvious clinical disease is usually between 20 and 50 years. The condition is gradually progressive. Phenytoin or procainamide sometimes helps the myotonia.

Myotonia congenita (Thomsen's disease)
This is an autosomal dominant disorder. An isolated myotonia, usually mild, occurs in childhood and persists throughout life. The myotonia is accentuated by rest and by cold. Diffuse muscle hypertrophy occurs and the patient appears to have well-developed muscles.

PERIODIC PARALYSES

These are rare membrane disorders characterized by intermittent flaccid muscle weakness and alterations in serum potassium.

Hypokalaemic periodic paralysis
This condition, usually inherited as an autosomal dominant trait, is characterized by generalized weakness (including the speech and bulbar muscles) which often starts after a heavy carbohydrate meal or after a period of rest after exertion. Attacks last for several hours. It is often first noted in the teenage years and tends to remit after the age of 35. The serum potassium is usually below 3.0 mmol·l^{-1} in an attack. The weakness responds to the administration of potassium chloride.

Similar weakness also occurs in hypokalaemia due to diuretics, and may occur during thyrotoxicosis.

Hyperkalaemic periodic paralysis
This condition, usually inherited as an autosomal dominant trait, is characterized by sudden attacks of weakness which are sometimes precipitated by exercise. Attacks start in childhood and tend to remit after the age of 20 years. They last from 30 min to 2 h. Myotonia may occur. The serum potassium is raised.

The attacks are terminated by intravenous calcium gluconate or chloride.

A very rare normokalaemic, sodium-responsive periodic paralysis also occurs.

SPECIFIC METABOLIC MYOPATHIES

This is a large group of rare, genetically determined muscle diseases. Two of these diseases will be mentioned here.

Myophosphorylase deficiency (McArdle's syndrome)
This is an autosomal recessive disorder in which there is a lack of skeletal muscle myophosphorylase. The disorder causes easy fatiguability and severe cramp on exercise, with myoglobinuria.

There is no rise in venous lactate during ischaemic exercise; this forms the basis of a test for the condition.

Malignant hyperpyrexia
Widespread skeletal muscle rigidity and hyperpyrexia developing as a sequel to general anaesthesia is due to an unknown muscle membrane defect. Sudden death during or after anaesthesia may occur in this rare condition, which is sometimes

inherited as an autosomal dominant trait. Dantrolene is useful in controlling the rigidity.

Further reading

Aids to the Examination of the Peripheral Nervous System, 3rd edn. (1986) London: Baillière Tindall.

Bannister R (1985) *Brain's Clinical Neurology*, 6th edn. Oxford: Oxford University Press.

Patten J (1977) *Neurological Differential Diagnosis*. London: Harold Starke.

Ross Russell RW & Wiles CM (1986) *Neurology* (Integrated Clinical Science Series). London: Heinemann.

Psychological Medicine

Introduction

Psychiatry is the branch of medicine that is concerned with the study and treatment of disorders of mental function. A substantial proportion of patients seen by a doctor suffer from psychiatric illness rather than organic disease. Some of these psychiatric problems occur as a consequence of individual social circumstances which may be difficult to alter. Physical and psychiatric disorders often coincide because:

- Patients with psychiatric problems can present with physical problems (e.g. the irritable bowel syndrome)
- Chronic or severe physical ill-health can result in psychiatric disorder (e.g. depression in the setting of a chronic painful disorder)
- Psychiatric symptoms can be part of a physical disease complex (e.g. depression in hypothyroidism)
- Patients with established psychiatric disorders can also develop physical disease

For these reasons, the psychological aspects of disease cannot be the exclusive preserve of psychiatrists but must be the concern of all doctors.

Approximately 15% of attenders at general practices suffer from psychiatric ill-health. Most of the illnesses are minor mood disorders, taking the form of various combinations of depression and anxiety, and about two-thirds are short-lived in nature and clear within 6 months. However, about 5% of general practice consultations involve patients suffering from major depression requiring energetic treatment. The major psychoses—schizophrenia and manic-depressive illness—are much less common in this setting. The general hospital physician and surgeon will tend to see psychiatric disorders that are associated with physical disease or caused by certain physical treatments as well as disorders related to alcohol and other forms of drug use and abuse.

In Britain, as in the rest of the Western World, there has been a shift away from the long-stay mental hospital as the focus of psychiatric treatment and towards acute units in district general hospitals. The number of beds in England occupied by mentally ill people fell from 100 000 to 70 000 between 1973 and 1983, while the proportion of inpatients who were discharged within 1 month rose from 42% to 58%. This reflects more effective assessment, treatment and rehabilitation. In addition, much mental illness can now be treated without admission to hospital.

About 25% of all those referred to psychiatric departments are aged 65 years and over; this includes patients with disorders such as depression and confusional states, which may be reversible, and dementias, which usually are not. It has been estimated that in England about half a million people over 65 years suffer from moderate or severe dementia, and about one-quarter of these are aged 85 years or more.

THE PSYCHIATRIC INTERVIEW

The interview is of prime importance in making a psychiatric diagnosis:

- It is a technique for obtaining information.
- It serves as a standard situation in which to assess the patient's emotions and attitudes.
- The first interview serves to establish an understanding with the patient which will be the basis of any subsequent therapeutic relationship.

The psychiatric history

The history records data from several sources. It is concerned with the patient's complaints, his recent and remote past, and the patient's present life situation up to the time of referral or admission.

The history consists of:

- *Reason for referral*—a brief statement of why and how the patient came to the attention of the doctor
- *Complaints*—reported by the patient in his own words
- *Present illness*—a detailed account of the illness

from the earliest time at which a change was noted until the patient came to the attention of the doctor

- *Family history*—this should focus on the family atmosphere in the patient's childhood, early stresses (including death or separation), and the occurrence of mental illness in family members
- *Personal history*—a short biography which covers childhood and school, jobs held and lost, marriage and divorce, children, and the present housing, social and financial situation
- *Personality*—this consists of a person's attitudes and beliefs, moral values and standards, leisure activities and interests, and usual reaction to stress and setback
- *Medical history*—this includes health during childhood, menstrual history, previous mental health and the use and abuse of alcohol, tobacco and drugs

Supplementary information should be obtained from a close relative or friend who can provide corroboration and additional details.

The mental state examination

Appearance and general behaviour
The patient's clothes, posture, facial expression, general grooming, and demeanour are noted. Posture and movement may also reflect mood. Any inappropriate activity or gross physical signs should also be noted. In the case of the mute or non-cooperative patient, this aspect of the examination should be quite detailed.

Speech
The form of the patient's speech (its rate and quantity) is assessed. Disorders of flow (e.g. whether there are interruptions, rapid shifts or sudden blocks) are relevant. Particularly unusual disturbances can be illustrated by recording typical excerpts.

Mood
This is the least objective part of the examination. Obvious misery, elation or anxiety should be noted. The patient's general feelings are explored (e.g. 'How do you feel in yourself?' 'How is your mood?'). Suicidal feelings are enquired about at this stage if a depressive mood is suspected (e.g. 'How desperate do you feel?' 'Have you ever felt like ending your life?' 'Have you found that you have been thinking of ways to do it?' 'Have you made an attempt?'). Likewise, where an expansive mood is noted, questions concerning elation, including the presence of excessive self-confidence, inflated self-assessment and extravagant plans, are raised. The constancy of mood during the interview, its appropriateness and its impact on the interviewer should be noted.

Enquiries should also be made concerning sleep, appetite, libido, fatigue and irritability.

Thought content
The patient's answers to questions such as 'What do you see as your main worries?' should be summarized. Questions should be asked concerning anxieties or preoccupations with the present life situation, with the future, with the past, and with the safety of themselves or others, and whether the worries interfere with concentration or sleep. Information should also be sought concerning the presence of phobias, obsessional ruminations, compulsions or rituals.

Abnormal beliefs and interpretations of events
The content, mode of onset and degree of fixity are noted of any abnormal beliefs:

- In relation to the environment (e.g. ideas of reference, misinterpretations or delusions). The patient is asked about beliefs that he is being persecuted, being treated in a special way or is the subject of an experiment.
- In relation to the body (e.g. ideas or delusions of bodily change)
- In relation to the self (e.g. delusions of passivity, influence, thought-reading or intrusion)

Abnormal experiences referred to the environment, body or self
The patient should be directly asked whether he/she has experienced unusual, odd or abnormal experiences related to:

- The environment (e.g. hallucinations and illusions, which may be auditory, visual, tactile, olfactory or gustatory; feelings of familiarity or unfamiliarity; derealization; déjà-vu)
- The body (e.g. feelings of deadness, pain or other alterations of bodily sensation)
- The self (e.g. depersonalization; awareness of disturbance in the mechanism of thinking, or blocking, retardation or autochthonous ideas)

Cognitive state
This should be briefly assessed in every patient and related to his general intelligence. It may be impaired in organic mental illness. However, the patient who can give a clear and accurate history is unlikely to have cognitive impairment. Aspects to be tested are shown in Table 19.1.

Insight
The degree to which a patient recognizes that he is ill should be assessed at the end of the mental state examination.

Summary

The psychiatric history, present state and mental state examination can now be summarized in order to provide a differential diagnosis. In psychiatry, the term 'the formulation' is used to describe a concise assessment of the case, which includes a discussion of alternative ideas about diagnosis, aetiology, treatment and prognosis and the arguments for and against each alternative.

Table 19.1 Assessment of cognitive functions.

Function	Questions
Orientation	What is the time/day/month/year? Where are you? What is this place? Whom do you recognize?
Concentration	Repeat months of the year backwards. Take 7 serially from 100 (serial 7s). Repeat a span of digits (e.g. 5-figure: 43701; 6-figure: 732156)
Memory:	
Short-term	Recall test name and address after 2 and 5 min.
Medium/long-term	Current affairs (e.g. name of the prime minister, occupant of the throne, events in the news) Dates of World War II
Intelligence	Simple arithmetic sums Meanings of words Meanings of proverbs Ability to read and write
Higher cortical function	Spatial awareness—drawing 3D objects Naming of objects Right – left discrimination ('Touch your left ear with your right hand'.)

SIGNS AND SYMPTOMS OF PSYCHIATRIC DISORDER

Appearance and general behaviour

Facial appearance, posture and movement provide information about a patient's mood. Patients with retarded depression sit with shoulders hunched, immobile, and with the gaze directed at the floor. Agitated depressives are often tremulous and restless, adjusting their clothing and pacing up and down, while manic patients are often overactive and disinhibited.

Certain uncommon disorders of behaviour are encountered, mainly in schizophrenia. These include:
- *Stereotypy*, which is repetition of movements that do not appear to have a purpose; the movement may be repeated in a regular sequence (e.g. rocking backwards and forwards)
- *Mannerisms*, which are repeated movements that appear to have some functional significance (e.g. saluting)
- *Negativism*, when patients do the opposite of

what is asked and actively resist efforts to persuade them to comply
- *Echopraxia*, when patients automatically imitate the interviewer's movements despite being asked not to do this

Speech

Disorders of thinking are usually recognized from the patient's speech.

Disorders of the stream of thought
There are abnormalities in the amount and speed of the thoughts experienced. At one extreme, there is *pressure of thought*, in which ideas arise in remarkable abundance and variety and pass rapidly through the mind. *Poverty of thought* is the opposite experience, when there appears to be a lack or absence of any thoughts whatsoever and the patient reports his mind to be blank or starved of ideas. Pressure of thought characteristically occurs in mania, and poverty of thought in depression; either may be experienced in schizophrenia. The stream of thought can also be suddenly interrupted. Minor degrees of this phenomenon are not uncommon, especially in normal people who are tired or tense. Severe *thought blocking*, in which there is a particularly abrupt and complete interruption of the stream of thought, strongly suggests schizophrenia. The patient often describes the experience as a sudden and complete emptying of his mind and may interpret the experience in an unusual way (e.g. as having had his thoughts removed by some alien person, presence or machine).

Disorders of the form of thought
These include flight of ideas, perseveration, and loosening of associations.

Flight of ideas. The patient's thoughts and speech move quickly from one topic to another, such that one train of thought is not completed before another appears. It is often accompanied by *clang associations* (the tendency to use two or more words with a similar sound), *punning* (the use of one word with two or more different meanings), rhyming, and responding to distracting cues in the immediate surroundings. Flight of ideas is characteristic of mania.

Perseveration. This is the persistent and inappropriate repetitions of the same thoughts or actions. It is often associated with dementia but can occur in other conditions.

Loosening of associations. This is manifested by a loss of the normal structure of thinking. The most striking impression is an extreme lack of clarity. There are several forms. *Knight's move* or *derailment* denotes transition from one topic to another, either between sentences or within a sentence, with no logical relationship between the two topics and no evidence of flight of ideas as described above. When this abnormality is extreme and disrupts not merely the connections between sentences but also the finer grammatical structure of speech, it is termed *word salad* or *verbigeration*. One effect of loosened associations is sometimes termed 'talking past the point'; the patient always seems to get near to talking about the matter in hand but never quite gets there.

Mood

In psychiatric disorders, mood may be altered in three ways:
- Its nature may be changed.
- It may fluctuate more than usual.
- It may be inconsistent either with the patient's thoughts and actions or with occurrences in the patient's immediate environment.

Changes in the nature of mood
Changes in the nature of mood may be towards depression, elation or anxiety. *Depression* may mean the symptom of feeling sad, melancholic or low in spirits, or it may mean the syndrome of depression as characterized by low mood, lack of enjoyment, reduced energy and changes in appetite, sleep and libido. *Elation* refers to a subjective feeling of high spirits, vitality and even ecstasy, which may or may not be accompanied by exuberant behaviour, increased energy and overactivity. *Anxiety* is a common symptom of worry or apprehension that is often accompanied by physical symptoms such as palpitations, trembling, 'butterflies in the stomach' and hyperventilation.

Anxiety and depression can occur separately or together and may be associated with an obvious cause or may appear to arise without reason.

A *phobia* is an intense fear of a specific object, activity or situation coupled with a wish to avoid it. The fear is irrational in that it is out of all proportion to the real danger. The patient recognizes that it is an exaggerated fear but finds it difficult to control. Objects that provoke such fear include insects, spiders and other animals (e.g. dogs, cats, horses) or natural phenomena such as lightning or the dark. Situations which provoke phobic reactions include open spaces (agoraphobia), closed spaces such as lifts and underground trains (claustrophobia), high places, and crowds.

Changes in the fluctuation of mood
These may result in a total loss of emotion or an inability to experience pleasure. The former is termed *apathy*. When the normal variation of mood is reduced rather than lost, the mood is described as *blunted*. Emotions that are changeable in a rapid, abrupt and excessive way are termed *labile* emotions.

Inconsistent or inappropriate mood
This occurs when the normal emotional expression of the person fails to match his thoughts and actions. For example, a patient may laugh when describing the death of a close and loved relative. Such incongruity needs to be distinguished from laughter that indicates that someone is ill at ease when talking about a distressing subject.

Changes of mood are found in a variety of psychiatric disorders, including depression, mania, anxiety, organic psychoses and schizophrenia.

Thought content

As discussed earlier, thought content refers to the worries and preoccupations manifested by the patient and elicited on interview. Abnormal beliefs and experiences are, of course, part of the thought content, but are regarded as sufficiently important to be discussed separately (see below).

An important disorder of thought content is an *obsession*, which is a recurrent, persistent thought, impulse or image that enters the mind despite the individual's effort to resist it. The individual recognizes that the obsession is his own and is not implanted by anyone or arising from elsewhere.

A *compulsion* is a repetitive and seemingly purposeful action performed in a stereotyped way, referred to as a *compulsive ritual*. Compulsions are accompanied by a subjective sense that they must be carried out and by an urge to resist. Common obsessions concern dirt, contamination, orderliness and dread of illness, while corresponding compulsions would be repeated hand-washings and checkings.

Abnormal beliefs and interpretations of events

The main form of abnormal belief is the *delusion*.
Delusions can be:
- *Primary* or *autochthonous*, i.e. they appear suddenly and with full conviction but without any preceding or related mental events. For example, a patient on being offered a cup of tea suddenly believes that this indicates that the Russians have landed at Dover.
- *Secondary*, i.e. derived from some preceding morbid experience, such as a depressed mood or an auditory hallucination.

Delusions are classified according to their content, and include persecutory delusions (also called paranoid delusions), delusions of reference, guilt, worthlessness or nihilism, religious delusions, and delusions of grandeur, jealousy or control. These are further defined when discussed in relation to specific conditions.

Particular delusions concerning thought control can occur. Patients who have delusions of *thought insertion* believe that some of their thoughts are not

> **Delusion**
>
> This is defined as an abnormal belief arising from distorted judgements and which is:
> - Held with absolute conviction
> - Not amenable to reason or modifiable by experience
> - Not shared by those of a common cultural or social background
> - Experienced as a self-evident truth of great personal significance
> - False

their own but have been implanted by some outside force or agency. The same or other patients may believe that thoughts are taken out of their minds by external forces or agencies (*thought withdrawal*), while in delusions of *thought broadcasting* the patient believes that his unspoken thoughts are known to other people through radio, television, telepathy or some other way. Feelings and actions may also be interpreted by the individual as being under the influence or control of some external, usually alien, power. Such *passivity* experiences, occurring in the absence of clear-cut brain disease, are regarded as diagnostic of schizophrenia. The patient may merely assert that his behaviour is controlled from without and may be unable to give any further explanation. This is usually described as an *experience of passivity*. The patient may develop secondary delusions which explain this alien control as a result of witchcraft, hypnosis, radio waves, television, etc.—so-called *delusions of passivity*. The disturbances of thought control discussed above are examples of passivity experiences involving the thought processes.

Delusions should be distinguished from *overvalued ideas*, i.e. deeply held personal convictions that are understandable when the individual's background is known. *Ideas of reference* that fall short of delusions are held by people who are particularly self-conscious. Such individuals cannot help feeling that people take particular notice of them in public places, pass comment about them and/or observe things about them that they would prefer were ignored. Such feelings are not delusional in that the individual who experiences them realizes that they originate within him and that he is no more noticeable or noteworthy than anyone else, but nevertheless he cannot dismiss the feelings.

Abnormal experiences referred to the environment, body or self

Illusions are misperceptions of external stimuli and are most likely to occur when the general level of sensory stimulation is reduced.

Hallucinations are perceptions that are experienced in the absence of any external stimulus to the sense organs in the outside world (and are not within one's mind as in imagery). Normal people

occasionally experience hallucinations, mainly auditory in type, particularly when tired and during the transition between sleeping and waking.

> **Hallucination**
>
> This is defined as thorough conviction of a sensation when no external object to excite or provoke such a sensation is present. It is:
> - A false perception and not a distortion
> - Perceived as inhabiting objective space
> - Perceived as having qualities of normal perceptions
> - Perceived alongside normal perceptions
> - Independent of the individual's will

Hallucinations can be *elementary* (e.g. bangs, whistles) or *complex* (e.g. faces, voices, music), and may be auditory, visual, tactile, gustatory, olfactory or of deep sensation.

A change in self-awareness such that the person concerned feels unreal is termed *depersonalization*. In this state the person feels detached or remote from his/her own experience and unable to feel emotion. The individual is aware of the subjective nature of this alteration. The feeling that the external environment has become unreal and/or remote is termed *derealization*. Both these phenomena occur in healthy people when they are tired, after sensory deprivation, during the use of hallucinogenic drugs, and also occur in certain conditions such as anxiety, depression, schizophrenia and temporal lobe epilepsy.

Cognitive state

There are four processes involved in normal memory:
- Registration—the ability to add new material to the existing memory stores
- Retention—the ability to retain the memory
- Recall—the ability to bring it back into awareness
- Recognition—the feeling of familiarity indicating that a particular person, event or object has been encountered before

Some patients describe the recognition of a situation, person or event as having been encountered before when it is in fact novel—the so-called *déjà vu* experience, whereas others report the reverse experience (*jamais vu*) when there is failure to recognize a situation, person or event that has been encountered before. Déjà vu experiences occur in healthy people as well as in anxiety states. Both types of experience can occur in epilepsy (see p. 823).

Patients with Wernicke–Korsakoff syndrome, who have extreme difficulty in remembering recent and past events, sometimes report remembering past events that have not actually taken place; this is known as *confabulation*. Failure of memory is termed *amnesia*.

Consciousness can be defined as the awareness of the self and the environment. Attention, concentration and memory are impaired and orientation is disturbed in any condition in which a disturbance of consciousness occurs. This subject is considered on p. 822.

CAUSES OF PSYCHIATRIC DISORDER

A single psychiatric disorder may result from several causes.

Predisposing factors

These are factors, often operating from early life, that determine a person's vulnerability to psychological distress. Such causes include:
- Genetic endowment
- Environment in utero
- Personality
- Childhood trauma

There is evidence for a strong genetic factor in the psychoses, and a weaker genetic factor in the neurotic disorders. Intrauterine disturbances may result in minor organic damage to the brain and central nervous system, which in turn may render the individual liable to develop serious mental disorder in later life in response to particular kinds of stress.

Personality results from the interaction of genetic endowment, uterine development, early childhood experience and various physical, psychological and social influences manifesting themselves up to and including adolescence. Certain personalities are believed to be particularly prone to develop certain disorders. For example, individuals who manifest certain obsessional traits as part of their personality have an increased risk of developing depressive and obsessional illnesses, while anxious, apprehensive individuals are prone to develop a variety of neurotic disorders. When taking the history, particular care should be taken to assess whether the individual's personality was well developed and mature *prior* to the development of the illness, as this will be a major factor in determining the outcome of treatment and the prognosis.

Precipitating factors

These are factors that occur shortly before the onset of a disorder and that appear to have caused it. They may be physical, psychological or social in nature. Whether they produce a disorder depends partly on their severity and partly on the presence of predisposing factors.

Physical precipitating factors include physical diseases (e.g. hypothyroidism, tumours, metabolic disorders) or drugs (e.g. steroids, hypotensives, alcohol). Psychological factors include loss of self-esteem due to a setback or misfortune such as marital infidelity or financial disaster. Social factors include moving house, job difficulties and family disturbances.

Occasionally, the same factor can act in more than one way. A head injury can induce psychological disturbances either through physical changes in the central nervous system or through the stress it provokes in the individual, while marital breakdown may lead to overindulgence in alcohol with secondary impairment of mental processes and psychiatric illness.

Perpetuating factors

These are factors that prolong the course of a disorder after it has occurred. For example, some psychiatric disorders lead to secondary demoralization. A medical student who suffers a depressive illness may well find it difficult to accept the diagnosis, may regard himself as weak and flawed, and may withdraw from social activities. Such a response could prolong the original disorder.

PSYCHIATRIC ASPECTS OF PHYSICAL DISEASE

Psychological and physical symptoms commonly occur together; surveys have shown that they tend to 'cluster' in some people, while others remain relatively free from illnesses. The commonest presentation of psychiatric ill-health in physically ill patients is as affective disorders or acute organic brain syndromes. The relationship between psychological and physical symptoms may be understood in one of three ways:
- Psychological distress and disorder can provoke and precipitate physical disease.
- Physical distress and disease can cause psychological ill-health (see Table 19.2), as can the medication given for the disease.
- Physical and psychological symptoms and disorders coexist because both are common, particularly in the elderly.

Physically ill patients often respond to their illness by feeling depressed, anxious, angry and/or unable to cope. Such reactions are very often transient and require little in the way of management other than recognition, reassurance and support. Sometimes, however, they persist after the acute stage of the physical illness has passed. Certain factors also increase the risk of a psychiatric disorder occurring in the setting of physical disease (Table 19.3). Treatment is the same as for physically healthy, psychiatrically ill patients, but care must be taken

Table 19.2 Psychiatric symptoms commonly associated with physical diseases.

Symptom	Examples of physical disease
Depression	Carcinoma
	Infection
	Thyroid disorders
	Adrenal disorders
	Diabetes mellitus
Anxiety	Hyperthyroidism
	Phaeochromocytoma
	Hypoglycaemia
	Partial seizures
	Alcohol/drug withdrawal
Irritability	Head injury
	Premenstrual tension
	Early dementia
	Hypoglycaemia
Fatigue	Anaemia
	Sleep disorders
	Infections
	Carcinoma
Behavioural	Epilepsy
disturbance	Toxic confusional states
	Dementia
	Porphyria
	Hypoglycaemia

Table 19.3 Factors increasing the risk of psychiatric illness in physically ill patients.

Patient
Previous history of psychiatric illness
History of difficulty in coping with stress
Disturbed personal, family or social circumstances

Setting
Intensive care units
Coronary care units
Renal dialysis units

Physical illness
Carcinoma
Endocrine disorders
Infections
Metabolic disorders
Head injury
Mutilating surgery

Physical treatment
Drugs (e.g. steroids)
Radiotherapy

when prescribing psychotropic drugs to avoid drug interactions.

One symptom that can be thought of as both a physical and a psychological symptom is *pain*. It is the commonest medical symptom, can cause considerable psychological distress and can arise from psychological disturbance. The main sites of psychologically determined pain are the head, the neck, the lower back, the abdomen and the genitalia.

Psychologically determined pain is often con-tinuous for lengthy periods and responds poorly to analgesics. It is often described by the patient as waxing and waning in response to emotional stress and, despite its severity, does not necessarily wake the patient from sleep. A particularly dramatic form of chronic, atypical pain is facial pain; antidepressant therapy has been found to be effective in up to 50% of such patients. Another common painful condition in which depression is often present but is 'masked' by the physical symptoms is the irritable bowel syndrome.

CLASSIFICATION OF MENTAL ILLNESS

The concept of mental illness is complicated. The diagnosis is only made when:
- There is a recognizable disturbance in one or more psychological functions, e.g. perception, emotion, thought.
- The disturbance is not under the comprehensive control of the individual concerned.
- The disturbance usually (though not invariably) causes distress to the affected individual.
- The disturbance usually (though not invariably) requires expert, professional assessment and treatment for recovery.

Particular problems in psychiatry are posed by such conditions as sexual disorders, drug and alcohol dependence and personality disorders.

The most widely used and inclusive classification of mental disorders is the World Health Organization's *Glossary of Mental Disorders* which is part of the 9th revision of the International Classification of Diseases. In 1980, the third edition of the *Diagnostic and Statistical Manual* of the American Psychiatric Association (DSM III) was published. This scheme has five axes. The two main axes are:
- Psychiatric syndromes
- Personality disorders

The others are:
- Physical disorders
- Severity of psychological stressors
- Highest level of adaptive functioning

A simple classification of psychiatric disorders is shown in Table 19.4. The term *psychosis* is usually applied to a psychiatric disorder that significantly impairs insight, involves a substantial break with reality, exercises a major impact on the individual's personality and functioning, and usually requires specialized, inpatient treatment. Certain symptoms that by definition involve an impairment of reality, such as delusions, hallucinations and formal thought disorder, are often termed psychotic symptoms. In contrast, the term *neurosis* is applied to psychiatric disorders in which psychotic symptoms and features are absent, the patient's personality is relatively

Table 19.4 A classification of psychiatric disorders.

Organic disorders (ICD 290–294)*

Functional psychosis
  Schizophrenia (ICD 295)
  Manic-depressive disorder (ICD 296)

Neurotic disorders
  Anxiety neurosis (ICD 300)
  Phobic neurosis (ICD 300.2)
  Obsessional neurosis (ICD 300.3)
  Hysteria (ICD 300.1)
  Hypochondriasis (ICD 300.7)

Personality disorders (ICD 301)

Sexual deviations and disorders (ICD 302)

Alcohol and drug dependence (ICD 303–305)

Other disorders e.g. anorexia nervosa (ICD 307.1)

* Three-digit numbers refer to the numbers of the diagnostic categories in the *Glossary of Mental Disorders*, part of the 9th revision of the International Classification of Diseases produced by the World Health Organization.

undamaged, and contact with reality is unimpaired. Neuroses can be thought of as exaggerated forms of the normal reactions to stressful events. Anxiety, depression, irritability and physical symptoms lacking an organic cause are experienced by many people in response to stressful circumstances and events. In the neuroses these symptoms become so intense as to be highly unpleasant and distressing and out of proportion to the severity of the stress.

Organic psychiatric disorders

Organic brain diseases result from structural pathology, as in senile dementia, or from disturbed central nervous system function, as in fever-induced delirium. A classification of organic brain syndromes, derived from the American classification, DSM III, is shown in Table 19.5.

Delirium

Delirium, also termed 'toxic confusional state', is an acute or subacute condition in which impairment of

Table 19.5 Classification of organic brain syndromes.

Delirium

Dementia

Amnestic syndrome

Organic delusional syndrome

Organic affective syndrome

Intoxication and withdrawal syndromes

consciousness is accompanied by abnormalities of perception and mood. The impairment of consciousness can range from mild befuddlement to serious disorientation and confusion. The degree of impairment classically fluctuates, so that there are intermittent lucid periods. Confusion is usually worse at night. During the acute phase, thought and speech are incoherent, memory is impaired and misperceptions occur. Transient hallucinations, usually visual, and delusions may occur and, as a consequence, the patient may be frightened, suspicious, restless and uncooperative. A large number of diseases may be accompanied by delirium; this is particularly so in elderly patients. Some causes of delirium are listed in Table 19.6. Delirium usually clears within a few days as the underlying illness resolves. If the delirium runs a subacute course, more permanent disorders of cognition, memory or personality may occur.

Investigation and treatment of the underlying physical disease should be undertaken. The patient should be carefully nursed and rehydrated. Pain relief should be adequate and sedation provided if necessary. If a high fever is present, the temperature should be reduced with fans, ice-packs and antipyretic drugs. All current drug therapy should be reviewed and, where possible, stopped. Benzodiazepines are the drugs of choice in the management of minor restlessness, but in severe delirium haloperidol is probably a more effective choice, the daily dose usually ranging between 10 and 60 mg. If necessary, the first dose of 2–10 mg can be administered intramuscularly.

Table 19.6 Some causes of delirium.

Systemic infection
  Any infection, particularly with high fever
    (e.g. malaria, septicaemia)

Metabolic disturbance
  Hepatic failure
  Renal failure
  Disorders of electrolyte balance

Vitamin deficiency
  Thiamine (Wernicke – Korsakoff syndrome, beriberi)
  Nicotinic acid (pellagra)
  Vitamin B_{12} deficiency

Endocrine disease
  Hypoglycaemia

Brain damage
  Trauma
  Tumour
  Abscess
  Subarachnoid haemorrhage

Drug intoxication
  Anticonvulsant
  Anticholinergic
  Anxiolytic/hypnotic
  Opiates
  Industrial poisons

Drug/alcohol withdrawal

Dementia

Dementia is defined as an acquired global impairment of intellect, memory and personality without impairment of consciousness. Usually, its onset is gradual, although a sudden change of environment, such as admission to hospital or an intercurrent illness, may bring it to light.

The symptoms and signs of dementia include:
- Memory impairment
- A decline in intellectual ability
- Coarsening of the personality
- A deterioration in social skills
- Disinhibition of behaviour
- Mood changes
- Paranoid delusions and hallucinations

Memory impairment, which affects short-term rather than long-term memories, is usually an early symptom. The intellectual decline is often gradual and alterations in personality follow. Depression, anxiety and irritability often accompany the intellectual and behavioural deterioration, while in the later stages paranoid delusions, which may be accompanied by auditory and visual hallucinations, appear.

About 25% of the elderly population suffer from a psychiatric disability, mainly anxiety and depression. However, dementia affects about 10% of those aged over 65 years and 20% of those over 80 years of age—a total of 650 000 people in England and Wales. The causes are many and are, for the most part, irreversible. Among elderly patients, degenerative and vascular causes predominate.

The main causes of dementia are given in Table 18.49, p. 853.

Amnestic syndrome

The amnestic syndrome is characterized by a marked impairment of memory occurring in clear consciousness and not as part of a delirium or dementia. Long-term memory is affected but the typical feature is impairment of short-term memory. Often the patient is blandly unconcerned and commonly displays confabulation. The disturbance is due to bilateral damage in the area of the mamillary bodies, fornix and hippocampus. When there are associated neurological signs and symptoms (e.g. ataxia, ophthalmoplegia, disorientation and impairment of consciousness), the term Wernicke–Korsakoff syndrome is sometimes used. The commonest cause is severe thiamine deficiency secondary to chronic alcoholism but other, less common causes occur (Table 19.7).

Organic delusional syndrome

The organic delusional syndrome is characterized by a mental state dominated by delusions which are

Table 19.7 Causes of amnestic syndrome.

Alcohol (Wernicke–Korsakoff syndrome)
Head injury (severe)
Anoxia
Posterior cerebral artery occlusion (bilateral)
Herpes simplex encephalitis
Chronic sedative abuse
Bilateral invasive tumours
Arsenic poisoning
Following hypoglycaemia

often accompanied by a persistent and distressing misperception of the environment, sometimes referred to as 'delusional tone'. The delusions are very often persecutory but may also be hypochondriacal, pathologically jealous, grandiose or erotic.

Organic affective syndrome

The organic affective syndrome consists of marked mood changes which result from organic brain damage. There are depressive and manic phases, often occurring suddenly, or there may be a persistently dysphoric state. There is no significant intellectual loss, delusions or hallucinations, and a family history of affective disorder is uncommon.

Intoxication and withdrawal syndromes

These are discussed on p. 892.

Schizophrenia

The term 'schizophrenia' was coined by the Swiss psychiatrist Eugen Bleuler in 1908 as a 'rending (disconnection) or splitting of the psychic functions'. The normal integration of emotional and cognitive functions is ruptured in schizophrenia. The annual prevalence of the condition ranges between 2 and 4 per 1000. The lifetime risk of contracting schizophrenia is 1%, but for first degree relatives of sufferers it is 12%. High rates have been reported in north-west Yugoslavia, the Tamils of south India and the Irish Republic.

CAUSES

No one cause has been identified to date. A number of possible causes have been implicated and are currently the subject of research. Biological causes are indicated in Table 19.8. Psychological theories suggest that schizophrenics have an impaired ability

Table 19.8 Possible biological causes of schizophrenia.

Genetic
40% risk for children of 2 affected parents
50% risk for monozygotic twin of affected individual
Nature of transmission unclear

Dopamine
Dopamine agonists (e.g. amphetamine) exacerbate the
  condition
The therapeutic potency of neuroleptics is directly
  related to their ability to block dopamine receptors
  in the brain
Withdrawal of dopamine antagonists causes rebound
  of symptoms in some patients
Post-mortem studies show increased dopamine-
  binding sites in the brains of affected patients

Brain damage (e.g. in utero from long-acting virus)
Enlargement of lateral ventricles and widening of
  cerebral fissures and sulci on CT scans of a
  subgroup of patients

Other
Disturbance in transmethylation
Abnormalities in monoamine oxidase function

to handle the amount and speed of incoming perceptual stimuli and/or that some schizophrenics have a left hemisphere limbic dysfunction. A popular social theory suggests disturbances in family relationships or communication are the cause, but the evidence is poor. Studies of so-called 'expressed emotion' suggest that schizophrenic patients are particularly vulnerable to highly expressed emotions, and such family atmospheres increase the chances of relapse in treated patients as do intensive psychotherapy and social demands.

CLINICAL FEATURES

The illness can begin at any age but is rare before puberty; the peak age of onset is in late adolescence and the early twenties. The overall sex incidence is about equal. Schizophrenia is probably not a specific condition but rather a number of clinical syndromes. The symptoms that have been considered as diagnostic of the condition have been termed 'first-rank' symptoms and were described by the German psychiatrist Kurt Schneider. They consist of:
- Auditory hallucinations—the patient hears his own thoughts spoken aloud and/or he hears one or several voices referring to himself in the third person or referring to him by name, and/or he hears voices commenting on his behaviour
- Thought withdrawal, insertion and interruption
- Thought broadcasting
- Delusional perceptions
- External control of emotions
- Somatic passivity and feelings—the patient believing that thoughts or acts are due to the influence of others

The World Health Organization's *International Pilot Study of Schizophrenia* has shown that the presence of any one of these symptoms, in the absence of physical disease, is highly discriminating for the diagnosis in a variety of countries and cultures. Other symptoms of acute schizophrenia include behavioural disturbances, thought disorder, hallucinations, delusions and mood abnormalities.

Chronic schizophrenia is characterized by thought disorder and the so-called 'negative' symptoms of underactivity, lack of drive, social withdrawal and emotional emptiness. Motor disturbances can occur but they are extremely rare. Such disorders are often described as catatonic and include stupor, excitement, mannerisms, stereotypies and automatic obedience. Delusions in chronic schizophrenia are often held with little emotional response (the so-called 'systematized' delusions) and may be 'encapsulated' from the rest of the patient's beliefs and behaviour.

DIFFERENTIAL DIAGNOSIS

Schizophrenia must be distinguished from
- Organic psychiatric disorders
- Affective disorders
- Personality disorders

The most important organic disorders, particularly in young patients, are drug-induced psychoses and temporal lobe epilepsy. Some of the drugs that can produce psychosis are listed in Table 19.9.

In older patients, any acute brain syndrome as well as dementia can present in a schizophrenia-like manner. A helpful diagnostic point is that clouding of consciousness and disturbances of memory do not occur in schizophrenia and visual hallucinations are unusual.

Affective disorders present with a more sustained disturbance of mood and any delusions and hallucinations that are detected are usually understandable in terms of the mood disturbance. 'First-rank' symptoms are not normally a feature of

Table 19.9 Drugs causing psychosis.

Glucocorticoids
Anticholinergic agents
Sympathomimetic central stimulants
Phenytoin
Carbamazepine
Disulfiram
Metronidazole
Cardiac glycosides
Hallucinogens, e.g. LSD, mescaline
Amantadine

Table 19.10 Prognostic factors in schizophrenia.

	Good factors	Bad factors
Premorbid state	No family history of schizophrenia	Family history of schizophrenia
	Stable personality	Withdrawn, solitary, eccentric personality
	Warm personal relationships	Poor work record; poverty of relationships
	Stable home relationships	Stormy domestic situation
Features of illness	Identifiable precipitating factor or 'life event'	No obvious triggering factor or 'life event'
	Acute onset	Insidious onset
	Few first rank sympoms	Many first rank symptoms
	Disturbance of mood	No mood disturbance
	Initiative, interest and motivation maintained	Blunting of emotional responses; initiative, motivation and interest impaired
	Prompt treatment	Treatment delayed

affective disorders. Differentiating insidiously arising schizophrenia from a personality disorder in a young person can be exceptionally difficult and the passage of time may be needed for the condition to be clarified.

COURSE AND PROGNOSIS (Table 19.10)

The prognosis of schizophrenia is highly variable. The patient's psychosocial environment appears important in that in an understimulating environment negative symptoms worsen whereas in an excessively stimulating environment positive symptoms may emerge or worsen. Some patients only suffer acute episodes which leave them relatively unimpaired, whilst others insidiously develop chiefly negative symptoms. The most common presentation and course is an initial acute episode of floridly positive symptoms followed by the emergence and persistence of negative symptoms.

A recent review of treatment studies suggests that between 15 and 25% of schizophrenics recover completely, another two-thirds will have relapses and may develop mild to moderate negative symptoms, while about 1 in 10 will become seriously disabled.

TREATMENT

The best results are obtained by combining drug and social treatments.

Antipsychotic (neuroleptic) drugs
These reduce psychomotor excitement and control many of the symptoms of schizophrenia without causing disinhibition, confusion or sleep. Such drugs are most effective against acutely occurring, positive symptoms and least effective in the manage-

ment of chronic, negative symptoms. Complete control of positive symptoms can take up to 3 months and premature discontinuation of treatment can result in prompt relapse.

The phenothiazines are the most extensively used group of neuroleptics. Chlorpromazine (100–1000 mg daily) is the drug of choice when a more sedating drug is required. Trifluoperazine is used when sedation is undesirable. Fluphenazine decanoate is used as a long-term prophylactic to prevent relapse (25–100 mg i.m. every 1–4 weeks). Promazine or thioridazine is useful in the elderly when it is desirable to reduce the risk of extrapyramidal and anticholinergic side-effects.

Antipsychotic drugs block dopamine receptors. Their action on the basal ganglion may produce extrapyramidal side-effects. This limits their use in the maintenance therapy of many patients. They also block adrenergic and cholinergic receptors and thereby cause a number of unwanted effects (Table 19.11).

In patients manifesting good prognostic features and responding well to drugs, treatment may be discontinued under supervision after several months. Poor prognosis schizophrenia, on the other hand, usually requires regular maintenance therapy for many months or even years.

Social treatment
Social treatment involves attention being paid to the patient's environment and social functioning. Patients with any degree of residual impairment and negative symptoms usually require rehabilitation in a structured work and social environment. Parents and relatives need advice concerning the optimum amount of emotional and social stimulation to be provided for the patient. Some patients can manage a normal job, whereas others require a sheltered

Table 19.11 Unwanted effects of neuroleptic drugs.

COMMON EFFECTS

Extrapyramidal
Acute dystonia
Parkinsonism
Akathisia
Tardive dyskinesia

Autonomic
Hypotension
Failure of ejaculation

Anticholinergic
Dry mouth
Urinary retention
Constipation
Blurred vision

Metabolic
Weight gain

RARE EFFECTS

Hypersensitivity
Cholestatic jaundice
Leucopenia
Skin reactions

Other
Precipitation of glaucoma
Galactorrhoea
Amenorrhoea
Cardiac arrhythmias
Seizures
Retinal degeneration (with thioridazine in high doses)

workshop. A very small number of severely disabled patients require long-term residential medical and nursing care.

Psychological treatment
This consists of reassurance, support and a good doctor–patient relationship. Psychotherapy of an intensive or exploratory kind is contraindicated.

Manic-depressive disorder

The central feature of this disorder is an abnormality of mood, either depression or elation or both. Mood is best considered in terms of a continuum ranging from severe depression at one extreme to severe mania at the other, with normal, stable mood at the centre (Fig. 19.1).

Manic-depressive disorders are divided into bipolar manic-depression, in which patients suffer attacks of both depression and mania, and unipolar disorders, in which there is either mania alone or, more commonly, depression alone. First-degree relatives of patients suffering from bipolar illness have an increased risk of manic-depressive illness but not those of patients with unipolar illness.

Depression is classically divided into endogenous depression and reactive depression, although the validity of this distinction is doubtful.

The criteria of endogenous depression include:
● Pervasive and unresponsive depression
● Early morning waking
● Diurnal variation of mood (worse in the morning)
● Profoundly depressive ideas (e.g. guilt, suicidal feelings)
● The lack of an obvious precipitating cause
● A stable premorbid personality

The criteria of reactive depression include:
● A fluctuating depression responsive to environmental change
● Self-pity rather than self-blame
● A clear precipitating cause
● A vulnerable or predisposed personality
● Absence of the criteria of endogenous depression

A mixture of both types is a commoner presentation than a pure form of either.

CLINICAL FEATURES

The clinical features of *mania* reflect a marked elevation of mood (Table 19.12). The term *hypomania* refers to a mild form of mania characterized by euphoria, overactivity and disinhibition. It can be difficult to distinguish this from simple exuberance, enthusiasm and good humour.

At the opposite pole of the affective continuum, *major depressive illness* is also characterized by disturbances of mood, talk, energy and ideation (Table 19.13). The mood may be described by the patient in physical terms, e.g. like a weight in the head, a tightness of the chest, or a feeling of almost physical

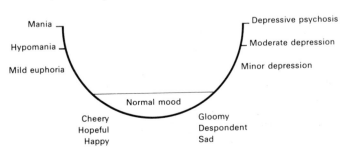

Fig. 19.1 Continuum of normal and abnormal mood.

Table 19.12 Clinical features of mania.

Mood	Elevated, infectious, labile
Talk	Fast, pressurized, flight of ideas, punning, rhyming
Energy	Excessive, restless, distractible
Ideation	Grandiose, self-confident, delusions of wealth, power, influence or of religious significance, persecutory delusions
Cognition	Formal testing difficult, disturbance of retrieval of memories
Physical	Insomnia, mild to moderate weight loss
Behaviour	Disinhibition, increased sexual interest, excessive drinking or spending
Hallucinations	Fleeting auditory or, more rarely, visual

Table 19.13 Clinical features of depression.

Mood	Depressed, miserable, unhappy
Talk	Impoverished, slow, monotonous, incomplete
Energy	Lacking, retarded (in some cases agitation), apathetic
Ideation	Feelings of futility, guilt, self-reproach, unworthiness, hypochondriacal preoccupations, worrying, suicidal thoughts, delusions of guilt, nihilism, persecution
Cognition	Verbal memory impaired, 'pseudodementia' in elderly patients
Physical	Early waking, appetite and weight loss, constipation, loss of libido, impotence, fatigue, bodily aches and pains
Behaviour	Retardation or agitation, poverty of movement and expression
Hallucinations	Auditory — often abusive, hostile, critical

pain. Depressed patients describe the world as grey, themselves as lacking a zest for living, and their bodies as devoid of pleasure and feeling. Anxiety is common, obsessional symptoms may emerge and, in the severer forms, delusions of guilt, persecution and of bodily disease are not uncommon. In severe depression apparent organic impairment, detectable on cognitive testing, can result in disorientation.

Depression is a common experience. It occurs in the setting of physical disease, social stress, personal problems and life crises. It is important to distinguish the more severe and potentially life-threatening *major* form, requiring energetic treatment, from the less severe *minor* form, which, with simple support, sympathy and reassurance, usually lifts (see Table 19.14).

The aetiological factors in manic-depressive disorders are listed in Table 19.15.

DIFFERENTIAL DIAGNOSIS

This is shown in Table 19.16.

Occasionally, doctors are called upon to distinguish between 'normal' grief following a separation or bereavement, and depressive illness. A number of symptoms that commonly occur in depressive illness also follow bereavement, most notably sleep disturbance, appetite and weight loss, and tearfulness. However, a number of distinguishing features can usually be identified (see Table 19.17).

Two conditions presenting in women and characterized by disturbance of mood may well be related to manic-depressive disorders. These are the premenstrual syndrome and puerperal affective disorders.

The premenstrual syndrome
Symptoms consist of irritability, depression and tension during the 7- to 10-day premenstrual period. These symptoms are often accompanied by breast tenderness, a subjective feeling of weight gain and bloatedness, and headache, and are usually dramatically relieved with the onset of the period. Women

Table 19.14 Features that help distinguish major from minor depression.

	Minor	Major
Mood	Transiently low Responsive to environment	Persistently low Unresponsive to environment
Behaviour	Capable of being lifted out of gloom and sadness	Persistently agitated and/or retarded
Suicidal feelings	Fleeting	Persistent
Delusions	Absent	Often present
Physical symptoms	Vague aches and pains, some appetite and sleep loss	Persistent bowel changes, appetite and weight loss, sleep disturbance and early waking
Hallucinations	Absent	Occasionally present

Table 19.15 Possible aetiological factors involved in manic-depressive disorders.

BIOLOGICAL

Genetic
10–15% of first degree relatives have an affective disorder (risk in community is 1–2%).
68% of monozygotic twins reared together or apart are concordant for manic-depressive disorder.
23% of dizygotic twins are concordant.
Possible links with genetic markers.

Biochemical
Imbalance in neurotransmitters (e.g. monoamine neurotransmitters are depleted in depression, but increased in mania)
Loss of diurnal rhythm of plasma cortisol in depression
Hormonal factors (e.g. depression is more common after childbirth, in premenstrual phase, with use of oral contraceptives, and around the menopause)
Electrolytes — intracellular sodium is high in affective disorders

PSYCHOLOGICAL

Maternal deprivation
Psychoanalysts initially suggested that loss of maternal affection in early life predisposes individuals to affective disorder in later life. This association has more recently broadened to include any significant loss in early childhood.

Learned helplessness
Experimental animals put in a position where they cannot escape nor control punishing stimuli develop a behavioural syndrome that resembles depression in humans. It has led to the suggestion that a similar mechanism is at work in humans.

SOCIAL

Stressful events
An excess of life events is found in the months before the onset of depression. Life events include bereavement, loss of a job, moving house, marriage and going on vacation.

Vulnerability factors
In women, it has been claimed that certain factors render them vulnerable to become depressed. These include lack of a job outside the home, the presence of three or more young children in the family, and lack of a confiding, intimate relationship

Table 19.16 Differential diagnosis of manic-depressive disorders.

Condition	Comments
Mania	
Drug-induced psychosis	Screen for suspected drugs (most notably amphetamines, cannabis)
Acute schizophrenia	Other classical (i.e. 'first rank') schizophrenic symptoms usually present or eventually emerge
Dementia	Global cognitive impairment may present with euphoria and irritability; in mania, any cognitive impairment improves with treatment
Hyperthyroidism	

Depression
Systemic physical disease
  Malignancy
  Hypothyroidism
  Hyperparathyroidism
  Cushing's syndrome
  Vitamin and mineral disorders
  Post-infection
  Multiple sclerosis
  Collagen disorders
  Cerebral ischaemia
  Congestive heart failure
  Porphyria

Drug-induced depression
  Corticosteroids
  Hormones
    Oestrogen
    Progesterone
  Antihypertensives
    Reserpine
    Methyldopa
    Clonidine
    Guanethidine
  Antiparkinsonian drugs
    Levodopa
    Amantadine hydrochloride
  Anticancer drugs
    Vincristine
    Vinblastine

Psychiatric disorders
  Schizophrenia
  Alcohol abuse
  Drug abuse
  Anxiety neurosis
  Dementia

who suffer from affective disorders may be more prone to experience premenstrual symptoms and to have exacerbations of their psychiatric disorder during the premenstrual phase.

The cause or causes of the premenstrual syndrome remain unclear and the various treatments proposed, which include the use of vitamin B_6, diuretics, progesterone, oral contraceptives, oil of evening primrose and oestrogen implants, remain empirical.

Puerperal affective disorders
In postpartum women, affective disorders also occur. Such disturbances are divided into 'maternity blues', postpartum ('puerperal') psychosis and chronic depression. Maternity blues is used to describe the brief episodes of emotional lability, irritability and tearfulness that occur in 65–90% of women 2–3 days postpartum and that resolve spontaneously

Table 19.17 Bereavement reaction versus depressive illness following bereavement ('morbid grief reaction').

	Normal bereavement	Depressive illness
Onset	Immediately follows loss	Delay for weeks or months
Duration	Lasts weeks rather than months	Persists for weeks/months/years
Pattern	Person slowly accepts loss and adjusts accordingly	Patient denies loss and refuses to accept implications
Grief	Expressed openly	Difficulty in expressing grief
Guilt	Mild regret in early stages	Marked guilt often present

in a few days. Postpartum psychosis occurs once in every 500–1000 births. Over 80% of cases are affective in type and the onset is usually within the first 2 weeks following delivery. In addition to the classical features of an affective psychosis, disorientation and confusion are often noted. Severely depressed patients may have delusional ideas that the child is deformed, evil or otherwise affected in some way, and such false ideas may lead to attempts to kill the child and to suicide. The response to speedy treatment is generally good. The recurrence rate for a depressive illness in a subsequent puerperium is 15–20%.

Less severe depressive disorders occur during the first postpartum year in 10–20% of mothers. Most patients recover after a few months. Social and psychological factors are important but the underlying aetiological factor is unknown.

TREATMENT

The treatment of affective disorders involves physical, psychological and social therapies. Hospitalization is usually required in the case of severely depressed, potentially suicidal patients and in mania. In general, neither severe depression nor mania respond to psychotherapy, and both require energetic physical treatment. Simple support, reassurance, sympathy and the opportunity to express distress and negative feelings are often sufficient to bring about relief of minor depressive episodes.

Physical treatment of depression
The most frequently used drugs are the tricyclic and related antidepressants. Imipramine and amitriptyline are the two most commonly used. Many related compounds have been introduced, some having fewer autonomic and cardiotoxic effects. Imipramine and amitriptyline are given by mouth in initial doses of 25–75 mg daily, building up over a week to 150–250 mg daily. The full therapeutic impact takes up to 2 weeks to occur. These drugs potentiate the action of monoamines, noradrenaline and serotonin by inhibiting their reuptake into nerve terminals. Other tricyclics in common use include nortriptyline, doxepin, mianserin and trazodone. Tricyclic antidepressants have a number of side-

Table 19.18 Unwanted effects of tricyclic antidepressants.

Anticholinergic effects
Dry mouth
Constipation
Tremor
Blurred vision
Urinary retention
Postural hypotension

Cardiac effects
ECG changes
Arrhythmias

Convulsant activity
Lowered seizure threshold

Other effects
Weight gain
Sedation
Mania

effects (see Table 19.18); in patients with established cardiac disease mianserin or nomifensine are preferred over the more cardiotoxic compounds.

A second group of antidepressants, the monoamine oxidase inhibitors (MAOIs), act by inhibiting the intracellular enzyme monoamine oxidase, leading to an increase of noradrenaline, dopamine and 5-hydroxytryptamine in the brain. There are two types:
- Hydrazine derivatives, e.g. isocarboxazid, phenelzine (toxic to the liver)
- Amphetamine related, e.g. tranylcypromine (potentially addictive)

The most widely used is phenelzine, which is given orally in doses of 30–60 mg daily. The onset of action of MAOIs is within 24–48 h. Unwanted effects include increased appetite and weight gain and difficulty in sleeping. MAOIs also produce hypertensive reactions with foods containing tyramine or dopamine. These amines are normally broken down by monoamine oxidase in the gut mucosa and the liver. Tyramine is present in cheese, pickled herrings, yeast extract, certain red wines and any food, such as game, that has undergone partial decomposition. Dopa is present in broad beans. This 'tyramine reaction' is treated with intravenous phentolamine. MAOIs interact with drugs such as pethidine (see p. 657) and cause liver damage. Particular caution should be taken when changing from a MAOI to a tricyclic or vice versa; it is safest to allow a 2 week drug-free interval between the two types of drug.

MAOIs are used in depressions which present with marked anxiety and obsessional or hypochondriacal features, and which lack marked biological symptoms characteristic of severe depression.

ECT (electroconvulsive therapy) is the most rapidly acting of the available physical treatments of depression. It can be the treatment of first choice in those cases where:
- The patient is dangerously suicidal
- A delay in treatment represents a serious risk to health
- The patient is refusing food and drink
- The patient is in a depressive stupor

The treatment involves the passage of an electric current, usually 80 V for a duration of 0.1–0.3 s, across two electrodes applied to the anterior temporal areas of the scalp. Before the treatment is given, the patient is anaesthetized (usually by means of thiopental 125–150 mg) and receives a muscle relaxant (usually suxamethonium 30–50 mg). A modified convulsion is produced. A course of six to eight treatments over 3 weeks has been shown to be superior to placebo treatment in severe depression characterized by retardation and delusions.

ECT is sometimes used in the management of acute schizophrenia, but the evidence of its effectiveness in this condition is less clear.

ECT is a controversial treatment, yet it is remarkably safe and free of serious side-effects. Serious complications are rare. However, post-ictal, short-term retrograde amnesia and a temporary defect in new learning can occur but these are short-lived effects. The mode of action of ECT in depressive illness is unclear.

Physical treatment of mania
The main physical treatment in mania is the use of neuroleptic drugs such as chlorpromazine, haloperidol and pimozide. Doses similar to those used in schizophrenia are used. Excitement and overactivity are usually reduced within days, but elation, grandiosity and associated delusions often take longer to respond. If improvement does not occur rapidly, larger doses of haloperidol (up to 120 mg daily) may be required. First attacks of mania usually require treatment for up to 3 months. Subsequent attacks, especially if they occur rapidly on cessation of treatment, may need drugs for at least a year after hypomanic features have disappeared.

Lithium carbonate is used but it can take up to 10 days to take effect. Lithium is more commonly used as a prophylactic agent in patients who have a history of repeated episodes of mania and/or depression. In the body it substitutes for sodium and potassium ions and thus can exercise profound effects on a number of metabolic processes. Toxic symptoms begin to occur when the serum concentration exceeds 1.5 mmol·l^{-1} and regular serum estimations are required. Persistent vomiting or diarrhoea with fluid and electrolyte imbalance (e.g. due to diuretic therapy) can precipitate toxic levels of lithium.

Lithium is rapidly absorbed from the gastrointestinal tract and more than 95% is excreted by the kidney, small amounts being found in the saliva and sweat. Renal clearance of lithium correlates with renal creatinine clearance. Its mode of action is unknown. Unwanted effects include:
- Gastrointestinal symptoms
- A fine tremor
- Polyuria and polydipsia
- Weight gain

At higher concentrations, toxic effects include drowsiness, blurred vision, a coarse tremor, ataxia and dysarthria. Such symptoms progress to delirium and convulsions, and coma and death can occur. Long-term effects include non-toxic goitre, hypothyroidism and nephrogenic diabetes insipidus.

Social treatment
Many patients with depression, particularly of the milder form, have associated social problems. Assistance with such social problems can make a significant contribution to clinical recovery. Other social interventions include the provision of group support, social clubs, occupational therapy and training to cope with particularly stressful situations.

Psychological treatment
The psychological treatments in affective disorders can be divided into:
- *Supportive.* Sympathy, reassurance and information should be part of every patient's treatment.
- *Dynamic psychotherapy* (see p. 890). This form of psychotherapy has a limited value in the treatment of affective disorder. In general, its use is restricted to the less severe cases.
- *Cognitive therapy.* This is a behavioural form of therapy which combines behavioural tasks with questioning and arguments designed to alter some of the ideas that are common among depressed patients and that appear to prolong their depression. Among these are negative interpretations of events and maladaptive assumptions (e.g. assuming that because a friend does not telephone it means he no longer cares about the patient). In treatment, the patient is required to record such ideas and examine the evidence for and against them. Patients are also encouraged to undertake some of the pleasurable activities they gave up when they became depressed. There is some evidence that the effects of cognitive therapy are about the same as those of antidepres-

sant drugs in the treatment of mild to moderate depression.

COURSE AND PROGNOSIS

Virtually all manic patients recover and the major problem is the prevention of relapse. Estimates of the proportion of patients who have only a single episode of mania have varied widely between 1 and 50%! Subsequent depressive disorder is common.

In general, manic-depressive illnesses have a marked tendency to recur. Episodes requiring hospital admission are likely to have a total duration of several months. Most people recover completely from the first episode (70–90%), but a majority of these will relapse. There may be a subpopulation of non-relapsing patients who are more likely to be depressive than manic. Between 5 and 10% develop a chronic disability which may follow the first episode. Between 5 and 10% become long-term hospital inpatients and an additional 25% have persistent affective symptoms that are to some degree incapacitating. The continuation of antidepressant therapy for up to 6 months after recovery from a depressive episode does reduce the probability of recurrence, while the use of lithium carbonate as a prophylactic therapy to prevent recurrence of bipolar manic-depressive swings is widely recommended.

Suicide and attempted suicide (deliberate self-harm) (see also p. 661)

Between 11 and 17% of people who have suffered a severe depressive disorder at any time will eventually commit suicide. About 1% of deaths in England and Wales each year are due to suicide, yielding a rate of 8 per 100 000. The rate increases with age, peaking for women in their sixties and for men in their seventies. The highest rates of suicide have been reported in Hungary (40 per 100 000) and East Germany (36 per 100 000), while the lowest are those of Spain (3.9 per 100 000) and Greece (2.8 per 100 000), but such variations may reflect differences in reporting as much as genuine differences in frequency of suicide.

Factors that increase the risk of suicide are indicated in Table 19.19.

A distinction must be drawn between those who attempt suicide ('parasuicides') and those who are determined and eventually succeed. The following points should be considered:
- Suicide is commoner in men, while parasuicide is commoner in women.
- The majority of parasuicides occur in people under 35.

Table 19.19 Factors that increase the risk of suicide.

Living alone
Immigrant status
Recent bereavement, separation or divorce
Recent loss of a job or retirement
Living in a socially disorganized area
Male sex
Older age
Family history of affective disorder, suicide or alcohol abuse
Previous history of affective disorder, alcohol or drug abuse
Previous suicide attempt
Addiction to alcohol or drugs
Severe depression or early dementia
Incapacitating, painful physical illness

- The majority of suicides occur in people over 60.
- Approximately 90% of parasuicides involve self-poisoning.
- A formal psychiatric disorder is unusual in parasuicide.

There is, however, overlap between the two groups and between 1 and 2% of people who attempt suicide will kill themselves in the year following their original attempt. In Britain, over 100 000 suicide attempts are made each year, and the overwhelming majority of these are seen and treated within accident and emergency departments.

The guidelines given below for the assessment of such patients will help to ensure that the important 'risk' factors relating to suicide are covered.

In general, it is worth trying to interview a family member or other close associate and check the above points with him or her. Requests for immediate re-prescription or discharge should be denied, except in cases of essential medication (e.g. epileptics). In such cases, however, only 3 days' supply of medication should be given and the patient should be instructed to report to their general practitioner or to their psychiatric outpatient clinic for further supplies.

Neuroses and personality disorders

These disorders constitute the largest portion of psychiatric disorders, accounting for 50% of admissions to psychiatric hospitals, 75% of patients seen in

---

Guidelines for possible psychiatric referral in deliberate self harm

Identification of the precipitant
- Was there a clear precipitant?
- What was the patient's state of mind at the time?
- Was the act premeditated or impulsive?
- Did the patient leave a suicide note?
- Had the patient taken pains not to be discovered?
- Did he make the attempt in familiar or strange surroundings (i.e. at home or away from home)?
- What are the patient's feelings about the attempt now?
- Was the patient under the influence of alcohol or drugs?

Present state examination
- Has the precipitant or crisis resolved?
- Is there continuing suicidal intent?
- Does the patient have any psychiatric symptoms?
- What is the patient's social support system?
- Has the patient harmed himself before?
- Has anyone in the family ever taken their life?
- Does the patient have a physical illness?

Indications for referral to a psychiatrist
Absolute indications include:
- Clinical depression
- Psychotic illness of any kind
- Clearly pre-planned suicidal attempts which were not intended to be discovered
- Persistent suicidal intent (the more detailed the plans, the more serious the risk)
- A violent method used

Other common indications include:
- Alcoholics and drug abusers
- Older patients over 45, especially if male
- Those with a family history of suicide
- Those with serious (especially incurable) physical disease
- Those living alone or otherwise unsupported
- Those in whom there is a major unresolved crisis
- Persistent suicide attemptors

---

psychiatric outpatient clinics, and over 90% of the psychiatric disorders seen and managed by general practitioners. There is an overlap between neuroses and personality disorders, although in general they can be distinguished.

Neurosis is defined below. Personality disorders are deeply ingrained maladaptive patterns of behaviour generally recognizable by the time of adolescence and often becoming less obvious in middle or old age. The personality is abnormal either in the balance of its components, its quality or expression, or in its total aspect, and this deviation has an adverse effect upon the individual or on society. A personality disorder includes what is sometimes called the psychopathic personality, a disorder characterized by a marked disregard for social obligations, lack of feeling for others and impetuous violence or callous unconcern.

Anxiety neurosis

An anxiety neurosis is a condition in which anxiety dominates the clinical symptoms.

CLINICAL FEATURES

The patient looks worried, has a tense posture, restless behaviour, a pale skin, and sweaty hands, feet and axillae. The physical and psychological symptoms (Table 19.20) result from either overactivity of the sympathetic nervous system or increased tension in the skeletal muscles. Sleep is disturbed: the patient has difficulty in getting to sleep because of worry and restlessness, and when he does sleep he wakes intermittently and may have unpleasant dreams. Another complication is the *hyperventilation syndrome*.

Sometimes the anxious patient has the conviction

Table 19.20 Physical and psychological symptoms of anxiety.

PHYSICAL
Gastrointestinal Dry mouth Difficulty in swallowing Epigastric discomfort Flatulence Diarrhoea
Respiratory Feeling of chest constriction Difficulty in inhaling Overbreathing
Cardiovascular Palpitations Awareness of missed beats Feeling of pain over heart
Genitourinary Increased frequency Failure of erection Lack of libido
CNS Tinnitus Blurred vision Dizziness
Other Headache Sleep disturbances
PSYCHOLOGICAL
Apprehension and fear Irritability Difficulty in concentrating Distractability Restlessness Sensitivity to noise Depression Depersonalization Obsessional symptoms

---

The hyperventilation syndrome

Features
Panic attacks—fear, terror and impending doom—accompanied by some or all of the following:
- Dyspnoea
- Palpitations
- Chest pain or discomfort
- Choking sensation
- Dizziness
- Paraesthesiae
- Sweating
- Carpopedal spasms

Cause
Overbreathing leading to a decrease in $PaCO_2$ and an increase in arterial pH.

Diagnosis
A provocation test—voluntary overbreathing for 2–3 min—provokes similar symptoms; rebreathing from a paper bag relieves them.

Management
- Explanation and reassurance is given.
- The patient is trained in relaxation techniques and slow breathing.
- The patient is asked to breathe into a closed paper bag.
- Antidepressant drugs are often helpful.

Table 19.21 The differential diagnosis of anxiety neurosis.

Psychiatric disorder
Depressive illness
Schizophrenia
Presenile dementia
Alcohol dependence
Drug dependence
Benzodiazepine withdrawal
Physical disorder
Hyperthyroidism
Hypoglycaemia
Phaeochromocytoma

that he suffers from heart disease. The conviction is accompanied by palpitations, fatigue, breathlessness and inframammary pain. The terms 'cardiac neurosis', 'effort syndrome' and 'neurocirculatory asthenia' used to be applied to the disorder. Betablockers are sometimes useful in controlling these symptoms.

Types of anxiety
Anxiety may be divided into the following categories:
- A more or less continuous *state of anxiety* which fluctuates to some extent in response to environmental circumstances
- Sudden and unpredictable attacks of anxiety which are usually accompanied by severe physical symptoms—the so-called *panic attacks*
- *Phobic anxiety*, which is anxiety triggered by a single stimulus or set of stimuli which are predictable and which normally cause no particular concern to others
- An *anxious personality*—an individual who has a lifelong tendency to experience tension and anxiety, and to have a worrisome attitude towards life and a constant anticipation of setback and stress

DIFFERENTIAL DIAGNOSIS

This is given in Table 19.21.

AETIOLOGY

Genetic factors
Anxiety neurosis occurs in 15% of relatives of affected patients compared with 3% of the general population. (The genetic role is less important in phobic anxiety.)

Psychodynamic theory
This is a theoretical explanation which suggests that anxiety neurosis reflects overwhelming stress, anxiety and difficulties in the child–parent relationship in early childhood or even at birth. Psychoanalysts also interpret phobic neurosis as an unconscious avoidance of unacknowledged feelings of temptation (usually sexual), the phobia representing a displacement of the real fear (e.g. the agoraphobic patient is really afraid of the feelings of temptation aroused when meeting people in the street).

Learning theory
Anxiety is regarded as a fear response that has been attached to another stimulus through conditioning.

TREATMENT

Psychological treatment
For many brief episodes of anxiety neurosis, a discussion with a doctor involving explanation and reassurance concerning the nature of physical symptoms of anxiety is usually sufficient. Relaxation training can be as effective as drugs in relieving mild or moderate anxiety. Such an approach uses an elaborate system of exercises designed to bring about relaxation of individual groups of skeletal muscles and to regulate breathing. A further development is anxiety management training, which involves two stages. In the first stage, verbal cues and mental imagery are used to arouse anxiety. In the second stage, the patient is trained to reduce this anxiety by relaxation, distraction and reassuring self-statements. Both of these approaches are forms of behaviour therapy.

The term behaviour therapy is applied to psychological treatments derived from experimental psychology and intended to change symptoms and behaviour. A behavioural therapy used in the treatment of phobias is desensitization. Patients are required to imagine the fear-provoking situations or objects, starting with those that evoke little fear, and progressing through carefully planned steps or a hierarchy to the most severe phobic stimulus. At each stage, anxiety is neutralized, usually by relaxation. Improvement in phobias is greater after this approach than after group or individual psychotherapy.

Flooding treatment is based on the finding that conditioned fear responses dissipate when experimental animals are prevented from running away from fear-provoking situations; if the animals are kept in the situation, the fear dies away. In flooding treatment, patients are required either to imagine or to enter feared situations in a way that maximizes anxiety. They continue to do this until the fear exhausts itself. In a variation on this approach, anxiety is increased still further by requiring the patient to imagine exaggerated scenes or situations; for example, a patient fearful of spiders might be required to imagine having hundreds of them crawling over his naked body. This procedure is termed implosion. There is little evidence that it is superior to the more straightforward desensitization.

The treatment of choice for agoraphobia is programmed practice. This combines exposure to real rather than imagined anxiety-provoking situations, with measures to control any anxiety experienced in these situations. The therapist teaches the patient how best to return to the feared situation and how to cope with the anxiety that results. This is carried out for at least one hour each day using situations chosen that give rise to moderate anxiety. Emphasis is placed on providing the patient with the knowledge required to plan his own treatment.

Non-behavioural treatments include individual and group-based psychotherapies. In general, however, behavioural therapy has replaced such approaches in the treatment of anxiety and phobias.

Physical treatment

Drugs used in the treatment of anxiety can be divided into two groups: those that act primarily on the central nervous system and those that block peripheral autonomic receptors. The main group of centrally acting anxiolytic drugs are the benzodiazepines. They appear to bind to specific receptors on neuronal cell membranes, producing a facilitation of the effects of the inhibitory transmitter gamma-aminobutyric acid (GABA). Diazepam (5 mg twice daily to 10 mg three times daily in severe cases) and nitrazepam have relatively long half-lives (20–40 h) and are more suitable as anti-anxiety drugs than as hypnotic drugs, whereas oxazepam, temazepam and lorazepam have shorter half-lives and may be used as hypnotics.

Adverse effects include overdosage, which may be accidental or deliberate, and produces drowsiness, sleep, confusion, incoordination, ataxia, diplopia and dysarthria. Physical as well as psychological dependence has been described, and convulsions have occurred on withdrawal of such drugs after long-term administration. The withdrawal syndrome (Table 19.22) is particularly severe when high doses have been given, e.g. 30 mg of diazepam daily or more. Tolerance can occur with repeated doses and can lead to an escalation of dosage. Thus, if a benzodiazepine drug is prescribed for anxiety, it should be given in as low a dose and for as short a time as possible (i.e. for not more than 3–4 weeks).

Many of the symptoms of anxiety are due to an increased release of adrenaline and noradrenaline from the adrenal medulla and the sympathetic nerves. Thus adrenergic blocking drugs such as propranolol (20–40 mg two or three times daily) are effective in reducing symptoms such as palpitations, tremor and tachycardia.

Table 19.22 Withdrawal syndrome with benzodiazepines.

Insomnia
Anxiety
Tremulousness
Muscle twitchings
Perceptual distortions
Frank convulsions

Obsessional neurosis and personality

Obsessional neuroses are characterized by obsessional thinking and compulsive behaviour (see p. 871) together with varying degrees of anxiety, depression and depersonalization. They account for some 2% of referrals to psychiatrists and have a prevalence in the general population of about 1 in 1000.

CLINICAL FEATURES

The obsessions and compulsions are so persistent and intrusive that they greatly impede the patient's functioning and cause considerable distress. There is a constant need to check that things have been done correctly and no amount of reassurance can remove the small amount of doubt that persists—the so-called 'folie de doute'. Some rituals are derived from superstitions, such as repetitive actions done a required number of times, with the need to start again at the very beginning if interrupted. When severe, obsessional neuroses last for many years and are very resistant to treatment. However, obsessional symptoms commonly appear in the setting of other disorders, most notably anxiety neurosis, depression, schizophrenia and organic cerebral disorders, and disappear rapidly with the resolution of such disorders.

Minor variants of morbid obsessional symptoms can be noted fairly frequently in people who are not regarded as ill or in need of treatment. The mildest grade is that of obsessional personality traits such as over-conscientiousness, tidiness, punctuality and other attitudes and behaviours indicating a strong tendency towards rigidity, conformity and inflexibility. Such individuals are perfectionists, have a poor tolerance of shortcomings in others and take pride in their high standards. When such traits are so marked that they override and dominate other aspects of the personality, in the absence of clear-cut obsessional thinking and compulsive rituals, the picture becomes that of an obsessional personality disorder.

AETIOLOGY

Genetic factors

Obsessional neuroses are found in 5–7% of the parents of obsessional patients. Such a finding may of course reflect environmental as well as genetic causes.

Organic factors

Symptoms have been seen following encephalitis lethargica and it has been suggested that organic factors may be involved. In most cases, however, there is no evidence of disease of the CNS.

Psychodynamic factors

Freud suggested that symptoms result from repressed impulses of an aggressive or sexual nature. He also suggested that they occur as a result of regression to the anal stage of development—an idea consistent with the obsessional patient's frequent concern over excretory functions and dirt.

Learning theory

This suggests that obsessional rituals are the equivalent of avoidance responses. However, anxiety actually increases rather than falls after some rituals, which is against such a theory.

PROGNOSIS

Two-thirds of cases improve within a year. The remainder run a fluctuating course. The prognosis is worse when the personality is obsessional and the symptoms are severe.

TREATMENT

Psychological treatment

A form of behaviour therapy that is particularly effective in the treatment of obsessional rituals is response prevention. Patients are instructed not to carry out their rituals; initially there is a rise in distress but with persistence both the rituals and the distress diminish. Patients are encouraged to prac-

tise keeping them under control while returning to situations that normally make them worse.

Another approach known as 'modelling' involves demonstrating to the patient what is required and encouraging the patient to follow this example. In the case of hand-washing rituals, this might involve holding an allegedly 'contaminated' object and carrying out other activities without washing, the patient being encouraged to follow suit. When obsessional thoughts accompany rituals, thought stopping is advocated. In this procedure the patient is taught to arrest the obsessional thought by arranging a sudden intrusion (e.g. snapping an elastic band, clicking the fingers).

Physical treatment

Anxiolytic drugs provide short-term symptomatic relief. Any coexisting depression should be treated with an antidepressant. One tricyclic antidepressant believed to have a specific action against obsessional symptoms is clomipramine, but studies suggest that the drug effects are modest and only occur in patients with definitive depressive symptoms.

Psychosurgery is sometimes recommended in cases of severe obsessional neurosis. The development of stereotactic techniques has led to the replacement of the earlier, crude leucotomies with more precise surgical interventions such as subcaudate tractotomy and limbic leucotomy, with lesions placed in the cingulate area and the ventromedial quadrant of the frontal lobe. These are undertaken to relieve patients of obsessional symptoms unresponsive to other treatments. Psychosurgery is now only performed in specialist centres, and formal and detailed consent requirements are laid down in England and Wales in the Mental Health Act 1983.

Hysterical neurosis and personality

Hysterical neurosis or hysteria is a condition in which there are symptoms and signs of disease with three characteristics:
- They occur in the absence of physical pathology.
- They are produced unconsciously.
- They are not caused by overactivity of the sympathetic nervous system.

The lifetime prevalence has been estimated at 3–6 per 1000 in women, with a lower incidence in men. Most cases begin before the age of 35 and it occurs rarely after 40 years. However, hysterical symptoms commonly occur after this age as part of some other disorder.

CLINICAL FEATURES

The various symptoms are usually divided into dissociative and conversion categories (Table 19.23). The term 'dissociative' indicates the seeming dissociation between different mental activities, and

Table 19.23 Common hysterical symptoms.

Dissociative (mental)
Amnesia
Fugue
Pseudodementia
Ganser syndrome
Somnabulism
Multiple personality
Psychosis
Conversion (physical)
Paralysis
Disorders of gait
Tremor
Aphonia
Mutism
Sensory symptoms
Repeated vomiting
Globus hystericus
Hysterical fits
Dermatitis artifacta

covers such phenomena as amnesia, fugues, somnambulism and multiple personality. The term 'conversion' derives from Freud's theory that mental energy can be converted into certain physical symptoms. Such symptoms include paralysis, fits, sensory loss, aphonia, blindness, deafness, disorders of gait and abdominal pain.

The main characteristics of hysterical symptoms include the following:
- They are not produced willfully or deliberately.
- They often reflect a patient's ideas about illness.
- They may imitate symptoms of a relative/friend who has been ill.
- There are obvious discrepancies between hysterical signs and symptoms and those of organic disease.
- The symptoms usually confer some advantage on the patient (so-called secondary gain).
- They are often accompanied by less than the expected amount of emotional distress ('belle indifference').

Hysterical amnesia commences suddenly. Patients are unable to recall long periods of their lives and may even deny any knowledge of their previous life or personal identity. A proportion who present thus have concurrent physical disease, especially epilepsy, multiple sclerosis or the effects of head injury. In a hysterical fugue, the patient not only loses his memory but wanders away from his usual surroundings, and when found, denies all memory of his whereabouts during his wandering. Apart from hysteria, fugue states are associated with epilepsy, depression and alcohol abuse.

Hysterical pseudodementia involves a memory loss and behaviour that initially suggest severe and generalized intellectual deterioration. Simple tests are answered wrongly but in such a way as to suggest that the correct answer is in the patient's

mind. The Ganser syndrome is a rare condition composed of four features:
- The giving of 'approximate answers' (i.e. almost correct)
- Physical or mental symptoms of hysteria
- Hallucinations
- Clouding of consciousness

The relation of somnambulism, or sleepwalking, to other forms of hysteria is unclear, but its similarity to the condition arising through hypnosis suggests that it may be a form of dissociation.

In multiple personality, there are rapid alterations between two patterns of behaviour, each of which is forgotten by the patient when the other is present. Each 'personality' appears to be a complex and integrated set of emotional responses. The condition is rare.

A variation of hysteria is the epidemic or mass hysteria, seen mainly in institutions for girls or young women in which the combined effects of suggestion and shared anxiety produce explosive outbreaks of sickness or other disturbed behaviour. Another variant is Briquet's syndrome, which is said only to occur in women, follows an intractable course, runs in families and involves multiple somatic symptoms occurring in several different bodily systems for which no organic cause is found.

Patients with a hysterical personality are those who exhibit a particular set or cluster of personality traits that include a remarkable egocentricity, a manipulative skill and an ability to attract attention to themselves by dramatic initiatives, often of a sexually provocative or emotionally exaggerated fashion. Their emotions are described as shallow and labile and there is an 'acting' quality attached to much of what they do and say. Their personal relationships are often transient yet full of dramatic intensity. Such individuals, when they do develop genuine physical illness, may be dubbed 'hysterical' because they describe their symptoms and complaints in such an exaggerated manner.

DIFFERENTIAL DIAGNOSIS

The diagnosis of hysteria may be erroneously made because:
- The symptoms may be those of an as yet undetected physical disease. For example, 'globus hystericus' (see p. 156) may actually be difficulty in swallowing secondary to an oesophageal cancer.
- Undetected brain disease (e.g. a tumour in the frontal lobe or early dementia) may in some way 'produce' hysterical symptoms.
- Physical disease may provide a non-specific stimulus to hysterical elaboration or an exaggeration of symptoms by a somewhat dramatic or histrionic patient.

Physical disease must be excluded. The distinction between hysteria and malingering (i.e. the conscious pretence of illness) should be considered but is difficult to make.

AETIOLOGY

Genetic factors
Studies have been inconclusive but reported rates in relatives of affected patients do appear higher than in the general population.

Psychodynamic factors
Central to the theory of psychoanalysis is the view that hysteria is the result of emotionally charged ideas lodged in the unconscious at some point in the past. Symptoms are explained as the combined effects of repression and the 'conversion' of psychic energy into physical channels.

Organic disease
Hysteria is sometimes associated with physical disease. However, it also quite clearly occurs in the absence of such pathology.

PROGNOSIS

Most cases of recent onset recover quickly. Those that last longer than a year are likely to persist for a very long time.

TREATMENT

Psychological treatment
Psychotherapy of a psychodynamic kind often uncovers striking memories of early childhood sexual experiences and other problems relevant to the patient's presenting condition. Psychodynamic psychotherapy is derived from psychoanalysis and is based on a number of key analytical concepts. These include Freud's ideas about psychosexual development, mechanisms of defence (including repression, projection and denial), free association as the method of recall, and the therapeutic technique of interpretation including that of transference, defences and dreams. Such therapy usually involves once-weekly 50-minute sessions, the length of treatment varying between 3 months and 2 years. The long-term aim of such therapy is two-fold: symptom relief and personality change. Psychodynamic psychotherapy is classically indicated in the treatment of the neuroses and personality disorders, but to date there is a remarkable lack of convincing evidence concerning its superiority over other forms of treatment.

Simpler forms of psychotherapy involving more straightforward reassurance and explanation, greater involvement of the therapist in the actual sessions, and the elimination of factors that appear to reinforce symptoms, are as effective and probably more so than the more complex and time-consuming forms. Group psychotherapy involving six to eight patients, which facilitates the development of confidence, the recollection of painful experiences and the growth of social and interpersonal skills, is also useful in a number of neurotic and personality disorders, although its usefulness in hysterical neuroses is doubtful.

Abreaction brought about by hypnosis or by intravenous injections of small amounts of amylobarbitone with or without amphetamine may produce a dramatic, if short-lived, recovery. In the abreactive state, the patient is encouraged to relive the stressful events that provoked the hysteria and to express the accompanying emotions, i.e. to abreact. Such an approach has been useful in the treatment of acute hysterical neuroses in war time, but appear to be of much less value in civilian life.

Physical treatment
Drug treatments have no part to play in hysteria unless the symptoms are secondary to a depressive illness or anxiety neurosis requiring treatment.

Hypochondriacal neurosis

This is a neurotic disorder in which the conspicuous features are an excessive concern with one's health in general, in the integrity and functioning of some part of one's body or, less frequently, one's mind. Hypochondriasis may coexist with actual physical disease; the important point is that the patient's concern is out of all proportion and is unjustified. The symptoms of hypochondriasis occur in a variety of psychiatric disorders, particularly in depression and anxiety. When hypochondriacal tendencies are lifelong, the condition is more usually termed 'hypochondriacal personality'.

Alcohol abuse and dependence

There are a number of different types of alcohol abuse, and a wide range of physical, social and psychological problems is associated with excessive drinking. Until recently, much attention was devoted to the syndrome of alcohol dependence. In fact, doctors should be concerned with the health problems caused by alcohol abuse whether or not such abuse is related to actual physiological dependence on alcohol. The term 'alcoholism' is a confusing one with off-putting connotations of vagrancy, 'meths' drinking and social disintegration. It has recently been replaced by the term 'alcohol dependence syndrome', which has seven essential elements:

- A compulsive need to drink
- A stereotyped pattern of drinking. Whereas the ordinary drinker varies his daily pattern, the addicted drinker drinks at regular intervals to avoid or relieve withdrawal symptoms.
- Drinking takes primacy over other activities
- Tolerance to alcohol is altered. The dependent drinker is ordinarily unaffected by blood alcohol levels that would incapacitate a normal drinker. Increasing tolerance is an important sign of increasing dependence. In the later stages of dependence, tolerance falls.
- Repeated withdrawal symptoms. These occur some 8–12 h after cessation of drinking or after a sharp fall in blood alcohol in people who have been drinking heavily for many years. They characteristically appear on waking as a result of the fall in the blood alcohol level during sleep.
- Relief drinking. Many dependent drinkers take a drink early in the morning to stave off withdrawal symptoms. In most cultures, early morning drinking is diagnostic of alcohol dependence.
- Reinstatement after abstinence. A severely dependent drinker who drinks again after a period of abstinence is likely to relapse quickly and return to his old addictive pattern.

The 'problem drinker' is one who causes or experiences physical, psychological and/or social harm as a consequence of drinking alcohol. Many problem drinkers, while heavy drinkers, are not physiologically addicted to alcohol. Heavy drinkers are those who drink significantly more in terms of quantity and/or frequency than the average drinker. Binge drinkers are those who drink excessively in short bouts, usually 24–48 h long, separated by often quite lengthy periods of abstinence. Their overall monthly or weekly alcohol intake may be relatively modest. The interrelationship between these types of drinking is shown in Fig. 19.2.

Extent of the problem

A conservative estimate is that there are at least 300 000 people in Britain with alcohol-related problems. A recent survey on drinking in England and Wales found that 5% of men and 2% of women reported alcohol-related problems. People with serious drinking problems have an increased risk of dying which is between two and three times greater than that of members of the general population at the same age and sex. Approximately one in five male admissions to acute medical wards are directly or indirectly due to alcohol. Between 33 and 40% of casualty attenders have blood alcohol concentrations above the present legal limit for driving. Up to one in five seemingly healthy men attending health screening programmes are found to have biochemical evidence of heavy alcohol consumption, though they are a selected population coming mainly from the upper social classes. Of the 2000 patients on the practice list of the average general practitioner, about 100 will be heavy drinkers, 40 will be problem drinkers and 10 will be physically dependent on alcohol.

Over the past 20 years, the average British adult has almost doubled his alcohol consumption (from 5.2 l of absolute alcohol per year in 1950 to 9.9 l in 1983). Over that same time period, admissions to psychiatric hospitals for treatment of alcoholism have increased more than 25-fold, cirrhosis rates have doubled, and drunkenness offences have risen from 60 000 to over 100 000 per year.

Detection

Many doctors still fail to recognize the heavy drinker and even the problem drinker. Greater awareness is urgently needed to allow intervention at a stage when something can still be achieved, and to provide better statistics.

Alcohol abuse should be suspected in any patient presenting one or more physical problems commonly associated with excessive drinking (see Chapter 3, p. 147). Alcohol abuse may also be associated with a number of psychological symptoms and social problems (see Table 19.24). Certain features in the

Table 19.24 Common alcohol-related psychological and social problems.

Psychological
Depression
Anxiety and phobias
Memory disturbances
Personality disturbances
Delirium tremens
Attempted suicide
Pathological jealousy

Social
Marital and sexual difficulties
Family problems
Child abuse
Employment problems
Financial difficulties
Accidents at home, on the roads, at work
Delinquency and crime
Homelessness

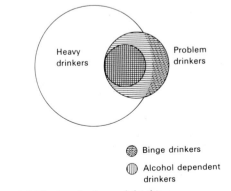

● Binge drinkers

◍ Alcohol dependent drinkers

Fig. 19.2 The terminology of drinking.

history should also raise suspicion, most notably:
- Absenteeism from work
- Frequent attendances for unexplained dyspepsia or gastrointestinal bleeds
- Hospital admissions for accidents of all kinds
- 'Fits', 'turns' or 'falls'

Certain signs may be helpful, if present, in detecting alcohol abuse in patients. These include:
- Plethoric face with/without telangiectases
- Bloodshot conjunctivae
- Smell of stale alcohol
- Facial appearance resembling Cushing's syndrome
- Marked tremor
- Signs of alcohol-related diseases

The patient's frequency of drinking and quantity drunk on typical occasions should be established. Patients can assess their alcohol consumption on the basis of units of alcohol. One standard unit of alcohol is equivalent to 8 g of absolute alcohol. This amount is found in:
- Half a pint of average strength beer
- One standard UK measure of spirits
- One glass of sherry
- One glass of table wine

The following are useful guidelines:
- Drinking up to 20 units of alcohol a week for men and 13 units for women carries no long-term health risk.
- There is unlikely to be any long-term health damage between 21–36 units (men) and 14–24 units (women) provided that the drinking is spread throughout the week.
- Beyond 36 units a week in men and 24 units a week in women, damage to health becomes increasingly likely.
- Drinking above 50 units a week in men (35 units in women) is currently regarded as a definitive health hazard.

A number of questionnaires, such as the CAGE questionnaire (see Table 19.25), have been devel-

Table 19.25 The CAGE questionnaire.

1 Have you ever felt you ought to CUT down on your drinking?
2 Have people ANNOYED you by criticizing your drinking?
3 Have you ever felt bad or GUILTY about your drinking?
4 Have you ever had a drink first thing in the morning (an 'EYE-OPENER') to get rid of a hangover?

From Mayfield D, McLeod G and Hall P (1974) *American Journal of Psychiatry* **131**: 1121–1123. With permission.

oped to help identify patients with alcohol-related problems. Two or more positive replies to the CAGE questionnaire are said to identify problem drinkers.

It is important to remember that there are a number of key 'at risk' factors involved, which include:
- Marital difficulties. These may conceal heavy drinking or may be used to justify it.
- Work problems. Alcohol abusers have $2\frac{1}{2}$ times as many days off work as more sober colleagues.
- An affected relative. Twenty-five per cent of the male relatives of alcohol abusers have similar problems.
- High-risk occupations. Examples of these include company directors, salesmen, doctors, journalists, publicans and seamen.
- Associated physical and mental conditions

A number of laboratory tests are helpful in the identification of excess chronic alcohol consumption:
- *Blood alcohol.* This is useful in anyone suspected of but who denies drinking; most people have no detectable alcohol in their blood in the middle of the day.
- *Urinary alcohol.* A value exceeding 120 mg·dl^{-1} is suggestive of chronic alcohol abuse, and a value over 200 mg·100 ml^{-1} (44 mmol·l^{-1}) is said to be diagnostic.
- *Gamma glutamyl transferase.* Elevated serum γ-GT activity is observed in about 75% of hospitalized alcoholics; in outpatients and heavy drinkers, the prevalence reaches 90%. Acute alcohol consumption does not lead to abnormal levels except in patients with pre-existing liver disease. Levels return to normal with abstention from alcohol.
- *Mean corpuscular volume.* An MCV of more than 96 fl is found in about 60% of alcohol abusers. The response to abstinence is a return to normal over a period of about 2 months.

Alcohol dependence syndrome

The alcohol dependence syndrome is usually very much easier to identify than problem-related drinking. Fig. 19.3 outlines the main characteristics of the syndrome but these do not necessarily present in any particular order. Symptoms of alcohol dependence in a typical order of occurrence are shown in Table 19.26.

COURSE

The course of the alcohol dependence syndrome comprises three linked stages. The first stage is 'heavy' social drinking, i.e. the ingestion of three to five standard drinks (units) of alcohol a day for several years. This stage can continue asymptomatically for a lifetime or, because of a change of circumstances or peer group, it can revert to a more moderate pattern of drinking or can progress to the second

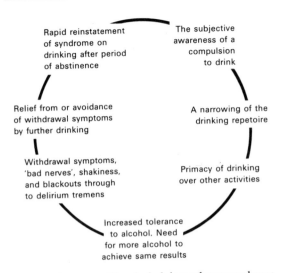

Rapid reinstatement of syndrome on drinking after period of abstinence

The subjective awareness of a compulsion to drink

Relief from or avoidance of withdrawal symptoms by further drinking

A narrowing of the drinking repetoire

Withdrawal symptoms, 'bad nerves', shakiness, and blackouts through to delirium tremens

Primacy of drinking over other activities

Increased tolerance to alcohol. Need for more alcohol to achieve same results

Fig. 19.3 Elements of the alcohol dependency syndrome.

Table 19.26 Symptoms of alcohol dependence.

Unable to keep to a drink limit
Difficulty in avoiding getting drunk
Spending a considerable time drinking
Missing meals
Memory lapses, 'blackouts'
Restless without drink
Organizing day around drink
Trembling after drinking the day before
Morning retching and vomiting
Sweating excessively at night
Withdrawal fits
Morning drinking
Decreased tolerance
Hallucinations, frank delirium tremens

stage of alcohol abuse. This stage is usually associated with frequent ingestion of more than eight drinks a day and there are associated medical, legal, social and/or occupational complications. About half of such abusers either return to asymptomatic (controlled) drinking or achieve stable abstinence. In a small number of cases, such alcohol abuse can persist intermittently for decades with minor morbidity and become milder with time. About 25% of all cases of alcohol abuse will lead to chronic alcohol dependence, withdrawal symptoms and the eventual need for detoxification. This last stage most commonly ends in social incapacity and death or abstinence.

Evidence suggests that alcohol-dependent drinkers do not develop their dependence after a few drinks but that the disorder requires up to 10 years of heavy drinking to evolve (3–4 years in women). In some individuals who use alcohol to alter consciousness, obliterate conscience and defy social canons, dependence and apparent loss of control may appear in only a few months to a few years.

Withdrawal symptoms
Mild tremor, headache, nausea and general malaise are characteristic of the 'hangover'. Chronic alcoholics often do not have these symptoms, partly because they are tolerant to alcohol and tend to continue to consume alcohol on the next day. In the chronic alcoholic, withdrawal causes
- Prominent tremor
- Insomnia
- Agitation
- Fits
- Delirium tremens (DTs)

Delirium tremens is the most serious withdrawal state and occurs 1–5 days after alcohol (or barbiturate) withdrawal. Patients are disorientated, agitated, and have a marked tremor and visual hallucinations ('pink elephants').

Signs include sweating, tachycardia, tachypnoea and pyrexia. Additional signs include dehydration, infection, hepatic disease or the Wernicke–Korsakoff syndrome. If delirium tremens is not treated promptly, death can occur.

CAUSES

Genetic factors
Sons of alcoholics adopted away from home are four times more likely to develop drinking problems than the adopted away sons of non-alcoholics.

Environmental factors
A Boston follow-up study showed that 1 in 10 of boys who grew up in a household where neither parent abused alcohol subsequently became alcohol dependent compared with 1 in 4 of those reared by alcohol-abusing fathers and 1 in 3 of those reared by alcohol-abusing mothers.

Biochemical factors
Several factors have been suggested, including abnormalities in alcohol dehydrogenase or in neurotransmitter mechanisms, but no firm evidence exists.

Personality
Follow-up studies have failed to identify any trait or tendency that significantly distinguishes those who subsequently abuse alcohol from those who do not.

Psychiatric illness
This is not a common cause of addictive drinking but it is a treatable one. Some depressed patients drink

excessively in the hope of raising their mood. Patients with anxiety states or phobias are also at risk.

Excess consumption in society

Recently, the idea has grown that rates of alcohol dependence and alcohol-related problems are related to the general level of alcohol consumption in society and, in turn, to factors that may control overall consumption, including price, licensing laws, the number and nature of sales outlets, and the customs and moral beliefs of society concerning the use and abuse of alcohol.

TREATMENT

Psychological treatment

Successful identification at an early stage constitutes an important treatment in its own right. It should lead to:

- The provision of information concerning safe drinking levels
- A recommendation to cut down where indicated
- Simple support and advice concerning associated problems

Such an approach has been found to be as effective as more expensive and specialized forms of psychotherapy in the treatment of moderate to heavy non-addictive drinking. With addictive drinking, the most favoured psychological treatment is group therapy, which involves identification, confession, emotional arousal, the implantation of new ideas, and the long-term support by fellow-members of the group. Family and marital therapy involving both alcoholic and spouse may also be important.

Behaviour therapies involving teaching patients how to drink in a more controlled way are currently the subject of much study.

Physical treatment

Addicted drinkers often experience considerable difficulty when they attempt to reduce or stop their drinking. Withdrawal symptoms are a particular problem and delirium tremens needs urgent treatment (Table 19.27). Drugs that show

Table 19.27 Management of delirium tremens.

1 The patient should be hospitalized.
2 Chlormethiazole 4 g daily for 2 days then reduced over 5 days or diazepam 40–100 mg for 2 days then reduced over 5 days should be given.
3 Any dehydration should be corrected.
4 Any electrolyte imbalance should be corrected.
5 Any systemic infection should be treated.
6 B vitamins should be given parenterally.

cross-tolerance for alcohol, such as diazepam or chlormethiazole, may be used in a regimen that involves a steady reduction over 5–7 days. A useful chlormethiazole regimen is 4 g daily for 2 days, 3 g daily for 3 days and 2 g daily for a final 2 days. However, long-term treatment with drugs should not be prescribed in those patients who continue to abuse alcohol. Many alcohol abusers add dependence on diazepam or chlormethiazole to their problems.

Drugs such as disulfiram (Antabuse) and citrated calcium (Abstem) react with alcohol to cause very unpleasant acetaldehyde intoxication and histamine release. A daily maintenance dose of such a drug means that an alcohol-dependent drinker must wait until the disulfiram or calcium carbimide is eliminated from the body before he can drink safely. Such drugs, therefore, can provide a 'chemical fence' around the drinker for at least 24 h. Disulfiram implants have been developed which have a treatment life of 6 months. As yet there is doubt as to whether their benefit is psychological rather than pharmacological.

OUTCOME

Whereas in the case of non-dependent heavy drinkers the goal of normal drinking within safe limits can be a very reasonable one, the alcohol-dependent drinker must be persuaded to abstain. Abstention, particularly after many years drinking, is a difficult goal and not surprisingly many fail in the attempt. Research suggests that between 40 and 50% of alcohol-dependent drinkers are abstinent or drinking very much less up to 2 years following intervention. Specialized treatment units, psychiatric treatment, group therapy and attendance at meetings of Alcoholics Anonymous—the self-help organization that provides members with a social structure to fill the gap previously occupied by drinking—are all potential elements in the attempt to keep the alcohol-dependent individual abstinent and healthy. To date, however, there is little convincing evidence that highly expensive, time-consuming and specialized modes of treatment are superior in their efficacy to straightforward advice, support, encouragement and monitoring.

Drug dependence

In addition to alcohol and nicotine, there are a number of psychotropic substances which are used for their effects on mood and other mental functions (Table 19.28).

Table 19.28 Commonly used drugs of dependence.

Stimulants
Methylphenidate
Phenmetrazine
Phencyclidine ('angel dust')
Cocaine
Amphetamine derivatives

Hallucinogens
Cannabis preparations
Solvents
LSD
Mescaline

Narcotics
Morphine
Heroin
Codeine
Pethidine
Methadone

Hypnotics
Barbiturates
Benzodiazepines

Solvents

Adolescents engage in glue-sniffing for the intoxicating effects produced by the solvents inhaled. The glue is sniffed directly from tubes, plastic bags or smears on pieces of cloth. Tolerance develops over weeks or months. Intoxication is characterized by:

- Euphoria
- Excitement
- A floating sensation
- Dizziness
- Slurred speech
- Ataxia

Acute intoxication can cause amnesia and visual hallucinations. The habit is dangerous because:

- There is a risk of tissue damage, including damage to bone marrow, brain, liver and kidneys. Death can occur.
- Acute intoxication can also result in aggressive and impulsive behaviour.

Amphetamines and related substances

These have temporary stimulant and euphoriant effects that are followed by depression, anxiety and irritability. Psychological rather than true physical dependence is the rule. In addition to restlessness, overtalkativeness and overactivity, amphetamines can produce a paranoid psychosis indistinguishable from acute paranoid schizophrenia

Cocaine

Cocaine is a CNS stimulant with similar effects to amphetamines. It is injected as well as sniffed; the latter practice can cause perforation of the nasal septum. The clinical picture is of excitation, dilated pupils, tremulousness and dizziness; a paranoid psychosis can occur. Cocaine abuse is currently a major problem and chronic use can lead to severe dependence.

Hallucinogenic drugs

Hallucinogenic drugs such as lysergic acid diethylamide (LSD), cannabis and mescaline produce distortions and intensifications of sensory perceptions as well as frank hallucinations.

Cannabis

A widely used drug in some subcultures is cannabis, derived from the plant *Cannabis sativa*. It is not thought to cause physical dependence. The drug, when smoked, seems to exaggerate the pre-existing mood, be it depression, euphoria or anxiety. There is no definite withdrawal syndrome or tolerance. There is disagreement over whether it can produce a psychosis.

Hypnotics

Other drugs of dependence include barbiturates and benzodiazepines. Discontinuing treatment with benzodiazepines may cause withdrawal symptoms such as anxiety, restlessness, tachycardia and sensory disturbances (see Table 19.22); for this reason, withdrawal should be supervised and gradual.

Narcotics

Morphine-type physical dependence occurs with morphine, heroin and codeine as well as with synthetic and semi-synthetic narcotic analgesics such as methadone and pethidine. These substances display cross-tolerance—the withdrawal effects of one are reduced by administration of one of the others. The psychological effect of such substances is of a calm, slightly euphoric mood associated with freedom from physical discomfort and a flattening of emotional response. This is believed to be due to the attachment of morphine and its analogues to receptor sites in the CNS normally occupied by endorphins. Tolerance to this group of drugs is rapidly developed and marked. Following abstinence it is rapidly lost. The abstinence syndrome consists of a constellation of signs and symptoms (see Table 19.29) that reach peak intensity on the second or third day after the last dose of the opiate. These rapidly subside over the next 7 days. Withdrawal is dangerous in patients with heart disease, tuberculosis or other chronic debilitating conditions.

Narcotic addicts are reported to have a high mortality rate due to acute illness associated with drug abuse. Heart disease (including infective

Table 19.29 Narcotic abstinence syndrome.

Yawning Rhinorrhoea Lacrimation Pupillary dilatation Sweating Piloerection Restlessness	12–16 h after last dose of opiate
Muscular twitches Aches and pains Abdominal cramps Vomiting Diarrhoea Hypertension Insomnia Anorexia Agitation Profuse sweating Weight loss	24–72 h after last dose of opiate

endocarditis), tuberculosis and glomerulonephritis are common causes of death, while tetanus, malaria and acute viral hepatitis B are also causally related to addiction.

TREATMENT

The treatment of a narcotic drug overdose requires immediate action. If opioid overdose is suspected, naloxone given intravenously (see p. 666) can be life-saving and diagnostic. There should be an immediate recovery of consciousness or a lightening of the comatose state if the offending agent is an opioid. Care must be taken, however, as opiate antagonists can precipitate violent abstinence symptoms. A constant infusion of naloxone hydrochloride may be required in methadone overdoses.

The treatment of chronic dependence is usually directed towards helping the addict to live without drugs. Some who cannot manage such a regimen may be maintained on oral methadone. In the UK, only specially licensed doctors may legally prescribe heroin and cocaine to an addict for maintenance treatment of addiction.

Causes of drug dependence

There is no single cause of drug dependence. Three factors appear important:
- Availability of drugs
- A vulnerable personality
- Social, particularly peer, pressures

Once regular drug taking is established, pharmacological factors are particularly important in determining dependence.

Eating disorders

Obesity (see p. 140)

The majority of cases of obesity are caused by a combination of constitutional and social factors that encourage overeating. It is relatively infrequent for psychological causes to be involved. However, even when obesity is not due to definite psychological causes, it may itself produce a psychological reaction of depression and tension, particularly if attempts by the patient to lose weight are repeatedly ineffective.

TREATMENT

Behavioural methods of treatment that make use of positive rewards for weight loss or for behaviour likely to lead to a reduction of weight have been attempted, but their efficacy is doubtful.

Anorexia nervosa

The main clinical criteria for diagnosis are:
- A body weight more than 25% below the standard weight
- An intense wish to be thin
- A morbid fear of fatness
- Amenorrhoea in women

Clinical features may include:
- Onset usually in adolescence
- A previous history of chubbiness or fatness
- A relentless pursuit of low body weight
- Usually a distorted image of her own body size
- The patient generally eating little
- Particular avoidance of carbohydrates
- Vomiting, excessive exercise and purging
- Amenorrhoea—an early symptom; in 20% it precedes weight loss
- Binge eating
- Usually a marked lack of sexual interest
- Lanugo

The physical consequences of anorexia include sensitivity to cold, constipation, hypotension and bradycardia. In most cases, amenorrhoea is secondary to the weight loss. Vomiting and abuse of purgatives may lead to hypokalaemia and alkalosis.

PREVALENCE

Case register data suggests a rate ranging from 1–10 per 100 000 females aged between 15 and 34 years. Surveys have suggested a prevalence rate of 1–2% among schoolgirls and university students. Many more young women have amenorrhoea accompanied by less weight loss than the 25%

required for the diagnosis. The condition is much less common among men. The onset in women is usually between 16 and 17 years of age and it seldom occurs after 30 years.

AETIOLOGY

Biological factors
Genetic. Six to ten per cent of siblings of affected girls suffer from anorexia nervosa. No study of monozygotic twins has been made so this increase could be due to environmental as much as genetic factors.

Hormonal. There could be a disturbance of hypothalamic function in that:
- Amenorrhoea precedes weight loss in 20% of sufferers.
- Hormonal disturbances include low luteinizing hormone levels with impaired response to luteinizing hormone releasing hormone and to clomiphene. However, such findings could be due to the effect of prolonged fasting.

Psychological factors
Individual. Patients usually have:
- A disturbance in body image
- Dietary problems in early life

Anorexia is seen as an escape from the emotional problems of adolescence and a regression into childhood.

Family. The specific pattern of relationships described is characterized by:
- Overprotectiveness
- Rigidity
- Lack of conflict resolution

Anorexia serves to prevent dissension in families. However, evidence in favour of such patterns is conflicting.

Social factors
There is a higher prevalence in higher social classes, and a high rate in certain occupational groups (e.g. ballet students and nurses) and in societies where cultural value is placed on thinness.

COURSE AND PROGNOSIS

The condition runs a fluctuating course, with exacerbations and partial remissions. Long-term follow-up suggests that about two-thirds of patients maintain normal weight and that the remaining third are split between those who are moderately underweight and those who are seriously underweight. Indicators of a poor outcome include:
- A long initial illness
- Severe weight loss
- Bulimia, vomiting or purging

- Difficulties in relationships

Suicide has been reported in 2–5% of patients with chronic anorexia nervosa. More than one-third have recurrent affective illness, and various family, genetic and endocrine studies have found associations between eating disorders and depression.

TREATMENT

Treatment can be conducted on an outpatient basis, but if the weight loss is severe it is accompanied by marked physical symptoms of lassitude, dizziness and weakness and/or electrolyte and vitamin disturbances; hospital admission may then be unavoidable. Rarely, the patient's weight loss may be so severe as to be life-threatening. If the patient cannot be persuaded to enter hospital, compulsory admission may have to be used.

Treatment goals include:
- Establishing a good relationship with the patient
- Restoring the weight to a level between the ideal body weight and the patient's idea of what her weight should be
- The provision of a balanced diet of at least 3000 calories in three to four meals per day
- The elimination of purgative and/or laxative use and vomiting

Treatment can be conducted on behavioural or dynamic psychotherapeutic lines or on a combination of both. The usual behavioural approach is to remove privileges on the patient's admission and to restore them gradually as rewards for weight gain. Intense psychoanalytically-derived psychotherapy is not helpful. Family therapy involving the exploration of problems in family relationships and their modification through counselling has been recently explored; however, evidence that it is superior to simple supportive psychotherapy is lacking.

Bulimia nervosa

This refers to episodes of uncontrolled excessive eating, which are also termed binges. There is a preoccupation with food and a habitual adoption of certain behaviours which can be understood as the patient's attempts to avoid the fattening effects of periodic binges. These behaviours include:
- Self-induced vomiting
- Laxative abuse
- Misuse of drugs—diuretics, thyroid extract or anorectics

Additional clinical features include:
- Physical complications of vomiting:
  Cardiac arrhythmias ⎫
  Renal impairment ⎬ Consequences of low K^+
  Muscular paralysis ⎭
  Tetany—from hypokalaemic alkalosis

Swollen salivary glands ⎰ From vomiting
Eroded dental enamel ⎱

- Associated psychiatric disorders:
  Depression in reaction to vomiting
  Alcohol dependence
- Fluctuations in body weight
- Menstrual function—periods irregular but amen-
  orrhoea rare
- Personality—neurotic traits present premorbidly

The prevalence of bulimia in community studies is high; it affects between 5 and 30% of girls attending high schools, colleges or universities in the US. Bulimia is often associated with anorexia nervosa. The prognosis is uncertain.

TREATMENT

As the condition has only recently been recognized, it is not yet clear what is the most effective form of treatment. Admission to hospital with careful control over eating has been advocated, while a behavioural approach involving careful diary-keeping regarding eating and making patients responsible for control is under extensive study. In this approach, patients attempt to identify and avoid any environmental stimuli or emotional changes that regularly precede the desire to binge. Preliminary results of this approach are promising.

Psychosexual disorders

Sexual disorders can be divided into sexual dysfunctions, sexual deviations and gender role disorders (see Table 19.30).

Sexual dysfunctions

Sexual dysfunction in men refers to repeated inability to achieve normal sexual intercourse, whereas in women it refers to a repeatedly unsatisfactory quality of sexual satisfaction. Problems of sexual dysfunction can be usefully classified into those affecting sexual desire, those affecting sexual arousal and those affecting orgasm. Among men presenting for treatment of sexual dysfunction, impotence is the most frequent complaint. The prevalence of premature ejaculation is low, while ejaculatory failure is rare.

Sexual drive is affected by constitutional factors, ignorance of sexual technique, anxiety about sexual performance, medical conditions and certain drugs (see Tables 19.31 and 19.32).

The treatment of sexual dysfunction involves

Table 19.30 Classification of sexual disorders.

Sexual dysfunction
Affecting sexual desire:
Low libido
Impaired sexual arousal:
Erectile impotence
Failure of arousal in women
Affecting orgasm:
Premature ejaculation
Retarded ejaculation
Orgasmic dysfunction in women
Sexual deviations
Variations of the sexual 'object':
Fetishism
Transvestism
Paedophilia
Bestiality
Necrophilia
Variations of the sexual act:
Exhibitionism
Voyeurism
Sadism
Masochism
Frotteurism
Disorders of the gender role
Transsexualism

Table 19.31 Medical conditions affecting sexual performance.

Endocrine
Diabetes mellitus
Hyperthyroidism
Hypothyroidism
Cardiovascular
Angina pectoris
Previous myocardial infarction
Hepatic
Cirrhosis, particularly alcoholic
Renal
Renal failure
Neurological
Neuropathy
Spinal cord lesions
Musculoskeletal
Arthritis
Respiratory
Asthma
Chronic bronchitis and emphysema

careful assessment, the participation where appropriate of the patient's partner, and specific therapeutic techniques including relaxation, behavioural training and supportive counselling.

Table 19.32 Drugs adversely affecting sexual arousal.

Male arousal
Alcohol*
Benzodiazepines
Neuroleptics
Cimetidine
Narcotic analgesics
Methyldopa
Clonidine
Spironolactone
Antihistamines

Female arousal
Alcohol*
CNS depressants
Oral combined contraceptives
Methyldopa
Clonidine

* Alcohol 'increases the desire but diminishes the performance'.

Sexual deviations

Nowadays, sexual deviations are more likely to be regarded as unusual forms of behaviour than as illnesses and doctors are only likely to be involved when the behaviour involves breaking the law (e.g. paedophilia or bestiality) and when there is a question of an associated mental or physical disorder. Homosexuality was formerly classified as an illness but today it is increasingly accepted as an alternative sexual lifestyle.

Transvestism is a form of sexual deviation in which individuals, usually men, dress in clothes of the opposite sex. The cross-dressing may either be a symptom of some other sexual deviation or may be employed as a means of fetishistic sexual excitement. It usually begins about puberty and the transvestite experiences sexual excitement and may masturbate when indulging in this behaviour. The overwhelming majority of cross-dressers believe that they are of the correct gender, in contrast to transsexuals (see below).

Gender role disorders

Transsexualism involves a disturbance in sexual identity. The criteria for establishing sexual identity are described on p. 707.

In transsexualism, there is no evidence as yet of abnormality in the chromosomal or phenotypic sex and social sex conforms to biological sex. There is, however, a severe disturbance in psychosexual differentiation. A person's gender identity refers to the individual's sense of masculinity or femininity as distinct from sex. It is thought to arise from a biological component (prenatal endocrine influences), psychological imprinting and social conditioning. Disturbances in these three areas have variously been blamed for the cause of transsexualism. The four key features of transsexualism are:

- A sense of belonging to the opposite sex and of having been born into the wrong sex
- A sense of estrangement from one's own body; all manifestations of anatomical sexual identification are regarded as repugnant
- A strong desire to resemble physically the opposite sex and seek treatment, including surgery, towards this end
- A wish to be accepted in the community as belonging to the opposite sex

For males treatment includes hormonal administration (oestrogen is used to produce some breast enlargement and fat deposition around hips and thighs) and, if surgery is to be recommended, a period of living as a woman as a trial beforehand. In the case of female transsexuals treatment involves surgery and the use of methyl testosterone.

Psychiatry and the law

At the heart of the relationship between psychiatry and the law is the issue of responsibility. Mental disorder, by virtue of its severity and/or quality, may impair the individual's responsibility for his thinking and actions. The law in most Western countries provides for the compulsory admission and/or treatment of the mentally disordered person for his own protection and/or the protection of others and for mitigation in the case of the mentally disordered individual who commits a criminal offence.

In England and Wales the law relating to the care and control of the mentally ill has evolved out of common law. The Act of Parliament that is crucially involved is the Mental Health Act of 1983. This Act is concerned not merely with provisions governing the compulsory admission and treatment of mentally disordered persons, but also with patients' rights, appeals tribunals and the overall supervision of the use of compulsory powers. The Act is divided into a number of sections, each of which deals with a different aspect of the process.

Apart from one provision of the National Assistance Act 1948, the Mental Health Act 1983 is the only method whereby individuals can legally be deprived of their liberty without having committed a crime or being suspected of committing a crime. It is, therefore, very important that doctors understand the seriousness of their responsibility and the details of the legislation.

There are only three conditions that need to be met before an appropriate compulsory section form is signed. The patient must:
- Be suffering from a defined mental disorder
- Be at risk to his/her and/or other people's health or safety

Table 19.33 Important sections of the Mental Health Act 1983.

Section	Duration	Signatures required	Purpose
2	28 days	Two doctors (one approved) plus nearest relative or social worker	Assessment and treatment
3	6 months	Two doctors (one approved) plus nearest relative or social worker	Treatment
4	72 h	One doctor plus relative or social worker	Emergency admission
5(2)	72 h	Doctor in charge of patient's care	Emergency detention of patient already in hospital
5(4)	6 h	Nurse (RMN)	Emergency detention of a patient already in hospital
136	72 h	Police officer	Psychiatric assessment of those in public places thought by police to be mentally ill and in need of a place of safety

- Be unwilling to accept hospitalization voluntarily

The reasons why there is no alternative approach to the treatment suggested for the patient should be outlined.

Sexual deviance or alcohol or drug dependence are *not* mental disorders, but otherwise the definition of mental disorder is broad and includes:
- Mental illness
- Mental impairment
- Severe mental impairment
- Psychopathy

Any registered medical practitioner may sign a 'medical recommendation' under the Act, but the added signature of a specialist psychiatrist approved under Section 12 is needed for compulsory orders lasting for more than 72 h. Unless the patient is already in hospital, the nearest relative or an approved mental health social worker is also required to sign the application form. Important sections of the Act are detailed in Table 19.33.

Sections 4, 5(2), 5(4) and 136 cannot be extended by repetition. They must be converted to a Section 2 or 3 if prolonged detention is necessary. Likewise, Section 2 should be converted to a Section 3 if required. Patients on the longer orders (2 and 3) can appeal to a Mental Health Review Tribunal. The Act also deals with consent to treatment, guardianship, mentally abnormal offenders and hazardous treatments. A Mental Health Act Commission supervises the Act, provides second opinions and regularly visits hospitals. Although much of the process of detention against one's will is formalized, there is no liability for a doctor who acts in good faith with a patient's best interests at heart. Clearly written medical notes, accepted forms of treatment and common sense remain the basis of good practice.

Further reading

Clare AW (1980) *Psychiatry in Dissent*, 2nd edn. London: Tavistock Publications.

Gelder M, Gath D & Mayou R (1983) *Oxford Textbook of Psychiatry*. Oxford: Oxford University Press.

Goldberg D & Huxley P (1980) *Mental Illness in the Community*. London: Tavistock Publications.

Silverstone T & Turner P (1978) *Drug Treatment in Psychiatry*, 2nd edn. London: Routledge & Kegan Paul.

Dermatology

e.g. the Ehlers–Danlos syndrome. Skin disease may present as part of a systemic disease, e.g. the rash associated with systemic lupus erythematosus, or alternatively a severe skin disease may cause systemic symptoms, e.g. pemphigus. Geographical factors are also important; in particular, skin conditions due to certain fungi and bacteria are more prevalent in the tropics.

Structure of the skin (Fig. 20.1)

The skin is divided into three layers:
- The epidermis
- The dermis
- The subcutaneous layer

The epidermis
The epidermis consists of stratified epithelium and is divided into two layers. The inner malpighian layer contains the germinal basal layer (stratum germinativum), above which lies the stratum spinosum or prickle cell layer; above this is the stratum granulosum. The outer layer consists of anucleate cornified cells (stratum corneum). The stratum lucidum lies between the granular and the cornified layers. The cells in the germinal basal layer give rise to successive layers of cells which lose their nuclei and die as they reach the surface.

Introduction

Skin diseases are extremely common but their exact prevalence is unknown. There are over 1000 different entities described, but two-thirds of all cases are due to fewer than 10 conditions. These common conditions include acne, warts, dermatitis, infections due to bacteria, viruses and fungi, and psoriasis.

Some conditions, e.g. acne, may be part of normal development, whilst others may be inherited,

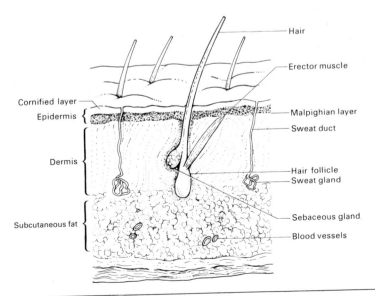

Fig. 20.1 The structure of the skin.

The cells in the epidermis consist of those synthesizing keratin (keratinocytes) and clear cells. The latter cells appear in the basal and suprabasal levels and consist mainly of:

- *Melanocytes*. These are dendritic cells which arise from the neural crest. They synthesize melanin and transfer it as pigment granules to the epidermal keratinocytes.
- *Langerhans' cells*. These are also dendritic cells. They are thought to be macrophages and are directly involved in allergic contact hypersensitivity, and with the uptake and processing of antigenic material.

The dermis

The dermis contains connective tissue fibres, amorphous ground substance, blood vessels, nerves, lymphatics and muscles. The connective tissue fibres consist mainly of collagen (75%), but some are elastic or reticulin fibres. These are embedded in a mucopolysaccharide ground substance. Fibroblasts lie between the collagen bundles and elastic fibres run parallel and enclose the bundles. This gives the skin its elasticity. The cells within the dermis include leucocytes, histiocytes, fibroblasts and mast cells.

The sweat glands

The sweat glands are of two varieties:

- The eccrine glands are present all over the skin, particularly the palms, but not in mucous membranes. The glands are situated in the dermis and secrete a watery fluid containing chloride, lactic acid, fatty acids, urea, glycoproteins and mucopolysaccharides.
- The *apocrine glands* are large sweat glands whose ducts open into the hair follicles. They are found in the axillae, anogenital areas, nipples and areolae. They do not function until puberty. Modified glands produce wax in the ears, and also occur on the eyelids. They produce a white secretion containing proteins and complex carbohydrates.

The sebaceous glands

Sebaceous glands occur all over the skin (except on the palms and soles) but are most numerous on the scalp and face. They have no lumen and their secretion is due to decomposition of the cells. The secretion, called sebum, consists mainly of fatty acids and cholesterol and is discharged into the pilosebaceous follicle.

Hair

Each hair consists of a shaft of keratinized cells which is produced by the hair bulbs, deep in the dermis and projects through the skin from the hair follicle. It is richly supplied by nerves and blood vessels and contains melanin. There are three types of hair:

- Terminal—coarse hair, e.g. scalp, mole, beard, eyebrows, pubic
- Vellus—short, fine, downy hair, e.g. on the face of women and prepubertal boys
- Lanugo—hair covering the fetus

Hair growth varies depending on the type. Every follicle has a phase of involution (catagen phase), a shedding phase (telogen phase), and a growth phase (anagen phase), which may last up to 3 years in scalp hair.

Nails

Nails are hard, translucent plates of keratin which grow from beneath the nail fold. A fingernail takes up to 6 months to replace itself and its growth is affected by disease and malnutrition.

The subcutaneous layer

This contains fat, sweat glands and blood vessels.

Functions of the skin

The skin acts as a protective covering to the body. Its functions are as follows:

- It forms a physical barrier to antigens or bacteria.
- It prevents excessive absorption or loss of water.
- Its pigmentation prevents injury from ultraviolet light.
- Vitamin D is synthesized by sunlight in the epidermis.
- It is involved in temperature regulation.
- Sensations of pain, touch and temperature can be distinguished.
- It is involved in immunological reactions.

Terminology

The terms used to describe skin diseases are shown in Table 20.1.

History

This should include questions on the patient's general health, past medical history, family history, and any drugs being taken. A description of the skin lesion should be obtained, including its site of origin, spread, length of time it has been present, whether it is itchy or painful, if it forms blisters or if any ointment or medicines have helped.

Examination

A careful examination of the whole skin should be made as clues to the diagnosis may be apparent in distant sites. If the nature of the skin disease is not obvious, a full general examination should be performed, as the skin disease may be a manifestation of a systemic disorder.

Table 20.1 Terminology used in skin diseases.

Annular lesions	Lesions occurring in rings
Atrophy	Thinning of skin
Bulla	A large vesicle
Crust	Dried exudate on the skin
Ecchymoses	Bruises more than 3 mm in diameter
Erythema	Redness
Erythroderma	Widespread redness of the skin with scaling
Excoriation	Linear marks due to scratching
Macule	A flat circumscribed area of discoloration
Maculopapule	A raised and discoloured circumscribed lesion
Nodule	A circumscribed large palpable mass >1 cm in diameter
Papule	A circumscribed, raised, palpable area
Petechiae	Bruises less than 3 mm in diameter
Plaque	A disc-shaped lesion; can result from coalescence of papules
Purpura	Extravasation of blood into the skin; does not blanch on pressure
Pustule	A pus-filled blister
Scales	Dried flakes of dead skin from horny layer (keratin)
Telangiectasis	A visible small dilated vessel on the skin
Vesicle	A small, visible, fluid-filled blister
Weal	A transiently raised, reddened area associated with scratching

---

Pruritus

This is an itch occurring in many skin conditions, including:
- Scabies
- Atopic eczema
- Candidiasis
- Urticaria
- Insect bites (e.g. flea, bed-bug)

It also occurs with systemic conditions, often without obvious skin involvement. These include:
- Metabolic disease—hyperthyroidism, carcinoid syndrome
- Malignant disease—chronic lymphatic leukaemia lymphoma, some carcinomas
- Haematological disease—polycythaemia vera
- Renal disease—chronic renal failure with uraemia
- Liver disease—cholestasis, particularly primary biliary cirrhosis
- Miscellaneous—senile pruritus, psychogenic, drugs, e.g. opiates

---

Investigation

- Skin scrapings for fungi. Scrapings from areas of involved skin are placed on a slide with 20% potassium hydroxide to clear extraneous material. Fungal mycelia, as well as parasites, lice, etc., may be seen under the microscope.
- Skin biopsy. Skin should be removed in the shape of an ellipse along lines of stretch (Langer's lines). Biopsies should either be fixed in formalin or frozen immediately for immunofluorescence.
- Wood's light. This is an ultraviolet light which is shone on the skin. Normal hair and skin fluoresce bluish-white. Certain types of ringworm (*Microsporum audouini* and *M. canis*) fluoresce a greenish colour; erythrasma due to *Corynebacterium minutissimum* fluoresces pink/red.
- Patch tests. These are used to confirm allergic contact dermatitis (see p. 907).
- Laboratory tests for the exclusion of bacterial and fungal infections. Tests for SLE or thrombocytopenic purpura, for example, should be performed as appropriate.
- Routine tests such as blood counts and ESR and also urine testing, e.g. for glucose in diabetes, should be performed.

Eczema and dermatitis

Dermatitis implies inflammation of the skin and can be due to many causes. It is usual to prefix the term with the causal agent, e.g. solar dermatitis or seborrhoeic dermatitis.

The following inflammatory changes are seen:
- *Redness* (erythema)
- *Heat*, which is associated with the erythema
- *Pain*. This is an uncommon feature of skin disease. Irritation is more common and can be so severe that the patient gouges the skin, thereby stimulating pain fibres in an attempt to alleviate the discomfort associated with itching. Most patients with eczema produce secondary thickening or lichenification of their skin from chronic scratching or rubbing, with exaggerated surface markings (Fig. 20.2).
- *Swelling*. Extracellular fluid is difficult to accommodate in the thin epidermal layer, so that excess fluid tends to move to the surface of the skin. Oozing of fluid or crusting may be seen in the acute phase of eczema, with scaling in more chronic disease. On sites where the epidermis is thicker, for example on the palms and soles, small collections of fluid may be trapped in superficial layers of the skin as vesicles or larger lesions (bullae).
- *Loss of function*. This is evident when large areas of

Fig. 20.2 Lichenification seen with chronic flexural eczema.

skin are erythematous, scaled or denuded. Thermoregulation is prevented by intense erythema, and the increased blood flow may lead to high-output cardiac failure. Both of these are not uncommon in elderly patients with erythroderma.

Denuding of the skin limits the ability to contend with invasion by bacteria, and increased catabolic changes may be seen with bullous diseases, toxic epidermal necrolysis and chronic widespread eczema.

The meaning of the word 'eczema' is 'flowing over', which describes some of the above inflammatory changes. The words eczema and dermatitis are used somewhat interchangeably as in both conditions similar inflammatory changes occur in the skin. Use of the term eczema avoids the word 'dermatitis', which often conjures up ideas in the patient's mind of external irritants, such as cause contact dermatitis.

Eczema occurs following a variety of stimuli.

ENDOGENOUS ECZEMA OR ATOPIC ECZEMA

PATHOGENESIS

The word 'atopy' implies a capacity to overreact to common environmental factors. It can be demonstrated by multiple positive skin-prick tests (see p. 570). A positive test to a specific antigen does not necessarily indicate that this antigen is involved in causation of the skin disease, and removal of the antigen, e.g. from the diet, often does not improve the skin condition.

Serum levels of the IgE antibody are elevated in atopic eczema as in all atopic diseases; higher values are seen when eczema is combined with asthma. The significance of these raised levels in the pathogenesis of the eczema is unclear.

Diet

Most research on causative factors in eczema has involved dietary manipulation in children. Sensible parents may be able to correlate the onset of itching and exacerbation of eczema with dietary factors such as eggs or milk. When such a clear-cut relationship between the two is found, the removal of the food item will often improve the skin condition. The number of patients in whom the two events can be clearly related is, however, small. The role of diet may need to be assessed over a prolonged period, and the reintroduction of foods that have been excluded over a long interval may cause severe generalized reactions. Serious attempts at dietary restriction should ideally be supervised by a trained dietitian in collaboration with a paediatrician.

Genetic factors

There is a hereditary predisposition; when both parents have the disease, the risk of their offspring developing eczema is approximately 60%.

Exacerbating factors

Non-specific stimuli such as heat, humidity, drying of the skin and contact with woollen clothing may cause a flare-up of disease, and patients should be advised to avoid these trigger factors.

PATTERNS OF DISEASE

Infantile eczema

Erythema, weeping or scaling usually appear first on the facial skin. Other body sites are less commonly affected.

Irritation produces restlessness and the child may rub his face or scalp on a pillow or the cot-side. With time there is a gradual spread of the eczema to the flexures.

Flexural or childhood eczema

In toddlers and older children the skin folds are typically involved. Facial involvement may persist, partly due to climatic factors, e.g. sunlight and low humidity.

Adult eczema

In those whose disease continues into adult life, the flexures at the neck, elbow, wrist, ankle or knee, and the limbs are often involved. Chronic eczematous changes are common on the face, although any body site may be involved.

PROGNOSIS

With a typical pattern of involvement and an early onset, the prognosis is good. Some children will lose their disease in infancy, whilst others improve gradually, so that by the early teens more than 90% will be clear of disease. Localized recurrence may occur in adult life if the skin is unduly stressed, e.g. the hands of nurses or hairdressers. An unusual pattern of eczema over extensor surfaces (reversed pattern) coming on later in childhood may represent more recalcitrant disease and the prognosis should be guarded.

TREATMENT

About a third of atopic children have a dry skin in addition to eczema, so that the regular use of emollients such as aqueous cream or emulsifying ointment applied to a damp skin after bathing or used instead of soap is fundamental to a treatment regimen. The use of perfumed soaps and 'bubble baths' should be avoided. Non-perfumed oils and gels should be used for washing, with the use of soap limited. Sunny holidays at the sea will often stabilize the skin condition and a course of ultraviolet light treatment may bring a similar benefit.

For widespread regular use over months or years a mild topical corticosteroid (Table 20.2), e.g. 1% hydrocortisone, is suitable; the cream base is the form best tolerated. Localized disease may require short courses of more potent topical corticosteroids on some occasions, especially when the skin is markedly thickened. The addition of tar as an alcoholic solution or as crude coal tar may also improve lichenified skin.

Bacterial infection seen with gross excoriation or with fissuring of the skin is treated with a steroid/antibiotic combination.

The treatment of associated atopic disease, e.g. asthma, may in turn improve the state of the skin, the child's well-being and sleep pattern. Sedative antihistamines, such as promethazine hydrochloride

Table 20.2 Topical steroids.

Actions
Anti-inflammatory
Immunosuppressive
Decrease rate of epidermal turnover

Types
Many. Available in cream, ointment or lotion form.
 Vary in potency:

Mild, e.g. hydrocortisone 1%
Moderate, e.g. clobetasone butyrate 0.05%
Potent, e.g. betamethasone 0.1% (as valerate),
 hydrocortisone butyrate, fluocinolone acetonide
 0.2%
Very potent, e.g. clobetasol propionate 0.05%

Compound preparations with, for example,
 antibacterials, are available.

Uses
In general, the least potent effective preparation
 should be used. The use of potent preparations on
 the face should be avoided.

Side-effects
Thinning of skin
Spread of local infection
Telangiectasia and striae
Hair growth
Acne
Adrenal suppression with long-term use of potent
 preparations

Side-effects are chiefly associated with the more
 potent forms.

elixir at night, will also help to prevent restless sleep and ceaseless scratching.

POMPHOLYX (Fig. 20.3)

This pattern of eczema commonly affects the sides of the fingers, palms, the toes or soles of the feet. Irritant vesicles are the initial feature, though with acute and more serious attacks bullae may be seen.

The patients are usually in their twenties or thirties when they develop the disease. A previous history of atopy is not elicited in the majority of patients.

Some normal individuals develop irritant vesicles on the sides of the fingers in warm weather, but there is no clear-cut relationship to sweating. Endogenous factors which trigger this type of eczema are not known. The role of dietary nickel provoking the disease in nickel-sensitive patients is controversial. Attacks may occur frequently and at regular intervals or merge.

TREATMENT

Drying and bacteriostatic solutions such as potassium permanganate 0.01% are used daily until

Fig. 20.3 Pompholyx.

weeping is controlled. Potent topical corticosteroids containing antibiotics or antiseptics may be necessary to control severe attacks, e.g. betamethasone 0.1% cream with neomycin (Betnovate-N) or fluocinolone acetonide 0.025% cream with cetomacrogol (Synalar C).

Systemic treatment with steroids, e.g. tetracosactrin, given at regular intervals over weeks or even months, or prednisolone by mouth in doses of between 10 and 15 mg daily, may be necessary to break the frequency of attacks and heal the skin.

DISCOID OR NUMMULAR ECZEMA

Annular patches of eczema may appear in association with other patterns of disease during early life, but the majority of individuals with this type of disease are middle-aged or elderly and have no previous history of skin disease. Papules and coin-shaped raised lesions associated with extreme itching occur on the limbs, most commonly on the lower leg; they may merge to form plaques. The cause is unknown but bacterial antigens have been implicated. Eczematous lesions on the legs are sometimes partly due to venous incompetence and support bandages may be necessary. Patients with irritation of the skin are not, however, enthusiastic about having the limbs covered.

TREATMENT

Occlusive bandages containing zinc paste or ichthammol may help to alleviate itching and prevent the trauma of incessant scratching. Impregnated steroid tape containing flurandrenolone 0.0125% may produce the same effect; intralesional triamcinolone or local potent topical corticosteroids improve the condition of the skin and give relief from itching. The disease often improves when the patient retires from work.

EXOGENOUS ECZEMA

Exogenous eczema can be divided into primary irritant dermatitis and true contact dermatitis associated with a cell-mediated immune response.

Primary irritant dermatitis

This is essentially a degreasing of the skin with a subsequent water loss followed by dryness, fissuring and cracking. It can occur both at work and in the home. Industrial solvents which remove greasy coatings covering metal components in industry can with equal efficiency remove surface lipids from the skin if they are not handled with care.

Housewives are also at risk; the changes in the skin occur in parallel with the extent of immersion of their hands in water, e.g. washing of kitchen utensils, personal garments or napkins. Initially the skin beneath a ring is often involved, as neat detergent or soap powder tends to lodge there and erode the skin, which becomes eczematous. This spreads to the thin skin on the sides of the fingers, the webs and the backs of the hands; the palms are only affected in more severe and chronic disease. A similar type of disease may be seen in other occupations that involve wet work and the use of cleaning and detergent solutions, such as bar work and hairdressing.

Asteatotic eczema or eczema cracquele
This is a condition often seen in long-stay elderly hospital patients. Older patients often lack sufficient surface lipids to prevent their skin from becoming dry. This can be made worse by an unusual amount

of washing with soap. The eczema can result in a 'crocodile skin' appearance, which is most noticeable on the lower limbs.

This condition may also be seen in hypothyroidism.

Although the skin may appear inflamed, the use of emollients and creams for washing instead of soap has the greatest beneficial effect and topical corticosteroids are often unnecessary.

Allergic contact dermatitis

This is a good example of a cell-mediated immune disease or type IV reaction. Lymphocytes are sensitized to the antigen, sometimes after the first contact. All areas of the skin may be involved and so the back can conveniently be used as a site for patch testing. The sensitivity lasts for life.

Small molecular weight substances passing through the skin need to be linked to skin proteins in order to sensitize. Langerhans' cells present in the dermis appear to fulfil the role of macrophages elsewhere in the body and present the antigen to lymphocytes.

CLINICAL FEATURES AND INVESTIGATION

An unusual pattern of rash with clear-cut demarcation or odd-shaped areas of erythema and scaling should arouse suspicion and in combination with a careful history indicate a cause. The suspected allergen is then placed in contact with the skin as a patch test. If the causative agent cannot be clearly defined, e.g. in hand eczema, then a range of known everyday antigens can be tested, including materials

---

Patch testing

The original skin disease should be in a quiescent phase before patch testing is done.

Systemic steroid therapy may alter the cutaneous response to an allergen.

- The back is a convenient site for testing.
- Sites for application of the antigen are clearly labelled and a map of their whereabouts is made.
- Materials are diluted in order to prevent irritant reactions and suspended in white soft paraffin.
- White soft paraffin should be used alone in some sites as a control.
- Each substance is then placed within an aluminium disc and kept in place next to the skin by adhesive strapping.
- The patches are taken off and an initial reading made after 48 h.
- A positive reaction is indicated by an area of eczema.
- Further readings are taken at 96 h.
- Blistering may indicate a non-specific irritant effect but it can occur with soap or detergent materials.

---

such as rubber, nickel and medicaments. Positive readings will need to be interpreted with caution and may not have an obvious relevance when considering the patient's history or occupation.

If the major distribution of an eruption appears to involve exposed skin, then photo-patch testing may be required. Two identical sets of likely allergens are placed on the back and one set is exposed to long wave ultraviolet light with the second non-exposed set acting as a control.

TREATMENT

Treatment is to remove the known irritant or allergen if this is possible. Steroid creams are helpful for short periods when the disease is severe. Anti-pruritic agents may be necessary for symptomatic relief.

Erythematous squamous eruptions

PSORIASIS

Psoriasis occurs throughout the world; in the temperate zones 2% of the population are affected. It is less common in some pigmented skins. This chronic skin disease is seen most commonly as erythematous well-demarcated silvery scaled plaques over extensor surfaces such as the elbows and knees, and in the scalp. In this common pattern the onset of the disease is unusual before 15 years of age, and the initial presentation may occur in old age.

Genetic factors are important in the aetiology of the disease, and certain triggers initiate or exacerbate the condition. Characteristically there are periods of activity and remission that are often impossible to predict.

Arthropathy occurs in association with the skin disease in about 8–10% of individuals, but pathogenetic factors which link the two conditions are not clear.

AETIOLOGY

Genetic factors
The mode of inheritance of the disease is not known but certain HLA markers are recognized. HLA-B13 and HLA-B17 are associated with an increased relative risk, but a more recently recognized association is with HLA-CW6, where the risk is increased up to 15 times that of the general population. It is now known that both of the B loci occupy an area adjacent to the gene which expresses CW6. HLA-B27 is seen in up to 90% of individuals with ankylosing spondylitis and in 70% of individuals who develop a similar spinal arthropathy with psoriasis.

Infection

The role of infection as an exacerbating factor is suggested by the following observations:

- In children, superficial small patterned lesions of guttate psoriasis may appear over the trunk and limbs 10–14 days following a throat infection with beta-haemolytic streptococci, and up to 75% of these individuals have the HLA-CW6 marker.
- Patients with Reiter's syndrome (see p. 350) may develop skin lesions which are identical to those seen in psoriasis. Reiter's disease can occur after dysentery or after venereal contact, again suggesting an infective aetiology which might apply to psoriasis itself.

Emotional trauma

It is a commonly expressed layman's view that many skin diseases are 'nervous' in origin. The role of emotional trauma in triggering psoriasis in a particular individual is best assessed over a long interval. For example, a child followed through to adolescence may be seen to have an exacerbation of the disease with the stress of school examinations. Patients can also develop a reactive psychological state owing to the severity of their skin disease. However, most patients appear as well-balanced individuals.

Mechanical trauma

Repeated trauma to the skin over the elbows and knees as part of everyday activity may explain the common involvement of these sites with psoriasis. In sedentary occupations, e.g. chauffeurs, there may be intractable disease over the lumbosacral region. Scratching the skin when the disease is in an active phase may induce lesions along the line of trauma—the isomorphic response or Koebner phenomenon. Irritant types of psoriasis such as that affecting the scalp may be made worse by scratching.

Drugs

It is well recognized that lithium carbonate may induce intractable psoriasis. This agent inhibits adenylate cyclase activity, which may alter epidermal cell kinetics. Beta-receptor antagonists such as propranolol may exacerbate psoriasis through similar mechanisms.

PATHOGENESIS

The pathogenesis is unclear but a number of factors play a role.

Epidermal cell proliferation is seen in both the lesions and the uninvolved skin of psoriatics. There is a shortening of the epidermal cell cycle time and an increase in the number of proliferative cells in the growth fraction of the epidermis. Division is normally limited to the basal layer in normal skin, but may extend over several layers within psoriatic plaques. Polyamines are known to be important in regulating cellular proliferation, and the levels of these substances and of their rate limiting enzyme ornithine decarboxylase are elevated in psoriasis.

Arachidonic acid levels are greatly elevated in both uninvolved and lesional skin. Many stimuli which affect the cell membrane may cause a release of phospholipase and arachidonic acid and a number of inflammatory mediators are formed from arachidonic acid via the lipoxygenase pathway (see Fig. 12.27, p. 588). The major initial metabolite in the lipoxygenase pathway is 5-hydroperoxyeicosatetraenoic acid (5-HPETE). This is the precursor of a family of peptido-HETEs, including the leukotrienes, which can alter enzyme pathways that control cell kinetics. Leukotrienes also have marked chemo-attractant properties.

Leukotriene B_4 (LT B_4) levels are elevated in lesional skin and the injection of this substance causes an increase in polymorphonuclear infiltration. Polymorphonuclear cell infiltration of the epidermis and the formation of Munro micro-abscesses are an important pathological feature in this disease. A variety of immune factors may also attract polymorphonuclear leucocytes; these include immune complexes and complement fragments.

Both humoral and cellular abnormalities have been demonstrated in psoriasis, including elevated IgA and alteration of T cell function. The relative lack of sensitization to the common sensitizer dinitrochlorobenzene (DNCB) in patients with psoriasis supports the concept of a decrease in the cell-mediated immune response.

CLINICAL FEATURES

Lesions are well demarcated, salmon pink in colour and are surmounted by silvery scaling which may be exaggerated by lightly traumatizing the skin with the edge of a fingernail.

The majority of patients with a plaque type of psoriasis show involvement of the skin over the extensor surfaces of the limbs such as the elbows and knees, with scattered smaller lesions on the limbs and trunk that increase with exacerbation of the disease. Involvement of the scalp with thickened hyperkeratotic scale is common. This is most clearly seen at the hair margin or over the occiput.

The arthropathy associated with psoriasis is described on p. 355.

Flexural psoriasis

This is a less common type of psoriasis which may be seen together with plaques or may occur alone. Lesions have a pinkish glazed appearance, are clearly demarcated and non-scaly. The groin, perianal and genital skin are principally involved. Other sites include inframammary folds and the umbilicus. The condition may prove intractable in situations such as the inframammary fold of elderly females with large and pendulous breasts, or when associated with incontinence.

Nail involvement

This can occur in isolation with no evidence of psoriasis elsewhere. The changes most commonly seen include pitting and onycholysis, when separation of the distal edge of the nail from the underlying vascular bed produces a whitish appearance. A red/brown, salmon pink or 'oil stain' coloration may be seen over the nail proximal to the onycholysis. Less commonly the nails are ridged or furrowed. Hyperkeratosis beneath the nail is a pattern of the disease most often seen on the toe-nails, especially in association with pustular variants of psoriasis. When only one or two toe-nails are affected it may be difficult to distinguish from a fungal infection.

Pustular psoriasis

This may occur in various patterns and in children it is often an isolated finding involving a single digit. The nail dystrophy most commonly seen is yellow discoloration and thickening. Scaling may be pronounced over the digit and, in association with erythema, may spread over the finger.

In its most common form, pustular psoriasis affects the palms or soles with areas of well-demarcated scaling and erythema (Fig. 20.4). Pustules may appear white, yellow or greenish in colour and when dried are deep brown. Pustulation may not always be evident and it is often associated with increased disease activity. When the condition is grossly hyperkeratotic and occurs in a conical or papular form it is termed 'rupioid'; identical lesions

Fig. 20.4 Pustular psoriasis of the palm.

are seen as one of the cutaneous features of Reiter's syndrome (keratoderma blennorrhagica).

The trunk and limbs may be involved by an almost universal scaling as exfoliative or erythrodermic psoriasis. When this condition is seen in association with superficial pustule formation it is termed 'generalized pustular psoriasis'. This is a serious and life-threatening condition with all the problems that are inherent in managing a patient with widespread burns. Such a disease may occur spontaneously but it is seen more frequently after the use of potent corticosteroid therapy given orally or by topical application.

MANAGEMENT

The majority of patients can cope with the chronic nature of the disease but the physician must take an active role in treating exacerbations. Tolerance and understanding are required in helping patients to overcome the social stigma that may be associated with this disease.

Active treatment can be divided into regimens suitable for hospital inpatient or day care centres and treatment which can be prescribed for use in the home. It is unreasonable to expect patients to go through lengthy rituals involving the application of messy topical agents routinely or for any length of time at home. The discoloration of personal garments and bed linen may cause further social or domestic upset and so medicaments containing tar or dithranol, which stain, should be confined to hospital use where possible.

Inpatient regimens

Dithranol in concentrations of between 0.05% and 0.5% in zinc and salicylic acid paste (Lassar's paste) is applied to the lesional skin and is protected by wearing a tubular stockingette suit for 12 to 24 h. Repeated treatments are necessary. The application of this paste is preceded by a tar bath and minimal erythema doses of UVB (ultraviolet light of short wavelength). The intensity of the ultraviolet irradiation is gradually increased throughout the treatment period. Coal tar and salicylic acid ointment containing dithranol in concentrations of between 0.05% and 0.1% is applied overnight to the scalp and removed in the morning with a tar-containing shampoo.

Outpatient treatments

Short contact (minutes therapy) consists of applying dithranol at increasing concentrations of between 1% and 3% mixed with 5% salicylic acid in white soft paraffin. The ointment is left on the skin for up to 20 min and is then washed off. This type of short application enables these messy preparations to be confined to the bathroom of the patient's home. Regular use is quite often prevented by the degree of irritancy experienced and by the marked staining of the skin that is seen with the increasing dithranol concentration.

Dithranol becomes unstable when mixed with creams but it may be combined with some steroid ointments. Steroids can also be mixed with an alcoholic solution of coal tar. These combined preparations are especially valuable at low concentrations in the treatment of flexural psoriasis, or for patients with widespread lesions who experience irritation with dithranol applied in a paste form. They are cosmetically acceptable for use in the home. In the early stages topical steroids can be used but long-term usage of strong steroids should be avoided.

Pustular psoriasis on the palms and soles is often an unremitting disease which may respond to prolonged courses of low dose tetracycline. This treatment tends to limit the accumulation of polymorphonuclear leucocytes, a prominent feature in the pathology of the disease. The retinoic acid derivative etretinate, taken by mouth ($1 \text{ mg} \cdot \text{kg}^{-1}$ daily), is helpful in managing this disease; however, long-term treatment may be required and this can cause loss of hair, hepatic disturbance, hyperlipidaemia and hyperostoses. As it is teratogenic it should not be given to pregnant women.

PUVA therapy may improve or clear most patterns of psoriasis. Photosensitizing agents, e.g. psoralens, are taken orally 2 h before or applied topically 30 min before the long-wave ultraviolet light (UVA). Exposure for 8–15 min on two to three occasions each week usually results in clearance of the psoriasis in 10–12 weeks. Maintenance treatment is required every 2–3 weeks.

Troublesome joint disease may respond to non-steroidal anti-inflammatory drugs. If widespread intractable disease is seen in older patients together with painful joints, cytotoxic drugs may help alleviate both conditions. Methotrexate is the most effective agent for severe chronic psoriasis of the skin, and azathioprine has a greater effect on arthropathy. Patients may experience complete and long-term clearing of their skin whilst taking methotrexate once a week in doses of up to 30 mg. There is, apart from the risk of bone-marrow suppression, a relationship between cumulative dosage of this drug and hepatic fibrosis. It is unfortunate that liver fibrosis cannot be detected by routine blood testing, so that liver biopsies are required prior to commencing the drug and annually for those who continue this treatment.

SEBORRHOEIC DERMATITIS

Seborrhoeic dermatitis affects those areas of the skin where there is a high density of sebaceous glands. The cause is unknown and no alteration in the function of the sebaceous glands has been demonstrated. For many years observers have attempted to link the disease to lipophilic yeasts which are present on the normal skin as saprophytes, e.g. *Pityrosporon orbiculare* and *P. ovale* which occur on the trunk and scalp respectively. Bacterial infection has also been considered in the pathogenesis, but infection is probably secondary to the skin maceration. Neurogenic factors play a role in that patients with Parkinson's disease may develop similar clinical features over their facial skin and continuing mental stress often exacerbates the disease. Patients are often fair-skinned types of Celtic origin, and so genetic factors may also be relevant.

CLINICAL FEATURES

The scalp is principally involved and shows diffuse scaling and erythema. Papules and pustules may accompany these changes, or present as the only manifestation of the disease. The spread locally is to the eyebrows, nasolabial folds, the ears and neck. Blepharitis and otitis externa can occur as single features, or they may accompany more widespread disease. Other skin sites affected include the sternal region, the thoracic spine and the paraspinal skin, the axillae, the groin folds and the perianal region. Greasy scales, weeping and maceration are seen with more severe or acute disease. On the back a folliculitis may be the predominant feature.

On occasions the condition may be seen together with more typical eczematous changes elsewhere on the skin; the term 'seborrhoeic eczema' is often used to describe this.

TREATMENT

Shampoos that contain substances with a cytostatic action, e.g. selenium sulphide or pyrithione zinc, can give initial benefit to patients with a scaly and greasy scalp. With time the beneficial effect may be lost and it is a good principle to change the shampoo after 6–8 weeks. These shampoos tend to aggravate the scalp if there are marked inflammatory lesions and in these situations antiseptic preparations such as cetrimide or povidone-iodine in shampoo forms can be added.

A course of tetracycline in a dose of 250 mg twice daily before meals given for 2–3 months may lower the intensity of the inflammatory patterns of the disease.

Creams or antiseptic powders may help to improve areas of maceration of the skin involving body folds. Steroid creams should be those of relatively low potency, and preferably they should be combined with an antibiotic or antiseptic such as tetracycline or clioquinol.

Candidiasis may accompany chronic disease and imidazole/hydrocortisone combination creams often help.

LICHEN PLANUS

This describes a condition in which the lesions are:
- Purplish in colour
- Polygonal in outline
- Planar or flat-topped papules

The cause is unknown but some gross forms of lichen planus may occur in association with diseases in which there is a profound immunological abnormality such as myasthenia gravis with thymoma, and with graft-versus-host disease. Lichen planus occurs with certain drugs such as sulphonamides (most commonly taken as sulphasalazine), sulphonylureas and thiazide diuretics. Patients with rheumatoid arthritis treated by agents that alter immune function such as antimalarials, gold, levamisole or penicillamine may also develop lichen planus-like lesions or lichenoid rashes.

PATHOLOGY

A marked chronic lymphocytic infiltrate is seen on light microscopy at the epidermo-dermal junction. This infiltration consists principally of T cells and suggests an immunological reaction to an epidermal antigen. On immunofluorescence, immunoglobulin deposits (mainly IgM) are seen at the epidermo-dermal junction of most patients.

CLINICAL FEATURES

The distribution of the lesions is peripheral, involving the wrists and ankles, usually symmetrically. The genitalia are less frequently involved. Pruritus is a common feature. Less commonly the scalp or nails may be affected; with chronic disease the scarring that occurs may permanently damage the growth of the hair or nails. Scarring may also accompany the less frequent annular patterns of the disease. Linear lesions may follow trauma or scratching (Koebner phenomenon) or may occur in children in a naevoid fashion along a limb. Trauma to the mucosa overlying the bite margin in the mouth commonly induces involvement at this site, producing distinctive pale white linear markings or patterns. Erosive changes may also be seen on the buccal mucosa or tongue.

The presence of Wickham's striae—fine white lacy patterning coursing over the papule—helps to distinguish this disease. Post-inflammatory hyperpigmentation is also a useful diagnostic sign if the disease is beginning to fade at the time of first presentation.

TREATMENT

Untreated, common patterns of the disease may last for 18–24 months. Hypertrophic lesions on the legs or annular patterns may be rather more persistent.

Widespread acute disease is often associated with intractable itching and this may require oral prednisolone for control, given over several months. Less acute disease may be managed with the topical application of potent corticosteroids together with a sedative antihistamine given at night to control the itching.

PITYRIASIS ROSEA

This is a self-limiting scaling maculopapular eruption occurring principally in children and young adults. It has a characteristic distribution with lesions being predominant on the trunk and the proximal aspect of the limbs. The disease is less common in the summer, and current epidemiological evidence suggests an infective cause, most probably viral. Males and females are equally affected.

CLINICAL FEATURES

Commonly, a larger and more conspicuous lesion, 2–6 cm in diameter, will precede the more widespread rash by 5–7 days (the herald patch). Individual lesions are reddish-brown in colour, macular, scaled and discrete. They often course over the chest wall, following the line of the ribs in a linear fashion. The proximal limb girdle is also affected, but the face and scalp are rarely involved. Individual lesions, especially over the neck, may show a collarette, i.e. a border composed of a rim of scales that point towards the centre. Florid inflammatory papules may occasionally be seen, and individual lesions may be rather more hyperkeratotic on black or Asian skins. The eruption is only mildly pruritic and usually clears in 6–8 weeks without treatment.

Constitutional upset may be noticed prior to the onset of the rash or within the first few days of its appearance. This should help to distinguish the condition from secondary syphilis, which it may closely resemble but in which systemic features are usually more severe. Other common features of secondary syphilis are involvement of the palms and soles and associated malaise, pharyngitis and alopecia.

Acne vulgaris

This chronic condition is associated with the blockage of the pilo-sebaceous duct and appears on areas of the skin, such as the face, chest and back, where sebaceous glands are most numerous and active.

Superficial blocking of the pilo-sebaceous orifice at the surface of the skin is manifest commonly as a comedo or 'blackhead'; this may be associated with or followed by a variety of inflammatory changes.

INCIDENCE

The incidence of acne vulgaris appears to be the same for both sexes; lesions are evident at a younger age in girls and occur with their earlier sexual maturation. The disease is usually more extensive and serious in males. The majority of patients are clear of acne lesions by their early twenties, but about 6% of patients will have disease continuing between the ages of 25 and 40 years.

PATHOGENESIS

There is at the present time no unifying concept with which to explain the pathogenesis of the most common patterns of this disease.

Alteration of the sebaceous glands

The principal age of onset is at puberty when, under the influence of androgenic hormones, sebaceous glands hypertrophy and increase the production of sebum. A greasy skin and scalp usually accompany the polymorphic lesions, which are distributed on the face, chest and back. The secretion of sebum may, however, remain the same or even be increased in the twenties when the acne has cleared.

Microbiology

Propionibacterium acnes, an anaerobic diphtheroid, is present within the pilo-sebaceous duct, and has lipolytic enzymes capable of altering the local lipid constituents. The products of this organism's enzyme activity, principally fatty acids, have been obtained from within the duct; however, they have little inflammatory properties when applied to the skin of acne subjects.

P. acnes has been shown to alter the cell-mediated immune response and to stimulate the classical and alternate complement pathways. The local accumulation of complement found in and around the duct may thus be due to the presence of *P. acnes*. Pro-inflammatory mediators, also induced by the organism, are chemo-attractant and are capable of producing many of the clinical features seen with active disease.

The sebaceous gland becomes decreased in size and activity when isotretinoin (13-*cis*-retinoic acid) is used in the treatment of acne, and the numbers of *P. acnes* diminish in parallel.

There is no convincing evidence, however, that the numbers of this organism are altered effectively by any of the oral antibiotics that are used in the treatment of the disease.

Keratinization

The superficial portion of the follicular duct undergoes keratinization and an early finding in acne is an increase in the amount of keratin material at this site. It is probable that one of the several effects of isotretinoin, which can so dramatically improve serious acne, is that it alters this abnormal production of keratin.

Androgens

The effect of androgens on the disease are clearly seen in a number of young women in whom the disease continues beyond the teens. Up to 50% of such patients may show evidence of increased circulatory androgen levels, with raised total and free testosterone and/or lowered sex hormone binding globulin. The alteration of these abnormal findings with treatment may lead to the clinical improvement of seemingly intractable disease.

CLINICAL FEATURES

The 'blackhead' or comedo is the common first-stage lesion, the pigmentation being provided by melanin from the hair. In the absence of such lesions the diagnosis of acne vulgaris is less likely. Closed comedones or 'whiteheads' are flesh coloured lesions which are most commonly seen on the cheeks or chin, especially with incidental light or when the skin is slightly stretched. Such lesions represent a very firmly obstructed follicle and are often the forerunners of more actively inflamed papules and pustules. Alteration of the water content of the keratin plugs may occur with hormonal changes during the menstrual cycle or with the application of moisturizing creams, e.g. in 'pomade acne', when whitehead lesions become predominant.

The development of inflammatory papules and pustules will follow the release into the skin of the contents of a blocked follicle and the diffusion of chemo-attractant materials across the wall. The pustules are sterile and produce no growth of organism with routine culture. More marked clinical inflammatory changes may lead to large cysts, scarring and keloid formation.

Increased local trauma may cause exacerbation of the disease; this may occur with head-gear, the pressure of strapping across the shoulders or trunk or on special sites, e.g. beneath the chin in professional violin players ('fiddler's neck').

When unusual sites are involved, such as the forearms and thighs, with eruptions that resemble acne on a superficial inspection, it will be seen that there is essentially a folliculitis on closer examination; this can be produced by substances such as cutting oils in industry.

TREATMENT

Diet

The role of diet is not important in the vast majority of patients. If, however, any individual experiences a worsening of their disease after eating chocolate, for example, this should be removed from their diet.

Local applications

Mild peeling agents may be required for acne that is principally comedonal and not resolved by tetracycline. These agents are compounds that contain benzoyl peroxide in concentrations of between 2.5 and 10%, presented as lotions, creams or gels, alone or in combination with sulphur. Treatment should initially be with low concentrations (usually applied at night) with the concentration being increased with time and as tolerance develops. Erythema, dryness and scaling or peeling of the skin are often seen in the first few weeks of treatment and diminish with time.

Sunshine or artificial ultraviolet light also help the comedonal stage of the disease. Mildly abrasive and particulate materials are of benefit to a very few patients with non-inflammatory patterns of disease.

Topical retinoic acid in concentrations of 0.025% in a lotion or a gel or at 0.05% concentration as a cream is helpful in the treatment of disease which is principally comedonal in pattern. Washing with povidone-iodine surgical scrub, which contains a surfactant, may 'freshen' the skin and give short-term relief from greasiness.

Systemic therapy

Pustular and inflammatory disease will respond to oral antibiotics such as tetracycline, oxytetracycline, erythromycin and co-trimoxazole. Treatment with tetracycline 250 mg two or three times daily is often not effective until the drug has been taken for 2 weeks and courses should extend over months. Iron and calcium will markedly diminish the absorption of oxytetracycline or tetracycline, which should therefore be given at least 30 min before food. The absorption of minocycline (100 mg daily) is less affected by food but the drug is more expensive.

Topical antibiotics are an effective form of treatment popular in the USA. The only preparation which has been demonstrated in clinical trials to be effective and is used in the UK is 1% clindamycin in alcohol.

The alteration of abnormal hormone levels in women may often improve acne. The use of a suitable oral contraceptive pill in which the progestogen component does not produce androgenic effects in the skin may help over the course of 6–8 months or more. Cyproterone acetate, an anti-androgen, has been combined at a low dosage (2 mg) with ethinyl oestradiol (50 μg) to produce an oral contraceptive; this needs to be prescribed for periods of up to a year in order to gain full benefit in terms of the skin.

Severe cystic acne which is unresponsive to the treatments outlined above is the current indication of the use of isotretinoin. Four months of therapy in doses of 0.5–1.0 mg·kg^{-1} per day by mouth will produce a remission of the disease in more than 80% of patients for periods of up to 6 years. The side-effects are described on p. 910.

Erythematous lesions

URTICARIA

The term 'urticaria' implies intermittent transient swelling of the skin with a loss of fluid from vessels into the extravascular space. Dermal swelling is associated with weals, whilst subcutaneous fluid collection is associated with brawny lesions around the lips and orbit (angio-oedema) or the genitalia. Attacks may be associated with pruritus. The skin appears completely normal afterwards (within minutes or hours).

The passage of fluid out of the vessel may accompany the dilatation caused by mediators such as histamine released from neighbouring mast cells or by other vasoactive compounds such as kinins or prostaglandins. More severe vessel damage, e.g. the vasculitis associated with diseases such as systemic lupus erythematosus or allergic vasculitis, may produce weals in association with purpura and necrosis. On occasions, rather ordinary looking weals may be accompanied by quite marked vessel damage seen on histological examination. Biopsies should therefore be obtained when weals:

● Last longer than 2 days
● Are accompanied by purpuric staining
● When antibodies and circulating immune complexes are present in the sera
● When attacks are accompanied by systemic features such as fever or arthralgia

An aetiological classification of urticaria is given in Table 20.3.

Table 20.3 An aetiological classification of urticaria.

Idiopathic
Immunological mechanisms
IgE mediated:
Atopy
Physical, e.g. cold, dermographism
Antigen sensitivity, e.g. pollens, foods, drugs, helminths
Complement mediated:
Hereditary angio-oedema
Serum sickness
Blood transfusion reactions
Necrotizing vasculitis
Non-immunological mechanisms
Mast cell-releasing agents:
Opiates
Radiological contrast media
Antibiotics
Prostaglandin inhibitors:
Aspirin
Non-steroidal anti-inflammatory drugs
Azo dyes
Benzoates

Fig. 20.5 Urticaria.

Chronic urticaria

This is arbitrarily defined as disease lasting for more than 6 weeks. Weals that irritate are seen on the trunk or limbs and usually last for several hours (Fig. 20.5). There may be accompanying angio-oedema, and this feature may predominate in some patients; swelling of the genitalia is less common.

PATHOGENESIS

Many trigger factors have been implicated, including salicylates, indomethacin, tartrazine dyes in food substances or benzoates used as preservatives. Such substances may exacerbate the disease when it is in an active phase in up to 40% of patients. Cross-reactivity between substances, e.g. tartrazine and salicylates is seen, but searching for a food allergen is often unrewarding. A direct pharmacological effect on vessel reactivity is probable, and both aspirin and indomethacin are known to affect prostaglandin metabolism. Agents which can liberate histamine include morphine and codeine.

Type I hypersensitivity is more commonly seen with acute disease, in atopic individuals, and may be triggered, for example, by penicillin in milk. Even when no obvious trigger factor is found there is a tendency towards resolution of the attacks over weeks or months in the majority of patients. In a recalcitrant case an exclusion diet may be used as a last resort but this is often unhelpful.

TREATMENT

Many patients can be managed as follows:
- A sedative antihistamine is given at night, such as long-acting chlorpheniramine maleate 8–12 mg, or brompheniramine (long-acting) 12–24 mg, or hydroxyzine hydrochloride 10–50 mg.
- Non-sedative antihistamines such as terfenadine 60 mg twice daily or astemizole 10 mg daily are useful for daytime use.
- Angio-oedema will often respond better to agents with a wider spectrum of action such as hydroxyzine or cyproheptadine hydrochloride than to routine H_1-receptor blocking agents.
- The combination of an H_1-receptor antagonist with an H_2-blocker such as cimetidine or ranitidine may stop attacks when other treatments fail.

Acute urticaria accompanied by anaphylaxis (see p. 651), for example from bee stings, snake bites or less frequently from food ingestion or drugs, will require the use of adrenaline. Intravenous hydrocortisone or antihistamines may be given to limit the swelling when the crisis is over, for their effect is not seen for up to 20 min.

Physical urticarias

These may be produced by pressure, sweating, touch, heat, ultraviolet light or cold. These patterns of urticaria are uncommon and are most likely to be misdiagnosed. This is particularly true of conditions that are not easily reproduced in the clinic, e.g. pressure urticaria.

Cholinergic urticaria

This is not an uncommon pattern of disease and is seen in young adults. The weals are usually small, are often associated with erythema, and last 5–20 min. Attacks are triggered by exercise, hot baths, showers or emotional upset. Such factors may also cause itching but no obvious weals (especially in blacks) and induce stress and panic reactions. Large quantities of histamine may be liberated during attacks and cause difficulty with breathing.

Patients should be advised to avoid histamine liberators such as codeine or aspirin. If attacks can be anticipated, pre-dosing with hydroxyzine, cyproheptadine or a non-sedative antihistamine such as terfenadine during the day may abort a reaction.

Dermographism (factitious urticaria)

This reaction represents an exaggeration of the third component of Lewis's triple response. A livid weal is produced in response to scratching in about 5% of the population; it is usually asymptomatic. Symptomatic disease occurs when symptoms of itching or discomfort occur after trauma to the skin. Patients may experience marked erythema and wealing when, for example, towelling dry after a bath. Complaints of generalized pruritus with, on occasions, nothing to see may prompt doctors to label the patient as neurotic.

Cold urticaria

This may be triggered by wind over the surface of the skin, e.g. when cycling, or by cold objects in contact with the skin, e.g. taking articles from a freezer. The weals may be reproduced in many patients by the application of an ice-cube to the flexor aspect of the forearm. Anaphylaxis may accompany submersion of the body in cold water and patients need to be warned against bathing unaccompanied.

Solar urticaria

Ultraviolet light-induced weals may be seen on sites that are not normally exposed such as the upper arm, especially during the early summer; the weals appear within minutes of sun exposure. The action spectra is variable between patients and it may need to be assessed in order to provide adequate sunscreens.

Aquagenic urticaria

Contact of the skin with water may induce itching with or without weals. Symptoms may be reproduced by touching the skin with wet gauze.

HEREDITARY ANGIO-OEDEMA

This is a familial disease inherited in an autosomal dominant manner, and many patients can give an account of crises occurring in relatives.

AETIOLOGY

The disease is associated with C1 esterase inhibitor deficiency (see p. 117) which may be qualitative or quantitative. Clinical features may not appear until adult life. Another form of disease, which is not familial, has recently been described in association with lymphoproliferative disorders.

CLINICAL FEATURES

Severe airways obstruction that is unresponsive to antihistamines may lead to death, and visceral oedema may produce attacks of abdominal pain. Attacks may be preceded by a prodromal rash evident as mild erythema or erythema marginatum. Trauma to the skin, e.g. knocking an arm on a doorpost, may trigger an attack, for C1 esterase inhibitor is involved in the fibrinolytic cascade as well as in complement pathways. The disease must be differentiated from non-hereditary angio-oedema by identifying a causative agent. Swellings may last for up to 72 h and are painful rather than irritant. Purpuric staining may occur, but pitting oedema is not seen.

An analysis of complement levels will demonstrate a low level of C1 esterase inhibitor or its deficient functional activity on laboratory testing; C2 and C4 levels are also reduced. The disease can be differentiated from that associated with lymphoma, when C1 levels are also low and there is no family history.

TREATMENT

Inhibitors of plasmin such as epsilon amino caproic acid and stanozolol (2.5–5 mg daily) or danazol (100–200 mg daily) may be used for long-term treatment. Long-term usage in females may cause menstrual irregularity, fluid retention and androgenicity. Acute attacks may also require the use of fresh frozen plasma.

MASTOCYTOSIS

Mast cells are normally distributed in the connective tissue of the skin and other organs. There is variation in the morphology of the cells and some types are concentrated in and around the vascular adventitia. An increase in the number of mast cells is referred to as mastocytosis. It may be confined to the skin, or, less frequently, may be widespread through all tissues including the viscera (systemic mastocytosis).

Cutaneous mastocytosis

Cutaneous disease is seen principally in children, whereas associated systemic disease is more common in adults. There is a positive correlation between a late onset in adult life, extent of skin involvement and systemic disease.

Clinical forms of the disease which affect principally the skin are varied. Cells may be concentrated into a tumour, often a solitary nodule of yellow/brown colour (mastocytoma). This occurs on the trunk or limbs in the first few years of life and regresses after an interval of 3–4 years.

In urticaria pigmentosa, macular or papular pigmented red/brown lesions are widely distributed on the trunk and are more sparse on the limbs. These lesions urticate on scratching. Trauma to the non-lesional skin may produce dermographism in many patients. Attacks of flushing or irritation of the skin may follow emotional upset, change of temperature or be precipitated by drugs that release histamine, such as codeine or aspirin. The majority of cases occur in children and the lesions fade in late childhood, but those patients with an onset in adult life tend not to lose their disease.

Children may be born with or develop in early infancy diffuse cutaneous mastocytosis, and blistering may be the first indication of the disease. Later in childhood the skin may be thickened and leathery when markings and folds are exaggerated. Individual lesions are not seen and very rarely erythrodermic forms occur. Hepatomegaly and splenomegaly may occur with diffuse disease.

In adults an uncommon variant of urticaria pigmentosa occurs in which the predominant skin change is widespread telangiectasia. Pigmented lesions are small and macular and are associated with erythema.

Adults may show systemic involvement, with a spread most commonly to the bone marrow or skeletal system. Widespread dissemination may be associated with headache, bronchospasm, hypotension, tachycardia or intestinal symptoms, depending on the organ involved. The treatment is symptomatic and the prognosis is good in the majority.

ERYTHEMA NODOSUM

This is an acute and sometimes recurrent panniculitis which produces painful nodules or plaques on the shins (Fig. 20.6), with occasional spread to the thighs or arms. Adult females are principally affected.

Histological features suggest that this is a cell-mediated immune reaction. Immune complex deposition within dermal vessels is an important component in the production of the symptom complex.

A wide range of antigenic stimuli may produce this pattern of reaction. Infectious conditions in which erythema nodosum may be seen include streptococcal infections, tuberculosis, leprosy (papules rather than nodules which are disseminated widely over the skin), yersiniosis, tularaemia, blastomycosis, coccidioidomycosis, histoplasmosis, lymphogranuloma venereum, psittacosis and cat scratch disease. Sarcoidosis is the commonest association in the UK. Erythema nodosum also occurs in 5–10% of cases of inflammatory bowel disease. Drugs that may produce this reaction include sulphonamides, bromides and possibly oral contraceptives. In half the cases no cause is found.

CLINICAL FEATURES

Painful nodules or plaques up to 5 cm in diameter appear in crops over 2 weeks and slowly fade to leave bruising and staining of the skin. Systemic upset is common, with malaise, fever and arthralgia; the condition is especially debilitating when it is recurrent.

Fig. 20.6 Erythema nodosum on the shins.

INVESTIGATION

Investigations should attempt to exclude streptococcal disease, sarcoidosis and viral causes. The association with sarcoidosis is discussed on p. 603.

TREATMENT

Bedrest helps when systemic features and arthralgia are present. Non-steroidal, anti-inflammatory drugs such as indomethacin should be given to lessen the pain associated with the cutaneous and joint symptoms. Recovery may take weeks and recurrent attacks may occur.

ERYTHEMA MULTIFORME

This is an acute self-limiting and often recurrent condition affecting the skin and mucosal surfaces. There is evidence suggesting that circulating immune complexes are important in triggering the reaction in the skin, which occurs from 7–14 days following, for example, recurrent herpes simplex infection.

AETIOLOGY

Children, adolescents or young adults are principally affected. It is associated with:

- Herpes simplex infection (usually type 1) in about one-third of cases. The virus is a common trigger factor for recurrent attacks.
- *Mycoplasma pneumoniae*
- Drugs, e.g. sulphonamides, sulphonylurea derivatives (chlorpropamide) and, less commonly now, barbiturates
- Other infections, including vaccinia or orf, streptococci, yersiniosis, tuberculosis and histoplasmosis
- Connective tissue diseases or neoplasia (rare precipitating factors)
- Topical applications triggering allergic reactions over the areas of skin on which they are placed —erythema multiforme lesions occur at the peripheries

In half of the cases no cause can be found.

CLINICAL FEATURES

Symmetrically distributed erythematous papules evolve into concentric rings of varying colour. These are commonly seen on the back of the hands and forearms, but may also be seen on the feet or toes. The lesions may show central pallor associated with oedema, bullae formation or peripheral erythema. Alternatively, pallor may be accompanied by central erythema or purpura. Frank bullae represent epidermal necrosis and the separation of this layer. Lesions often spread proximally along the limbs or affect dependent parts in prostrated patients.

In the Stevens–Johnson syndrome there is severe erythema multiforme with a widespread bullous disease associated with oral and genital ulceration. Severe mucosal disease is seen with *Mycoplasma pneumoniae* infection. Peripheral lesions in the Stevens–Johnson syndrome may be few in number and difficult to discern.

Eye changes include conjunctivitis, ulceration of the cornea, uveitis or panophthalmitis, so that the opinion of an ophthalmologist should be sought in the early stages of disease. These latter features are often the most serious of the complications associated with erythema multiforme.

TREATMENT

The disease is usually self-limiting, but death can occur with the Stevens–Johnson syndrome. The withdrawal of offending drugs and the prompt treatment of associated disease is important. It is unlikely that systemic steroid therapy alters the outcome, and such treatment has been shown to be disadvantageous in children. Care of the eye and mucosal

Fig. 20.7 Pyoderma gangrenosum.

ulceration are important, and in severe cases intravenous fluids and feeding may be required.

PYODERMA GANGRENOSUM (Fig. 20.7)

The term pyoderma gangrenosum is used to describe characteristic ulceration of the skin that occurs in association with underlying systemic disease or blood dyscrasia in 50% of patients.

AETIOLOGY

The term 'pyoderma' was used to imply a role for pathogenic cocci in the aetiology of the disease but this has not been proved. Associated diseases are described in Table 20.4; these are diverse and give no obvious clue to a common pathogenesis. Paraproteinaemia, hypergammaglobulinaemia and hypoproteinaemia have all been described, but no constant abnormality of humoral or cell-mediated immunity has been demonstrated.

The pathological features include a massive polymorphonuclear cellular infiltrate but, despite the marked necrosis, no primary vascular damage is evident, nor have consistent abnormalities of leucocyte function been demonstrated.

Table 20.4 Conditions associated with pyoderma gangrenosum.

Multiple myeloma
Other paraproteinaemias, especially IgA
Sero-negative and sero-positive arthropathy
Inflammatory bowel disease
Acute leukaemia
Polycythaemia vera

NB   No cause is found in 50% of cases.

CLINICAL FEATURES

Lesions most commonly arise as inflammatory pustules or papules which appear on the trunk and limbs. They may rapidly enlarge over several days to produce large necrotic ulcers with a crescentic or polycyclic outline and sloughy base, which undermines a raised purplish prominent rim. Other patients may have a more slowly progressive indolent ulcer.

Less frequently, but especially in association with acute leukaemia, ulceration may be superficial and arise as necrotic bullae.

TREATMENT

Lesions usually regress with the treatment of the underlying cause, e.g. colectomy in ulcerative colitis. Rapidly progressive and painful lesions are accompanied by systemic symptoms and require doses of prednisolone 80–100 mg. Azathioprine may be used in combination or alone.

Tetracyclines, colchicine and clofazimine have all been shown to alter polymorph function and each has been shown to be of benefit in a few patients.

Indolent ulcers may respond to topical therapy and intralesional steroid injections.

ROSACEA

This chronic inflammatory facial eruption is manifest as erythema, often accompanied by papules, pustules and telangiectasia.

AETIOLOGY

Those most commonly affected are fair-skinned, middle-aged females, who often give a history of a ready flushing tendency which is triggered by a warm atmosphere, emotional upset, hot drinks, spicy foods or alcohol. Males often have more severe disease, but blacks are rarely affected with rosacea.

PATHOGENESIS

There is no cohesive view which can explain the combination of clinical findings and pathological changes. Gastritis and other gastrointestinal diseases were once thought to play a role in pathogenesis, but intensive investigation, experiment and therapeutic trials have found little support for this.

Histological sections frequently show changes which are interpreted as folliculitis, but a more constant feature is hyperplasia of the connective tissue around dilated blood vessels of the superficial dermis. This suggests that actinic (i.e. sunlight-induced) damage to the skin is an important component of the disease. The possibility that affected persons might be unduly sensitive to the effect of vasoactive mediators such as sympathomimetic amines, histamine and acetylcholine has not been substantiated.

CLINICAL FEATURES

Patients demonstrating the most florid aspects of the disease will have an intense erythema of the skin overlying the flush areas of the face, i.e. the cheeks, nose and chin. The presence of papules and pustules distinguish rosacea from the facial eruptions of systemic lupus erythematosus. The lesions are intermittent initially, but with chronic disease the erythema is persistent and marked telangiectasia appears. Other less common features include lymphoedema of the cheeks or lower eyelids and rhinophyma. In the latter condition there is irregular thickening of the skin of the nose and the follicular orifices are enlarged. The skin of the nose is bright or purplish red. In severe cases there is marked thickening of the skin on the surrounding cheeks. Rhinophyma can occasionally be the only manifestation of rosacea.

Approximately one-half of the patients with rosacea have a variety of ocular lesions. Blepharitis and conjunctivitis are the most common findings, but episcleritis, iritis and keratitis also occur, the latter being a potentially serious complication.

TREATMENT

- Factors that provoke facial flushing should be avoided.
- Tetracycline in doses of 250 mg two or three times daily for periods of at least 12 weeks will improve the inflammatory aspect of the eruption in most patients.
- Metronidazole may be of help when tetracycline is not effective, but care must be taken with the use of this drug over prolonged periods. Three months treatment at doses of 200 mg three times daily is often adequate.
- Hydrocortisone combined with 0.5–1% sulphur as a cream may bring some relief of facial discomfort. Recently, isotretinoin (13-cis-retinoic acid) at doses of 0.5–1 mg·kg^{-1} for a period of 4 months has been shown to clear resistant disease.

Rhinophyma is improved by shaving hypertrophic tissues from the nose, although regrowth of tissue frequently occurs.

Bullous diseases

Bullae or blisters are seen on occasions as an accompanying feature of common skin diseases such as eczema and as a reaction to insect bites or infection.

The dermatoses in which bullae form the primary lesions, though rare, are important because a significant mortality is associated with both the diseases and the types of treatment that are required for their control. Immunopathological findings are important in the confirmation of diagnosis, in monitoring disease activity, and for understanding the pathogenesis.

PEMPHIGUS

Pemphigus is a rare disease in which antibody, usually of the IgG class, reacts with an antigen at the surface of the epidermal cell that forms part of the intercellular cement substance. The interaction of the two causes proteases and plasmin to be released and the cells lose their adhesion and become rounded (acantholysis). Such cells may be seen when blister fluid obtained from skin lesions is spread onto a slide (Tzanck smear) and examined under the microscope.

The zone of separation within the epidermis may vary; in pemphigus vulgaris it appears just above the basal layer, whilst in superficial forms of pemphigus clefts occur adjacent to the granular layer. Nikolsky's sign consists of extending the zone of separation by light pressure or rubbing the skin.

Pemphigus vulgaris

Patients are usually between the ages of 40–60 years and are often Jewish. It is also common in India. Antigen–antibody complexes have been shown, on immunofluorescence, to localize within the intercellular substance of the epidermis, adjacent to clefts. Animal and human keratinocytes lose adhesion when cultured in the presence of sera from patients with pemphigus vulgaris.

CLINICAL FEATURES

Lesions may be confined to the mucosal surfaces in the early stages of the disease and in the mouth may present as bright-red, sore and denuded mucosa. In a few patients this may be the only site involved; more commonly, however, thin-walled blisters appear over normal looking skin elsewhere on the body. Such lesions soon rupture to leave moist eroded areas and secondary bacterial infection is common. When large areas of the skin are denuded, fluid loss and catabolic changes may produce severe metabolic disturbance. These metabolic changes may be compounded in the early stages of systemic steroid treatment.

Blisters may never be evident clinically in the more superficial patterns of pemphigus.

INVESTIGATION

The diagnosis is confirmed by the cytological examination of blister fluid, and by direct immunofluorescent staining of a skin sample obtained from the edge of a fresh blister. Fluorescent anti-human IgG and anti-human C3 outline the intercellular substance between the epidermal cells and the edges of the cleft in the skin which forms the blister.

Indirect immunofluorescence demonstrates the presence of circulating antibodies; the titres often reflect disease activity.

TREATMENT

Treatment includes general measures of controlling bacterial infection and fluid loss. Air beds are useful for nursing such patients. Prednisolone in doses of 60–100 mg daily or more may be needed to prevent new blisters forming, and drugs such as azathioprine or methotrexate may be required to enable the dose of steroid to be lowered at the earliest opportunity.

Bullous pemphigoid

Bullous pemphigoid tends to affect older people; most are more than 60 years old at the time of presentation. Direct immunofluorescence demonstrates staining of the basement membrane zone, and on electron microscopy specific antibodies are seen at the level of the lamina lucida (Fig. 20.8). Circulating antibodies can be detected in the sera.

Fig. 20.8 Section of skin to show sites of damage or immune deposition in lupus erythematosus and some bullous diseases.

CLINICAL FEATURES

The disease may begin with irritation and erythema of the skin occurring for weeks or months before blistering appears. Bullae then develop, often on an erythematous background but also on normal skin. These tense bullae, which are often secondarily infected, may be localized to one area of the skin (often the legs of elderly patients) or may be more widespread. Involvement of mucosae is rare.

INVESTIGATION

The diagnosis may be confirmed by the immunofluorescent staining of the basement membrane.

TREATMENT

Smaller doses of prednisolone than those required for pemphigus (40–60 mg daily) are needed to control this disease. Steroid-sparing or substitution may again be achieved with azathioprine or methotrexate and in some patients with dapsone 75–100 mg.

It is possible to stop all medication in many patients after 2–3 years of treatment.

EPIDERMOLYSIS BULLOSA

This is the name given to a group of rare and largely genetically determined diseases which vary from localized disease on the soles of the feet in one form, to infants born with a loss of skin from large areas of their body surface at the other extreme.

PATHOGENESIS

In epidermolysis bullosa simplex, the defect is within the anchoring fibrils of the basal layer cells of the epidermis, while in junctional epidermolysis bullosa the area of cleavage is within the lamina lucida. In the dystrophic form of the disease, separation occurs beneath the lamina densa within the superficial dermis.

CLINICAL FEATURES

Epidermolysis bullosa simplex
This presents within the first year of life, when blisters appear over contact areas of the skin such as the palms and knees; the soles often become affected when walking commences. Scarring is unusual.

Epidermolysis bullosa dystrophica
There are two forms of this disease:
● In the autosomal dominant form, bullae occur on the limbs in infancy.
● In the recessive form, bullae occur at birth and large areas of the skin are denuded with sub-

sequent scarring; contractures and fusion of the skin between the fingers and toes leads to syndactyly.

Epidermolysis letalis (junctional epidermolysis bullosa)
Epidermolysis letalis presents at birth with both mucosal disease and widespread erosions of the skin which often fails to heal. The child dies in infancy.

TREATMENT

There is a tendency for non-lethal forms of the disease gradually to improve through childhood. Protection of the skin and the prompt care of newly eroded skin may lessen scarring, but at this time there is no good evidence that drugs will alter the extent of blistering.

DERMATITIS HERPETIFORMIS

Dermatitis herpetiformis (DH) is an extremely itchy, papulovesicular rash which is symmetrically distributed over the extensor surfaces of the body. The unusual feature of this condition is that most patients also have a gluten-sensitive enteropathy, which is usually asymptomatic.

PATHOLOGY

The dermal papillae are infiltrated with neutrophils, eosinophils and fibrin. Later subepidermal vesicles develop. The major diagnostic factor is IgA deposits in the normal skin which can be seen on immunofluorescence. These deposits are usually granular, but in 10–20% of patients they may be linear, with the deposits lying within the basal lamina. Linear deposits may also be seen in some other subepidermal blistering conditions. The small bowel lesion is similar to that seen in coeliac disease (see p. 178) except that it is less severe and varying degrees of villous atrophy are seen; small bowel lesions are associated with the granular skin deposits.

Immunogenetic findings
The HLA markers and changes in humoral and cellular immunology are similar to those found in coeliac disease (see p. 178).

CLINICAL FEATURES

DH can occur at any age but is seen chiefly in the second, third and fourth decades. Erythematous plaques, excoriations, urticarial papules, crusts or vesicles appear on elbows, knees, shoulders, buttocks and scalp; the mucous membranes are occasionally affected. The lesions are extremely itchy and the vesicles have usually been burst by scratching, leaving encrusted lesions. The course of the disease is one of remissions and exacerbations. Patients can often predict an eruption 8–12 h before its onset because of localized itching. Gastrointestinal symptoms are rare, even with small intestinal lesions. Malabsorption is seen in less than 5% of patients.

INVESTIGATION

The diagnosis is made on the clinical and histological appearance of the skin, by finding IgA deposits in normal skin, and by the response to dapsone.

TREATMENT

Dapsone 50–200 mg daily will usually control the rash within hours, and on stopping the drug the symptoms promptly recur. Occasionally higher doses of dapsone are required. Maintenance doses vary, but patients can adjust their own medication to the minimal dose required to control the rash. Complications of dapsone therapy are rare and include haemolytic anaemia and methaemoglobulinaemia. Sulphapyridine 1–1.5 g daily may be used in patients who are intolerant of dapsone.

A gluten-free diet not only improves the intestinal lesions but also helps the skin lesions, leading to a reduction or cessation of medication.

Other conditions that produce blistering include porphyria and drug eruptions; these are discussed on pp. 936 and 937.

Infections

Some of the bacterial, viral and fungal infections that affect the skin are considered in this section. Most skin infections are considered under the individual causative organisms in Chapter 1.

BACTERIAL INFECTIONS

An important role of the intact skin is to prevent the entry of infective organisms. This is achieved by the following:
- The cornified surface on many body sites is difficult to breach and has a dessicating effect on some microorganisms.
- Surface long-chain fatty acids inhibit the growth of staphylococci.
- The resident flora on the skin surface can limit the growth of potential pathogens by the production of antimicrobial substances. This is especially useful on continually moist surfaces such as the flexures when the opportunity for invasion is increased.

AETIOLOGY

- Trauma, or abrasion of the skin removes the stratum corneum and allows infection to occur much more readily; *Staphylococcus aureus* or *Streptococcus pyogenes* are the usual invaders. A cleft in the skin can often be seen at the site of entry of streptococci, e.g. below the ear lobe when erysipelas ensues, causing cellulitis affecting the face.
- Viral disease or primary dermatoses may allow secondary bacterial infection, e.g. impetigo can follow a 'cold sore' or eczema.
- Other organisms which breach the skin include fleas and lice, and with subsequent itching and excoriation bacterial infection may spread. In patients with continuing bacterial infection (particularly children) an underlying disease such as infestation should always be sought.
- *Staphylococcus aureus* may form part of the flora of the nose in 20% of individuals. It can also be carried on perianal skin, especially in males. In the majority of infections, invasion of the skin remains localized to, for example, a hair follicle as a furuncle or boil. Toxins produced by staphylococci, e.g. exfoliatin are released by certain phage types and will cause separation of epidermal cells to produce toxic epidermal necrolysis. Toxic shock syndrome is associated with staphylococcal infection, serious systemic disease, widespread erythema and subsequent peeling of the skin. Erythrogenic toxins may produce a disease that resembles scarlet fever, which is induced by streptococci.

Staphylococcal infection (see p. 19)

Boils
Boils or furuncles are painful, erythematous, tender, papular lesions that are related to infection of the hair follicle and can occur on any part of the hair-bearing skin. They are most commonly seen on the neck, axillae, buttocks and thighs. Spread to involve several follicles will produce a carbuncle. Superficial infection of the follicle causes pin-point pustules over the face or legs, especially in children.

Follicular impetigo. Papular lesions may occur when the whole follicle is inflamed to produce sycosis. Sycosis barbae occurs when the beard area is involved. Less commonly, crusted, necrotic or scarred lesions occur on the scalp or face. Staphylococci can sometimes be isolated from these but the pathogenesis of such lesions is not clear.

Treatment of boils. Acute lesions should only be treated with systemic antibiotics if there is marked surrounding erythema or associated constitutional symptoms. When the lesion is beginning to 'point' then the overlying skin may be broken with a sterile needle and the area gently swabbed with an antiseptic, such as chlorhexidine or povidone-iodine.

Recurrent boils will require the long-term use of an antiseptic regimen over several months, including bathing with povidone-iodine added to the bath or washing water. Affected sites and areas of carriage such as the nose or perianal skin will require the application of an antiseptic cream or dusting powder. Family members may also require treatment if, despite the above measures, chronic sepsis continues. Similar treatment may be required for staphylococcal infection associated with sycosis barbae.

Impetigo

This crusted eruption commonly seen on the face of children may be caused by staphylococci, streptococci or a combination of the two organisms. Staphylococcal infection induces superficial bullae, which are seldom evident because they quickly rupture to leave a moist yellow crusted surface with surrounding inflammation. Typically the facial skin is involved and children are most frequently affected. Bullous lesions are less commonly seen and are associated with the same phage type of staphylococcus which produces toxic epidermal necrolysis. The reason why the disease is limited in some children whilst it becomes disseminated in others, is not clear.

Treatment. Care should be taken to prevent or limit spread of the disease in families or institutions. Areas should be gently bathed with an antiseptic solution such as hexachlorophane or povidone-iodine. Similar preparations in a paint or powder form should be applied to the skin after cleansing. Systemic antibiotics are prescribed if infection is widespread and there is uncertainty about the organism. Rarely, nephrotoxic strains of streptococci are associated with impetigo. Erythromycin or cephalosporins both give adequate levels in the skin when given by mouth.

Streptococcal infection

Erysipelas

This is most commonly seen in the skin as widespread erythema and cellulitis. The organisms gain entry through fissures in the skin, e.g. in a toe-cleft, and the skin becomes red, swollen and tender. Constitutional symptoms of fever, malaise and hallucinations often accompany the cutaneous features. With recurrent disease the area affected, e.g. the foot and lower leg, may become lymphoedematous.

Treatment. It is important to treat any underlying skin disease that may be associated with maceration or fissuring of the skin. Local antiseptics applied as paints or dusting powder should be used on areas of chronic fissuring. Foot soaks which are bacteriostatic and astringent, e.g. potassium permanganate 0.01% solution, might be prescribed when maceration of the toe-clefts is associated with excessive sweating. Recurrent erysipelas may require long-term prophylaxis with oral penicillin or erythromycin.

Ecthyma

This disease is not common nowadays in the UK. Chronic ulceration is produced by infection of the dermis and both *Streptococcus pyogenes* and *Staphylococcus aureus* may be isolated from the same wound.

Debilitation, poor hygiene or nutrition are important contributing factors. Often prolonged and intensive local antiseptic treatment combined with systemic antibiotics will be needed to heal the skin.

Erysipeloid

This is an acute infective disease of the skin. It is most often localized to areas which have been traumatized by contact with carcasses and bones of pigs, chickens or fish. The condition is therefore seen in butchers, meat porters, fishermen or rarely housewives. The causative organism is *Erysipelothrix insidiosa*, which also causes swine erysipelas, a serious and systemic disease of pigs. In humans well-demarcated blue/red discoloration is noticed on the hands, fingers or arms. This follows several days after laceration or abrasion and clears without sequelae. Rarely, fever and malaise accompany the common cutaneous presentation and cases of systemic and cutaneous disease resembling swine erysipelas have been recorded.

The disease is self-limiting and lasts about 7–10 days. If treatment is required then penicillin given for a week is effective.

Gram-negative infection

This type of infection may occur in moist wounds such as leg ulcers treated with occlusive bandages. *Pseudomonas aeruginosa* is the most frequent contaminant of such wounds. Astringent solutions such as acetic acid (1–2% solution) will often dry the skin sufficiently to discourage the growth of gram-negative organisms. Potassium permanganate 0.01% can be used as an alternative for bathing the limb or may be applied as a compress.

Debilitated or immunocompromised patients may rarely develop necrotic skin lesions (from which *Pseudomonas* may be isolated) when local vasculitis follows *Pseudomonas aeruginosa* septicaemia (ecthyma gangrenosum).

Erythrasma

Chronic localized pigmented scaled lesions of the skin occur over skin flexures such as the axillae, groin, toe-webs and beneath the breasts.

The organism isolated from such sites is often a normal commensal of the skin, *Corynebacterium minutissimum*. It is not clear therefore why some adults are especially prone to the disease. Excessive sweating and poor hygiene are frequent accompanying features. Wood's light examination causes the organism to fluoresce, producing a pink-red colour.

Treatment. Oral erythromycin will eradicate extensive disease, and the drying of macerated skin with imidazole powders or topical fucidic acid cream will clear more limited infection.

Mycobacterial infection

Cutaneous disease can be due to *Mycobacterium tuberculosis or M. leprae*; it is also associated with atypical mycobacteria, including *M. ulcerans*, which causes tropical Buruli ulcer, and *M. marinum*, which causes fish tank or swimming pool granuloma.

Infection of the skin with M. tuberculosis

This is infrequently seen in Western society where pulmonary tuberculosis is now less common.

Lupus vulgaris. This condition is the most common form of skin disease associated with tuberculosis. Two forms are recognized:

- Haematogenous spread from a reactivated primary lesion
- More rarely, following scrofuloderma, which occurs when the skin is ulcerated by the spread of infection from an adjacent infected lymph gland

Histologically, the cutaneous lesions show granulomas with central caseation. It is unusual to be able to demonstrate the organism from the skin lesions.

Sites of involvement are usually on cooler areas of the skin, with the face being most frequently involved. Erythema, scaling and scarring plaques are seen (Fig. 20.9). In severe intractable disease subcutaneous tissues appear 'gnawed' and hence the term 'lupus' (meaning 'wolf').

Tuberculosis verrucosa cutis. Primary inoculation of the skin with *M. tuberculosis* may give rise to warty lesions on the skin of young children who come into contact with infected sputum or on the fingers of surgeons or pathologists who handle infected tissue.

Secondary inoculation of the skin occurs from endogenous sources, e.g. at the site of the mouth from infected sputum (tuberculosis orificalis cutis); it appears as a plaque or papule.

Tuberculides. Tuberculides form a group of poorly defined eruptions and our knowlege of their pathogeneses is incomplete. It is probable that they represent a reaction in the skin to the haematogenous spread of *M. tuberculosis*. They have declined in parallel with pulmonary tuberculosis. Included under this general heading are papulonecrotic tuberculide, lichen scrofulosorum and erythema induratum or Bazin's disease.

Treatment. Lupus vulgaris and other forms of tuberculosis of the skin should be treated with standard chemotherapy for 6–9 months (see p. 602). Tuberculides such as erythema induratum will clear on the same regimen.

Atypical mycobacterial infections

The only infection which will be considered is swimming pool or fish tank granuloma. The organism causing this infection is *M. marinum*.

Skin granulomas develop where the skin is

Fig. 20.9 Lupus vulgaris with active granuloma formation at the margins.

traumatized against the rough surface of the lining or surround of a swimming pool, or over a digit, hand or forearm abraded against the side of an aquarium during cleaning. The latter is the more common nowadays, when the patient presents with a chronic papular lesion on the finger, usually with scaling and less frequently with atrophic changes. On occasions more than one lesion may be seen following spread along cutaneous lymphatics.

Lesions may clear over the course of months and routine antituberculous treatment is ineffective. Minocycline in doses of up to 100 mg twice daily for 6–8 weeks may hasten resolution of the lesions.

Leprosy (see p. 38)

M. leprae infection of the skin gives rise to leprosy. However, in order to lessen the stigma associated with the disease, the term Hansen's disease is often applied.

Tuberculoid leprosy. The organism may be confined to the primary site of involvement in neural tissue and from here there is a spread to the skin. Lesions are few and typically there are plaques with an elevated rim, dusky red in colour and with some central pallor. The surface of the skin is often dry over the lesion, hairless and insensitive. Local peripheral nerves may be enlarged.

Biopsy shows tuberculoid granulomas but no bacilli.

Lepromatous leprosy. Evidence of nerve involvement in the skin is often lacking and presenting signs may be in the respiratory system with nasal congestion. The plaques, nodules, macules and papules which occur are usually erythematous and multiple and have no appreciable loss of sensation. With untreated disease, the facial skin may become thickened and the remainder of the integument is often scaly and dry. Increasing nerve damage leads to loss of sensation, ulceration of limbs, loss of digits and muscle wasting.

Diagnosis and treatment are discussed on p. 40.

VIRAL INFECTIONS

Herpes simplex (see p. 52)

There are two types of herpes simplex virus (HSV) infection. HSV type I infection is most commonly seen on the lip or facial skin as a cold sore (herpes labialis). Type II infection occurs frequently on genital skin and is transmitted by sexual contact (herpes genitalis). However, genital infection can be due to HSV type I.

CLINICAL FEATURES

Primary herpes gingivostomatitis may be asymptomatic in children, but others can experience severe stomatitis associated with buccal ulceration, marked local lymph node enlargement and systemic features. Trauma to the skin may introduce the virus, as in gladiatoral or 'scrum-pox'. Damage to the skin over a finger may produce a herpetic whitlow.

Type II genital infection may not cause symptoms in females, especially if it is intravaginal. Vulvovaginitis causes burning irritation, dysuria and lymph node enlargement. Extragenital infection on the thigh or buttock can occur with myalgia and dysaesthesiae of the affected overlying skin.

Recurrent disease may induce systemic upset, with fever, headaches and meningeal irritation associated with the spread of the virus into the central nervous system. There is local dysaesthesiae followed after hours by vesiculation, weeping and crusting; less commonly there is local erythema and papule formation but no blistering. Depending on the degree of secondary bacterial infection, attacks clear, with separation of the crust, in 10–14 days.

Complications

Ocular complications. More serious and chronic disease can occur when the eye is the site of primary herpes infection or of recurrent attacks. Ulceration may give rise to marked local pain and oedema, and produce keratitis, scarring and visual impairment.

Cutaneous complications. Recurrent herpes simplex type I infection is probably the most common cause of erythema multiforme, which occurs 10–14 days following vesiculation over the lips, face or mucous membranes.

Typical target or iris lesions appear usually over acral skin on the fingers, toes, arms or soles.

Eczema herpeticum. Atopic individuals can develop widespread disseminated viral infection at any time. This does not only occur when their eczema is in an active phase, nor does it occur on every occasion of contact. Nurses and parents with active cold sores should avoid nursing children with atopic eczema.

DIAGNOSIS

This is usually clinical. Rarely the virus may need to be cultured from the vesicles and differentiated immunologically from varicella zoster virus.

TREATMENT AND MANAGEMENT

Local drying agents such as ether or surgical spirit will promote crusting and diminish pain and discomfort.

Povidone-iodine has a mild antiviral action. In an alcoholic solution or paint form (10% w/v) the astringent effect is a useful adjunct and secondary infection may not occur so readily.

Specific measures include the use of idoxuridine, acyclovir or adenosine arabinoside. Infection of the eye is improved by the use of local application of eye drops containing 0.1% idoxuridine or an ointment containing 0.5% idoxuridine. Adenosine arabinoside is available as 3% ointment. Idoxuridine 5–20% is applied to the skin in a vehicle such as dimethyl sulphoxide (DMSO), which aids the absorption of the active ingredient into the skin. The local applications need to be made at the onset of discomfort and for the ensuing few days.

Acyclovir, a thymidine analogue, is activated in the presence of HSV thymidine kinase. Toxicity to normal tissues is therefore reduced and treatment with this agent in severe local infection or disseminated disease in neonates, atopic individuals or those with immune deficiency may greatly reduce morbidity and mortality. The compound is available for local use as a 2% cream. In tablet form, acyclovir 200 mg five times daily for 5 days is a normal dosage for type I infection. This may need to be increased or doubled when treating type II disease. Parenteral forms of the drug are also available for severely ill patients and for disseminated disease.

Women with genital herpes should undergo cervical screening as there may be a link with carcinoma of the cervix. This should always be performed if their sexual partners have recurrent disease.

Varicella (chicken pox)

This is a common infectious disease of childhood occurring in the winter and spring and caused by the varicella zoster virus (VZV) (see p. 52).

Herpes zoster (shingles)

This infection usually represents the re-emergence of the varicella zoster virus from posterior nerve roots in the spinal cord or cranial nerves into the skin (see p. 838).

AETIOLOGY

This is a disease principally of patients in their middle years or old age. Factors which cause the re-emergence of the virus are often unknown and probably represent changes in the immune status of the host. The induction of an attack by local spinal disease or concomitant malignancy is unusual.

CLINICAL FEATURES

The prodromal symptoms of pain, tingling and dysaesthesia may precede by days the re-emergence of the virus into the skin. It then produces characteristic vesicles, papules or bullous lesions throughout the dermatome. Unusual sites of involvement such as sacral nerve disease may give rise to visceral changes and lead to, for example, bladder dysfunction.

Complications

Secondary infection increases discomfort, and in an elderly person intractable post-herpetic neuralgia may follow an attack of shingles. Trophic ulcers are sometimes seen over the face in association with cranial nerve involvement. Trigeminal nerve disease (ophthalmic division) can lead to infection of the eye. Swelling of the eyelid, conjunctivitis or blistering at the side of the nose require an ophthalmic opinion.

TREATMENT

- Drying solutions such as calamine cream or lotion are soothing.
- Antiseptic powders containing povidone-iodine or hexachlorophane may help to limit secondary infection.
- Idoxuridine 20–40% in dimethyl sulphoxide (DMSO) may be applied where practical to the affected dermatone on dressings which are kept moist with the compound for the first 3–4 days of infection. This treatment should be limited to immunocompromised or elderly patients with severe disease.
- Acyclovir 400–800 mg orally five times daily for 7 days, is now becoming the treatment of choice. Acyclovir cream 5% may be applied for less severe attacks.
- Prednisolone in doses of 40–60 mg decreasing over 3 weeks may prevent post-herpetic neuralgia in those over 60 years of age. Dissemination of disease is not seen with systemic steroids.
- Management of post-herpetic neuralgia is discussed on p. 838.

Orf

This disease is due to a pox virus infection which commonly affects young sheep, producing a pustular dermatitis. Vesiculopustular lesions appear around the mouth or feet of lambs, and persons coming into contact with the fluid from these may develop papular lesions on traumatized skin. Veterinary surgeons, farmers or their families and butchers are among those principally at risk.

Milker's nodes are produced by a pox virus which is morphologically identical to that of orf. Lesions are seen in farm workers handling the mouths or teats of cattle, and the organism may be carried by domestic cats.

CLINICAL FEATURES

Hands are usually affected. The lesions consist of red/blue papules, 1–2 cm in diameter, with a grey edge and surrounding erythema. Misguided incision of such a swelling may release antigen and produce erythema multiforme. Lesions settle in 6–8 weeks and immunity appears to be life-long.

Molluscum contagiosum

AETIOLOGY

This infection is usually grouped with other diseases caused by the pox viruses, but the virus is antigenically different. Atopic individuals appear to be especially prone to infection and in such persons lesions may be more numerous and difficult to eradicate.

CLINICAL FEATURES

Flesh coloured, umbilicated papules are seen. They are usually more than 5 mm in diameter, but the size may vary. Children are most commonly infected. In adults, spread often occurs with sexual contact. Irritation over the surrounding skin may induce scratching and further spread. Single lesions may occur and become quite large and inflammatory; the diagnosis may not be easy.

TREATMENT

The papules need only to be opened and the contents expressed; this often occurs with scratching. Silver nitrate or phenol may be applied or electrocautery or a hyfrecator (which seals blood vessels using a small charge of electricity but without heat) used. Associated changes in the skin, such as eczema, need to be treated in order to prevent scratching and further spread of lesions.

Warts

AETIOLOGY

The human papillomavirus (HPV) is within the genus papovavirus, which includes other species-specific viruses that infect domestic animals such as the dog, rabbit, horses or cattle. It has long been recognized that tumours induced in animals by this group of viruses may undergo malignant transformation, and the oncogenic potential for man is of increasing concern.

Types of virus
DNA hybridization techniques have demonstrated 32 different virus types, and immunocytochemical methods have identified virus particles in human tumours.

Previously warts have been classified according to the clinical appearance or anatomical site which they infect. It is now recognized that one or several viral types can be found in each of the clinically different lesions, e.g. plantar warts are caused by HPV-1 and HPV-4. The genus is divided into types according to the homology of the DNA pattern.

PATHOGENESIS

Viral DNA can be isolated from the basal cells of the epidermis, but the fully infective virion is only evident in more superficial epidermal cells. Cytology or histology shows gross disruption of the cells of the granular layer or below, which have intranuclear and cytoplasmic eosinophilic inclusions. Gross hyperkeratosis and parakeratosis are also associated with viral infection.

CLINICAL FEATURES

Common warts
Common warts are individual papular lesions with a coarse or roughened surface which are seen on the palmar aspect of the fingers and on the knees; other sites are less commonly affected. Children between the ages of 11–16 years are principally affected. Spread is associated with trauma. Many periungal warts are seen in nail biters, who may also have warts on or around their lips.

Plantar warts (verrucae)
These lesions are often solitary and are distributed over contact areas of the foot. When they overlie a bony prominence and are associated with marked hyperkeratosis, pain and tenderness when pressure is applied may be severe. Squeezing a plantar wart or verruca may more readily induce pain than pressing on the lesion and this is a useful test in differentiating a verruca from a callosity. Paring down the skin over a verruca will demonstrate a pit in the skin at which the surface markings come to an abrupt halt; they are, however, continuous over a callus. Maceration of the skin associated with sweating may induce many superficial lesions which form a mosaic wart.

Single filiform warts
These lesions occur on the face and at the nasal vestibule or around the mouth; they may also be seen over the face or neck of older patients.

Plane warts
Plane warts are flat topped and slightly rough on the surface, which is often pigmented. They are usually 2–3 mm in diameter and may require incidental lighting to discern their outline. The face, around the mouth and chin are the sites most commonly involved, and the hyperpigmentation may give children an unwashed appearance. Young women are also affected and lesions may persist for years. The backs of the hands and knees are sometimes involved and trauma may demonstrate the Koebner phenomenon at these sites.

Genital warts
Genital warts often have a fleshy consistency. Maceration of the overlying keratin mass may produce whitish vegetations. There is evidence for venereal transmission and for malignant transformation in both sexes.

In the female the vulva is most frequently involved at the introitus and over the labia; the perineum and perianal skin are less commonly involved. A thorough vaginal inspection should be undertaken in women with persistent genital infection or in those whose consorts have genital warts. There is increasing evidence to link HPV-6, -11, -16 and -18 with cervical dysplasia or frank malignant change.

Male infection involves the glans penis, prepuce, frenulum and coronal sulcus; the shaft and scrotum may bear sessile or flat-topped, papular warts.

TREATMENT

Spontaneous resolution is common and this makes it difficult to assess the value of therapy.

Keratolytics containing salicylic or lactic acid may lessen the unsightly appearance of common warts, which is peculiarly loathsome to so many patients.

Drying preparations may speed resolution if maceration of the skin over the hands and feet is associated with excessive sweating. Glutaraldehyde 10% w/v may be applied twice daily with a brush to individual lesions or wiped over the surface of mosaic warts. Soaks include formaldehyde as a formalin solution at concentrations of between 2 and 5%, or potassium permanganate 0.01%. Too strong solutions or too frequent applications may induce cracking or fissuring over areas of the skin such as the toe-clefts.

Destructive methods may hasten resolution by producing local inflammatory changes and enhancing immune reactions. These include chemical cautery, electrocautery and cryosurgery.

On some occasions curettage may prompt the resolution of painful verrucae but any scarring which accompanies such procedures may give rise to chronic pain, particularly when situated over pressure points.

FUNGAL INFECTIONS

Fungal infections of the skin can be divided into those associated with yeasts such as *Candida albicans* and others caused by dermatophytes or ringworm fungi.

Candidiasis

AETIOLOGY

Use of drugs such as corticosteroids, cytotoxics, antibiotics and oral contraceptives can predispose to candidiasis.

Local factors in the skin, such as maceration, may predispose to secondary invasion at sites such as the groin or breast fold, particularly if obesity is present.

CLINICAL FEATURES

Oral candidiasis
This is discussed on p. 155.

Cutaneous candidiasis
Maceration of the skin in body folds, especially in the obese, induces erosion and intertrigo (Fig. 20.10). In a similar fashion the wet napkins of infants may encourage opportunistic infection with *C. albicans*.

Paronychia
Chronic maceration of the skin is important in the development of paronychial infection. Commonly the seal or eponychium at the proximal nail fold is lost by continual immersion of the hands in water. A space is opened up beneath the nail fold and the continuing moist environment suits the growth of *C. albicans*.

Disease is manifest by a swelling or bolstering of the nail fold, erythema, pain and deformity of the nail plate. Greenish black discoloration of the nail plate often indicates concomitant infection with organisms such as *Pseudomonas aeruginosa*.

Fig. 20.10 Intertrigo with the typical satellite pustules seen with secondary candidiasis.

TREATMENT

An attempt to dry areas of skin, e.g. beneath the breasts by interposing an absorbent material between the two skin surfaces, is important. The routine use of a fine powder containing antifungal agents such as miconazole or clotrimazole as a talc after washing is helpful.

Specific antifungal agents used are nystatin, which has only topical activity, and an imidazole (e.g. clotrimazole or miconazole) cream, lotion, spray or powder.

In severe intertrigo it is important to incorporate a low potency steroid together with the antifungal agent in order to allay the inflammatory changes, itching and excoriation.

More serious and widespread disease in infants or those who are immunocompromised by disease or therapy may be effectively treated with oral keto-conazole 200–400 mg daily. The unusual but potentially serious hepatotoxic effects of this drug require that it should be reserved for very intractable or life-threatening disease.

Infection with dermatophytes or ringworm fungi

Dermatophytes or ringworm fungi are able to invade the keratinized tissue of the skin, nails or hair and include *Epidermophyton*, *Microsporum* or *Trichophyton*. The descriptive term 'tinea', which means 'moth-eaten', is an apt one and may be used in a generic sense to denote the pattern of involvement, e.g. tinea capitis.

The source of the fungus may be zoophilic (animal-to-man), arthrophilic (man-to-man) or geophilic (soil-to-man).

Scrapings taken from the skin and dissolved in 20% potassium hydroxide should reveal the presence of hyphae. A second sample is plated on a culture medium and incubated. Samples from nail clippings and hairs may be analysed in the same way.

Tinea capitis

This is now an uncommon disease in the UK. The organism most commonly involved is *Microsporum canis*, which is transmitted from the coats of dogs and cats.

Clinical features. Areas of scaling and hair loss are evident in children infected by *M. canis*, but at puberty changes within the hair itself limit infection. On occasions more marked inflammatory changes are seen with a boggy swelling in the scalp, surmounted by crusting and loss of or matting of the hair; this is called kerion. Scarring of the scalp which may follow such infection can lead to permanent hair loss.

Trichophyton species, *T. tonsurans* and *T. viola-ceum*, invade the hair shaft (endothrix) and often cause the hair to break off at the level of the scalp, producing a black dot appearance. More widespread and severe hair loss associated with a characteristic pattern of scaling in which yellowed keratin scale passes upwards along the hair shaft forming a scutulum or 'shield shape' is seen with the infection favus, which is caused by *T. schoenleini*. This organism is seen in the Middle East, southern Africa, Greenland and, less frequently, in Pakistan.

Diagnosis. Wood's light examination produces a greenish fluorescence of the scalp when it is infected with *M. canis* and other species that invade the surface of the hair (ectothrix).

Treatment. It is important to treat the animal source of infection. Spread from human to human is unusual with infection produced by *M. canis*. Griseofulvin is given by mouth and treatment may need to be prolonged for up to 3 months. Antibacterial treatment may be required for suppurative disease (kerion), either topically or by mouth, in order to lessen the risk of scarring.

Tinea pedis

This refers to infection which involves principally the toe webs or the soles of the feet.

Aetiology. The infecting organism is most commonly *Trichophyton rubrum* (colonies produce red coloration on culture). *Epidermophyton floccosum* and *T. mentagrophytes* are less commonly seen.

Occupations which produce maceration of the skin and communal spread include coal mining and working on a submarine, where warm decks and rubber soled shoes encourage infection. Athletic pursuits (athlete's foot infection), the wearing of occlusive footwear and swimming also encourage spread of these infections.

The disease is often intractable and *T. rubrum* infection may be especially difficult to eradicate, with the organism showing resistance to both topical and systemic fungicides.

Clinical features. Infection is mostly seen as:
- Scaling, maceration and erythema of the lateral toe webs
- Blistering lesions, often few in number on the plantar surface of the toes or foot
- Confluent erythema and scaling on the soles

Spread may occur to the palms (Fig. 20.11) or to the medial aspect of the thigh or perianal skin of males.

Treatment. Traditional foot powders often contain antifungal agents of low potency, but their drying effect is useful when they are regularly applied. Drying foot soaks such as potassium permanganate 0.01% solution may discourage infection by preventing maceration.

Fig. 20.11 Trichophyton rubrum infection of the right palm.

Specific measures include oral griseofulvin. This may need to be given for periods of up to 3 months for disease associated with *T. rubrum* in doses of 500 mg twice daily. Imidazoles (clotrimazole or miconazole) can be applied overnight as a cream and used as a talc in powder form by day.

Tinea unguium

This most commonly affects the great toe-nails but several nails may be affected. It causes discoloration, chalky deposits, subungual hyperkeratosis and fragmentation of the nail plate. Infected fingernails show similar changes (Fig. 20.12) but are less frequently involved.

Unusual trauma associated with occupations and hobbies, congenital changes or malalignment may also produce dystrophic changes of the great toe-nail. When several toe-nails are involved the differential diagnosis includes psoriasis.

Diagnosis. Clippings taken from the free edge of the nail should be sent for culture. Usually the same organisms that cause tinea pedis are found.

Treatment. Nail-plate infection will require systemic treatment for up to 9 months for fingernails and 2 years for toe-nails. Griseofulvin 0.5–1 g daily given for such a length of time is seldom associated with serious side-effects, but it may fail to eradicate the infection, even though the cosmetic appearance is improved.

Tinea corporis

Infection of the skin of the groin (tinea cruris) is not infrequently seen in males with chronic infection of the feet, so that both areas should be examined at the same time. An area of erythema and scaling is surrounded by a well-defined edge and is often studded with pustules or papules. Infection may extend over the perianal skin (Fig. 20.13).

Tinea corporis may be evident in older members of the family, while children are infected on the scalp. Annular, erythematous and scaled lesions are then seen on the trunk or limbs. More inflammatory, pustular and indurated plaques affect the neck or shoulders of farm workers who come into contact with cattle infected with *Trichophyton verrucosum*.

Diagnosis is by direct microscopy and culture of skin scrapings.

Treatment is with griseofulvin and local antifungal cream.

INFESTATIONS

Scabies (the itch)

This is a highly irritant condition occurring on the skin of an individual sensitized to the female mite of *Sarcoptes scabiei* or its products.

Mode of transmission

Transmission is by skin to skin contact with an affected individual and usually occurs in bed. Holding hands is a less common mode of spread from infested children. Warmth is necessary for the mite

Fig. 20.12 Dystrophy of the fingernails associated with dermatophyte infection (tinea unguium).

Fig. 20.13 Tinea cruris extending to perianal skin and buttocks.

or acarus to remain mobile, and thereby pass from one person to another.

Most individuals will only harbour about a dozen mature female acari. However, many thousands of mites may be associated with crusted or Norwegian scabies, and the affected individuals seem unable to mount the same sensitizing responses. This condition is more common in mentally subnormal individuals and those with Down's syndrome. Other immunocompromised individuals may also have large numbers of mites and this imposes a hazard for those who come into casual contact with them whilst inpatients in hospital.

CLINICAL FEATURES

Sites of predeliction for burrows include the finger webs, wrists, elbows, ankles, breasts and genitalia. Linear or curved tracts may be seen with a tiny vesicle at one end which contains the mite. The mite can be removed on the end of a needle, or the burrow scraped to reveal eggs, mite fragments or faeces as firm evidence of infestation.

Sensitivity to the mite products occurs after 4–6 weeks, when individuals develop most commonly a widespread, highly irritant, excoriated and often secondary infected folliculopapular eruption. Secondary eczematous changes may be evident, or the patient (especially children) may present with impetigo.

The diagnosis should be suspected if symptoms of itching are severe, when papules appear over genitalia and the history indicates that bed fellows, family or friends are also complaining of irritation. Infants develop papules on the palms, soles or the

axillary folds and some adults suffer post-scabetic papules for up to several months after sensitization. Mites from dogs or birds may produce vesicular lesions, crusting or urticaria but infestation from these sources is not associated with burrows.

TREATMENT

All infested individuals and their close contacts should be treated. A lotion containing gamma-benzene hexachloride (lindane 0.1–1%) must be applied to all parts of the skin surface save the face and kept in contact with the skin for a full 24 h, so that hand washing must be followed by re-application. The process is then repeated 24 h later and all personal garments and bed-linen should then be laundered in a washing machine.

Pediculosis capitis (head lice)

This condition is prevalent in school children in the UK, with infestation also occurring (though less commonly) in those who have close contact with the children, i.e. mothers. The head louse itself is difficult to find within a thick head of hair but evidence of its presence is seen in the many eggs or 'nits' laid along the hair shafts. The initial lesions occur close to the scalp, especially over the occipital region and the nape of the neck. In children, infestation should be suspected when excoriation is seen and impetigo is evident around the hair margin. Infestation occurs from the close touching of heads and is often widespread within a class of school children.

TREATMENT

The mite is now resistant in many cases to gamma-benzene hexachloride so that more certain cure follows the application of malathion 0.5%. This is left on for 12 h overnight and removed with malathion shampoo. Cutting the hair facilitates the use of local applications. Thereafter a second application may be necessary at an interval of 7 days. Eggs are killed by this treatment and it is not necessary to continually attempt to remove them.

Pediculosis corporis (body lice)

This condition is seldom seen now; it is usually found only in those with a gross lack of hygiene such as vagrants. The skin of affected individuals is often thickened, pigmented and excoriated; lice, often few in number, may be evident on the seams of clothing worn next to the skin.

Pediculosis pubis (pubic lice)

Infestation is evident over the pubic hair, with occasional spread in hairy individuals on to the body or even the eyebrows. Contracting the disease is often related to promiscuity. Irritation is the initial symptom and patients are able to detect movement of the louse over relatively sparse hairs. Treatment of the infestation is the same as that for head lice.

Arthropod-borne diseases

Development of these diseases depends on contact with the animals or birds who form the primary host for the causative organisms. These include *Cheyletiel-liae*, most commonly *C. yasgouri* or *C. parasitovorax*, from dogs, cats, rabbits and other pets. On close inspection of their coats such animals will often have evidence of scaling and thickening of the skin, on which mites are sometimes evident by their movement. Brushings are taken onto dark paper, which is then scanned for evidence of mites, fleas or their products. Bites should be suspected in those who have close contact with animals; the area of skin affected shows grouped vesiculopapular lesions.

TREATMENT

This must first begin with the elimination of the arthropod at its source. All other manoeuvres which attempt to produce symptomatic relief of itching associated with bites, such as repellants, calamine lotion, cream or antihistamines, give only temporary relief.

Cutaneous manifestations of systemic diseases

CONNECTIVE TISSUE DISEASES (see p. 339)

These systemic diseases often have cutaneous manifestations which are described here.

Systemic lupus erythematosus (SLE)

Photosensitivity is a presenting feature in about one-fifth of patients and may occur with a greater frequency as the disease progresses.

The nose, cheeks, forehead, ears and the backs of the hands are affected by the non-specific changes of diffuse erythema or maculopapular lesions; blistering may accompany more acute disease.

Alopecia occurs in three different patterns:
● Broken hairs, most noticeable over the frontal region, are the typical change and are the consequence of thinning of the hair shaft.
● Diffuse hair loss is associated with more severe generalized disease. There is an increase in the number of telogen hairs over the scalp and these are shed in the ensuing 3–4 months.
● Marked inflammatory disease of the scalp may induce scarring and a permanent hair loss.

More chronic changes on the backs of the hands or fingers include blue/red discoloration of the skin, reticulate patterning or poikiloderma (i.e. scarring, atrophic changes and vessel prominence combined with erythema). Nail fold capillary dilatation and ragged cuticles with haemorrhages are seen in this disease, as well as in dermatomyositis and systemic sclerosis. Loss of tissue over finger pads associated with Raynaud's phenomenon is seen, although this is a more prominent feature in systemic sclerosis or mixed connective tissue disease. Purpura and urticaria may be presenting features of SLE or they may accompany a more widespread vasculitis.

Cutaneous lupus erythematosus
This condition represents disease which is almost totally confined to the skin. There are two different patterns:
● Discoid lesions involving principally facial skin
● Widespread cutaneous disease, when the hands, feet, limbs and trunk may also be affected.

Arthropathy, Raynaud's phenomenon, haematological abnormalities, a raised ESR and normal serological findings are sometimes seen with disease which is seemingly limited to the skin. Patients with widespread cutaneous disease may develop SLE, whilst patients with SLE may develop chronic discoid lesions. It may be difficult therefore to decide whether a patient has just cutaneous disease or a systemic illness. Obvious ill health, high levels of DNA binding, hypocomplementaemia and a positive lupus band test (typical immunofluorescent changes seen on a biopsy, suitably stained and taken from normal unexposed skin) are important findings in SLE that may help to differentiate the two conditions.

Clinical features. Women are more frequently affected (female to male ratio of 2:1) and the peak incidence is between 40 and 50 years. In discoid LE the face, neck and, less commonly, the scalp are the principal sites of involvement. Erythematous scaled plaques, oval or round or contoured in outline may be seen on the nose, cheeks (Fig. 20.14), chin, sides of the face, or neck. Characteristically follicular plugging is seen; this may be demonstrated as spikes of keratin seen

Fig. 20.14 Discoid lupus erythematosus.

on the undersurface of a removed scale. Atrophy and scarring are common features and when these occur on the scalp, permanent hair loss follows. Although sunlight is an exacerbating factor in most patients, other forms of trauma to the skin, such as cold injury, may trigger the onset of new lesions or reactivate areas of previously involved skin.

Widespread, cutaneous disease may demonstrate similar morphological features, although scaling is not so pronounced. Reticulate patterning or smooth, shiny red/blue atrophic skin is seen, especially on the fingers or plantar aspect of the toes. Chilblain-like lesions may be seen at the same sites and on the heels or earlobes.

Treatment. Suitable protection from strong sun or cold should be worn. High protection factor sunscreens need to be regularly applied.

Hydroxychloroquine in doses of 200–400 mg daily during spring and summer gives extra protection from sunlight and settles inflammatory changes. Prolonged treatment at high dosage can produce permanent retinal damage so that an ophthalmic opinion should be sought prior to starting treatment and at regular intervals thereafter. Oral prednisolone is given for more florid cutaneous disease.

Potent topical corticosteroids may improve cutaneous lupus erythematosus; this disease is one indication for their application to facial skin. Treatment may need to be intensified when acute inflammatory changes affect the scalp so that scarring and permanent hair loss are prevented.

Other agents which have been used for recalcitrant patterns of disease include thalidomide, vitamin E and retinoids.

Systemic sclerosis and morphoea (scleroderma)

The term scleroderma means a thickening or hardening of the skin associated with an increase in its collagen content. Thickening of the skin also occurs in association with other conditions such as porphyria or the carcinoid syndrome. In these conditions the lesion is called pseudoscleroderma. The generic term 'scleroderma' should therefore not be used, as systemic sclerosis and morphoea are distinct entities. Systemic sclerosis has both cutaneous and systemic features, whilst morphoea is confined to the skin.

Morphoea

Females are more frequently affected, in a ratio of 3:1. It most commonly presents in young patients as a plaque of thickened red or blue skin, sometimes showing central pallor; the skin over the trunk or limbs is most frequently involved. A more superficial and widespread pattern of disease affects the trunk of middle-aged females. Children are affected by linear lesions seen on the skull and over the face; tissues underlying the skin may also be involved, producing facial hemiatrophy.

Plaques evolve to produce waxy, thickened skin which cannot be easily separated from the underlying tissue. Individual plaques may enlarge or new lesions appear over an interval, and resolution is associated with hyperpigmentation which may never totally fade. Involvement of the limb may be associated with widespread and severe induration of the skin, muscle pain and joint stiffness.

Generalized cutaneous disease is rare. It can, however, give rise to difficulties in bending and locomotion, and movements of the chest wall may be limited during deep inspiration. Softening of the skin occurs after months or years and is accompanied by slowly fading hyperpigmentation. The affected skin may show scaling, loss of hair and loss of sweating when the sweat glands are damaged by early inflammatory changes or by thickening of collagen.

Treatment. The early inflammatory changes, if severe and associated with oedema and induration, as for example in the leg, may be limited by systemic steroids and azathioprine. It is difficult to treat well-established disease.

Systemic sclerosis (see p. 342)

In two-thirds of patients, Raynaud's phenomenon may be present for years or even decades prior to the development of other clinical features. Severe ischaemia associated with this disease may lead to severe ulceration, gangrene and a loss of digits.

Typically the skin in systemic sclerosis is bound down to underlying structures and the fingers taper (known as sclerodactly or acrosclerosis). Fibrotic changes around the joints may produce flexion deformities and prevent fine movements. A binding down of facial skin may produce beaking of the nose, a fixed facial expression, radial furrowing of the lips and limitation of mouth opening. Mat-like telangiectases on the face or hands and some proximal spread of skin thickening complete the usual picture. Calcium deposits are sometimes extruded from the skin over digits (CR(E)ST syndrome, see p. 344). Thickening of the skin and pigmentary changes are often seen at the base of the neck or over the cervical spine and shoulders.

The disease may sometimes present as puffiness or oedema of the hands or feet, with preceding or accompanying attacks of Raynaud's phenomenon. A more explosive onset with widespread or universal skin thickening and more extensive visceral disease is less common.

Treatment. Severe Raynaud's phenomenon may be helped by charcoal glove warmers or electrically heated gloves. Nifedipine may limit the attacks. Severe ulceration or imminent gangrene may be prevented by the intravenous infusion of prostaglandin E_1 or prostacyclin. Dryness of the skin associated with hair loss, damage to sweat glands and sebaceous glands may respond to emollients and soap substitutes.

Dermatomyositis and polymyositis (see p. 344)

These uncommon diseases affect blood vessels, muscle and skin in a varying fashion.

Dermatomyositis when seen in childhood often has a marked vascular component, whilst disease in adults aged 40–60 years affects the skin and muscle tissue together. Proximal myopathy, often associated with malignant disease per se, and non-specific skin changes have sometimes been mislabelled as dermatomyositis. This misdiagnosis has probably given a falsely high incidence of associated malignant disease (10–25%), which can be seen in adults with dermatomyositis.

CLINICAL FEATURES

The rash is often very distinctive and may display features of photosensitivity. Fingers show ragged cuticles and haemorrhages with dilated and altered nail-fold capillary changes. Erythematous, blue plaques are evident over the dorsal aspect of the fingers, more especially over the small joints, with a similar but streaked appearance over the metacarpophalangeal joints (Fig. 20.15). Mild scaling may accompany these findings.

Scaling and erythema are seen at the elbow, and on occasions blue/red discoloration and reticulate

Fig. 20.15 Ragged cuticle and nail fold capillary dilatation associated with dermatomyositis.

patterning of the skin over the wrists, knees, feet, arms or thighs are seen.

Facial changes may include a marked erythema resembling sunburn, but inflammation of the eyelids or heliotrope coloration suggest the true diagnosis. Other exposed skin, e.g. the 'V' of the neck or the upper arms, may show erythema and sunburn-like changes which may also cause confusion. Marked cutaneous changes may occur in the absence of muscle disease. Typically, however, patients experience a proximal muscle weakness, noticeable when getting off a lavatory or combing the hair; dysphagia and respiratory muscle involvement are more rare.

INVESTIGATION

An underlying malignancy should be looked for. The malignancy may precede, accompany or follow the rash. Measurement of muscle enzyme levels and electromyogram (EMG) studies are helpful in the diagnosis and in following disease progress (see p. 863).

TREATMENT

The prevention of joint contractures is very important in the childhood pattern of disease and soft tissue calcification may regress with time. In adults, prednisolone with or without azathioprine or methotrexate is given (see p. 345). Sun screening and topical corticosteroid therapy may help to limit changes in the skin in those patients with predominantly cutaneous disease.

SARCOIDOSIS

The non-specific changes of erythema nodosum often accompany a mild systemic form of this disease in adults (see p. 603). More specific forms of cutaneous sarcoidosis occur in about one-quarter of patients with chronic disease.

The facial skin appears to be the site of predilection for limited forms of sarcoidosis as with other granulomatous diseases such as leprosy and tuberculosis. Red/blue or brown plaques, papules or nodules may be seen with chronic sarcoid or, less commonly, macular, annular or hypopigmented lesions. Micropapular lesions are common in blacks.

An uncommon variant of cutaneous sarcoidosis known as lupus pernio principally affects the nose with a diffuse bluish plaque, which, on close examination, will often reveal small papules within the bulk of the swelling or at the periphery. These are frequently accompanied by plaques or papules on the cheeks.

Brownish red plaques or papules may be seen on the forehead or cheeks. This is the most common specific form of cutaneous sarcoidosis in caucasians. In West Indians, the micropapular lesions are the normal skin colour for that group or darker and are distributed around the nasal alae within the vestibule, on the lips or cheeks, or over the periorbital skin (Fig. 20.16).

Widespread cutaneous sarcoidosis is often papular or nodular. Less commonly, subcutaneous nodules are found. Involution, occurring spontaneously or following treatment, may produce brownish annular forms.

Sarcoidosis of the skin may appear in old scars or on recently traumatized skin such as venepuncture sites.

Blue, nodular lesions, especially those occurring on the face, will need to be differentiated from lymphomas, particularly when general symptoms of weight loss or pyrexia are present.

TREATMENT

Most cutaneous forms of sarcoidosis will improve with increasing doses of systemic steroids. Drugs such as methotrexate or chloroquine may help in reducing the dose of steroid required. Intralesional steroids can aid resolution on occasions. Lesions may recur on withdrawal of drugs.

METABOLIC DISEASE

Diabetes mellitus (see p. 744)

Cutaneous abnormalities occur in more than 25% of patients with diabetes mellitus. They may be non-specific, such as infection with candidiasis, or so distinctive that the dermatologist may be able to predict the diagnosis of diabetes mellitus before symptoms have occurred.

Secondary causes of diabetes (see p. 746), e.g. haemochromatosis and liver disease, may in themselves have cutaneous manifestations and these features are described under the appropriate disease heading.

Necrobiosis lipoidica (diabeticorum)

The association of this condition with diabetes is unpredictable; 50% of such cutaneous changes occur in non-diabetic patients. Necrobiosis lipoidica is an unusual complication of diabetes and is not necessarily related to other vascular complications. Nevertheless, small vessel damage is thought to be a central feature of the pathogenesis. There is partial necrosis of dermal collagen and connective tissue cells and a histiocytic cellular response. It is more common in females, and presents in young adults or early middle life.

The skin over the shins is the site principally involved and pigmentary changes may cause the casual observer to associate the eruption with

Fig. 20.16 Micropapular sarcoidosis affecting the eyelids.

Fig. 20.17 Necrobiosis lipoidica.

venous incompetence. On close examination the features are characteristic; erythematous plaques are seen which gradually develop a brown waxy discoloration that is more evident when stretching the skin. The skin's blood vessels are prominent because of the associated atrophic changes in the dermis. Fibrosis and scarring from previous ulceration may also be seen (Fig. 20.17).

Treatment is with support bandaging. The use of an antiseptic powder or spray such as povidone-iodine is useful when the skin is broken. Non-adhesive dressings should be used. Low dose aspirin may help to improve the healing of such lesions.

Diabetic dermopathy
This is also a common finding on the shins of diabetics. Initially the lesions are erythematous and papular, but tend with time to become flat, hyperpigmented and atrophic. The changes are often seen in association with microangiopathy elsewhere. The pathogenesis of these lesions, which are not specific to diabetes mellitus, is unclear, although intimal thickening of small blood vessels has been demonstrated.

Diabetic stiff hands
This condition was first described in patients with juvenile-onset diabetes, but similar changes have been seen in middle-aged diabetics.

Tight waxy skin principally affects the dorsum of the fingers and is associated with joint stiffness that can limit extensor movements of the small joints. Histological sections demonstrate thickening of dermal collagen.

Scleroedema
This condition is seen as a spreading erythema and induration of the skin that starts on the upper trunk of middle-aged diabetics. These changes are often heralded by a respiratory illness or by streptococcal infection. The lesion may become generalized over the trunk, limbs, hands and feet, although the genitalia tend to be spared. There is a spontaneous resolution with time.

Diabetic bullae
This is an unusual complication of diabetes. Blisters usually develop over the lower limb, though in a few cases lesions have been described on the hands. They are of an acute onset and occur without any obvious preceding trauma. The disease has been described in patients with extensive peripheral neuropathy complicating their diabetes but the association is not universal. Histological section shows a cleft in the region of the lamina lucida but the cause is not known.

Granuloma annulare
This presents as flesh-coloured papules in annular or crescentic configurations, principally over the extensor surface of the joints of the fingers (Fig. 20.18). The feet, ankles, hands and wrists may be similarly affected. A disseminated pattern involves principally sun-exposed skin and is probably triggered by sunlight.

The association of such lesions with diabetes mellitus remains controversial; a few cases do not

Fig. 20.18 Granuloma annulare.

have overt diabetes but only impaired glucose tolerance. The pathology is similar to necrobiosis lipoidica.

Eruptive xanthomas

These may appear suddenly as crops of yellow papules on the knees, elbows, back and the buttocks. They are associated with hyperlipidaemia (see p. 771) and are particularly common in diabetics. They resolve with the control of the diabetes and hyperlipidaemia.

Other skin disorders

Infections and lipodystrophies are often seen in diabetes mellitus; they are discussed on p. 766.

Porphyria cutanea tarda (see p. 779)

Only the changes seen in porphyria cutanea tarda are considered here. Similar changes in the skin may be seen with variegate porphyria and hereditary coproporphyria (see p. 779).

Cutaneous lesions occur on exposure to sunlight. These consist of increased fragility of the skin over the dorsum of the hands, fingers and face and are associated with erythema, blistering and scarring (Fig. 20.19). Hypertrichosis on the sides of the face and between the eyebrows and hair margin is common and may be associated with facial skin thickening and loss of hair (pseudoscleroderma). Hyperpigmentation or loss of pigment may also be seen on the facial skin. Itching may be troublesome.

The diagnosis and treatment are discussed on p. 779.

Cutaneous amyloidosis

Amyloidosis is discussed on p. 323.

Cutaneous forms of the disease may be widespread on the skin and mucosal surfaces or localized to particular areas. The skin is involved in about 40% of patients who have systemic amyloidosis in association with diseases such as myelomatosis.

The gums may appear nodular and waxy and bleed easily on trauma. Pale yellow-brown papules may appear over the basal conjunctivae and at other mucosal sites and purpura is seen following mild trauma.

Sites of predilection elsewhere on the skin include the eyelids, the nasolabial folds, the sides of the neck, and the flexural surfaces. Thickened indurated plaques may rarely affect the chest, abdomen or hands. Cutaneous disease is rare in the hereditofamilial patterns of disease.

Cutaneous disease where there is no evidence of systemic spread is seen in two forms: macular and lichen amyloidosis.

Macular amyloidosis

Macular amyloidosis is quite commonly seen on the shoulders, neck or upper back of patients of Asian origin. The hyperpigmented macular changes have a rippled appearance likened to the changes seen on a sandy beach at low tide. Patients are only normally concerned about the appearance of the lesions, which are dark grey/black in colour. The amyloid material is difficult to demonstrate on histology using routine methods.

Lichen amyloidosis

Lichen amyloidosis is an uncommon papular eruption which is often pruritic and occurs on the lower limbs. There is no explanation for the appearance of the amyloid material at this site. Other pruritic diseases on the lower legs are often hypertrophic, especially in patients of African or Asian origin. Diseases such as hypertrophic lichen planus and lichen simplex may resemble the disease on routine

Fig. 20.19 Scarring and blister formation seen with porphyria cutanea tarda.

inspection. Close examination should, however, distinguish these diseases. The shiny warty close-set papules of lichen amyloidosis are characteristic of the disease.

CNS-RELATED DISEASES

The number of dermatoses that have been associated with diseases of the nervous system is large but most are extremely rare.

Neurofibromatosis (see p. 854)

This condition is inherited as an autosomal dominant disease but spontaneous mutation is not uncommon. Incomplete forms are seen, and the clinical features tend to follow a familial pattern.

The neurofibromas arise from peripheral or cranial nerves and from the spinal roots. They are composed of proliferating Schwann cells and fibroblasts.

CLINICAL FEATURES

The characteristic features are cutaneous hyperpigmentation (café-au-lait spots) and flesh-coloured smooth polypoid swellings, i.e. neurofibromas. Molluscum fibrosum (skin tags) are sessile pink-coloured tumours which are often numerous over the trunk. Plexiform neuromas are uncommon and tend to follow the course of a nerve, usually on the face or neck. In some areas there is overgrowth of skin and subcutaneous tissue in addition and this may give rise to gross disfigurement (elephantiasis neuromatosa).

Oral lesions occur in up to 10% of patients; skeletal abnormalities, e.g. kyphoscoliosis, may also be present. The formation of neurofibromas within cranial nerves may result in space-occupying lesions, e.g. an acoustic neuroma. Sarcomas may occur within such lesions and there is an increased incidence of all neural tumours. Associated endocrine diseases include phaeochromocytoma, Addison's disease, hyperparathyroidism and acromegaly.

Café-au-lait spots may suggest the diagnosis in children, but there should be more than five in number to support it. The pigmentary changes must be differentiated from those seen in Albright's syndrome (see p. 696). In neurofibromatosis the café-au-lait spots show histologically the presence of giant melanosomes; these are rare in Albright's disease.

Tuberous sclerosis (epiloia) (see p. 854)

The cutaneous lesions in tuberous sclerosis are derived from connective tissue and are of several different types.

CLINICAL FEATURES

Adenoma sebaceum are erythematous papules or nodules on the cheeks or within the folds at the sides of the mouth or nose. The tumours are vascular and fibrous in origin; the term 'adenoma' used to describe them is therefore inappropriate. Periungual fibromas occur as pink firm claw-like tumours arising from and around the nail folds.

Shagreen patches are flesh-coloured tumours which are firm and plaque-like. They often have a wrinkled surface and are most frequently seen over the lumbosacral region.

Areas of macular hypopigmentation occur in ovoid or leaf-like shapes. They may be seen over the trunk or back and are most easily detected by Wood's light examination. They appear early in childhood, associated in many cases with mental retardation, so that their presence may help to suggest the diagnosis of epiloia in a retarded infant. Some degree of mental deficiency is present in up to 60% of cases; this feature is often associated with epilepsy.

TREATMENT

Small erythematous papules on the face and cheeks may be treated with an electrical hyfrecator or cautery.

Other CNS-related diseases

Naevoid lesions may be seen in conjunction with neurological disease; for example in the epidermal naevus syndrome pigmented naevi occur in a linear fashion on the limb or trunk and may be associated with epilepsy or mental retardation.

Gross ichthyotic changes may occur on the skin of patients with spastic diplegia and mental retardation in the Sjögren–Larsson syndrome.

Drug eruptions

Skin rashes account for one-third of all side-effects of drugs. It is sometimes difficult to differentiate an eruption due to a drug from one produced by the underlying illness itself. On occasions the effects of both are relevant to the onset of the rash, for example patients prescribed ampicillin for infectious mononucleosis will almost always develop a widespread eruption.

Patients often take many drugs together and it may be difficult to incriminate one agent in the production of the rash. In vitro testing of drugs in these situations is inadequate in establishing or predicting the likelihood of the drug causing the cutaneous side-effect.

Only common eruptions or conditions in which there is some understanding of underlying mechanisms will be considered here.

Urticaria (see p. 913)

Urticaria may be associated with a type I reaction and anaphylaxis in patients who are hypersensitive, for example, to penicillin. Some drugs and diagnostic agents may release histamine directly. These include:

- Codeine, opiates, and tubocurarine
- Radiological contrast media
- Aspirin and non-steroidal anti-inflammatory drugs, e.g. indomethacin may trigger blood vessel hyper-reactivity by affecting the metabolism of arachidonic acid metabolites

Allergic vasculitis

Allergic vasculitis may accompany a wide range of diseases, including streptococcal infection, connective tissue diseases and malignancy. Drugs that produce this condition may activate the alternative pathway of complement or produce cryoglobulins and immune complexes in the serum. Antibody, principally IgA, may be deposited around damaged vessels in the kidney and skin. Purpuric lesions appear most frequently on the extremities and may be accompanied by urticaria, blisters, necrosis of the skin and ulceration.

Drugs that have been associated with this disease include allopurinol, sulphonamides, gold, hydralazine, quinidine and methyldopa.

Purpura

Purpura may be seen following drug-induced thrombocytopenia (p. 296) or severe bone marrow suppression. Drugs may combine with the platelets to form an antigen; antibody formation follows, leading to platelet destruction.

Erythema nodosum and erythema multiforme

Erythema nodosum and erythema multiforme may be induced by drugs; these are considered on p. 916.

Morbilliform eruptions

These are the commonest type of drug eruption. They usually occur 1 week after starting the medication and are widespread on the trunk and over pressure sites such as the thighs, knees and elbows. Diffuse erythema may be accompanied by pruritus and followed by desquamation. An accompanying fever may cause confusion with viral illnesses. Paired sera for viral antibodies may help to establish the correct diagnosis in retrospect.

Ampicillin, amoxycillin, sulphonamides and barbiturates are agents most likely to induce this type of reaction.

Lichen-planus-like or lichenoid eruptions

These are discussed on p. 911.

Photo-sensitizing agents

These are discussed on p. 945.

Toxic epidermal necrolysis

This is the most serious type of drug-induced disease. It can be distinguished on histological grounds from the condition seen in children which produces a similar clinical picture and is induced by staphylococci (see p. 921). The agents most likely to cause such disease are sulphonamides, allopurinol and barbiturates.

Fixed drug eruption

The pathogenesis of this type of reaction is unknown. The face, hands and genitalia are most commonly affected. Bright red, sometimes purpuric or even blistered plaques or annular lesions are seen. An accompanying burning discomfort is present. The lesions are fixed in site and appear within hours of the offending drug's administration. They will occur at exactly the same sites if the drug is given again at another time. Post-inflammatory hyperpigmentation is a striking feature.

Phenolphthalein in laxatives or as a colouring in sweets is a common cause. Other agents include tetracycline, sulphonamides, phenacetin, salicylates and the oral contraceptive pill.

Pigmentation

Pigmentation that occurs with oral agents is considered below (see p. 944).

Exacerbation of pre-existing skin diseases

Pre-existing skin diseases may be exacerbated by drugs. Examples include lithium carbonate, which will exacerbate psoriasis.

Lupus erythematosus-like rash

This can be produced by drugs such as hydralazine, phenytoin, penicillamine and isoniazid. The lesions are often reversed on stopping the drug.

Skin tumours

The skin is a prime target for aberrant growth and tumour formation. It may be in direct contact with ionizing radiation and many chemical substances that act as inducers of abnormal cellular activity. There are also a large number of different cell types within the skin.

Many skin tumours are rare and in practice are confined to a few types.

Melanocytic naevus (naevocytic naevus)

This is a tumour produced by cells of neural crest origin, usually melanocytes. Schwann cells may also contribute to the dermal aspect of these lesions. This is the most common type of skin tumour. It is pigmented and is referred to as a 'mole' in lay terms.

These tumours originate as a proliferation of melanocytes at the epidermo-dermal junction, so that clinically little growth above the skin surface is seen at this stage (junctional naevus). Such lesions may be present in childhood but they appear more obvious and increase their numbers with puberty. Sun-sensitive individuals tend to produce greater numbers, particularly on exposed areas of skin. There is therefore a greater number over the lateral aspect of the arm compared with the medial side. Pregnancy will also increase the numbers of naevi and the degree of hyperpigmentation. With time, cells migrate downwards into the dermis and their bulk increases so that tumours become elevated above the skin surface. Both an epidermal and dermal component are now seen (compound naevus). Gradually the epidermal component becomes less evident and the tumour becomes a cellular naevus; fibrotic changes and a loss of pigment may then cause a lesion to become less evident or disappear. The average count of melanocytic naevi on a caucasian from the Western hemisphere is more than a dozen by the third decade. Junctional naevi and malignant melanomas should be differentiated by the even degree of pigmentation, the smoothness of the overlying epidermis and lack of symptoms in the former.

Congenital melanocytic naevi may cover large areas of the skin as a bathing trunk naevus. These have an irregular surface and an irregular degree of pigmentation. There is an increased potential for malignant change with larger lesions.

Juvenile melanoma (Spitz naevus)

These are solitary pink or reddish brown lesions on the face or limbs of children. A history of rapid growth is given and for this reason they are often removed.

A proliferation of naevus cells in the dermis may give rise to blue discoloration of the skin. The 'mongolian spot' in children represents a more diffuse spread of such cells. When these are localized to form a slightly elevated papule, especially in adults, they are called a 'blue naevus'.

Lentigo maligna

Lentigo maligna represents an increased number of melanocytes at the epidermo-dermal junction. It is a premalignant condition and begins as a flat freckle-like lesion which in time changes colour and pattern as it grows. It is a precursor of malignant melanoma.

Basal cell papilloma (seborrhoeic wart)

This is a benign proliferation of basal cells which produces a raised lesion with a varying degree of pigmentation. The numbers of these tumours increase with age. The consistency is often greasy and this aspect has led to the misnomer 'seborrhoeic wart'—the lesions are *not* related to sebaceous tissue growth. 'Senile wart' is another unacceptable term because the lesions may be seen in young adults.

The face and trunk are the sites most commonly affected. Marked hyperpigmentation may cause confusion with malignant melanoma. Maceration of these tumours from sweating may, in summer-time, lead to irritation. The numbers present on the trunk may prohibit their removal in some patients, but readily traumatized or irritant lesions can be removed with a curette and the base cauterized, or they may be frozen with liquid nitrogen.

Keratoacanthoma

This rapidly growing tumour of the epidermis arises most commonly on the skin of the hand and face. The aetiology is unknown; it is possible that trauma initiates the event and there is often evidence of chronic actinic damage of the surrounding skin (Fig. 20.20).

The lesions are often pale or flesh-coloured, well demarcated papules and on occasions appear inflammatory. Usually 0.5–1 cm in diameter, they may reach 3–4 cm across in giant lesions. The increase in size is rapid and often alarming to the patient. The greatest diameter is attained in 4–8 weeks; involution then occurs and the centre becomes a keratinous crater. Regression may then become complete over several months but, since a ragged scar may be left, it is often better to remove the tumour by curettage.

Fig. 20.20 Keratoacanthoma occurring on chronically sun-damaged skin.

Histological sections may reveal changes that are difficult to differentiate from a squamous carcinoma.

Angiomas

Capillary naevus (naevus flammeus)

This is associated with a proliferation of capillaries in the superficial dermal capillary plexus. The salmon-coloured patch may be seen on the face or more commonly on the nape of the neck in up to 40% of infants. They may be slow to fade from the latter site and are often covered by hair. Facial lesions occur on the glabella, forehead and eyelids and tend to fade away in the first year of life.

Port-wine stain

This is a tumour present at birth that consists of dilated capillary vessels with endothelial cell lining. The face and neck are most commonly affected and there is no natural regression with age. Those patients who experience such growths around the orbit may have in addition a proliferation of vessels on the meninges (Sturge–Weber syndrome) and neurological defects.

Camouflage is the only practical method of managing such lesions. Laser therapy is time consuming, is only available at a few centres and the best results appear to follow the treatment of such naevi in adults.

Cavernous haemangioma (strawberry naevus)

This tumour is not present at birth, but usually appears in the first month of life. Lesions are often well circumscribed, round and lobulated and are usually seen on the face, neck or trunk. Growth continues in the first year in many patients; this is followed by slow involution which is complete in the majority by 4–5 years, so that reassurance is often all that is required. Gross lesions warrant attempts at treatment when, for example, they obstruct the eye and threaten the development of binocular vision. The bulk of such tumours may be reduced by systemic steroids. Some naevi show features of both capillary and cavernous tissue within a single tumour.

Cherry angioma (Campbell de Morgan's spot)

Campbell de Morgan's spots are angiokeratomas that appear as pin-point lesions or naevi of several millimetres in diameter on the trunk or limbs with an increasing frequency throughout middle-age. Treatment is only required for cosmetic reasons; cautery or diathermy is effective.

Pyogenic granuloma

This tumour is a proliferation of dermal vasculature so that the term pyogenic granuloma is a misnomer. Often trauma will initiate this growth on the finger or elsewhere on the skin. In children the trunk is a common site of involvement and there is a tendency for recurrence here from a deep-feeding vascular channel. Bleeding after trauma is a troublesome and worrying feature for some patients, and older lesions may become fibrotic. Treatment is by curettage and cautery.

Epidermal naevus

This may appear as a single lesion unassociated with any other developmental abnormality or may occur in association with, for example, neurological defects as part of a syndrome. Histologically, there is a proliferation of epidermal structures that are often mixed, so that verrucous, sebaceous, apocrine, eccrine or follicular changes may all occur. The predominant component will determine the clinical appearances. Some types of naevi may undergo malignant transformation, though this is not common.

Sebaceous naevi appear most frequently on the scalp as flesh-coloured, leaf-shaped tumours, which may with time undergo malignant transformation.

Histiocytoma (dermatofibroma)

This tumour is composed of blood vessels, histiocytes or dense fibrous tissue, according to the age of the tumour. It usually arises from trauma such as insect bites and is a common tumour on the legs or buttocks of adults, especially females. A firm tender papule develops, forming a button-like tumour on the surface of which the overlying skin can be wrinkled. The brown pigment or rapid growth may cause alarm and confusion with melanoma.

MALIGNANT TUMOURS

There is increasing concern about the increased numbers of malignant tumours of the skin and their association with sun exposure. The malignant transformation of pre-existing naevi or chronic inflammatory lesions on the skin are less common events.

Basal cell carcinoma (rodent ulcer)

This is the most common cancer of the skin and is frequently seen on the face of middle-aged or elderly people in the UK, especially those with fair hair and blue eyes who are sun-sensitive and often of Celtic origin. Such tumours are seen at a younger age in those living nearer to the equator, but the reasons why tumours appear with such frequency on sites such as the peri-orbital skin, which is to some degree protected from sunlight, is not clear.

Other types of ionizing radiation such as x-rays, for example given to young adults for ankylosing spondylitis, have in the past produced sufficient stimulus for the development of basal cell car-

Fig. 20.21 Basal cell carcinoma.

cinomata at the irradiated site after a prolonged interval of 10–20 years. Arsenicals have only recently been abandoned as oral medication and may also cause cutaneous malignancy after a similar induction time.

CLINICAL FEATURES

Lesions are most commonly seen at the sides of the nose and around the orbit as flesh-coloured translucent papules or plaques with superficial dilated blood vessels coursing over the surface; central necrosis with ulceration or crusting is frequent (Fig. 20.21). Scarring or cystic or pigmented lesions are less common. There is a tendency for basal cell carcinomas to be locally invasive, but metastasis is extremely rare.

The differential diagnosis includes pigmented papules, which are generally more numerous and are seen in the basal cell naevus syndrome. Superficial scarring or morphoeic basal cell carcinomas are more difficult to discern at their margins from normal skin; although uncommon they are important as they tend to follow tissue planes and invade an orifice such as the orbit. Treatment with x-rays is less effective for such tumours.

TREATMENT

Tumours are normally removed surgically, by cryotherapy or x-irradiation. However, lesions which become invasive or are less accessible to normal treatments may be removed by chemosurgery. In Mohs' method the tissue is fixed in situ and excised in a systematic fashion and examined immediately under a microscope to determine the presence or absence of tumour.

Squamous carcinoma

This invasive tumour with the ability to metastasize arises from the epidermis or skin appendages. It is most commonly seen on previously damaged or chronically irritated skin. It has also been associated with certain occupations, e.g. chemical carcinogens inducing cancer of the scrotum, or with certain social customs, e.g. tumours on the legs from radiant heat from fires. Albinism and xeroderma pigmentosum may produce severe actinic damage to the skin and frank malignancy at an early age. Viral disease may predispose to squamous carcinoma and the human papilloma virus may be isolated from the skin of patients with epidermodysplasia verruciformis.

CLINICAL FEATURES

Tumours are hyperkeratotic and crusted and are usually seen over sun-damaged skin, e.g. on the pinna. Induration of the tissues provides a further clue to the diagnosis. Ulceration may occur if the lesion is on sites such as the lip or genitalia. Papilliferous and more friable tumours may appear on relatively normal skin.

TREATMENT

Treatment is usually by excision. Tumours on the head and neck may also be treated by radiotherapy. Superficial lesions may be treated with cryosurgery.

Malignant melanoma

This tumour, formed by epidermal melanocytes, is rising in incidence throughout the world. This increase has been seen particularly in light-skinned people of Celtic origin. The latitude and length of residence of these people in places such as Australia suggest that ultraviolet light exposure is important. An increase in tumours on skin that has not until recent years been commonly exposed, such as the legs of females, also indicates that chronic sun exposure is a significant factor. Inheritance is also important in the dysplastic naevus syndrome, when large multiple and atypical naevi on the trunk show a familial trait and patients may develop multiple primary melanomas.

Malignant change is recognized in pre-existing naevi, especially pigmented naevi, which cover a large surface of the skin, e.g. bathing trunk naevi, and in lentigo maligna, as seen on the cheeks of elderly patients.

Malignant change in a mole should be suspected with a change in size, outline, colour, surface or elevation. Symptoms that include itching, bleeding after minor trauma or an increasing awareness of the tumour should also arouse suspicion.

The prognosis is directly related to the thickness of the tumour assessed at histological examination;

patients with a tumour less than 1 mm thick have a 5-year survival rate of more than 90%, but for tumours greater than 3.5 mm thick the 5-year survival rate is less than 50%.

The prognosis is also related to site; patients with a tumour on the trunk fair better than those with facial lesions, but melanomas on the trunk have a worse prognosis than those on the limbs. The depth of invasion of skin (Clark's level) and local cellular reactions on histological section also indicate the prognosis.

TREATMENT

Excision is performed according to the depth of invasion with a wide excision of deeper invasive lesions followed by skin grafting. Deeply invasive lesions on a limb may be further treated by isolation and arterial perfusion with cytotoxic agents such as mustine hydrochloride. Radiotherapy, chemotherapy and immunotherapy have not yet been shown to materially alter the outlook for those with disseminated disease.

Mycosis fungoides

This is a lymphomatous invasion of the skin by T lymphocytes (see p. 315) which may eventually form cutaneous tumours. In the final stages of the disease there is spread to lymph nodes and other organs. The name implies mushroom-like growths on the skin but these are a rare and often terminal event.

In the Sézary syndrome the skin infiltration is greater; this condition is classified as a T cell chronic lymphatic leukaemia.

CLINICAL FEATURES

The most common presentation of patients seen in the UK is with a pattern of scaling and erythema which may remain confined over areas such as on the buttocks, thighs or trunk as rather fixed patches for many years. Tumours may then develop initially as plaques (Fig. 20.22) and then as ulcerating nodules or masses; dissemination follows with visceral spread and death. With an onset in middle life or old age, patients will often die of other causes. Presentation with advanced disease and spread to local lymph nodes is uncommon in the UK but has been described more frequently in the USA.

TREATMENT

Topical mustine hydrochloride or PUVA (psoralens and ultraviolet A) therapy may control widespread disease and plaque forms of the disease. The combination of prednisolone and chlorambucil may limit the spread of more advanced disease, but dissemination to the viscera is associated with the terminal

Fig. 20.22 Figurate erythema and plaque formation seen with mycosis fungoides.

phase of the disease. Multiple chemotherapeutic regimens are disappointing in their effect.

Disorders of pigmentation

There are many factors which alter the hue of a normal skin. The principal pigments are melanin and haemoglobin or its breakdown products. Carotene, if taken in large amounts in the diet, is concentrated in subcutaneous fat and in keratin, giving a yellow coloration to the skin. The skin can also change its colour by deposition of abnormal substances or by alteration of melanogenesis. These substances include drugs, bilirubin, haemosiderin, heavy metals and the deposition of metal salts, dyes and inks in tattooing. In practice, patients are most concerned with alterations in the degree of melanin pigmentation. This is especially so in those races who have a greater deposition of melanin in their skin as a normal characteristic. Alteration in the degree of pigmentation in those with pigmented skins may be striking and give rise to much personal and social stress.

HYPOPIGMENTATION

Generalized hypopigmentation (albinism)

Albinism is inherited as an autosomal recessive disorder of melanin synthesis. This disorder produces a milky white skin, white hair, blue eyes and photophobia. There are different types, but in the commoner type there is a defect or inhibition of tyrosinase biosynthesis. In phenylketonuria (see p. 775) there is a failure to convert phenylalanine to tyrosine and hypopigmentation of the skin, hair and eyes occurs.

Localized hypopigmentation

Localized absence of melanocytes is seen in vitiligo. In post-inflammatory hypopigmentation some melanocytes are seen but these have reduced activity. In pityriasis versicolor the lipophilic yeast *Pityrosporon orbiculare* produces substances that have an inhibiting effect on melanocytes.

Industrial processes may expose the skin and melanocytes to substances such as phenols which are also toxic to these pigment-producing cells.

Vitiligo

This is a common skin disease affecting approximately 1% of the population. It has a familial incidence. Melanocytes are lost from affected areas of skin. The reason is unclear but hypotheses include the following:

- There may be autodestruction of melanocytes by the products of melanin synthesis.
- There may be autoimmune damage to melanocytes. Antigens have been detected on the surface of melanocytes and antimelanocyte antibodies have been detected in the sera of some patients. There is also an association of vitiligo with other diseases that demonstrate organ-specific antibody production, such as diabetes mellitus, thyroiditis and pernicious anaemia.
- Neurogenic dysfunction has been invoked as an important factor in the production of rare naevoid patterns of the disease which tends to affect the limbs.

CLINICAL FEATURES

More than half the patients notice a loss of pigment before the age of 20 years. Areas of pigment loss are usually symmetrical and often annular in outline, though other shapes and patterns may be evident. These areas tend to enlarge peripherally and present a convex edge to the normal pigmented skin. The initial areas of involvement often include the fingers, hands, face and genitalia. These regularly traumatized areas of skin may show evidence of the Koebner phenomenon (see p. 908) when the disease is in an active phase.

TREATMENT

This is unsatisfactory. Traditional therapy in places such as the Middle East include the use of psoralens obtained from plant sources and applied topically or taken in tablet form. These substances enter into the skin and are then activated by sunlight. PUVA therapy used in the treatment of psoriasis is derived from these observations. Many treatments with PUVA therapy are required for vitiligo and there is concern over the long-term effects of the continuing use of high-intensity ultraviolet light for long periods, especially in younger patients. Potent topical corticosteroids, probably through their action as anti-inflammatory agents, may induce repigmentation when applied to new lesions of vitiligo, and a trial over a limited area of skin for a period of 6–8 weeks is warranted. There may be spontaneous recovery, especially in children.

Post-inflammatory hypopigmentation

This may follow trauma to the skin from chemicals or physical agents or following inflammatory skin diseases. It is a noticeable feature in some patients with eczema. Mild hypopigmentation on the cheeks of children may be associated with scaling and erythema. These inflammatory changes are usually more evident in winter time and are associated with conditions of low humidity and drying winds.

The tanning of surrounding skin in summer will often make the eruption appear more striking, especially in dark-skinned children (pityriasis alba). Pityriasis versicolor may also tend to present in the summer for similar reasons.

TREATMENT

The intensity of local inflammatory changes will be reduced with topical corticosteroids. Soap substitutes and emollients should be used when excessive drying seems to be a causative factor.

HYPERPIGMENTATION

Hyperpigmentation is most commonly seen following sun exposure but may also follow inflammatory changes in the skin. It is often much more evident in those races whose skins are already heavily pigmented.

Epidermal naevi may contain an increased number of melanocytes and be pigmented. Melanin deposited in the dermis will often produce a blue discoloration of the skin which is seen in the following:

- Mongolian blue spot on the backs of children, more especially those of Asian origin
- Naevus of Ito (on the neck)

- Naevus of Ota (on the face)
- Blue naevus

Brown-coloured naevoid lesions

In neurofibromatosis, café-au-lait patches and axillary freckling are seen.

Albright's syndrome (see p. 696) produces extensive light brown discoloration of the skin over the trunk, buttocks and thighs which is often asymmetrical and affects children of pre-school age.

Xeroderma pigmentosum is associated with a freckling type of hyperpigmentation on the face or other sun-exposed sites. In those patients with severe disease it is associated with solar damage and cutaneous malignancy, which may be evident early in childhood.

Freckling on the skin of fair-skinned and otherwise normal persons increases with the length of sun exposure. Histological sections appropriately stained demonstrate an increase in the size and shape of melanosomes within the melanocyte.

Lentigines

These are circumscribed dark brown macules that are less than 0.5 cm in diameter. There is a localized increase in the number of melanocytes seen on light microscopy and the degree of pigmentation is often much more intense clinically than that seen with freckles. A generalized distribution of lentigines may be seen as part of a syndrome that includes cardiac defects (Leopard or Moynahan's syndrome). In the Peutz–Jegher syndrome (orofacial lentiginosis) (see p. 206) lesions are localized to the face and hands and there is an association with intestinal polyposis.

Generalized hypermelanosis

Liver disease
In haemochromatosis there is a grey/black component to the hyperpigmentation which is more evident in sun-exposed areas of skin. Hypermelanosis may also be pronounced in patients with primary biliary cirrhosis.

Endocrine disease
In Addison's disease pigmentation may be diffuse but it is often much more pronounced on sun-exposed or traumatized skin, e.g. beneath bra straps or over the buccal mucosa in the mouth. Both ACTH and melanocyte stimulating hormone (MSH) are increased, but it is uncertain which plays the dominant role in producing the pigmentation. Hyperthyroidism may rarely produce a similar pattern of hyperpigmentation.

Acromegaly, Cushing's syndrome and ACTH therapy may also be associated with pigmentation which may be particularly pronounced in patients with sella turcica enlargement following adrenalec-tomy (Nelson's syndrome), when multiple lentigines and oral hyperpigmentation are also seen.

Pregnancy and the oral contraceptive pill may both produce an increase in pigmentation on the neck, the areolae of the breasts, over the abdominal skin and genitalia. Involvement of the face (melasma) may cause the patient to seek medical advice.

Neoplastic disease and cachexia can produce a general darkening of the skin colour; more marked changes occur with ectopic ACTH production.

Other diseases
Acanthosis nigricans is most commonly seen as localized hyperpigmentation of the axillae (Fig. 20.23), groins or facial skin, but the changes may be generalized and profound. Velvety overgrowth of the skin at the flexures may be accompanied by filiform growths around the face, mouth or over the tongue, and by a curious roughness of the palmar or plantar skin (tripe palms). These changes are seen in middle-aged patients with visceral malignancies such as carcinoma of the stomach, but other types of neoplasia such as lymphomas have also been reported in association with these typical cutaneous features. Acanthosis nigricans can, however, occur without an underlying malignancy.

Renal failure is associated with hypermelanosis

Fig. 20.23 Acanthosis nigricans.

and an increase in MSH-like reactive hormone production is seen in some patients. A yellow/brown, widespread coloration of the skin often occurs; scaling and irritation may also be seen. The relief of itching is difficult to achieve in such patients.

Systemic sclerosis may produce localized pigmentary changes in sites such as the nape of the neck or over the shoulder girdle but hyperpigmentation may be profound and generalized in some patients. Thickening of the skin is usually present and should offer a clue as to the primary diagnosis.

Chemical deposition in the skin may occur as an occupational hazard, e.g. in those who process silver.

Mercurials may produce hypermelanosis, and gold taken by mouth may cause blue/black pigmentation most evident on sun-exposed sites (chrysiasis).

The iron-containing pigment *haemosiderin* may also stimulate localized melanin production. This occurs on sites such as the legs of patients with varicose eczema following the loss of red cells into the skin. Mucocutaneous discoloration may also be seen with chrome lead poisoning.

Drugs

Mepacrine imparts a yellow colour to the skin but the sclera are spared. Chloroquine and chlorpromazine may produce bluish/grey coloration of the skin, especially in areas exposed to the sun. Arsenicals ingested over a long interval cause macular hyperpigmentation together with areas of hypopigmentation (rain-drop appearance).

Sunlight and the skin

The effects of ultraviolet light on the skin may be beneficial or damaging. The formation of vitamin D from sterol precursors in the skin is dependent on sunlight, and ultraviolet light exposure may be used with benefit in the treatment of chronic skin conditions such as acne, eczema and psoriasis.

Damaging effects, however, occur with chronic irradiation, giving rise to changes in connective tissues which produce ageing, wrinkling, altered texture, dryness and changes in skin pigmentation. Epidermal changes include hyperkeratosis, dysplasia and malignancy.

PHOTODERMATOSES

These can be divided into:
- Eruptions in which sunlight has a primary role
- Diseases where sunlight is a trigger or an exacerbating factor

Primary photosensitivity

Polymorphic light eruption

The term 'polymorphic' refers to the difference in the morphology of the eruption between patients: lesions may be erythematous, papular or vesicular. The lesions tend, however, to be monomorphic in any one individual.

Lesions are usually papulovesicular. Eczema, urticarial plaques or purpuric changes are less common. The rash is seen after a few hours of sun exposure and is most common on the chest and arms, the backs of the hands or lower legs. The eruption usually occurs in spring and early summer and improves as summer progresses and the skin 'hardens'. Fair-skinned individuals are most commonly affected by intense sunlight, but those who have previously tanned easily and are of a darker complexion can also be affected. The papules may be associated with weeping and intense pruritus lasting for 5–10 days. The reaction can be readily produced in the clinic or laboratory using high-intensity ultraviolet light at a wavelength of 320–420 nm.

Pretreatment during spring-time with 10–12 treatments of PUVA may prevent the disease. Hydroxychloroquine given in doses of 400 mg daily for 2–3 weeks before and during sun exposure may prevent attacks. Topical corticosteroids such as betamethasone and high-factor sun-blocking creams (factors 15–18) also help to minimize the disease.

Hutchinson's summer prurigo

This rare disease usually has its onset before puberty. It affects both exposed and unexposed skin and may last throughout the year. Lesions are often excoriated and the necrotic papules may be quite disfiguring. The wavelengths responsible are usually in the sunburn range (290–320 nm). Sun-screen creams should be used but these do not offer sufficient protection in most cases. Beta-carotene given by mouth may help a few patients.

Actinic reticuloid (chronic actinic dermatitis)

This is a rare condition affecting older men in which the gross thickening, coloration and texture of exposed skin may resemble lymphomatous infiltration, both clinically and on microscopy. Many patients have had eczema previously and a significant proportion of these patients also have a positive patch test to materials such as rubber or plants. Clinical features include eczematous and purpuric lesions on non-exposed skin such as the legs, arms and trunk. Light sensitivity may be such that during active phases of the disease the only respite for patients is found in a darkened room. Protective clothing, sun-barrier creams, systemic steroid therapy, azathioprine, cytotoxic drugs and hydroxychloroquine may be required in combination to produce improvement.

Secondary photosensitivity

Topical agents

The application of perfumes (e.g. those containing bergaptine), sulphonamides and antimicrobial agents (e.g. halogenated salicylanilide) may produce photosensitive reactions. The latter group of compounds have been largely withdrawn.

Plant extracts such as psoralens commonly found in the family Umbelliferae are used in photochemotherapy (PUVA therapy). However, phytophotodermatitis may occur when the leaves of such plants (e.g. giant hogweed, wild parsley) abrade the skin surface. Psoralen compounds are absorbed into the skin and then activated by natural long-wavelength ultraviolet radiation.

Systemic agents

Systemic agents associated with photosensitivity include tetracyclines (chiefly dimethylchlortetracycline), thiazides, frusemide and phenothiazines.

Disease states

Sunlight can exacerbate systemic lupus erythematosus. Antibodies formed against DNA denatured by ultraviolet light form immune complexes in the skin and other organs.

In porphyria, porphyrins deposited in the skin are activated by ultraviolet light, producing systemic disease.

Collagen diseases

The term 'collagen disease' refers to inherited abnormalities of both collagen and elastic tissue. These diseases are due to enzyme defects affecting chiefly post-translational changes in the development of collagen. Further defects will undoubtedly be defined with the isolation of collagen genes and DNA hybridization techniques.

Abnormalities of collagen

Collagen has a molecular weight of approximately 290 000 and is composed of three alpha polypeptide chains, each containing over 1000 amino acids. Each alpha chain has its own mRNA and genetic make-up; defects at various points of the process of formation of these chains will lead to abnormalities such as the Ehlers–Danlos syndrome, osteogenesis imperfecta and Menkes' syndrome. After a complex series of metabolic steps, a cross-linked fibre consisting of three helical collagen molecules is formed.

There are five genetically different types of collagen which occur in different parts of the body. The skin contains collagen types I, III and V within the dermis and type IV in the basement membrane.

Breakdown of collagen leads to excretion in the urine of amino acids such as hydroxyproline and hydroxylysine; their excretion rate indicates the rate of collagen turnover.

Glycosaminoglycans are mucopolysaccharides that are involved in collagen synthesis. A number of separate enzyme defects have been described that alter the rate of turnover of glycosaminoglycans, resulting in skeletal abnormalities (see p. 776).

The end result of this abnormal collagen or elastic tissue formation is a loss of tensile strength. A variety of tissues or organs may be affected by these structural protein changes, and these include the eye, blood vessels, bone and the skin. Cutaneous features are seen in cutis laxa, Ehlers–Danlos syndrome, pseudoxanthoma elasticum and in Marfan's syndrome.

Ehlers–Danlos syndrome

This is a heterogeneous group of diseases where at least nine different varieties have been described. Hyperextensibility, fragility and bruising of the skin occurs to a varying degree with each of the diseases and it is accompanied by the hypermobility of joints. Fragility of blood vessels occurs and rarely aortic rupture.

The patterns of inheritance are varied and can be autosomal recessive, autosomal dominant or X-linked recessive.

The skin is velvety to the touch and hyperextensible but recoils normally on stretching. Trauma or laceration of the skin can lead to tissue-paper scars and poor wound healing. Pseudotumours may occur over the elbows and knees; they consist principally of fat, but may show signs of calcification.

Abnormalities of elastic tissue

Solar elastosis

Degradation of elastic fibrils in the skin normally occurs with ageing. This usually begins in early adult life, but changes are more noticeable in the sixties and seventies. The clinical features are characterized by yellowish papules or plaques and wrinkling, and are usually associated with pigmentation and keratoses on exposed skin.

Cutis laxa (generalized elastolysis)

This is a rare disease in which there are a number of variants. These are inherited as autosomal recessive, X-linked recessive or dominant traits. A defect in the cross-linking of elastin is suggested, but other abnormalities, including copper deficiency, have been reported. The subsequent changes in the skin, sometimes gross, may be evident at birth or arise at the time of puberty. The disfiguring changes may be severe, with extreme laxity of the facial skin and massive folds over the trunk which have no recoil on stretching. Joint hypermobility is not a common feature.

Pseudoxanthoma elasticum

This is a generalized disorder of elastic tissue. The pathogenesis is unknown, and both autosomal dominant and recessive modes of transmission are seen. The skin, eye and vascular structures are involved.

Cutaneous features are seen in childhood and are most evident over flexural surfaces and at the sides of the neck. Initially there is an accentuation of skin lines or folds and this is followed by thickening around yellowish diamond-shaped papules, producing a peau d'orange or plucked chicken appearance. The skin may be lax and hang in folds. The skin demonstrates very little elastic recoil on stretching. The mucous membranes may also be affected. Long-term and high-dose treatment with D-penicillamine produces similar cutaneous features.

Widespread vascular changes are associated with fibrous proliferation and the deposition of calcium in the media of the arteries. Intermittent claudication and angina pectoris occur at an early age as a result. Gastrointestinal bleeding may be a troublesome feature. Splits in Bruch's membrane, which contains both elastin and collagen and separates the choroid from the retina, are demonstrated as angioid streaks on ophthalmoscopy.

Marfan's syndrome

A biochemical defect for this disease has not been identified, and some features of the condition may be seen in association with the Ehlers–Danlos syndrome or with homocystinuria. Inheritance is usually in an autosomal dominant manner.

Striae distensae are the only common dermatological sign, and the most impressive changes affect the skeleton. The facial appearance of affected patients may be distinctive, with elongation and asymmetry. A high-arched palate, although frequently described, is not a common feature. A tall stature, long thin digits and alteration in the body proportions are seen; the distance from the soles to the pubis (lower segment) is greater than the distance from the pubis to the vertex (upper segment). The arm span, measured from the extended fingers, often exceeds the height of the patient.

Joints. A laxity of ligaments may give rise to dislocation of joints such as the jaw or patellae. Steinberg's sign occurs when the thumbs are adducted over the palm and their tips are seen to cross the ulnar border of the hand. Inguinal or femoral hernias are often seen.

Respiratory system. Pulmonary changes include hernia of the diaphragm, emphysema and spontaneous pneumothorax.

Cardiovascular system. Cardiovascular symptoms follow the degeneration in the media of vessel walls. The aortic valve ring may dilate and produce an incompetent valve, and less commonly the mitral valve is similarly involved, producing the 'billowy valve syndrome' (see p. 517). Aneurysm formation may occur, usually in the ascending aorta, and may be followed by dissection and/or rupture.

Eyes. Weakness of the suspensory ligament of the lens may cause dislocation; this is a common clinical feature of the disease.

Diseases of the hair and nails

Both hair and nails are composed of keratin and are derived principally from the epidermal layer. Each may be affected by the same type of disease process, e.g. lichen planus, or altered by conditions that affect primarily the epidermis.

DISORDERS OF HAIR GROWTH

The extent and distribution of body hair is largely determined genetically. At the time of puberty, terminal hair growth occurs in males on the beard area, over the upper lip, chest, abdomen and thighs. Androgens determine the extent of secondary sexual patterns of hair growth during adolescence in both sexes. In females any marked alteration in the extent of hair growth or hair loss at times other than at puberty or the menopause may reflect serious endocrine disturbance.

Hirsuties (see p. 702)

Hirsuties is defined as an excessive growth of hair of male type and distribution in females. In many parts of the world an excess of body hair is accepted as a racial characteristic or may, in addition, be seen as a family trait. In the Western World, excess body hair in females is considered less acceptable and women may become self-conscious about the extent of their hair growth.

Most hirsute females do not have recognizable clinical or biochemical evidence of endocrine disease, though this must be excluded by a careful history, examination and hormone profile where appropriate.

Some drugs alter the texture and extent of hair growth; these include cortisone, minoxidil, diazoxide and hydantoins.

The problem should not be lightly dismissed as most women who are affected are not prepared to accept these cutaneous manifestations of androgenicity.

Methods of hair removal include removal by abrasion with mittens that have a roughened surface, shaving and plucking, but these give short-term relief. Depilatory creams and waxing should not be frequently used on facial hair, but may be used elsewhere, such as on the legs.

Bleaching facial hair with peroxides will produce an acceptable appearance for fine hair. Coarse hairs are best dealt with by electrolysis, but this needs to be performed by skilled personnel and may produce scarring, especially if acne is a concurrent problem on the chin. With severe hirsutism, anti-androgens (e.g. cyproterone acetate) or prednisolone (5 mg at night and 2.5 mg in the morning) may be used to produce a slowing of hair growth so that mechanical removal need not be so frequent or vigorous.

Hair loss

Hair loss which occurs to the extent that scalp skin becomes abnormally visible is termed alopecia. It may be permanent, when the hair follicles are damaged by scarring (e.g. in lichen planus or discoid lupus erythematosus), or may recover if the follicles are left intact, e.g. in some endocrine diseases or alopecia areata.

Alopecia areata

This occurs in both sexes and all races and is usually seen in young adults or children as a well-defined patch of hair loss. Only 25% of cases are seen over the age of 40 years and 25% of patients give a family history of the condition.

Aetiology. There is often a personal or family history of atopy. Alopecia areata occurs in association with autoimmune diseases such as thyrotoxicosis, Addison's disease, pernicious anaemia and chronic active hepatitis.

The association of alopecia areata with such diseases suggests that immune changes are important in the pathogenesis. It is also seen in association with Down's syndrome, vitiligo and hypogammaglobulinaemia.

Clinical features. Patients are often dark-skinned and patches of hair loss can occur over any part of the body, e.g. the beard area or eyebrows, but the scalp is most frequently affected. Asymptomatic loss may first be noticed by a relative or hairdresser. Patches tend to regrow over the course of several months within the scalp margin in adults. An extension into the margin (ophiasis) is often less quick to recover. Children with an atopic background may lose all their scalp hair (alopecia totalis) and the prognosis in such patients should be guarded; alopecia totalis is seen less frequently in adults. Loss of hair from all body sites (alopecia universalis) may occur by exten-sion from other sites but can also occur acutely.

Diffuse loss of hairs in alopecia areata is an infrequent occurrence and may be difficult to differentiate from other causes of hair loss. The extension of hair loss occurs in a peripheral fashion; at the advancing edge, broken hairs (exclamation mark hairs) provide evidence of disease activity.

Regrowing hair appears as a fine, depigmented downy growth. Areas of alopecia principally affect pigmented hair and premature greying is seen after diffuse hair loss.

Treatment. Large doses of corticosteroids will produce a regrowth of hair, but relapse occurs after treatment is stopped. Topical corticosteroids may also help to speed the rate of regrowth of hair. Other treatment modalities, effective in small numbers of patients, include PUVA therapy and topical minoxidil.

Diffuse hair loss

Hairs are lost in the telogen phase. Normally about 100 hairs are shed each day. In severe illness or following pregnancy there is an increase in the number of hairs entering the telogen phase (telogen effluvium). Hair loss is seen 3–4 months after the event. Nail growth may be affected in the same way.

Other causes of diffuse hair loss include endocrine disease such as hyperthyroidism or hypothyroidism and androgen overactivity in both males and females. Iron deficiency, rapid weight loss associated with dieting, and drugs such as lithium or vitamin A and its derivatives also produce diffuse and treatable hair loss.

Premature male pattern baldness

Recession of the hair margin is an ageing characteristic of primates. This may appear early in males but such a pattern of loss in young females may indicate serious androgenicity. Vertical thinning is seen in association with margin recession in both sexes. In young women there is often evidence of androgen excess which may be treated by anti-androgen therapy over an interval of a year with some recovery. The primary defect is atrophy of the hair follicle. It is due to a number of factors other than excess androgen activity, for anti-androgen therapy is not always effective in stimulating strong terminal hair growth in females.

Abnormalities of the hair shaft

The hair shaft may become twisted, beaded or broken, leading to hair loss. Short, unruly or broken hair is then the primary complaint. Similar patterns of loss will be seen with drying of the hair or the effect of weathering, cosmetics, bleaching agents or grooming.

Traction

Traction associated with fashion, traditional or ethnic practices, such as hot combing, braiding or plaiting, may also cause a localized hair fall, especially over the temporal region. Straightening or relaxing the hair, undertaken by those with naturally curly hair may, in addition, produce permanent root damage.

DISEASES OF THE NAILS

The nail plate grows continuously although the rate varies with age, slowing with advancing years, and with some generalized diseases. Growth of fingernails is normally at a rate of about 1 cm every 3 months, so that renewal of a fingernail may take 6 months and toe-nails, which grow slower, may take from 18 months to 2 years. An increase in the rate of growth of the nail plate occurs in psoriasis and other skin diseases.

The nail plate arises from the matrix and lies on the nail bed. The hard outer layer is formed from the proximal matrix and the bulk of the nail, composed of soft keratin, is produced by the distal matrix.

The nail matrix lies within a fold of epidermis, so that dermatoses or infections that involve the posterior nail fold may also cause abnormalities of the nail plate; these include chronic paronychia, fungal disease, eczema and psoriasis. These nail changes have been discussed in the appropriate sections.

Congenital defects of the nail occur in conjunction with abnormalities of the epidermis, teeth or skeleton.

Nail disorders in generalized diseases

Clubbing
This is discussed on p. 562.

Connective tissue diseases
Short and brittle nails occur in severe circulatory disorders, e.g. Raynaud's phenomenon (see p. 548), especially in association with systemic sclerosis. Pterygium formation also occurs when a thin skin fold merges with the cuticle, widening it by several millimetres. Chronic paronychia may persist despite all therapeutic manoeuvres in patients with severe digital ischaemia. Nail fold capillary dilatation and distortion or the absence of capillaries, usually with severe Raynaud's phenomenon, is seen in systemic sclerosis. Ragged cuticles containing haemorrhages are often most pronounced in patients with dermatomyositis.

Yellow nail syndrome
The nail plate is thickened, yellow in colour, smooth and with an increased lateral curvature. The rate of growth of the nail is reduced. Such nails are seen in association with chronic oedema of the hands, feet, ankles or face, congenital lymphoedema, pleural effusions, chronic sinus infection and thyroid disease.

White bands
Distal white bands that are parallel to the lunula and separated from the rest of the nail by a normal pink coloured portion are seen in patients with hypoalbuminaemia. The nails return to normal when the level of protein is restored.

Half-and-half nails
This is the name given to nails where the proximal nail is pale or white and the distal portion is red or brown in colour; these nails may indicate renal failure.

Brown streaks
Longitudinal brown streaks are commonly seen in black patients when pigment cells are incorporated into the nail matrix. Alteration of pigment beneath the nails which is localized and not related to obvious trauma in white-skinned patients may require a biopsy of the nail to exclude subungual melanoma.

Onycholysis
Onycholysis or separation of the distal edge of the nail from the vascular nail bed will cause whiteness of the free edge and this most commonly follows trauma or faulty or excessive manicure. Psoriasis is another common cause and similar changes may be seen in thyrotoxicosis or following photo-onycholysis produced by photoactive drugs such as tetracycline or psoralens, as well as in porphyria.

Splinter haemorrhages
These are most frequently caused by trauma to the nail; subacute infective endocarditis, systemic lupus erythematosus and psoriasis are less common causes.

Koilonychia
Spoon-shaped nails or koilonychia is seen in association with iron-deficiency anaema, but it may also follow trauma, e.g. in garage mechanics who regularly fit tyres.

Chronic paronychia
This is due to chronic infection from bacteria or fungi. It is rarely a manifestation of an underlying systemic disease such as hypoparathyroidism, multiple endocrine disease or chronic iron deficiency.

Transverse lines
Transverse lines (Beau's lines) related to acute physical or psychiatric illness or the use of cytotoxic drugs represent a temporary arrest of growth. They may be associated with an arrest of hair growth and subsequent fall (telogen effluvium).

Blue discoloration of the nail
This may be seen in hepatolenticular degeneration (Wilson's disease) as blue lunulae.

Effects of drugs

A number of drugs including antimalarials such as chloroquine may cause a blue/black discoloration of the nail plate. Mepacrine may stain the nail plate blue and fluoresces green on Wood's light examination. Argyria occurring as an occupational disease or following, for example, the use of silver-containing nose drops will stain the nails a grey/blue colour. Phenothiazine produces a blue/black coloration which is often accentuated in summer-time. Phenolphthalein, used in purgatives, will also give rise to blue nails.

Cytotoxic drugs
Diffuse, longitudinal or horizontal melanonychia affecting the nail base or nail plate may occur in association with pigmentary changes of the surrounding skin with doxorubicin, bulsulphan, cyclophosphamide and daunorubicin therapy.

Further reading

Fitzpatrick TB (ed.) (1979) *Dermatology in General Medicine*, 2nd ed. New York: McGraw Hill.

Kirby J (1986) *Roxburgh's Common Skin Diseases*. London: Lewis.

Mackie R (ed.) (1984) *Current Perspectives in Immunodermatology*. Edinburgh: Churchill Livingstone.

Moschella S (ed.) (1979) *Dermatology Update*. New York: Elsevier.

Appendices

Diets

These diets were compiled by Jasmine Challis, Senior Dietitian, St Bartholomew's Hospital, London.

DIABETIC DIET

The basic principles of the diabetic diet are given below:
- Sugar and foods with a high sugar content, e.g. sweets, chocolate, honey, preserves, sweet biscuits, cakes, ordinary fruit squashes and fizzy drinks, and sweet alcoholic drinks, should be avoided.
- Fats should be used sparingly.
- Fibre intake should be increased by the use of wholemeal bread and high fibre cereals, pulses and fruit.
- Salt should be used sparingly.
- Protein intake should be normal.
- Most vegetables, herbs, spices, condiments (except salt), tea, coffee, sugar-free squashes and fizzy drinks, and soda water are allowed freely.
- Carbohydrate foods with a low sugar content should provide a high proportion of the energy intake. Carbohydrate intake should be spread throughout the day to include between-meal and bedtime snacks.
- Alcohol can be taken in moderation.

Patients who are overweight are given an appropriate reducing diet until they achieve ideal weight.

To provide variety in the diet, a system of carbohydrate exchanges is used, some of which are listed below. Each of the following contains approximately 10 g of carbohydrate (CHO) and is equal to one 'exchange':
- 1 small slice bread
- 2 crackers or plain biscuits
- 1 digestive biscuit
- 1 Weetabix
- 1 small potato ('egg-sized')
- 1 heaped tablespoon boiled rice
- ⅓ pint (175 ml) milk
- 1 small carton plain yoghurt
- 2 tablespoons dried beans
- 1 apple, orange, pear or peach
- 1 small banana
- 1 small glass orange juice (100 ml)

SAMPLE MEAL PLAN

For a lean patient maintaining weight on 2000 kcal (8400 kJ) and 260 g of CHO (i.e. 50% of total energy as CHO).

	CHO (g)
Daily	
175 ml semi-skimmed milk for tea or coffee	10
20 g polyunsaturated margarine	
Breakfast (60 g CHO)	
2 Weetabix	20
175 ml semi-skimmed milk	10
2 slices wholemeal bread	20
Margarine from allowance	
100 ml orange juice	10
Mid-morning (20 g CHO)	
Large banana	20
Lunch (60 g CHO)	
4 slices wholemeal bread for sandwiches— with lean meat, and salad vegetables	40
Low-fat plain yoghurt	10
Pear	10
Mid-afternoon (20 g CHO)	
2 digestive biscuits	20
Evening meal (60 g CHO)	
Beef and butter bean casserole	10
Jacket potato	30
Vegetables	
Baked apple with dates	20
Bedtime (30 g CHO)	
Wholemeal fruit bun	30
	Total 260 g CHO

It should be remembered that patients will have to be instructed how to maintain their carbohydrate intake during illness, cope with their diet while travelling, and adjust their intake prior to exercise.

GLUTEN-FREE DIET

This is used for the treatment of coeliac disease and dermatitis herpetiformis.

The diet involves the exclusion of wheat, rye, barley and oats. *Any* food containing gluten—either as an obvious constituent (e.g. flour, bread) or as a 'hidden' ingredient (e.g. stock cubes, dessert mixes)—must be avoided.

Foods allowed

- Gluten-free (GF) bread*, GF crispbread*, GF pasta*
- GF flour*, soya flour, potato flour, pea flour, rice flour
- Soya bran, rice bran
- GF biscuits, GF cakes
- Rice Krispies, cornflakes
- Rice, tapioca, sago, arrowroot, buckwheat, millet, maize
- Fresh or frozen meat, poultry, offal
- Plain fresh or frozen fish, fish canned in oil
- Eggs, plain cheeses
- Milk, cream, butter, margarine, oils
- Plain fresh, frozen or tinned vegetables and potatoes
- Tinned fruit in syrup or natural juice, fresh or frozen fruit
- Nuts
- Tea, coffee, fruit juice, fruit squash, fizzy drinks
- Sugar, glucose, boiled sweets, syrup, honey, jam, marmalade, jelly, gelatine
- *Pure* herbs, spices, mustard, vinegar, salt, pepper
- Monosodium glutamate
- Wine, beer, spirits, liqueurs

* Products prescribable on the National Health Service in the UK for coeliac disease and dermatitis herpetiformis.

In addition any homemade items, e.g. soups or sauces, made with GF ingredients are obviously suitable.

Foods forbidden

- Ordinary bread, crispbreads, pasta
- Ordinary flour, rye flour, barley flour
- Wheat bran
- Ordinary biscuits and cakes
- Breakfast cereals made with wheat or oats
- Barley, oatmeal, semolina
- Meat pies, most beefburgers, most sausages, most tinned meats
- fish with breadcrumbs or batter, fish cakes, fish in sauce

- Potato croquettes
- Fruit pies
- Ovaltine, barley water
- Most stock cubes and gravy mixes

The lists above are *not* comprehensive and it is not always possible to tell from a 'label' whether or not a manufactured product is gluten-free. In the UK The Coeliac Society produces a comprehensive list of manufactured foods which are gluten free, and patients prescribed such a diet are advised to join:

The Coeliac Society
PO Box 220
High Wycombe
Bucks HP11 2HY

RENAL DIETS

Low-protein diet

This contains approximately 24 g of protein, 2800 kcal, (11 760 kJ), 40 mmol of sodium and 50 mmol of potassium. This is the minimum acceptable protein restriction for uraemic patients.

SAMPLE MEAL PLAN

Breakfast
Fruit in syrup, drained
Low-protein bread with salt-free butter
Jam, marmalade or honey

Mid-morning
Low-protein biscuits

Lunch
25 g meat or 40 g fish
100 g potato ⎫
Vegetable ⎬ with salt-free butter
Low-protein pasta ⎭
Fruit and double cream

Mid-afternoon
Low-protein bread with salt-free butter
Jam, marmalade or honey

Evening meal
1 egg ⎫
100 g potato ⎬ with salt-free butter
Vegetable ⎭
Fruit and double cream

Bedtime
Low-protein biscuits

Daily
175 ml milk ⎫
1 bottle Hycal or ⎬ as part of fluid allowance
  equivalent ⎭

Suitable drinks
Tea
Lemonade
Coca-Cola
Bitter lemon
} as part of fluid allowance

Allowed freely
Sugar
Jam, honey, marmalade
Boiled sweets
Salt-free butter
Low-protein products

In general, a small amount of salt may be used in cooking, but none added at table. See 'no added salt' diet for further restrictions.

Restricted protein diet

This contains approximately 40 g of protein, 2900 kcal (12 180 kJ), 65 mmol of sodium and 55 mmol of potassium. It is used in the treatment of patients with moderate uraemia or prophylactically in patients with asymptomatic moderate renal failure (creatinine clearance < 40 ml·min^{-1}).

SAMPLE MEAL PLAN

Breakfast
1 egg
2 slices white bread with salt-free butter
Jam, marmalade or honey

Mid-morning
Low-protein biscuits

Lunch
25 g meat or 40 g fish
100 g potato
Vegetable } with salt-free butter
Low-protein pasta
Fruit and double cream

Mid-afternoon
1 slice white bread with salt-free butter
Jam, marmalade or honey

Evening meal
25 g meat or 40 g fish
100 g potato } with salt-free butter
Vegetable
Fruit and double cream

Bedtime
Low-protein bread or low-protein biscuits

Daily
175 ml milk
1 bottle Hycal or } as part of fluid allowance
   equivalent

Suitable drinks
Tea
Lemonade
Coca-Cola
Bitter lemon
} as part of fluid allowance

Allowed freely
Sugar
Jam, honey, marmalade
Boiled sweets
Salt-free butter
Low-protein products

In general, a small amount of salt may be used in cooking, but none added at table. See 'no added salt' diet for further restrictions.

High-protein, no added salt diet

This contains approximately 90 g of protein and 100 mmol of sodium. It is used for patients with the nephrotic syndrome.

SAMPLE MEAL PLAN

Breakfast
Cereal with milk
2 slices toast with butter or margarine
Jam or marmalade

Main meal
150 g meat or 200 g fish
Potatoes or rice
Vegetables
Milk pudding, or pudding with custard, or fruit and ice-cream

Snack meal
75 g meat or 100 g fish or 3 eggs
Bread or potatoes
Vegetables or salad
Fruit

Daily
At least 1 pint of milk

A small amount of salt may be used in cooking, but none added at table. See 'no added salt' diet for further restrictions.

Low-calcium, low-oxalate diet

This is required in hypercalciuric or hyperoxaluric stone formers, in combination with a high fluid intake (> 2 l daily).

SAMPLE MEAL PLAN

Breakfast
1 egg
1 slice white bread with butter
Cereal

Main meal
Average helping of meat or fish
Potatoes or rice
Vegetables
Fruit or jelly

Snack meal
Average helping of meat or fish
2 slices white bread with butter

Daily
150 ml milk

Avoid:
Foods rich in calcium, e.g. cheese, ice-cream, yoghurt, extra milk
Foods rich in oxalate, e.g. rhubarb, spinach, beet-
root, beans

Tea intake is restricted to 4 cups daily.

DIET IN LIVER DISEASE

40 g protein, no added salt diet

This is used in the treatment of liver disease. See 'no
added salt' diet for additional instructions.

SAMPLE MEAL PLAN

Daily
150 ml milk

Breakfast
Fruit juice
1 egg
1 slice bread or toast with butter and jam or
marmalade
Tea or coffee with milk from allowance

Mid-morning
Fruit juice
Tea or coffee with milk from allowance

Lunch
25 g meat or 40 g fish or 1 egg or 1 small yoghurt or 3 tablespoons pulses
1 slice bread or equivalent
Vegetables or salad
Fruit

Mid-afternoon
1 slice bread with butter and jam or honey
Tea or coffee with milk from allowance

Evening meal
25 g meat or 40 g fish or 1 egg or 1 small yoghurt or
3 tablespoons pulses
1 slice bread or equivalent
Vegetables or salad
Fruit

Bedtime
1 slice bread or equivalent
Tea or coffee with remainder of milk allowance

Fat and fatty foods must be restricted if poorly
tolerated. Alcohol must be avoided.

1 slice of bread may be exchanged for any of the
following:
3 plain biscuits
2 crispbreads
1 small bowl breakfast cereal or porridge
2 tablespoons cooked rice or cooked pasta
2 small potatoes
1 small slice cake
1 tablespoon flour
1 tablespoon ice-cream

Extras
Sugar
Glucose
Boiled sweets
Mints
Fruit squash
Fizzy drinks
Fruit
Fruit juice

These are 'encouraged' in order to increase energy
intake.

SALT RESTRICTION DIETS

No added salt diet

This restricts sodium intake to between 60 and
100 mmol daily depending on energy intake. A small
amount of salt may be used in cooking, but none
must be used at table.

The following foods contain considerable amounts
of sodium and *must be avoided*:
Bacon, ham, sausages, pâté
Cheese
Tinned fish and meat
Smoked fish and meat
Salted fish and meat
Fish and meat pastes
Tinned vegetables
Tinned and packet soups
Sauce mixes
Bottled sauces and chutneys
Meat and vegetable extracts, stock cubes
Salted nuts and crisps
Soya sauce
Monosodium glutamate

40 mmol sodium diet

This is used in the treatment of ascites or severe oedema associated with salt and water retention. It is often used in conjunction with fluid restriction and/or diuretics.

In addition to avoiding the foods listed under 'no added salt' diet, the following restrictions apply:
- No salt to be used in cooking or at table.
- Salt-free butter must be used.
- Milk should be restricted to 300 ml daily.
- Only 4 slices ordinary bread are permitted daily—extra bread must be salt-free.
- All-Bran, cornflakes and Rice Krispies must be avoided.

LOW-FAT DIET

If the body's ability to digest and/or absorb fat is impaired, a diet low in fat is indicated. In this case *all* fats, i.e. both animal and vegetable in origin, must be restricted.

Where fat tolerance is low it is better to distribute the fat intake throughout the day.

Care should be taken to check the fat content of manufactured foods.

SAMPLE MEAL PLAN

Daily
Low-fat milk as required
10 g butter or margarine or oil or 20 g 'low-fat' spread

Breakfast
Fruit or fruit juice
Breakfast cereal or porridge
Bread or toast with butter or margarine from allowance
Jam, marmalade or honey

Snack meal
Lean meat, chicken, low-fat cheese, egg, fish or baked beans
Bread, toast or crispbread
Vegetables or salad
Fruit or low-fat yoghurt

Main meal
Clear soup, fruit juice, melon or grapefruit
Lean meat, chicken or fish cooked without fat, beans or pulses
Potato, rice or pasta cooked without fat
Vegetables or salad
Fruit, jelly or pudding made with low-fat milk

Beverages
Tea, coffee, fruit juice, fruit squash or fizzy drinks

Extras
Boiled sweets, mints, fruit gums, meringues, water ice, ice lollies
Plain or semi-sweet biscuits
Herbs, spices, mustard, vinegar, pickles, oil-free salad dressings

REDUCING DIET

This diet is also suitable for obese diabetics, although distribution of carbohydrate-containing foods may need modification for those on oral hypoglycaemic agents or insulin. Energy restriction is achieved by reducing *fat*, *sugar* and *alcohol*, while maintaining a modest intake of fibre-containing carbohydrate foods.

SAMPLE MEAL PLAN

Breakfast
Small cupful of breakfast cereal or porridge with low-fat milk, no sugar
1 slice wholemeal bread or toast with a little butter or margarine*

Snack meal
Average helping of lean meat, poultry, fish, eggs, cheese or small tin baked beans
Salad vegetables
2 slices wholemeal bread or 4 crispbread or 2 small potatoes
Fresh fruit or sugar-free, low-fat yoghurt

Main meal
Average helping of lean meat, poultry, fish, eggs, cheese or pulses
Cooked vegetable and/or side salad
1 small potato or 1 tablespoon boiled rice or 1 slice wholemeal bread
Fruit, fresh or tinned in natural juice

Low-fat milk (skimmed or semi-skimmed) should be used in tea and coffee. Artificial sweeteners may be used if necessary. Other suitable drinks include sugar-free squashes and fizzy drinks, soda water, and mineral water.

Not more than 100 g of butter or margarine is allowed per week.

Avoid:
Sweets, chocolate, honey, preserves, sweet biscuits, cakes, tinned fruit in syrup, puddings
Ordinary fruit squash and fizzy drinks
Malted milk drinks and drinking chocolate
Fried foods, cream, mayonnaise, salad dressing, crisps, cream cheese, pastry, dumplings, avocado pear, nuts
Diabetic or 'slimming' foods except sugar-free drinks
Alcohol

CHOLESTEROL-LOWERING DIET

The diet involves reducing total fat intake (particularly saturated fat) and restricting foods high in cholesterol. Foods high in fibre are encouraged.

Overweight patients would normally be given a suitably modified reducing diet.

SAMPLE MEAL PLAN

Breakfast
Fruit or fruit juice
Cereal (preferably wholegrain) or porridge with low-fat milk
Bread (preferably wholemeal) with polyunsaturated margarine
Jam, marmalade or honey

Snack meal
Sandwich or salad with *lean* meat, fish or low-fat cheese
Bread or crispbread with polyunsaturated margarine
Or baked beans on toast
Fresh fruit or low-fat yoghurt

Main meal
Clear soup, fruit juice, melon or grapefruit
Lean meat or fish or low-fat cheese
Vegetables
Potatoes—jacket (with polyunsaturated margarine or low-fat yoghurt), boiled, mashed or fried in polyunsaturated oil, or pasta or rice
Fruit, jelly or pudding made with low-fat milk

Avoid:
Butter, lard, suet, cooking fats, other margarines, 'vegetable oils', coconut oil, salad cream, mayonnaise, egg yolk, whole milk, dried milk with added vegetable fat, cream, yoghurt made with whole milk
Duck, goose, offal, sausages, pâté, luncheon meat, salami-type sausages
Fish roe, prawns, shrimps
Avocado pear, nuts, crisps
Ice-cream, tinned and packet desserts, chocolate spread, lemon curd, chocolate, toffee, butterscotch, cocoa, drinking chocolate, malted milk drinks
All biscuits (except crispbreads, water biscuits, plain and semi-sweet biscuits), cakes, pastries, pies (unless made with suitable ingredients)

CHOLESTEROL- AND TRIGLYCERIDE-LOWERING DIET

In addition to the restrictions listed under the cholesterol-lowering diet, sugar and foods with a high sugar content must be avoided. The intake of other carbohydrate-containing foods is controlled.

Foods with a high fibre content are encouraged. Alcohol intake should be restricted.

For overweight patients a modified reducing diet is advised.

DIETS FOR SPECIFIC URINE COLLECTIONS

Diet for 5HIAA collections

The following items may need to be avoided prior to 5-hydroxyindole acetic acid (5HIAA) urine collections:
- Tomatoes and tomato products
- Broad beans
- Bananas
- Plums
- Pineapple
- Avocado pears
- Aubergines
- Plantain
- Papaw, passion fruit
- Nuts

Diet for VMA collections

The following foods may need to be avoided prior to vanillylmandelic acid (VMA) urine collections:
- Vanilla essence
- Vanilla-containing foods
  Ice-cream
  Cakes
  Biscuits
  Puddings
  Desserts and dessert mixes
  Custard
- Bananas
- Nuts
- Chocolate and bedtime beverages
- Coffee
- Cola-flavoured drinks and foods

STANDARD TOTAL PARENTERAL REGIMEN FOR A 24-h PERIOD

This regimen provides:
- 35–45 kcal·kg^{-1} (150–190 kJ·kg^{-1}) daily
- 35% of the non-protein energy as fat
- 65% of the non-protein energy as carbohydrate
- 14–20 g of nitrogen

The following are mixed in a 3 l bag under laminar flow conditions in the pharmacy:

1 l Synthamin 14 with electrolytes	348 kcal
0.5 l 20% Intralipid	900 kcal
1.5 l 20% dextrose	1200 kcal
	2448 kcal

+ 10 ml Vitlipid Adult (fat-soluble vitamins)
+ 10 ml Addamel (minerals)
+ 1 vial Solivito (water-soluble vitamins)
+ 15 units soluble insulin

Careful biochemical monitoring is essential.

STANDARD ENTERIC DIET

This is given in Table 3.14 (see p. 143).

Normal values

These normal values were compiled by Ruth Halliday SRN, St Bartholomew's Hospital, London

HAEMATOLOGY

Basophil granulocytes	$0.01–0.1 \times 10^9/l$
Eosinophil granulocytes	$0.04–0.4 \times 10^9/l$
Erythrocyte sedimentation rate (ESR)	<20 mm in 1 h
Haemoglobin—male	$14.0–17.7$ g·dl^{-1}
—female	$12.2–15.2$ g·dl^{-1}
Leucocytes	$4.3–10.8 \times 10^9/l$
Mean corpuscular haemoglobin (MCH)	27–33 pg
Mean corpuscular haemoglobin concentration (MCHC)	32–35 g·dl^{-1}
Mean corpuscular volume (MCV)	80–96 fl
Monocytes	$0.2–0.8 \times 10^9/l$
Neutrophil granulocytes	$3.5–7.5 \times 10^9/l$
Packed cell volume (PCV)—male	$0.42–0.53$ l·l^{-1}
—female	$0.36–0.45$ l·l^{-1}
Plasma volume	45 ± 5 ml·kg^{-1}
Platelet count	$150–400 \times 10^9/l$
Red cell folate	>160 μg·l^{-1}
Red cell mass—male	30 ± 5 ml·kg^{-1}
—female	25 ± 5 ml·kg^{-1}
Reticulocyte count	0.5–2.5% of red cells
Serum B$_{12}$	150–675 pmol·l^{-1} (160–925 ng·l^{-1})
Serum folate	5–63 nmol·l^{-1} (3–20 μg·l^{-1})
Total blood volume—male	75 ± 10 ml·kg^{-1}
—female	$70 \pm$ ml·kg^{-1}

Coagulation

Bleeding time (Ivy method)	3–8 min
Partial thromboplastin time (PTTK)	30–40 s
Prothrombin time	10–14 s

BIOCHEMISTRY

Acid phosphatase	$1–5 \text{ U·l}^{-1}$
Alanine aminotransferase (ALT)	$5–30 \text{ U·l}^{-1}$
Albumin	$34–48 \text{ g·l}^{-1}$
Alkaline phosphatase	$25–115 \text{ U·l}^{-1}$
Alpha-1-antitrypsin	$2–4 \text{ g·l}^{-1}$
Alpha-fetoprotein	$<10 \text{ kU·l}^{-1}$
Amylase	$70–300 \text{ U·l}^{-1}$
Angiotensin-converting enzyme	$204–360 \text{ U·l}^{-1}$
Aspartate aminotransferase (AST)	$10–40 \text{ U·l}^{-1}$
Bicarbonate	$22–30 \text{ mmol·l}^{-1}$ $(22–30 \text{ mEq·l}^{-1})$
Bilirubin	$<17 \text{ μmol·l}^{-1}$ $(0.3–1.5 \text{ mg·dl}^{-1})$
Calcium	$2.2–2.67 \text{ mmol·l}^{-1}$ $(8.5–10.5 \text{ ng·dl}^{-1})$
Chloride	$100–106 \text{ mmol·l}^{-1}$ $(100–106 \text{ mEq·l}^{-1})$
Cholinesterase	$2.25–7.0 \text{ U·l}^{-1}$
Copper	$12–25 \text{ μmol·l}^{-1}$ $(100–200 \text{ mg·dl}^{-1})$
Complement—total haemolytic	$150–250 \text{ U·ml}^{-1}$
Creatinine	$0.06–0.12 \text{ mmol·l}^{-1}$ $(0.6–1.5 \text{ mg·dl}^{-1})$
Creatinine kinase (CPK)	$24–195 \text{ U·l}^{-1}$
Ferritin	$5.8–120 \text{ nmol·l}^{-1}$ $(15–250 \text{ μg·l}^{-1})$
Gamma glutamyl transferase (γ-GT)	$10–40 \text{ iu·l}^{-1}$
Glucose	$4.5–5.6 \text{ mmol·l}^{-1}$ $(70–110 \text{ mg·dl}^{-1})$
Glycosylated haemoglobin (Hb_1Ac)	$3.8–6.4\%$
Hydroxybutyric dehydrogenase (HBD)	$40–125 \text{ U·l}^{-1}$
Iron	$13–32 \text{ μmol·l}^{-1}$ $(50–150 \text{ μg·dl}^{-1})$
Iron binding capacity (total)	$42–80 \text{ μmol·l}^{-1}$ $(250–410 \text{ μg·dl}^{-1})$
Lactate dehydrogenase	$240–525 \text{ U·l}^{-1}$
Lead	1.8 μmol·l^{-1}
Magnesium	$0.7–1.1 \text{ mmol·l}^{-1}$
Osmolality	$280–296 \text{ mmol·kg}^{-1}$ $(280–296 \text{ mosmol·kg}^{-1})$
Phosphate	$0.8–1.4 \text{ mmol·l}^{-1}$
Potassium	$3.5–5.0 \text{ mmol·l}^{-1}$ $(3.5–5.0 \text{ mEq·l}^{-1})$
Protein (total)	$62–80 \text{ g·l}^{-1}$ $(6.2–8.0 \text{ g·dl}^{-1})$
Sodium	$135–146 \text{ mmol·l}^{-1}$ $(135–146 \text{ mEq·l}^{-1})$
Urate	$0.18–0.42 \text{ mmol·l}^{-1}$ $(3.0–7.0 \text{ mg·dl}^{-1})$
Urea	$2.5–6.7 \text{ mmol·l}^{-1}$ $(8–25 \text{ mg·dl}^{-1})$
Vitamin A	$0.5–2.1 \text{ μmol·l}^{-1}$ $(0.15–0.6 \text{ μg·ml}^{-1})$
Vitamin D—25-hydroxy	$19.4–137 \text{ nmol·l}^{-1}$ $(8–55 \text{ ng·l}^{-1})$
—1,25-dihydroxy	$62–155 \text{ pmol·l}^{-1}$ $(26–65 \text{ pg·l}^{-1})$
Zinc	$7–18 \text{ μmol·l}^{-1}$

Lipids and lipoproteins

Cholesterol	3.9–7.8 nmol·l^{-1}
Triglyceride	0.5–2.1 nmol·l^{-1}
Phospholipid	2.9–5.2 nmol·l^{-1}
Non-esterified fatty acids—male	0.19–0.78 nmol·l^{-1}
—female	0.06–0.9 nmol·l^{-1}
Lipoproteins—VLDL	0.128–0.645 nmol·l^{-1}
—LDL	1.55–4.4 nmol·l^{-1}
—HDL—male	0.7–2.0 nmol·l^{-1}
—female	0.95–2.15 nmol·l^{-1}
Lipids (total)	4.0–10 g·l^{-1} (400–1000 mg·dl^{-1})

Blood gases

Arterial $P\text{co}_2$	4.8–6.1 kPa (36–46 mmHg)
Arterial $P\text{o}_2$	10–13.3 kPa (75–100 mmHg); for every year over 60 *add* 0.13 kPa
Arterial [H$^+$]	35–45 nmol·l^{-1}
Arterial pH	7.35–7.45

Urine values

Calcium	7.5 mmol daily or less (300 mg daily or less)
Copper	0–1.6 µmol daily (0–100 µg daily)
Creatinine	0.13–0.22 mmol·kg^{-1} body weight daily (15–25 mg·kg^{-1} body weight daily)
5-Hydroxyindole acetic acid	10–45 µmol daily (2–9 mg daily); amounts lower in females than males
Lead	0.39 µmol·l^{-1} or less (0.08 µg·ml^{-1} or 120 µg daily or less)
Protein (quantitative)	< 0.15 g per 24 h (< 150 mg per 24 h)

Tests in endocrinology

These tests were compiled by Dr Paul Drury, Consultant Physician, King's College Hospital, London.

General

Different laboratories will have different normal ranges for many of these tests, and slightly different protocols—*always* consult the laboratory before performing or interpreting these tests. Also check whether plasma or serum is required, and whether any special handling is needed.

Time, date, stage of test and date of last menstrual period when appropriate should always be noted on the request form as they are critical for interpretation.

GONADAL AXIS

Basal levels

Basal levels are often sufficient to indicate the site of the problem; they can always indicate the stage of the menstrual cycle.

Male adult

Testosterone	10–35 nmol·l^{-1}
Luteinizing hormone (LH)	1–10 u·l^{-1}
Follicle-stimulating hormone (FSH)	1–7 u·l^{-1}

Female adult

	Follicular	Mid-cycle	Luteal	Postmenopausal
LH ($u \cdot l^{-1}$)	2.5–21	25–70	1–10	> 50
FSH ($u \cdot l^{-1}$)	1–10	6–25	0.3–21	> 25
Oestradiol ($pmol \cdot l^{-1}$)	< 110	500–1100	300–750	< 150
Progesterone ($nmol \cdot l^{-1}$)	< 12	—	> 30	< 3
Testosterone ($nmol \cdot l^{-1}$)		0.5–3.0		

LHRH test

100 µg of luteinizing hormone releasing hormone (LHRH) is given intravenously into an indwelling catheter at time 0; samples are taken at time 0, +20 and +60 min for LH and FSH. Normal responses are:

	20 min	60 min
Female (follicular phase)		
LH ($u \cdot l^{-1}$)	15–42	12–35
FSH ($u \cdot l^{-1}$)	1–11	1–25
Male		
LH ($u \cdot l^{-1}$)	13–58	11–48
FSH ($u \cdot l^{-1}$)	1–7	1–5

Sperm counts

Volume	0.1–11 ml
Density	1.5–375×10^6 ml
Motility	5–95%

Prolactin

Stress can affect prolactin levels. To establish a definite abnormality several samples should be taken, ideally through an indwelling venous catheter.

Normal levels are < 400 mu·l^{-1} in most laboratories. The significance of minor increases (400–600 mu·l^{-1}) is disputed. Levels above 2000–3000 mu·l^{-1} *suggest* the presence of a prolactinoma.

GROWTH AXIS

Basal levels

Growth hormone (GH) release is episodic; however, an undetectable or very low level (< 1 mu·l^{-1}) on a random sample excludes acromegaly.

Acromegaly

In normal subjects, GH levels are suppressed to below 1–2 mu·l^{-1} during an oral glucose tolerance test (for details see Chapter 17).

GH deficiency

In children, exercise and arginine are often used to stimulate GH secretion; a level above 20 mu·l^{-1} is a normal response. The insulin tolerance test is, however, the optimal test for adults and children.

Insulin tolerance test for GH reserve

After an overnight fast, a rapid-acting (ideally human) insulin is administered at 0900 via an indwelling intravenous catheter. The dose is usually 0.15 u·kg^{-1} body weight but should be 0.1 u·kg^{-1} for hypopituitarism and 0.2–0.3 u·kg^{-1} in cases of insulin resistance (e.g. acromegaly, Cushing's syndrome). Clinical hypoglycaemia and a blood glucose < 2.2 mmol·l^{-1} should be produced; if not, repeat the dose at 45 min. Samples are collected at 0, +30, +45, +60, +90 and +120 min. A normal response for GH is > 20 mu·l^{-1}. A large breakfast should be given afterwards.

The test should not be used in patients with epilepsy, heart disease or profound hypopituitarism—a normal ECG and a cortisol result > 180 nmol·l^{-1} should be seen before the test. Syringes loaded with 50% dextrose and hydrocortisone must always be available during the test.

This test is also used to measure ACTH reserve (see below).

THYROID AXIS

Basal levels

Levels of the thyroid hormones vary very little by hour or day unless patients are acutely ill; basal levels thus usually suffice.

Total serum thyroxine (T_4)	60–160 nmol·l^{-1}
Total serum triiodothyronine (T_3)	1.2–3.1 nmol·l^{-1}
Free serum thyroxine (T_4)	13–30 pmol·l^{-1}
Thyroid-stimulating hormone (TSH)	0.5–5.0 mu·l^{-1} (lower limit not definable on older assays)

TRH test—now much less used

200 µg of thyrotropin-releasing hormone (TRH) is given via an indwelling intravenous catheter at time 0 after a basal sample is collected; subsequent samples are taken at +20 and +60 min. Normal responses are:

0 min	0.5–5.0 mu·l^{-1}
20 min	3.4–20 mu·l^{-1}
60 min	< 20 min level
Increment	> 2.0 mu·l^{-1}

An excessive response indicates hypothyroidism; an inadequate one indicates either primary hyperthyroidism or pituitary disease.

ADRENAL AXIS

Basal levels

Adrenocorticotrophic hormone (ACTH) and cortisol levels vary episodically and with a circadian rhythm; single untimed samples are of *very* little value. Normal values are as follows for circadian studies:

	0900	2400 (must be asleep)
ACTH	10–80 ng·l^{-1}	< 10 ng·l^{-1}
Cortisol	180–700 nmol·l^{-1}	< 180 nmol·l^{-1}

Short ACTH stimulation test

This test is used to exclude Addison's disease. After taking a first sample for cortisol, 0.25 mg of tetracosactrin is given at time 0. Further samples are taken at +30 and +60 min. Normal values are:

30 min	550–1160 nmol·l^{-1}
60 min	690–1290 nmol·l^{-1}
Increment	330–850 nmol·l^{-1}

Dexamethasone suppression tests

These are used to exclude Cushing's syndrome. They are described on p. 724.

Insulin tolerance test—for ACTH reserve

This can be used to measure ACTH reserve; details are given above. It should only be performed if the 0900 cortisol is > 180 nmol·l^{-1}.

A normal response to hypoglycaemia is a cortisol level ≥ 550 nmol·l^{-1}; most authorities also demand an increment of > 180 nmol·l^{-1}.

ENDOCRINOLOGY OF BONE

Calcium levels only change abruptly after surgery or other therapy. They are, however, dependent on protein concentration and should be measured in uncuffed samples. The values given below are for albumin levels of 47 g·l^{-1}; to correct, add or subtract 0.02 mmol·l^{-1} for each g·l^{-1} of albumin below or above 47 g·l^{-1}.

Serum calcium	2.20–2.65 mmol·l^{-1}
Serum phosphate	0.80–1.40 mmol·l^{-1}
Alkaline phosphatase	25–115 U·l^{-1}
Serum parathormone (PTH)	Very variable between assays
Vitamin D	Very variable between assays

ENDOCRINOLOGY OF BLOOD PRESSURE AND THIRST

Blood pressure

Plasma renin activity (PRA) varies very widely according to method—your own laboratory should be consulted.

Aldosterone (and PRA) should be measured after at least 30 min recumbency and, possibly, after 4 h ambulation. Normal values are:

| Lying | 100–500 pmol·l^{-1} |
| Standing | 200–1000 pmol·l^{-1} |

Thirst

As a screening test, early morning plasma and urine osmolalities are measured. Normal values are:

| Plasma | 275–290 mosmol·kg^{-1} |
| Urine | Above 600 mosmol·kg^{-1} suggests good concentration |

Plasma and urine osmolalities must be interpreted together. Further study requires a water deprivation test.

WEIGHT AND HEIGHT CHARTS

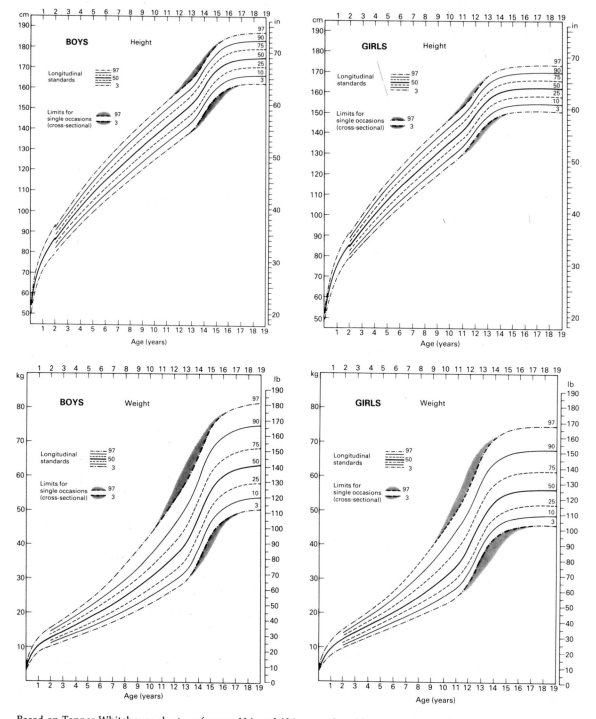

Based on Tanner-Whitehouse charts, reference 11A and 12A, reproduced by permission of Castlemead Publications.

Guidelines for body weight

Values given are weights without clothes.

Height (m)	Men (kg)			Women (kg)		
	Acceptable average	Acceptable weight range	Obese*	Acceptable average	Acceptable weight range	Obese*
1.45				46.0	42–53	64
1.48				46.5	42–54	65
1.50				47.0	43–55	66
1.52				48.5	44–57	68
1.54				49.5	44–58	70
1.56				50.4	45–58	70
1.58	55.8	51–64	77	51.3	46–59	71
1.60	57.6	52–65	78	52.6	48–61	73
1.62	58.6	53–66	79	54.0	49–62	74
1.64	59.6	54–67	80	55.4	50–64	77
1.66	60.6	55–69	83	56.8	51–65	78
1.68	61.7	56–71	85	58.1	52–66	79
1.70	63.5	58–73	88	60.0	53–67	80
1.72	65.0	59–74	89	61.3	55–69	83
1.74	66.5	60–75	90	62.6	56–70	84
1.76	68.0	62–77	92	64.0	58–72	86
1.78	69.4	64–79	95	65.3	59–74	89
1.80	71.0	65–80	96			
1.82	72.6	66–82	98			
1.84	74.2	67–84	101			
1.86	75.8	69–86	103			
1.88	77.6	71–88	106			
1.90	79.3	73–90	108			
1.92	81.0	75–93	112			
Body mass index†	22.0	20.1–25.0	30.0	20.8	18.7–23.8	28.6

* Value and above for all entries.
† Body mass index = weight (kg)/height^2(M).

From Bray GA (ed) (1979) *Obesity in America*. Proceedings of the 2nd Fogarty International Centre Conference on Obesity, No. 79. Washington: US DHEW.

Abbreviations and symbols used in respiratory medicine

A–a	Difference of a gas pressure between alveolus (A) and pulmonary artery (a)
ARDS	Adult respiratory distress syndrome
C_aO_2	Arterial oxygen content
C_L	Lung compliance
FEV_1	Forced expiratory volume in 1 s
FRC	Functional residual capacity
FVC	Vital capacity during forced full expiration
IPPV	Intermittent positive pressure ventilation
LAP	Left atrial pressure
P_ACO_2	Partial pressure of carbon dioxide in alveolar gas
P_aCO_2	Partial pressure of carbon dioxide in arterial blood
PAEDP	Pulmonary artery end diastolic pressure
P_AO_2	Partial pressure of oxygen in alveolar gas
P_aO_2	Partial pressure of oxygen in arterial blood
PAP	Pulmonary artery pressure
$PD_{20-FEV1}$	Provocation dose producing a 20% reduction in FEV_1
PCO_2	Partial pressure of carbon dioxide
PCWP	Pulmonary capillary wedge pressure
PEFR	Peak expiratory flow rate; measured in litres per minute

P_Ico_2	Partial pressure of carbon dioxide in inspired air	So_2	Percentage saturation of haemoglobin with oxygen
P_Io_2	Partial pressure of inspired oxygen	TLC	Total lung capacity
PEEP	Positive end-expiratory pressure	$\dot{V}_{max}$	Maximal rate of air flow during forced expiration
Po_2	Partial pressure of oxygen		
$P_{\bar{v}}o_2$	Partial pressure of mixed venous oxygen	V_A	Volume of alveolar gas
		VC	Vital capacity
$\dot{Q}_t$	Total cardiac output	VT	Tidal volume
RV	Residual volume	$\dot{V}/\dot{Q}$	Ventilation:perfusion ratio

Index